First Aid®
Clinical Pattern Recognition
for the USMLE® Step 2 CK

Asra R. Khan, MD
Associate Professor of Clinical Medicine
University of Illinois College of
 Medicine-Chicago
Chicago, Illinois

Christopher R. Fernandes, MD
Assistant Professor of Clinical Medicine
University of Illinois College of
 Medicine-Chicago
Chicago, Illinois

Radhika Sreedhar, MD, MS
Associate Professor of Clinical Medicine
University of Illinois College of
 Medicine-Chicago
Chicago, Illinois

Joseph R. Geraghty, MD, PhD
University of Illinois College of
 Medicine-Chicago
Chicago, Illinois

Ananya Gangopadhyaya, MD
Associate Professor of Clinical Medicine
University of Illinois College of
 Medicine-Chicago
Chicago, Illinois

New York   Chicago   San Francisco   Athens   London   Madrid
Mexico City   Milan   New Delhi   Singapore   Sydney   Toronto

ISBN 978-1-264-28596-9
MHID 1-264-28596-5

This book was set in Minion Pro by KnowledgeWorks Global Ltd.
The editors were Bob Boehringer and Peter J. Boyle.
The production supervisor was Catherine Saggese.
Project management was provided by Tasneem Kauser, KnowledgeWorks Global Ltd.

This book is printed on acid-free paper.

Library of Congress Control Number: 2023938928

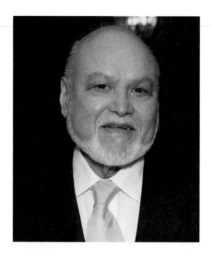

My brilliant father, M. A. Rahman Khan, was my everything—my first teacher/tutor, role model, guide, and cheerleader. He taught computer sciences at Kennedy King College and other city colleges of Chicago for many years. In addition to possessing both intelligence and a sharp sense of humor, he was a truly gifted storyteller, writer, and teacher. He used his gifts to impart knowledge in a practical and digestible format to his busy students, who often juggled family and job responsibilities while learning new skills. He strongly believed in making education accessible, and in its power to connect people. His mission carried me through completing this book. We all love and miss him dearly.

—Asra R. Khan

Contents

About the Editors

Asra R. Khan, MD
Editor-in-Chief

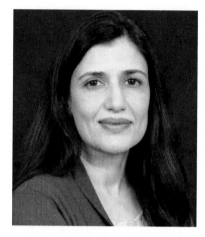

Asra is an Associate Professor of Clinical Medicine and Director of the Internal Medicine Clerkship and Internal Medicine Sub-Internship at the University of Illinois College of Medicine (UICOM)-Chicago. She is a former Associate Program Director of the Internal Medicine Residency Program and Course Director of the Doctoring and Clinical Skills Course. She earned her B.A. at the University of Chicago and was inducted into Phi Beta Kappa. She received her M.D. at The University of Chicago-Pritzker School of Medicine and completed her internal medicine residency at Northwestern Memorial Hospital in Chicago. Since joining UICOM-Chicago, she has been involved in teaching residents and students and has received a Golden Apple Award, was inducted into the Alpha Omega Alpha Honor Society, has been named Castle and Connolly's Top Regional Doctor in Internal Medicine, and has been featured in *Chicago Magazine*, Top Doctors edition. She enjoys working in teams and has recruited and led a top-notch team consisting of brilliant faculty, fellows, residents, and students to develop this product. In addition to editing, she helped create many of the tables, algorithms, and cases throughout the book. Her vision for the book was to create a product that would help students become better clinicians and be successful on the USMLE Step exams and beyond.

Christopher R. Fernandes, MD
Editor

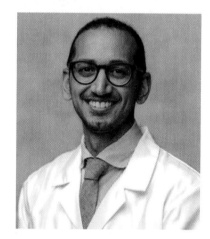

Christopher is an Assistant Professor of Clinical Medicine, Assistant Course Director of the Doctoring and Clinical Skills Course at the University of Illinois College of Medicine (UICOM)-Chicago, Associate Program Director of the Internal Medicine Residency, and Director of Hospital Medicine at University of Illinois Hospital. He earned his B.S. at the University of Michigan. He received his M.D. at UICOM-Chicago and graduated with honors, and received the William J. Grove Award and induction into the Alpha Omega Alpha Honor Society. He completed his internal medicine residency at University of Chicago Hospital, where he received the Arnold P. Gold Foundation Humanism and Excellence in Teaching Award. He completed his Chief Residency at Mercy Hospital and Medical Center in Chicago. Since joining the faculty at UICOM-Chicago, he has enjoyed working closely with medical students and residents to provide excellent clinical care to patients. He has received the Academic Internal Medicine Attending of the Year Award, New Attending Physician of the Year Award, a Golden Apple Award and Alpha Omega Alpha Faculty Teacher of the Year Award. In his clinical teaching, he prioritizes organization of clinical information and has incorporated many of these principals into this book. In his spare time, he enjoys pop music and modern art.

Radhika Sreedhar, MD, MS
Editor

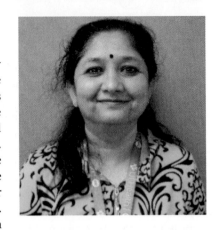

Radhika is an Associate Professor of Clinical Medicine, Director of Curricular Integration, and Assistant Internal Medicine Sub-Internship Director at the University of Illinois College of Medicine (UICOM)-Chicago. Dr. Sreedhar works in both the outpatient clinics and inpatient wards at UI Health. She leads the Evidence-Based Medicine (EBM) Subtheme for all three campuses of UICOM and has helped create and integrate the EBM curriculum into the organ system blocks. She has held positions as Associate Program Director at several internal medicine residency programs, including University of Illinois-Chicago. She has been the Course Director for Body Systems and Homeostasis block and Co-director for electives in Artificial Intelligence in Medicine and Pharmacogenomics at UICOM. She earned a master's degree in Preventive Medicine and Environmental Health from University of Iowa, received her M.D. degree from the University of Madras, and completed her internal medicine residency at Rush-Westlake Hospital in Illinois. She has received awards for outstanding teaching from several institutions and has been involved in teaching residents and students since 1999, prioritizing physical examination skills, critical thinking, application of evidence at the bedside, and engaging in safe transitions of care. She has been engaged in several interprofessional projects and collaborates with other disciplines to take medical education to the next level.

Joseph R. Geraghty, MD, PhD
Editor

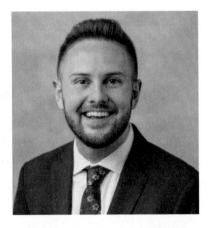

Joseph is a resident in the neurology program at the Hospital of the University of Pennsylvania in Philadelphia. He graduated from the Medical Scientist Training Program (MSTP) at the University of Illinois College of Medicine (UICOM)-Chicago in 2023, earning his MD and PhD. He earned his bachelor's degree in biochemistry at the State University of New York (SUNY) College at Geneseo in 2014, graduating summa cum laude and being inducted into Phi Beta Kappa. For his neuroscience PhD, he characterized inflammatory and electroencephalographic responses following subarachnoid hemorrhage, and how these contribute to downstream changes in brain activity, cognition, and overall neurological function. His academic interests are in neurocritical care and medical education. While at UICOM, he was inducted into the Alpha Omega Alpha and Gold Humanism Honor Society. He has published several peer-reviewed papers in neuroscience, neurology, and medical education. He was also the recipient of the Granville A. Bennett Award for Excellence in Contributions to Medical Education. He co-founded the UICOM Student Curricular Board, which seeks to engage medical students as agents of change in medical education, developed a USMLE strategies series for students, and currently serves as the first-ever trainee member of the editorial board of the journal *Academic Medicine*. Along with Dr. Asra Khan, he served as editor of *First Aid Clinical Pattern Recognition for USMLE Step 1*. He served as author, reviewer, and editor for this current book and ensured the trainee voice went into each page. In his spare time, he enjoys running and traveling.

Ananya Gangopadhyaya, MD
Editor

Ananya (Ani) is an Associate Professor of Clinical Medicine in the Division of Academic Internal Medicine at the University of Illinois College of Medicine (UICOM)-Chicago. She completed undergraduate and medical school training at UICOM Chicago and residency training in internal medicine at the University of Chicago. Dr. Gangopadhyaya works in both the outpatient clinics and inpatient wards at UI Health. She is a Tri-Campus Lead and Course Director for the Phase 1 Doctoring & Clinical Skills Course, which focuses on history-taking, interpersonal communication, physical exam, and clinical reasoning. She is an Associate Clerkship Director for the M4 Sub-Internship in internal medicine and has also served as a Co-Course Director for the Phase 1 Cardiology and Respiratory Educational Blocks. She has been awarded the Attending of the Year Award by the Internal Medicine Residency Program, the Gold Humanism Award, the C. Thomas Bombeck Award for Excellence in Medical Education, a Department of Medicine Rising Star Award, was inducted into the Alpha Omega Alpha Honor Society, and is a three-time recipient of the Golden Apple Award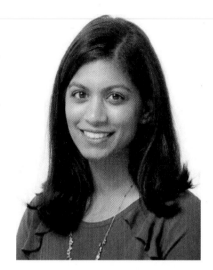
for Excellence in Teaching. When not on campus, she can often be found under a pile of dinosaurs and construction vehicles with her two boys, trucking along long distance-runs, or asking her awesome husband to take care of the dishes.

Fred A. Zar, MD
Content Consultant

Fred is a Professor of Clinical Medicine, Co-Course Director of the Synthesis Course, Course Director of the Immunology Course, and Director of Integrated Science Education at the University of Illinois College of Medicine (UICOM)-Chicago. He earned his B.S. at the University of Iowa where he was inducted into Phi Beta Kappa. He received his M.D. at UICOM-Chicago, graduating with honors, and was inducted into the Alpha Omega Alpha Honor Society. He also received the Granville Bennett Award for Outstanding Contributions to Medical Education as a medical student. He completed his internal medicine residency at Illinois Masonic Medical Center in Chicago, where he was Chief Resident, followed by an Infectious Diseases Fellowship at the University of Illinois at Chicago. He has been an Internal Medicine Residency Program Director for 34 years and is currently the Internal Medicine Res-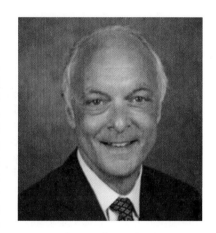
idency Senior Associate Program Director at the University of Illinois at Chicago. He practices as a hospitalist at the University of Illinois Hospital. His medical school awards include an Alpha Omega Alpha Outstanding Faculty Award, a College of Medicine Faculty of the Year Award, and is a two-time recipient of a Gold Humanism Award, a three-time recipient of the C. Thomas Bombeck Award for Excellence in Medical Education, and a 14-time recipient of a Golden Apple Award for Excellence in Teaching. The Internal Medicine residents have selected him 16 times as the Attending Physician of the Year. He is a firm believer that patients teach us medicine, and it is through pattern recognition of how they present themselves to us that we become excellent diagnosticians. He is a 12-time finisher of the Chicago Marathon, and a former chess master who is still active online most evenings.

Chapter Leads

All are current or former faculty members at University of Illinois College of Medicine (UICOM) in Chicago, Illinois unless otherwise indicated.

Mina Al-Awqati, MD
Division of Rheumatology
Department of Medicine
UICOM-Chicago

Leslie Ballard, MD
Department of Obstetrics and Gynecology
UICOM-Chicago

Amelia Bartholomew, MD
Department of Surgery
UICOM-Chicago

Sean M. Blitzstein, MD
Department of Psychiatry
UICOM-Chicago

Claudia C. Boucher-Berry, MD
Department of Pediatrics
UICOM-Chicago

Christie Brillante, MD
Division of Pulmonary/Critical Care
Department of Medicine
UICOM-Chicago

Julia Brown, MD
Division of Nephrology
Department of Medicine
UICOM-Chicago

Linda Chang, PharmD, MPH
Department of Clinical Family Medicine
UICOM-Rockford
Rockford, Illinois

Euna Chi, MD
Division of Academic Internal Medicine
Department of Medicine
UICOM-Chicago

Jared Davis, MD
Division of Neurocritical Care
Department of Neurology and Rehabilitation
UICOM-Chicago

Colin D. Goodman, MD
Division of Academic Internal Medicine
Department of Medicine
UICOM-Chicago

Shikha Jain, MD
Division of Hematology/Oncology
Department of Medicine
UICOM-Chicago

Mayank Kansal, MD
Division of Cardiology
Department of Medicine
UICOM-Chicago

Fazal R. Khan, MD, JD
University of Georgia School of Law
Athens, Georgia

Yasaman Kianirad, MD
Department of Neurology
UICOM-Chicago

Nathaniel Koo, MD
Division of Pediatric Surgery
Department of Surgery
UICOM-Chicago

Christy Ky, MD
Department of Psychiatry
UICOM-Chicago

Amy Lin, MD
Department of Pathology
UICOM-Chicago

Julie Loza MD
Department of Family and Community Medicine
UICOM-Chicago

Sarah Messmer, MD
Division of Academic Internal Medicine
Department of Medicine
UICOM-Chicago

Vinay Mikkilineni, MD
Department of Emergency Medicine
Department of Medicine
UICOM-Chicago

Adam E. Mikolajczyk, MD
Division of Gastroenterology/Hepatology
Department of Medicine
UICOM-Chicago

Samuel Ohlander, MD
Division of Urology
Department of Surgery
UICOM-Chicago

Mahesh C. Patel, MD
Division of Infectious Diseases
Department of Medicine
UICOM-Chicago

Alejandra M. Perez-Tamayo, MD
Division of Colon and Rectal Surgery
Department of Surgery
UICOM-Chicago

Eshana E. Shah, MD
Division of Hematology/Oncology
Department of Medicine
UICOM-Chicago

Asim Shuja, MD
Division of Gastroenterology/Hepatology
Department of Medicine
UICOM-Chicago

Radhika Sreedhar, MD, MS
Division of Academic Internal Medicine
Department of Medicine
UICOM-Chicago

Sai S. Sunkara, MD
Division of Pulmonary/Critical Care
Department of Medicine
UICOM-Chicago

Daniel Joseph Toft, MD, PhD
Division of Endocrinology
Department of Medicine
UICOM-Chicago

Stephanie M. Toth-Manikowski, MD
Division of Nephrology
Department of Medicine
UICOM-Chicago

Maria M. Tsoukas, MD, PhD
Department of Dermatology
UICOM-Chicago

Daphne L. Vander Roest, MD
Division of General Pediatrics
Department of Pediatrics
UICOM-Chicago

Catherine Wheatley, MD
Department of Obstetrics & Gynecology
UICOM-Chicago

Fred A. Zar, MD
Department of Medicine
UICOM-Chicago

Contributors

All are current or former students, residents, fellows, post docs, or faculty members at University of Illinois College of Medicine (UICOM) in Chicago, Illinois.

Javaneh Abbasian, MD

Saba Ahmad, MD

Sofia Ahmed, MD

Jonathan Alcantar, MD

Waddah Alrefai, MD

Lisa Anderson-Shaw, DrPH, MA, MSN

Jacquelyne Anyaso, MD, MBA

Amer Ardati, MD

Ajit Augustin, MD

Meghana Babu, MD

Carolina Baz, MD

Rachel Bernard, MD

Ryan Bolton, MD

Nicolas Bonamici, MD

Scott Borgetti, MD

Claudia Boucher-Berry, MD

Alan B. Carneiro, PhD

Anthony Carrera, MD

Robert Carroll, MD

Michael Charles, MD

Rozina Chowdhery, MD

Maya Cloyd, MD

Julia Conrad, MD

Mary B. Coomes, MD

Kathryn Cushing, MD

Matthew Del Pino, MD

Farheen Dojki, MD

Tessa Eckley, MD

Suzanne Falck, MD

Christopher Fernandes, MD

Benjamin David Follman, MD

John Galvin, MD, MS, MPH

Ananya Gangopadhyaya, MD

Joseph R. Geraghty, MD, PhD

Tara Gill, MD

Artemis Gogos, MD, PhD

Sophie Gough, MD

Anna Marie Gramelspacher, MD

Ethan Harris, MD

John Hickernell, MD

Yonatan Hirsch, MD

Samantha Hunt, MD

Nuzhath Hussain, MD

Jonwei Hwang, MD

Vanessa Jerger, MD

Eitan Katz, MD

Asra R. Khan, MD

Esther Kim, MD

Seoyeon Kim, MD

Soobin Kim, MD

Yoo Jin Kim, MD

Haley Kittle, MD

George T. Kondos, MD

Brittany Kotek, MD

Laura Krivicich, MD

Samantha Lagestee, MS

Hwa-Pyung (David) Lim, MD

Amy Lin, MD

Natalia Litbarg, MD

Rachel Lombard, MD

Claudia Lora, MD

Sherin Mahrat, MD

Maya McKeown, MD

Natalie Meeder, MD

Alfredo Mena Lora, MD

Jonathan Meyer, MD

Adam J. Miller, MD

Andrew Mudreac, MD

Olivia Murray, MD

Pooja Nayak, MD

Noreen Nazir, MD

Elsa Nico

Kimberly Orozco, MD

Kathryn Ospino, MD

Philip B. Ostrov, MD

Srinivas Panchamukhi, MD

Aashutos Patel, MD

Kruti H. Patel, MD

Saavan Patel, MD

Katherine Petrovich, MD

Nikita Pillai, MD

Anne Polick, MD

Azizur Rahman, MD

Nimmi Rajagopal, MD

Diana Rapolti, MD

Jorge W. Rivera, MD

Ashima Sahni, MD

Manpreet Samra, MD

Hoda Sayegh, MD

Logan Schwarzman, MD

Minji Seok, MD

Neelofer Shafi, MD

Dillon Sharp, MD

Ardaman Shergill, MD

Zafar Siddiqui, MD

Arjun Singh, MD

Divya Singh, MD

Mahi K. Singh, MD

Jasmine Solola, MD

Nidhi Suthar, MD

Arjun Tambe, MD

Zachary Taub, MD

Analisa Taylor, MD

Margaret M. Van Der Bosch, MD

Anthony Vergis, MD

Claire Wilson, MD

Helena Xeros, MD

R. Deepa Yohannan, MD

Alexandria N. Young, MD, PhD

Helen Zhang, MD

Acknowledgments

We would like to thank many of the faculty, fellows, residents, and students at the University of Illinois College of Medicine for their collaboration, contributions, and valuable input. We are grateful to our publishing/editorial team led by Bob Boehringer, Peter Boyle, and Rachel Norton at McGraw Hill, Tasneem Kauser at KnowledgeWorks Global Ltd., and Mastan Basha and Ankita Mapwal at MPS Limited for helping us throughout this process.

Asra R. Khan
I am grateful to God for blessing me with so much.

I want to thank and acknowledge my incredible team: Joe, Radhika, Ananya (Ani), Chris, and Fred for their valuable input, contributions, and support. I give special thanks to my husband Ali Nawaz and my sons Saif and Sohail for their love, encouragement, and patience. I'm also blessed to have so many wonderful supporters including my father (Rahman), mother (Zehra), sisters (Saera and Amera), brothers (Mujeeb and Fazal), parent-in-laws (Khader Nawaz and Sultana), brother- and sister-in-laws (Mehdi, Maliha, Matt, and Nadia), nephews (Raihan, Samad, and Sultaan), nieces (Ameera, Anya), and my entire extended family. Finally, I am grateful and privileged to have so many amazing friends, colleagues, teachers, students, and patients who have brought joy to my life and from whom I have learned so much over the years.

Radhika Sreedhar
I would like to express my heartfelt gratitude to Dr. Khan for her visionary leadership in bringing this book to fruition, and for entrusting us with the responsibility of making it a reality. Working alongside my colleagues on this book has been an enriching experience, and I am grateful to them for this. I would like to extend a sincere thank you to my husband, Madhu, and my children, Hari and Siva, for their unwavering love and support. I am also thankful to my parents, Sivadas and Sowmini, for instilling in me a sense of curiosity and providing a nurturing upbringing that has shaped the person I am today. A special shoutout to my sister, Renuka, and sister-in-law, Latha, for their constant presence and unwavering support. Last but not least, I am deeply grateful to all my teachers, colleagues, and students for inspiring me to continue learning and growing. Thank you all for being a part of my journey.

Christopher R. Fernandes
Thank you to Asra for asking me to join this project, to Ani, Radhika, Joe, and Fred for being an excellent team, and to all the faculty and students who put in countless hours of work to bring this to life. Thanks to my parents, Hubert and Diana, my siblings, Carlo and Caroline, and my family and friends for always supporting me. A special thanks to Grace for the constant encouragement to keep working. Lastly, thanks to all the patients I have met who are always teaching me new things!

Joseph R. Geraghty
I would like to thank Dr. Khan for inviting me to be a part of this project and for being such a great educator and mentor. I would also like to thank Dr. Gangopadhyaya, Dr. Sreedhar, and Dr. Fernandes for their mentorship and support throughout this process. Finally, I am grateful to all my medical student peers and friends at the University of Illinois College of Medicine for instrumental feedback on the contents of this book and for helping make sure that students played a key role in its development. Finally, I would like to thank my friends and family who have supported me throughout this journey. Cheers!

Ananya Gangopadhyaya
Thank you to Dr. Asra Khan for this opportunity to work with such a wonderful team on this project! To my parents, for their bravery and belief in us. To Pavan, for keeping me on my toes, for the laughs, and for always being ready for the next adventure. To Anuj and Claire, for being my sounding boards and board game people. To Abhi, Anshu, and Isabel, for being the reason why we always try harder. And always, to our teachers and our students, for keeping us humble and asking the hard questions.

Fred A. Zar

I would like to thank the amazing editorial leadership (Asra, Chris, Radhika, and Ani) for giving me the honor of contributing to this scholarly work, the hundreds of colleagues who are contributors that shared their knowledge, time, and passion, and the thousands of medical students, residents, and faculty who have educated me over the last several decades. Lastly, I want to thank my wife Lisa, and my daughters, Rachel and Danielle, who have stood by me during many busy educational endeavors in my career, including the development of this book.

Introduction

Why Use This Book?

- United States Medical Licensing Examination (USMLE) uses clinical case–based approaches to questions, translating into a need for medical students to rapidly recognize clinical patterns, to develop a prioritized differential diagnosis, and to use clinical reasoning and basic science skills to answer questions. Cases or vignettes provided on the Step exams are usually given in their most classic presentation. Given the goals and sheer volume of material necessary to include in Step prep books, many of the existing Step exam preparation materials often only provide a list of signs, symptoms, tests, and findings for a given condition without providing the clinical context that ties all of these features together. They often do not discuss the subtle similarities and differences between conditions that initially may not seem related.

- The *First Aid Clinical Pattern Recognition for the Step 2 CK* (Clinical Knowledge) book aims to present classic "textbook" vignettes of high-yield syndromes and cases that are clinically relevant and frequently tested on USMLE Step 2 CK, NBME subject ("shelf") exams for core clerkships, and encountered in clinical practice. This resource aims to provide context that ties different symptoms, signs, and conditions together. It encourages medical students to consider a differential diagnosis for a given chief concern and the relationships between different conditions. It explains what tests will help establish a diagnosis as well as rule out "can't miss" differentials. It includes high-yield cases that highlight major buzzwords and findings, as well as schematics, tables, and algorithms. Ultimately, this book will help medical students learn to recognize patterns and start building illness scripts for various high-yield conditions encountered in the clinical years.

- This text is an extension of the *First Aid Clinical Pattern Recognition for USMLE Step 1* book, focuses specifically on advanced diagnosis and management of disease and injury, and is designed to be used in tandem with other resources throughout the clinical years and leading up to the USMLE Step 2 CK exam. We have added chapters corresponding to both major organ systems and fields of practice, including surgery, pediatrics, and emergency medicine.

- By reinforcing the importance of obtaining a focused history and physical examination, developing a differential diagnosis, and understanding the purpose of common diagnostic tests and general treatment concepts for various conditions, students will recognize common patterns, build illness scripts, and improve their clinical reasoning skills.

How Should Students Use This Book?

- Start using this book as early as possible and definitely during your clinical years.

- This book will serve as your go-to resource for identifying what features of a given condition are the most commonly tested on "shelf" exams and USMLE Step 2 CK. As such, this book is a great accompaniment to your clinical experiences throughout the last 2 years of medical training.

- When you learn about a particular condition or encounter a patient with a particular illness in the clinic or hospital, it is helpful to go back to this book for reference of what a classic "textbook" manifestation of disease would look like. Did your patient have all of these findings? Did they have a unique or unusual presentation? Annotate this into the book!

- Keep in mind that this is not a question book. Instead, the vignettes highlight what a classic presentation of a particular case would look like: who gets the disease, the common symptoms and physical exam findings, other conditions that may present similarly, tests that will help confirm the diagnosis (and what will the typical findings be) or help refute the other conditions, and what the standard treatments are. The discussion portion reinforces the common presentations and discusses the underlying pertinent basic science principles.

- You may find it helpful to cover up specific boxes as you read through the cases to help quiz yourself. For example, cover the "Conditions with Similar Presentations," or "Initial Diagnostic Tests" sections for each vignette to see if you can generate these lists.

- Compared to USMLE Step 1, Step 2 CK builds upon basic science knowledge by emphasizing application to clinical practice. Questions will focus on screening and diagnosis, interpretation of labs and imaging, and approaches to management. In Step 2 CK exam items, there may be multiple choices that you would do in a real clinical setting; however, the exam expects you to reason through which ones are the most important or significant in order to rule in or rule out certain diagnoses.

- Many of the cases build upon each other. Simple, more straightforward cases are often followed by less common and more complex vignettes.
- Given the volume of potential conditions you may come across on NBME Subject exams and USMLE Step 2 CK, we have also added "mini-cases," which provide only the most high-yield, relevant information that you need to know.
- When you are first starting your clinical rotations, consider reading the applicable chapter, including the discussion section, thoroughly. This will help guide you as you are developing your assessments and plans for your written and oral case presentations.
- When reviewing for the exam, you may want to test yourself by primarily focusing on initial diagnostic tests and next steps in management.

Anatomy of the Cases

CASE 1	Actual Case (eponyms in parenthesis)
Vignette	
The vignette includes classic demographics (who gets the disease), common symptoms and signs, other relevant history, and physical exam findings.	
Conditions with Similar Presentations	This section highlights common and Step 2 CK-relevant differential diagnoses, including clues within the case that make other diagnoses more or less likely
Initial Diagnostic Tests	• This section includes important initial tests to begin the diagnostic work-up or to help confirm the diagnosis. • Tests to help rule out alternative diagnoses are also included.
Next Steps in Management	This section includes standard treatment and management for the actual case in an abbreviated format.
Discussion	**Overview:** This section reinforces the salient features of the case, including a discussion of high-yield terms or buzzwords, pathophysiology, and epidemiology **History:** Includes common presenting symptoms, risk factors, and other important historical findings **Physical Exam:** Includes common signs and important physical exam findings **Diagnostics:** Includes more detailed discussion (including important findings) on diagnostic testing and more advanced workup beyond initial diagnostic tests. When multiple diagnostic tests are available, discussion of the benefits and drawbacks of each will be discussed, including sensitivity and specificity. Particular attention will also be paid to screening guidelines and the potential adverse effects associated with diagnostic workup. **Management:** Includes more detailed recommendations on how to treat the condition or disease, including prognosis, options for monitoring the disease, and important considerations related to pharmacologic and/or surgical treatment options. Particular attention will be paid to potential adverse effects of treatments as well as when more conservative approaches (including no treatment at all!) may be warranted.
Additional Considerations	This section may include the following additional important information related to the clinical case: screening, complications, or considerations for surgery or specific patient populations (e.g., pediatric, obstetric, or hospitalized patients).

Example Full Case

Case X	Alcohol-Associated Cirrhosis
A 55-year-old woman with a history of alcohol use disorder presents with worsening abdominal distension and lower extremity edema for the past 3 weeks. She has been drinking about 10 beers daily for the past 18 years. She has no shortness of breath or orthopnea. She has no other drug use. Two months ago, she had an esophageal variceal bleed that was treated with banding. Patient's temperature is 37°C (98.6°F), pulse 90/min, respirations 20/min, and BP 100/64 mmHg. BMI is 21 kg/m². On exam, she is cachectic, has slow speech, icteric conjunctiva, multiple spider angiomas, palmar erythema, asterixis, and decreased breath sounds and dullness to percussion at bilateral lung bases. Her abdomen is distended with caput medusae, a positive fluid wave, and bilateral lower extremity pitting edema.	

Conditions with Similar Presentations	**Heart failure decompensation:** Presents with shortness of breath, possibly orthopnea, and other signs of hypervolemia; however, would not have jaundice, asterixis, or cutaneous signs of liver disease. **Nephrotic syndrome:** Presents with signs of hypervolemia but would not have jaundice, asterixis, or spider angiomas.
Initial Diagnostic Tests	• Obtain abdominal ultrasound with Doppler, transaminases, albumin, complete blood count, PT/INR • Check HBV and HCV serologies
Next Steps in Management	Diagnostic and therapeutic paracentesis with ascites fluid protein, albumin, and neutrophil count

Discussion	Alcohol-associated cirrhosis is the culmination of progressive liver injury from sustained alcohol use and comprises a substantial portion of the overall cirrhosis burden worldwide. Heavy alcohol use results in accumulation of fat in the liver, which triggers steatohepatitis and fibrosis. Fibrosis increases portal venous pressure, which increases the pressure and size of paraesophageal and periesophageal veins, producing varices which may then bleed. Increased portal pressures may also cause dilation of the umbilical vein, resulting in a caput medusa. Loss of hepatocyte function leads to hypoalbuminemia (decreased synthesis), coagulopathy (decreased coagulation factor production), and signs of increased estrogens (decreased catabolism in liver), such as spider angiomata, palmar erythema, and gynecomastia in men.
	History:
	• Prolonged (often decades-long) history of daily alcohol use (~1 standard drink per day for a woman and ~2 standard drinks per day for a man)
	• Nonspecific symptoms (weakness, fatigue), altered mental status, pruritis
	Physical Exam:
	• Jaundice, peripheral edema, spider angiomas, palmar erythema, gynecomastia, nail changes, Dupuytren contractures, or testicular atrophy
	• Signs of decompensated cirrhosis include abdominal distension, GI bleed, confusion, asterixis, renal failure, and hypoxemia
	Diagnostics:
	• The following can help establish a diagnosis of cirrhosis:
	  • Low platelet count, low albumin, and elevated PT/INR
	  • Ultrasound or cross-sectional imaging revealing nodular contour to the liver and/or evidence of portal hypertension (e.g., splenomegaly, recanalized umbilical vein)
	  • Elastography (a noninvasive radiographic assessment of the stiffness of the liver) showing high liver stiffness
	  • Ascitic fluid with serum-ascites albumin gradient (SAAG) >1.1 g/dL
	  • Liver biopsy is not needed if the clinical picture, labs, and imaging strongly suggest cirrhosis
	• The following can be suggestive of a diagnosis of alcohol-associated cirrhosis:
	  • Elevated AST and ALT levels with AST:ALT ratio >2 and macrocytosis
	  • Detectable biomarkers for alcohol use (e.g., phosphatidylethanol)
	  • Biopsy demonstrating steatohepatitis
	• Without a known significant alcohol use history or if you suspect a less common etiology of cirrhosis, consider alpha-1 antitrypsin level (if low, genotypic confirmation of a deficient variant), antinuclear antibodies (ANA), antismooth muscle antibodies (ASMA), antimitochondrial antibodies (AMA), iron studies, serum copper, and ceruloplasmin.
	• Also rule out chronic viral hepatitis B and C, because their presence may accelerate the development of cirrhosis.
	Management: Primarily focused on symptom relief but should also include measures to treat and prevent complications.
	• Alcohol cessation and avoidance of other hepatotoxins; offer pharmacotherapy for those with alcohol use disorder
	• **Vaccinations:** HAV, HBV, and 23-valent pneumococcal vaccines
	• **Ascites:** Low-salt diet, diuretics (spironolactone and/or furosemide), prophylactic antibiotics to prevent spontaneous bacterial peritonitis (SBP)
	• **Varices:** Upper endoscopy to evaluate for esophageal varices (can be life-threatening if ruptured); nonselective beta blockers and/or endoscopic variceal ligation (banding) for prophylaxis
	• **Hepatic encephalopathy:** If present, treat with lactulose ± rifaximin
	• **Hepatocellular carcinoma:** Screen with liver US and alpha fetoprotein (AFP) every 6 months
	• **Nutrition:** Vitamin and micronutrient repletion, especially folate, thiamine, and pyridoxine in setting of heavy alcohol use, high-protein diet
	• Definitive treatment for eligible patients is liver transplantation

Additional Considerations	**Screening:** USPSTF recommends screening for unhealthy alcohol use in adults ≥18 years old, with brief behavioral counseling interventions for those engaged in risky or hazardous drinking (Grade B).

Example Mini-Case

Condition	Key Findings
Non-Alcoholic Fatty Liver Disease (NAFLD)	**Hx:** • Risk factors include obesity, diabetes, and/or insulin resistance, and certain medications, including steroids, antiretrovirals for HIV, methotrexate, and amiodarone • Most are asymptomatic, but symptoms may include fatigue, RUQ fullness/pain, and jaundice **PE:** • Often obese, with increased waist circumference • May have hepatomegaly and signs of cirrhosis (e.g., jaundice, ascites, spider angiomas, gynecomastia) **Diagnostics:** • Often incidental finding of elevated AST and ALT (2-5 times upper limit of normal) on blood tests, or steatosis on imaging • Rule out other etiologies of chronic liver disease (e.g., alcohol, alpha-1 antitrypsin deficiency, Wilson disease, hemochromatosis) • Liver biopsy considered for patients at high risk of advanced fibrosis and/or with indeterminate initial testing **Management:** • Exercise, restrict caloric intake, advise ≥3–10% weight loss • Counsel on reducing risk of developing cirrhosis from other etiologies, including avoidance of alcohol and treatment of concomitant viral hepatitis • Pioglitazone, vitamin E, and GLP-1 agonists can be considered in certain patients after weighing individual risks vs. benefits **Discussion:** • NAFLD is the most common cause of elevated liver tests in adults in the United States, with a reported prevalence of 24–45%. This continues to increase in the setting of increased incidence of obesity. • Some patients with NAFLD can progress from steatosis to steatohepatitis to fibrosis and eventually cirrhosis and hepatocellular carcinoma.

We hope that this book is helpful to medical students as they master the material needed to find success on the USMLE Step 2 CK examination, NBME Subject exams, and beyond. Most of the information in this book was confirmed using online resources and references such as Dynamed, UpToDate, CDC.gov, United States Preventative Services Task Force (USPSTF), and other national society guidelines. As medicine is an ever-evolving discipline where new diagnostic tests and management options are developed every year, we welcome suggestions to improve the clarity, accuracy, and completeness of this work. Good luck!

How to Contribute

First Aid Clinical Pattern Recognition for USMLE Step 2 CK is a novel, innovative study resource assembled by hundreds of medical students and faculty. We welcome suggestions from readers to improve content, study strategies, diagrams, and images throughout the book to enhance the ability to ensure student success on the USMLE Step 2 CK exam. All submissions should be supported by relevant sources or hyperlinks from resources including UpToDate, AccessMedicine, or PubMed. We also welcome potential errata on grammar and style that can help improve the readability of the book. If you would like to submit an entry, clarification, or correction with appropriate references, please email our team at facprstep2@gmail.com. All efforts will be made to respond to your submission, including editor decision to include in the subsequent version of the book.

1

Health Care Ethics, Law, and Patient Safety

Lead Author: Fazal Khan, MD, JD
Contributors: Claire Wilson, MD; Sarah M. Russel, MD, MPH;
Kathryn Cushing, MD; Lisa Anderson-Shaw, DrPH, MA, MSN

It is important to understand the fundamentals of medical ethics and how to apply them in common situations. On USMLE Step 2 CK and throughout your medical school clerkships, you will encounter numerous ethical scenarios that may not always have a single, clear answer. When working through these scenarios, think about the ethical principles involved in the situation at hand. If the concern is over autonomy, pick the option that allows for the most patient autonomy possible while considering the patient's decision-making capacity. Remember that a provider's personal beliefs should not interfere with the patient's autonomous decisions. The correct decision is often the most patient-centered, open-ended one that allows for the least judgmental, most unbiased approach to patient care. Recent changes to USMLE have also increased the percentage of questions testing your knowledge of core principles related to health care ethics and communication skills, demonstrating an increasing recognition of the importance of the principles of clinical ethics.

CORE ETHICAL PRINCIPLES AND SITUATIONS

CASE 1 | Autonomy

A 19-year-old undomiciled man presents to clinic with an inguinal abscess. He has a temperature of 101°F and blood pressure of 100/75 mmHg, but is alert and oriented to person, place, and time. He is advised to proceed to the emergency department (ED) for further evaluation and treatment due to concerns for sepsis. The patient says he understands that if not treated appropriately, his infection could have dire consequences, yet he still refuses to go to the ED. He has had prior poor experiences with ED providers and is also concerned about the wait time and the cost.

Considerations and Next Steps	The patient should demonstrate a clear understanding of the physician's recommendation and the benefits of seeking care as well as the risks associated with refusing treatment. It should be confirmed that he has decision-making capacity, that the decision is his own, and that he is not being influenced by others. His wishes should be respected by his treating physician; however, the provider should engage in a conversation addressing the barriers to care.
Clinical Decision	The patient has a right to refuse the provider's recommendation to proceed to the ER, and if feasible, should be provided with alternative methods of treatment and care.
Discussion	Autonomy is the ability of a person to make their own decisions through agency and non-interference of others. If a patient who has agency and has been given all the information to make an informed decision makes a decision, there is generally an obligation to respect and honor their preference in accepting or refusing medical care. This patient demonstrates a desire to not proceed with physician recommendations. Furthermore, the patient has decision-making capacity. The patient can communicate his preferred option, he understands the information provided and potential consequences, and he provides a clear rationale behind his decision. Therefore, his wish must be respected, and the patient should be provided with alternative options to treat his condition, appropriate follow-up, and information should he change his mind or if his condition worsens.
Additional Considerations	Most institutions have policies to cover many scenarios including the following: **Minors** whose parents refuse life-saving treatment (e.g., blood transfusion, treatment for a curable cancer) should still receive treatment regardless of parental wishes. **Unconscious patients** whose wishes are unknown and are unable to provide consent should still receive treatment. A surrogate decision-maker would make decisions for this person if there is one to be found. **Jehovah's Witnesses** believe that a human must not sustain life with another creature's blood and therefore may refuse blood transfusions. Some may carry a blood refusal card. However, if they do not have this card and present in a medical emergency unable to articulate their wishes, the physician can give a life-saving blood transfusion.

CASE 2 | Beneficence

A 28-year-old woman presents to the ED with profuse vaginal bleeding. She notes that she is 20 weeks pregnant and is worried she may be having a miscarriage. While performing an abdominal ultrasound, the patient loses consciousness. Two large-bore IVs are placed, and lab results show a hemoglobin of 6 g/dL. A blood transfusion is necessary for the safety of the mother.

Considerations and Next Steps	The patient is unconscious and therefore unable to communicate or provide consent. The medical indications for blood transfusion are clear. ER staff should review her health record to see if there is any contact information for a friend or family member who may act as a legal surrogate decision-maker for the patient while she is not able to make decisions for herself. If no surrogate decision-maker is identified and the patient's condition requires emergency treatment to save her life, such treatment should be rendered.

CASE 2 | Beneficence *(continued)*

Clinical Decision	The patient should receive the blood transfusion.
Discussion	Beneficence refers to a physician's duty to act in a patient's best interest. A blood transfusion is medically indicated and there is no evidence that she would refuse treatment. Therefore, under the principle of beneficence, this patient should receive a life-saving transfusion. However, if the patient was conscious with decision-making capacity, her pregnancy would not supersede her right to bodily autonomy should she choose to refuse treatment. Though the practitioner may experience moral hazard as they attempt to do what is best for the fetus, a pregnant patient with capacity is able to refuse treatment.

CASE 3 | Nonmaleficence

A 23-year-old woman presents to the dermatology clinic seeking a renewal of her isotretinoin prescription, which previously resolved her acne. She is frustrated with her primary care doctor who did not renew her prescription because the patient is now trying to conceive and has had her intrauterine device removed. The dermatologist concurs with the primary care physician and refuses to renew the prescription.

Considerations and Next Steps	Isotretinoin can cause birth defects, and the patient is not on reliable birth control and is trying to conceive. The patient should be informed of the risks and benefits of the treatment and possible alternatives.
Clinical Decision	The patient should not be given isotretinoin due to potential teratogenic effects, and safer alternatives should be explored with the patient.
Discussion	Nonmaleficence means "do no harm" and refers to a physician's obligation to balance the risks and benefits of action to best treat the patient. In this case, isotretinoin may treat her acne, but can cause serious fetal harm if she becomes pregnant. Females of reproductive age who are prescribed isotretinoin should demonstrate use of at least two methods of contraception. For those seeking to conceive, alternative methods of acne treatment that involve non-teratogenic medications should be sought.

CASE 4 | Justice

Five patients have been waiting for over an hour in the ED. They were all triaged by the nurse, and their vital signs were stable, and their chief concerns were as follows: ankle pain, penile discharge, dysuria, cough, and rash. As staff prepares to bring the next patient back, an ambulance arrives with a patient from a motor vehicle collision. The patient is alert but is complaining of neck and chest pain. The provider decides to attend to the patient brought by the ambulance first.

Considerations and Next Steps	It is important to recognize and treat patients requiring urgent or emergent conditions first.
Clinical Decision	The physician should first attend to the potentially unstable or serious patient. In this case, the incoming patient from the ambulance should be attended to first. Once this patient has been stabilized, the provider may then attend to those patients in the waiting room who were not in critical condition.
Discussion	Justice is the principle of treating patients fairly and equitably. This does not imply that patients will be seen at the same time. Some patients may need to wait a longer time for care if the medical condition of another patient demands the physician's immediate attention. All patients will receive medical care (fairness). *Triage* is the method clinicians must use when vital resources are limited. Those with the greatest need take priority. During the height of the COVID-19 pandemic, physicians had to make extremely difficult decisions every day on how to distribute ventilators, medications, or even allocate a bed in a hospital.

CASE 5 | Confidentiality

An 18-year-old man comes to the clinic and claims he cut his left arm while cooking. The provider notes a 5-cm horizontal laceration across the wrist and several healed lacerations proximally. On further probing, the patient tearfully admits that he has been self-harming. He also reports thoughts of ending his life, and has plans to shoot himself once the gun permit he applied for is approved. The provider expresses concern for his safety and notes that he will need to hospitalize the patient. The patient insists that the provider not inform others, as the patient believed he shared this information in confidence.

CASE 5 | Confidentiality *(continued)*

Considerations and Next Steps	Confidentiality must be maintained unless there is risk of harm or death to self or others.
Clinical Decision	The presence of a clear and imminent risk to the patient's safety creates an exception to the principle of confidentiality. The patient should be evaluated and treated emergently in a hospitalized setting if he is assessed to be at high risk for suicide.
Discussion	If the patient presented with lacerations but denied a plan to end his life and did not present a continuing risk of imminent self-harm, then confidentiality should be maintained based on the principles of patient privacy and autonomy. In some states, extreme risk protection or "red flag" laws allow physicians, law enforcement, or household members to petition a court to prevent a person from possessing or buying a gun if they present a risk of harm to self or others. Due to the large variation in state laws, this specific issue is highly unlikely to appear on a national exam.
Additional Considerations	**Other exceptions to patient confidentiality** include mandatory reporting of positive sexually transmitted infection (STI) results where potential contacts may need to be informed, risk of harm to others (e.g., homicide; child or elder abuse), epileptic patients, and other causes of impaired driving. Of note, epileptic patients who are seizure-free for a predetermined period and have regular physician evaluations can be deemed eligible to drive, depending on state laws. How long they must be seizure-free varies in different states, but it is usually between 6 months and 1 year. **Adolescent patients:** Protecting confidentiality in adolescents patients is appropriate for sensitive issues such as sexuality, mental health, and substance use disorder in certain situations. For example, if an adolescent patient presents with symptoms concerning for an STI, they have the right to consent for diagnosis and treatment without breaking confidentiality (this is important to maintain a healthy patient–physician relationship). **Access to medical records:** Patients may also at times request for their medical record to be shared with other providers. The Health Insurance Portability and Accountability Act (HIPAA) established federal guidelines to safeguard protected health information (PHI) from being disclosed without the patient's knowledge or consent. Documentation of patient authorization should be obtained, and the transfer of patient information should ideally be done directly from the old to the new provider to reduce intermediaries with access to sensitive medical information.

CASE 6 | Fidelity (Professional Conduct)

A representative from a pharmaceutical company offers a resident physician free tickets to a football playoff game at a research conference. The company is handing out free tickets to various professional sporting events to all attendees. The resident is trying to decide whether it is appropriate to take the tickets since he is only a casual football fan and cannot conceive that accepting this gift would have any impact on his clinical decision-making.

Considerations and Next Steps	Regardless of the perceived or actual monetary value of the gift, accepting the football tickets does not directly benefit his patients and may influence the physician to prescribe this pharmaceutical company's medications.
Clinical Decision	The physician respectfully declines the free gift.
Discussion	Professional conduct falls under the principle of fidelity, and many institutions have policies regarding gifts from industry representatives and patients. Accepting gifts from external parties as a physician has important implications on the physician–patient relationship. Many patients would be less likely to take prescribed medications from their doctor if their physician had recently accepted a gift in exchange for listening to a pharmaceutical company's drug information. According to the American Medical Association, accepting small nonmonetary gifts (e.g., unbiased educational materials for patient care, drug samples) is appropriate, but no gifts of cash or gifts that do not directly benefit patients should be accepted. When accepting gifts from patients directly, physicians should be sensitive to the gift's value relative to the patient's means, and decline gifts that are disproportionately large. Physicians should not allow the gift to affect their relationship with the patient or the care that patient receives. Physicians may also suggest making a charitable donation instead to patients wishing to do so.

HEALTH CARE LAW

While detailed knowledge of health care law is beyond the scope of this book, it is important for physicians to understand that particular principles, responsibilities, and tasks are regulated based on local, state, and federal law. Even though health care laws vary from state to state, it is also important to recognize some guiding principles that apply across the nation. USMLE questions will focus on more universal principles (discussed here) rather than those that may differ based on local and state laws.

CASE 7 | Informed Consent

An 87-year-old widow with Alzheimer's dementia is brought to the ED after her daughter observed her fall to the ground after losing consciousness. The patient is now alert but disoriented to place, time, and location. The physician recommends that the patient have a head CT, electrocardiogram, labs, and possible admission for further evaluation and treatment. The patient's daughter agrees with admission, but the patient becomes very agitated and refuses hospitalization and imaging. She insists she needs to go home to take care of her baby.

Considerations and Next Steps	The process of obtaining informed consent requires that the risks and benefits of a procedure be disclosed to the patient after the patient has been assessed to retain decisional capacity to make their own health care decisions. In addition, there should be no coercion or manipulation of the patient with regard to the process of consent. This patient has documented dementia and has been assessed to lack decisional capacity.
Clinical Decision	As the patient lacks decision-making capacity, the physician should obtain informed consent from a designated health care power of attorney (POA) or surrogate decision-maker. If there is a spouse, they would be the next person in line to act as a surrogate decision-maker under most state laws. However, since the patient is a widow, the patient's daughter is an appropriate surrogate.
Discussion	Obtaining informed consent involves a discussion of the nature of the proposed treatment or procedure, reasonable alternatives to the proposed treatment, the risks/benefits of each option and of obtaining no treatment, and an evaluation of patient understanding and preference. A patient can revoke consent at any time if they have maintained their decision-making capacity. Ideally, the treating physician provides informed consent to the patient, or at the very least, a provider who has in-depth understanding of the procedure/treatment and would be able to answer patient questions. Informed consent can be waived by patients (if this happens, a legal decision-maker must be available) and is not legally required in emergency situations.

CASE 8 | Consent for Minors

A 15-year-old girl presents to clinic as she believes she may be pregnant. She notes she has had consensual sex with her partner and a home pregnancy test was positive. She is unsure of what to do next and asks if she needs her parents to sign anything for her to receive obstetric care. If not, she requests that you do not tell anyone she is pregnant.

Considerations and Next Steps	Although the patient is a minor (<18 years old; there are exceptions), parental consent is usually not required in the context of STIs, contraception, and pregnancy.
Clinical Decision	The physician is not required to inform the parents. Routine testing and counseling for an initial pregnancy visit should be performed.
Discussion	A minor is any person <18 years of age. Parental consent should be obtained for most medical procedures and treatments except for issues related to sex (contraception, STIs, pregnancy), drugs (substance abuse treatment), in emergency situations (life-saving treatments such as blood transfusions or emergency surgeries), or if the minor is legally emancipated from guardians. In these situations, the provider is not required to obtain parental consent and can honor the patient's wishes of confidentiality. Even when the minor's assent is not required and parents or guardians have given consent, the physician should still seek assent from the minor as this promotes patient autonomy and a healthy patient–physician relationship. In cases where a child is put at significant risk for harm due to parental refusal, physicians can obtain a court injunction or involve Child Protective Services (CPS) to proceed with life-saving medical treatment of a minor.

CASE 9 | Decision-Making Capacity

A 29-year-old man with history of intravenous drug use is brought to the ED by his partner due to fluctuating mental status and fevers. At the time of evaluation, he is alert and oriented to person, place, time, and location. He has a fever of 102°F, blood pressure of 80/55 mmHg, heart rate 102/min, pinpoint pupils, a holosystolic murmur at the left sternal border, multiple pink macular lesions on his palms, and subungual splinter hemorrhage on multiple digits. Urine toxicology is positive for fentanyl. Admission for treatment of endocarditis is advised but the patient refuses to be admitted, despite informing him of the risk of death without proper treatment.

Considerations and Next Steps	Fluctuating mental status is consistent with delirium, and the patient's vital signs and exam are consistent with sepsis/endocarditis. Also, pinpoint pupils and urine toxicology support current narcotic intoxication. Therefore, the patient does not currently have decision-making capacity. A surrogate decision-maker should be asked to consent for this patient until patient regains the capacity to make his own decisions. On rare occasions, a legal guardian may be sought to make medical decisions for a person who lacks capacity and has no surrogate decision-maker.
Clinical Decision	The patient should be admitted and treated with IV antibiotics. Once the patient is no longer intoxicated or delirious, he should be reassessed for decision-making capacity. After a conversation about the risks/benefits of treatment, alternatives, or refusal of treatment, and patient demonstration of understanding of his condition and options, he can refuse treatment.
Discussion	Decision-making capacity refers to the real-time determination, made by health care professionals, that dictates whether a patient can make a medical decision. Capacity is something that can change throughout a patient's care (e.g., they become unconscious, delirious, or sober). This is different from *competency*, which is determined by a judge and relates to whether an individual can make any health care-related decisions at all. A common scenario is one in which a patient has some degree of cognitive decline (e.g., mild cognitive impairment) but can understand and explain back the risks and benefits of a medical procedure fully. If a patient can do this and understands the consequences of their decision as well as give a rationale, they are considered to possess decision-making capacity despite their cognitive decline.

CASE 10 | Advance Directives

A daughter brings her 88-year-old mother with Alzheimer's dementia for an outpatient visit to follow up after an inpatient hospitalization for aspiration pneumonia. The patient was diagnosed with Alzheimer's 15 years ago, and in the last 4 months she has been admitted twice for aspiration pneumonia. The daughter noted that the patient becomes extremely agitated whenever she is in the hospital and must be heavily sedated. The daughter considers further aggressive inpatient treatment, including intubation, to be against her mother's best interests, and asks what can be done to prevent this from continuing to recur. The patient is a widow, and her daughter is her only child and caregiver.

Considerations and Next Steps	The care team should determine if the patient has some form of official advance directive on file. This could include a written living will, oral advance directive, a designated medical POA (health care proxy), or documentation of a do not resuscitate (DNR), do not intubate (DNI) order, or physician order for life-sustaining treatment (POLST).
Clinical Decision	If there is an official advance directive on file, it should guide any pertinent medical decisions. If there is no official advance directive available, in an acute setting a surrogate decision-maker (see next case), in this case, the daughter, must be consulted. The most common types of advance directives are the living will and the durable **power of attorney** for health care (medical POA). The living will is a legal document used to state future health care decisions only when a person becomes incapacitated and is unable to do so. This may apply to certain treatments such as dialysis, tube feedings, or the use of ventilators. A POA makes a person's health care decisions according to their wishes when they become unable to do so.
Additional Considerations	**POLST form:** An advance care directive that has a set of specific medical orders that a seriously ill person can fill in and ask their health care provider to sign. Without a POLST form, emergency personnel are required to provide every possible treatment to help keep a patient alive in the absence of other directives. POLST forms are available in all 50 states and the District of Columbia. Patients may change their mind/revoke at any time about what is written in their advance directive. **DNR/DNI orders:** Orders that notify the health care team of a patient's wishes in life-threatening emergencies. DNR means no cardiopulmonary resuscitation (CPR) will be performed, and DNI means no breathing tube will be placed. There are situations where a patient may be amenable to certain aspects of resuscitation and not others, and their preferences should always take priority.

CASE 11 | Surrogate Decision-Maker

A 27-year-old man struck by a car while riding his bike becomes unconscious and must be intubated. Attempts at weaning the patient off the ventilator over subsequent days are unsuccessful, and the patient has no official advance directive on file. Numerous family members, including the patient's wife, sister, and parents are present.

Considerations and Next Steps	The patient is unconscious and does not have an official advance directive on file. Thus, the patient's own preferences regarding treatment cannot be communicated, and a surrogate decision-maker or POA should be consulted.
Clinical Decision	The patient's family must be consulted to decide the course of treatment. Priority of the surrogate decision-maker is, from highest to lowest: 1) guardian of the person, 2) spouse, 3) adult children, 4) parents, 5) siblings, 6) adult grandchild, 7) close friend, 8) guardian of the estate.
Discussion	The purpose of a surrogate decision-maker is to have someone make medical decisions on behalf of the patient if the patient has become non-decisional. Under the substituted judgment standard, decisions should be made *based on what the patient would have wanted*. In this case, the patient's wife is the primary decision-maker, but the physician should encourage an open dialogue among the family. People who are alone in the hospital with no one to reach are far more likely to receive a court-appointed guardian. If it is not clear who should make decisions for the patient, doctors may need to consult the hospital ethics committee.
Additional Considerations	**Medical guardianship** is different from POA documents. In many cases where a patient has no family or friends to act as legal surrogate decision-maker, the hospital petitions the state court to have a legal guardian appointed to make health care decisions on behalf of the patient. A guardian can only be appointed in cases where a judge finds a patient does not retain decisional capacity such that it prevents the patient from being able to effectively make decisions or manage their health. The appointment of a guardian removes a patient's rights to make decisions for themself and and names a court-appointed individual to be personally legally responsible for the patient medical decisions.

CASE 12 | Elder Abuse

An 80-year-old woman with Parkinson's disease with dementia and type 2 diabetes mellitus presents to clinic with her son for medication refills. Her husband passed away 2 years ago, and she now lives at home with her adult son, her son's wife, and their three teenage children. Her vital signs are within normal limits. On physical exam, the patient has scattered bruises across her back, some of which appear new and others old. The patient has limited communication and masked facies, which is her baseline. Her diabetes had been well-controlled for the past several years, but today her hemoglobin A1c is 10%. Per chart review, it is noted that her medications have not been picked up from the pharmacy for several months. The patient's son tells the physician that "the old lady" takes her own medications and did not tell them she needed refills. He reports that her bruises are from falling and does not understand why the physician would be worried, as "old people" are "always tripping over things."

Considerations and Next Steps	The patient is examined alone but is unable to provide much history due to her limited communication. Prior to his death, the husband used to assist his wife with her medications and would accompany her to her appointments. The physician suspects that the patient is being neglected and is concerned that she is in an unsafe living environment.
Clinical Decision	The physician should file a report with Adult Protective Services to investigate the living situation. Concurrently, they should educate family about this patient's condition(s) and need for supervision and assistance with medications and activities of daily living. In addition, they should offer social work, home physical/occupational therapy, and home safety assessment/assistance.
Discussion	Based on the patient's physical appearance and lack of medication usage after having well-controlled conditions for some time, there is concern for abuse and/or neglect, which is a form of elder abuse. Elder abuse is more common in elderly women, and risk is increased in those with cognitive, social, and/or functional impairment. This patient is especially vulnerable to abuse because of her inability to provide an adequate history and to relay information to the physician. Other risk factors for elder abuse include financial dependence, caretaker perception of the elderly patient as a burden, and caretaker substance use disorder. Potential signs to look out for include poor hygiene, injuries (fractures, lacerations, burns) without appropriate or consistent explanations, or changes in behavior, especially when the caretaker is in the room compared to outside of the room. If the patient is in immediate danger, they should be admitted to the hospital. Health care providers can refer patients and their families to social work or respite care, which can be arranged for just an afternoon or several days or weeks. **Respite care** helps ease the burden for caregivers through many different services such as in-home care services, day centers, and residential facilities.

CASE 13 | Child Abuse

A 9-year-old boy is brought into the ED for pain with urination. The child said it hurts when he pees and when people touch his penis. On exam, the physician notices various bruises on the boy's body, some of which appear well healed and others more recent.

Considerations and Next Steps	The comment that other people are touching the patient's penis, as well as the bruising on the boy's body, are concerning for child abuse.
Clinical Decision	Health social work should be notified and Child Protective Services (CPS) should be contacted to ensure that the child is in a safe environment at home or if removal from home is warranted. Further, the child should be screened for STIs and urinary tract infection.
Discussion	The most common form of child maltreatment is **neglect**, or failure of a parent or guardian to provide a child with adequate food, shelter, supervision, education, and/or affection. **Physical abuse** can be seen at any age, but it occurs more frequently in young children aged 9–12 years old. Child abuse should be suspected in cases where the history does not match the physical findings, in children with repeated hospitalizations, or in unstable family situations. On exam, look for bruises in different stages of healing or spiral fractures, parent or guardian stories that are inconsistent with the type of injury sustained by the child, or delay in seeking care. **Sexual abuse** should be suspected if a child has genital trauma, bleeding, discharge, or an excessive preoccupation or knowledge of adult sexual behaviors. If sexual abuse is suspected, testing for gonorrhea, syphilis, chlamydia, and HIV is warranted. Physicians are required by law to report all reasonable suspicions of child abuse or endangerment. The child abuse reporting system for doctors is designed to be *sensitive*, not *specific*, which means that it is acceptable if some false positive reports are filed.
Additional Considerations	In **infants**, abuse may present as failure to thrive, irritability, somnolence, seizures, or apnea. A parent or guardian may state that a child did something that is incongruent with their developmental stage (such as rolling off the bed at 2 months when this is typically achieved by infants at 4–6 months). **Shaken baby syndrome** is from repetitive acceleration–deceleration leading to subdual hematomas with coup–contrecoup injury. Ophthalmologic exams are useful to examine for retinal hemorrhages. Non-contrast CT may show subdural hematomas, while MRI can visualize white matter changes associated with violent shaking. **Immersion burns** can be a sign of child abuse caused by forcing a child into hot water. Burn injuries may be observed on the buttocks and/or in a stocking-glove distribution that spares flexural skin creases.

CASE 14 | Intimate Partner Violence (IPV)

A 32-year-old woman with no significant past medical history presents for her well adult visit. She lives at home with her husband and her three young children. She expresses interest in a new form of contraception, as she is currently on oral contraception pills but is worried about how this would appear on her insurance statement. The physician inquires as to why she is concerned, and she expresses that her partner wants her to get pregnant again and has been withholding her birth control. She then shares that sex has started to become coercive and her husband has started to become physically aggressive during sex.

Considerations and Next Steps	The patient is describing a situation of domestic abuse, or IPV. The physician listens to the patient's story and confirms that currently she is safe as her husband is traveling for work. Interfering with birth control can be a form of reproductive control within a relationship. Despite the patient and her husband previously having a sexual relationship, both partners need to consent to sex.
Clinical Decision	The physician should offer the patient assistance including referral to social work but should not pressure the patient to leave the partner. The physician is not legally obligated to report the behavior to authorities.

CASE 14 | Intimate Partner Violence (IPV) *(continued)*

Discussion	IPV is unfortunately a common occurrence that is underreported. IPV risk factors include alcohol consumption, psychiatric illness, and a history of violent relationships in childhood. Risk is highest in younger females, including pregnant women; however, it can occur in anyone at any age. Suspect IPV when injuries (e.g., fractures, lacerations, burns) lack appropriate or consistent explanations, are repetitive in nature, or have signs of both acute and chronic injury. Other signs include changes in behavior, especially when the partner is in the room compared to outside of the room. Signs to look out for in a potential abuser include refusal to leave the patient alone with a provider or let the patient answer provider questions. Therefore, it is important to try to examine and talk to the patient alone and ensure confidentiality and shared decision-making. Physicians are not required by federal law to report incidents of domestic violence. The physician should support the patient, ensure their safety, and provide resources the patient may need such as contact information for a social worker, a domestic abuse hotline number, and appropriate close follow-up. The discussion should also include a plan of what the patient can do in the event of an emergency. The US Preventative Services Task Force guidelines recommend *all women of childbearing age be screened annually for IPV* as there is a low risk of negative effects from screening. Unfortunately, IPV is associated with increased risk of homicide, unintended pregnancies, complications associated with pregnancy, and psychiatric illness.

CASE 15 | Medical Aid in Dying (MAID)

A 64-year-old man with stage 4 pancreatic cancer presents with rapid deterioration of his condition. He no longer enjoys spending time with his family or friends. He describes excruciating 10/10 pain that keeps him bedridden and unable to cook or take his dog on walks—activities he used to enjoy doing. He relies on his daughter, who is a single mom of three young children, to drive him to doctor appointments and buy him groceries. The patient has tried multiple chemotherapy and radiation therapy treatments with no response. He tells his physician, "I need you to promise me that you will help me end my suffering when the time comes. I do not want to discuss this with my family because I know they will disagree, but I am tired of this, and I know this cancer will kill me. Please help me end my life."

Considerations and Next Steps	The initial response to such a request should include exploring the patient's reasoning and identifying their fears and concerns so that the provider can work to improve their quality of life.
Clinical Decision	The physician should empathize with the patient and ask how they came to this decision of wanting to end their life. The physician should assess the bases for the patient's fears and determine if interventions such as hospice care, comfort care, or more aggressive pain control can address their concerns.
Discussion	MAID or provider aid in dying (PAD) is the process by which a physician helps competent patients voluntarily end their lives when faced with end-of-life suffering. In states where this is legal, physicians may provide medication or information to patients knowing that they will use it to end their life. However, MAID remains a controversial ethical topic and is legal in only a few states. Physicians are required to confirm the diagnosis as terminal and if the patient has the mental capacity to make such a decision. The primary physician must also make the patient aware of all the alternatives, including hospice care, comfort care, and pain control options. Many practices now use the term "physician-assisted death" rather than "suicide." The specific method in each state varies. The exam is unlikely to make you choose MAID as an option for the patient because it is still controversial and only legal in a few states; the key point in this case is to find out how the patient ended up wanting to make this decision to end his life. Finding out his reasoning may help the team optimize the patient's remaining quality of life and give him the power to ask for what he needs.
Additional Considerations	**Euthanasia** should be differentiated from physician-assisted suicide; euthanasia involves the physician administering a lethal substance, and is illegal in all states.

CASE 16 | Involuntary Psychiatric Hospitalization

A 43-year-old undomiciled man with a history of schizophrenia is brought into the ED by police for wandering outdoors looking lost and shouting to himself and others. He appears unkempt, and is malodorous and extremely thin. He has been hospitalized more than 10 times in the past for his schizophrenia and has tried to commit suicide by walking in front of oncoming traffic. He is not taking any of his antipsychotic medication. When probed about suicidal ideations or plan, the patient asks to leave the hospital immediately because "CIA agents are out to get me" and he is hearing voices telling him to go to the White House and warn the president. On mental status exam, the patient makes poor eye contact, has tangential speech, and is responding to internal stimuli throughout the interview. He makes an elopement attempt and when unsuccessful, threatens the ED staff and becomes agitated.

CASE 16 | **Involuntary Psychiatric Hospitalization** *(continued)*

Considerations and Next Steps	This patient is suffering from a severe chronic mental illness, has a history of a suicide attempt (which increases future risk of successful suicide attempt), and therefore is not safe to be discharged back onto the streets. This patient has not been able to care for himself, is unable to converse with the physician, and is a threat to himself and others.
Clinical Decision	The patient requires inpatient psychiatric hospitalization due to high acute risk of harm to himself and others.
Discussion	Safety of the patient and others is paramount when deciding whether a patient requires inpatient psychiatric hospitalization. The team should try to have the patient sign into admission voluntarily, but involuntary admission should be implemented if he refuses. The general predicates for involuntary psychiatric hospitalization include the presence of a mental illness with danger to self or others, and/or grave disability (inability to provide oneself with clothing, food, and/or shelter) due to mental illness.

QUALITY CARE AND PATIENT SAFETY

The Institute of Medicine defines health care quality as "the degree to which health care services for individuals and populations increase the likelihood of desired health outcomes and are consistent with current professional knowledge." The Institute of Medicine further defines quality in terms of having the following domains: effectiveness, efficiency, equity, patient centeredness, safety, and timeliness. Patient safety is an essential component of quality health care. Several system tools are in place to detect causes of safety errors in health care such as the Plan-Do-Study-Act (PDSA) cycle and root cause analysis. Preventing errors relies on a safe culture and human factors engineering (HFE) to identify and address risks. It is important for health care workers to be aware of cognitive biases to avoid future mistakes in taking care of patients. These concepts are all high yield for the USMLE exam and are essential in future practice as well.

CASE 17	**Medical Error Disclosure**
	A 21-year-old woman is admitted to the medicine service with a hemoglobin of 4.5 g/dL. She is extremely fatigued and dizzy, and recently passed out at work. She is about to receive a second blood transfusion. The treating physician notices that the patient was admitted to the hospital about a year ago and given the diagnosis of paroxysmal nocturnal hemoglobinuria, but the patient was never given the test results and never followed up in the hematology clinic due to miscommunication between team members.
Considerations and Next Steps	This presents a difficult and awkward situation for the provider who noticed this miscommunication; they may feel a need to clarify the situation before notifying the patient. However, this patient did not receive the necessary care she needed for a year and is now needing at least two blood transfusions and a hospitalization because no one followed up with her or informed her of the diagnosis.
Clinical Decision	The provider discloses the situation to the patient in an honest and concise manner and tells the patient they will look closely into the situation to provide a more definitive answer as to how this happened. The provider then gives the patient information about her condition and allows her to ask any questions she may have. The provider expresses empathy and tells the patient they are there to support her, and documents the medical record accordingly.
Discussion	Physicians have a legal fiduciary duty to act in the patient's best interests. When a mistake is discovered, the facts should be disclosed to the patient immediately. Patients are less likely to sue their physicians if their physicians are upfront and honest about the error. Preventing harm to future patients is the primary goal of error disclosure. Most institutions have a safety/risk department that keeps track of medical errors (as well as providing root cause analysis) and can provide support and resources when medical errors occur.

CASE 18	**Plan-Do-Study-Act (PDSA) Cycle**
	The director of an inpatient medicine floor notices an increased rate of catheter-associated urinary tract infections (CAUTI) among patients. He decides to design a quality improvement project with the goal to reduce CAUTI by 50%. The primary issue with the increased infections seems to be a lack of standardized catheter removal strategies. The director leads a team focused on quality improvement to write a checklist and standardized protocol which will be the key component of the plan. He organizes training sessions for physicians and staff to attend and administers exams after the sessions to ensure understanding. Based on the PDSA paradigm, what should be the director's next steps?

CASE 18 | Plan-Do-Study-Act (PDSA) Cycle (continued)

Considerations and Next Steps	The director should implement the new strategy for catheter removal and evaluate infection rates after a predetermined period of time.
Discussion	The PDSA cycle is an important tool in quality improvement. It is a four-step process that consists of the following: **Plan:** Identify an area that needs improvement and plan a change or action to bring about such improvement. It helps to have realistic, clear objectives that can be implemented in a timely manner. **Do:** Test the new action; document any problems/issues. **Study:** Analyze data before and after the change and its impact on the quality of health care. **Act:** Action consists of either implementating a new plan according to the data or determining any changes that need to be made to the current plan followed by preparing a new plan and beginning the cycle again. In this example, the director should implement the plan and make sure to collect data and document any observations or unexpected problems. The goal of the PDSA cycle is continual improvement.

CASE 19 | Root Cause Analysis

During a complicated laparoscopic hernia repair, sterile surgical towels were used to soak up excess blood inside the patient's abdomen. Throughout the procedure, the surgeons verbally expressed their discontent with the student's ability to appropriately retract to create better visibility. The resident and attending surgeon spend a long time suturing the inside of the abdominal cavity and are about to close and finish the operation. The student realizes the towels are still inside the patient's abdomen and thinks they are supposed to be removed, but is unsure and is too afraid to speak up for fear of being reprimanded. The scrub technician miscounts the number of towels used during the procedure and informs the resident they can complete closure/suturing. The mistake is noted several days post op when the patient develops fevers and abdominal pain and must be taken back to the operating room (OR).

Considerations and Next Steps	Conduct a root cause analysis after the patient is appropriately treated.
Discussion	Root cause analysis is a retrospective review used to identify the root causes of an error or near miss and develop methods to prevent it from happening again. Root cause analysis answers three main questions: what happened, why did it happen, and what can be done to prevent it from happening again in the future. The goal is to not place blame on a single individual, but to take a closer look at the error and improve patient care. The **Swiss cheese model of error causation** depicts how catastrophic safety failures are almost never caused by isolated events but rather result from multiple smaller errors. The model depicts how a series of unlikely errors (i.e., holes in health care) ultimately lead to dangerous and sometimes life-threatening situations. For instance, in this scenario the surgeon and resident mistakenly left the towel in the abdominal cavity, the medical student noted the error but was afraid to speak up, and the scrub nurse miscounted the towels.

CASE 20 | Human Factors Engineering (HFE) Strategies

A 30-year-old woman is brought to the OR and is awaiting a laparoscopic cholecystectomy. In preparation for the surgery, the anesthesiologist prepares the local anesthetic, pain management, and prophylactic antibiotics. The medications are in similar appearing bags. The nurse in the OR connects the patient's intravenous line and begins infusion, believing it is the antibiotics when it is actually the anesthetic. Within a few minutes, the patient's breathing slows and she experiences a cardiac arrest. The patient is resuscitated but suffers multiple rib fractures, bruises, and pain as a consequence of cardiopulmonary resuscitation.

Considerations and Next Steps	Treat the patient, disclose the error, and consider what else could be done in the future to prevent such an error from happening again.
Discussion	The goal of HFE is to reduce errors based on common human behaviors. Key HFE measures include forcing functions, standardization, simplification, effective communication, and morbidity and mortality reviews. In this patient example, **forcing functions** (hard stops) in design would have prevented this error. Designing an anesthetic bag that would be incompatible with a peripheral line would have prevented the possibility of the wrong infusion in the first place. The health care setting is a busy, fast-paced environment with a heavy workload. HFE anticipates the human desire to try to work around certain protocols that may be ultimately harmful for patients and thus facilitates efficient design strategies. An example of standardization and simplification would be for every hospital unit to follow the same protocol for deep venous thrombosis prophylaxis so that no patient is forgotten after surgery. Institutional best practices often include mandatory checklists and/or physical safeguards that do not require much human effort so that the possibility of such an error is eliminated.

CASE 21 | Closed-Loop Communication

A 68-year-old man who recently suffered an ST-segment elevation myocardial infarction is found to be pulseless and in ventricular fibrillation. A code is called, and compressions are initiated. The physician running the code directs the nurse, "Administer 1 mg of epinephrine." After the pharmacist has drawn up the medication and passed it to the nurse, how should the nurse respond?

Considerations and Next Steps	The nurse should respond, "Administering 1 mg of epinephrine," and, after the medication is given, "One milligram of epinephrine given."
Discussion	This is an example of closed-loop communication. The nurse responded by repeating the order back to the physician, which ensures that the proper instructions were heard. This is particularly important in loud settings with many providers present, such as codes, to confirm that one provider heard the other correctly. This limits the possibility of errors due to misunderstandings. Elements of closed-loop communication include repeating all elements of the order as the initial provider stated it and speaking clearly and loudly enough for the first provider to hear. Poor communication would include saying nothing at all or simply saying "It's in."

CASE 22 | Biases

The overnight on-call pediatric surgeon receives a call from an outside hospital stating that they want to transfer a 14-year-old girl with right-sided abdominal pain and bedside ultrasound findings consistent with acute appendicitis. When the patient arrives in the ED, the on-call physician obtains surgical consent from the patient's mother for a laparoscopic appendectomy. The operation proceeds without complication, but intraoperatively, the surgeon finds diffusely inflamed bowel and an appendix that is only mildly edematous—findings more consistent with gastroenteritis. However, the appendix is removed, and the case concludes without complication.

Considerations and Next Steps	Acute appendicitis can sometimes be confused with gastroenteritis on ultrasound if the technician fails to examine sufficient surrounding bowel, for they will fail to recognize that the inflamed appendix is consistent with findings throughout the rest of the bowel rather than inflamed in isolation.
Discussion	Cognitive or diagnostic errors can occur due to various biases (see table below). These errors are often due to known associations and patterns they have witnessed before, which prevents physicians from considering other possibilities. These errors can occur for anyone, but physicians who are fatigued or overworked are particularly prone to making these errors. This case is an example of an **anchoring bias**, which is when a physician sees a patient with a particular diagnosis in mind and either A) fails to explore other differential diagnoses, or B) fails to change from an initial diagnosis despite evidence refuting the original diagnosis. This case exemplifies the first of these in which the on-call surgeon proceeded with surgery without obtaining their own history and physical exam and/or reviewing studies. Consequently, the surgeon's anchoring bias led to an unnecessary operation.

Common Cognitive Errors in Medicine

Bias	Definition	Example
Anchoring	Failing to entertain additional differential diagnoses after a diagnosis has been made	Continuing to reassure parents for more than a week that their child's nausea, vomiting, and diarrhea is gastroenteritis, without exploring potential alternative causes
Availability	Choosing a diagnosis based on previous similar presentations, i.e., what comes to mind first, without considering other possibilities	Attributing the pain of a patient with sickle cell disease to a sickling crisis without ruling out other possible causes
Confirmation	Assigning preference to evidence or findings that support a physician's view and ignoring/minimizing findings that refute this idea	Continuing to believe that a patient's sore throat and lymphadenopathy are due to streptococcal pharyngitis despite a negative antigen test and throat culture, causing a delay in diagnosing what was actually squamous cell carcinoma of the throat
Framing	Narrowing history-taking based on a certain potential diagnosis and failing to broaden the history to rule out other possibilities	Asking a pregnant woman with abdominal pain about only her obstetric and gynecological history, failing to discuss gastrointestinal issues, and subsequently missing acute appendicitis
Premature Closure	Failing to obtain additional information about the patient and/or additional tests after reaching a diagnostic conclusion and treating that diagnosis	Failing to test for osteoporosis and/or failing to consider secondary causes (e.g., vitamin D deficiency, multiple myeloma) when a fracture is likely a fragility fracture; failing to conduct a tertiary trauma survey 24–48 hours after the initial presentation and subsequently missing injuries

CASE 23 | Physician Misconduct and Medical Malpractice

An ED physician completes her 12-hour shift and wants to sign her patients out to her colleague. However, her colleague does not answer any of the pages or texts and shows up 2 hours late. She learns from her staff that this colleague has been late on several occasions and often does not return texts or pages in a timely fashion. When her colleague finally shows up, she notices that she looks unkempt, has some slurred speech, and her breath smells of alcohol. How should the ED physician handle the situation?

Considerations and Next Steps	Her colleague is showing signs concerning for alcohol intoxication and alcohol use disorder and is not in the proper condition to take care of patients. The physician should inform her superiors and continue managing the patients until backup coverage arrives.
Discussion	The impaired physician should be pulled from clinical duties and referred for further evaluation and treatment. They may also be referred to the state medical board, which has Physician Health Programs (PHPs). These programs can assess whether an impairment is present and offer a treatment plan. If the physician refuses treatment, the PHP can inform the state medical board, and the physician's licensure may be in jeopardy.
Additional Considerations	If the physician was found to have caused patient harm through her intoxication, this would be an example of **medical malpractice**. Additionally, if the ED doctor discovered a medical error occurred due to her colleague's intoxication, she is obligated to report this error to the hospital authorities or state medical board.

2

Epidemiology and Biostatistics

Lead Authors: Linda Chang, PharmD, MPH; Radhika Sreedhar, MD, MS
Contributors: Vanessa Jerger, MD; Kruti H. Patel, MD; Tara Gill, MD; Nicolas Bonamici, MD

INTRODUCTION

On the USMLE Step 2 CK exam, EBM questions focus on

- Application: interpreting medical literature
- Choosing between diagnostic tests
- Determining statistical and clinical significance

To this end, there is emphasis on methods of analysis such as Kaplan-Meier survival curves, systematic reviews and meta-analyses, and receiver–operator characteristic curves. Like the Step 1 exam, foundational concepts including sensitivity/specificity, 2×2 tables, and study designs are tested on Step 2 CK.

Addressing an EBM question:

1. Recognize the direction the question is taking: Does it involve reading/interpreting an abstract *or* does it involve determining the better diagnostic test for a patient?
2. Read the last sentence of the question stem and skim the answer choices to further identify the direction of the question.
3. Focus on the area of the abstract that will answer the question, as given below.

Anatomy of an Abstract

> **Introduction:** Look for the following:
>
> Is the description relevant to your clinical problem?
>
> Does PICO (population, intervention, comparison, outcomes) match your patient?

> **Methods:** Look for the following:
>
> Study design and study setting
>
> Inclusion/exclusion criteria
>
> Patient demographics match your patient profile
>
> Data/statistical analysis
>
> Primary and secondary outcomes

> **Results:** Look for the following:
>
> Outcomes (efficacy and side effects)
>
> Statistical significances
>
> Clinically significant for your patient?

> **Conclusion:** Look for the following:
>
> Do conclusions match what was seen in the study or goes beyond the study findings?
>
> What are the study limitations?

STUDY DESIGN

Types of Studies

Determining the type of study is best done by looking at the following:

- What is the starting point of the study?
- What is the study direction?

- When the exposure (e.g., risk factor, drug treatment, procedure) is assessed?
- When the outcome of a particular event (e.g., disease, adverse effect, cure) is assessed?

Based on this:

- If both exposure and outcome were determined at the same point in time, it is a *cross-sectional study*.
- If the study starts with cases and controls and the presence/absence of exposure is then determined in them, it is a *case-control study*.
- If exposure occurs first and the frequency of an event is studied among subjects at a later point in time, it is a *cohort study*.
- If the subjects are randomized to experimental treatment or placebo and frequency of events in the study subjects is assessed at a later point in time in a controlled setting, it is an *experimental study*. The gold standard of experimental studies is a *randomized control trial*.

Study Direction	Description	Study Design Measure of Association
Starts at one point in time Ends at the same point in time	Assesses the frequency of an outcome (disease) and/or the frequency of risk factor in a population at one point in time	**Cross-sectional** Prevalence of outcome and/or risk factor Does not show causality
Starts in the present where cases and controls are selected Exposure to risk factors is assessed in the past in both groups **Direction of inquiry: present to past**	Retrospectively compares the exposure in people with and without the outcome (disease)	**Case control** Odds ratio—compares the odds of exposure among cases to the odds of exposure among controls
Starts in the present with groups of people who are exposed and not exposed Ends in the future when the frequency of outcome is assessed in both groups **Direction of inquiry: present to future**	Compares outcomes (disease) among people with and without exposure to a risk factor (treatment)—can be prospective or retrospective	**Cohort** Incidence and relative risk **Prospective cohort**
Starts in the past with groups of people who are exposed and not exposed Ends in the present when the frequency of outcomes is assessed in both groups **Direction of inquiry: past to present**		**Retrospective cohort**
Starts in the present with people randomized to treatment (exposed) and to placebo (not exposed) Ends in the future when the frequency of outcome is assessed in both groups **Direction of inquiry: present to future**	Prospective study comparing outcomes among people with and without exposure (treatment) after randomization to minimize bias	**Randomized controlled trial** Incidence Relative risk Absolute risk Number needed to treat/harm

Types of Study Vignettes

CASE 1 | Case Series

A neurologist observes that eight patients who presented with stroke had taken an unknown supplement "clotamin" for the past 4 months. She plans to publish a report of these patients.

Discussion	A case series is a collection of similar cases presented in one report often used for rare or unique clinical presentations of a disease.
Strengths	• Cost-efficient • Easy to conduct • Generate hypotheses for more formal testing
Weaknesses	• No comparison or control group • No specific research questions • Results are based solely on interesting observations

CASE 2 | Cross-Sectional Study

An 18-year-old woman presents to clinic with swelling and discoloration of toes during the height of the COVID pandemic. She reports that the skin color on her toes changed to purple, and this was followed by the appearance of red to brown spots. She wishes to know if these changes in her toes are related to COVID infection (exposure), given the media reports of "COVID toes" (outcome). To answer her question, an article is reviewed in which all adolescents who had a COVID test in the prior month in the state of Illinois were surveyed as to whether they experienced changes in the color of their toes.

Discussion	Cross-sectional studies are used to examine the frequency of an event in a population at **one point** in time. The research question focuses on the prevalence of disease in a population. • Exposures and outcomes are assessed at the **same time**. • The measure of association used is the **prevalence ratio**. • Prevalence ratio is the proportion of patients with the outcome divided by the proportion of patients with the exposure.
Diagram	 Cross-sectional study.
Strengths	• Cost-efficient. • Easy to conduct and implement. • Large size permits estimation of risk factors in populations.
Weaknesses	• Not possible to distinguish cause and effect. • Inferences are limited to the specific time. • Not generalizable to other times or places. • Sampling bias is present (not everyone agrees to participate).

CASE 3 | Case-Control Study

To study the effectiveness of the use of masks against COVID-19, an investigator reviewed the medical records of patients admitted to the hospital and identified 100 patients with and 100 without a positive COVID test. Each patient was interviewed to assess if they used a mask or not prior to the COVID test. The purpose of the study was to see if there was an association between use of a mask and the diagnosis of COVID-19.

Discussion	Case-control studies begin with determining if the outcome of interest is present or not. Once the cases and controls are identified, the proportion of persons with exposure to the risk factor is assessed in both groups to determine whether there is an association between the exposure to the risk/protective factor and the occurrence of disease. • In this study the outcome of interest is a person with a positive COVID test (case). • Persons with (COVID cases) and without the outcome (controls) are then evaluated to determine if they have had the exposure of interest (use of mask). • The study is retrospective in its assessment of exposures (use of mask).

CASE 3 | Case-Control Study (continued)

Discussion	• A difference in the proportions of persons with the exposure of interest will help determine if there is an association between the exposure and outcome. • **Odds ratios** (ORs) are used as the measure of association. • OR indicates the odds of a disease or event occurring in an exposed population compared to the unexposed population.
Diagram	 Case control study.
Strengths	• Cost- and time-efficient. • Can study significant numbers of cases, which is useful for rare conditions. • Can minimize ethical problems since potential harmful exposure such as identifying drug side effects is not allocated to any study group.
Weaknesses	• Study is retrospective. • Potential sources of bias include confounding factors, selection bias, and recall bias, as cases may remember exposures better than controls. • Over-/underestimation of association is possible since sampling relies heavily on outcome. Both exposure and disease have already occurred, making it difficult to establish a temporal relationship.

CASE 4 | Cohort Study

An investigator wants to assess whether the use of adenoviral vector–based vaccines for COVID-19 is associated with immune thrombotic thrombocytopenia. The investigator reviewed records and identified 500 patients who were given the mRNA vaccine and 500 similar patients who were given the adenoviral vector–based vaccines. All patients were followed up for 6 months after they received the vaccine to determine if there was a difference between these two groups in the number of patients who developed immune thrombotic thrombocytopenia.

Discussion	Cohort studies begin with persons who do not have the disease. They are either exposed or not exposed to a potential risk factor. Individuals are followed in time to determine how many develop the disease in the exposed and unexposed group. • In a **prospective cohort study**, a group of people with similar baseline characteristics except for exposure (vaccine type) are followed in time to determine if there is a difference in the incidence of outcome (immune thrombotic thrombocytopenia) between the exposed and unexposed groups. • In a **retrospective cohort study**, researchers use data that have already been collected on a defined group of people (immunized against COVID) to identify their exposure status (type of vaccine) and then determine if the outcome occurred (immune thrombotic thrombocytopenia) because of their exposure.

CASE 4 | Cohort Study *(continued)*

Diagram	
	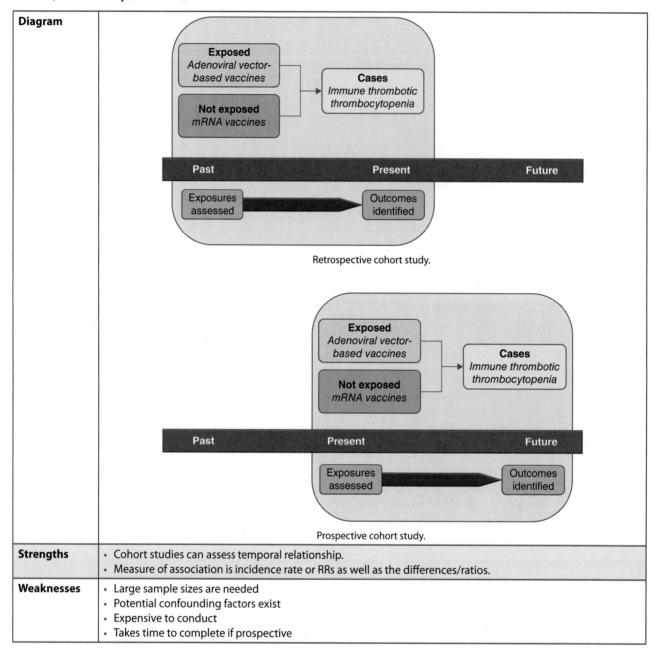

Retrospective cohort study.

Prospective cohort study.

Strengths	• Cohort studies can assess temporal relationship. • Measure of association is incidence rate or RRs as well as the differences/ratios.
Weaknesses	• Large sample sizes are needed • Potential confounding factors exist • Expensive to conduct • Takes time to complete if prospective

CASE 5 | Randomized Clinical Trial (RCT)

A randomized double-blind study of 5000 participants compares the efficacy of two medications in reducing death due to COVID-19: The first is a novel drug, and the second is remdesivir with dexamethasone. Over the 1-month study period, participants will be monitored for all-cause mortality and the major sequela of COVID-19. Participants will not be informed which drug they are taking. In addition, the physician and other individuals responsible for collecting all outcome measures will not be aware of what medication the patient is taking. The average reduction in mortality and risk of major sequela will be compared between the medications at the end of the 1-month study.

Discussion	In an RCT, the researcher plans the experiment in such a manner that the two groups differ only in the exposure to the treatment. This helps minimize bias and confounding so that the results we see can be directly ascribed to the treatment. • People are randomized to receive either the novel treatment, *or* • the placebo/standard of care (remdesivir + dexamethasone). • Blinding helps minimize bias.

CASE 5 | Randomized Clinical Trial (RCT) *(continued)*

Diagram	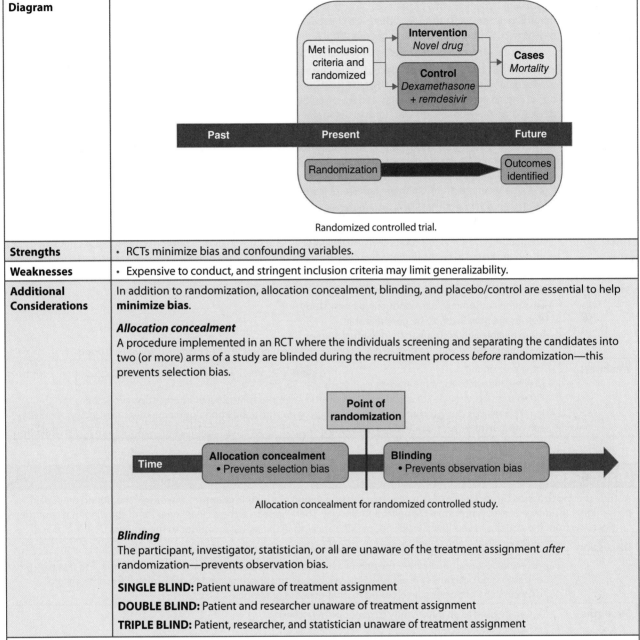<div align="center">Randomized controlled trial.</div>
Strengths	• RCTs minimize bias and confounding variables.
Weaknesses	• Expensive to conduct, and stringent inclusion criteria may limit generalizability.
Additional Considerations	In addition to randomization, allocation concealment, blinding, and placebo/control are essential to help **minimize bias**. ***Allocation concealment*** A procedure implemented in an RCT where the individuals screening and separating the candidates into two (or more) arms of a study are blinded during the recruitment process *before* randomization—this prevents selection bias. Allocation concealment for randomized controlled study. ***Blinding*** The participant, investigator, statistician, or all are unaware of the treatment assignment *after* randomization—prevents observation bias. **SINGLE BLIND:** Patient unaware of treatment assignment **DOUBLE BLIND:** Patient and researcher unaware of treatment assignment **TRIPLE BLIND:** Patient, researcher, and statistician unaware of treatment assignment

Clinical Phase	Purpose	Population	Number of Subjects	Duration of Clinical Phase
I (Not blind)	Drug safety and pharmacokinetics	Healthy volunteers	20–100	Several months
II (Single or double blind)	Drug efficacy and safety	Patients with target disease	Few hundred	Months to 2 years
III (Double blind)	Drug efficacy and safety	Patient with target disease	Few hundred to few thousand	1–4 years
IV (Post-marketing surveillance trials)	Safety monitoring	This safety monitoring phase takes place after FDA approval of the new drug. The goal is to monitor drug safety over a long period of time.		

Source: https://www.fda.gov/patients/drug-development-process/step-3-clinical-research

CASE 6 | Systematic Review and Meta-Analysis

A 62-year-old woman with hyperlipidemia presents to clinic to discuss her medications. She was recently prescribed rosuvastatin and has trouble affording it. She wants to know if there is a cheaper cholesterol-lowering medication. The physician searches the topic and finds a systematic review to best answer her question. A sample of the abstract is as follows.

Objective: This systematic review compares the efficacy and safety profiles of different statins.

Methods: Publications of RCTs of statins were collected (using the search terms dyslipidemia, LDL lowering, and statin therapy) from the Oregon state database from 1966–2004, MEDLINE from 2005–2006, and EMBASE 2005–2006. The publications were selected based on set criteria based on study quality and reviewed by a team of three reviewers. The mean change in cholesterol per statin was calculated and a meta-analysis was done to determine the estimates of the statins' efficacies and differences.

Results: Seventy-five RCTs comparing statins were included. The pooled results showed that daily doses of atorvastatin 10 mg, simvastatin 20 mg, fluvastatin 80 mg, and lovastatin 40–80 mg decreased LDL-C by 30–40%. Daily doses of pravastatin 20–40 mg, fluvastatin 40 mg, and lovastatin 10–20 mg decreased LDL-C by 20–30%. Rosuvastatin and atorvastatin at a daily dose of 20 mg or higher were the only two statins that could reduce LDL-C more than 40%. There was a statistically significant but clinically minor difference (<7%) between the statins in their cholesterol-lowering effect.

Modified from: Weng TC, Yang YH, Lin SJ, Tai SH. A systematic review and meta-analysis on the therapeutic equivalence of statins. J Clin Pharm Ther. 2010 Apr;35(2):139-51.

Discussion	Systematic reviews provide a comprehensive review of all relevant studies on a health-related topic or clinical question and are considered to be the highest level of evidence if done well. A meta-analysis is a way to systematically combine relevant qualitative and quantitative data to develop a single conclusion of higher statistical power.
Strengths	• Less costly • Less time consuming than conducting a new study • Results are more likely to be generalizable • More reliable and accurate than individual studies • Systematic review with meta-analysis is considered the highest level of evidence when well done
Weakness	• Time consuming • May be difficult to combine studies • Often does not provide specific details about study demographic data or intervention protocol • In meta-analysis the inclusion of studies of different design/populations/outcome measures and poor quality can result in heterogeneity, making it less reliable.

CASE 7 | Ecologic Study

A study is done to assess the incidence of skin cancer in the population of multiple countries. The researcher found that Spain had a higher incidence of skin cancer than Denmark and Norway. There appears to be a clear linear trend showing that countries farther away from the equator have a lower incidence of skin cancer than those that are closer to the equator.

Discussion	In these studies, the unit of observation is a population or entire community, not an individual person. An *ecologic study* is one where the unit of assessment is the population rather than a person. The rate of exposure and outcomes are assessed in populations and are compared to determine if the differences in exposure at a population level results in differences in outcomes.
Strengths	• Can be used as an initial study to generate hypothesis • Faster data collection • Less costly • Larger data pools for population data
Weaknesses	• Cannot be generalized to individuals in a population (see "Ecological Fallacy") • Discrepancies in regional data collection • Limited data available on confounding factors

STUDY BIASES

Bias is a systematic deviation from the truth that occurs in a study resulting in erroneous conclusions. It can occur in

- Data collection
- Data analysis
- Interpretation
- Publication

As we appraise studies, we should be aware of these biases and ensure that the results we see are not due to these biases. Lead time and length time biases are the most frequently misinterpreted, so pay close attention to the nuances in Cases 11 and 12.

Description	Name	Strategies to Reduce Bias
Systematic error in which participants selected for a study group all have a similar characteristic as compared to the other group that is unintended by the researchers.	Selection bias	Randomization
If individuals experienced a disease or adverse outcome they are more likely to think about possible "causes" of the outcome, so they are more likely to remember their previous exposures.	Recall bias	Measure exposures before outcomes occur
Systemic issue in the collection of the data such that it does not capture the information accurately.	Measurement bias	Use objective criteria for measurement of exposures and outcomes
Outcomes are assessed in greater detail among those who have the disease as compared to those who do not have the disease.	Ascertainment bias	Blinding of assessors to outcomes and using objective measures to assess outcomes
Factor that is: • Associated with the exposure • Associated with outcome independent of exposure • Not in causal pathway of exposure to outcome	Confounding	Randomization
Diagnosis as the result of early screening may result in an overestimation of survival duration when survival is measured from the time of diagnosis. This is not a true increase in survival, but rather an artifact caused by an earlier diagnosis.	Lead time bias	Use mortality rates instead of survival rates
Overestimation of survival duration caused by the relative excess of slowly progressive cases among screen-detected cases.	Length time bias	Assess all outcomes regardless of method of detection

CASE 8 | Selection Bias

A 65-year-old woman with a history of breast cancer presents for follow-up. She brings an article she found on the relationship between the use of acetaminophen and occurrence of breast cancer. She has used acetaminophen intermittently over the years for joint pains and would like to know if this could have contributed to her cancer. On review of the abstract, it is noted that for this study the cases were recruited from hospital records, and controls were recruited by cold calling a list of random phone numbers between 10 a.m. and 4 p.m. on weekdays.

Discussion	• Selection bias is a systematic error in which participants selected for a study group all have a similar characteristic that is unintended by the researchers. • The cases and controls differ in baseline characteristics because of the manner in which participants were recruited for the study or assigned to their study groups. • This may limit generalizability of findings beyond the specific population selected.

CASE 9 | Recall Bias

A 56-year-old man who was recently diagnosed with polyps on screening colonoscopy brings in a study showing a link between the use of instant coffee and colon cancer. He wishes to know if he should stop drinking instant coffee to reduce his risk of developing colon cancer. In the study, the cases were people who had colon cancer and the controls were people without colon cancer. They were asked whether they used instant coffee, with the intention of determining whether instant coffee was associated with colon cancer.

Discussion	If individuals experienced a disease or had an adverse outcome, they are more likely to think about the possible "causes" of the outcome, and so are more likely to remember their previous exposures.

CASE 10 | Measurement Bias

A local meat packing plant hopes to decrease the rate of contaminated products. An observational study on handwashing by employees is done. A researcher is stationed in each hallway and records how many employees washed their hands before entering the work area.

Discussion	• Measurement bias occurs when there is a systemic issue in the collection of the data such that it does not capture the information accurately. • The above example represents a particular type of measurement bias called the **Hawthorne effect**, in which subjects of a study are likely to change their actions if they know they are being observed.

CASE 11 | Lead Time Bias

A 64-year-old woman with lung cancer diagnosed on low-dose lung computed tomography (CT) 2 months ago presents for a second opinion. She brings an advertisement for a new sputum cytology test which claims to detect lung cancer earlier than low-dose CT scan. She asks if her life expectancy would have been longer had she had the sputum cytology test rather than the low-dose lung CT. The abstract is as follows:

A new test for sputum cytology for lung cancer detection was tested in patients over age 45 attending a pulmonary clinic. The survival duration of patients with lung cancer detected by the sputum test is 20 years versus 15 years with detection of lung cancer by symptoms. There is no difference in the quality-of-life measures annually between the two groups. At autopsy, the extent of progression of lung cancer is the same in both groups of patients despite treatment.

Discussion	Because survival is measured from the time of diagnosis, early diagnosis as the result of early screening may result in an overestimation of survival duration.
Diagram of Lead Time Bias	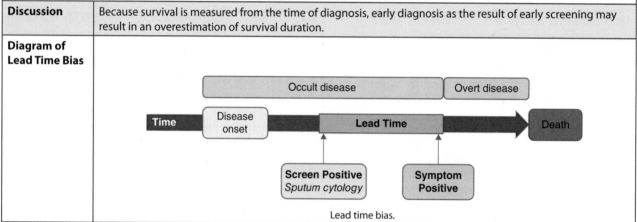 Lead time bias.

CASE 12 | Length Time Bias

A 45-year-old man brings in an abstract about a new stool test for colon cancer. The study compared the survival of asymptomatic people who were diagnosed with colon cancer using the new stool-based screening test with the survival of patients with colon cancer detected by colonoscopy when they presented with cough and weight loss. It found that patients whose colon cancer was detected by the stool test lived longer than those detected by colonoscopy when they presented with symptoms. Autopsy results showed that the stool test–positive colon cancers were less aggressive and more slow growing when compared to the colonoscopy-detected colon cancer.

Discussion	Length time bias refers to the overestimation of survival duration caused by the relative excess of slowly progressive cases among screen-detected cases.

CASE 12 | Length Time Bias *(continued)*

Diagram of Length Time Bias	
	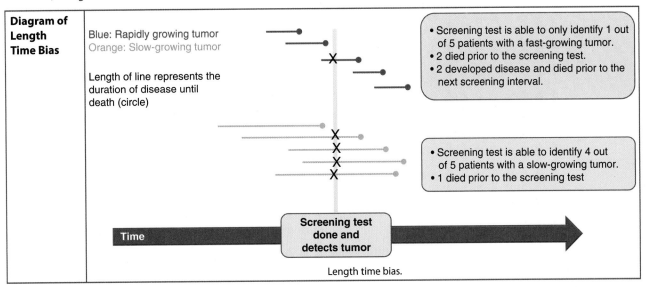

Length time bias.

CASE 13 | Ecological Fallacy

A 75-year-old woman with hypertension and hyperlipidemia comes to the physician's office for her annual visit. She recently read an article that showed that the number of cell phones per capita was negatively associated with rates of death from stroke. She does not own a cell phone and wonders if her risk of mortality from stroke has been decreased.

Discussion	• Ecological fallacy is an interpretive error where individual interpretations are made based on population level data. • It assumes that individuals within a group have the same characteristics as the average of the whole group.

EVALUATION OF TEST RESULTS

Step 2 CK generally provides abstracts about screening and diagnostic tests and assesses your ability to determine and interpret the following:

- Sensitivity
- Specificity
- Positive Predictive Value (PPV)
- Negative Predictive Value (NPV)

Sensitivity and specificity are two qualities of screening and diagnostic tests that clinicians use to capture the test's ability to correctly identify those who have and don't have the disease. The following abbreviations will be used in this section:

True Positive -TP; False Positive - FP; False Negative - FN; True Negative - TN.

Let us look at the performance of a new screening test for diabetes to get a conceptual understanding of what these terms mean.

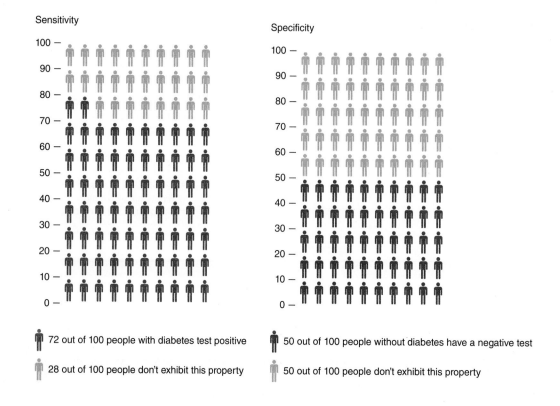

Sensitivity

🚹 72 out of 100 people with diabetes test positive

🚹 28 out of 100 people don't exhibit this property

Specificity

🚹 50 out of 100 people without diabetes have a negative test

🚹 50 out of 100 people don't exhibit this property

Sensitivity of a test reveals the proportion of patients with a positive result among all the patients who have the disease. Tests with high sensitivity are used to rule out disease when they are negative as they have low false negative rates. SnNout- highly Sensitive tests when Negative rule out disease. This is a stable property of test that *does not* change with prevalence of the disease.

In this study, 72 out of 100 people with diabetes test positive with the new screening test

Sensitivity = Positivity in Disease (PID) = Test positive/Disease positive = TP/ (TP + FN) = 72%
Sensitivity (Sn) = 72% of people with diabetes will have a positive test result

Specificity of a test reveals the proportion of patients with a negative result among all the patients who do not have the disease. Tests with high specificity are used to rule in disease when positive as the false postive (FP) rates are low. SpPin- highly Specific tests when Negative help rule in disease. This is a stable property of test that *does not* change with the prevalence of the disease.

In this study, 50 out of 100 people without the diabetes test negative with the new screening test.

Specificity = Negative in Health (NIH) = Test negative/Disease negative = TN/ (TN + FP) = 50%
Specificity (Sp) = 50% of people without diabetes will have a negative test result.

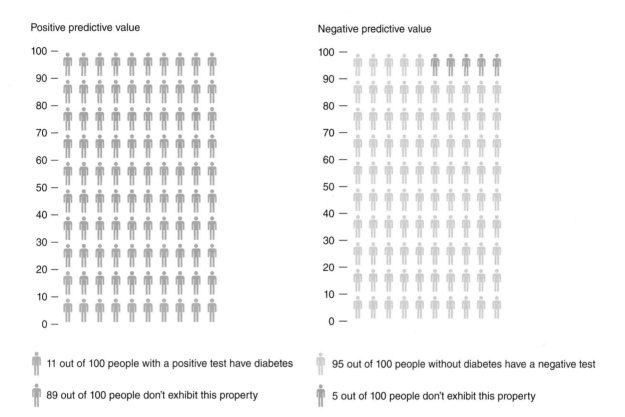

Positive predictive value

Negative predictive value

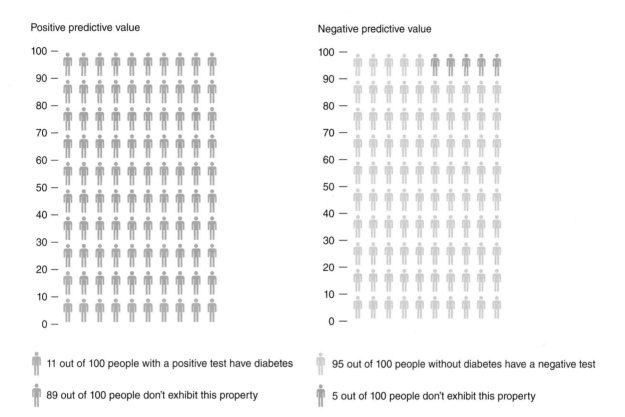

11 out of 100 people with a positive test have diabetes

95 out of 100 people without diabetes have a negative test

89 out of 100 people don't exhibit this property

5 out of 100 people don't exhibit this property

The **PPV** tells us the proportion of patients with the disease among all patients with a positive test result. This value *changes* with disease prevalence: as prevalence or pre-test probability increases, PPV increases.

In the same study, 11 out of 100 people with a positive screening test have diabetes based on the gold standard.

$$PPV = \text{True positives/all positives} = TP/TP + FP = 11$$
$$PPV = 11\% \text{ of people with a positive test result.}$$

The **NPV** tells us what the proportion of patients without the disease is among all the patients with a negative test result. This value *changes* with disease prevalence: As prevalence or pre-test probability increases, NPV decreases.

In this study, 95 out of 100 people with a negative screening test do not have diabetes.

$$NPV = \text{True negative/all negatives} = TN/TN + FN = 95\%$$
$$NPV = 95\% \text{ of people with a negative test will not have the disease.}$$

VIGNETTE

A 51-year-old woman brings in the following abstract about the use of fecal immunochemical test (FIT) for screening for colon cancer. She heard the FIT is less invasive and wondered if it may be equally accurate or better for her as a screening test.

ABSTRACT

Purpose

The FIT screening test is less invasive and more convenient than the traditional colonoscopy. We wish to determine the diagnostic characteristics of FIT testing in the detection of colon cancer in patients older than 50 years.

Materials and Methods

Stool samples were sent in by 173 participants to be analyzed by the FIT. Participants then underwent colonoscopies with subsequent biopsies to histologically diagnose colon cancer. Sample results were evaluated independently by three pathologists who did not know the results of the biopsy.

Results

Cancer was confirmed histologically in 145 participants, and the FIT was positive in 120 of these patients. Among the 28 patients without cancer, the FIT was negative in 21. The results of testing are provided in the table that follows. Of patients with a positive FIT, 94% were found to have colon cancer.

Conclusion

FIT has good diagnostic characteristics in detecting colon cancer in patients older than 50 years. Further studies should be done to determine if this test is a good screening test for colon cancer in a large patient population.

	Disease + Colon Cancer	Disease – No Colon Cancer	Total
Screen positive test result FIT positive	120 TP	7 FP	127 All screen positive
Screen negative test result FIT negative	25 FN	21 TN	46 All screen negative
Total	145 All disease positive	28 All disease negative	173

Abbreviations: TP, true positive; FP, false positive; FN, false negative; TN, true negative.

Source: Chen H, Lu M, Liu C, et al. Comparative Evaluation of Participation and Diagnostic Yield of Colonoscopy vs Fecal Immunochemical Test vs Risk-Adapted Screening in Colorectal Cancer Screening: Interim Analysis of a Multicenter Randomized Controlled Trial (TARGET-C). *Am J Gastroenterol.* 2020 Aug;115(8):1264-1274. [PMID: 32282342].

CASE 14 | Sensitivity

Based on the abstract, how many patients will have a positive FIT among all patients with colon cancer?

Equation	$$\text{Sensitivity} = \frac{\text{True Positives}}{\text{True Positives + False Negatives}}$$
Discussion	This question is asking about sensitivity, **the true positive (TP) rate**. Among all patients with the disease, sensitivity reveals how many patients will have a positive test result ("positive in disease"). This is $\frac{120}{145} = 83\%$
Diagram	

Sensitivity			
	Disease +	Disease –	Total
Screen positive test result	TP True Positive	FP False Positive	All screen positive
Screen negative test result	FN False Negative	TN True Negative	All screen negative
Total	All Disease Positive	All Disease Negative	Total population

Sensitivity.

CASE 15 | Specificity

Based on the abstract, how many patients will have a negative FIT among all patients without colon cancer?

Equation	$$\text{Specificity} = \frac{\text{True Negatives}}{\text{True Negatives + False Positives}}$$

CASE 15 | Specificity (continued)

Discussion	This question is asking about specificity, **the true negative [TN] rate**. Among all patients without disease, specificity reveals how many will have a negative test result ("negative in health")? This is $\frac{21}{28} = 75\%$
Diagram	 Specificity.

The diagram table for Specificity:

	Disease +	Disease −	Total
Screen positive test result	TP True Positive	FP False Positive	All screen positive
Screen negative test result	FN False Negative	TN True Negative	All screen negative
Total	All Disease Positive	All Disease Negative	Total population

---

CASE 16 | Positive Predictive Value (PPV)

Based on the abstract, how many patients truly have colon cancer among all patients with positive FIT results?

Equation	$$PPV = \frac{True\,Positives}{True\,Positives + False\,Positives}$$
Discussion	This question is asking about PPV. Among all patients with a **positive test result**, how many will **truly have the disease**? This is $\frac{120}{127} = 94\%$
Diagram	Positive predictive value.

The diagram table for PPV:

		Disease +	Disease −	Total
PPV	Screen positive test result	TP True Positive	FP False Positive	All screen positive
	Screen negative test result	FN False Negative	TN True Negative	All screen negative
	Total	All Disease Positive	All Disease Negative	Total population

---

CASE 17 | Negative Predictive Value (NPV)

Based on the abstract, how many patients truly do not have colon cancer among all patients with negative FIT results?

Equation	$$NPV = \frac{True\,Negatives}{True\,Negatives + False\,Negatives}$$
Discussion	The patient is asking about the NPV of the test. Among all patients with a **negative test** result, how many truly **do not have the disease**? This is $\frac{21}{46} = 45\%$
Diagram	Negative predictive value.

The diagram table for NPV:

		Disease +	Disease −	Total
	Screen positive test result	TP True Positive	FP False Positive	All screen positive
NPV	Screen negative test result	FN False Negative	TN True Negative	All screen negative
	Total	All Disease Positive	All Disease Negative	Total population

CASE 18 | Prevalence

The patient states that there is no history of any cancer in her family, and she wonders how many people in the study had colon cancer.

Equation	$\text{Prevalence} = \dfrac{\#\,\text{new cases}}{\text{Total}\,\#\,\text{people}}$ at a point in time
Discussion	The **total number of cases** of a disease in a population **divided by the total population** gives the prevalence rate. It is a measure of disease occurrence at a specific point in time. This will help answer the patient's question about how many people in the study had colon cancer. $\text{Prevalence} = \dfrac{\text{TP + FN}}{\text{TP + FN + FP + TN}} = \dfrac{145}{173} = 83\%$
Diagram	

	Disease +	Disease −	Total
Screen positive test result	TP True Positive	FP False Positive	All screen positive
Screen negative test result	FN False Negative	TN True Negative	All screen negative
Prevalence	All Disease Positive	All Disease Negative	Total population

Prevalence.

CASE 19 | Incidence

The study had a high prevalence of colon cancer. How many new cases of colon cancer occur every year?

Equation	$\text{Incidence rate} = \dfrac{\#\,\text{new cases}}{\#\,\text{people at risk}}$ during a specific time period

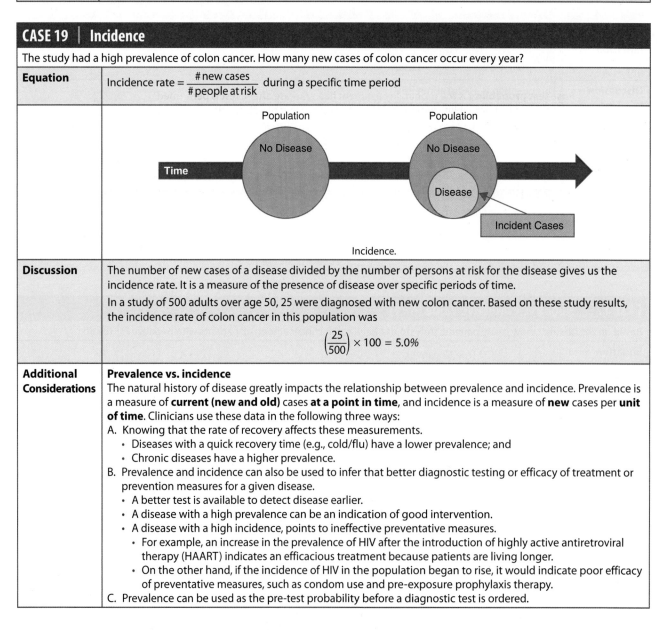

Incidence.

Discussion	The number of new cases of a disease divided by the number of persons at risk for the disease gives us the incidence rate. It is a measure of the presence of disease over specific periods of time. In a study of 500 adults over age 50, 25 were diagnosed with new colon cancer. Based on these study results, the incidence rate of colon cancer in this population was $\left(\dfrac{25}{500}\right) \times 100 = 5.0\%$

Additional Considerations	**Prevalence vs. incidence**
	 The natural history of disease greatly impacts the relationship between prevalence and incidence. Prevalence is a measure of **current (new and old)** cases **at a point in time**, and incidence is a measure of **new** cases per **unit of time**. Clinicians use these data in the following three ways:
	 A. Knowing that the rate of recovery affects these measurements.
	 • Diseases with a quick recovery time (e.g., cold/flu) have a lower prevalence; and
	 • Chronic diseases have a higher prevalence.
	 B. Prevalence and incidence can also be used to infer that better diagnostic testing or efficacy of treatment or prevention measures for a given disease.
	 • A better test is available to detect disease earlier.
	 • A disease with a high prevalence can be an indication of good intervention.
	 • A disease with a high incidence, points to ineffective preventative measures.
	   • For example, an increase in the prevalence of HIV after the introduction of highly active antiretroviral therapy (HAART) indicates an efficacious treatment because patients are living longer.
	   • On the other hand, if the incidence of HIV in the population began to rise, it would indicate poor efficacy of preventative measures, such as condom use and pre-exposure prophylaxis therapy.
	 C. Prevalence can be used as the pre-test probability before a diagnostic test is ordered.

Factors used to determine whether a test is warranted include its:

- Diagnostic characteristics
- Cost
- Harms
- Pre-test probability (prevalence) of disease
- Likelihood ratios

VIGNETTE

Two patients arrive at the emergency department with similar presentations of right lower quadrant (RLQ) abdominal pain. One patient is a 25-year-old man (assigned male at birth) and the other is a 21-year-old woman (assigned female at birth). Two life-threatening causes of RLQ abdominal pain are acute appendicitis and ectopic pregnancy.

CASE 20	Pre-Test/Post-Test Probability
	To rule out ectopic pregnancy, a pregnancy test can be ordered. However, a pregnancy test would not be ordered for the male patient because the probability of being pregnant is 0%. Because the pre-test probability is zero, a positive test would be a false-positive test and the positive predictive value is zero. Therefore, a pregnancy test should not be ordered in a male patient.
Discussion	**Pre-test probability** is the probability the patient has a disease before the test is performed (usually provided by population prevalence in the Step Exam). If the pre-test probability (prevalence) is low: • A positive test is more likely to represent a FP. 　• This could lead to more unnecessary testing. 　• It would not change management. **Post-test probability** is the probability a patient has a disease after a test is performed. • If the post-test probability is extremely low it helps rule out the diagnosis. • If the post-test probability is in the indeterminate zone, further testing will be needed to confirm the diagnosis. • If the post-test probability of disease is high, a positive test is sufficient to make a diagnosis.

After ordering a pregnancy test for the 21-year-old woman and confirming it is negative, imaging tests must be ordered to rule out acute appendicitis. Review the results of the following meta-analysis that was done to determine if an abdominal CT is an appropriate test to diagnose acute appendicitis.

Study Purpose

To compare the accuracy of CT and ultrasonography (US) in the detection of acute appendicitis in adults.

Materials and Methods

Two investigators performed literature searches on PubMed, Embase, Google Scholar, and OVID using the search terms acute appendicitis, CT abdomen, ultrasound (US) abdomen, and diagnostic accuracy. Studies were selected if they were high quality randomized controlled trials or cohort studies and all patients had either both diagnostic tests or one imaging test and surgery. Five prospective cohort studies met these criteria and were selected. Data from these studies were pooled and summary estimates of sensitivity and specificity were calculated. These values were then used to determine the summary likelihood ratios (LRs).

Results

CT: sensitivity 0.95, specificity 0.90, +LR 9.50, −LR 0.06.

US: sensitivity 0.80, specificity 0.85, +LR 5.33, −LR 0.24.

Conclusion

Compared to US, CT is a more accurate test for diagnosing acute appendicitis.

Doria A, Moineddin R, Kellenberger C, et al. US or CT for diagnosis of appendicitis in children and adults? A meta-analysis. Radiology 2006 Oct;241(1):83-94.

CASE 21	Likelihood Ratios (LRs)

The patient is worried about the radiation exposure from the CT scan and inquires whether this test will change the care she receives as compared to the US, which does not expose her to any radiation.

Discussion	LRs are used in clinical practice to:

- Determine how much a test can change the post-test probability of disease
- Use the change in post-test probability to decide whether to do the test
- Compare different tests to choose which test is most helpful in making a diagnosis

Definition: The likelihood of a specific test result in a patient with the target disorder compared to the likelihood of the same result in a patient without the target disorder is the LR.

The formula for +LR and its interpretation is given below.

$$\text{Positive LR} = \frac{\text{sensitivity}}{(1 - \text{specificity})} = \frac{\text{TP rate}}{\text{FP rate}}$$

Values of +LR
- >10 very useful as it increases post-test probability by 45%
- 5 moderately useful as it increases the post-test probability by 30%
- 2 less useful as it increases the post-test probability by 15%
- 1 useless as it does not change the post-test probability

In the study above,
+LR for abdominal CT is $\frac{0.95}{(1 - 0.90)} = 9.5$

This +LR is between 5 and 10, meaning it will increase the post-test probability between 30% and 45%, which places it in the *moderately useful* category. To determine the usefulness of this test for our patient we will also consider the negative LR.

$$\text{Negative LR} = \frac{(1 - \text{sensitivity})}{\text{specificity}} = \frac{\text{FN rate}}{\text{TN rate}}$$

Values of −LR
- <0.1 very useful as it decreases the post-test probability by 45%
- 0.2 moderately useful as it decreases the post-test probability by 30%
- 0.5 less useful as it decreases the post-test probability by 15%

In the study above,
−LR for abdominal CT is $\frac{(1 - 0.95)}{0.90} = 0.06$

This −LR is <0.1, placing it in the *very useful* category, indicating a negative CT will decrease the post-test probability by 45%.

Based upon the positive and negative LRs calculated above, the results from the CT scan will impact the management of this case. While a positive test is only moderately useful according to the LR of 9.5, a negative result will successfully rule out the condition (LR 0.06). Thus, these values indicate the CT scan is useful in the management of this patient and should be ordered.

Overall, a clinically useful **+LR should be as high as possible** (at least >5) and a **−LR should be as low as possible** (at least <0.2).

TEST CUTOFFS

Test cutoff:

- Is an arbitrary point value
- Is used to determine when a screening or diagnostic test is positive or negative for a given disease condition
- Is chosen at a point that maximizes the diagnostic value of the test
- Considers the cost of the test and its consequences

Changes in the cutoff values of tests can impact the number of people classified as having the disease.

CASE 22 | Lowering a Test Cutoff

A 54-year-old woman with type 2 diabetes mellitus returns to clinic for diabetes management. She has been trying to lower her blood sugars with lifestyle modifications, and today her fasting blood glucose is 122 mg/dL. She wants to know if she still has diabetes and if she needs any additional treatment to prevent long-term diabetic complications.

A study was recently published in which physicians determined that patients with fasting blood glucose >116 mg/dL are at increased risk for vascular complications. As a result, they suggested that screening cutoffs for diabetes be changed from 126 mg/dL to 116 mg/dL to identify people with increased risk earlier. Based on the lowered cutoff score of 116, what will happen to the sensitivity, specificity, and predictive values of a blood glucose measurement used to diagnose diabetes mellitus and how may this impact the management for this patient?

Diagram	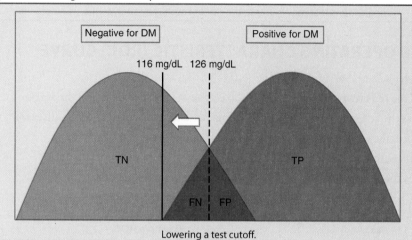

Lowering a test cutoff.

Discussion	Lowering the positive cutoff value for the test (126–116 mg/dL) will:

- Increase the number of positive tests (both TP and FP)
- Decrease the number of negative tests (both TN and FN)
- **Increase the sensitivity** (by decreasing FN in the denominator)
- **Decrease the specificity** (by increasing FP in the denominator)
- **PPV will decrease** because FP (only in the denominator) increased
- **NPV will increase** because FN (only in the denominator) decreased
- Identify more patients with diabetes

Options for this patient include continuing lifestyle modifications or supplementing with an oral medication to increase her sensitivity to insulin to reduce type 2 DM-related vascular complications.

CASE 23 | Raising a Test Cutoff

A week later, the patient brings her father (a 76-year-old male with type 2 diabetes mellitus) to clinic. His fasting blood glucose is 132 mg/dL. In the same study described in Case 22, researchers found that fasting blood glucose <136 mg/dL was sufficient in those older than age 70 to balance the risk of diabetes complications and treatment risks (e.g., hypoglycemia) and recommended changing screening cutoffs in this population to 132. How would this change affect the sensitivity, specificity, and predictive values of a blood glucose measurement and how may this impact the management for this patient?

Diagram	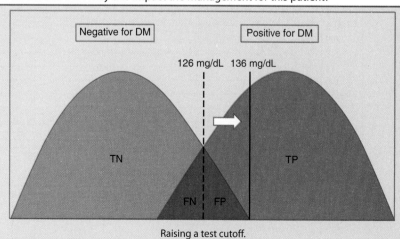

Raising a test cutoff.

CASE 23 | Raising a Test Cutoff *(continued)*

Discussion	Increasing the positive cutoff value for the test (126–136 mg/dL) will: • Increase the number of negative tests (both TN and FN) • **Decrease the sensitivity** (by increasing FN in the denominator) • **Increase the specificity** (by decreasing FP in the denominator) • **PPV will increase** because FP (only in the denominator) decreased • **NPV will decrease** because FN (only in the denominator) increased • Reduce the number of patients like him who tested positive for type 2 DM
	Options for this patient include being less aggressive in treating his blood sugars and discontinuing any medications that may increase the risk of causing hypoglycemia.

RECEIVER OPERATING CHARACTERISTIC (ROC) CURVE

The ROC curve:

- Is a plot of the sensitivity of the test on the *y* axis against (1 – specificity) on the *x* axis
- Helps assess the accuracy of the test in classifying patients as diseased and non-diseased
- Demonstrates the relationship between the TP rate and FP rate
- Helps compare the accuracy of similar tests
- Determines the LR at any given cut point to identify optimal test cutoffs

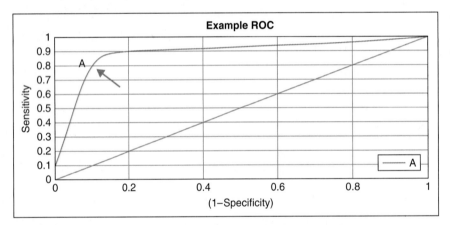

Figure 1. Receiver operating characteristic curve.

The point near the top left-hand corner (*arrow*) is the **optimal compromise** between sensitivity and specificity.

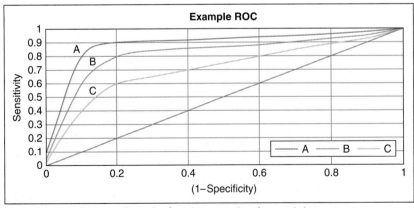

Figure 2. Example of receiver operating characteristic curve.

Tests A, B, and C represent different diagnostic tests plotted on the ROC curve. Test A, with the **greatest area under the curve (AUC)** also has the most favorable tradeoff since its curve is closest to the upper left-hand corner. Test C is closer to the 45-degree line and is the least accurate in identifying a disease.

CASE 24	ROC Curve	
A new set of tests are available to detect disease X as illustrated in Figure 2. The new chief medical officer in the hospital is wondering which test to adopt for this community hospital.		
Discussion	The accuracy of a test: • Depends on how well the test separates the group into who has the disease and who do not. • Is measured as the AUC for the ROC curve. • AUC = 1 represents a perfect test, which is one that best discriminates between patients who have disease and those who do not. • AUC = 0.5 represents (the diagonal line in the middle) a test that does not give any useful information and does not help differentiate those who have the disease from those who do not. • The best cutoff test has the value closest to the left-hand upper corner (*arrow*). The chief medical officer adopts the "A" test in Figure 2. **Note:** The positive LR is the $\dfrac{\text{sensitivity}}{(1 - \text{specificity})}$ and can be determined from the ROC curve as it is a plot of sensitivity against (1 − specificity).	

QUANTIFYING RISK

When discussing the efficacy of a treatment it is important to understand:

- The concepts of relative and absolute risk as it helps us assess the impact of the treatment, relative to no treatment and the impact of the treatment on the individual patient.
- The NNT and number needed to harm (NNH) to compare the risks and benefits of treatment and decide whether to use the treatment.

Example	Formula	Definition	Explanation
8/10 people exposed to ivermectin develop liver failure while 1/10 exposed to placebo develop liver failure	Relative risk (RR) = Experimental event rate (EER) divided by the Control event rate (CER) RR = 8/10 divided by 1/10 = 8	Risk of events in exposed group relative to the risk in the unexposed group	Used in cohort studies RR >1 means that the exposure is associated with more disease RR <1 means that the exposure is associated with less disease RR = 1 means no association between exposure and disease
Of the treatment group, 5% develop a stroke while on drug A and 15% of the control group develop a stroke while on the placebo drug	Relative risk reduction (RRR) RRR = 1 − RR RRR = (EER − CER)/CER	The proportion of risk reduction in the intervention arm relative to the control arm	RR = 5%/15% = 0.33 RRR= 1 − 0.33 = 0.66 or 66%
	Absolute risk reduction (ARR) = CER − EER	The absolute difference in event rates between the intervention and control arms	ARR = 15% − 5% = 10%
	Number needed to treat (NNT) = 1/ARR	The number of people who need to be treated for one additional patient to benefit	1/ARR = 1/10% = 10
The risk of skin cancer is 12% in high sun-exposure population vs. risk of skin cancer is 2% in minimal sun-exposure population	Attributable risk AR = Risk (i.e., proportion with an outcome) in exposed group − Risk (i.e., proportion with the outcome) in nonexposed group (baseline risk in the population)	Attributable risk (AR) is used in prospective cohort studies and measures the excess risk accounted for by exposure to a particular factor	AR = 12% − 2% = 10% Excess risk of skin cancer from sun exposure

VIGNETTE

A 26-year-old G3P2 woman at 10 weeks' gestation presents for prenatal care. She has a history of preeclampsia and asks what her risk of preeclampsia is, and what she can do to minimize the risk during her current pregnancy. To better answer her question, you review the following article.

Background

Preterm preeclampsia represents a common and important cause of maternal and fetal complications during pregnancy, particularly among those with a significant history. This study aims to determine the efficacy of daily low-dose aspirin at reducing the complications of preterm preeclampsia.

Methods

This was a multicenter, double-blind randomized controlled trial in which 17,187 patients with singleton pregnancies at high risk for preterm preeclampsia were randomized to placebo or 160 mg/day aspirin from weeks 11–36 gestation.

Results

Preterm preeclampsia occurred in 804/8587 (9.4%) patients randomized to the aspirin group vs. 1016/8600 (11.8%) patients randomized to the placebo group (OR: 23%; p <0.0001). The RR for all deaths with aspirin vs. placebo was 0.80 (95% confidence interval [CI]: 0.75–0.95).

Conclusions

160 mg aspirin daily appears to be associated with decreased preterm preeclampsia compared to placebo.

Modified from Rolnik DL, Wright D, Poon LC, et al. Aspirin versus placebo in pregnancies at high risk for preterm preeclampsia. N Engl J Med 2017 Aug 17;377(7):613-622. doi: 10.1056/NEJMoa1704559. Epub 2017 Jun 28. PMID: 28657417.

It is helpful to make a **2 × 2 contingency table**. These tables are useful for assessing disease rates and comparing those who received a particular intervention (e.g., drug vs. placebo) or those exposed to a risk factor (e.g., smoking vs. no smoking).

	Preterm Preeclampsia	No Preterm Preeclampsia	Totals
Aspirin (ASA) experimental group	804	8587 – 804 = 7783	8587
Placebo control group	1016	8600 – 1016 = 7584	8600
Totals	804 + 1016 = 1820	7783 + 7584 = 15367	17187

CASE 25	Event Rates	
Explanation	Event rates are measures of how often a particular event—typically the outcome or endpoint of a study—occurs within a group of people, typically within the experimental group. In this case, the event is preterm preeclampsia, and the two groups are the aspirin (ASA) and placebo groups. Event rates can subsequently be used to calculate other measurements such as RR that are more useful when interpreting a study.	
Calculation(s)	**Experimental Event Rate (EER)** = Absolute risk of preterm preeclampsia ASA group = $\dfrac{\text{risk of preterm preeclampsia in ASA group}}{\text{total number of patients in ASA group}} = \dfrac{804}{8587} = 9.4\%$	
	Control Event Rate (CER) = Absolute risk of preterm preeclampsia in placebo group = $\dfrac{\text{risk of preterm preeclampsia in placebo group}}{\text{total number of patients in placebo group}} = \dfrac{1016}{8600} = 11.8\%$	
Discussion	The CER can be used in this case to help the patient understand her risk of developing preeclampsia during her pregnancy.	

CASE 26 | Relative Risk (RR)

Explanation	The RR is a ratio of event rates between two groups: the risk of an event in the exposed group vs. the risk in the unexposed group. Because the calculation of RR requires the experimental and control event rates, it requires knowledge of each patient's exposure to either drug or placebo.
Calculation(s)	$RR = \dfrac{EER}{CER}$
Discussion	In this trial, the RR of preterm preeclampsia among those given aspirin as compared to placebo is 9.4/11.8 = 0.796. Because the RR is <1, aspirin is a protective factor, or exposure associated with a decrease in disease occurrence. The **relative risk reduction (RRR)**, which is the proportion of RR attributable to the intervention compared to control, calculated by RRR = 1 − RR. In this study the RRR of preterm preeclampsia among those given aspirin is 1 − 0.796 = 0.2. In other words, aspirin reduces the risk of preterm preeclampsia by 20% when compared to placebo.

CASE 27 | Absolute Risk Reduction (ARR)

Explanation	The ARR is the absolute difference in the proportions (percentage) of patients in the experimental arm and the control arm with the outcome of interest
Calculation(s)	ARR = (CER − EER)
Discussion	The ARR in preterm preeclampsia among those given aspirin was 11.8% − 9.4% or 2.4%. This study demonstrated that treatment with ASA reduces the risk of preterm preeclampsia by 2.4%.

CASE 28 | Number Needed to Treat (NNT)

Explanation	The NNT: • Is the inverse of the ARR expressed as a decimal. • Is a direct measure of intervention effect. • Considers the underlying risk—what would happen without the treatment. • Tells us whether the treatment works and how well it works compared to placebo/another treatment. NNT • Tells us how many patients must receive the treatment for one additional patient to experience the benefit of treatment. • NNT of *x* means that for every *x* patients treated with the experimental drug, one patient will respond specifically because of the experimental drug. The others will respond because of placebo-related mechanisms, and the rest will not respond. • A lower NNT means fewer people need to be treated for an additional patient to derive benefit, indicating a greater treatment effect. • The ideal NNT is 1, meaning that for every person treated an additional person will derive the benefit of treatment.
Calculation(s)	$NNT = \left(\dfrac{1}{ARR}\right) \times 100$ where the ARR is expressed as a percentage or $\left(\dfrac{1}{ARR}\right)$ where ARR is expressed as a decimal.
Discussion	The number of patients with a history of preterm preeclampsia who needed to be treated with aspirin 160 mg to prevent further preterm preeclampsia is (1/2.4) × 100 = 41. This means that for every 41 people with a history of preeclampsia treated with aspirin, one additional preterm preeclampsia is prevented when compared to placebo. **Number needed to harm (NNH)** Conversely, if the study found that aspirin increased the risk of preterm preeclampsia, the NNH could be calculated. • NNH represents the number of people who need to be exposed to the detrimental factor to result in one additional adverse event. • Higher numbers indicate treatment or exposure associated with fewer adverse events. • NNH is calculated as: $NNH = \left(\dfrac{1}{ARI}\right)$, where ARI is the absolute risk increase expressed as a percentage. • ARI = EER − CER

CASE 28 | Number Needed to Treat (NNT) *(continued)*

Discussion	NNT vs. NNH • In general, a good NNT is as low as possible and a good NNH is as high as possible. • The NNT and NNH are useful measures to help determine the balance of benefits vs. harms of treatment, with the goal of every treated patient experiencing improvement but not adverse events. • NNT is commonly used in clinical discussions with patients because it helps convey tangible conclusions from medical literature in a way that is readily understood.

The patient then asks if preterm preeclampsia could lead to preterm delivery. To help her understand her risk of preterm delivery, you review a study investigating the link between preterm preeclampsia and preterm delivery. The abstract follows:

Background

Preterm delivery is the leading cause of newborn mortality. Preterm preeclampsia has previously been shown to contribute to the risk of spontaneous or iatrogenic preterm delivery. This study aims to aid evidence-based prioritization of resources by quantifying the contribution of preeclampsia toward preterm delivery.

Methods

This was large population-based case-control study using a multi-hospital database to analyze data on women with singleton pregnancies who delivered between 2006 and 2016.

Results

21,640 patients were identified, of whom 20,366 had normal blood pressure throughout pregnancy. Of these patients, 1330 had a preterm delivery (6.5%). Of the 1274 patients with preeclampsia, 262 had a preterm delivery (20.6%). Preterm preeclampsia was found to be associated with higher rates of preterm delivery OR = 3.76 95% CI: (3.30–4.76).

Conclusions

Preterm preeclampsia is a contributing factor to preterm delivery in our hospital system and therefore potentially a useful condition to target to reduce preterm delivery.

Davies EL, Bell JS, Bhattacharya S. Preeclampsia and preterm delivery: A population-based case-control study. Hypertens Pregnancy 2016 Nov;35(4):510-519. doi: 10.1080/10641955.2016.1190846. Epub 2016 Jun 20. PMID: 27322489.

2 × 2 Contingency Table

	Preterm Delivery (Outcome)	No Preterm Delivery (No Outcome)	
Preeclampsia (exposure group)	a 262	b 1012	1274
No preeclampsia (no exposure group)	c 1330	d 19,036	20,366
	1592		21,640

CASE 29 | Odds Ratio (OR)

Explanation	Odds compares events with non-events. The OR tells us how strongly an event is associated with an exposure. It is the ratio of the odds of exposure to a risk factor among cases to the odds of exposure to the risk factor among controls. This is mathematically equivalent to the odds of an event in the exposed group (cases) to the odds of an event in the unexposed group (controls). OR is typically used in case-control studies where the incidence of disease cannot be determined, as the cases are not randomly sampled from the population, but instead selected by the investigator using a set of criteria.
Calculation(s)	$OR = \dfrac{\text{Odds of event in exposed group (cases)}}{\text{Odds of event in unexposed group (controls)}} = (a/b)/(c/d) = ad/bc$

CASE 29 | Odds Ratio (OR) *(continued)*

Discussion	Because this is an example of a case-control study, the OR can be calculated and is an appropriate measure of risk in the exposed population compared to the general population. It can be calculated as:
	OR = (262/1012) / (1330/19036) = 0.25889 / 0.06987 = 3.70
	Therefore, those who experienced preterm preeclampsia had 3.7 times greater odds of preterm delivery than those with normal blood pressure. • OR <1 indicates a decreased frequency of disease in someone with a given exposure. • OR >1 indicates an increased frequency of disease in someone with an exposure. • OR = 1 indicates no correlation between exposure and incidence of disease. • OR can be used to determine correlation between exposure and disease. • OR **does not imply causation**. • For diseases that have a low prevalence and are considered "rare," OR is similar to RR.
	In this study a diagnosis of preterm preecclampsia correlates with preterm delivery. There is a four times greater risk of preterm delivery in the group with preeclampsia as compared to the group without preecalmpsia. Based on this information, treatment for preterm preeclampsia can be considered to help reduce risk of preterm delivery.

SURVIVAL ANALYSIS AND PROPORTIONAL HAZARDS

Survival analysis is:

- Used to assess the time between entry into a study and a subsequent event
- Used to determine a patient's prognosis after an intervention
- Used to depict the average time from an event (diagnosis, disease presentation, disease treatment) to a given outcome using a survival curve

The most published survival analysis is the **Kaplan-Meier** analysis.

Proportional Hazards Ratio

- Compares the survival percentage at a given time between two or more survival curves
- Is a relative measure and does not reflect absolute risk
- Are analyzed *within a given time period*, making the study's length of follow-up critical in evaluating clinical significance

Estimation and interpretation of hazards ratio appear on the USMLE Step 2 CK, but quantification of the proportional hazards is beyond the scope of the exam.

VIGNETTE

A 72-year-old man with a history of atrial fibrillation treated with rivaroxaban is concerned about future stroke risk. To address this concern, you review the following abstract.

Background

Anticoagulation is the standard of care for patients with atrial fibrillation to reduce strokes and other thromboembolic events. In this study, rivaroxaban and a placebo control group were compared with respect to stroke.

Methods

This was a retrospective cohort study done between 2010 and 2020 of 1494 patients in one hospital system who were started treatment with rivaroxaban or placebo within a month of a diagnosis of atrial fibrillation. Kaplan-Meier stroke survival curves were constructed and analyzed.

Results

After mean follow-up of 27.2 months, 12 rivaroxaban-treated and 29 placebo-treated patients developed stroke. Proportional hazards showed that treatment with rivaroxaban reduced stroke risk by 22% (hazard ratio [HR], 0.78 [95% CI 0.72–0.90]).

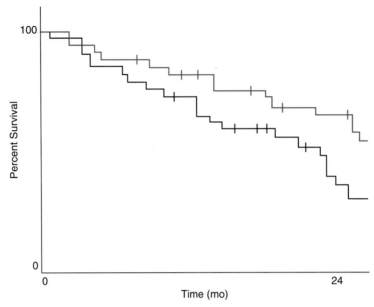

Kaplan-Meier stroke survival curve of placebo treated (■) and rivaroxaban treated (■) patients with atrial fibrillation.

CASE 30 | Kaplan-Meier (KM) Survival Curve

Explanation	The KM curve shows patient survival over time while on treatment intervention. In this study, at 24 months 60% of patients were stroke-free while on rivaroxaban, while only 35% were stroke-free on placebo. Therefore, rivaroxaban helps reduce the risk of stroke.
Diagram	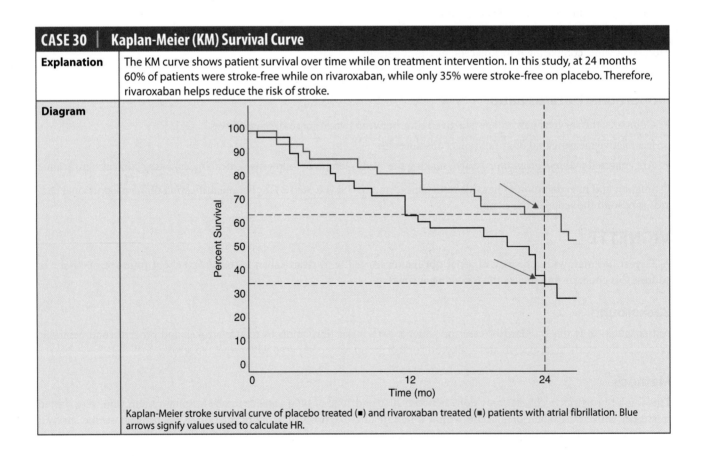 Kaplan-Meier stroke survival curve of placebo treated (■) and rivaroxaban treated (■) patients with atrial fibrillation. Blue arrows signify values used to calculate HR.

CASE 30 | Kaplan-Meier (KM) Survival Curve (continued)

Discussion	This patient is concerned about his risk of developing stroke due to atrial fibrillation. Interval survival—that is, the likelihood of survival within a time interval—can easily be extrapolated from a KM curve. • As shown in the figure above, drawing intersecting lines at 24 months shows that the rivaroxaban-treated cohort has an approximate stroke rate of 55–60%, while the placebo-treated cohort only has a stroke rate of approximately 35–40%. • In this study, the researchers compared their KM curves by use of a proportional HR. A HR of 0.78 (<1) signifies a survival benefit in the experimental group. • This means there is a 0.78 × risk of stroke in those treated with rivaroxaban compared to placebo. • Since this is <1, we can say that rivaroxaban imparted a 22% reduced stroke risk when compared to placebo.
Comment	The KM survival curve provides a probability of an event at a certain time interval.

STATISTICAL TESTS, ERRORS, AND VALIDITY

When appraising a research study, it is important to consider whether appropriate methods of analysis, including statistical tests have been used.

- Hypothesis testing is an **objective** way of making **inferences** from sample data to predict outcomes in the population.
- Sample data are used to assess which **hypotheses** or statements about the difference between two or more groups in a population is correct.
- Statistical tests are used to determine if we should reject or fail to reject the **null hypothesis (H_o)**, or the hypothesis of no difference between two or more groups of data.
- When a difference exists between the groups, this is referred to as the **alternative hypothesis (H_A)**.

Imagine a new antidepressant, Drug X, was developed, and researchers wanted to know how effective it is at reducing depression while comparing it to a placebo or control group.

- Null hypothesis: There is no difference between Drug X and placebo in depression symptoms reduction.
- Alternative hypothesis: There is a difference between Drug X and placebo group, resulting in improvement of depression symptoms.

To help envision these possibilities, use the following table.

	TRUTH	
Study Decision	**H_A (Alternate Hypothesis)** **There is a difference between groups**	**H_o (Null Hypothesis)** **There is no difference between groups**
Rejects null hypothesis (study finds there is a difference between groups)	**Power** Alternative hypothesis true ***Good decision*** (Probability = $1 - \beta$)	**Type 1 error** (False positive) **(Probability = α)**
Does not reject null hypothesis (study finds no difference between groups)	**Type 2 error** (False negative) **(probability = β)**	Alternative hypothesis false ***Good decision*** (Probability = $1 - \alpha$)

Power type 1 and type 2 errors.

As interpreting the results of clinical studies can have important consequences on the health and wellbeing of patients, it is important to ensure that the study results accurately describe what is going on in the population.

- If no difference exists between groups in the population, the statistical test should fail to reject the null hypothesis.
- If a difference does exist, the statistical test should reject the null hypothesis.

The following terms help us identify how well the study is designed to determine whether a difference exists between the groups or not:

- **Power** $(1 - \beta)$
  - Probability of correctly rejecting the null hypothesis in favor of the specific alternative when there is a difference between the groups.

- **p-value**
  - Probability of obtaining the study results by chance if the null hypothesis is true.
  - Is the probability of type 1 error or alpha level.
  - **If the p-value is less than alpha, the predetermined level of statistical significance, the null hypothesis is rejected** in favor of the alternative.
  - A p-value of <0.05 or <0.01 is often used in medical studies.
- **Type 1 error**
  - Occurs when a null hypothesis is rejected when it is true.
  - Also called "false positive" or "alpha error."
  - The lower the significance level alpha, the less likely it is to commit a type 1 error.
- **Type 2 error**
  - Occurs when a null hypothesis is not rejected when it is false.
  - Also called "false negative" or "beta error."
  - Occurs because the sample size is small and the study is underpowered to detect the difference between the groups

Statistical Tests

Most statistical tests are designed to test whether a true difference or relationship exists between two or more groups. Examples of commonly encountered statistical tests are shown in the table.

Example	Variable	Number of Groups	Measures	Test
Mean blood pressure before and after using a drug	Continuous	Two	Difference in means	T test
Cholesterol levels in patients with type 1, type 2 diabetes, and healthy adults	Continuous	Three or more	Difference in means	Anova
Percentage of patients on two different anticoagulants who develop subarachnoid hemorrhage	Categorical	Two or more	Difference in percentages	Chi-square
Relationship between body mass index and body fat	Continuous	Two or more	Compares relationship *Correlation coefficient r can be* between −1 (negative correlation) and +1 (positive correlation)	Correlation

CASE 31	Type I Error

In a study of 200 adults, those who lived within 5 miles of a paint factory had increased odds of developing cancer when compared to those who lived over 5 miles away. However, when this OR was adjusted for water quality in the home, the p-value was greater than 0.05 (α level chosen for this study), so there was no difference in the number of patients diagnosed with cancer living within 5 miles or greater than 5 miles of the paint factory. When the data was not adjusted for water quality in the home, the investigators would have incorrectly rejected the null hypothesis.

Discussion	This is an example of a type I error.
	• A type I error occurs when the null hypothesis is true, but the data in the study leads us to reject H_0.
	• In this study, if the correction for water quality was not done, the study would have incorrectly rejected the true null hypothesis and found increased odds of developing cancer among those who lived within 5 miles of the paint factory.
	• Type I error is denoted by the symbol α which is the level of significance of a test.
	• A result is considered statistically significant if the p-value is less than α, indicating that the role of chance in explaining the results of the study is less than the value of α (very small), and so the study result is likely to be true.
	• A p-value that is greater than α suggests that the result is not statistically significant, and the null hypothesis is true.
	• Typically, an **α-value** of **0.05** is used in medical studies.

CASE 32	Type II Error
A trial of 38 patients with COVID-19 found no difference in reducing death from COVID-19 when comparing monoclonal antibody treatment, casirivimab, and placebo. The significance level alpha is set at 0.05. The authors conclude that the study is underpowered to detect the difference in outcomes between casirivimab and placebo, as the sample size fell short of the 300 patients needed for 80% power.	

Discussion	This is an example of a type II error.
	 • In this study, because the sample size is very small and the study is underpowered, it is possible to fail to reject the incorrect null hypothesis even if casirivimab were truly able to reduce death due to COVID-19.
	 • Type II error occurs when the null hypothesis (casirivimab does not reduce death due to COVID-19) is not rejected when it should be rejected, and the alternative hypothesis is true (casirivimab reduces death due to COVID-19).
	 • Type II error is denoted by the symbol β.
	 • Type II errors occur:
	    • When the **sample size is small**
	    • When the **difference between the two groups is small**

Statistical and Clinical Significance

- A result is statistically significant when it is found to be unlikely to have occurred by chance. Common methods to assess statistical significance are p-value and confidence interval.

- A result is clinically significant when the magnitude or "effect size" is large enough to consider changes to clinical care. Effect size and NNT are methods commonly used to describe clinical significance.

- NOT all statistically significant results are clinically significant in a study.

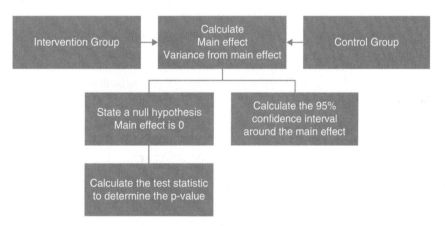

Approaches to determine statistical significance.

Confidence intervals (CIs)

- The range of values within which the "true population" effect is likely to reside.

- A CI gives us the same information as a p-value in terms of whether the results are statistically significant or not.

- In addition, CIs give us information about the sample size and variations in the sample.

CIs and statistical significance

- The CI is statistically significant when it doesn't cross the **"point of no difference."**

- If you are **subtracting** two results and they are equal, then the **point of no difference is zero** (If a = b, then a−b = 0).

Example: Absolute risk reduction

- If **you are creating a ratio** (such as in relative risk) then the **point of no difference is 1**. (If a = b, then a/b = 1)

CI and precision

- **Narrow CIs are more precise**

- Studies with **larger sample sizes** tend to have a **narrower CIs**

- Studies with **smaller sample sizes** often tend to have **wider CIs**
- Studies with **greater standard deviations** tend to have **wider CIs**

p-value

- Probability of obtaining the study results by chance if the null hypothesis is true.
- **If the p-value is less than alpha, the predetermined level of statistical significance**, the **null hypothesis is rejected** in favor of the alternative hypothesis.
- Typically, p-values <0.05 are set to be the threshold of statistical significance.
- If the statistical test to determine if there is a relationship between two variables gives a p-value <0.05, the probability of observing those same results due to chance if the null hypothesis was true would be <5%, and so you reject the null hypothesis. Based on this, you infer the results suggest that there is likely a relationship between the two variables being studied.

VIGNETTE

A 30-year-old woman brings in the following abstract about the use of mindfulness-based stress reduction (MBSR) to treat migraine headaches. She is wondering whether this treatment can help her reduce the number of migraines she experiences per month.

Purpose

To determine whether MBSR improves outcomes for adults with migraine headaches compared with headache education.

Materials and Methods

This RCT studied 200 adult patients (18 and older) who experience greater than 15 migraine days per month. Participants were randomized to the following groups: MBSR, headache education, and standard of care. Patients in the MBSR and headache education group received treatment for a total of 3 hours a week over an 8-week period. Patients were monitored for number of migraine days per month and quality-of-life at baseline and at 2 months.

Results

At 2 months, participants in each group saw a significant decrease in migraine headache days per month (MBSR: −2.0 days of migraine per month; 95 % CI, (−0.5 to −3.0); headache education: −3.0 days of migraine per month; 95% CI, (−1.0 to −3.5) compared to the standard of care. Participants in the MBSR group saw a significant improvement in quality of life 6.0; 95% CI (1.0 to 9.0); P = .01 compared to headache education.

Conclusion

While both MBSR and headache education saw significant decreases in headache days per month, headache education was more effective than MBSR. However, MBSR significantly increased quality of life, while headache education did not. This suggests that while MBSR does not decrease the number of headache days as effectively as headache education, it can help decrease the level of disability experienced by patients with migraines.

Wells RE, O'Connell N, Pierce CR, et al. Effectiveness of mindfulness meditation vs headache education for adults with migraine: A randomized clinical trial. JAMA Intern Med 2021 Mar 1;181(3):317-328. doi: 10.1001/jamainternmed.2020.7090. PMID: 33315046; PMCID: PMC7737157.

CASE 33	Statistical Significance vs. Clinical Significance
The patient expresses an interest in using mindfulness as a treatment option for her migraine headaches. The concepts of statistical significance and clinical significance can help clinicians decipher if a treatment is appropriate for their patients.	
Discussion	Statistical significance can be determined by examining the CI and p-value of a study. • The p-value in the abstract above is <0.01, indicating that <1% of the results were due to chance and so it is statistically significant. • All three CIs in the abstract do not cross the point of no difference of 1 and thus are considered statistically significant. • The width of the CI for quality of life is from 1.0 to 9.0 and it is wide, meaning the results are less precise. A decrease in migraine headache days of half a day to as much as three and a half days per month is clinically significant for the patient.
Additional Considerations	• Statistical significance identifies that the study result is "NOT due to chance." • Clinical significance identifies whether the study result is meaningful or not in terms of effect size and the balance of benefits and harms for the patient to make a change in medical care.

VIGNETTE

A 21-year-old man with a past medical history of depression and ADHD arrives at the office with the following abstract about the treatment of major depression with selective serotonin reuptake inhibitors.

Purpose

Selective serotonin reuptake inhibitors (SSRIs) have been used for the treatment of depression, but the effectiveness of SSRIs has not been researched in real-world settings. The objective of this study is to determine the efficacy of escitalopram for the treatment of depression in an outpatient setting.

Materials and Methods

1500 patients 18 years or older with major depressive disorder (MDD) who were being treated at 50 outpatient clinics across the United States were recruited for the study. After assessing their baseline depression score according to the 17-item Hamilton Depression Scale (HAM-D), patients were prescribed flexible doses of escitalopram according to FDA guidelines for up to 3 months. Patients were permitted to continue other psychiatric medications for the treatment of comorbid mental health conditions. Follow-up visits were conducted monthly for 3 months to monitor response to treatment (HAM-D Score). Remission of depression is defined as an exit HAM-D score <7. Completion of 80% or more of escitalopram therapy was considered adequate adherent to recommended intervention.

Results

Overall, 30% of patients achieved remission after 3 months of using escitalopram. Out of 1500, 1000 (66%) completed 80% or more of escitalopram therapy. Among the patients who achieved remission, 90% were adherent with the drug therapy regimen.

Conclusion

Escitalopram therapy is 30% effective in achieving remission in patients with MDD in real-world outpatient settings. Remission rates were higher in those who completed 80% or more of the drug therapy regimen.

Yates WR, Mitchell J, Rush AJ, et al. Clinical features of depressed outpatients with and without co-occurring general medical conditions in STAR*D. Gen Hosp Psychiatry 2004 Nov-Dec;26(6):421-9. doi: 10.1016/j.genhosppsych.2004.06.008. PMID: 15567207.

CASE 34	Intention to Treat vs. per Protocol Analysis
	Based on the results of the study above, the patient is prescribed escitalopram. Today he presents for a 3-month follow-up visit and states he has only completed 50% of his medication and wants to know if the treatment is still effective.
Discussion	In intention-to-treat (ITT) analysis, data from all participants is included, regardless of whether they followed the protocol or not. • In the above study, ITT analysis was done because it included all 1500 patients in its final analysis, even though only 66% of patients were compliant with the drug therapy. • In this study, ITT analysis found that only 30% of the patients achieved remission. • ITT analysis tends to **underestimate an effect, identify loss to follow up, and captures side effects**. • Matches a real-life clinical setting, as not all patients follow through with the recommended intervention. In per-protocol (PP) analysis, only data from patients who followed the protocol are included in the analysis. • If the study above followed the PP principle, the final analysis would have consisted of only the 1000 patients who completed 80% or more of the drug therapy.

Validity

Even when the results of a statistical test are correct, it is still important to consider the validity of a given study. **Validity** can be thought of as how accurately the results of a study reflect the truth. Two broad types of validity are internal and external validity.

Internal validity describes whether a study is free of bias and if its conclusions accurately reflect the actual or true relationship between the variables in the study. A study is considered internally valid if:

• it uses appropriate techniques or methodology,

• it is adequately powered to detect differences between groups,

• and there are no biases.

External validity (or generalizability) describes whether the results of a study can be applied to the general population. A study is considered generalizable if:

- it has a spectrum of patients similar to the general population or the patient a clinician is taking care of,
- the treatment is feasible in most similar settings,
- and the potential benefits of treatment should outweigh potential harms for most patients.

CASE 35 | Internal Validity

The patient comes in for a 6-month follow-up and states he is feeling better. He continued his stimulant medication for ADHD and wonders if it may have contributed to the remission of his symptoms. By questioning confounding factors, he is questioning the internal validity of the study.

Discussion	The internal validity of the study above reflects the true relationship between escitalopram treatment and the remission of MDD. The following factors found in the abstract compromise the internal validity of this study. • The **duration of the study** decreases the internal validity because it was only conducted for 3 months. MDD is episodic in nature and can be influenced by seasonal changes. To reflect the true effect of escitalopram treatment on MDD, the study should follow response for at least 12 months to account for fluctuations of the disease and seasonal changes. • **Confounding factors** also decrease the internal validity of the study. A confounding factor is an outside variable that *could* influence the variable being studied. In the study above, patients were permitted to continue the use of other psychiatric medications for comorbid mental health conditions. These medications could positively or negatively affect a patient's response to escitalopram. The fact that these medications were not discontinued weakens the internal validity of the study because we are unsure how much of the response was due to escitalopram alone. • The lack of **placebo group** in this study also weakens the internal validity. Placebo groups in drug trials consist of a control group that is given a sugar pill or saline injection instead of the actual drug treatment being studied. Both the experimental and placebo group are followed, and their response is analyzed. By comparing the differences in findings between the two groups, researchers can determine how much of the response to treatment is due to the drug *alone*. For example, if 80% of patients who received escitalopram reached remission but 20% of those who received the placebo achieved remission, only 60% of the response was due to escitalopram.
Additional Considerations	Look for the study process that involves participant demographic data, selection, randomization, study outcomes, or any variables that could affect the validity of the study design

CASE 36 | External Validity

The patient's sister, a 24-year-old woman, presents to the office for treatment of depression. She heard from her brother that escitalopram was an effective treatment for depression and wonders if it would be a good fit for her.

Discussion	The external validity of a study determines how generalizable a study is to the general population. To determine if the results of the study are generalizable to our new patient, a 24-year-old woman, we can look at the sample characteristics of the study. • The **sample characteristics** of this study include all adult patients 18 years or older with a diagnosis of MDD. While this study would not be generalizable to teens with depression because they were not included in the study, it is generalizable to all ages of adults, including our new patient. It is also necessary to review the sample characteristics in detail when determining the generalizability of a study. In most research papers there is a table that summarizes the characteristics. This is important because while the study may be open to all adults, the sample may have consisted of 80% female patients, which would decrease the external validity of the study for the general population. • The **setting** of the study also helps to determine the external validity of the study above. The study took place in 50 different outpatient clinics located across the United States. Because the clinics were in various regions of the United States, it is more generalizable to the population, which increases its external validity. • We must assess if the treatment is feasible in our setting; and escitalopram is available in the United States so the treatment is feasible. • Our patient will likely accept the use of escitalopram.
Additional Considerations	Consider if the study is applicable to the clinical setting, patient, and feasibility of providing similar treatment.

3

General and Preventive Medicine

Lead Author: Julie Loza, MD
Contributors: Divya Singh, MD; Logan Schwarzman, MD

INTRODUCTION

Prevention is better than cure
        —Desiderius Erasmus, 1500

Preventive medicine focuses on promoting and maintaining health at both the individual and community levels.

   The following section covers the high-yield topics that are often tested on the USMLE Step 2 CK exam. In recent years, an increasing number of questions have focused on areas such as risk factors, screening recommendations, and vaccinations. In this chapter, we explore primary prevention strategies and recommendations for patients in various age groups. Some screening tools are recommended for all adults; others are recommended based on age and sex. The term *sex* in this book refers to a reproductive category, while *gender identity* refers to an inner sense of self. The sex of an individual is referred to when it is relevant to screening or treatment based on the risks associated with a specific gamete-producing body type. This terminology permits avoidance of sex stereotyping and ensures that sex-based screening/treatment is addressed. It is important to remember that in providing patient-centered care for transgender patients, natal organ–based cancer screening is recommended, regardless of hormone use.

   Guidelines from this section are from U.S. Department of Health and Human Services, United States Preventive Services Task Force (USPSTF), and United States Centers for Disease Control and Prevention (CDC). Guidelines are up-to-date as of the publication of this book. Varying governmental and medical organizations may differ in their guidelines; thus we recommend checking the organization or society-specific websites for the most current recommendations.

PRIMARY, SECONDARY, AND TERTIARY PREVENTION

Disease prevention can occur at both the population and individual level. The three levels of prevention are primary, secondary, and tertiary, and each level is important in decreasing the burden of disease states on the individual and on society.

Level of Prevention	Examples
Primary	• Vaccination • Smoking cessation, alcohol reduction • Education on weight loss, exercise, drugs • Legislation to mandate safety measures (e.g., seat belts) • Legislation to ban harmful substances (e.g., lead paint)
Secondary	• Screening for cancer • Screening for chronic conditions (e.g., hypertension [HTN]) • Screening for acute conditions (e.g., sexually transmitted infections [STI])
Tertiary	• Treatment of current disease states • Providing accessibility (e.g., wheelchair access) • Treatment of cancer (e.g., chemotherapy)

Obesity: Examples of Interventions Highlighting Different Levels of Preventive Care

Level of Prevention	Intervention
Primary prevention Aims to prevent disease before it occurs ***Most cost-effective form of prevention***	**45-year-old *without* obesity** • Education on weight loss and exercise to prevent obesity
Secondary prevention Aims to identify disease states early or before patients are symptomatic	**45-year-old with obesity** (body mass index [BMI] ≥30) • Screening for elevated blood pressure, diabetes, hyperlipidemia • Education on weight loss and exercise to prevent diabetes and other complications
Tertiary prevention Aims to prevent complications of current disease states and to improve quality of life or restore function ***Most expensive form of prevention***	**45-year-old with obesity and diabetes** • Treatment of current disease states including obesity and diabetes • Checking urine microalbumin and use of ACE-inhibitors to prevent further progression of diabetic nephropathy • Performing a foot exam and fundoscopic exam to assess for neuropathy and retinopathy, respectively

COMMON MODIFIABLE RISK FACTORS

Modifiable risk factors are important for counseling patients and are commonly tested. The following table contains the most important modifiable risk factors associated with common diseases.

Condition	Modifiable Risk Factor
Coronary artery disease Myocardial infarction	Smoking, diabetes, hyperlipidemia, HTN
Stroke	HTN, smoking, physical inactivity
Abdominal aortic aneurysm	Smoking, HTN
Osteoporosis	Low BMI, smoking, nutritional deficiencies, estrogen deficiency
Obstructive sleep apnea	Obesity, smoking, alcohol use
Osteoarthritis	Obesity, occupational/sports
Bladder cancer	Smoking
Lung cancer	Smoking, asbestos exposure
Acute pancreatitis	Gallstones, alcohol abuse
Head and neck cancer	Human papilloma virus (HPV), smoking
Cervical cancer	HPV, smoking
COPD	Smoking
Chronic kidney disease	Diabetes, HTN
***Clostridium difficile* infection**	Antibiotic use
Aortic dissection	HTN
Atrial fibrillation	Obesity, obstructive sleep apnea, diabetes, alcohol use
Hepatocellular carcinoma	Hepatitis B infection, hepatitis C infection, cirrhosis

Live Attenuated	Inactivated	Toxoid, Conjugate	Subunit	Covid 19
• Measles • Mumps • Rubella • Polio • Varicella • Influenza • Yellow fever • Zoster • Typhoid (oral) • Cholera • Yellow fever • BCG	• Influenza • Polio (Salk) • Rabies • Hepatitis A • Cholera	• Toxoid: Diptheria & Tetanus • Conjugate: Hemophilus influenza B	• Hepatitis B • Pertussis • Pneumococcal • HPV • Meningococcal (MenACWY and MenB) • Shingles/(VZV) • Typhoid	• mRNA • Adenovirus vector

Routine immunizations

Adult Vaccines

Vaccine	Routine Indications	Special Indications/Considerations
Tdap or Td	Td or Tdap every 10 years	One dose Tdap each pregnancy One dose Td for tetanus-prone wounds if >5 years since last dose Tdap should be given once in adults
Pneumococcal vaccination (Pneumococcal polysaccharide [PPSV23] or Pneumococcal conjugates [PCV15 and PCV20])	≥65 years	≥65 years: One dose PCV 20 or PCV 15. If PCV 15 given, also give PPSV23 one year later 19–64 years: Chronic heart, lung or liver disease, splenectomy, diabetes, immunocompromising conditions,* cerebrospinal fluid (CSF) leak, cochlear implant, smoking, alcohol use disorder, immunocompromising conditions,* CSF leak, cochlear implant See current clinical practice guidelines for regimen, which varies by previous PCV vaccination status
Recombinant zoster vaccine (RZV)	≥50 years	≥18 years: Consider if immunodeficiency or immunocompromising conditions*
Varicella	Health care workers if no immunity Adults who did not have chicken pox or were never vaccinated	(Live vaccine; avoid in pregnancy and in HIV if CD4 <200)
Hep A	Chronic liver disease	• Travel to or adopting from countries with high endemic hep A • Alcohol use disorder, illicit drug use • HIV • Men who have sex with men • Undomiciled
Hep B	Chronic liver disease Health care workers	• HIV, high-risk sexual exposure, recent or current injection drug use • End-stage renal disease (ESRD) • Travel in countries with high endemic hepatitis B
Meningococcal ACWY	First-year college-students who live in residential housing	Asplenia, HIV, complement component deficiency, use of complement inhibitor, travel to endemic area, military recruits
Meningococcal B (Men B)	Shared decision-making 16–23 years	Shared decision-making Asplenia, complement component deficiency, use of complement inhibitor
Influenza	6 months and older, yearly	
Measles, mumps, rubella (MMR)	Health care workers with no evidence of immunity	(Live vaccine, avoid in pregnancy and in HIV if CD4 <200)
Hemophilus influenza B		• Anatomic or functional asplenia • Hematopoietic stem cell transplant
HPV	All persons ages 9–26 years	Two to three doses based on age at initial vaccination Shared decision making for ages 27–45 years
COVID-19	All persons over 6 months of age	This is still evolving based on data; check current CDC guidelines

Based on information from https://www.cdc.gov/vaccines/schedules/hcp/imz/adult.html#table-age.
*Immunocompromising conditions include human immunodeficiency virus (HIV), iatrogenic immunosuppression, solid organ transplants, chronic renal failure, nephrotic syndrome, immunodeficiency, generalized malignancy, Hodgkin disease, leukemia, lymphoma, multiple myeloma, congenital or acquired asplenia, sickle cell disease, or other hemoglobinopathies.

Vaccine Contraindications in Adults

Vaccine	Contraindication*
Varicella-zoster	Pregnancy, severely immunocompromised state**
	HIV patients with a CD4+ T lymphocyte count <200
MMR	Pregnancy, severely immunocompromised state**
	HIV patients with a CD4+ T lymphocyte count <200
DTaP	Encephalopathy within 7 days of administration

*Prior severe allergic reaction to a vaccine is a contraindication to that particular vaccine.
**Severely immunocompromised state examples include blood dyscrasias (i.e., lymphoma, leukemia), severe concurrent illness, receiving high-dose systemic immunosuppressive medications.

BEHAVIORAL COUNSELING

Counseling, when done correctly, is a powerful tool that can encourage positive behaviors and build trust between physicians and patients. In order to provide appropriate counseling, it is important to meet the patient where they are and recognize the phase of change a patient is currently in.

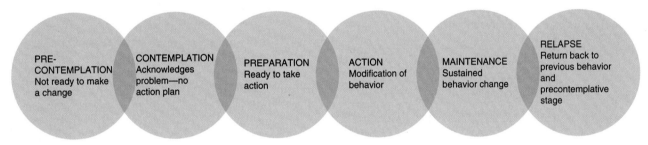

PRE-CONTEMPLATION
Not ready to make a change

CONTEMPLATION
Acknowledges problem—no action plan

PREPARATION
Ready to take action

ACTION
Modification of behavior

MAINTENANCE
Sustained behavior change

RELAPSE
Return back to previous behavior and precontemplative stage

Behavioral counseling.

An Example of Phases of Change for a Patient Based on Tobacco Use

Phases of Change	Description	Patient Behavior
Precontemplation	Denial or ignorance of the problem	Has not yet thought about cessation
Contemplation	Ambivalence or conflicted emotions toward the problem. It is important to assess barriers to change in this stage.	Considers reducing the number of cigarettes used per day
Preparation	Trying small changes or obtaining information about change	Actively seeks advice about quitting
Action	Taking action toward achieving a goal	Quits smoking with the help of nicotine patches and medications
Maintenance	Sustaining a new behavior/avoiding temptation and triggers	Continues cessation journey by seeking social support and avoiding known triggers

SCREENING

Cancer

The cancer screening guidelines that follow are adapted from the USPSTF recommendations and apply to patients without increased risk factors for particular conditions or diseases. Please note that recommendations may vary among different professional organizations and based on an individual's risk factors. For the most current recommendations, please refer to each professional organization's website.

Type of Cancer	Screening	Frequency	Risk Factors	Other Considerations
Breast	Women 50–74 years		• First-degree relative with breast cancer • High risk based on risk calculators	Twofold risk for breast cancer; consider starting annual screening at 40 years or younger
	• Screening mammography	Every 2 years		
Cervical	Women 21–29 years		• High-risk HPV types (hrHPV) exposure • HIV infection • Compromised immune system • In utero exposure to diethylstilbestrol • Previous high-grade precancerous lesion	Stop screening if patient had a hysterectomy with removal of cervix for benign reasons
	• Cervical cytology alone	Every 3 years		
	Women 30–65 years			
	• Cervical cytology alone	Every 3 years		
	• High-risk human papillomavirus (hrHPV) testing	Every 5 years		
	• hrHPV testing in combination with cytology (co-testing)	Every 5 years		
Colorectal	Adults 45–75 years		• Inflammatory bowel disease • Familial cancer syndromes • History of colon cancer in the family	Earlier screening if risk factors are present
	• High-sensitivity guaiac fecal occult blood test (HSgFOBT) or fecal immunochemical test (FIT)	Every year		
	• Stool DNA-FIT	Every 1–3 years		
	• Computed tomography colonography	Every 5 years		
	• Flexible sigmoidoscopy	Every 5 years		
	• Flexible sigmoidoscopy + annual FIT	Every 10 years		
	• Colonoscopy	Every 10 years		
Lung	Adults 50–80 years	Every year	Smoking and older age	Stop screening when patient has quit smoking ≥15 years or limited life expectancy or inability to tolerate surgical treatment for lung cancer
	With a 20 pack-year smoking history **and** currently smoke **or** have quit within the past 15 years • Low-dose computed tomography (LDCT)			
Prostate	Men 55–69 years	Shared decision-making		
	Periodic prostate-specific antigen (PSA)-based screening			

Risky Alcohol Use in Adults

Male	• More than 15 alcoholic drinks in a week, *or* • More than 5 alcoholic drinks in one occasion
Female	• More than 8 alcoholic drinks in a week, *or* • More than 4 alcoholic drinks in one occasion

≥18-Year-Old Female Well Visit and Standard Screening

Interventions	Descriptions
Vaccinations	
HPV	Ages 18–26 years: If did not receive in adolescence (Ages 27–45 years: Shared decision-making)
Td, Tdap	Td booster every 10 years, Tdap one of those times and during each pregnancy
Meningitis	Starting at age 18, if indicated
Influenza	Yearly
COVID-19	All adults with boosters as recommended by CDC
Pneumococcal (PPSV23)	Age ≥65 years, or earlier if other chronic conditions (DM, COPD) or immunocompromising conditions
Pneumococcal (PCV13)	Case-by-case basis for age ≥65 years, or earlier if immunocompromising conditions, CSF leak, or cochlear implant
Hepatitis B	If chronic liver disease, DM, high-risk (e.g., health care workers)
Screening Tests	
STI screening	Ages ≤24 years (sexually active): Yearly gonorrhea, chlamydia screening Age >24 yearly if at increased risk* Ages 15–65 years: HIV screening at least once
Chronic Conditions	
Hyperlipidemia	Ages 40–75 years (younger if risk factors): Lipid profile American College of Cardiology (ACC)/American Heart Association (AHA) recommends starting screening at 35
Diabetes	Blood glucose (fasting or random) or HgA1c in adults aged 40–70 years with BMI >25 or with HTN
Hepatitis C	One-time hepatitis C virus (HCV) antibody screening, in all adults 18–79 years, may repeat if increased risk for hepatitis C infection
Osteoporosis	Dual-energy x-ray absorptiometry (DXA) at age 65, or younger if risk factors present
Cancer Screening	
Cervical cancer	Ages 21–65 years (see cancer screening table)
Breast cancer	Biennial screening aged 50–74 years (may start at age 40; see cancer screening table)
Colon cancer	Screen adults aged 45–75 years (see cancer screening table)
Screening Tools	
Depression	Patient Health Questionnaire (PHQ)-2
Obesity	Screen adults at office visits
Hypertension	Adults 18+ years, screen with in-office measurement; frequency varies
Substance Use	
Tobacco use	Screen all adults, recommend cessation, and offer behavioral/medication strategies to quit
Alcohol use	Alcohol Use Disorders Identification Test-Concise (AUDIT-C) or other screening tool

*Factors increasing risk for STIs: Prior STI, new partner, multiple partners, partner found via internet, contact with sex workers, injection drug use, recent jail or detention facility, exchanging sex for drugs/money, Men who have Sex with Men (MSM).

≥18-Year-Old Male Well Visit and Standard Screening

Interventions	Descriptions
Vaccinations	
HPV	Ages 18–26: If did not receive in adolescence Ages 27–45 years should discuss with their physician
Td, Tdap	Td booster every 10 years, Tdap one of those times
Meningitis	Starting at age 18
Influenza	Yearly
COVID-19	All adults with boosters as recommended by CDC
Pneumococcal (PPSV23)	Age ≥65 years, or earlier if other chronic conditions (DM, COPD) or immunocompromising conditions
Pneumococcal (PCV13)	Case-by-case basis for age ≥65 years, or earlier if immunocompromising conditions, CSF leak, or cochlear implant
Hepatitis B	If chronic liver disease or DM, high-risk (e.g., healthcare workers)
Screening Tests	
STI screening	Men who have sex with men (MSM) yearly Men who have sex with women (MSW) yearly if at risk* Ages 15–65 years: HIV screening at least once
Chronic Conditions	
Hyperlipidemia	Lipid profile screening in adults aged 40–75 years, or younger if risk factors American College of Cardiology (ACC)/American Heart Association (AHA) recommends starting screening at 35
Diabetes	Blood glucose (fasting or random) or HgA1c in adults aged 40–70 years with BMI >25 or with HTN
Hepatitis C	One-time HCV antibody screening in all adults 18–79 years; may repeat if increased risk for hepatitis C infection
Cancer Screening	
Colon cancer	Screen adults aged 45–75 years (see cancer screening table)
Prostate cancer	Males aged 55–69 years; discuss PSA screening with their doctor (selectively recommended)
Screening Tools	
Depression	PHQ-2
Obesity	Screen adults at office visits
Hypertension	Adults 18+ years, screen with in-office measurement; frequency varies
Substance Use	
Tobacco	Screen all adults, recommend cessation, and offer behavioral/medication strategies to quit
Alcohol	AUDIT-C or other screening tool

*Factors increasing risk for STIs: Prior STI, new partner, multiple partners, partner found via internet, contact with sex workers, injection drug use, recent jail or detention facility, exchanging sex for drugs/money, MSM.

CASE 1 | Wellness Visit for 18- to 40-Year-Old Male

A 40-year-old man presents for an annual checkup. He has no acute concerns. He has a desk job, has not had any occupational exposures, and smoked one-half pack per day ages 20–25. He currently is not using any tobacco products, drinks five alcoholic beverages per week, and denies any other drug use except for occasional marijuana few times per year. He is sexually active with one partner and is in a monogamous relationship. He consistently uses condoms and denies history of STI. He eats a standard "American diet," does not have time to exercise, and received the standard childhood immunizations. His last tetanus shot was 13 years ago. He got the flu shot last winter and his COVID booster 1 month ago. He had blood work done 8 years ago and does not recall ever getting tested for HIV. On exam, patient is afebrile, pulse is 70 bpm, blood pressure is 128/79 mmHg. Body mass index (BMI) is 32 kg/m^2 and the rest of the physical exam is normal.

CASE 1 | Wellness Visit for 18- to 40-Year-Old Male *(continued)*

Immunizations	Tdap today, then Td every 10 years, influenza annually, COVID booster when recommended by CDC
Screening	Check blood glucose or A1c, lipids, HIV test
Counseling/ Prevention	Advise weight loss, diet, exercise
Discussion	Performing a thorough social and family history, review of systems and physical exam can help identify areas that should be addressed with counseling. This patient has obesity (BMI >30). His reported use of alcohol of five drinks per week is not concerning for risky alcohol use.

Diagnostics:

Screen for diabetes: A1c, blood glucose or oral glucose tolerance test (GTT) (typically used for screening pregnant patients)
- Prediabetes: A1c 5.7–6.4% or fasting plasma glucose level of 100–125 mg/dL
- Diabetes: A1c ≥6.5% or fasting plasma glucose level ≥126 mg/dL

Screen for hyperlipidemia: Lipid profile
- Consider low–moderate intensity statin in adults 40–75 years to prevent coronary vascular disease (CVD) if ≥1 risk factors for CVD and calculated 10-year risk of a CVD event ≥10%.

  (American College of Cardiology/American Heart Association [ACC/AHA]) risk calculator is commonly used to calculate 10-year risk of CVD events).

Screen for HIV: Combination antigen/antibody testing, ELISA
- Confirmatory with HIV-1 and HIV-2 immunoassay, western blot, viral RNA detection.
- USPSTF recommends at least one-time screening for HIV in 15- to 65-year-old patients.

Screen for unhealthy alcohol use:
- Initial brief screening tools are appropriate: (e.g., Alcohol Use Disorders Identification Test-Consumption [AUDIT-C]).
- If positive screen, perform more in-depth assessment and consider brief behavioral intervention.

Screen for depression:
- Recommended in the general adult population.
- Performed at a routine wellness visit, or if appropriate given the patient's presenting concern.
- Common screening instruments include the Patient Health Questionnaire (PHQ). A brief initial screen can be done with the two-question PHQ-2, and if positive then followed up with the full nine-question PHQ-9.

Counseling:
- General heart-healthy diet (mostly vegetables, fruits, fibers, whole grains; less salt, fat, red/processed meats).
- Exercise (moderate intensity for 150 minutes or vigorous intensity exercise 75 minutes per week).
- Encourage smoking cessation (if applicable).

CASE 2 | Wellness Visit for 50- to 65-Year-Old Female

A 57-year-old woman presents for an annual exam. She has no concerns but requests a flu shot. She drinks two glasses of wine per week and has never smoked. She denies other drug use. She went through menopause at the age of 52 and is not currently sexually active. Her last gynecologic exam was 5 years ago. She does not recall ever being tested for HIV or hepatitis C. Her father passed away from an MI at the age of 75; her mother is alive and has hypertension. Her paternal aunt had breast cancer. Given her father's cardiac history, she tries to follow a plant-based diet. She walks for exercise, about 20 minutes 5 days a week. She does not recall when her last tetanus shot was and has never received a zoster vaccine or a COVID vaccine. On exam, patient is afebrile, pulse is 65 bpm, blood pressure is 130/78 mmHg. Her BMI is 26.7 kg/m². The rest of her physical examination is unremarkable.

Immunizations	Tdap now and Td every 10 years, Recombinant zoster now and second dose in 2–6 months, influenza annually, COVID now and booster when recommended by CDC
Screening	Mammogram, colonoscopy, hrHPV testing, blood glucose or A1c, lipid profile, HIV, Hep C Ab
Counseling/ Prevention	Healthy diet, exercise, osteoporosis prevention

CASE 2 | Wellness Visit for 50- to 65-Year-Old Female *(continued)*

Discussion	This patient has a family history of CAD and given her family history of breast cancer, an additional familial risk assessment tool can be performed in office to determine if earlier screening and/or genetic testing is indicated.
	Diagnostics:
	Screen for hyperlipidemia: Lipid profile
	• Consider low- to moderate-intensity statin in adults 40–75 years to prevent CVD if ≥1 risk factors for CVD and calculated 10-year risk of a CVD event ≥10%.
	(ACC/AHA risk calculator is commonly used to calculate 10-year risk of CVD events.)
	Screen for breast cancer: Biennial screening with mammography ages 50–74 years.
	• If patients have a first-degree relative with breast cancer or multiple relatives, consider using a brief familial risk assessment tool to determine if earlier screening or further genetic testing is indicated.
	• Other guidelines may recommend different intervals and ages to initiate screening.
	Screen for cervical cancer: Cervical cytology and/or high-risk human papillomavirus (hrHPV) testing starting at age 21
	• 21–29 years: Cervical cytology every 3 years.
	• 30–65 years: Cervical cytology alone every 3 years, hrHPV only every 5 years *or* cytology and hrHPV (cotesting) every 5 years.
	• Discontinue screening at age 65 if three prior negative cervical cytology tests, or two negative cervical cytology tests with negative hrHPV co-testing.
	Screen for colorectal cancer: All adults aged 45–75 years. Several recommended screening tests are available.
	• Colonoscopy every 10 years *or*
	• Sigmoidoscopy every 5 years with high-sensitivity FOBT every 3 years *or*
	• High-sensitivity FOBT annually.
	Screen for diabetes: A1c, blood glucose or oral GTT (typically used for screening pregnant patients).
	• Prediabetes: A1c 5.7–6.4% or fasting plasma glucose of 100–125 mg/dL
	• Diabetes: A1c ≥6.5% or fasting plasma glucose ≥126 mg/dL
	Screen for HIV: Combination antigen/antibody testing, ELISA
	• Confirmatory with HIV-1 and HIV-2 immunoassay, western blot, viral RNA detection.
	• USPSTF recommends at least one-time screening for HIV in 15- to 65-year-old patients.
	Screen for unhealthy alcohol use:
	• Initial brief screening tools are appropriate (e.g., AUDIT-C).
	• If positive screen, perform more in-depth assessment and consider brief behavioral intervention.
	Screen for depression:
	• Recommended in the general adult population.
	• Performed at a routine wellness visit, or if appropriate given the patient's presenting concern.
	• Common screening instruments include the PHQ. A brief initial screen can be done with the two-question PHQ-2, and if positive then followed up with a full nine-question PHQ-9.
	Counseling:
	• Osteoporosis prevention with regular weight-bearing exercise, calcium (1200 mg daily, ideally from diet), vitamin D (600–800 IU daily or higher if deficient).
	• General heart-healthy diet (mostly vegetables, fruits, fibers, whole grains; less salt, fat, red/processed meats).
	• Exercise (moderate intensity for 150 minutes or vigorous intensity exercise for 75 minutes a week
	• Encourage smoking cessation (if applicable).

CASE 3 | Wellness Visit for 65+ Year-Old Male

A 68-year-old man presents for annual checkup and reports no concerns. He denies any past medical history or medications that he takes regularly. He is retired and lives with his wife. He smokes cigarettes (per calculation, he has a 45-year-pack history). He drinks alcohol occasionally and denies other drug use. His family history is notable for a history of hypertension and diabetes in his father, and high cholesterol in his brother. He has not seen a physician in years, and suspects he is due for all vaccines. On exam, patient is afebrile, pulse is 82 bpm, blood pressure is 145/85 mmHg. BMI is 31 kg/m². His physical examination is otherwise unremarkable.

Immunizations	Tdap now and Td every 10 years, zoster now and second dose in 2–6 months, influenza annually, COVID now and booster when recommended by CDC, pneumococcal (PCV20)

CASE 3 | Wellness Visit for 65+ Year-Old Male *(continued)*

Screening	Blood glucose or A1c, lipid profile, abdominal ultrasound for abdominal aortic aneurysm (AAA), low-dose lung CT, colonoscopy, hepatitis C
Counseling/ Prevention	Healthy diet (low salt), tobacco cessation, weight loss, fall and osteoporosis prevention
Discussion	This patient is 60+ and an active smoker with a significant smoking history. Counseling on cessation and screening for complications related to long-term tobacco use is imperative in a patient such as this. **Diagnostics:** Screen for diabetes: A1c, blood glucose or oral GTT (typically used for screening pregnant patients). • Prediabetes: A1c 5.7–6.4% or fasting plasma glucose level of 100–125 mg/dL • Diabetes: A1c ≥6.5% or fasting plasma glucose level ≥126 mg/dL Screen for hyperlipidemia: Lipid profile. • Consider low-moderate intensity statin in adults 40–75 years to prevent CVD if ≥1 risk factors for CVD and calculated 10-year risk of a CVD event ≥10%. (ACC/AHA risk calculator is commonly used to calculate 10-year risk of CVD events.) Screen for AAA: Abdominal aorta ultrasound. • Refer males aged 65–75 years who have ever smoked once for an ultrasound. "Ever smoker" is someone who has smoked 100+ cigarettes in their life. Screen for lung cancer: Screen annually for lung cancer with a LDCT. • Recommended for adults 50–80 years of age with a 20-pack-year smoking history and are currently smoking, *or* who have quit smoking within the last 15 years. • Shared decision-making regarding this testing should be discussed. Screen for colorectal cancer: All adults aged 45–75 years. Several recommended screening tests are available. • Colonoscopy every 10 years *or* • Sigmoidoscopy every 5 years with high-sensitivity FOBT every 3 years *or* • High-sensitivity FOBT annually Screen for prostate cancer: PSA. • In men aged 55–69 years, the decision to screen for prostate cancer is an individual decision. • The benefits and harms of screening should be discussed with the patient prior to testing. Screen for hepatitis C. • Recommend screening individuals aged 18–79 years. • Can be repeated if increased risk, though there is not clear guidance on interval frequency. Screen for HIV: Combination antigen/antibody testing, ELISA. • Confirmatory with HIV-1 and HIV-2 immunoassay, western blot, viral RNA detection. • USPSTF recommends at least one-time screening for HIV in 15- to 65-year-old patients. Screen for unhealthy alcohol use. • Initial brief screening tools are appropriate (e.g., AUDIT-C). • If positive screen, perform more in-depth assessment and consider brief behavioral intervention. Screen for depression. • Recommended in the general adult population. • Performed at a routine wellness visit, or if appropriate given the patient's presenting concern. • Common screening instruments include the PHQ. A brief initial screen can be done with the two-question PHQ-2, and if positive then followed up with a full nine-question PHQ-9. • In geriatric populations, the Geriatric Depression Scale (GDS) is also a useful tool. Screen for fall risk: A timed Get-Up-and-Go Test should be administered in patients aged 65 years and older who are at increased risk of falls. • Increased risk criteria: Two falls in the past year, gait or balance difficulties, acute fall episode. • How to perform: Have the patient rise from an armchair, walk 10 feet, turn, walk back, and sit down. • Normal results are <12 seconds.

CASE 3 | **Wellness Visit for 65+ Year-Old Male** (*continued*)

Discussion	Screen for elder abuse: There is no reliable screening tool to identify elder abuse or neglect. Instead, be sure to take a thorough history and physical examination.
	• Risk factors include social isolation, functional impairment, poor physical health, a shared living environment with numerous household members other than a spouse.
	• Types of elder abuse include physical, sexual, emotional/psychological, neglect, abandonment, financial/material exploitation.
	Management/Counseling:
	Smoking cessation
	• All adults should be asked about tobacco use.
	• This patient should be counseled to stop using tobacco and offered behavioral and medication strategies to help quit.
	Hypertension
	• This patient's blood pressure is elevated.
	• Confirm with a repeat measurement, preferably one obtained out of office.
	• Counsel regarding diet and exercise. The Dietary Approaches to Stop Hypertension (DASH) has been shown to help lower blood pressure.
	• Exercise and tobacco cessation counseling is further discussed below.
	• Reassess in a few months.
	Obesity
	• BMI ≥30 kg/m² is obesity.
	• Offer intensive behavioral interventions to help patient achieve weight loss, with a goal of 5% or greater weight loss.
	• Weight loss is often achieved through a combination of diet changes and physical activity.
	• Appropriate exercise goals: moderate intensity for 150 minutes or vigorous intensity exercise for 75 minutes a week
	Osteoporosis prevention
	• Regular weight-bearing exercise, calcium (1200 mg daily, ideally from diet), vitamin D (600–800 IU daily or higher if deficient), and tobacco cessation.

CASE 4 | Wellness Visit for 65+ Year-Old Female

A 67-year-old woman presents for annual checkup. She has no concerns but wanted to make sure her immunizations were up-to-date. She denies any previous medical problems or surgeries. Her family history is significant for heart disease. She works as a social worker and enjoys her job. She is married and has two healthy adult children. She has never smoked; she drinks alcohol, one to two glasses of wine only on weekends with friends, and has no other drug use. She follows a Mediterranean diet, and mostly does yoga for exercise. She is up-to-date on her cervical cancer screening and has no history of abnormal results. Her last test was done 2 years ago. She has received her flu shot and recommended COVID vaccinations. On exam, patient is afebrile, pulse is 80 bpm, blood pressure is 120/75 mmHg. BMI is 24 kg/m². Physical examination is otherwise unremarkable.

Immunizations	Tdap now and Td every 10 years, zoster now and second dose in 2–6 months, influenza annually, next COVID booster when recommended by CDC, pneumococcal (PCV20).
Screening	Blood glucose or A1c, lipid profile, hepatitis C, mammogram, cervical cancer screening, colon cancer screening, bone density testing.
Counseling/ Prevention	Healthy diet (low salt), fall and osteoporosis prevention.
Discussion	This patient is due for multiple age-based screening tests. In addition, this well visit is a good opportunity for counseling on exercise recommendations as well as osteoporosis prevention. Given her previous normal cervical cancer screening results, she will no longer need cervical cancer screening.
	Diagnostics:
	Screen for hyperlipidemia: Lipid profile.
	• Consider low- to moderate-intensity statin in adults 40–75 years to prevent CVD if ≥1 risk factors for CVD and calculated 10-year risk of a CVD event ≥10%.
	(ACC/AHA risk calculator is commonly used to calculate 10-year risk of CVD events.)

CASE 4 | Wellness Visit for 65+ Year-Old Female *(continued)*

Discussion	Screen for breast cancer: Biennial screening with mammography ages 50–74 years.
	• If patients have a first-degree relative or multiple relatives with breast cancer, consider using a brief familial risk assessment tool to determine if earlier screening or further genetic testing is indicated.
	• Other guidelines may recommend different intervals and ages to initiate screening.
	
	Screen for osteoporosis: Females age 65 years and older should undergo a DXA scan of hip and lumbar spine to assess their bone density and risk for osteoporosis.
	• Can also consider screening younger than 65 years if additional risk factors for osteoporotic fractures are present.
	• DXA results are given as T-scores, which compare the patient's results to that of an average 30-year-old of the same sex.
	  • Normal: T ≥1.0
	  • Osteopenia: −2.5 ≥T ≤ −1.0
	  • Osteoporosis: T ≤ −2.50
	  • Severe osteoporosis: T ≤ −2.50 with a fragility fracture
	
	Screen for cervical cancer: Discuss discontinuing screening with this patient.
	• Discontinue screening at age 65 if three prior negative cervical cytology tests or two negative cervical cytology tests with negative hrHPV co-testing.
	
	Screen for colorectal cancer: All adults aged 45–75 years. Several recommended screening tests are available.
	• Colonoscopy every 10 years *or*
	• Sigmoidoscopy every 5 years with high-sensitivity FOBT every 3 years *or*
	• High-sensitivity FOBT annually
	
	Screen for diabetes: A1c, blood glucose or oral GTT (typically used for screening pregnant patients).
	• Prediabetes: A1c 5.7–6.4% or fasting plasma glucose of 100–125 mg/dL
	• Diabetes: A1c ≥6.5% or fasting plasma glucose ≥126 mg/dL
	
	Screen for unhealthy alcohol use:
	• Initial brief screening tools are appropriate (e.g., AUDIT-C).
	• If positive screen, perform more in-depth assessment and consider brief behavioral intervention.
	
	Screen for depression:
	• Recommended in the general adult population.
	• Performed at a routine wellness visit, or if appropriate given the patient's presenting concern.
	• Common screening instruments include the PHQ. A brief initial screen can be done with the two-question PHQ-2, and if positive then followed up with a full nine-question PHQ-9.
	• In geriatric populations, the GDS is also a useful tool.
	Screen for hepatitis C:
	• Screen individuals aged 18–79 years.
	• Test can be repeated if increased risk, though there is not clear guidance on interval frequency.
	
	Screen for fall risk: A timed Get-Up-and-Go Test should be administered in patients 65 years and older at increased risk of falls.
	• Increased risk criteria: Two falls in the past year, gait or balance difficulties, acute fall episode.
	• How to perform: Have the patient rise from an armchair, walk 10 feet, turn, walk back, and sit down.
	• Normal results are <12 seconds.
	
	Screen for elder abuse: There is no reliable screening tool to identify elder abuse or neglect. Instead, be sure to take a thorough history and physical examination.
	• Risk factors include social isolation, functional impairment, poor physical health, a shared living environment with numerous household members other than a spouse.
	• Types of elder abuse include physical, sexual, emotional/psychological, neglect, abandonment, financial/material exploitation.
	Counseling:
	• General heart-healthy diet (mostly vegetables, fruits, fibers, whole grains; less salt, fat, red/processed meats).
	• Exercise: moderate intensity for 150 minutes or vigorous intensity exercise for 75 minutes a week.
	• Osteoporosis prevention with regular weight-bearing exercise, calcium (1200 mg daily, ideally from diet), vitamin D (600–800 IU daily or higher if deficient).

BEERS CRITERIA

Beers criteria were developed to help reduce the potentially inappropriate prescription and polypharmacy in the geriatric population. The full list of Beers Criteria can be found in the 2019 American Geriatric Society Beers Criteria® table. Medications included on this list should be avoided, or at least used with caution due to a potentially increased risk of harm in older populations. In addition, medications on this list may have harmful drug-drug interactions, harmful side effects, or may need dose adjustments due to reduced kidney function.

The full list includes over 30 individual medications or medication classes. A brief list is provided here.

Medication Class	Rationale
α-Blockers	Increased risk of hypotension
Anticholinergics, antidepressants, first-generation antihistamines	Increased risk of delirium, falls, sedation, urinary retention, and constipation
Benzodiazepine receptor agonists	Increased risk of delirium, sedation, and fall
Chronic NSAIDs	Increased risk of gastrointestinal bleeding
Proton pump inhibitors	Increased risk of *C. difficile* infection, decreased bone density

LEADING CAUSES OF DEATH

According to the CDC, the following table lists the leading causes of death in the United States by age group in 2019.

Leading Causes of Death in Adults

Rank	Adults 18–34 years	Adults 35–44 years	Adults 45–64 years	Adults 65 years and older
1	Unintentional injury	Unintentional injury	Malignant neoplasm	Heart disease
2	Suicide	Malignant neoplasm	Heart disease	Malignant neoplasm
3	Homicide	Heart disease	Unintentional injury	Chronic lower respiratory disease

Leading Causes of Death in Children

Rank	Infant	Children 1–4 years	Children 5–9 years	Children 10–14 years	Adolescent 12–17 years
1	Congenital anomaly	Unintentional injury	Unintentional injury	Unintentional injury	Unintentional injury
2	Short gestation and low birthweight	Congenital anomaly	Cancer	Suicide	Suicide
3	Unintentional injury	Cancer	Congenital anomaly	Cancer	Homicide

CASE 5 | Obesity

A 50-year-old man presents with continued weight gain. He has struggled with his weight for years, trying fad diets without much success. He currently is not following any particular diet or exercise regimen because he does not know where to start and is frustrated. On exam, patient is afebrile, pulse is 75 bpm, blood pressure is 132/85 mmHg. BMI is 36 kg/m². His abdominal circumference is 45 inches (114 cm).

Conditions with Similar Presentations	Hypothyroidism, Cushing syndrome, genetic obesities, behavioral (i.e., binge-eating disorder)

CASE 5 | Obesity *(continued)*

Initial Diagnostic Tests	Thyroid-stimulating hormone (TSH), A1C, lipid profile
Next Steps in Management	Multifactorial approach consisting of nutritional and physical activity counseling, and behavior therapy

Discussion	Overweight/obesity is a concern when an abnormal/excessive amount of fat presents a health risk. Obesity results from an imbalance between energy intake (determined by factors such as diet and appetite) and energy expenditure (determined by metabolic activity and physical activity) and results from both genetic and environmental influences. Obesity is a clinical diagnosis defined as BMI ≥30 (calculated as weight in kg/height in m²).
	• BMI of 25 to 29.9 is "overweight"
	• BMI of 30.0 to 34.9 is Class 1 obesity
	• BMI of 35.0 to 39.9 is Class 2 obesity
	• BMI of ≥40 is Class 3 obesity
	
	History: Risk factors for obesity include medical conditions (Cushing syndrome, hypothyroidism, polycystic ovary syndrome [PCOS]) in females, medications (glucocorticoids, antiepileptics, antipsychotics), sleep disturbances, and stress.
	• Inquire about diet, physical activity, decreased sleep, social support, access to healthy food, weight changes, and prior attempts to lose weight.
	• Inquire about cold intolerance (thyroid), easy bruising (cortisol excess), and medications, which may all be secondary causes of weight gain.
	
	Physical examination: May be normal other than elevated BMI and central adiposity.
	• Measure waist circumference. Elevated waist circumference suggests increased cardiometabolic risk.
	  • Men: >40 inches (>102 cm)
	  • Women: >35 inches (>88cm)
	• Check blood pressure.
	
	Diagnostics: A1c or fasting blood glucose level, lipid profile, TSH (to evaluate for secondary causes of obesity).
	
	Consider additional tests, such as comprehensive metabolic panel (electrolytes, kidney function, liver function).
	Management: Multifactorial and should include nutrition, physical activity, and behavior therapy counseling. Some patients may be interested in and benefit from pharmacotherapy and/or bariatric surgery.
	
	Nutrition:
	• Dietary interventions should be safe, effective, and easy for the patient to maintain.
	• Many fad diets may lead to quick but non-sustained weight loss.
	• Generally, patients should be encouraged to maintain a negative calorie balance. Highly processed junk food is high in calories but of little nutritional value and should be limited.
	• While considering the patient's dietary preferences, encourage lean proteins, vegetables and leafy greens, fruits, nuts and beans, and whole grains.
	
	Physical activity: Assess the patient's current activity level and mobility prior to recommending a particular physical activity plan.
	• Moderate intensity exercise for 150 minutes *or*
	• Vigorous intensity aerobic exercise for 75 minutes weekly.
	• Higher levels of activity often result in greater weight loss and improved weight loss maintenance.
	• Anaerobic resistance exercise is also encouraged.
	
	Behavioral therapy:
	• High-intensity counseling combined with behavioral interventions produces modest, sustained weight loss.
	• A structured program often has many components. This may include goal setting, self-monitoring, meal planning, and other techniques.
	
	Weight loss medications (such as phentermine, buproprion, naltrexone, topiramate, and GLP-1 agonists) can be considered if:
	• BMI ≥30 kg/m² without comorbidity *or*
	• BMI ≥27 kg/m² with obesity-related risk factors or diseases.
	Bariatric surgery (see below).

CASE 5 | Obesity *(continued)*

Additional Considerations	Negative stereotypes and obesity bias can lead to stigma against obesity, including from health care providers. This can lead to undue stress and anxiety, avoidance of care, and mistrust of the health care system.
	Complications: Complications from obesity are a result of either fat mass disease or adiposopathy.
	• Fat mass disease results from abnormal biomechanical and physical forces from excess fat deposition (e.g., obstructive sleep apnea, osteoarthritis, obesity hypoventilation).
	• Adiposopathy refers to the adipose tissue dysfunction that occurs in obesity and can result in elevated blood sugar, blood pressure, cholesterol, and other metabolic conditions.
	Metabolic syndrome: Patients with metabolic syndrome are at increased risk of atherosclerotic cardiovascular disease, and aggressive risk factor modification is recommended. A patient is diagnosed with metabolic syndrome if they have at least three of the following five conditions:
	• Increased waist circumference (see above)
	• Triglycerides ≥150 mg/dL
	• Low HDL: <40 mg/dL in men or <50 mg/dL in women
	• Blood pressure >130/85
	• Fasting blood glucose >100 mg/dL
	Pediatric considerations:
	• Prevalence is rising in recent years.
	• In pediatric populations, classification is by using BMI percentiles.
	Surgical considerations: Bariatric surgery is an effective means of weight loss and can be considered in patients with:
	• BMI ≥40 without comorbidity, *or*
	• ≥35 with comorbidity (i.e., diabetes).
	Surgical options include: Sleeve gastrectomy, laparoscopic adjustable gastric banding, Roux-en-Y gastric bypass, or biliopancreatic diversion with duodenal switch.

CASE 6 | Unintentional Weight Loss

A 65-year-old man without any significant past medical history presents for an annual checkup. He is not on any medications and on review of symptoms reports considerable weight loss in the last 6 months. He notes that his clothes are fitting more loosely. He denies any changes in his diet, exercise, or activity levels. He has no other symptoms and no other concerns. His vital signs are within normal range. His BMI is 20 kg/m². His prior visit BMI 6 months ago was 25 kg/m². Physical exam is otherwise unremarkable.

Conditions with Similar Presentations	Differential diagnosis of unintentional weight loss should include, but not be limited to the following:
	• Malignancy
	• Non-malignant gastrointestinal disease: Celiac disease, chronic pancreatitis, IBD, chronic mesenteric ischemia
	• Psychiatric: Depression, eating disorders
	• Infections: HIV, AIDS, tuberculosis
	• Endocrine: Uncontrolled diabetes, hyperthyroidism, chronic adrenal insufficiency
	• Neurologic: Dementia, stroke, Parkinson disease
	• Medications, alcohol, tobacco use, illicit drugs
	• Food insecurity
	• Chronic illness: Heart failure, COPD
Initial Diagnostic Tests	• Confirm diagnosis by checking body weight and comparing to previous body weights.
	• Check CBC, CMP, TSH
	• Age-appropriate cancer screening
Next Steps in Management	Follow up on any concerning patient history, abnormal labs, or abnormal diagnostic findings.

CASE 6 | Unintentional Weight Loss *(continued)*

Discussion	Significant unintentional weight loss is defined as >5% loss of usual body weight in the last 6–12 months. The underlying cause for unintentional weight loss may include decreased food intake, increased metabolism due to malignancy, infection or thyroid disorders, and caloric loss due to malabsorption or proteinuria. It is seen in one-third of frail elderly patients, and most common causes include: • Cancer (most commonly gastrointestinal, lung, or lymphoma) ~29% • Depression and alcoholism ~16% • Nonmalignant gastrointestinal diseases ~13% • Unknown ~22% **History:** Inquire about the following: • Access to and availability of food • Anorexia • Chewing or swallowing difficulties • Fever, palpitations, neuropsychiatric symptoms, weakness • Changes in diet, exercise, or activity level • Diarrhea or constipation, malodorous stool or change in stool texture, color, consistency, or smell • History of mood disorders, eating disorders, or history of weight loss pattern • Smoking, alcohol, or drug use history • Associated symptoms such as loss of appetite, fatigue, night sweats, lymphadenopathy **Physical examination:** Thorough tracking of weight loss over time is important to determine possible correlation and causation. Perform a comprehensive examine including oropharynx, thyroid, lymph nodes, abdomen. **Diagnostics:** Based on the patient's history, physical exam, lab work, and diagnostic testing, pursue further testing for any abnormalities observed. Consider: • CBC with differential • Renal and hepatic function • Urinalysis • Calcium level • Fasting glucose levels • Erythrocyte sedimentation rate (ESR) • TSH • Chest x-ray • FOBT • Age-appropriate cancer screening **Management:** Treat the underlying cause (in ~25% of cases, no definitive cause will be found). • Modify diet to include foods the patient likes and can consume. • Medications to stimulate appetite have significant side effects and there is inconsistent evidence that they improve patient-centered outcomes in older adults. • If no cause is found, continue to monitor and track weight, perform close follow-up exams, and consider additional testing based on shared decision-making.

EDEMA

- Edema (swelling) is noted when excess interstitial body fluid is present.
- Occurs due to an imbalance between the hydrostatic pressure in the capillaries and the colloid oncotic pressure in the interstitial space.
- Imbalance may be due to:
  - Obstruction of lymphatic drainage
  - Increase in the intracapillary hydrostatic pressure
  - Increase oncotic pressure in the interstitium
  - Decrease in the plasma oncotic pressure
  - Damage to capillary endothelium

- When approaching edema, it is important to determine if it is generalized or localized.
- If localized, identify the local pathology causing the edema:
  - Obstruction of lymphatic flow (e.g., cellulitis, resection of the lymph nodes, filariasis)
  - Increased venous hydrostatic pressure (e.g., varicose veins, thrombophlebitis, venous thromboembolism)
- If generalized, evaluate the patient for:
  - Decreased oncotic pressure from hypoalbuminemia: Cirrhosis, protein malnutrition, protein-losing enteropathy, nephrotic syndrome
  - Increased hydrostatic pressure:
    - Venous: Right heart failure
    - Arterial: Calcium channel blockers
    - Increased intravascular volume: Hypercortisolism (e.g., steroids), renal failure, NSAIDs, cyclosporine

Differential Diagnosis for Lower Extremity Edema

Bilateral	Unilateral
Pitting	*Pitting*
Generalized edema causes (see above)	Deep venous thrombosis
Venous insufficiency	Ruptured Baker cyst
Inferior vena caval obstruction	Pelvic tumor
Nonpitting	Pelvic lymphadenopathy
Severe hypothyroidism (myxedema):	Venous insufficiency
Deposition of hyaluronic acid	*Nonpitting*
Hyperthyroidism (Graves disease):	Lymphedema
Pretibial edema	Regional lymph node dissection
Lipedema	Filariasis

CASE 7 | Venous Thromboembolism: Deep Venous Thrombosis

A 58-year-old man with colon cancer presents with left lower extremity pain and swelling. He reports no leg trauma, chest pain, or shortness of breath. On examination, his vital signs are temperature 37.5°C, pulse 100/min, respirations 16/min, and pulse oximetry 99% on room air. Lung exam is clear. There is asymmetric 2+ pitting edema of the left leg from the foot up to the knee. Pulses are palpable on both extremities. Skin exam is normal.

Conditions with Similar Presentations	**Cellulitis:** Can present with pain and swelling, but would have abnormal skin findings, and commonly fever.
	Ruptured popliteal (Baker) cyst: Seen in the setting of arthritis or trauma. The cyst originates from the popliteal fossa, and thus swelling is behind the knee and does not extend down to the foot.
	Venous insufficiency: Usually present with bilateral swelling and may have visible varicosities, hyperpigmentation +/− ulcerations.
Initial Diagnostic Tests	Lower extremity venous compression ultrasound with Doppler
Next Steps in Management	Therapeutic anticoagulation (LMWH, heparin, or direct oral anticoagulant [DOAC])
Discussion	Virchow's triad (stasis, hypercoagulability, vessel wall injury) characterizes the various clinical states that may predispose a patient to venous thromboembolism (VTE).
	History:
	• Risk factors:
	• Immobility, bed rest, long flight, post-surgery
	• Known hypercoagulable states (e.g., defect in coagulation cascade proteins, malignancy)
	• Trauma or surgery
	• Symptoms: swelling, pain, and warmth of the leg.

CASE 7 | Venous Thromboembolism: Deep Venous Thrombosis *(continued)*

Discussion	**Physical examination:**
	• Unilateral edema occurs if DVT is at or proximal to the popliteal vein (the definition of a "proximal DVT"). This leads to a difference in measured circumference of the calves.
	• Palpable posterior cord (the thrombosed vein) is seen in <50% of patients but has a specificity >85%.
	• Warmth, redness, and tenderness of the calf may be seen.
	• Homan sign (calf pain with dorsiflexion of the foot) is neither sensitive nor specific and should not be performed.
	Diagnostics:
	• Lower extremity compression Doppler ultrasound is the test of choice. It has a >95% sensitivity and specificity for proximal venous thrombosis.
	Management:
	• **Proximal DVTs** should be treated with immediate-acting oral anticoagulants (rivaroxaban, apixaban) or bridging with heparin (LMWH or unfractionated) or fondaparinux while starting other oral anticoagulants.
	• **Distal DVTs** can be observed with serial Doppler ultrasounds *unless* any of the following is true:
	• DVT was unprovoked
	• Prior DVT or pulmonary embolus (PE)
	• D-dimer is >500 ng/mL
	• Continued risk factors for DVT (cancer, immobility)
Additional Considerations	**Complications:**
	• Pulmonary embolism: See Pulmonary Chapter.
	• Post-thrombotic (postphlebitic) syndrome: Continued constant or intermittent pain and swelling of the leg.
	Obstetric considerations: Certain anticoagulants (e.g., warfarin and DOACs) are contraindicated in pregnancy.

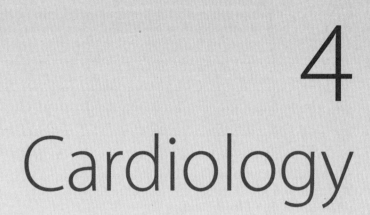

4

Cardiology

Lead Authors: Mayank Kansal, MD; Colin D. Goodman, MD
Contributors: Sophie Gough, MD; Hoda Sayegh, MD; Rachel Lombard, MD

HYPERTENSION

Hypertension (HTN) is a major risk factor for myocardial infarction (MI), ischemic and hemorrhagic strokes, and aortic dissection. It is initially asymptomatic and most patients have primary (aka essential) HTN. Significantly elevated blood pressure (>180/120) is categorized as either hypertensive emergency (signs of vital end-organ damage) or hypertensive urgency (no end-organ damage) and managed accordingly.

Classification of Blood Pressure

Blood Pressure Category	Systolic mmHg		Diastolic mmHg
Normal	<120	and	<80
Elevated blood pressure	120–129	and	<80
Hypertension stage 1	130–139	or	80–89
Hypertension stage 2	>140	or	>90 +
Hypertensive crisis	>180	or	>120 +

Secondary HTN related to an underlying cause is present in 5–10% of patients. Evaluation for secondary HTN should be considered in the following patients:

- Onset <30 years old
- Abrupt onset over a period of months
- Resistant HTN (defined as uncontrolled on three medications including a diuretic)
- An acute rise in blood pressure from previously stable readings

Tests to Consider for Evaluation of Secondary Hypertension

Tests	Pathology
Sleep study	Obstructive sleep apnea
Serum creatinine	Renal parenchymal disease
Echocardiogram	Aortic regurgitation, coarctation of the aorta
Renal ultrasound	Renal artery stenosis, Polycystic kidney disease (PCKD)
Elevated 24-hour urine cortisol	Cushing syndrome
Renin:Aldosterone	Hyperaldosteronism (Conn syndrome)
Plasma metanephrines	Pheochromocytoma
TSH/T4	Hyperthyroidism
Serum calcium	Hypercalcemia

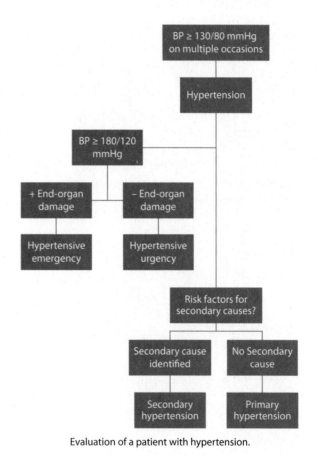

Evaluation of a patient with hypertension.

Classes of Antihypertensives

Class of Medication	Mechanism of Action	Side Effects/Contraindications	Additional Notes
Thiazide Diuretics			
Hydrochlorothiazide (HCTZ) Chlorthalidone	Antagonist of the Na-Cl transporter in the distal convoluted tubule	Side effects: Hypokalemia, hypercalcemia, hyponatremia hyperuricemia (caution in gout)	First line for HTN
ACE Inhibitors (ACEi)			
Lisinopril Enalapril Benazepril	Inhibit conversion of angiotensin I to angiotensin II	Side effects: Dry cough (switch to an ARB), angioedema, hyperkalemia Contraindicated in pregnancy, renal artery stenosis	First line for HTN Used in patients with DM and/or CKD, prevents nephropathy
Angiotensin Receptor Blockers (ARB)			
Losartan Valsartan Candesartan Irbesartan	Block the action of angiotensin II at the receptor	Side effects: Hyperkalemia, much less likely to have cough, angioedema Contraindicated in pregnancy, renal artery stenosis	First line for HTN Used in patients with DM and/or CKD, prevents nephropathy
Mineralocorticoid Receptor Antagonists			
Spironolactone Eplerenone	Block aldosterone	Side effects: hyperkalemia, gynecomastia	Not First line unless patient has primary hyperaldosteronism
Calcium Channel Blockers (CCB)			
Dihydropyridine (DHP) Amlodipine Nifedipine	Inhibit the dihydropyridine receptors, decreasing vascular resistance	Side effects: Lower extremity edema	First line for HTN
Non-DHP Verapamil Diltiazem	Decrease vascular resistance and AV nodal blocker	Side effects: lower extremity edema, bradycardia	Not used as commonly for HTN as DHP-CCBs
Beta-Blockers (BB)			
Cardioselective (β_1) Atenolol Metoprolol	Antagonist of β_1 and/or β_2 receptors to decrease contractility and O_2 demand	Side effects: Bradycardia	Not first line unless also have CHF and/or post MI
Non-selective (β_1 and β_2) Propranolol		Side effects: Bradycardia Bronchospasm can be seen with non-selective BB Caution in patients with frequent or active asthma and COPD exacerbations (β_2 antagonism can worsen bronchoconstriction)	Not first line unless also have CHF and/or post MI
Mixed α- and β-blocker Carvedilol Labetalol		Side effects: Bradycardia	Not first line unless also have CHF and/or post MI
Alpha Blockers			
Prazosin	Peripherally acting alpha-1 blocker that causes vascular smooth muscle relaxation	Side effects: Postural hypotension, dizziness, headaches, weakness	Not first line due to increased risk of side effects and limited HTN outcome data

Classes of Antihypertensives (*Continued*)

Class of Medication	Mechanism of Action	Side Effects/Contraindications	Additional Notes
Central Alpha-2 Agonists			
Methyldopa Clonidine	Clonidine is a centrally acting alpha-2 agonist that results in decreased sympathetic outflow	Sudden stopping can cause rebound hypertensive urgency or emergency	Not first line but can be added when combination therapy needed Methyldopa used to treat HTN in pregnancy Clonidine is a very potent anti-HTN med
Direct Vasodilators			
Hydralazine Minoxidil Sodium nitroprusside	Dilate vessels by relaxing smooth muscle cells in blood vessels	Side effects: tachycardia, fluid retention, headaches	Not first line Used for resistant HTN

Important Drug Classes to Consider Based on Comorbid Conditions

Indication	Treatment Choices
Heart failure	(ACE-I or ARB) + BB + spironolactone + loop diuretic
Coronary artery disease (CAD) or Post-myocardial infarction	(ACE-I or ARB) + BB
Diabetes	(ACE-I or ARB), CCB, SGLT2 inhibitor (SGLT2i)
Chronic kidney disease	ACE-I or ARB, SGLT2i
Recurrent stroke prevention	ACE-I, thiazide diuretic
Pregnancy	Labetalol, nifedipine, methyldopa
Atrial fibrillation	BB, non-dihydropyridine CCB
Benign prostatic hypertrophy	Alpha-1 blockers

CASE 1 | Primary (Essential) Hypertension (HTN)

A 55-year-old woman with no past medical history presents for routine health maintenance. She is feeling well and has no concerns. Three months ago, at a dental checkup, her blood pressure was noted to be 150/88 mmHg. The patient's temperature is 36.2°C, pulse is 75/min, blood pressure is 156/80 mmHg (154/84 on repeat measurement 10 minutes later), and respirations are 14/min. Blood pressure is equal in both arms and the rest of the physical exam is unremarkable.

Conditions with Similar Presentations	**Secondary HTN:** HTN due to another medical condition; see table below for details. **White coat HTN:** HTN only in the clinical setting due to anxiety; normotensive at home and in the community.
Initial Diagnostic Testing	• Confirm diagnosis: Elevated BP readings on three separate occasions • Consider additional testing for complications and comorbidities
Next Steps in Management	• Lifestyle modifications and Dietary Approaches to Stop Hypertension (DASH) diet • Antihypertensive medications
Discussion	95% of HTN is primary (essential) HTN with no identifiable cause. **History:** Usually asymptomatic • Symptoms may present when complications develop, including shortness of breath, chest tightness, headache, vision changes, or urinary changes • Risk factors: Age, obesity, diabetes, physical inactivity, alcohol intake, tobacco use, and family history of HTN **Physical exam:** Elevated blood pressure (>130/90) • Exam may reveal signs of end-organ damage/hypertensive complications, including laterally displaced point of maximal impulse (PMI), loud S2, or an S4 • Eye exam with arteriovenous nicking and copper wire changes to the arterioles, flame hemorrhages, papilledema

CASE 1 | Primary (Essential) Hypertension (HTN) *(continued)*

Discussion	**Diagnostics:** • Elevated blood pressure at two to three different visits • Consider evaluation for secondary HTN if onset <30 years old, 65 years old with new diastolic HTN, abrupt onset over a period of months, resistant HTN, or acutely worsening blood pressure **Tests to consider:** • Fasting blood glucose, lipid profile to evaluate for comorbid diabetes and dyslipidemia • Creatinine to assess for chronic kidney disease (CKD) • Electrocardiogram (ECG) may show left ventricular hypertrophy (LVH) • Urinalysis (UA) may reveal microalbuminuria/proteinuria/hematuria • CBC for anemia • Electrolytes—hypokalemia may be associated with hypercortisolism, hyperaldosteronism, and pheochromocytoma • Thyroid-stimulating hormone (TSH) for hyperthyroidism **Management:** • For all patients, start with lifestyle modifications: Weight loss, exercise, abstain from alcohol, salt restriction, decreased fat intake, DASH diet. • DASH diet: Rich in fruits, vegetables, low-fat milk products, whole grains, fish, poultry, beans, seeds, and nuts. Encourages less sodium, sweets, added sugars, and beverages containing sugar, fats, and red meats than the typical American diet. • Initiate pharmacologic therapy if stage 2 HTN (>140/90) or stage 1 HTN (>130/80) with elevated cardiovascular disease (CVD) risk. Thiazide diuretics, ACE-inhibitors/ARBs, and calcium channel blockers are all considered first line. Choice may depend on patient's comorbid conditions; see the table above.
Additional Considerations	**Screening:** USPSTF recommends screening for HTN in adults 18 years or older. **Complications:** Coronary artery disease, renal failure (hypertensive nephropathy), stroke (HTN is the most important risk factor for hemorrhagic and ischemic stroke), cerebral aneurysm, congestive heart failure (CHF) (both systolic and diastolic), hypertensive retinopathy, hypertensive emergency, and peripheral vascular disease. **Pediatric considerations:** Secondary HTN workup indicated in this patient population.

CASE 2 | Hypertensive Emergency

A 66-year-old man with poorly controlled HTN presents with a severe headache and blurry vision. The patient's temperature is 36.2°C, pulse is 82/min, blood pressure is 210/125 mmHg (no change on repeat measurements) in both arms, and respirations are 16/min. Fundoscopic exam demonstrates arteriolar narrowing and arteriovenous nicking and papilledema; remainder of the physical exam is normal.

Conditions with Similar Presentations	**Hypertensive urgency:** presents with BP >180/120 mmHg; however, there will be no symptoms, signs, or laboratory findings of vital end-organ (brain, heart, kidney) damage. **Acute ischemic or hemorrhagic stroke:** may present with severe headache and HTN but the patient will have evidence of stroke by history and physical and CT or MRI imaging.
Initial Diagnostic Testing	• Confirm diagnosis: BP >180/120 mmHg on repeat examinations • Check UA, serum creatinine, ECG and troponin • Non-contrast head CT if focal neurologic findings, urine tox screen if clinical presentation concerning for substance use (e.g. cocaine, amphetamines) and CXR if concern for pulmonary edema
Next Steps in Management	Admit to ICU, reduce BP by 10–20% within first hour using IV antihypertensive (labetalol, esmolol, nicardipine, nitroprusside, nitroglycerin).

CASE 2 | Hypertensive Emergency *(continued)*

Discussion	Hypertensive emergency occurs when there is a failure of autoregulatory mechanisms in the vascular supply which leads to inappropriately increased vascular resistance and/or inappropriate activation of the renin-angiotensin-aldosterone system (RAAS). History or physical exam will reveal signs of end-organ damage which should be investigated with further testing. **History:** Headache, visual changes, chest pain, dyspnea, focal neurologic deficit, encephalopathy, nausea/vomiting, or seizures may be symptoms of end-organ damage. **Risk factors:** Poorly controlled HTN, unable to adhere to medication regimen. **Physical exam:** Severely elevated blood pressure (>180/120 mmHg) with evidence of end-organ damage (papilledema/flame hemorrhages/cotton wool spots, focal neurologic deficit, S3/JVD [Jugular venous distension], pulmonary crackles). **Diagnostics:** Blood pressure >180/120 mmHg with evidence of end-organ damage. Check for end-organ injury with: • Serum creatinine, UA—AKI • ECG, troponin—ACS • CXR—pulmonary edema • Non-contrast CT of the head—intracranial hemorrhage **Management:** • Admit to ICU. • Reduce BP 10–20% within first hour, down to 160/100 mg over next 2–6 hours, and normal in next 24–48 hours. • Use IV antihypertensives including labetalol, esmolol, nicardipine, nitroprusside, nitroglycerin. • Once stabilized, transition to outpatient regimen with close follow-up.
Additional Considerations	For patients with **hypertensive urgency** and *no* evidence of end-organ damage: • Management goals are to lower blood pressure gradually over the next 24–48 hours with oral medications. • Antihypertensive medication titration and close follow-up indicated.

Secondary Hypertension Mini-Cases

Cases	Key Findings
Obstructive sleep apnea (OSA)	**Hx:** Fatigue, daytime sleepiness, snoring, morning headache, male > female **PE:** Obesity, micrognathia **Diagnostics:** Sleep study **Management:** • Lifestyle (weight loss, exercise, sleep position change) • Continuous positive airway pressure (CPAP) **Discussion:** • Excess pharyngeal tissue reduces airflow despite respiratory drive • HTN a multifactorial complication from increased sympathetic activity and RAAS activation
Coarctation of the aorta	**Hx:** Poor feeding (infants) or fatigue, dyspnea on exertion (children, adolescents). • Associated with bicuspid aortic valve, monosomy X (Turner syndrome), Williams syndrome. **PE:** Elevated blood pressure in upper extremities, delayed femoral pulses, systolic or continuous murmur. **Diagnostics:** • Transthoracic echocardiogram shows accelerated and delayed flow in proximal descending thoracic aorta. • Collateral circulation causes intercostal arteries to enlarge causing rib notching on chest x-ray. **Management:** • Prostaglandin E in neonates with coarctation to maintain patent ductus arteriosus (PDA) for systemic perfusion. • Consider surgical or transcatheter repair in adults or children with HTN. **Discussion:** • Etiology either post-ductal (adult type) in which narrowing occurs distal to the ductus arteriosum or pre-ductal (infantile type) in which narrowing occurs proximal to the ductus arteriosum.

Secondary Hypertension Mini-Cases (continued)

Renal artery stenosis (RAS)	**Hx:** Treatment-resistant HTN without other clear cause, young onset without family history, renal asymmetry. **PE:** Abdominal bruit over renal arteries. **Diagnostics:** • Initial imaging—ultrasound with Doppler. • CT angiography and MR angiography more sensitive/specific. • Gold standard—catheter angiography. **Management:** • ACE-inhibitor or ARB (contraindicated if bilateral RAS or single kidney). • Revascularization indicated if severe complications (heart failure, pulmonary edema, CKD, uncontrolled HTN). **Discussion:** Secondary to atherosclerosis (older patient with smoking history and fatty diet) or fibromuscular dysplasia (young women).
Polycystic kidney disease (see Chapter 13)	**Hx:** Family history of kidney disease or hemorrhagic stroke at an early age, flank pain, hematuria. **PE:** May have bilateral flank masses on physical exam. **Diagnostics:** • Ultrasound (renal cysts) and consistent clinical picture (HTN in a young adult). • *PKD1* (chromosome 16) or *PKD2* (chromosome 4) mutations, however genetic testing not recommended for diagnosis. **Management:** • ACE-inhibitors or ARBs. • Manage complications (hematuria, nephrolithiasis, urinary tract infections, HTN, and intracranial aneurysms). **Discussion:** Autosomal dominant (presents in adulthood) or autosomal recessive (presents in childhood).
Cushing syndrome (see Chapter 9)	**Hx:** Symptoms of cortisol excess: Weight gain, easy bruising, new diagnosis of diabetes **PE:** • Abdominal adiposity, thin skin with purple striae, buffalo hump, excessive hair growth, moon facies (cannot see ears when looking directly from the front) **Diagnostics:** • Initial 24-hour urinary free cortisol (3× upper limit of normal) • Then dexamethasone suppression testing and/or ACTH levels • Obtain imaging based on suspicion of pituitary adenoma, adrenal disease, or ectopic ACTH secretion **Management:** • Resectable lesions (pituitary/adrenal malignancies) should be localized and resected if possible **Discussion:** Cushing syndrome is a state of excess cortisol from the pituitary gland (adenoma), adrenal gland (adenoma, bilateral hyperplasia, carcinoma), exogenous glucocorticoids, or paraneoplastic ACTH secretion
Primary hyperaldosteronism (Conn syndrome) (see Chapter 9)	**Hx/PE:** HTN and symptoms of aldosterone excess: Muscle cramps, weakness, fatigue, excessive thirst. **Diagnostics:** • Plasma aldosterone to plasma renin ratio >30 (screen), saline infusion test (definitive diagnosis), adrenal venous sampling (determine bilateral vs. unilateral hyperplasia). • CT indicated to differentiate hyperplasia, adenoma, carcinoma. **Management:** • Resectable lesions of the adrenal should be localized and resected if possible. • Treat HTN from hyperaldosteronism with eplerenone or spironolactone (aldosterone receptor antagonist). **Discussion:** Primary hyperaldosteronism is a syndrome of increased aldosterone secretion from the adrenal cortex due to aldosterone-secreting adrenal adenoma, bilateral adrenal hyperplasia, or adrenal carcinoma (very rare). Abnormal aldosterone secretion causes hypokalemia and metabolic alkalosis (due to loss of H^+).

Secondary Hypertension Mini-Cases *(continued)*

Pheochromocytoma (see Chapter 9)	**Hx:** Episodic (may be constant) HTN, headache, palpitations, diaphoresis. **PE:** HTN, tachycardia, diaphoresis, loud S1 and S2. **Diagnostics:** • Screen with increased free plasma metanephrines. • Confirm with 24-hour urine metanephrines (↑) and vanillylmandelic acid (VMA) (↑). • MRI or CT to localize source prior to surgery; unilateral adrenal in 80%, bilateral in 10%, and 10% are extra-adrenal (**paragangliomas**). **Management:** • Alpha-antagonist (phenoxybenzamine) to prevent unopposed alpha-action when beta receptors blocked, followed by beta-blocker and tumor resection. • Prognosis good with resection. **Discussion:** Pheochromocytoma is a catecholamine-secreting neuroendocrine tumor. Pheochromocytomas may secrete catecholamines (from adrenal chromaffin cells) in a pulsatile fashion leading to intermittent symptoms and signs.
Hyperthyroidism (see Chapter 9)	**Hx:** • Young, middle-aged females with family/personal history of autoimmune conditions. • Tachycardia, weight loss, tremulousness, frequent stools, warm moist skin, heat intolerance, eye pain. **PE:** Isolated systolic HTN, anti-gravity action tremor. In Graves' disease proptosis, exophthalmos, lid lag. **Diagnostics:** TSH and T4. Radioactive iodine thyroid scan can help differentiate specific thyroid etiologies. **Management:** • Propranolol (blocks beta-1 sympathetic effect of thyroid hormone). • Methimazole or propylthiouracil (prevents thyroid hormone synthesis). • Radioiodine ablation (indicated if patient fails antithyroid drugs). **Discussion:** Graves' disease vs. multinodular toxic goiter, toxic thyroid adenoma, and iatrogenic thyroid hormone excess.

CHEST PAIN

Chest pain has a broad differential that includes both cardiac and noncardiac etiologies. Chest pain can be classified as cardiac, possibly cardiac, or noncardiac based on the symptom characteristics by history and clinical presentation. "Do Not Miss" causes of chest pain include acute coronary syndrome (ACS), pulmonary embolism (PE), tension pneumothorax, and aortic dissection. An initial evaluation for possible ACS (which includes unstable angina, non ST-elevation myocardial infarction (NSTEMI), ST-elevation myocardial infarction (STEMI)) begins with an ECG and a serum troponin. Other testing is ordered based on the clinical situation and can include echocardiography, stress testing, cardiac magnetic resonance (CMR), coronary computed tomography angiography (CCTA), and left heart catheterization (LHC).

Differential Diagnosis

1. Skin—rash/herpes zoster, mastitis, fibromyalgia
2. Musculoskeletal—rib fracture, costochondritis, pectoral muscle strain, precordial catch syndrome, mastitis
3. Pulmonary/Pleura—pneumonia, tracheobronchitis, pulmonary embolism, pleural disease, pneumothorax
4. Cardiac—ACS, stable angina, pericarditis, myocarditis, Prinzmetal angina, stress-induced cardiomyopathy (Takotsubo)
5. Gastrointestinal—GERD, esophagitis, esophageal rupture, peptic ulcer, cholecystitis, pancreatitis
6. Vasculature—aortic dissection, Kawasaki disease
7. Neuropsychological—panic attack, anxiety disorder

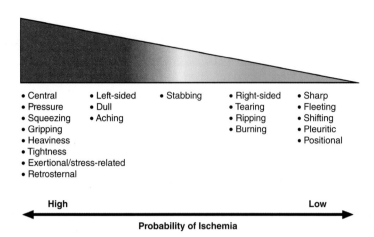

- Central
- Pressure
- Squeezing
- Gripping
- Heaviness
- Tightness
- Exertional/stress-related
- Retrosternal

- Left-sided
- Dull
- Aching

- Stabbing

- Right-sided
- Tearing
- Ripping
- Burning

- Sharp
- Fleeting
- Shifting
- Pleuritic
- Positional

High ← → Low

Probability of Ischemia

Chest pain or discomfort has many descriptors that can be more or less suggestive of being due to coronary disease. (Reproduced with permission from Gulati M, Levy PD, et al. 2021 AHA/ACC/ASE/CHEST/SAEM/SCCT/SCMR Guideline for the Evaluation and Diagnosis of Chest Pain: A Report of the American College of Cardiology/American Heart Association Joint Committee on Clinical Practice Guidelines. *Circulation*. 2021; 30:144(22):e368-e454.)

"Cardiac" chest discomfort (stable angina) is often characterized by the following:

1. Provoked by exercise or emotional stress
2. Relieved by nitroglycerin or rest
3. Description is most commonly substernal discomfort or pressure
4. Duration (lasts minutes with gradual onset and offset)

"Possible cardiac" and "noncardiac" chest discomfort may include some typical but also sharp or fleeting characteristics, or pain related to inspiration or positional changes that are less suggestive of coronary disease.

Pretest Probability of CAD	Characteristics	Next Steps
Low	No significant cardiac risk factors and symptoms consistent with noncardiac pain	No testing required
Intermediate	Concern for possible CAD. May have some symptoms consistent with possible cardiac pain	Stress test
High	Concern for ACS	Cardiac catheterization

"Do Not Miss" Diagnoses for Chest Pain

Diagnoses to Consider	Description of Pain	Associated History Findings	Key Physical Findings	Confirmatory Testing
Acute coronary syndrome (ACS)	Squeezing, pressure, may radiate to arm(s), neck, back	Worse with exertion and relieved by rest. Cardiovascular risk factors	Diaphoresis, pallor, S4, possible S3	ECG (ST elevation in STEMI), cardiac markers (troponin elevation in STEMI and NSTEMI)
Aortic dissection	Tearing or ripping pain, may radiate to the mid-back	HTN, connective tissue disease (Marfan syndrome)	Depends on location of dissection. Asymmetric blood pressures, weak, asymmetric peripheral pulses, possible diastolic murmur of aortic insufficiency	CXR (widened mediastinum), CT or TEE (widened mediastinum and intimal flap visualized)

"Do Not Miss" Diagnoses for Chest Pain (*Continued*)

Diagnoses to Consider	Description of Pain	Associated History Findings	Key Physical Findings	Confirmatory Testing
Cardiac tamponade	Chest discomfort, dyspnea, lighteadedness, syncope	Predisposing condition (MI, uremia, neoplastic, infection, trauma)	Beck's triad (elevated JVP, hypotension, muffled heart sounds), pulsus paradoxus, Kussmaul sign	ECG (low voltage QRS, electrical alternans), echocardiogram (pericardial effusion and diastolic collapse of right heart)
Pulmonary embolism	Pleuritic, sharp, cough/hemoptysis, shortness of breath	Recent surgery or immobilization, hypercoagulable states	Tachypnea (always present), tachycardia, hypoxia	CT angiography (pulmonary embolism) or V/Q scan (V/Q mismatch)
Acute pneumothorax	Sudden onset, sharp, pleuritic	Primary pneumothorax: no lung disease, commonly tall, thin male smoker Secondary pneumothorax: trauma, history of lung disease, or connective tissue disease (Marfan syndrome)	Tachypnea, decreased breath sounds and hyperresonance over affected lung field Tracheal shift toward affected side unless a tension pneumothorax where it shifts away from affected side	CXR: Radiolucency in pleural space with collapse of adjacent lung segment; possible tracheal shift if tension pneumothorax

		Acute Coronary Syndrome (ACS)		
	Stable Angina	**Unstable Angina**	**NSTEMI**	**STEMI**
Pathophysiology	Stable plaque, demand ischemia	Plaque rupture, thrombus causing new partial occlusion	Plaque rupture, thrombus causing subendocardial infarct	Plaque rupture, thrombus causing transmural infarct
Typical presentation	Substernal pressure worse with exertion/stress and relieved with rest	New onset angina or change in stable angina (requiring less exertion/stress, lasting longer, less responsive to medications)	Persistent chest pain with increased intensity or severity	
Diagnosis	Clinical diagnosis Order stress test or cardiac catheterization based on pre-test probability	Clinical diagnosis May have nonspecific ECG changes	Elevated troponin and characteristic ECG changes below	
ECG	Usually normal	Normal or nonspecific (occasionally dynamic ST depression and/or T wave inversion, more commonly in NSTEMI)		ST elevations in anatomic distribution +/− T wave inversions
Cardiac biomarkers (troponin)	Normal	Normal	Elevated Usually higher with STEMI	
Treatment	Antianginal medications (nitroglycerin, beta-blockers, ± calcium channel blockers), aspirin and statin	*M*orphine (only for uncontrolled pain), *O*xygen (if pO$_2$ <94), *N*itrates, *A*spirin/Antiplatelet (P2Y$_{12}$ inhibitor), *B*eta-blocker, *A*CE-inhibitor (for STEMI), *S*tatin, *H*eparin (MONA BASH) Urgent or emergent Left heart catheterization (LHC) for NSTEMI/STEMI Unstable angina: Risk stratify for stress test or cardiac catheterization based on "clinical presentation"		

CASE 3 | Stable Angina

A 75-year-old woman with HTN, type 2 diabetes mellitus, hyperlipidemia presents with intermittent chest discomfort for the past 2 months. She reports a squeezing pressure sensation mid-chest area radiating to her neck. The symptoms gradually begin each time she climbs two flights of stairs and improve after she rests for a few minutes. Her vital signs and heart, lung, and abdominal exam are normal. There is no reproducible chest wall tenderness or lower extremity edema.

Conditions with Similar Presentations	**Unstable angina:** Also causes chest pain, but pain occurs at rest or with less exertion than before, or is more severe/lasts longer compared to stable angina. New-onset angina is also considered unstable angina. **Vasospastic (aka variant/Prinzmetal) angina:** Similar to angina, but occurs at rest and in younger patients and may be triggered by substances such as triptans, cocaine, cannabis, ephedrine-based products, or alcohol. ECG may be normal or show ST elevations/depressions and/or hyperacute T waves.
Initial Diagnostic Testing	• Clinical diagnosis • ECG to rule out ST elevations and assess for prior MI • If history not typical, consider stress test to confirm diagnosis
Next Steps in Management	• Start aspirin, statin and treat symptoms with nitrates, beta-blockers and if needed, calcium channel blockers. • Optimize risk factors/lifestyle modifications.

Discussion	Stable angina occurs when there is an obstructive atherosclerotic lesion in the coronary arteries, usually over 70% stenosis. Symptoms occur when the blood supply cannot meet the requirements for oxygen demand.
	
	 History:
	 • Risk factors include age (male patients >45, female patients >55), male sex, HTN, DM, hyperlipidemia, family history of premature coronary artery disease (males <55, females <65), smoking, and abdominal obesity.
	 • Episodes of discomfort or pressure sensation rather than pain, provoked by exercise or emotional stress and relieved by rest or stress reduction.
	 • Additional symptoms include dyspnea, nausea, diaphoresis, lightheadedness, dizziness, and easy fatigability.
	 • Women will most commonly present with chest pain or pressure but are more likely than men to have presentations of nausea, fatigue, or dyspnea.
	
	 Physical Exam: Normal
	
	 Diagnostics:
	 • Pre-test probability and clinical diagnosis based on history.
	 • Resting ECG without ST elevations.
	 • If possible cardiac symptoms with intermediate pre-test probability, a stress test can be performed to further evaluate:
	   • Positive **exercise ECG** shows ≥1 mm horizontal or down-sloping ST depression in more than one contiguous lead.
	   • **Stress echo** demonstrates inducible regional wall motion abnormalities consistent with ischemia.
	 • If patient has typical cardiac symptoms with high-pretest probability, a cardiac catheterization can be performed to further evaluate.
	
	 Management:
	 • Treat with anti-anginal medications: nitroglycerin, beta-blockers, ± calcium channel blockers, and statins.
	 • Aspirin indicated for all CAD.
	 • Optimize risk factors (diabetes, HTN, dyslipidemia) and encourage lifestyle modifications (diet, exercise, smoking cessation).
	 • Persistent symptoms despite optimal medical therapy and affecting lifestyle should have cardiac catheterization and possible revascularization.

CASE 4 | Acute Coronary Syndrome (ACS): ST-Segment Elevation Myocardial Infarction (STEMI)

A 75-year-old woman with HTN, diabetes, and hyperlipidemia presents with worsening severe substernal chest pain and shortness of breath for the past hour. The pain radiates to her left arm and is accompanied by a feeling of light headedness and nausea. On exam, she appears anxious, distressed, and diaphoretic. Temperature is 37.3°C, pulse is 110/min, blood pressure is 150/76 mmHg, respirations are 24/min, and SpO$_2$ is 98% on room air. Blood pressure and pulse are equal in both arms. Cardiovascular exam is notable for an S4, and the rest of the exam is normal.

Conditions with Similar Presentations	**Stable angina:** Predictable chest pain (no significant change over time); worse with exercise or stress; improves with rest or nitroglycerin (see Case 3). **Vasospastic angina:** Recurrent chest pain often at rest with spontaneous resolution. **Pericarditis:** Chest pain worsens when lying flat and with inspiration; improves with sitting up and leaning forward; pericardial rub on exam.

CASE 4 | Acute Coronary Syndrome (ACS): ST-Segment Elevation Myocardial Infarction (STEMI) *(continued)*

Conditions with Similar Presentations	**Aortic dissection:** Tearing chest pain that radiates to back; difference in blood pressure and pulse intensity between right and left arm. **Pulmonary causes (PE, pneumothorax):** Pleuritic pain worsens with inspiration and is sharp/stabbing in nature; respiratory distress; hypoxia. **Costochondritis:** Reproducible chest wall tenderness; pain is pleuritic; persistent/prolonged pain. **Gastrointestinal/esophageal:** Pain worse after meals and when supine; improves with PPI/H2 blockers/antacids; associated with nausea, sour taste in mouth, hoarseness, or dysphagia. **Panic attack:** Associated with anxiety.
Initial Diagnostic Tests	Check ECG, troponin
Next Steps in Management	• Emergent cardiac catheterization and primary percutaneous intervention (PCI) for STEMI (within 90 minutes of first medical contact). • Initiate therapy: For patients with ACS (unstable angina, STEMI, NSTEMI), give aspirin, beta-blocker, high-intensity statin, ACE inhibitor, heparin, and $P2Y_{12}$ inhibitor, nitroglycerin. If pO_2 ≤94% start oxygen. If pain uncontrolled, give morphine.

Discussion	ACS most commonly occurs due to rupture of a thrombotic occlusion of a coronary artery with underlying atherosclerosis. ACS can be divided into the following:
	• **Unstable angina**—partial occlusion of the vessel resulting in supply ischemia (*in contrast to demand ischemia*) without necrosis or infarction of the myocardium.
	• **NSTEMI**—subtotal occlusion of the vessel that results in necrosis and infarct in the sub-endocardium (inner 1/3 of myocardium).
	• **STEMI**—complete occlusion of the vessel that results in a transmural infarct.
	
	History:
	• Risk factors include diabetes mellitus, HTN, hyperlipidemia, smoking, age (men >45 years old; women >55 years old), and family history of premature CAD or MI in a first-degree relative (if relative male <55 years old, and if female <65 years old). Other less traditional risk factors include HIV, inflammatory disorders such as rheumatoid arthritis, and prior history of mediastinal radiation.
	• Symptoms:
	  • Substernal chest pain often described as "intense pressure sensation" or "crushing" that may radiate to neck, jaw, arms, or back.
	  • Other symptoms include dyspnea, diaphoresis, nausea, vomiting, epigastric pain, fatigue, and syncope. Up to one-third of patients can be asymptomatic.
	
	Physical Exam: Usually normal CV exam
	• Occasionally includes S4 (ischemia-related diastolic "stiffening"), pulmonary crackles (acute pulmonary vascular volume overload from ischemic LV dysfunction), and/or mitral regurgitation secondary to ischemic papillary muscle rupture/dysfunction.
	
	Diagnostics: Check ECG and troponin
	• STEMI: ST elevation and elevated troponin
	• NSTEMI: Normal or nonspecific ST changes and elevated troponin
	• Unstable angina: Clinical diagnosis with normal or nonspecific ST changes and normal troponin

CASE 4 | Acute Coronary Syndrome (ACS): ST-Segment Elevation Myocardial Infarction (STEMI) *(continued)*

Discussion	In STEMI, pattern of ST elevation localizes infarct as follows:

Anatomic distributions:

Anterior MI (LAD): V1-V4
Lateral MI (LCX): I, avL, V5–V6
Inferior MI (RCA): II, III, avF

ECG Leads and Coronary Arteries

V1-V4	Anterior/Septal leads	Left Anterior Descending (LAD)
I, aVL, V5-V6	Lateral Leads	Left Circumflex (LCx) or Diagonal of LAD
II, III, aVF	Inferior Leads	RCA (and/or 10% LCx)

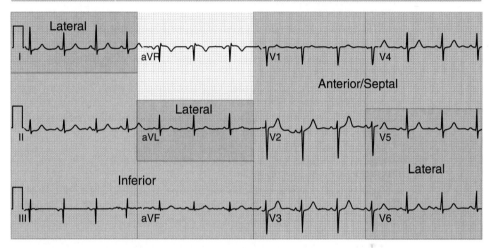

Reproduced with permission from Rebel Reviews. rebelem.com/rebel-review/rebel-review-29-coronary-anatomy-ecg-leads/coronary-anatomy-ecg-leads/.

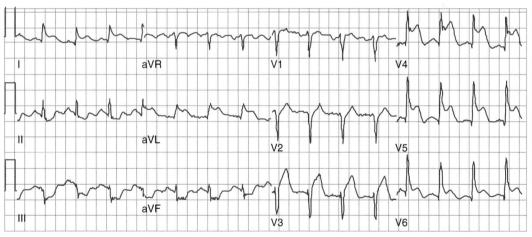

Example of anterolateral STEMI. (Reproduced with permission from Crawford MH, ed. *Current Diagnosis & Treatment: Cardiology.* 5th ed. New York: McGraw Hill; 2017.)

- Additional baseline tests: CBC, BMP, BNP, PT/PTT/INR, and CXR

CASE 4 | Acute Coronary Syndrome (ACS): ST-Segment Elevation Myocardial Infarction (STEMI) *(continued)*

Discussion	**Management:**
	• Everyone with ACS (unstable angina, STEMI, NSTEMI) should be placed on telemetry and receive treatment with **MONABASH**
	  • **M**orphine (only if pain uncontrolled)
	  • **O**xygen (if SpO$_2$ less than 94%)
	  • **N**itrates (decreases preload, dilates coronaries, improves symptoms)
	  • **A**spirin (antiplatelet activity prevents further thrombus propagation, lowers mortality, secondary prevention)/**A**ntiplatelet therapy with a PGY12 inhibitor (clopidogrel, ticagrelor)
	  • **B**eta-blocker (lowers mortality, secondary prevention, reduces cardiac remodeling); use caution in setting of acute heart failure, bradycardia, hypotension, heart block
	  • **A**CE inhibitor (lowers mortality; secondary prevention)
	  • **S**tatin (lowers mortality; secondary prevention)
	  • **H**eparin (prevents further thrombus propagation)
	• Treatment with cardiac catheterization and PCI:
	  • STEMI: Within 90 minutes of presentation and if not available within 120 minutes, give thrombolytics.
	  • NSTEMI: Within 24–48 hours. Sooner if ongoing signs of ischemia.
	  • Unstable angina: Risk stratify for stress testing vs. cardiac catheterization.
	• If three-vessel disease or left main CAD is present, PCI may be challenging and coronary artery bypass graft **(CABG)** should be considered.
	• If a drug-eluting stent is placed, then dual antiplatelet therapy (DAPT) with aspirin plus clopidogrel or ticagrelor is recommended for at least 1 year.
	• After ACS, patients should have long-term treatment with **ABC** to reduce the risk of future events in patients with known disease (secondary prevention):
	  • **A**spirin and **A**CEi or **A**RB
	  • **B**eta-blocker, especially if LV dysfunction persists after ACS
	  • **C**holesterol treatment (statin)
	• Most patients after ACS stabilization and treatment (e.g., PCI) can be discharged home 1 day after stenting. Referral to outpatient cardiac rehabilitation at time of discharge should be done.

Additional Considerations	**Screening:** The USPSTF recommends starting a statin for primary prevention of coronary vascular disease (CVD) in patients with an elevated 10-year risk or for any of the following reasons:
	• LDL ≥190 mg/dL
	• LDL 70–189 and age 40–75 and either one of
	  • Diabetes mellitus *or*
	  • Ten-year risk of atherosclerotic CVD of ≥7.5%
	
	Complications of MI: Risk factors for developing complications include no PCI or delayed presentation.
	• **Interventricular septum defect/rupture:** Within 24 hours of transmural MI if the infarcted myocardium is near the ventricular septum. This results in an acute left-to-right shunt and associated murmur (holosystolic murmur best heard at the sternal border). Presents as acute heart failure due to volume overload created by the shunt. Diagnose by echocardiogram.
	• **Papillary muscle rupture:** Within 3–5 days of MI resulting in acute mitral regurgitation and presents with pulmonary edema secondary to increased pulmonary venous pressures. Will have systolic murmur radiating to the apex. Diagnose by echocardiogram.
	• **Free wall rupture:** Five days to 2 weeks of transmural MI and can result in either pseudoaneurysm or cardiac tamponade.
	  • **Pseudoaneurysm** occurs when ventricular free wall rupture is contained by the pericardium and presents with recurrence of chest pain that is pericardial in nature.
	  • If the rupture is not contained, rapid blood accumulation in the pericardial space results in **cardiac tamponade** with pulsus paradoxus, jugular venous distension, and shock.
	• **Dressler syndrome:** Acute pericarditis following transmural MI, thought to be an autoimmune phenomenon resulting in fibrinous pericarditis. Occurs a few weeks after MI or heart surgery.
	• **Systolic heart failure** is related to the size of infarction and is usually associated with a proximal left anterior descending artery occlusion. Patients present either early or late after infarction with signs and symptoms of heart failure with reduced ejection fraction.
	
	Surgical considerations: CABG should be considered depending on results of catheterization (see above).

CASE 5 | Aortic Dissection

A 66-year-old man with HTN is brought to the emergency department (ED) with severe chest pain for 2 hours. Pain was sudden onset, tearing in nature, and radiates to his back. He has no shortness of breath, palpitations, or lightheadedness. On exam, pulse is 107/min, blood pressure is 174/94 mmHg in the left arm and 151/81 mmHg in the right arm. A decrescendo diastolic murmur is most prominent at the lower left sternal border. His lung and abdominal exams are normal.

Conditions with Similar Presentations	**Acute coronary syndrome, pulmonary embolus, tension pneumothorax, tamponade** (discussed in other cases) must be considered in the differential for sudden-onset severe chest pain.
Initial Diagnostic Tests	• Check CT angiogram to confirm diagnosis • Consider ECG to rule out other causes
Next Steps in Management	• Morphine, IV beta-blocker, then sodium nitroprusside (if systolic BP >120 mmHg) • Emergent surgical repair if type A (ascending) dissection. Type B (descending) dissection can be treated medically unless critical aortic branch occlusions occur.
Discussion	Aortic dissection is a life-threatening emergency. Without immediate therapy, morbidity and mortality are high. A tear in the intimal layer of the aorta results in a separation (dissection) of layers within the aortic wall creating a false lumen that may re-rupture back into the true lumen further down the aorta. Dissections are classified by location of aortic involvement, which guides treatment. The Stanford (Daily) system classifies dissections as: • *Type A dissections:* Dissection involving the ascending aorta (including and proximal to the brachiocephalic trunk). Are life-threatening dissections with mortality rates of 1–2% per hour after symptom onset. • *Type B dissections:* All other dissection locations. **History:** • Risk factors: HTN (strongest risk factor), advancing age, male sex, connective tissue disorder (e.g., Marfan syndrome), bicuspid aortic valve (as seen in some Turner syndrome patients), coarctation of the aorta, preexisting aortic aneurysm, cocaine use (especially in young patients), and risk factors for atherosclerosis. • Symptoms: Sharp, severe, sudden, "tearing" chest pain radiating to the back. **Physical Exam:** • Systolic blood pressure (SBP) difference of >20 mmHg between arms (especially if the false lumen involves one subclavian artery and true lumen involves the contralateral subclavian artery). Note that absence of this finding should not exclude aortic dissection as a diagnosis. • Hypotension/shock (more common in type A) or HTN (more common in type B). • Acute aortic regurgitation can occur if the dissection involves the aortic valve, presenting as new diastolic decrescendo murmur with wide pulse pressure. **Diagnostics:** • Confirm diagnosis with a CT angiography, transesophageal echocardiography (TEE), or MR angiography (chosen based on availability and patient factors) revealing a **double aortic lumen** or **intimal flap**: 1. CT angiography—definitive test in hemodynamically stable patients 2. TEE—if unable to obtain CT due to hemodynamic instability or renal insufficiency 3. MR angiography—if unable to obtain CT due to renal insufficiency but is time-consuming **Aortic dissection** 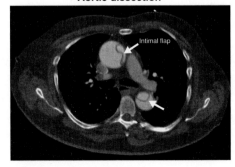 CT image of false and true lumen caused by an intimal tear. Note the true lumen is often the lumen smaller in size. 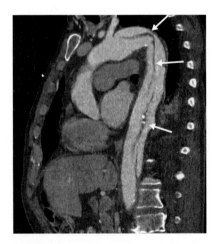 Sagittal CT image of a Type B aortic dissection: origin is distal to the brachiocephalic trunk. (Reproduced with permission from Sörelius K, Wanhainen A. Challenging Current Conservative Management of Uncomplicated Acute Type B Aortic Dissections. *EJVES Short Rep.* 2018;39:37-39.)

CASE 5 | Aortic Dissection *(continued)*

Discussion	Other tests: • Chest x-ray may show widened aortic silhouette/mediastinum. • ECG can be normal or with nonspecific abnormal changes. **Management:** • *Morphine:* For pain management. • *IV beta-blocker* (e.g. propranolol, labetalol, esmolol): Decreases SBP, heart rate, and LV contractility which reduces aortic wall stress. • *Sodium nitroprusside:* If SBP >120 mmHg despite beta-blocker. Do not give nitroprusside first because this will cause a reflex tachycardia and increased contractility, which can increase aortic sheer stress and worsen the dissection. • *Emergent surgical repair* for type A dissections.
Additional Considerations	**Complications:** Stroke (carotid artery involvement), acute aortic regurgitation (aortic root involvement), pericardial effusion/tamponade (dissection ruptures into the pericardium), mesenteric ischemia (celiac artery involvement), acute kidney injury (renal artery involvement). **Surgical considerations:** Emergent surgical repair (open repair) indicated for type A dissections. Type B dissections: Treat medically unless critical aortic branch occlusions occur.

CASE 6 | Pericarditis

A 56-year-old woman presents with sharp, non-radiating chest pain for 2 days. The pain is worse with inspiration and lying down and improved with leaning forward and ibuprofen. She has no shortness of breath but did note having a cold a few weeks ago. Patient's temperature is 37.5°C, respirations are 20/min, blood pressure is 102/85 mmHg, and SpO$_2$ is 98% on room air. Physical exam is notable for mild distress and a scratchy three-component pericardial friction rub on auscultation. Lungs are clear and there is no tenderness on palpation of the chest and no lower extremity edema.

Conditions with Similar Presentations	**Cardiac tamponade:** results from a rapidly accumulated pericardial effusion and patients are usually hemodynamically unstable and have pulsus paradoxus (Beck's triad). **MI:** chest pain is usually substernal pressure/tightness (not related to inspiration or position) and ECG shows focal ST elevations. It is not relieved by sitting up. **Pleural effusions/pleuritis:** can cause pleuritic chest pain but would not present with cardiac friction rub or abnormal ECG.
Initial Diagnostic Testing	ECG (diffuse ST elevation and PR depression).
Next Steps in Management	• NSAIDs or aspirin, and colchicine. • Treat underlying cause.
Discussion	Pericarditis is inflammation of the pericardium due to infection (viral most common), autoimmune disorders, drugs/toxins, metabolic causes (uremia, hypothyroidism), malignancy (metastatic, rarely primary), injury (post MI, Dressler syndrome), postoperative (after CABG), aortic dissection, radiation, or trauma. Most cases are idiopathic. Etiology will help guide treatment. **History:** • Risk factors: Viral illness (~2 weeks after initial illness) or any of the above potential causes. • Symptoms: Sharp pleuritic, positional chest pain 　• Improved by sitting up and leaning forward 　• Worse with inspiration and laying supine 　• May have shoulder pain (referred pain from phrenic nerve which innervates the pericardium). **Physical exam: Pericardial friction rub** (pathognomonic, from inflamed pericardial layers rubbing against each other), scratchy systolic and early and late diastolic heart sound (three-component) best heard at left lower sternal border (LLSB). Components correspond to maximum movement of the pericardium during ventricular systole, ventricular diastole, and atrial systole. • Possible fever and tachycardia • Look for signs of complications (constrictive pericarditis or tamponade) see Case 7

CASE 6 | Pericarditis *(continued)*

Discussion	**Diagnostics:** Clinical picture (sharp/pleuritic/positional chest pain, friction rub) and ECG with **diffuse ST elevations and PR depressions**.

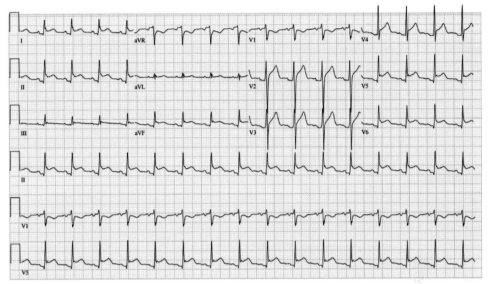

Electrocardiography findings in a patient with acute pericarditis. Note the widespread ST-segment elevation. This electrocardiogram also demonstrates PR-segment change with PR depression (best seen in lead II) and PR elevation in lead aVR. (Reproduced with permission from Fuster V, Harrington RA, Narula J, Eapen ZJ. *Hurst's The Heart*, 14e. New York: McGraw Hill; 2017.)

- Echocardiography can assess for presence of pericardial fluid but absence does not exclude pericarditis.

Additional tests to consider:
- Inflammatory markers (ESR, CRP) are elevated, but are not sensitive/specific for pericarditis.
- Chest x-ray helpful to rule out pneumonia or other pulmonary etiology.

Management:
- NSAIDS to reduce pain and inflammation.
- Colchicine shown to reduce symptoms and recurrence.
- Corticosteroids should not be given (unless an autoimmune origin) because they increase the relapse rate.
- Treat underlying cause as follows:

Etiology	Treatment
Uremia	Dialysis
Autoimmune (SLE or RA)	Steroids + immunosuppressants
Viral illness (e.g., coxsackievirus)	High-dose aspirin or NSAIDs; colchicine
MI complication (1–3 days after *and* several weeks after [Dressler syndrome])	High-dose aspirin or NSAIDs; colchicine
Rheumatic fever	Supportive
Tuberculosis	Treat tuberculosis
Malignancy	Treat underlying malignancy

Additional Considerations	**Complications:** Pericardial effusion, cardiac tamponade, and constrictive pericarditis. **Surgical considerations:** Pericardiectomy can be considered for severe, symptomatic, and recurrent pericarditis. **Inpatient considerations:** Mild symptoms with typical presentation can be treated as outpatient. Admit if concerns for tamponade, ACS, bacterial pericarditis, or presence of high-risk markers such as fevers, immunocompromise, hemodynamic instability, or large effusion.

CASE 7 | Cardiac Tamponade

A 46-year-old woman with newly diagnosed metastatic melanoma presents with chest pain, shortness of breath, and fever for the past 2 days. She is lightheaded and almost passed out, so her daughter brought her to the emergency department (ED). Her temperature is 37.4°C, respirations are 23/min, O_2 sat is 95%, pulse is 125/min, and blood pressure is 94/60 mmHg during expiration and 82/59 mmHg during inspiration (pulsus paradoxus). She is ill appearing, lethargic, has an elevated jugular venous pressure (JVP), muffled heart sounds, and her lungs are clear to auscultation.

Conditions with Similar Presentations	**Constrictive pericarditis:** may also present with chest pain and an increase in JVP with inhalation (Kussmaul sign), but usually presents in patients with a history of acute pericarditis or prior cardiac surgery, and exam may have pericardial friction rub. **Tension pneumothorax:** may also present with chest pain and signs of hemodynamic instability (hypotension), but physical exam would show unilateral decreased or absent breath sounds and hyperresonance to percussion. History usually involves penetrating trauma or lung disease. **Pericarditis with pericardial effusion:** may present with chest pain and pericardial effusion but without hemodynamic instability.
Initial Diagnostic Testing	• Confirm diagnosis with transthoracic echocardiogram (TTE). • Consider ECG, CXR.
Next Steps in Management	• Urgent pericardiocentesis • IV fluids to maintain preload
Discussion	Cardiac tamponade results from an acute increase in pericardial fluid which restricts the heart from normally expanding within the pericardium. Due to this constraint, filling of the right atrium, then right ventricle during inspiration results in shifting of the interventricular septum toward the left ventricle (interventricular dependence), restricting left ventricular filling, reducing left ventricular stroke volume, and leading to systemic hypotension. Acute cardiac tamponade occurs within minutes to hours due to trauma, cardiac/aortic rupture, or as a procedural complication, and causes hemodynamic instability. Subacute pericardial effusion occurs over days to weeks and can be associated with pericarditis, malignancy, uremia (CKD), SLE, TB, or penetrating trauma. This can still cause tamponade, but a larger volume of fluid can accumulate before causing hemodynamic instability.

History: Risk factors as above (e.g., trauma, uremia, infection, cancer).

Symptoms: Chest pain or discomfort, lightheadedness, dyspnea, syncope.

Physical Exam:
• **Beck's triad:** Elevated JVP, hypotension, muffled heart sounds.
• **Pulsus paradoxus:** Drop in systolic blood pressure >10 mmHg with inspiration.
• **Kussmaul sign:** Increase in JVP with inspiration.

Though all three components of Beck's triad only occur in a minority of patients, the finding of pulsus paradoxus should strongly signal that cardiac tamponade may be present.

Diagnostics:
• **Echocardiography** with pericardial effusion and diastolic collapse of the right heart, respiratory variation of flow into the ventricles, and a dilated inferior vena cava without collapse are signs of increased pericardial pressures.

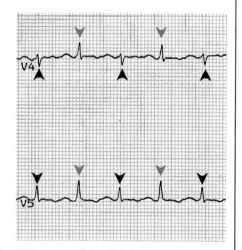

ECG example of electrical alternans. (Reproduced with permission from Knoop KJ, Stack LB, Storrow AB, Thurman RJ. *The Atlas of Emergency Medicine*. 5th ed. New York, NY: McGraw Hill; 2021.)

• **ECG** may show sinus tachycardia, low-voltage QRS complexes, electrical alternans (arrows in ECG shown point to variations in the QRS voltages as the heart swings within the pericardial effusion toward then away from the ECG leads).
• **Right/left heart catheterization (R/LHC)** can assess intracardiac hemodynamics if uncertain whether the pericardial effusion is causing hemodynamic instability. Characteristic findings are elevated filling pressures with diastolic equalization in all four chambers and signs of interventricular dependence (RV pressures increase during inspiration while LV pressures decrease, with the opposite occurring during expiration).
• CXR may show enlarged cardiac silhouette suggestive of pericardial effusion.
• BMP and additional labs to evaluate for uremia, malignancy, SLE and TB based on the clinical presentation.

CASE 7 | Cardiac Tamponade *(continued)*

Discussion	**Management:** • Urgent pericardiocentesis to reduce the pressure surrounding the heart and allow for LV filling. • IV fluids to maintain preload. • Treat underlying cause.
Additional Considerations	**Complications:** Cardiac tamponade is a medical emergency and must be diagnosed and treated immediately with pericardiocentesis to reduce the pressure surrounding the heart and allow for LV filling. **Surgical considerations:** Consider surgical drainage with pericardial window for patients with incomplete drainage from pericardiocentesis or with recurrent pericardial effusions.

Pericardial Disease Mini-Cases

Cases	Key Findings

Myocarditis	**Hx:** Acute or subacute onset of chest pain and shortness of breath, recent upper respiratory tract infection, pain worse with inspiration.
	PE:
	• Signs consistent with new heart failure (displaced PMI, elevated JVP, S3, bibasilar crackles, and bilateral lower extremity pitting edema).
	• +/− fever, tachycardia, +/− hypoxia.
	Diagnostics: Clinical presentation + elevated troponin.
	• ECG may show conduction defects and signs of associated pericarditis (diffuse ST segment elevation and PR depression).
	• CXR may show volume overload (vascular congestion, pulmonary edema), and cardiomegaly.
	• Echo may demonstrate reduced ejection fraction.
	• Cardiac MRI may reveal presence of myocardial edema/inflammation.
	• Definitive diagnosis with myocardial biopsy showing inflammation but only indicated if
	  • Cardiogenic shock
	  • Continued heart failure that does not improve over 1–2 weeks.
	Management: Directed at underlying cause and treating symptoms and complications (i.e., heart failure).
	Discussion: A common presentation includes viral prodrome with chest pain and elevated troponin without risk factors for ACS. Pathology, if biopsy performed, shows inflammation of the myocardium resulting in myocardial necrosis.
	Etiologies include viral (coxsackie, HIV, adenovirus, parvovirus B19), parasitic (*Toxoplasma gondii*, *Trypanosoma cruzi*), bacterial (*Borrelia burgdorferi*, *Mycoplasma pneumoniae*, *Corynebacterium diptheriae*), toxins (carbon monoxide, black widow venom), medications (doxorubicin, daunorubicin), autoimmune (Kawasaki, sarcoidosis, SLE).

Pericardial effusion	**Hx:** Dyspnea improving with sitting up; chest pain. History of malignancy, uremia, SLE, tuberculosis, pericarditis. **PE:** Distant heart sounds, pericardial friction rub may be present. No significant pulsus paradoxus if no hemodynamic compromise as seen in tamponade. **Diagnostics:** • TTE is the best diagnostic tool to visualize the effusion. • CXR may show a "boot-shaped" heart in a chronic effusion (higher volume). • ECG can range from normal to nonspecific ST changes to electrical alternans if a very large effusion. **Management:** • Small effusions with low risk for hemodynamic compromise may be monitored with serial echocardiograms. • Larger effusions causing dyspnea should be drained via pericardiocentesis. • Management also depends on etiology. **Discussion:** Pericardial effusions have the same etiologies as tamponade; the only difference between the two conditions is that in tamponade the cardiac chambers are unable to fill adequately during diastole and therefore stroke volume is decreased, reducing cardiac output and causing hemodynamic compromise.

Pericardial Disease Mini-Cases *(continued)*

Constrictive pericarditis	**Hx:** Volume overload (weight gain), decreased cardiac output (progressive fatigue, dyspnea), increasing abdominal girth/swelling.
	PE: Elevated JVP, **Kussmaul's sign** (paradoxical increased jugular venous pressure on inspiration), pericardial knock (from abrupt cessation of ventricular filling during diastole), ascites, edema.
	Diagnostics:
	• Echocardiography is the best diagnostic tool, similar hemodynamic respiratory changes as in tamponade.
	• Cardiac CT, MRI: Thickened pericardium.
	• Right/Left Heart Catheterization (R/LHC): Hemodynamics similar to those seen in tamponade (see above).
	• CXR: Pericardial calcifications may be present (eggshell pericardium).
	Management: Initially treated with NSAIDs/colchicine if acute inflammation, cautious diuretics if volume overloaded; if symptoms persist, the definitive treatment is pericardiectomy (high operative mortality).
	Discussion: Fibrosis of pericardium restricts diastolic filling. Often idiopathic (previous pericarditis) or due to radiation, cancer, uremia, TB, or autoimmunity.

Pleuritic Chest Pain Mini-Cases

Cases	Key Findings
Pleuritis	**Hx:** Sharp and localized thoracic and/or shoulder pain worse with inspiration.
	PE: May hear pleural friction rub.
	Diagnostics:
	• CXR: Pleural effusion; if pleuritis due to associated pneumonia would see lung consolidation.
	• Perform thoracentesis if etiology of effusion not clear to use Light's criteria to differentiate transudate from exudate.
	• Consider checking CBC (leukocytosis); CMP and lactate dehydrogenase (if calculating Light's criteria).
	Management: Treat underlying cause.
	Discussion: Pleuritis is inflammation of the pleura and can be caused by infection or disease that affects the pleural space (e.g., malignancy, infection, rheumatologic disease).
Pulmonary embolus (PE)	**Hx:** Sudden-onset shortness of breath. Minority have pleuritic chest pain. Risk factors are same as those for a deep venous thrombosis: prolonged immobilization, malignancy, thrombophilia, pregnancy, and hormonal contraceptives.
	PE: Tachypnea, tachycardia, loud P2, increased splitting of P2, hemodynamic instability.
	Diagnostics: Confirm diagnosis with CT angiography (CTA) of the chest (preferred) or VQ scan.
	• D-dimer has high sensitivity but poor specificity for PE and high negative predictive value (helpful in ruling out diagnosis).
	Management:
	• Anticoagulation (heparin, enoxaparin).
	• Thrombolytic therapy (tPA) if high-risk (massive) PE, which is defined as hemodynamically instability.
	• Catheter-based thrombectomy may be considered if systemic tPA is too high-risk.
	Discussion: See PE case in Pulmonology Chapter for full discussion.

PALPITATIONS/SYNCOPE/ARRHYTHMIAS

Palpitations are the unpleasant sensation of strong, rapid, or irregular heartbeats and can be due to excessive caffeine intake, smoking, stress/anxiety, hyperthyroidism, anemia, or arrhythmias. The first step is to identify whether the palpitations are due to an underlying cardiac or a noncardiac cause.

Syncope is defined as transient and abrupt loss of consciousness and postural tone secondary to decreased blood flow to the brain. The etiology can be cardiac, neurological, neurally mediated (reflex), or psychiatric. The etiology of syncope is not determined in up to 50% of individuals.

History: Ask about:

• Prodromal (warning) symptoms such as palpitations, chest pain, dyspnea, lightheadedness, dizziness, weakness, diaphoresis, nausea, and epigastric discomfort preceding the event.

- Postictal (after seizure) symptoms such as confusion, drowsiness, headache, tongue biting, and loss of bowel or bladder function noted after recovery. Postictal loss of consciousness is not true syncope because it is not due to decreased cerebral blood flow.
- Personal history of heart disease, seizures, and family history of sudden cardiac death.

Physical Exam:

- Vital signs, including orthostatic blood pressure and heart rate, and a thorough cardiac and neurologic exam.

Diagnostics:

- Initial important tests include checking blood glucose, ECG, electrolytes.
- If cardiac causes are suspected, patients should be placed on continuous telemetry monitoring or followed up with an outpatient Holter or event monitor and echocardiogram.
- Reflex syncope can be confirmed with tilt-table testing.
- If neurologic causes of syncope are suspected, consider EEG and brain imaging with MRI or CT scan.

Management: Treat underlying condition.

Approach to Syncope

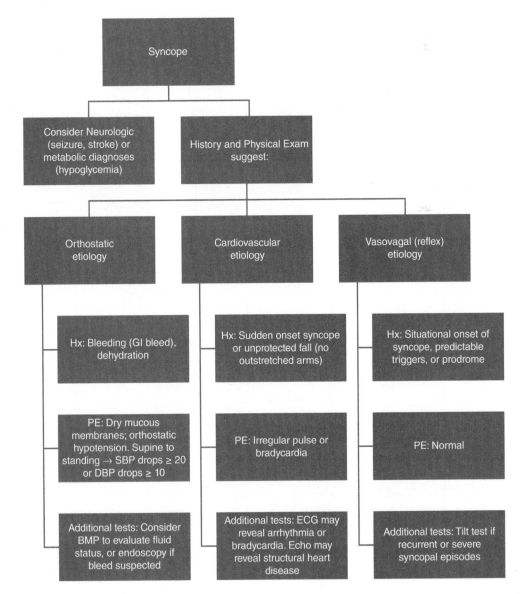

Arrhythmias may present as palpitations, syncope, tachycardia, lightheadedness, dyspnea, or may be asymptomatic. Recognizing the typical pattern of atrial fibrillation, atrial flutter, heart block, and supraventricular tachycardia (SVT) will help guide management of these conditions. Arrhythmias can be divided into supraventricular and ventricular arrhythmias.

- Supraventricular tachycardias (SVTs) arise in the AV node or atrium and have a narrow QRS complex:
  - AV node: AV nodal reentrant tachycardia (AVNRT), atrioventricular reentrant tachycardia (AVRT)
  - Atrium: Atrial fibrillation, atrial flutter, or multifocal atrial tachycardia (MAT)
- Ventricular arrhythmias arise below the AV node and have a wide QRS
  - Includes ventricular tachycardia and ventricular fibrillation, which are key to recognize as can be fatal if not defibrillated

On initial assessment, all patients should have an ECG. Further testing may include BMP, thyroid function studies, and ambulatory ECG monitoring.

High-risk features associated with arrhythmias include syncope, cardiac arrest, dyspnea, lightheadedness, angina, or signs of heart failure.

Eight-Step Approach to ECG Rhythm Interpretation

1. Rate	Is the rate normal, or is there tachycardia or bradycardia?	(Normal rate is 60–100 beats per min)
2. Rhythm and pattern of QRS complex	Is the rhythm regular or irregular?	
3. Axis	Is the axis normal, or is there left or right axis deviation?	 An approach to electrical axis. (Reproduced with permission from Loscalzo J, Fauci AS, Kasper DL, Hauser SL, Longo DL, Jameson JL, eds. *Harrison's Principles of Internal Medicine.* 21st ed. New York: McGraw Hill; 2022.)
4. Intervals	Measure the PR interval, QRS interval, and QT interval.	Normal PR interval is <0.2 sec Normal QRS interval is <0.12 sec Normal QT interval is <½ the RR interval
5. P waves	Are P waves present or absent? What is the morphology, amplitude, duration?	
6. QRS complex	Is the QRS complex wide or narrow?	Normal QRS (narrow) is <0.12 sec
7. Ischemia	Are there any ST elevations or depressions, T wave inversions, or Q waves? Are they in a vascular distribution?	
8. Overall Interpretation		

Approach to Tachycardia

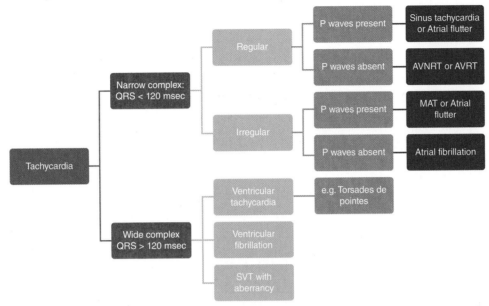

Supraventricular Tachycardia

SVT Type	ECG	Pathology/ Associations	Management
Atrial fibrillation (AF)	Irregular R-R intervals No clear p waves Chaotic/erratic baseline atrial activity Reproduced with permission from Elmoselhi A, ed. *Cardiology: An Integrated Approach.* New York: McGraw Hill; 2018.	• Multiple foci in atria firing in a chaotic pattern • Associated with HTN, CAD, rheumatic heart disease, catecholamine excess, hyperthyroidism, or anything that enlarges the atria	• Rate control and anticoagulation • Rhythm control with anti-arrhythmic and/or atrial fibrillation ablation in some cases
Atrial flutter	Regular "sawtooth" baseline, flutter waves Reproduced with permission from Elmoselhi A, ed. *Cardiology: An Integrated Approach.* New York: McGraw Hill; 2018.	• Re-entrant circuit in right atrium at 300 bpm resulting in regular atrial contractions w/ventricular rate of 150, 100, or 75 depending on AV node ability to conduct • Similar associations as AF	• Similar approach as atrial fibrillation • Atrial flutter ablation is first-line management
Multifocal atrial tachycardia (MAT)	Irregular Three or more morphologically distinct p-waves Variable RR and PR intervals Reproduced with permission from Jason Winter 2016-ECG Educator.	• Multiple ectopic foci in atrium firing and competing • Associated with severe pulmonary disease (e.g., COPD) or catecholamine excess	• Treat underlying disease (improve oxygenation and ventilation)

Supraventricular Tachycardia (*Continued*)

SVT Type	ECG	Pathology/ Associations	Management
Sinus tachycardia	Regular Clear p-waves before QRS and QRS after every p-wave Reproduced with permission from Elmoselhi A, ed. *Cardiology: An Integrated Approach*. New York: McGraw Hill; 2018.	• Associated with pain, infection, exercise, hypovolemia, fear, stress, catecholamine excess, hypoxia, anemia, pulmonary embolus	• Treat underlying cause
Atrioventricular nodal reentrant tachycardia (AVNRT)	Regular Narrow QRS No discernable p-waves (buried in QRS) or retrograde p-waves Short sudden onset with palpitations 150–250 bpm Reproduced with permission from Stone C, Humphries RL. *Current Diagnosis & Treatment: Emergency Medicine*, 8e. New York: McGraw Hill; 2017.	• Reentrant rhythm involving fast and slow pathways in the AV node	• Terminates quickly with • AV blocking maneuvers • (Valsalva, carotid massage, or adenosine)
Atrioventricular reciprocating tachycardia (AVRT)	Regular Narrow QRS complex P-waves may or may not be discernable depending on rate Reproduced with permission from Stone C, Humphries RL. *Current Diagnosis & Treatment: Emergency Medicine*, 8e. New York: McGraw Hill; 2017.	• Reentrant rhythm involving the AV node and an accessory pathway • Wolf-Parkinson- White syndrome is a type of AVRT	• Vagal manuevers (valsalva, carotid massage) • Adenosine
Wolf-Parkinson-White syndrome (WPW)	Delta waves Short PR interval Widened QRS complex Reproduced with permission from Knoop KJ, Stack LB, Storrow AB, Thurman RJ. *The Atlas of Emergency Medicine*. 5th ed. New York, NY: McGraw Hill; 2021.	• Type of AVRT; can conduct antegrade from the atrium to the ventricle resulting in a pre-excitation pattern on ECG (delta wave) • Can be familial or associated with atrial fibrillation	• Procainamide • Avoid AV node blockers

Types of Heart Block

AV Blocks	Main ECG Features and Example ECG	Pathology/Associations	Management
First-degree AV block *If R is far from P, then you have first-degree*	PR interval prolonged >200 msec Reproduced with permission from Elmoselhi A, ed. *Cardiology: An Integrated Approach*. New York: McGraw Hill; 2018.	• Most common cause: Fibrosis and sclerosis of the conduction system • Second most common cause: Ischemic heart disease • May present in young athletes due to increased vagal tone • Associated with the following medications: β-blockers, calcium channel blockers, adenosine, digoxin, amiodarone	• No treatment
Second-degree AV block Mobitz I Wenckebach *Longer, longer, longer, DROP, then you have Wenckebach*	PR progressively gets longer, then QRS "dropped" Reproduced with permission from Elmoselhi A, ed. *Cardiology: An Integrated Approach*. New York: McGraw Hill; 2018.	• Increased vagal tone • Can be seen in patients with drug intoxication (e.g., β-blockers and digitalis)	• No treatment unless symptomatic (atropine or temporary pacemaker)
Second-degree AV block (Mobitz II) *If some P's do not get through, then you have Mobitz II (two)*	Dropped QRS not preceded by PR lengthening Reproduced with permission from Elmoselhi A, ed. *Cardiology: An Integrated Approach*. New York: McGraw Hill; 2018.	• Increased vagal tone • Can be seen in patients with drug intoxication (e.g., β-blockers and digitalis) • Risk of progression to complete heart block	• If unstable: Beta-1 agonists (isoproterenol, dobutamine) and temporary pacing • Permanent pacemaker unless the cause is reversible (such as medications)
Third-degree AV block or Complete heart block *If P's and Q's do not agree, then you have Type III (three)*	P and QRS completely dissociated; more P's than QRS because atrial rate faster than ventricular rate Reproduced with permission from Elmoselhi A, ed. *Cardiology: An Integrated Approach*. New York: McGraw Hill; 2018.	• Can be a complication of late Lyme disease	• Atropine • Temporary pacing • Permanent pacemaker unless the cause is reversible (such as medications)

CASE 8 | Atrial Fibrillation

A 64-year-old man with HTN presents with palpitations, weakness, and fatigue for the last 2 weeks. Patient's vital signs are temperature 37.1°C, pulse 136/min, respirations 18/min, blood pressure 130/80 mmHg, and SpO$_2$ 98% on room air. On physical exam, patient has an S1 present with varying intensity and pulse is irregularly irregular on radial exam. No S3 or S4 and no murmurs are appreciated. The lungs are clear bilaterally, and there is no edema in the lower extremities.

Conditions with Similar Presentations	MAT, heart blocks, and frequent PACs or PVCs can present with irregular rhythm, which can be distinguished via ECG (see the preceding table).
Initial Diagnostic Tests	• Confirm diagnosis with ECG. • Consider checking CBC, TSH, troponin, BNP.

CASE 8 | Atrial Fibrillation *(continued)*

Next Steps in Management	• If hemodynamically stable: Slow the ventricular rate with AV nodal blockers such as beta-blockers (metoprolol) or non-dihydropyridine calcium channel blockers (diltiazem; verapamil). • If hemodynamically unstable: Synchronized cardioversion.

Discussion	Atrial fibrillation (Afib or AF) occurs due to multiple foci in the atria firing off in a chaotic pattern that results in an irregular and rapid ventricular rate.
	History:
	• Can be asymptomatic or have palpitations, fatigue, weakness, exertional dyspnea, lightheadedness, presyncope, and syncope.
	• Risk factors: HTN and CAD in developed world, and rheumatic heart disease in developing world.
	• Other associations include cardiomyopathy, valvular disease, history of cardiac surgery, MI, pulmonary disease, hyperthyroidism, excessive stress, systemic illness, obstructive sleep apnea, diabetes, and excessive alcohol or illicit drug use.
	
	Physical exam: Irregularly irregular pulse. Apical-radial pulse deficit (apical heart rate > radial pulse rate) due to some ventricular contractions having less forward stroke volume from shortened diastolic filling times. Loss of jugular A waves.
	Diagnostics:
	• ECG with irregularly irregular R-R intervals, absence of p-waves, chaotic/erratic atrial activity.
	• Test for possible etiologies of AF including BMP (hypokalemia) abnormalities, TSH and free T4 (hyperthyroidism), TTE (valvular disease, cardiomyopathy).
	Management:
	• If hemodynamically *unstable:* Immediate electrical cardioversion.
	• If hemodynamically *stable:* Rate control with beta-blockers (metoprolol; propranolol) or non-dihydropyridine calcium channel blockers (diltiazem; verapamil).
	• If duration <48 hours and patient low risk for stroke, consider cardioversion.
	• Long-term anticoagulation with direct oral anticoagulant (DOAC) or warfarin to prevent stroke based on $CHA_2DS_2VAS_c$ score:
	  • Score ≥2 then chronic anticoagulation recommended.
	  • Score ≤1 then consider anticoagulation (especially in males if risk factor is age 65–74), aspirin no longer recommended.
	  • Score is 0 or 1 in females then anticoagulation generally not recommended.
	
	<table><tr><th></th><th>Condition</th><th>Points</th></tr><tr><td>C</td><td>Congestive heart failure</td><td>1</td></tr><tr><td>H</td><td>Hypertension</td><td>1</td></tr><tr><td>A₂</td><td>Age >75</td><td>2</td></tr><tr><td>D</td><td>Diabetes</td><td>1</td></tr><tr><td>S₂</td><td>Stroke or transient ischemic attack or thromboembolism</td><td>2</td></tr><tr><td>V</td><td>Vascular disease <i>Prior MI, PAD, or aortic plaque</i></td><td>1</td></tr><tr><td>A</td><td>Age 65–74</td><td>1</td></tr><tr><td>Sc</td><td>Sex category (female)</td><td>1</td></tr></table>

Additional Considerations	**Complications:** Cardioembolic stroke is a complication from stasis and thrombosis in the left atrial appendage. **Inpatient Considerations:** Hospitalize if high-risk features such as syncope, cardiac arrest, dyspnea, lightheadedness, angina, or signs of heart failure.

CASE 9 | Complete Heart Block (Third-Degree Atrioventricular Block)

A 68-year-old man with HTN presents to the ED after sudden loss of conscious. He had prior lightheadedness and fatigue; witnesses did not see any abnormal movements after syncope, and exam reveals no tongue bites or bowel/bladder incontinence. He has had several pre-syncopal episodes in the last month. On exam, his vital signs are temperature 37.4°C, pulse 40/min and regular, blood pressure 90/70 mmHg, and respirations 18/min. Cardiac exam is notable for soft S1 and S2. Neurologic exam is normal.

Conditions with Similar Presentations	**Second-degree AV block Mobitz II:** is also a high-degree AV block and can present similarly to third-degree AV block with syncope, but ECG will distinguish. **Sinus node dysfunction (sick sinus syndrome):** is caused by fibrosis of the sinus node or surrounding tissue, resulting in delayed conduction to the ventricles. Presents with fatigue, syncope/presyncope, or intermittent palpitations. ECG patterns include sinus bradycardia with sinus pauses. **Sinus bradycardia:** is usually asymptomatic and ECG shows 1:1 ratio of p-waves and QRS complexes. History and physical can elicit the etiology such as a conditioned athlete, medications, eating disorders, or hypothyroidism.
Initial Diagnostic Tests	• Confirm diagnosis with ECG and place patient on telemetry. • Consider checking CBC, TSH, troponin, BNP.
Next Steps in Management	• Initial IV atropine, IV dopamine, and/or transcutaneous or transvenous pacing. • Discontinue medications that cause bradycardia. • Permanent pacemaker for long-term management.
Discussion	Complete heart block or third-degree atrioventricular (AV) block indicates that there is no conduction between the atria and the ventricles. When this occurs, the atria and ventricles beat independently and cause decreased cardiac output, which can lead to symptoms such as syncope. It commonly is due to degenerative conduction system disease in older patients with CV risk factors such as HTN and CAD. Other causes include inferior wall MI (Bezold–Jarisch reflex) which is usually transient, infiltrative disease (sarcoidosis and amyloidosis), medications (beta-blocker or digoxin), or electrolyte abnormalities (hyperkalemia, hypothyroidism). **History:** • Fatigue, dizziness/lightheadedness, dyspnea, angina, and syncope. • May be asymptomatic if there is a sufficient escape rhythm to maintain blood pressure. **Physical Exam:** Bradycardia *Cannon A waves* are secondary to right atrial contraction when the tricuspid valve is closed (ventricular systole), resulting in an intermittently increased JVP. Note that cannon A waves are seen also in ventricular tachycardia, premature atrial contractions, or any arrhythmia involving AV dissociation. **Diagnostics:** ECG shows bradycardia and complete atrial and ventricular dissociation (no relationship between p-waves and QRS complexes). 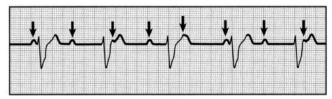 Reproduced with permission from Elmoselhi A, ed. Cardiology: An Integrated Approach. New York: McGraw Hill; 2018. **Management:** • Restore cardiac output by increasing the heart rate with atropine, dopamine, and/or electrical pacing. • Discontinue medications that may worsen AV nodal conduction such as beta-blockers, non-dihydropyridine calcium channel blockers (diltiazem, verapamil), and digoxin. • Permanent pacemaker if no clear reversible cause.
Additional Considerations	**Pediatric considerations:** Neonatal lupus can present with fetal AV block. **Other considerations:** Individuals with **first-degree AV block** or **second-degree (Mobitz I**/Wenckebach) are usually asymptomatic and require no treatment. **Second-degree Mobitz II** may progress to third-degree block and should be treated with a pacemaker if symptoms are present.

CASE 10 | Hypertrophic Cardiomyopathy (HCM)

A 19-year-old man presents after a collapsing on the basketball court during a game. He also reports occasional exertional chest pain, pre-syncope, and palpitations. On exam, there is a prominent, sustained PMI (LV impulse) and a harsh/mid- to late-systolic murmur best heard in left third to fourth intercostal space. The murmur increases with Valsalva/standing and decreases with rapid squatting/sustained hand grip. An S4 can be heard. He has a family history of sudden death in two maternal family members.

Conditions with Similar Presentations	**Restrictive cardiomyopathy:** can also present with exertional dyspnea and chest pain, however you may see Kussmaul sign (increased JVP with inspiration) on physical exam and low voltages on ECG. **Dilated cardiomyopathy:** can also present with exertional dyspnea and syncope; however, echocardiography will reveal reduced ejection fraction. **Congenital aortic stenosis:** can also present with exertional syncope, dyspnea, chest pain, and a systolic murmur; however, this rare condition is seen in children and confirmed with echocardiography. **Congenital long QT syndrome:** can present with sudden death during exercise due to torsades de pointes (TdP) and is associated with congenital sensorineural deafness. ECG will have prolonged QTc.

Initial Diagnostic Tests	• Confirm diagnosis with echocardiogram
	• Consider:
	  • ECG
	  • Cardiac MRI to further assess LV if not well seen by echo
	  • Genetic testing

Next Steps in Management	Beta-blocker or calcium channel blocker for symptomatic patients.
Discussion	Hypertrophic cardiomyopathy is characterized by asymmetric LVH and diastolic dysfunction. Asymmetric LV septal wall hypertrophy can result in left ventricular outflow tract obstruction (LVOTO) due to a dynamic interplay between the anterior mitral valve leaflet (systolic anterior motion of the mitral valve), septal hypertrophy, and myocardial hypercontractility. Familial, autosomal dominant disorder with mutations encoding sarcomere proteins, most commonly myosin binding protein c (MYBPC3) and beta-myosin heavy chain (MYH7). Similar appearance can be seen in Friedrich ataxia and Pompe disease. Most patients have a normal life expectancy, but some have an increased risk of sudden cardiac death. **History:** • Classic presentation is syncope during exertion in a young athletic patient. • Risk factors: Family history of sudden cardiac death. • Symptoms: Syncope during exercise, dyspnea on exertion, angina, palpitations, sudden death from ventricular arrhythmia. **Physical exam:** • S4 gallop (sign of LV hypertrophy). • Mid- to late-peaking systolic murmur that increases in intensity with Valsalva and standing up (decreased preload) and decreases in intensity with hand grip (increased afterload) and squatting (increased afterload). **Diagnostics:** Diagnosed by clinical presentation and imaging findings from echo and/or cardiac MRI. • Echocardiogram with normal ejection fraction, hypertrophy of ventricular walls and interventricular septum, LVOT obstruction due to systolic anterior motion of mitral valve which may also lead to mitral regurgitation. • ECG shows LVH and nonspecific ST changes. • Histology (on autopsy or biopsy) will show tangled and disoriented myofibrils (myofiber disarray). **Management:** • For *symptomatic* obstructive HCM: Beta-blockers or calcium channel blockers can improve LV filling time and blunt LV contractile force to improve obstructive gradient during exertion. • For *asymptomatic* obstructive HCM: Counseling and monitoring for symptoms. • Avoid dehydration. • Mild to moderate exercise okay. Avoidance of overexertion and caution in strenuous or high-level athletic activities. • Surgical septal myectomy and catheter-based alcohol septal ablation in select patients. • Implantable cardioverter defibrillator (ICD) for patients at elevated risk or personal history of sudden cardiac death.
Additional Considerations	**Screening:** Family screening indicated in first-degree relatives. No formal screening indicated in general population unless murmur noted on sports physical, ECG +/− echo is indicated. **Complications:** Sudden cardiac death. **Surgical considerations:** Surgical septal myectomy—consider if significant heart failure symptoms persist despite maximal medical therapy, or patients have recurrent syncope due to LVOTO. **Pediatric considerations:** Similar to adult management. **Other considerations:** All patients should have genetic counseling.

DYSPNEA

The differential for dyspnea is broad and begins with pulmonary and cardiac etiologies. One can also consider neuromuscular diseases (myasthenia gravis, ALS) and hematologic etiologies (anemia). Timing (chronic vs. acute), associated symptoms (e.g., chest pain, cough, wheezing, fevers, edema), and clinical context aid in discerning the etiology of dyspnea.

Focused pulmonary and cardiac exam in addition to assessment for edema and weakness will help further narrow the differential.

Initial useful labs and tests include assessing oxygen saturation (SpO_2) with pulse oximetry, CBC to check for anemia, basic metabolic panel (BMP), and TSH to check for hyper- or hypothyroidism. Troponin, brain natriuretic peptide (BNP), and D-dimer can also be useful in assessing for ischemia, heart failure, and pulmonary embolus, respectively. Imaging can show parenchymal pulmonary and cardiac abnormalities. Other testing may include ECG, and echocardiography. Arterial blood gas (ABG) can quantify the oxygenation of the blood and can indicate respiratory acidosis. Pulmonary function tests can identify obstructive or restrictive lung disease.

An Approach to Dyspnea

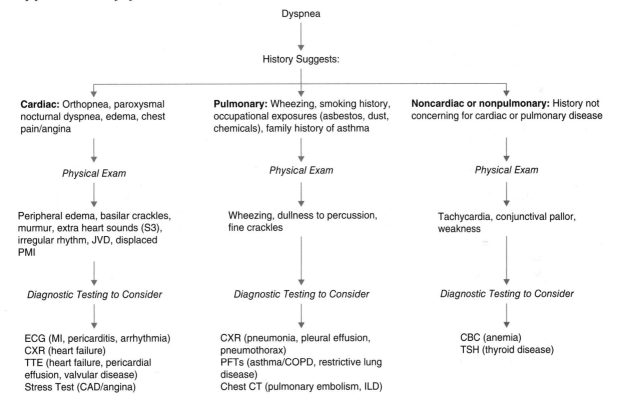

Heart Failure

Heart failure is a clinical syndrome resulting from the inability of the heart to fill and/or eject blood sufficiently to maintain health. Symptoms and signs are caused by a functional or structural cardiac abnormality and supported by elevated natriuretic peptide levels and/or signs of pulmonary or systemic congestion.

Symptoms: Dyspnea on exertion, fatigue, orthopnea, paroxysmal nocturnal dyspnea (PND), and/or edema.

Signs: Elevated (>8 cm) JVP, murmurs or abnormal heart sounds (S3 if systolic left-sided heart failure, S4 if diastolic dysfunction, loud P2 with increased splitting if pulmonary HTN, fixed split S2 if ASD), displaced PMI, bibasilar crackles on lung exam or dullness to percussion (pleural effusion), ascites, and bilateral lower extremity edema.

Diagnostics: TTE to confirm diagnosis of heart failure (HF).

Management: Centered around treating the underlying cause, reducing morbidity and mortality (management of chronic stable heart failure) and managing acute symptoms of volume overload (acute decompensated heart failure). Guideline-directed medical therapy (GDMT) helps in reducing HF hospitalization, mortality, and improving functional capacity.

Congestive heart failure (CHF) can be divided into:

- Heart failure with reduced ejection fraction (**HFrEF**, EF ≤40%)
- Heart failure with preserved ejection fraction (**HFpEF**, EF ≥50%)
- Heart failure with midrange or mildly reduced ejection fraction (**HFmrEF**, EF 40–49%).

As the etiology and management for HFpEF and HFmrEF is the same, many texts will combine this into one category as HFpEF (EF>40%). Causes of HFrEF include ischemic heart disease, HTN, valvular disease, and other causes of dilated cardiomyopathy (ethanol, uremia, peripartum, thiamine deficiency, catecholamine excess, Lyme disease, SLE). Causes of HFpEF include HTN, ischemic heart disease, restrictive cardiomyopathy, aortic stenosis, and hypertrophic cardiomyopathy.

High-output heart failure is due to hyperthyroidism, chronic severe anemia, AV fistulas, class III obesity, and pregnancy. Patients with high-output heart failure have a high cardiac output accompanied by low systemic vascular resistance compared to the usual forms of heart failure with low/normal cardiac output with elevated systemic vascular resistance as seen in MI, dilated cardiomyopathy, and HTN.

Restrictive cardiomyopathy can be due to infiltrative disorders (e.g., amyloidosis, sarcoidosis, scleroderma), endomyocardial disorders (carcinoid, metastatic cancer, radiation, or chemotherapy), storage diseases (e.g., Pompe disease, hemochromatosis, Gaucher disease), or idiopathic.

New York Heart Association (NYHA) Classification of Heart Failure Symptoms

Class I	No limitation of physical activity
Class II	Slight limitation of physical activity
Class III	Marked limitation of physical activity
Class IV	Symptoms occur even at rest and discomfort with any physical activity

Etiologies of Heart Failure and Next Steps

Type of Heart Failure	Etiology	Next Steps
HFrEF (LVEF ≤40%)	Ischemic heart disease	Medical management and revascularization if indicated
	Chronic hypertension	Manage HTN
	Dilated cardiomyopathy	Treat based on etiology: • Idiopathic (50% of dilated cardiomyopathies) • Familial/hereditary/genetic conditions (mutations in sarcomere proteins) • Myocarditis (parvovirus B19, HHV6, HIV, coxsackievirus, adenovirus, echovirus, influenza, CMV) • Infectious (HIV, Chagas disease, Lyme disease) • Toxins (alcohol, cocaine) • Medications (methamphetamines, adriamycin, cyclophosphamide, trastuzumab) • Stress-induced cardiomyopathy (also known as Takotsubo cardiomyopathy or transient left ventricular apical ballooning) • Peripartum cardiomyopathy • Tachycardia-mediated cardiomyopathy • Infiltrative cardiomyopathy (may present as a combination of dilated cardiomyopathy and restrictive cardiomyopathy—includes sarcoidosis, amyloidosis, hemochromatosis) • Autoimmune cardiomyopathy (SLE)
	Valvular disease	Consider valve replacement or repair

Etiologies of Heart Failure and Next Steps

Type of Heart Failure	Etiology	Next Steps
HFpEF *LVEF ≥50%* HFmrEF *LVEF 41–49%*	Chronic hypertension Ischemic heart disease Valvular disease	See above Hypertrophic Cardiomyopathy
	Hypertrophic cardiomyopathy	See Case10 "Hypertrophic Cardiomyopathy"
	Amyloidosis	Biopsy with Congo red staining with apple-green birefringence
	Sarcoidosis	Cardiac MRI and cardiac positron emission tomographic (PET) scan shows patchy areas of myocardial inflammation and fibrosis
	Hemochromatosis	Genetic testing gold standard for diagnosis (C282Y mutation in HFE gene) Iron chelation therapy to treat
	Rheumatic disease	Treat disease (refer to Chapter 10 for details)
	Radiation fibrosis	History of radiation to the chest and cardiac MRI to diagnose

CASE 11 | Heart Failure With Reduced Ejection Fraction (HFrEF)

A 62-year-old woman with CAD and HTN presents to clinic with a 4-month history of increased fatigue, dyspnea on exertion, and paroxysmal nocturnal dyspnea. She is still able to complete her daily activities. On exam, her vital signs are temperature 37.5°C, pulse 88/min, blood pressure 135/90 mmHg, respiration 22/min, and O_2 sat 94% on RA. She has bibasilar crackles and 1+ bilateral lower extremity pitting edema. She is sent for a TTE which reveals a left ventricular ejection fraction (LVEF) of 35%.

Conditions with Similar Presentations	**Anemia:** may present with dyspnea and fatigue, may also have conjunctival pallor and signs and symptoms of bleeding. **HFpEF** (EF ≥50%) and **HFmrEF** (EF 41–49%): can also present with dyspnea on exertion and fatigue, but the EF will be >40% on echocardiogram. **ACS/angina, pulmonary embolism,** and **pneumothorax:** may also present with dyspnea, but typically also have associated acute-onset chest pain. **Pneumonia, COPD, lung cancer,** and other pulmonary disease: can present with dyspnea, but LVEF is unaffected.
Initial Diagnostic Tests	• Obtain a TTE • Also check ECG, CXR, CBC, BMP, BNP
Next Steps in Management	• Initiate GDMT (see table) • Diuresis for initial symptom control • Left heart catheterization to evaluate for ischemic etiology • Educate patient on lifestyle modification

Discussion	The most common etiology of HFrEF is ischemic heart disease. Other etiologies include valvular heart disease, other cardiomyopathies, HTN, and smoking. The treatment of HFrEF is centered on GDMT and reducing hospital admissions.
	History:
	• Dyspnea, orthopnea, PND, fatigue, nonproductive cough (often at night).
	Physical exam: Volume overload
	• Increased JVP (>8 cm)
	• Positive hepatojugular reflux (>4 cm increase in JVP for >15 seconds after applying abdominal pressure)
	• S3
	• Displaced PMI
	• Bibasilar crackles
	• Pitting edema (lower extremities, abdominal wall, anasarca)
	Diagnostics:
	• TTE for establishing baseline ejection fraction and confirm diagnosis (HFrEF, **EF ≤40%**)
	• ECG to establish baseline rhythm and evaluate for ischemia
	• Left heart catheterization to evaluate for ischemic disease
	• Consider:
	  • CXR for signs of congestion (pulmonary edema, Kerley B lines)
	  • Pulmonary function tests if history/physical suggests pulmonary etiology of dyspnea

CASE 11 | Heart Failure With Reduced Ejection Fraction (HFrEF) *(continued)*

Discussion	**Management:**
	• Start GDMT (i.e., ACEi/ARB/ARNI, BB, aldosterone antagonist, SGLT2i) • Patient education on salt restriction and lifestyle management • Diuresis for symptomatic volume overload • If patient remains symptomatic after maximum GDMT, would consider device intervention (indications in table below).

Additional Considerations	**Inpatient considerations:** Patients with acute decompensated heart failure (**ADHF**) should be admitted for treatment. ADHF is a clinical diagnosis, and triggers include increased salt or water intake, missed diuretics, new decrease in contractility (new ischemic event).
	
	BNP typically elevated (consider checking when patient euvolemic to establish "dry" BNP for future admissions).
	• TTE often repeated to check for change in ejection fraction or wall motion abnormalities and ECG and troponins for arrhythmia and ischemic changes.
	• Initial treatment/management includes:
	  • IV loop diuretics (furosemide, bumetanide)
	  • Identify and treat trigger of the exacerbation (medication compliance, fluid/salt intake, new ischemia, arrhythmia)
	  • Continue beta-blocker if hemodynamically stable
	
	Severe ADHF can result in cardiogenic shock with hypotension, narrow pulse pressure, and cool or clammy extremities on exam. These patients may need ICU-level care and inotropic support.
	
	Surgical considerations: Temporary or surgically-placed mechanical support devices such as left ventricular assist device (LVAD) can be considered in select cases.
	
	Pediatric considerations: Heart failure in pediatrics is often due to underlying congenital heart disease.

Management of Chronic Stable HFrEF: The goal is to provide GDMT to help reduce HF hospitalization, morbidity and mortality, and improve symptoms and functional capacity.

Guideline Directed Medical Therapy (GDMT) for HFrEF

Therapy	Medication Examples	Indication	Mortality Benefit
ACEi	Lisinopril, enalapril	All patients with HFrEF	Yes
ARB	Losartan, valsartan	All patients with HFrEF if intolerant of ACEi due to side effects	Yes
Beta-blockers (BBs)	Only metoprolol succinate, carvedilol, bisoprolol	All patients with HFrEF	Yes
Aldosterone antagonists	Spironolactone, eplerenone	HFrEF with persistent symptoms on initial therapy	Yes
SGLT-2 inhibitors	Dapagliflozin	HFrEF with persistent symptoms on initial therapy	Yes
Loop diuretics	Furosemide, bumetanide	Volume overload	No
Angiotensin receptor-neprilysin inhibitor (ARNi)	Valsartan-Sacubitril	All patients with HFrEF; replaces ACEi or ARB	Yes
Hydralazine + isosorbide dinitrate		HFrEF with intolerance of ACEi, ARB, or ARNi or HFrEF with persistent symptoms on initial therapy	Yes
Ivabradine		HFrEF, sinus rhythm, pulse >70 bpm on max beta-blockers	No
Implantable cardioverter defibrillator (ICD)		HFrEF with NYHA II and III, and LVEF <35%	Yes
Cardiac resynchronization therapy (CRT)		HFrEF with LVEF <35%, left bundle branch block (LBBB), and QRS ≥150 ms	Yes
Cardiac transplant		Refractory heart failure despite maximum medical therapy	Yes

Heart Failure Mini-Cases

Cases	Key Findings
High-Output Heart Failure	**Hx/PE:** Symptoms and signs consistent with HF and may have well-perfused extremities, bounding pulses, and hyperkinetic precordium. If due to anemia will have pallor. **Diagnostics:** • TTE and BNP to confirm diagnosis of HF • Determine the cause of the high-output heart failure if not obvious (e.g., pregnancy) • Check TSH, CBC, transaminases, and consider checking vitamin B1 **Management:** • Manage symptoms (diuretics for pulmonary congestion) • Treat underlying etiology **Discussion:** Patients with high-output heart failure have a high cardiac output and low systemic vascular resistance. In addition to classic signs of heart failure such as dyspnea, swelling, and fatigue, patients may also have well-perfused extremities, bounding pulses, and hyperkinetic precordium. High-output heart failure should be considered in high metabolic states or states that cause low vascular resistance. Causes include the following: • Obesity • Chronic anemia • Wet Beri-Beri (vitamin B1 [thiamine] deficiency) • Pregnancy • Sepsis • Hyperthyroidism • Arteriovenous fistulas • Cirrhosis • Paget disease of bone • Myeloproliferative disorders
Restrictive Cardiomyopathy	**Hx/PE:** Symptoms and signs consistent with HF and may have Kussmaul sign (increase in JVP with inspiration). **Diagnostics:** • Clinical signs and symptoms of HF • Echocardiogram with normal EF and evidence of myocardial infiltration • ECG may show low voltage • Endomyocardial biopsy for definitive diagnosis of cause **Management:** • Manage symptoms (diuretics for pulmonary congestion) • Treat underlying etiology **Discussion:** Restrictive cardiomyopathy is defined by non-dilated ventricles with impaired filling. Systolic function is normal, at least early in the disease. Diastolic dysfunction occurs due to a rigid non-compliant myocardium, and therefore restrictive cardiomyopathy is considered a cause of HFpEF. Causes of restrictive cardiomyopathy include the following: • Idiopathic • Post-radiation fibrosis • Amyloidosis • Sarcoidosis • Fabry disease • Loeffler endocarditis (endomyocardial fibrosis with eosinophilic infiltrate) • Endocardial fibroelastosis (in children) • Scleroderma • Hemochromatosis (more commonly caused dilated but can also cause restrictive cardiomyopathy)

Valvular Disease

Valvular disease may present as many of the symptoms described elsewhere in this chapter (syncope, dyspnea, chest pain). Learning the valvular diseases collectively can provide valuable contextualization to diagnostic workup and management strategies. Echocardiography is critical to visualizing diseased valves. Repair and replacement of diseased valves is becoming increasingly safe when clinically indicated.

Symptoms: May be asymptomatic or present with dyspnea, orthopnea, PND, fatigue, palpitations, chest pain, dizziness, abdominal discomfort (due to an enlarged liver), and/or leg swelling.

Signs: Heart murmurs and/or signs of HF

- Murmurs may be classified as pathologic due to a leaky (regurgitant or insufficient) or stenotic cardiac valve, an abnormal communication between cardiac chambers (ASD, VSD), or a communication between the great vessels (PDA).

- A murmur may also be described as physiologic/functional, meaning that the murmur is caused by a physiologic condition outside of the heart (e.g., hypervolemic state of pregnancy, severe anemia, hyperthyroidism).

- Heart murmurs may be characterized by location (e.g., apical), by intensity (grade I–VI), by time of occurrence (systolic vs. diastolic), duration (early or late), shape/quality (crescendo-decrescendo, plateau-systolic), and radiation.

Diagnostics: Evaluate with TTE when:

1. Patients have possible cardiac symptoms and a murmur *or*
2. have a high-grade intensity (grade IV–VI) systolic or pansystolic murmur *or*
3. have a diastolic murmur or soft/absent S2.

Murmur Descriptions and Diagnoses

Murmurs with Key Associated Exam Findings		Diagnoses
Increased with inspiration.		Right-sided murmurs, particularly tricuspid regurgitation
Systolic Murmurs		
High-pitched blowing plateau holosystolic murmur, radiating to axilla. Best heard at apex.		Mitral regurgitation
Plateau holosystolic murmur, increases with inspiration. Best heard at LLSB.		Tricuspid regurgitation
High-pitched, holosystolic murmur. The smaller the VSD, the louder the murmur. Best heard at third left intercostal space (ICS).		Ventricular septal defect (left to right shunt)
Harsh, crescendo-decrescendo, ejection murmur, radiating to carotids (in severe cases: decreased A2, reverse splitting of A2, and a late peaking murmur), increases with squatting and decreases with Valsalva or standing. Best heard at right second ICS.		Aortic stenosis
Midsystolic, crescendo-decrescendo murmur (in severe cases: wide split S2 and decreased P2). Best heard at left second to third ICS.		Pulmonary stenosis
Harsh/mid- to late-systolic murmur, increases with Valsalva or standing (decreased preload) and decreases with squatting or sustained hand grip (increased afterload). S3, S4 may be present. Best heard at left third to fourth ICS.		Hypertrophic cardiomyopathy

Murmur Descriptions and Diagnoses

Murmurs with Key Associated Exam Findings		Diagnoses
Mid-systolic click (C) with late systolic murmur ("click-murmur syndrome"). Standing/Valsalva moves the systolic click and murmur earlier and increases loudness. Squatting or sustained hand grip moves the click and murmur later and decreases the loudness. Best heard at apex.	C S_1　S_2　S_1	Mitral valve prolapse
Systolic ejection murmur, crescendo-decrescendo, at the left upper sternal border (LUSB). Widely fixed S2. Best heard at LUSB.	A_2 P_2 S_1　S_2　S_1	Atrial septal defect
Diastolic Murmurs		
High-pitched, blowing, diastolic, decrescendo murmur, best heard sitting/leaning forward in end-exhalation. Best heard at left third ICS.	S_1　S_2　S_1	Aortic regurgitation
Decrescendo murmur. Best heard at LLSB.	S_1　S_2　S_1	Pulmonic regurgitation
Opening snap (OS), high-pitched sound, after S2 (heard best with the diaphragm) accompanied by a decrescendo diastolic rumble with pre-systolic accentuation. Best heard with a bell in left lateral decubitus position at apex.	OS S_1　S_2　S_1	Mitral stenosis
OS may be heard. Decrescendo diastolic murmur with pre-systolic accentuation, increased with inspiration and other maneuvers which increase venous return and blood flow across the tricuspid valve. Best heard at LLSB.	OS S_1　S_2　S_1	Tricuspid stenosis
Systolic and Diastolic Murmur		
Harsh, continuous, crescendo-decrescendo, machinery-like murmur, radiates toward clavicle. Best heard at left second ICS.	S_1　S_2　S_1	Patent ductus arteriosus

Source: Reproduced with permission from Khan AR, Geraghty JR, eds. First Aid Clinical Pattern Recognition for the USMLE Step 1. New York: McGraw Hill; 2022.

CASE 12 | Aortic Stenosis

A 70-year-old man with HTN and hyperlipidemia presents after he passed out while running to catch the bus today. Over the past 2 months, he has felt more fatigued and notes chest pain and lightheadedness with moderate exertion. On exam, vital signs are temperature 37.4°C, pulse 76/min, blood pressure 144/108 mmHg, respirations 18/min, and O₂ sat 97% on RA. Physical exam is notable for delayed and diminished carotid pulses and a sustained PMI. Auscultation reveals a late-peaking III/VI harsh systolic crescendo-decrescendo murmur at the right upper sternal border radiating to the carotids. Lungs are clear to auscultation.

Conditions with Similar Presentations	**Stable angina:** may also present with exertional chest pain and dyspnea on exertion, but systolic murmur and symptoms of lightheadedness and syncope are not present. **Mitral regurgitation (MR):** may also present with a systolic murmur, but the murmur would be holosystolic or plateau-systolic and radiates to the axilla (central MR) or to the aortic area (anteriorly-directed MR) and not the carotids. **Hypertrophic cardiomyopathy (HCM):** also presents with a crescendo-decrescendo murmur but can be differentiated by exam maneuvers (see table above). **Ventricular septal defect (VSD):** also presents with a systolic murmur but the murmur in VSD is holosystolic and best heard in the left third intercostal space.
Initial Diagnostic Testing	• Confirm diagnosis with TTE. • Consider ECG.
Next Steps in Management	Aortic valve replacement (surgical or transcatheter) because of symptoms.
Discussion	Aortic stenosis (AS) is seen in older patients (senile calcific valve disease), or in younger patients with early-onset calcification secondary to bicuspid valves (e.g., Turner syndrome, congenital abnormalities) or rheumatic disease. **Hx:** • Asymptomatic until stenosis is severe. • Symptoms include dyspnea with exertion, angina, syncope, decreased exercise tolerance, lightheadedness. **PE:** • Auscultation reveals a mid-peaking, crescendo-decrescendo, systolic ejection murmur best heard at the right second intercostal space (aortic area), with radiation to the carotids. • Intensity of the murmur is flow-dependent so may be less intense in the setting of decreased LV stroke volumes. • The timing of the peaking of the murmur can correlate with severity of stenosis of the valve. In severe cases, can have a late-peaking murmur and single, soft, or absent S2. S4 may be present. • **Pulsus parvus et tardus** refers to decreased carotid pulse (parvus) with a delayed upstroke (tardus). • The AS murmur can be differentiated from the murmur of hypertrophic cardiomyopathy. Maneuvers that increase LV preload (leg raising) will increase the intensity of the AS murmur because of increased flow through the stenotic valve. Increased preload in HCM will increase LV filling and cavity size which decreases the outflow obstruction resulting in decreased murmur. **Diagnostics:** TTE will show calcified aortic valve with reduced valve area. Bicuspid aortic valve may be present. Additional tests: ECG demonstrates LVH and left atrial enlargement. **Management:** • Aortic valve replacement (see below). • Manage risk factors including HTN, DM, hyperlipidemia.
Additional Considerations	**Screening:** Patients with known asymptomatic AS should be monitored using history, physical, and TTE to assess for disease progression. **Complications:** Include heart failure, pulmonary HTN, syncope, sudden cardiac death, arrhythmias, and increased risk of endocarditis. **Surgical considerations:** Aortic valve replacement. Patients with **SAD** symptoms (syncope, angina, or dyspnea) should have valve replaced via transcatheter aortic valve replacement (TAVR) or open-heart surgery. Without valve replacement, median survival is only 2–3 years. Other indications are aortic valve area <1 cm², peak velocity >4 m/s, or mean gradient >40 mmHg).

Murmurs Mini-Cases

Cases	Key Findings

Mitral Regurgitation (MR)	**Hx:** Unless acute, patients are often asymptomatic until LV dysfunction develops. Symptoms are initially those of left heart failure and include:
	• Shortness of breath (often exertional), orthopnea, PND, fatigue.
	• This can lead to right heart failure with LE edema.
	PE:
	• Holosystolic, harsh murmur at the apex that radiates to the axilla.
	• S1 is decreased and apical impulse is laterally displaced.
	• May be associated with signs of heart failure such as pulmonary crackles, pitting edema, and an S3.
	• If left atrial enlargement may develop atrial fibrillation.
	Diagnostics:
	• TTE to assess mitral valve.
	• BNP may be elevated and CXR may show pulmonary congestion.
	Management:
	• Mitral valve surgery for symptomatic severe mitral regurgitation (MR) or acute cases of MR.
	• Catheter-based repair may be an option in some cases.
	• Diuresis for congestive symptoms.
	• Guideline-directed medical therapy for LV dysfunction.
	Discussion: MR can occur due to various etiologies.
	• **Acute causes:** Papillary muscle rupture and/or LV dysfunction from MI, endocarditis. Sudden onset symptoms and may be hemodynamically unstable, requiring urgent surgery.
	• **Chronic causes:** Divided into:
	  • Valvular MR—mitral valve prolapse, rheumatic heart disease.
	  • Functional MR—LV dysfunction from dilated cardiomyopathy with mitral annular dilatation, left atrial dilatation.

Aortic Insufficiency (AI) or Regurgitation (AR)	**Hx:** Seen in older patients with cardiovascular risk factors. Often asymptomatic. • Symptoms may include shortness of breath (often exertional), orthopnea, PND, and fatigue. **PE:** • **Diastolic decrescendo murmur** at third to fourth left intercostal space, PMI, S3, **wide pulse pressure** (large difference between systolic and diastolic BP). • Other findings include **water-hammer/bounding/Corrigan pulse** (rapidly increasing pulse intensity that collapses suddenly), **de Musset sign** (head-bobbing with each heartbeat), **Müller sign** (bobbing of the uvula). **Diagnostics:** • Echocardiography to assess aortic valve and degree of regurgitation. • BNP may be elevated if left heart failure present. • CXR may show enlarged cardiac silhouette, a dilated aorta, and pulmonary edema. **Management:** • Aortic valve surgery for symptomatic severe AI. • Diuresis for congestive symptoms. • Guideline-directed medical therapy for LV dysfunction if present. **Discussion:** • **Acute causes:** Infective endocarditis, proximal aortic dissection with aortic valve involvement. Sudden onset symptoms and may be hemodynamically unstable requiring urgent surgery. • **Chronic causes:** Degenerative calcification, connective tissue diseases (e.g., Marfan syndrome), bicuspid aortic valve, rheumatic heart disease, or aortic root dilation from ankylosing spondylitis or syphilis.
Tricuspid Regurgitation (TR)	**Hx:** • Symptoms nonspecific and patients asymptomatic with mild to moderate regurgitation. • With severe TR, patients may experience symptoms of right-sided heart failure (distended neck veins, peripheral edema, fatigue, ascites) including painful hepatosplenomegaly.

Murmurs Mini-Cases *(continued)*

Tricuspid Regurgitation (TR)	**PE:**
	• Holosystolic murmur at the left lower sternal border that intensifies with maneuvers that increase preload (deep inspiration, leg raising).
	• Distended jugular vein with blunted x descent and prominent v wave, pulsatile hepatomegaly, peripheral edema, ascites, hepatojugular reflux.
	• If sufficient right atrial enlargement may have signs of atrial fibrillation.
	
	Diagnostics:
	• Echocardiogram reveals TV regurgitation. Pulmonary HTN often present.
	
	Management:
	• Treat underlying cause.
	• GDMT for right-sided HF and pulmonary HTN if present.
	• Tricuspid valve surgery considered if patient is undergoing left-sided valvular surgery.
	
	Discussion:
	• Primary causes (10%): Directly affect the valve
	  • Direct valve injury from an implantable pacemaker or cardioverter-defibrillator lead passing through the tricuspid valve into the right ventricle.
	  • **Ebstein anomaly:** Congenital heart disease characterized by downward displacement of tricuspid valve and commonly associated with tricuspid regurgitation, atrial septal defect, and/or patent foramen ovale.
	  • **Tricuspid endocarditis:** Seen in patients with IV drug use
	• Secondary causes (90%): Anatomically normal TV
	  • Dilatation of the RV/tethering of the TV leaflets: RV cavity enlargement due to volume or pressure increase most often secondary to right-sided HF.
		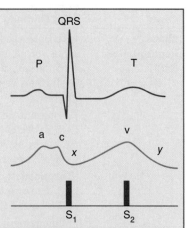
		Jugular venous pressure waveforms in relation to the electrocardiogram (P wave, QRS, and T wave) and the first and second heart sounds (S1 and S2). The bottom of the x descent occurs coincident with the first heart sound (S1). The v wave occurs just after the apical impulse is felt at the same time the second heart sound (S2) is heard. (Reproduced with permission from Hammer GD, McPhee SJ. *Pathophysiology of Disease: An Introduction to Clinical Medicine.* 8th ed. New York: McGraw Hill; 2019.)

Mitral Stenosis	**Hx:** • Progressive dyspnea on exertion, orthopnea, PND, and decreased exercise tolerance. • Cough and/or hemoptysis may occur. • Most common cause is rheumatic fever but patients may not know they had it. **PE:** • Opening snap preceding a diastolic rumbling murmur, best heard at the apex (in the lateral decubitus position). The closer the distance between S2 and the opening snap, the more severe the stenosis. **Diagnostics:** • Echocardiogram reveals left atrial enlargement, thickened mitral valve leaflets with elevated trans-mitral gradient, and a "fish-mouth" valve. **Management:** • Diuresis for congestive symptoms. • Beta-blockers to slow heart rate, allowing increased LV filling time. • Balloon valvuloplasty for severe disease. • Mitral valve replacement for severe stenosis if not amenable to balloon valvuloplasty. **Discussion:** • **Rheumatic fever** is the most common cause of mitral stenosis, in which the immune response against group A Strep cross-reacts with host antigens on cardiac valves leads to tissue inflammation. • Symptomatic mitral stenosis is a relative contraindication to pregnancy, as the hemodynamic changes of pregnancy may not be tolerated. • Left atrial enlargement increases the risk of developing atrial fibrillation.

Murmurs Mini-Cases *(continued)*

Atrial Myxoma	**Hx:** Presents with constitutional symptoms (fever, weight loss, fatigue, arthralgias) as well as SOB, dyspnea on exertion, syncope, and palpitations. **PE:** • Tumor "plop" heart sound is heard immediately after S2. • Low-pitched diastolic murmur following the "plop." **Diagnostics:** Most are in the left atrium. Echocardiogram reveals large atrial pedunculated mass with a "ball valve" obstruction of mitral valve inflow. **Management:** Surgical resection. **Discussion:** A myxoma is a pedunculated mass that can have a "wrecking ball" effect by intermittently obstructing the mitral valve, and can cause valvular dysfunction and/or embolize. It is the most common primary tumor of the heart and is benign. Pathology reveals myxoma cells in glycosaminoglycan matrix.

5

Pulmonology

Lead Authors: Christie Brillante, MD; Sai S. Sunkara, MD
Contributors: Esther Kim, MD; Srinivas Panchamukhi, MD; Arjun Tambe, MD; Yoo Jin Kim, MD

DYSPNEA

Dyspnea, or shortness of breath, can be a normal sensation after heavy exercise or abnormal when it is associated with mild exertion or rest. Physiologically, two major causes are:

1. Increased afferent input to the respiratory centers within the brainstem, due to stimulation of chemoreceptors in the setting of hypercapnia (elevated CO_2).
2. Impaired ventilatory mechanics due to increased workload on the chest (e.g., obesity, kyphoscoliosis) or neuromuscular weakness (e.g., myasthenia gravis, Guillain-Barré syndrome).

The differential for dyspnea is broad. Most causes are due to pulmonary and/or cardiac etiologies, and this chapter will focus on respiratory conditions.

Key History

- Chronicity, quality, and triggers of dyspnea
- Associated symptoms such as cough, hemoptysis, chest pain, wheezing, stridor, fevers, or edema
- Tobacco use, environmental and occupational exposures (asbestos, dust, chemicals)
- Family history of lung disease such as asthma

Key Focused Cardiac and Pulmonary Physical Exam

- General appearance: tachypnea, tripod position, accessory muscle use, and intercostal retractions
- Lung auscultation: Inspiratory or expiratory wheezing, decreased breath sounds, or crackles
- Signs of consolidation: Dullness to percussion, increased/decreased fremitus, egophony

Diagnostic Testing

- Pulse oximetry (SpO_2), CBC for anemia, serum creatinine, and bicarbonate to evaluate renal function and acid-base status
- May need arterial blood gas (ABG) for further interpretation of acid-base status
- Pulmonary function tests (PFTs) can identify obstructive and/or restrictive lung diseases
- Imaging begins with a chest x-ray. CT scan can show more detail if needed.
- If cardiac cause suspected: ECG, echocardiography, cardiac enzymes, brain natriuretic peptide (BNP)
- D-dimer can help rule out a pulmonary embolus (high negative predictive value)

An Overview of Pulmonary Function Tests

Spirometry:

- A low forced expiratory volume in the first second (FEV1)/forced vital capacity (FVC) (defined as <70%) is diagnostic of obstruction.
- The lower the FEV1 (normal is 80% of predicted), the worse the obstruction.
- Plateauing of the inspiratory and/or expiratory curves suggest large-airway obstruction in extrathoracic and intrathoracic locations, respectively.

Lung volumes:

- A low total lung capacity (TLC) (<80% of predicted) defines a restrictive defect.
- A symmetric decrease in both FEV1 and FVC is only *suggestive* of restrictive lung disease.

Diffusion capacity of carbon monoxide (DLCO):

- A low DLCO (<70% of predicted) suggests impaired gas exchange, such as in pulmonary vascular disease, anemia, emphysema, or pulmonary fibrosis.
- A significantly high DLCO can be seen in obesity, asthma, or pulmonary hemorrhage.

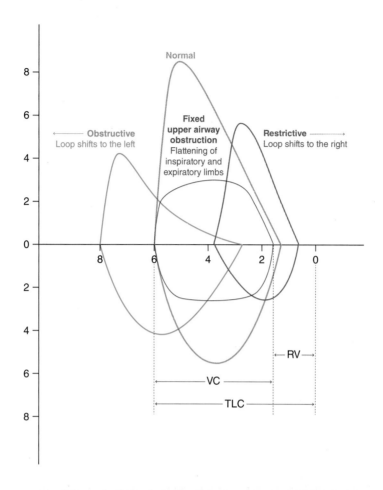

CASE 1	Chronic Asthma

A 40-year-old woman with asthma presents for increasing shortness of breath, wheezing, and cough for 3 months. She has been using her albuterol inhaler at least five to six times a week and notes night-time symptoms. She has been waking up about three to four times a month with these symptoms. Her asthma had previously been well-controlled with rare use of an albuterol inhaler. She has no prior hospitalizations for asthma, has seasonal allergies but no new exposures or environments, illness, or travel. She works as an administrative assistant at a local company. She does not use tobacco, alcohol, or other drugs. Her temperature is 37.5°C, blood pressure 120/80 mmHg, pulse 70/min, and respirations 20/min and O_2 Sat is 98% on room air. Her BMI is 30. Lung auscultation shows normal breath sounds bilaterally without wheezing. Heart sounds are normal.

Conditions with Similar Presentations	**Chronic obstructive pulmonary disease (COPD):** May also present with chronic dyspnea and wheezing. More commonly associated with tobacco use, chronic air pollution, or alpha-1-antitrypsin deficiency.
	Decompensated heart failure: Can also present with chronic dyspnea and wheezing, but patients usually will have other signs/symptoms of volume overload (peripheral edema, elevated jugular venous pressure [JVP], bibasilar crackles).
	Allergic bronchopulmonary aspergillosis (ABPA): Presents with difficult-to-control asthma, eosinophilia, and infiltrates on CXR. Patients with structural airway disease (e.g., asthma, cystic fibrosis) and history of recurrent infections/mucus hypersecretion are susceptible to chronic colonization by the *Aspergillus* species (ubiquitous in the environment) which leads to hypersensitivity reaction in the lungs with Th2-mediated Ig-E production and eosinophilia. Consider in patients with difficult-to-control asthma or illness (e.g., fever, thick sputum) that does not respond to treatment. Diagnosis is made if the patient has underlying asthma or cystic fibrosis, detectable IgG against *Aspergillus fumigatus*, increased total IgE, precipitating antibodies to *A. fumigatus*, and lung infiltrates on CXR. Treatment is with systemic glucocorticoids. In some cases, may need to treat with voriconazole.
Initial Diagnostic Tests	• If diagnosis established, further testing not needed and can treat symptomatically. • Diagnosis is confirmed with spirometry, PFTs, or methacholine challenge test.

CASE 1 | Chronic Asthma (continued)

Next Steps in Management	• Avoid triggers (allergens, temperature extremes). • Initiate or add medications depending on severity of symptoms (see below).

Discussion	Asthma is a chronic inflammatory condition that results in airway hyperresponsiveness. Triggers can cause the hyperresponsive airways to become swollen and narrow resulting in reversible airflow obstruction. Incidence of self-reported asthma is 7–19% of adults, and it usually begins in childhood but can present in adulthood.
	• Atopy increases the chances the individual will develop an IgE-mediated response to common allergens.
	• Allergen activation of mast cells and Th2 cells leads to production of bronchoconstrictor mediators, resulting in the reversible symptoms of asthma.
	• Repeated airway inflammation eventually leads to permanent changes in the airway structure such as smooth muscle hypertrophy, mucus hypersecretion, and angiogenesis.
	
	History:
	Symptoms:
	• Recurrent wheezing, difficulty breathing, chest tightness, dry cough.
	• Triggered/worsened with exposure to allergens, exercise, or at night leading to frequent nighttime awakenings.
	Risk factors/associations:
	• The strongest predisposing factor for asthma is atopy.
	• Allergic rhinitis, sinusitis, GERD, nasal polyps, obesity, ABPA.
	• Perinatal/childhood factors (preterm delivery, maternal smoking, RSV) and environmental factors (tobacco smoke, mold, and paints).
	
	Physical exam:
	• Exam may be normal between asthma symptoms.
	• Wheezing, prolonged expiration, tachypnea, tachycardia, hyperresonance, and increased accessory muscle use.
	• Findings of associated conditions such as atopic dermatitis, eczema, nasal polyps, increased nasal secretion/mucosal swelling from allergic rhinitis may be present.
	
	Diagnostics:
	• Diagnosis is confirmed with spirometry/PFTs showing obstructive pattern with reversibility after bronchodilator, short-acting beta-2 agonist (SABA) administration during an exacerbation OR positive methacholine challenge test.
	• Initial obstructive pattern:
	  • FEV1/FVC < 70%: ↓ FEV1, normal or ↓ FVC
	  • ↑ RV, high FRC
	  • Normal or ↑ DLCO
	• Reversibility: Beta-2-agonist results in significant ↑ FEV1 or FVC from baseline.
	• Consider methacholine challenge (measures hyperresponsiveness of airway) test if PFTs are normal or nondiagnostic but asthma is still suspected.
	• Chest x-ray may show hyperinflation of lungs but is only indicated in severe asthma to exclude other diagnoses.
	
	Management:
	1. Assess level of control.

A. Assessment of symptom control		Level of asthma symptom control		
In the past 4 weeks, has the patient had:		**Well controlled**	**Partly controlled**	**Uncontrolled**
Daytime symptoms more than twice/week?	Yes☐ No☐	None of these	1–2 of these	3–4 of these
Any night waking due to asthma?	Yes☐ No☐			
Reliever needed more than twice/week?	Yes☐ No☐			
Any activity limitation due to asthma?	Yes☐ No☐			

2. Nonpharmacologic interventions: Increased physical activity, healthy diet, avoid exposure to triggers, smoke (smoking cessation) and other noxious substances.
3. Management of comorbidities (rhinitis, GERD, chronic rhinosinusitis, obesity, OSA, depression, anxiety).
4. Worsening asthma control usually requires a "step up" in pharmacologic therapy. Treatments are usually divided into "Reliever" and "Controller" medications.

CASE 1 | Chronic Asthma *(continued)*

Discussion	**Asthma "Reliever" Medications** **– For treatment of exacerbations or acute worsening of symptoms**	**Examples**
	Inhaled short acting B$_2$ agonists (SABA)	Albuterol
	Inhaled short acting anti-muscarinics (SAMA)	Ipratropium
	Inhaled corticosteroid (ICS) and formoterol *Single Maintenance and Reliever Therapy (SMART): ICS-formoterol relieves asthma symptoms and reduces severe asthma exacerbations at an overall lower ICS exposure, when compared to SABA	Budesonide-formoterol Mometasone-formoterol
	Oral or Intravenous corticosteroids *onset requires several hours	Prednisone Methylprednisolone
	Asthma "Controller" Medications **– For prevention of exacerbations** **– Several combination inhaler therapies exist**	**Examples**
	ICS	Budesonide Mometasone
	Inhaled long acting beta-agonists (LABA)	Formoterol Salmeterol
	Inhaled long acting anti-muscarinics (LAMA)	Tiotropium Umeclidinium
	Leukotriene modulators	Montelukast
	Immunomodulator (aka Biologics)	Omalizumab – binds to IgE Mepolizumab - anti-IL5 Ab Dupilumab - anti IL-4 receptor alpha subunit Ab
	Methylxanthine *weak efficacy and high potential for side effects	Sustained release theophylline
Additional Considerations	**Complications:** **Respiratory failure** in acute asthma exacerbation manifests as altered mental status, absent/minimal wheezing, and/or cyanosis. On arterial blood gas (ABG), there will be persistent hypoxemia despite oxygen therapy, worsening hypercarbia, and respiratory acidosis. It is managed with endotracheal intubation and mechanical ventilation. **Secondary lower respiratory infections** and other complications related to chronic use of glucocorticoids are also possible. **Other Considerations** **Exercise-induced asthma:** • Asthma symptoms due to transient narrowing of bronchial airways during or after exercise • Symptoms peak 5–10 minutes after starting activity and spontaneously resolve within 30–90 minutes • Post-exercise cough is common, and intensity of symptoms may vary by season or location • Management includes SABA 15 minutes prior to exercise and avoiding training in extreme cold/pollution **NSAID-exacerbated respiratory disease:** • Characterized by chronic rhinosinusitis with nasal polyps and asthma symptoms, after COX inhibition (leukotriene overproduction results in airway constriction). **Occupational asthma:** • Results from allergen exposure at the workplace. • Initially asthma symptoms are closely linked/limited to the workplace, but after prolonged exposure, the symptoms may become persistent and cease only after long-term absence from work (e.g., vacation and/or traveling). • Diagnosis is made with a decline in peak expiratory flow rate measurement by ≥20% at workplace compared to home.

CASE 2 | Asthma Exacerbation

A 19-year-old man presents to the ED with acute shortness of breath and cough for 2 days, which developed after a recent cold. His symptoms are worse at night, and he is now experiencing mild chest discomfort. He has tried over-the-counter cough medications without improvement. His medical history is significant for chronic rhinosinusitis and occasional chest tightness and wheezing with the change of weather. He has no prior hospitalizations, smokes one to two cigarettes a day for the past year and has no other substance use. His temperature is 37.5°C, blood pressure 120/80 mmHg, respirations 30/min, and pulse 108/min, with O_2 saturation of 92% on room air. On exam, he appears to be in distress, talks in short sentences, and prefers sitting upright. Physical exam is notable for diffuse bilateral wheezing, increased expiratory phase, and use of accessory muscles.

Conditions with Similar Presentations	**Acute bronchitis:** May present similarly and is caused by viral pathogens (e.g., rhinovirus, adenovirus, influenza, parainfluenza, RSV, COVID-19). Patients initially experience upper respiratory tract symptoms such as cough, nasal congestion, sore throat, headache, and/or wheezing followed by persistent coughing for >5 days after other symptoms resolve.
	Pulmonary embolism: May also present with acute-onset shortness of breath, tachycardia, and tachypnea but lung exam is usually normal; rarely can include expiratory wheezing. Look for risk factors (estrogen use, immobility, smoking, prior venous thromboembolism).
	Panic attack: May present with acute shortness of breath and chest pain; exam would be normal.
	Pneumothorax: Presents with sudden pleuritic chest pain and shortness of breath but exam would include unilateral decreased breath sounds and hyperresonance to percussion.
	Anaphylaxis: May present with acute-onset shortness of breath but would also have other signs such as rash/urticaria, edema, or nausea, vomiting and diarrhea. Patients are often aware of the inciting event (bee sting, peanuts, medications).
	Foreign body aspiration: Is most often seen in the pediatric population and presents with sudden-onset respiratory distress and unilateral wheezing and/or stridor, even if there is no witnessed choking. Chest x-ray may show unilateral hyperinflation distal to obstruction and mediastinal shift away from obstruction. Treatment is immediate rigid or flexible bronchoscopy and removal of aspirated object.
Initial Diagnostic Testing	• Clinical diagnosis • Consider chest x-ray
Next Steps in Management	• Supplemental oxygen, albuterol (SABA), systemic corticosteroids • Consider noninvasive ventilation (BiPAP) or intubation if impending respiratory failure
Discussion	Asthma exacerbations are acute or subacute worsening of a patient's symptoms or lung function but may be the initial presentation for some patients. **History:** Symptoms include: • Difficulty breathing, cough, wheezing, or chest tightness • Often occur or worsen at night • Common triggers and/or family history may be present • Allergens (dust mites, pollen, pet dander, cockroaches), extremes of temperatures, and viral URIs Risk factors for *asthma-related deaths* include: • Prior asthma exacerbation requiring intubation and ventilation • Hospitalization in the past year for asthma • Recent discontinuation of an oral corticosteroid • Non-adherence to long-term asthma management • History of psychiatric or psychosocial problems • Absence of written asthma action plan **Physical exam:** • Respiratory distress, nasal flaring, use of accessory muscles, wheezing, tachycardia, hunched shoulders, tripod position, and/or cyanosis depending on the severity of exacerbation. • Associated findings suggestive of chronic asthma include atopic dermatitis, eczema, nasal polyps, increased nasal secretion/mucosal swelling from allergic rhinitis.

CASE 2 | Asthma Exacerbation *(continued)*

Discussion	**Diagnostics:** Clinical diagnosis based on history and exam
	• *Mild to moderate exacerbation*—talks in phrases, not agitated, no use of accessory muscles.
	• *Severe exacerbation*—talks in words, respiratory rate >30, agitated, +accessory muscle use, O_2 sat <90%, "silent chest," tripoding.
	• Although ABG is not necessary for diagnosis for asthma, normalization of CO_2 levels indicates impending respiratory failure.
	  • Tachypnea → respiratory alkalosis (low CO_2, high pH) → worsening tachypnea and obstruction → muscle fatigue → CO_2 normalizes.
	• Peak expiratory flow (PEF) rates below 200 L/min or <50% predicted suggests severe obstruction.
	
	Management: Treatment consists of administration of oxygen, inhaled β2-agonists, and systemic corticosteroids.
	• Short-acting β2-agonist (SABA) albuterol by nebulization or pressurized metered-dose inhaler with spacer.
	  • Ipratropium (SAMA) can be added if poor initial response to SABA.
	• Systemic corticosteroids, initially IV if severe, then PO for a total of 5–7 days.
	• Supplemental oxygen to maintain oxygen saturation >90%.
	• Magnesium sulfate IV if no response to initial treatment.
	• Frequently assess response to therapy to escalate care and/or readiness to discharge.
	• Consider non-invasive ventilation (BiPAP) or intubation if impending respiratory failure.
	• Nonpharmacologic preventative measures include avoidance of triggers, quitting smoking, and avoiding second-hand exposure.

CASE 3 | Chronic Obstructive Pulmonary Disease (COPD)

A 58-year-old woman with a 30-pack-year history of tobacco use presents to clinic with persistent cough for the past several months. The cough is productive with clear sputum, worse in the mornings. She reports increasing shortness of breath over the past year, having to frequently stop and rest before resuming daily activities. She has no orthopnea, paroxysmal nocturnal dyspnea, or leg swelling. Her temperature is 37.5°C, respirations 20/min, pulse 92/min, and blood pressure 140/80 mmHg, and O_2 Sat of 93% on room air. On exam, the patient has a barrel-shaped chest with prolonged expiratory phase, hyperresonance to percussion, and diminished breath sounds bilaterally with faint expiratory wheezes. There is no jugular venous distension or lower extremity edema. Heart sounds are distant without gallops or murmurs. CXR shows hyperinflation with flattening of the diaphragms.

Conditions with Similar Presentations	**Asthma:** May also present with chronic cough and dyspnea but often presents earlier, and COPD is more common than asthma in patients with smoking history. On PFTs, low DLCO and minimal responsiveness to bronchodilators suggests COPD over asthma. **Decompensated heart failure:** Can present with chronic dyspnea and wheezing, but patients have other signs/symptoms of volume overload (peripheral edema, elevated JVP, bibasilar crackles). **Tuberculosis:** May present with chronic cough and dyspnea, but patients have fatigue/malaise, weight loss, findings on CXR (hilar lymphadenopathy, pulmonary infiltrates/cavities, pleural effusions). Risk factors (incarceration, homelessness, birth in a TB-endemic area, immunosuppression, health care worker) may be present. **Bronchiectasis:** Can also present with chronic productive cough and has numerous etiologies including cystic fibrosis and pulmonary infections, but CT chest will have characteristic findings of airway dilation. **Alpha-1 antitrypsin (AAT) deficiency:** Suspect AAT deficiency in patients presenting with early-onset COPD (< age 45) with minimal smoking history or family/personal history of liver disease. Due to lack of AAT, these patients develop panacinar emphysema predominantly in the lower lobes (compared to patients with smoking history presenting with centriacinar emphysema in upper lobes) and may also have chronic liver disease.
Initial Diagnostic Tests	• Confirm diagnosis with spirometry (pre- and post-bronchodilator with non-reversible airflow obstruction): FEV1/FVC <70% • Consider CXR or CT chest, ABG, alpha-1 antitrypsin levels, TTE, ECG
Next Steps in Management	• Smoking cessation and vaccinations for respiratory pathogens • Oxygen therapy if indicated • Inhalers depending on disease severity by GOLD criteria

CASE 3 | Chronic Obstructive Pulmonary Disease (COPD) *(continued)*

Discussion	COPD is a progressive condition of significant airflow obstruction that is not completely reversible (unlike asthma), caused by chronic inflammation in the airways that leads to permanent destruction of the lung tissue. It commonly affects adults over 40 years old, with an estimated prevalence of 4–10% worldwide. The two major subtypes of COPD include chronic bronchitis and emphysema.

- **Chronic bronchitis** is a clinical diagnosis of productive cough for >3 months per year for 2 consecutive years.
- **Emphysema** is a pathologic diagnosis demonstrating destruction and dilation of structures distal to the terminal bronchioles due to smoking (centrilobular) or alpha-1 antitrypsin deficiency (panlobular).

COPD type	Definition	Characteristics
Chronic bronchitis aka Blue bloater	Productive cough >3 months for 2 consecutive years	Overweight, cyanotic Earlier onset of hypoxia and/or hypercarbia
Emphysema aka Pink puffer	Terminal airway destruction and dilation	Thin, pursed lips, minimal cough Later onset of hypoxia and/or hypercarbia

History:
- Chronic and progressive symptoms of dyspnea, cough, and sputum production, may be associated with wheezing, leading to significant limitation in activity.
- Risk factors: Cigarette smoking; occupational or environmental exposure.

Physical exam:
- Barrel chest, end-expiratory wheezing, muffled breath sounds, pursed-lip breathing, reduced chest expansion, hyperresonance to percussion.
- During exacerbation, look for use of accessory muscles, Hoover sign (paradoxical inward movement of the lower rib cage with inspiration).
- If cor pulmonale present, may see jugular venous distension and lower extremity edema.

Diagnostics:
- Diagnosis confirmed by the presence of non-reversible airflow obstruction on post-bronchodilator spirometry.
  - FEV1/FVC <70%
  - ↓/normal FEV1, ↓/normal FVC
  - ↑ RV and TLC
  - Minimal to no change in FEV1 with SABA
  - ↓ DLCO in emphysema, normal DLCO in chronic bronchitis
- ABG may show hypoxemia and hypercarbia (acute or chronic).
- CXR findings of COPD include hyperinflation, increased anteroposterior diameter, decreased lung markings with flattened diaphragm, and thin-appearing heart and mediastinum. Bullae/subpleural blebs may be seen with emphysema.

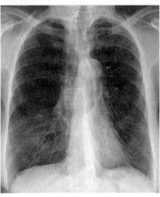
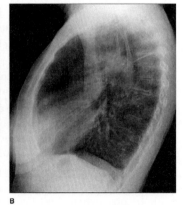

A   B

(A) PA and (B) lateral of a patient with severe emphysema-predominant COPD. Salient features are upper lobe predominant hyperinflation (denoted by flattening of the diaphragms and increased craniocaudal and anteroposterior diameters of the chest), hyperlucency of the parenchyma, and increased interstitial markings.
(Reproduced, with permission, from Grippi MA, Antin-Ozerkis DE, Dela Cruz CS, Kotloff RM, Kotton C, Pack AI. Fishman's Pulmonary Diseases and Disorders, 6e; 2023.Copyright © 2023 McGraw-Hill Education. All rights reserved.)

CASE 3 | Chronic Obstructive Pulmonary Disease (COPD) *(continued)*

Discussion	**Management:**
	• Therapies that decrease mortality:
	  • Smoking cessation
	  • Pulmonary rehabilitation including exercise and nutrition counseling for patients with high risk of exacerbation
	  • Long-term oxygen therapy (LTOT) if:
	    • SpO_2 ≤88% or PaO_2 ≤55 mmHg
	    • SpO_2 ≤ 89% or PaO_2 ≤59 mmHg in patients with evidence of right heart failure, cor pulmonale, or Hct >55
	  • Immunizations (influenza, COVID-19, pertussis, pneumococcal vaccines)
	• Therapies that do not decrease mortality but decrease symptoms and/or complications.
	  • Inhaled bronchodilator therapy (see table below)
	• Consider lung transplant for severe cases.

Additional Considerations	**Screening:** For asymptomatic patients, screening for COPD with spirometry is not recommended. **Surgical considerations:** Lung transplant for patients with very severe COPD with a history of multiple exacerbations, pulmonary hypertension, cor pulmonale, and FEV1 <20%. Complications include acute rejection, bronchiolitis obliterans, opportunistic infections (e.g., CMV, *Aspergillus*, Pneumocystis), and lymphoproliferative disease.

Choosing an Initial Inhaler for COPD based on Global Initiative for Chronic Obstructive Lung Disease (GOLD)

Group	Exacerbations or Hospitalizations	Functional Capacity	First Choice Inhaler Type
A	≤1 exacerbation/year	Good	A bronchodilator
B	≤1 exacerbations/year	Poor	LAMA (e.g., tiotropium, umeclidinium) and LABA (e.g., formoterol, salmeterol)
E	≥2 exacerbations/year *or* ≥1 hospital admission/year	Good or Poor	LAMA + LABA consider LAMA + LABA + ICS if blood eosionphils ≥300 cells/microliter

CASE 4 | Chronic Obstructive Pulmonary Disease (COPD) Exacerbation

A 60-year-old man with COPD and 45-pack-year tobacco history presents to the ED with worsening dyspnea and cough for the past 5 days. The cough is productive of thick sputum, which has increased in amount compared to his baseline. The severity of cough does not worsen with certain positions or at night when he is sleeping. Home albuterol and ipratropium bromide nebulizer treatments have not helped in the last few days. He recently recovered from an upper respiratory tract infection. He has no recent travel history or exposure to new allergens. His temperature is 37.0°C, blood pressure is 140/90 mmHg, pulse is 115/min and regular, and respirations are 22/min; his O_2 sat is 85% on room air. On exam, the patient is in moderate respiratory distress and is breathing through pursed lips. Auscultation of the lungs shows bilateral wheezing and prolonged expiration. There is no egophony or dullness to percussion. There is no jugular venous distension or peripheral edema.

Conditions with Similar Presentations	**Pneumonia:** Can also present with dyspnea and productive cough but would have fever, and x-ray would show an infiltrate. **Pulmonary embolism:** Can also present with dyspnea and cough but would be more acute in onset. Exam would generally not include wheezing, but PE can also trigger COPD exacerbation. **Pleural effusions:** Can present with dyspnea, but lung auscultation would reveal decreased breath sounds and dullness to percussion over the effusion, and CXR would show effusion. **Heart failure:** May present with dyspnea and signs of volume overload (e.g., JVD, edema, crackles on lung exam).
Initial Diagnostic Tests	• Would check arterial blood gas, pulse oximetry, CXR • Consider BNP to rule out cardiac causes
Next Step in Management	• Supplemental oxygen with goal SpO_2 of 88–92% • Inhaled bronchodilators (SABA or SAMA) • Systemic glucocorticoids • Antibiotics if ≥ two of three of the three cardinal symptoms (see discussion below)

CASE 4 | Chronic Obstructive Pulmonary Disease (COPD) Exacerbation *(continued)*

Discussion	Acute COPD exacerbation results from increased airway inflammation that leads to bronchoconstriction, airway wall edema and thickening, and increased mucus production. A COPD exacerbation is characterized as a change from baseline symptoms that requires further treatment.
	History:
	• The 3 *cardinal symptoms* are changes in cough severity or frequency, change in volume or character of sputum production, and change in level of dyspnea.
	• Other symptoms may include wheezing, chest discomfort/tightness, fatigue, cyanosis, confusion, somnolence, depression, or insomnia.
	• COPD exacerbation is often precipitated by an upper respiratory infection or exposure to air pollution, though cause may not always be identified.
	• Increased risk of exacerbation in patients with severe COPD, history of prior exacerbations, poor physical activity, inadequate social support, difficulty with medications, underuse of home oxygen.
	Physical exam:
	• Tachypnea, pursed-lip breathing, tachycardia, signs of respiratory failure (use of accessory muscles, acute mental status changes, paradoxical abdominal motion, intercostal retraction, cyanosis), wheezing, rhonchi, diminished breath sounds, prolonged expiratory phase
	Diagnostics:
	• Pulse oximetry to evaluate the need for supplemental oxygen.
	• ABG to identify hypoxemia and hypercarbia and determine adequacy of ventilation.
	• CXR to support (hyperinflation with increased anteroposterior diameter and flattened diaphragm) and exclude alternative diagnoses.
	• BNP, troponin, and ECG may be considered to rule out cardiac etiology.
	Management:
	• Hospital admission for patients with severe symptoms (e.g., resting dyspnea, decreased saturation, confusion, drowsiness), acute respiratory failure, lack of response to initial medical management, or serious comorbidities.
	• Supplemental oxygen with goal SpO_2 of 88–92%.
	• Inhaled bronchodilators such as SABAs (albuterol) and SAMAs (ipratropium).
	• Systemic glucocorticoids (prednisone 40 mg/day for 5 days) to shorten the recovery time and improve overall lung function.
	• Antibiotics if patient has ≥ two of three cardinal symptoms or requires mechanical ventilation.
	• Noninvasive positive pressure ventilation (NPPV), such as BiPAP, if unresponsive to standard medical treatments.
	• Intubation for patients who fail to improve on NPPV or who have contraindications for NPPV (e.g., unable to protect airway, facial fractures, hemoptysis).

CASE 5 | Pleural Effusion

A 65-year-old man with an extensive smoking history presents with right-sided chest pain and dyspnea for the past month. Pain is worse with deep inspiration, and he is having trouble taking deep breaths. Breathing worsens with exertion and when lying down. He has unintentionally lost 25 pounds in the last 5 months and reports decreased appetite and easy fatigability. On exam, he is cachectic and has dullness to percussion and decreased breath sounds on the right base. There is also decreased tactile fremitus on the right and slight crackles in the right upper lobe.

Conditions with Similar Presentations	**Lung cancer:** May present with pleuritic chest pain if the tumor involves the parietal pleura. If a malignant effusion is present, thoracentesis will show an exudate that is commonly hemorrhagic.
	Heart failure: Can present with dyspnea and can cause bilateral transudative pleural effusions. Unless very advanced, it is not associated with weight loss. Other symptoms of heart failure (orthopnea, PND, peripheral edema) are suggestive, and confirmed with echocardiography.
	Pneumonia: Present with fever and cough, and CXR would show an infiltrate and possible effusion.
Initial Diagnostic Tests	Confirm diagnosis with CXR or point-of-care ultrasound
Next Steps in Management	• Thoracentesis and pleural fluid analysis to determine exudate vs. transudate • Treat underlying condition(s)

CASE 5 | **Pleural Effusion** (continued)

Discussion	Pleural effusions are due to excess fluid in the pleural space. This is usually due to pleural fluid accumulating at faster rates than it is being reabsorbed or not being removed from the pleural space (via lymphatic drainage). Pleural effusions are divided into transudative and exudative effusions:

- **Transudative:** Fluid leaks into the pleural space due to high pulmonary intravascular pressure or low plasma oncotic pressure. Capillary permeability is generally unaffected, and the resulting pleural effusion has a low protein count and cell count. Causes include heart failure, hypoalbuminemic states (nephrotic syndrome, cirrhosis, protein losing enteropathy)
- **Exudative:** Pathologic process results in increased capillary permeability which allows fluid to leak into the pleural space. Exudative pleural effusions tend to have higher protein content and cell counts compared to transudative effusions. Causes include infection, cancer, vasculitides, hemorrhage, pulmonary embolism

History:
- Dyspnea, cough, and pleuritic chest pain but can also be asymptomatic

Physical exam:
- Reduced breath sounds, dullness to percussion, and decreased tactile fremitus on the affected side
- May have pleural friction rub, asymmetric chest expansion, and crackles

Diagnostics:
- Chest x-ray or point-of-care ultrasound to visualize effusion
- Thoracentesis for diagnostic (pleural fluid analysis) and therapeutic (large volume drainage for symptomatic relief)

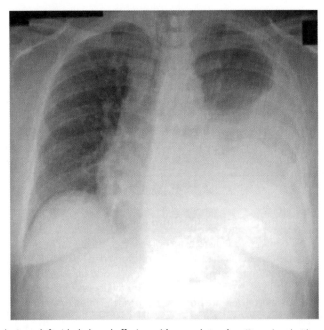

Chest radiograph displaying a left-sided pleural effusion with a meniscus sign. (Reproduced with permission from Imaging of the Critically Ill Patient: Radiology, Oropello JM, Pastores SM, Kvetan V. Critical Care. Copyright © 2017 by McGraw-Hill Education. All rights reserved.)

Pleural Fluid Analysis:

Use **Light's criteria** to differentiate transudate from exudate effusions. **Exudative effusions:**
- Ratio of pleural/serum total protein >0.5, *or*
- Ratio of pleural/serum LDH >0.6, *or*
- Pleural LDH > two-thirds the upper limit of normal serum LDH

CASE 5 | Pleural Effusion (*continued*)

Discussion	**Management:**
	• Thoracentesis to identify transudate vs. exudate and treat underlying cause when identified (e.g., antibiotics for pneumonia, diuretics for heart failure)
	• Recurrent effusions may need repeat thoracentesis, or surgical treatment (pleurodesis)
	• Chest tube may be indicated for:
	  • Recurrent symptomatic malignant effusions requiring repeated thoracentesis.
	  • Pleural fluid pH <7.2 or glucose <60 with concern for parapneumonic effusion or empyema.

Additional Considerations	**Complications:** Permanent lung damage, pleural thickening, and pneumothorax.

Causes of Pleural Effusions

Transudate	Exudate

Heart failure
  ↑ pulmonary capillary hydrostatic pressure
	Malignancy
	  Cytology will show malignant or suspicious cells. Immunohistochemical tests frequently needed

Cirrhosis, Nephrotic syndrome, Protein Losing Enteropathy
  ↓ plasma oncotic pressure
	Empyema or para-pneumonic
	  Fluid will be purulent or have +Gram stain/culture, ↓ pH, and ↓ glucose levels. AFB can be positive but has low NPV to r/o TB

	Chylothorax Milky appearance due to thoracic duct lymphatic obstruction or injury causing ↑ triglycerides

	Pseudochylothorax
	  ↑ cholesterol
	  Seen in TB, yellow nail syndrome

	Pancreatitis or esophageal perforation ↑ amylase
	Hemothorax ↑ hematocrit

CASE 6 | Primary Spontaneous Pneumothorax

A 21-year-old man with no significant medical history presents to the ED for evaluation of abrupt onset of chest pain while he was sitting at the computer. The pain is in his left chest and worsened by deep inspiration. There is no history of trauma. His temperature is 36.6°C, pulse is 90/min, respirations are 24/min, blood pressure is 126/82, and SpO$_2$ 94% on room air. On exam, the patient is taking short, shallow breaths, his trachea is slightly deviated to the left, and there are decreased breath sounds and hyperresonance over the left chest. There are no wheezes, rhonchi, rales, or chest wall tenderness.

Conditions with Similar Presentations	**Pulmonary embolism (PE), acute coronary syndrome (ACS),** and **aortic dissection:** Are less likely in a healthy young patient with no cardiac risk factors and would not cause unilateral decreased breath sounds and hyperresonance to percussion. **Pleural effusion:** May cause decreased breath sounds but would be dull to percussion (rather than hyperresonant) and would not cause sudden chest pain outside of the setting of trauma.
Initial Diagnostic Testing	Confirm diagnosis with CXR or point-of-care ultrasound
Next Steps in Management	• Supplemental oxygen • Chest tube only if pneumothorax is large or patient is unstable
Discussion	The pleural space is a potential space between the visceral and parietal pleura and normally has negative pressure relative to the alveolar pressure throughout the respiratory cycle. When air enters the pleural space (chest wall trauma or bronchopleural fistula), the lung is compressed.

CASE 6 | Primary Spontaneous Pneumothorax *(continued)*

Discussion	Classification:
	• **Primary spontaneous pneumothorax (PTX):** No known lung disease, usually tall, thin young men who are smokers. Caused by rupture of subpleural blebs.
	• **Secondary PTX:** Known lung disease (malignancy, COPD), trauma, infections (TB, *Pneumocystis jiroveci*) pneumonia, connective tissue disease (Marfan syndrome) or iatrogenic factors (thoracentesis, subclavian line placement, mechanical ventilation, bronchoscopy).
	• **Tension PTX:** Caused by either primary or secondary PTX. Occurs when the connection between the lung and pleura has a ball/valve mechanism allowing air to enter the pleural space during inspiration but not leave the pleural space during expiration. This leads to continued increase in size of PTX, shifting of the mediastinum away from the PTX and compression of great vessels, and requires immediate chest tube insertion. On exam, the trachea is shifted *away* from the PTX.
	
	History and physical exam: Clinical presentation varies depending on etiology (primary vs. secondary vs. traumatic pneumothorax) but the mnemonic P-THORAX is useful: **P**leuritic pain, **T**racheal deviation, **H**yperresonance, **O**nset sudden, **R**educed breath sounds (and dyspnea), **A**bsent fremitus (asymmetric chest wall), **X**-ray shows collapse.
	
	Diagnostics:
	• Chest radiograph (CXR): Standard for diagnosing PTX and shows absent lung markings on the side of the pneumothorax. However, if patient is supine, the only sign of PTX may be ***deep sulcus sign***.
	• Point-of-care ultrasound: May also be used to diagnose pneumothorax (absence of "sliding" pleura).
	• CT: Indicated if CXR not diagnostic and PTX still suspected.
	
	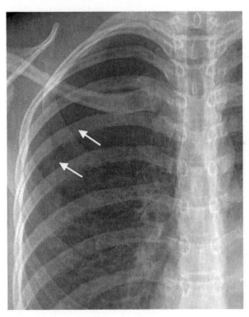
	
	Right-sided pneumothorax with collapsed lung (white arrows) with loss of normal lung markings. (Reproduced with permission from Chen MM, Pope TL, Ott DJ. Basic Radiology, 2e; Copyright © 2011 McGraw-Hill Education. All rights reserved.)
	
	Treatment:
	• Tension pneumothorax: Emergent needle decompression (second intercostal space at the midclavicular line) followed by chest tube placement.
	• Small pneumothorax (≤2 cm from periphery). If stable observation ± supplemental O_2, may resorb spontaneously. Stability defined as the presence of **all** of the following:
	  • RR <24
	  • HR 60–120
	  • BP normal
	  • Oxygen saturation >90%
	  • Able to speak in whole sentences
	If unstable, need aspiration ± chest tube insertion.
	• If large pneumothorax or unstable, need aspiration ± chest tube.
	• Recurrent pneumothorax: Common with secondary PTX. Usually requires chemical or physical pleurodesis.

CASE 7 | Idiopathic Pulmonary Fibrosis (IPF)

A 72-year-old woman presents to the clinic with increasing dyspnea and fatigue over the past 5 months. At baseline, she could walk 5–7 blocks without difficulty, but now is short of breath after walking 2–3 blocks. She has a persistent dry cough but no fever, night sweats, or weight loss. She has no leg swelling, orthopnea, or paroxysmal nocturnal dyspnea. She smokes a pack of cigarettes daily for the past 35 years but quit recently because of her dyspnea. She has no other substance use. She is a retired businesswoman and has no recent travel history or environmental exposures. On exam, temperature is 37.5°C, blood pressure 150/85 mmHg, pulse 90/min, respirations 20/min, SpO_2 95% on room air and, BMI is 28. Auscultation of the lungs reveals fine, high-pitched bibasilar inspiratory crackles. Cardiac examination is unremarkable. Digital clubbing is seen. Joints appear normal with full range of motion. CXR shows bilateral basal reticular markings. PFTs have normal FEV1/FVC, reduced TLC, and reduced DLCO.

Conditions with Similar Presentations	**Connective tissue disease (SLE, RA, dermatomyositis):** Can also develop interstitial lung disease but would see signs and symptoms of the respective disease (SLE: arthralgia, skin/mucous/membrane changes; RA: arthritis, rheumatoid nodules, skin changes; dermatomyositis: muscle pain and weakness, skin changes).
	Pneumoconiosis (asbestosis, silicosis, berylliosis): Can also develop interstitial lung disease but history would have an occupational exposure.
	Hypersensitivity pneumonitis (extrinsic allergic alveolitis): Presenting symptoms include flu-like illness with fever, chills, cough, and dyspnea, with chest x-ray or CT showing pulmonary infiltrates. History will include exposure to organic dusts from mold, birds (bird fancier's lung), or thermophilic bacteria (hot tub alveolitis). These antigens induce immune-mediated pneumonitis, and chronic exposure can lead to restrictive lung disease. Though serum IgG directed against known antigens (precipitins) has variable sensitivity and specificity, its presence and characteristic CT findings can help in differentiating the two. Infiltrates in IPF predominate in the lower lobes, and hypersensitivity pneumonitis is either more diffuse or upper lung fields.
Initial Diagnostic Tests	• Check CXR, high-resolution CT (HRCT), pulmonary function tests • Consider autoimmune panel (ANA, RF, anticyclic citrullinated peptide) to rule out other causes
Next Steps in Management	• Smoking cessation, pulmonary rehabilitation, supplemental oxygen (if needed) • Anti-fibrotic therapy (e.g., pirfenidone, nintedanib) • Evaluate for comorbidities (pulmonary hypertension, lung CA)
Discussion	IPF is a severe progressive disease affecting adults aged 55–75. It is a chronic idiopathic fibrosing pneumonia characterized histologically by usual interstitial pneumonia. Pathogenesis involves recurrent epithelial injury and inappropriate repair by myofibroblast proliferation and subsequent interstitial fibrosis. **History:** • Nonspecific pulmonary symptoms such as progressive dyspnea, fatigue, and nonproductive cough. • Risk factors include cigarette smoking, older age, and male sex, environmental exposures such as metal (e.g., brass, lead), livestock, stone cutting/polishing, and hair dressing. **Physical exam:** • Fine "Velcro" bibasilar inspiratory crackles and digital clubbing. • In late stages, may see signs of cor pulmonale (e.g., right ventricular heave, loud P2, increased splitting of S2, tricuspid regurgitation, parasternal lift, JVD, peripheral edema). **Diagnostics:** Diagnosis based on clinical presentation, exclusion of other causes, chest imaging, and sometimes histopathologic evaluation. • History and physical should focus on occupational history, rheumatologic signs/symptoms (Raynaud phenomenon, joint pain, digital ulcers, fevers, telangiectasia), medications (amiodarone, bleomycin, nitrofurantoin), and family history to rule out other conditions such as pneumoconiosis, hypersensitivity pneumonitis, rheumatologic diseases, COPD, or heart failure. • CXR shows increased bilateral basal reticular markings. • HRCT findings highly suggestive of IPF include subpleural, basilar predominant honeycombing.

CASE 7 | Idiopathic Pulmonary Fibrosis (IPF) *(continued)*

Discussion	
	• PFTs will show decreased TLC, FVC, and DLCO without a reduction in FEV1/FVC ratio, consistent with restrictive pattern. • Autoimmune panel to rule out systemic and connective tissue diseases (ANA, RF, anticyclic citrullinated peptide). **Management:** • Vaccination, smoking cessation, and oxygen therapy. • Anti-fibrotic drugs (pirfenidone, nintedanib) which target pro-fibrotic growth factors such as *TGF-β* initiated as soon as possible to prevent further disease progression. • Steroids have no role in treatment. • Lung transplantation is an option for advanced disease.

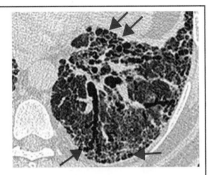

Red arrows show honeycombing. Blue arrows show bronchiectasis, or abnormally dilated airways. (Reproduced with permission from First Aid for the USMLE Step 1 2019. New York, NY: McGraw-Hill; 2019.)

Additional Considerations	
	Screening: Routine screening is not recommended for IPF. However, in patients diagnosed with IPF, TTE can evaluate for secondary pulmonary hypertension and cor pulmonale arising from chronic lung disease. The following tables provide non-idiopathic causes of pulmonary fibrosis.

Pneumoconioses	Associated Occupations	Comments/Associations
Coal Workers	Coal mining, foundry	• *Anthracosis* is the benign accumulation of carbon commonly seen in city dwellers
Asbestosis	Shipbuilding, roofing, plumbing	• CXR shows lower lobe fibrosis and calcified pleural plaques, commonly also has pleural effusion • Lung cancer more common than malignant mesothelioma • Bronchoalveolar lavage with Prussian Blue staining will show golden-brown fusiform rods "dumbbell shaped" asbestos (ferruginous) bodies.
Berylliosis	Aerospace, nuclear weapons, dental prosthesis	• Affects upper lobe • Beryllium lymphocyte proliferation test is the initial test
Silicosis	Mining, sandblasting, foundry	• "Eggshell" calcifications of hilar lymph nodes • Increased susceptibility to TB

Connective Tissue Diseases Associated with Pulmonary Fibrosis	Other Common Pulmonary Manifestations
Systemic Lupus Erythematosus (SLE)	Disappearing lung
Rheumatoid arthritis (RA)	Pleural effusions, bronchiolitis obliterans, lung nodules
Sjogren's	Lymphocytic interstitial pneumonia (LIP)
Scleroderma	Pulmonary hypertension, non-specific interstitial pneumonia (NSIP)
Polymyositis/Dermatomyositis	Bronchiolitis obliterans, NSIP

CASE 8 | Sarcoidosis

A 37-year-old woman with no previous medical history presents with a 2-month history of exertional dyspnea and non-productive cough. She has occasional chest pain that is not related to exertion and chronic generalized muscle aches. She has no orthopnea or PND. She has been using over-the-counter eye drops frequently to treat her red and occasionally dry eyes. She takes no other medications and is currently employed as a lawyer. She has not traveled and her substance use and family history is unremarkable. On physical exam, her vital signs are temperature 37.2°C, blood pressure 124/74 mmHg, pulse 82/min, respirations 20/min. BMI is 28. On exam, she has a purplish-red indurated plaque on the nose (lupus pernio). Her right eye demonstrates ciliary injection (uveitis). Cardiac examination is notable for a loud P2. There is no increased JVP. Auscultation of the lungs reveals bilateral fine diffuse crackles. She has no leg edema but has tender subcutaneous nodules along the extensor surface of both legs (erythema nodosum). CXR reveals bilateral hilar adenopathy and bilateral reticulonodular opacities.

Conditions with Similar Presentations	**Heart failure:** May also present with dyspnea on exertion but often have additional signs and symptoms (orthopnea, PND, increased JVP). **COPD:** May present with dyspnea and cough but usually have long history of smoking, and expiratory wheezing on exam. **Asthma:** May present with dyspnea and cough but may also have history of atopy or triggers and exam with expiratory wheezing. **Interstitial lung disease (ILD):** May present with dyspnea and cough and may be associated with other underlying conditions with systemic findings such as rheumatoid arthritis, SLE, and dermatomyositis. **Pneumoconiosis:** May present with dyspnea and cough but will have occupational exposure in their history.
Initial Diagnostic Testing	• Check CXR followed by CT chest without IV contrast • Rule out other diseases, including TB or HIV • Assess organ involvement (PFTs, ophthalmologic exam, ECG, echocardiogram) • Bronchoscopy/biopsy to confirm diagnosis in some cases (see Discussion)
Next Steps in Management	• For symptomatic patients, start glucocorticoids

Discussion	Sarcoidosis is an idiopathic disease characterized by noncaseating granulomas with widespread organ involvement. A small percentage of patients can develop restrictive lung disease characterized by parenchymal fibrosis. Other organs that can be affected include eyes (uveitis), heart (conduction abnormalities or cardiomyopathy), the cranial nerves (seventh nerve palsy), skin (lupus pernio, erythema nodosum), and joints (rheumatoid arthritis–like arthropathy).
	
	History:
	• Most common symptoms are cough and dyspnea.
	• Nonspecific constitutional symptoms include fatigue, fever, night sweats, and weight loss.
	• Higher incidence in women between the ages of 20 and 60, and is more common in those of African or Northern European descent.
	
	Physical exam:
	• May have reduced breath sounds.
	• Skin findings: Lupus pernio (discolored, indurated, raised lesions, usually on the face), erythema nodosum (tender raised areas, usually on the shins).
	• Involvement of other systems such as restrictive cardiomyopathy and arrhythmias, joint swelling and stiffness, cranial nerve palsies, uveitis.
	
	Diagnostics: There is no single test to diagnose sarcoidosis. Diagnosis can be made using the following principles:
	• Compatible clinical and CXR/CT findings.
	• Excluding other illnesses with similar presentations.
	• Biopsy (if needed) showing noncaseating granulomas. Biopsy is not needed if patients have the following two sarcoidosis-related syndromes:
	  • Lofgren syndrome: Fever, erythema nodosum, arthralgias, and bilateral hilar adenopathy.
	  • Heerfordt syndrome: Uveitis, parotid enlargement, fever, and lupus pernio.

CASE 8 | Sarcoidosis *(continued)*

Discussion	
	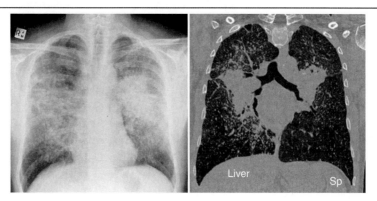 CXR showing mediastinal and hilar lymphadenopathy and bilateral air-space consolidations and septal thickening. (Reproduced with permission from First Aid for the USMLE Step 1 2019. New York, NY: McGraw-Hill; 2019.) • CXR findings are divided into four stages: • Stage I: Bilateral hilar adenopathy • Stage II: Bilateral hilar adenopathy and parenchymal infiltrates • Stage III: Parenchymal infiltrates with no hilar adenopathy • Stage IV: Fibrosis with or without cysts and masses • Noncontrast chest CT may better demonstrate the extent of lymph node and parenchymal involvement. • Pulmonary function tests can show restrictive defect and/or reduced DLCO. • Serum calcium may be elevated due to increased 1, 25-dihydroxyvitamin D3 production by macrophages in granulomas. • Serum ACE level is neither sensitive nor specific (can be used as a supportive test, but not confirmatory). **Management:** • Patients with asymptomatic bilateral hilar adenopathy can be observed with no biopsy or treatment. • Treatment is recommended for symptomatic pulmonary disease or other vital organ involvement (brain, eye, kidney, heart, liver). • First-line treatment for symptomatic patients is glucocorticoids (e.g., prednisone) followed by immunosuppressive agent (methotrexate, azathioprine, leflunomide). • If pulmonary involvement results in severe fibrosis, patient may require lung transplant. • Evaluate for and treat extrapulmonary involvement.
Additional Considerations	*Once a diagnosis is made, evaluation of extrapulmonary involvement should be completed, and include:* • Ophthalmologic exam (visual acuity, tonometry, slit lamp, and fundoscopic testing) to evaluate for optic neuritis or uveitis. • ECG to evaluate for heart block and arrhythmias. • Echocardiogram to evaluate for pericardial effusion, valve abnormalities, and right heart complications, including pulmonary hypertension.

HYPOXIA

Hypoxia refers to under-oxygenation of cells, tissues, and organs. It differs from hypoxemia, which refers to low partial pressure of oxygen in the blood.

The exact threshold of SaO_2 and/or PaO_2 that defines hypoxia has not been established and varies by context. Generally, a resting SaO_2 ≤95% in a healthy patient is considered abnormal. A PaO_2 <80 mmHg is generally considered abnormal in patients without any underlying lung disease.

An ABG is usually the first lab test performed to determine the etiology. The ABG allows us to calculate the difference in oxygen levels in the alveoli (PAO_2) versus the arteries (PaO_2), or the A-a gradient. In general, a normal A-a gradient is <10 mmHg, but it increases with age.

$$Normal\ Aa\ difference = \frac{Age\ (yrs) + 10}{4}$$

Alveolar CO_2 tension
(Use pCO_2 value from ABG)

$$Aa\ difference = P_AO_2 - P_aO_2$$

$$P_AO_2 = (FiO_2 \times [P_{atm} - P_{H_2O}]) - \left(\frac{PaCO_2}{Q}\right)$$

Atmospheric pressure   H$_2$O vapor pressure   Respiratory Quotient
(760 mmHg @ sea level)   (47 mmHg in the lungs)   (normally ~0.8)

Hypoxia has the following five main etiologies and is separated further based on A-a gradient, but usually only the first four are clinically relevant.

Normal A-a gradient:

1. Low inspired FiO_2 (normal $PaCO_2$): High altitude.
2. Hypoventilation (elevated $PaCO_2$): Opioid overdose, cervical spinal cord injury.

Elevated A-a gradient:

3. V/Q mismatch: Ventilation (COPD, pneumonia, pulmonary edema) or perfusion (pulmonary embolism) decreased. Corrects with supplemental oxygen.
4. Shunt: Extreme V/Q mismatch with no ventilation, not corrected with supplemental oxygen (ARDS, intracardiac shunt, atelectasis).
5. Diffusion defect: Alveolar and/or interstitial inflammation/fibrosis (emphysema, interstitial lung disease). Not usually clinically relevant because of reserve diffusion capacity at rest.

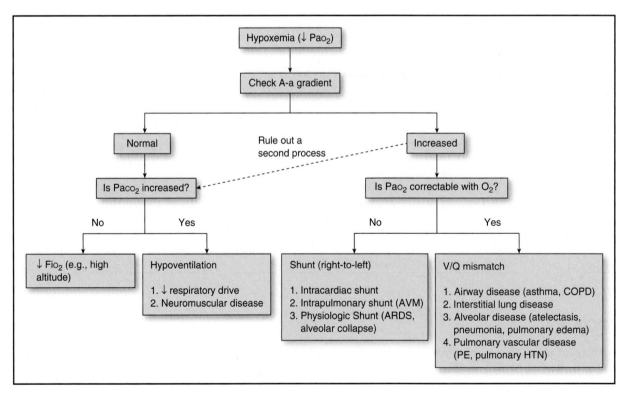

Reproduced with permission from Le T., Bhushan V., Deol M., Reyes G. First Aid For The USMLE Step 2 CK. 10th ed. New York: McGraw Hill; 2019.

Mechanical Ventilation

Patients with severe hypoxia may require invasive mechanical ventilation, which delivers positive pressure to the lungs, usually through an endotracheal tube. Other indications for mechanical ventilation include airway obstruction, hemodynamic instability, and altered mental status with inability to protect the airway.

Ventilators allow management of oxygenation by setting the FiO_2 and the positive end-expiratory pressure (PEEP), as well as ventilation (removal of CO_2) by setting the respiratory rate (RR) and tidal volume (TV).

Ventilator Settings

Oxygenation	Mechanism
FiO_2 (21% at room air)	Increased concentration of O_2 in inhaled gas → increased O_2 delivered to alveoli
PEEP	Stents open the alveoli → increase surface area for gas exchange
Ventilation (removal of CO_2)	**Mechanism**
Respiratory rate	CO_2 is exhaled
TV (volume of air inhaled or exhaled)	CO_2 is exhaled

There are complications associated with mechanical ventilation. Prolonged intubation is associated with an increased risk of aspiration and ventilator-associated pneumonia (VAP). Other serious complications include pneumothorax and right mainstem bronchus intubation, both of which may present with worsening respiratory failure and hemodynamic instability. Increased pressure readings on the ventilator may provide clues to these diagnoses.

Types of Pressure to Monitor in Volume-Controlled Mechanical Ventilation

	Peak Pressure	Plateau Pressure
Definition	Pressure in the airways and tubes	Pressure in the alveoli
Causes of Elevated Pressure	Pneumothorax, mainstem intubation, kink in ventilator tubing, secretions	Pulmonary edema, atelectasis

---

CASE 9 | Pulmonary Embolism (PE)

A 27-year-old woman presents with acute-onset chest pain and dyspnea that began 2 hours ago. The chest pain is worsened by deep inspiration. She also has pain and swelling in her left calf, which she first noticed 3 days ago after returning from a vacation overseas. She has no significant past medical history, and her only medication is a combined oral contraceptive that she started taking 6 months ago. Temperature is 37.2°C, pulse is 120/min, respirations are 28/min, blood pressure is 110/76 mmHg, and SpO_2 92% on room air. On exam, the patient is anxious and in respiratory distress. Cardiac examination is unremarkable, and the lungs are clear to auscultation bilaterally. Her left calf is tender, mildly erythematous, and larger than the right. A urine pregnancy test is negative.

Conditions with Similar Presentations	**Pneumothorax:** Can also present with acute pleuritic chest pain and dyspnea, but physical exam will have unilateral decreased breath sounds and hyperresonance to percussion.
	Pericarditis: Presents with pleuritic chest pain that improves with leaning forward and exam may have a pericardial rub and/or decreased heart sounds (if pericardial effusion present). ECG shows diffuse ST elevations and PR depressions.
	Myocardial infarction: Patients with cardiac risk factors and ECG may show ST elevations (if STEMI) and troponin levels will be elevated.
	Costochondritis: Chest pain is reproducible on exam by palpation.
Initial Diagnostic Tests	• Confirm diagnosis with CT pulmonary angiography. • Consider V/Q scan if contrast contraindicated (allergy, kidney disease)
Management	• Therapeutic anticoagulation (LMWH, heparin, or direct oral anticoagulant [DOAC])
Discussion	PE refers to an embolus to the pulmonary arterial vasculature, leading to partial or complete vascular occlusion and inability to perfuse the associated alveoli. Pulmonary thromboemboli usually originate from a deep vein thrombosis (DVT). Occlusion of the pulmonary artery results in a V/Q mismatch because ventilation remains the same, yet perfusion is absent ("dead space"). This can lead to respiratory distress (e.g., hypoxemia, tachypnea, tachycardia). Very large pulmonary emboli may cause acute right-sided heart failure accompanied by hemodynamic instability.

CASE 9 | Pulmonary Embolism (PE) *(continued)*

Discussion	
	History: • Sudden onset of symptoms (e.g., pleuritic chest pain, dyspnea, respiratory distress, cough) or may be minimally symptomatic. • Hemoptysis can be a presenting symptom in ~10% of cases. • Risk factors for venous thromboembolism include recent prolonged immobility, post-surgery, estrogen-based contraceptives, malignancy, smoking, obesity, prior DVT or PE, hypercoagulable states. **Physical exam:** • Patients with clinically significant PE will have tachypnea. • Additional symptoms may vary from none to obstructive shock. • May show evidence of a DVT (e.g., leg swelling, tenderness, erythema, palpable cord). • Lungs typically clear bilaterally but may hear wheezing (PF4-induced bronchospasm). • Cardiovascular exam may reveal signs of pulmonary hypertension (loud P2, increased splitting of S2), or right heart failure (increased JVP, S3, edema). **Diagnostics:** • Since PE can have a variety of presentations, Wells criteria is helpful in guiding whether imaging should be performed to detect a PE.

Wells Criteria for PE	
Factor	**Score**
Clinical signs and symptoms of DVT	+3
PE is #1 diagnosis OR equally likely	+3
Heart rate >100 bpm	+1.5
Immobilization at least 3 days *or* surgery in the previous 4 weeks	+1.5
Previous, objectively diagnosed DVT or PE	+1.5
Hemoptysis	+1
Malignancy with treatment within 6 months, or palliative treatment	+1

Wells Score	Interpretation and Management
<2	Low probability of PE Use PE Rule-Out Criteria (see below) or D-dimer (high negative predictive value) to r/o PE
2-6	Moderate probability of PE Check D-dimer and if high → CT pulmonary angiography or V/Q scan
>6	High probability of PE CT pulmonary angiography or V/Q scan

The Pulmonary Embolism Rule-Out Criteria
(If all are present, < 2% chance of a PE = PE ruled out.)
Age <50 years
Heart rate <100 bpm
Oxyhemoglobin saturation ≥95%
No hemoptysis
No estrogen use
No prior DVT or PE
No unilateral leg swelling
No surgery/trauma requiring hospitalization within the prior 4 weeks

CASE 9 | Pulmonary Embolism (PE) *(continued)*

Discussion	• Confirm diagnosis with CT pulmonary angiography.

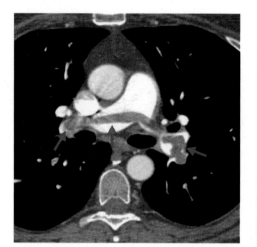

Image demonstrates axial cuts with contrast (white) filling the pulmonary arteries. Red arrows indicate filling defects (dark), representing the emboli. (Reproduced with permission from First Aid for the USMLE Step 1 2019. New York, NY: McGraw-Hill; 2019).

• ECG usually shows sinus tachycardia. In some cases, there may be an "$S_1Q_3T_3$" pattern, indicating right heart strain. The pattern is characterized by a large S-wave in lead I, a Q-wave in lead III, and an inverted T-wave in lead III.

Management:
• Supportive care (e.g., supplemental O_2).
• Therapeutic anticoagulation for at least 3 months (IV unfractionated heparin, subcutaneous low molecular weight heparin, DOACs).
• If hemodynamically unstable (aka "massive" or "high risk" PE), consider thrombolysis with systemic tPA, catheter-directed tPA, or embolectomy.

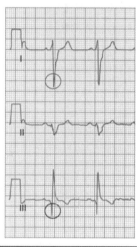

The S1Q3T3 pattern can be seen in right ventricular dysfunction such as acute PE. S-waves are observed in lead I (blue circle), Q-waves in lead III (red circle), and inverted T-waves also in lead III (yellow box). (Reproduced with permission from Timothy MF, PF. Fedullo, Pulmonary Thromboembolic Disease In: M A. Grippi, CS Dela; Fishman's Pulmonary Diseases and Disorders, 6ed; New York: McGraw Hill, 2023.)

Additional Considerations	**Prevention:** Appropriate anticoagulation of patients with **DVT** reduces risk of PE. **Virchow's triad** effectively characterizes the various clinical states that may predispose a patient to VTE. • Stasis (immobility, bed rest, long flight, post-surgical) • Hypercoagulability (malignancy, estrogen therapy, hypercoagulable states [e.g., factor V Leiden]) • Vessel wall injury (from trauma or surgery)

Pulmonary emboli are most commonly venous thromboemboli as discussed above, but they may also be fat, air, amniotic fluid, septic, or tumor.

Type of Embolism and Etiology	Mechanism and Clinical Presentation	Diagnosis and Treatment
Fat Caused by bone fractures, orthopedic surgery, sickle vaso-occlusive crisis, or liposuction	• The free fatty acids increase permeability, induce capillary leak syndrome, and trigger platelet aggregation. • Vague chest pain, shortness of breath; may have petechiae, particularly involving the conjunctiva, oral mucosa, and upper half of the body. Tachypnea and fever associated with disproportionate tachycardia. Neurological manifestations include drowsiness, confusion, decreased level of consciousness, and seizures.	Clinical diagnosis: CXR and CTA may be normal because emboli are numerous but too small to be detected. Supportive treatment. Prevention: Early immobilization of fractures.
Air Iatrogenic (e.g., central line placement/removal, positive pressure ventilation) or decompression sickness (seen in ascending deep-water divers)	• Large air emboli can obstruct the right ventricular outflow tract or pulmonary arterioles, leading to V/Q mismatch, dyspnea + tachypnea + hypoxemia ± obstructive shock.	Treat with high-flow or hyperbaric oxygen. Place patient in a position left lateral decubitus (Durant maneuver) or head down (Trendelenburg position). This places the right ventricular outflow tract inferior to the right ventricle so air migrates to apex of right ventricle where it is less likely to embolize.
Amniotic fluid Rare but catastrophic complication of labor/delivery: amniotic fluid enters maternal circulation	• Emboli to the heart and lungs cause cardiac dysfunction and respiratory distress. The debris and fluid activate the coagulation system, potentially leading to disseminated intravascular coagulation. • Abrupt onset of respiratory distress, hemodynamic instability, coagulopathy, and/or neurologic symptoms. May lead to cardiovascular collapse and death.	Treatment is supportive (e.g., respiratory, hemodynamic, and coagulation support). The fetus should be delivered as soon as the mother is stabilized.
Septic A complication of infective endocarditis or pelvic thrombophlebitis	• Right-sided endocarditis and pelvic thrombophlebitis (a complication of endomyometritis) can produce emboli that enter the pulmonary circulation, causing symptoms due to both vessel occlusion and infection. • Chest imaging will show bilateral and multifocal consolidations. Some consolidations may cavitate due to necrosis.	Antibiotics directed at organisms found in blood cultures.

CASE 10 | Acute Respiratory Distress Syndrome (ARDS)

A 44-year-old man with alcohol use disorder presents to the ED with nausea, vomiting, and severe epigastric pain that has been increasing in intensity over the past 2 days. He drinks a pint of vodka every day and has no other substance use. He is in moderate distress, his temperature is 38°C, blood pressure 100/80, pulse 130/min, respirations 22, and SpO_2 95%. BMI is 20 and there is tenderness to palpation in the epigastric region with normoactive bowel sounds. Lipase is elevated. He is admitted for treatment of acute pancreatitis. The next day, the patient reports feeling fatigued and short of breath. His respirations are 28/min and SpO_2 at 88% on room air, which does not improve with 100% supplemental oxygen. On exam, there are bilateral diffuse crackles but no JVD or peripheral edema. CXR shows diffuse bilateral infiltrates. During the evaluation, he decompensates further and requires endotracheal intubation and mechanical ventilation.

Conditions with Similar Presentations	**Cardiogenic pulmonary edema** and **iatrogenic volume overload:** Can cause respiratory failure but will have signs of fluid overload (peripheral edema, JVD, S3) on exam. **Diffuse alveolar hemorrhage:** Can also cause acute respiratory failure but will present with hemoglobin drop, cough, fever, and hemoptysis.
Initial Diagnostic Tests	• Check ABG, CXR • Consider ECG, BNP, CT chest
Next Steps in Management	• Maintain adequate oxygenation via mechanical ventilation and low tidal volume lung protective ventilation • Treat the underlying cause as well as associated complications

CASE 10 | Acute Respiratory Distress Syndrome (ARDS) *(continued)*

Discussion	ARDS is a diffuse lung injury causing severe hypoxia. ARDS results from either direct pulmonary insult (e.g., pneumonia) or release of inflammatory mediators from other organs (e.g., pancreatitis). Alveolar inflammation and damage lead to increased alveolar-capillary permeability, promoting leakage of fluid and cytokines into the interstitial space and alveoli. This leads to impaired gas exchange and hypoxemia due to profound V/Q mismatch. Because there is shunting there is minimal improvement with 100% supplemental oxygen. 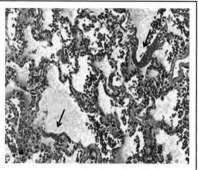 Arrow shows hyaline membrane. Note the pink proteinaceous edema fluid within alveoli. (Reproduced with permission from First Aid for the USMLE Step 1 2019. New York, NY: McGraw-Hill; 2019.)

A useful mnemonic for ARDS (based on Berlin 2012 criteria) is:
- **A**bnormal CXR (bilateral lung opacities) (see figure)
- **R**espiratory failure <1 week
- **D**ecreased PaO_2/FiO_2 (ratio <300) indicating hypoxia due to intrapulmonary shunting and diffusion abnormalities
- **S**ymptoms not due to cardiogenic edema or fluid overload

History:
- Respiratory distress, dyspnea, tachypnea, and tachycardia due to increased work of breathing.
- Causes include sepsis, aspiration pneumonitis, severe trauma, pancreatitis, pulmonary contusion, multiple fractures, burns, inhalation injuries (smoke, chlorine gas, near drowning), massive transfusion and transfusion-related acute lung injury (TRALI), drugs (amiodarone, bleomycin), radiation.

Physical exam:
- Pulse oximetry reveals hypoxia minimally responsive to supplemental oxygen.
- Bilateral diffuse crackles.
- Absent signs of volume overload (e.g., peripheral edema, JVD, S3).

Diagnostics:
- ABG to calculate PaO_2/FiO_2 and determine the severity of ARDS.
- CXR to demonstrate bilateral pulmonary infiltrates.
- ECG and BNP to rule out cardiogenic causes of pulmonary infiltrates.
- If patient is stable, CT chest can be obtained and can also consider bronchoscopy and bronchoalveolar lavage to identify pulmonary causes of ARDS and other complications.

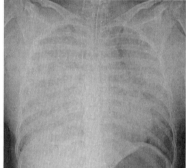 Reproduced with permission from First Aid for the USMLE Step 1 2019. New York, NY: McGraw-Hill; 2019.

Management: There is no direct treatment that is effective in decreasing the lung injury in ARDS. Management consists of supporting oxygenation with mechanical ventilation and treating the underlying cause.

Mechanical ventilation settings should be guided by:
- Low tidal volumes: 4–6 cc/kg ideal body weight.
- Use of higher PEEP (>5 cm H_2O).
- FiO_2 to <60% to avoid oxygen toxicity. |
| **Additional Considerations** | **Complications:** Pulmonary hypertension or pulmonary fibrosis. Other complications are related to mechanical ventilation (pneumothorax, VAP, tracheal stenosis) or critical illness (venous thromboembolism, GI ulcers).

Pediatric:

ARDS in children: Is most commonly precipitated by respiratory viral or bacterial pathogens. Other risk factors include pulmonary contusion, inhalational injury, near drowning, sepsis, trauma, and burns. Diagnostic criteria are similar in adult and pediatric groups.

Neonatal respiratory distress syndrome: Is primarily caused by surfactant deficiency, often seen in premature babies. With low to absent surfactant, the surface tension within alveolar walls is high. High surface tension results in low compliance, resulting in collapse of alveoli. This can be seen on chest x-ray as a characteristic ground-glass appearance.

Maternal diabetes (due to high fetal insulin) and C-section delivery (due to low fetal glucocorticoid release as compared to vaginal delivery) are additional risk factors. |

CASE 11 | Group I Pulmonary Arterial Hypertension (PAH)

A 58-year-old man with hypertension and obesity presents with new-onset bilateral lower extremity edema and abdominal bloating over the past 3 weeks. He has had generalized fatigue and progressive dyspnea on exertion over the last 6 months. He has not had fevers, chills, or cough. He has no history of substance use and is only on lisinopril for his hypertension. On exam, his vital signs are temperature 37.0°C, respiratory rate 26/min, pulse 104 beats/min, blood pressure 136/82 mmHg, BMI 34, and a pulse oximetry on room air showing blood oxygenation of 86% that increases to 94% after giving oxygen at 2 L/min via nasal cannula. Lungs are clear and cardiac exam is notable for JVD, a holosystolic murmur at the left sternal border that increases with inspiration, a loud P2, wide splitting of S2, and a parasternal heave. The PMI is not displaced. There is hepatomegaly and bilateral lower extremity pitting edema.

Conditions with Similar Presentations	**Left-sided heart failure:** Can also present with dyspnea on exertion, and eventual signs of right-sided heart failure (lower extremity edema, and elevated JVP) but exam also shows pulmonary crackles, S3, and a displaced PMI. **Cirrhosis:** Can also cause lower extremity edema, dyspnea on exertion, and abdominal bloating, but history (alcohol use, chronic viral hepatitis, non-alcoholic steatohepatitis (NASH)) and imaging (RUQ US or CT) and hypoalbuminemia or elevated INR will help differentiate. **ILD:** Can also present with worsening dyspnea on exertion in patients with rheumatologic diseases and signs of right-heart failure but CT chest findings show parenchymal disease.
Initial Diagnostic Testing	• Echocardiogram (Echo), followed by right heart catheterization to confirm. • Consider ECG, chest x-ray, and other tests to rule out other causes.
Next Steps in Management	• Supplemental oxygen. • Medical management of group I PAH consists of phosphodiesterase inhibitors, endothelin receptor antagonists, and prostacyclin analogs (see medication table). • Treat underlying causes of pulmonary hypertension if not idiopathic.
Discussion	PAH is high blood pressure in the pulmonary vasculature and has a variety of causes (see table). Group I is progressive and fatal without transplantation. The remaining groups are managed with medical therapies. • In all causes of Group I PAH, the pulmonary arteries become thickened and stiff. • In the case of hereditary pulmonary hypertension, inactivation of the *BMPR2* gene can cause unchecked proliferation of the vascular smooth muscle, resulting in increased arterial pressures. • Connective tissue diseases (e.g., scleroderma, lupus) can also cause narrowing of the lumen in the pulmonary arteries. • HIV-associated pulmonary hypertension does not correlate to the severity of HIV disease. **History:** • Progressive dyspnea. • Risk factors: Family history of pulmonary hypertension, obesity, congenital heart disease, history of the autoimmune conditions, HIV infection, diet pill use (aminorex, fenfluramine, and dexfenfluramine). **Physical exam:** • Parasternal heave, loud P2, initially normal splitting of S2, then increased splitting as RV fails. • RV failure, especially if there is RV dilation, can lead to tricuspid regurgitation and a holosystolic murmur that increases with inspiration. **Diagnostics:** • Initial transthoracic echo, then right heart catheterization demonstrating pulmonary arterial pressures (PAP) over 25 mmHg with normal pulmonary capillary wedge pressures. • Consider: ECG, chest x-ray, 6-minute walk test, PFTs, V/Q scanning, autoimmune serologies (Sjögren syndrome, scleroderma, SLE), HIV test to rule out other causes. **Management:** • Supplemental oxygen • Medical management (see table) • Manage underlying condition, if present
Additional Considerations	**Complications:** Related complications of pulmonary hypertension include cor pulmonale (right heart failure) and arrhythmias. **Cor pulmonale:** Right-sided heart failure that will cause pre-pulmonary fluid retention (elevated JVP, hepatomegaly, pitting edema) and signs of right heart strain such as a heave, loud P2, increased splitting of S2.

World Health Organization (WHO) Groups of Pulmonary Hypertension

Group I	Primary PAH (e.g., Sjögren, scleroderma, SLE, amphetamines, fenfluramine, HIV, hereditary [*BMPR2* gene])
Group II	Left heart failure
Group III	Pulmonary disease (e.g., COPD, IPF)
Group IV	Thromboembolic disease (e.g., chronic PE)
Group V	Other causes (where mechanism is unclear, e.g., sarcoidosis, sickle cell)

Medications Used to Treat Group 1 PAH

Medications	Mechanism of Lowering Pulmonary Artery Pressure	Side Effects/Contraindications
Dihydropyridine calcium channel blockers (amlodipine)	Blocks calcium channel leading to smooth muscle relaxation and vasodilation	Edema, headaches, reflex tachycardia Contraindicated in Hypertrophic cardiomyopathy (HCM) (reduces afterload which can increase outflow obstruction)
Endothelin receptor antagonists (bosentan, macitentan, ambrisentan)	Competitively inhibits endothelin-1 receptor and reduces vasoconstriction in pulmonary arteries	Hepatotoxicity Monitor transaminases, teratogenicity, and embryotoxicity
Prostacyclin analogs (epoprostenol, treprostinil, iloprost)	Long-acting prostacyclin that induces vascular smooth muscle relaxation, and vasodilation	GI upset, headaches, hypotension, jaw pain
Prostacyclin receptor agonist (selexipag)	Induces vascular smooth muscle relaxation	Do not take with CYP inhibitors
PDE5 inhibitors (sildenafil, tadalafil)	Increases levels of cGMP intracellularly and causes relaxation of smooth muscle	Headache, dizziness, flushing, dyspepsia, muscle ache, priapism Do not take with nitroglycerin because life-threatening hypotension may occur

CASE 12 | Aspiration Pneumonia

An 82-year-old man with dementia, two prior strokes, and chronic dysphagia is brought to the ED with 1 week of cough, dyspnea, and fevers. He has been producing green, foul-smelling sputum. Over the past 2 years, he has had three episodes of pneumonia. Temperature is 38.3°C, pulse is 108/min, respirations are 22/min, blood pressure is 138/86 mmHg, and SpO_2 92% on room air. On exam, the patient is in moderate respiratory distress. Pulmonary auscultation reveals crackles at the right lung base; cardiac and abdominal examinations are unremarkable. He is alert and oriented to person and place, but not time. A chest x-ray shows an infiltrate without air fluid levels in the right lower lobe.

Conditions with Similar Presentations	**Aspiration pneumonitis:** Is caused by aspiration of acidic gastroesophageal contents, causing direct injury to airways. Subsequent inflammation leads to pulmonary edema, presenting as possible respiratory distress, cough, and crackles on pulmonary auscultation. Chest imaging reveals new pulmonary infiltrates. In contrast to aspiration pneumonia, pneumonitis will have a more rapid onset (e.g., hours) after aspiration. Treatment is supportive. Antibiotics are not indicated. **Community-acquired pneumonia:** Can also present with fever, productive cough, dyspnea, hypoxia, and infiltrate on chest x-ray but history and risk factors for aspiration (see below) will be absent. **Viral respiratory infections (influenza, COVID-19):** Can also present with fever, cough, hypoxia, and dyspnea but chest x-ray may be normal or show diffuse ground-glass opacities.
Initial Diagnostic Tests	CXR

CASE 12 | Aspiration Pneumonia *(continued)*

Management	• Respiratory support (e.g., supplemental O_2) • Antibiotics

Discussion	Aspiration provides pathogens a route for colonizing oropharyngeal organisms to enter the lungs, leading to pneumonia. In many patients, a poor cough reflex prevents clearance of aspirated contents, which serve as a nidus for infection.
	• Common pathogens are colonizing anaerobes of the oropharynx and gastrointestinal tract (e.g., *Fusobacterium, Bacteroides*) and aerobes (e.g., *S. pneumoniae, S. aureus, P. aeruginosa, H. influenzae*).
	• Onset is *not* immediately after the aspiration (in contrast with aspiration pneumonitis), as the infection requires time to develop.
	• The most common site of aspiration is the right lung, whether sitting or supine, as the right main bronchus is more in line with the trachea.
	
	History:
	• Often in elderly patients (cough, fever) with the following risk factors: unconsciousness/sedation, esophageal disease (e.g., dysphagia, Zenker's diverticulum, esophageal cancer), poor cough reflex (intoxication, dementia, and post-stroke), mechanically ventilated patients.
	• Patients may experience recurrent aspiration pneumonia.
	
	Physical exam:
	• Fever (+/– accompanying tachycardia), tachypnea, and hypoxemia.
	• Lung exam: Crackles, dullness to percussion, increased tactile vocal fremitus, bronchophony, and/or egophony over the affected region.
	
	Diagnostics:
	• Clinical diagnosis: Combination of risk factors for aspiration, clinical features (e.g., fever, dyspnea, cough, purulent sputum production, and infiltrates on chest imaging).
	• Attempts to determine the causative organism(s) include sputum gram stain and cultures, blood cultures, COVID-19 and respiratory viral panel testing, CT chest if CXR normal, and MRSA screening.
	
	Management:
	• Supplemental oxygen.
	• Antibiotic regimen is determined in the same way as that for other pneumonias based on the risk of colonization with resistant organisms (MRSA, *P. aeruginosa*) and severity.
	  • Outpatient regimens
	    • No comorbidities: Doxycycline or amoxicillin
	    • Comorbidities: Quinolone or ceftriaxone + macrolide
	    • Penicillin allergy: Moxifloxacin or clindamycin
	  • Inpatient regimens
	    • Quinolone or beta-lactam + macrolide
	  • Severe pneumonia in the ICU
	    • No risk of *P. aeruginosa*: ceftriaxone + macrolide or levofloxacin
	    • Risk for *P. aeruginosa*: Piperacillin/tazobactam + either of
	      • Levofloxacin +/– gentamicin
	      • Azithromycin + gentamicin

Additional Considerations	**Complications:** Lung abscess, empyema. **Prevention:** Reduce aspiration risk factors; patients at risk for aspiration should be evaluated with a swallow study to determine safe and unsafe foods.

CASE 13 | Adult Obstructive Sleep Apnea (OSA)

A 57-year-old woman with hypertension presents for evaluation of fatigue and snoring. She sleeps 8 hours per night but wakes up tired and often with morning headaches and a dry cough. She snores loudly at night, and her partner notes that she sometimes appears to have stopped breathing. On occasion, she has fallen asleep while driving or working. She takes her prescribed hypertension medications consistently and has no substance use. Her vital signs include blood pressure 160/90 mmHg, pulse 90/min, respiration 16/min, and BMI is 40 kg/m². She has a neck circumference of 18″, and her oropharynx is crowded with large tonsils and tongue.

Conditions with Similar Presentations	**Primary snoring** and **insufficient sleep** (medical students and residents!): Are very common and require polysomnography (PSG) to differentiate from OSA (will not have apneas on PSG). **Central sleep apnea:** Apneas with **absent** respiratory effort (unlike OSA), at times associated with Cheyne-Stokes breathing (CSB), due to dysfunction within the brainstem respiratory centers. Most commonly seen in heart failure, cerebrovascular disease, or opioid usage. **Narcolepsy:** Is excessive daytime sleepiness due to impaired regulation of sleep–wake cycle, associated with cataplexy (loss of muscle tone after intense emotion), hallucinations before going to sleep or right before waking, and/or sleep paralysis (unable to move for minutes just prior to or just after sleep). PSG must be normal (to rule out OSA and insufficient sleep), and additional multiple sleep latency test would show decreased sleep latency and rapid REM onset. **Depression:** May have daytime sleepiness accompanied with feelings of hopelessness and chronic fatigue.
Initial Diagnostic Tests	Screening tests: STOP BANG.

STOP-BANG
Do you **S**nore loudly?
Do you often feel **T**ired, fatigued, or sleepy during the daytime?
Has anyone **O**bserved you stop breathing during sleep?
Do you have (or are you being treated for) high blood **P**ressure?
BMI ≥35
Age >50
Neck circumference > 40 cm (15.7 inches)
Male (**G**ender)
Score (1 point for each item)
<3: Low risk of OSA
≥3: High risk of OSA

Confirm diagnosis with **PSG**.

Next Steps in Management	Continuous positive airway pressure (CPAP) and lifestyle modification for weight loss.
Discussion	OSA is a sleep disorder caused by repetitive collapse of the upper airway during sleep. Characteristic features include: obstructive apneas, hypopneas, and/or respiratory effort–related arousals. During sleep, upper airway structures lose tone and collapse, causing physical obstruction of the airway. The patient will continue to have abdominal and chest respiratory movements, but the lack of airflow (due to obstruction) causes apnea or hypopnea, which can lead to brain cortical arousal (although the patient may not remember waking up). Each episode of apnea or hypopnea represents a reduction in breathing for at least 10 seconds that commonly results in a ≥3% drop in oxygen saturation and/or a brain cortical arousal. **History:** • Excessive daytime sleepiness, may have even been involved in motor vehicle accidents. • Sleep witnesses may note snoring, choking or gasping arousals, and apneas. • Risk factors: Obesity, large neck circumference, and family history of sleep apnea. **Physical exam:** Thick neck and crowded airway.

CASE 13 | Adult Obstructive Sleep Apnea (OSA) *(continued)*

Discussion	**Diagnostics:** • Diagnosed with PSG ("sleep study"). • Criteria for diagnosing OSA from a PSG utilizes the number of times during the study that apnea (reduction of airflow ≥90% from baseline) or hypopnea (a drop in airflow by ≥30%) occurs. Combined, these are apnea-hypopnea events and the number of times they occur per hour when averaged over the entire study is the **apnea-hypopnea index** (AHI). Sleep apnea can be diagnosed if: 1. AHI ≥5/hour with symptoms 2. AHI ≥15/hour without symptoms **Management:** • Discuss options for weight loss management, including lifestyle modifications, medications, possible bariatric surgery. • CPAP machine. • Upper airway surgery, hypoglossal nerve stimulator, or oral appliance can be considered in select patients if not tolerating CPAP, or as adjunctive therapy.
Additional Considerations	**Complications:** Increased risk of developing systemic and pulmonary hypertension. OSA may also cause a variety of cardiac arrhythmias and metabolic conditions including type 2 diabetes mellitus. There is an association between uncontrolled OSA, sudden cardiac death, MI, and stroke.

COUGH AND HEMOPTYSIS

Cough

Cough is a common symptom but also a necessary reflex to prevent retention of respiratory secretions and to clear aspirated material. Although commonly thought of as a pulmonary issue, the cough receptors can be found in the esophagus, diaphragm, and even the eardrums.

Determining the etiology of a cough is facilitated by the duration of symptoms (see table below). Obtaining a history of occupational exposures (pneumoconiosis), use of cigarettes/e-cigarettes (COPD, vaping use-associated lung injury [VALI]), family history of lung diseases (asthma, bronchiectasis), or recent history of viral infection (post-infectious cough) will also help narrow the differential diagnoses. Other symptoms or pertinent positives/negatives, such as heartburn (GERD), worse with exposure to strong smells (asthma), use of ACE-I (ACE-I–induced cough) will also guide diagnosis.

Differential Diagnosis of Cough Based on Duration of Symptoms

	Acute	Subacute	Chronic Cough
Duration	<3 weeks	3–8 weeks	>8 weeks
Common etiologies	Viral, COPD/asthma, pneumonia, irritants or foreign bodies	Postinfectious, COPD/asthma	COPD/asthma, GERD, ACE-I, ILD, cancer, infections (TB, MAI), bronchiectasis

Management of cough is primarily dependent on identifying and treating the etiology, as cough is frequently the body's defense mechanism. However, there are many over-the-counter medications that are commonly used to decrease coughing.

Medication	Mechanism
Antihistamine (loratadine)	Histamine H1 receptor antagonists
Expectorants (guaifenesin)	Decrease bronchial mucus production, making secretions easier to remove through cough or ciliary transport
Mucolytics (carbocisteine)	Decrease viscosity of bronchial secretions, making them easier to clear through coughing
Opiates and opiate derivatives (codeine)	Stimulates opiate receptors which suppress cough
Local anesthetic (benzocaine)	Anesthetizes the oropharynx
Dextromethorphan	NMDA antagonist: Inhibits medullary cough center

Management of cough secondary to chronic conditions such as COPD, asthma, or GERD includes optimization of treatment of those etiologies. For management of cough where the etiology is unclear, imaging studies such as a chest radiograph may be helpful. If imaging studies are nondiagnostic, a trial of empiric treatment for the most common causes of cough such as upper airway cough syndrome, asthma, or GERD should be done.

Evaluation of Subacute or Chronic Cough in Adults

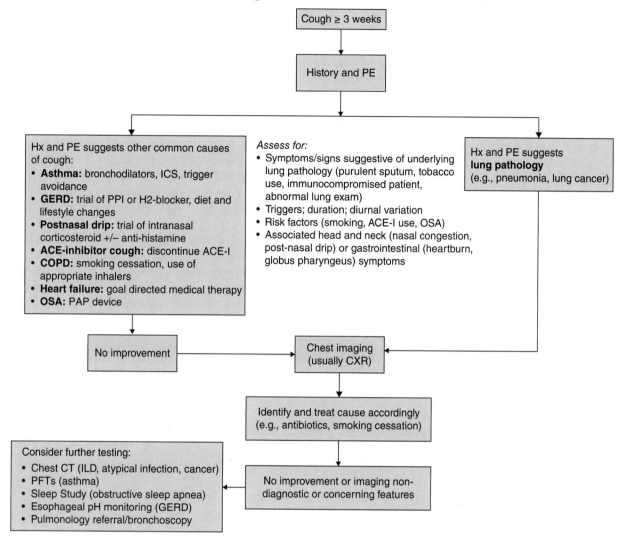

Hemoptysis

When a patient presents with hemoptysis (expectoration of blood or blood-streaked sputum), it is crucial to identify whether the expectoration of blood is significant. Significant hemoptysis can impair gas exchange, obstruct the airways, or result in hemodynamic instability. Bleeding to this extent is defined as expectoration of blood >100 mL/hour or >500 mL within 24 hours and is labeled as "life-threatening" or "massive" hemoptysis.

Etiologies of hemoptysis are summarized below. Differential alveolar hemorrhage (DAH) is a medical emergency and characterized by hemoptysis, anemia, respiratory failure, and diffuse radiographic infiltrates. It is commonly associated with autoimmune vasculitides.

Etiologies of Hemoptysis

Infectious/Inflammation	• Bronchitis (most common) • Bronchiectasis • Tuberculosis • Aspergilloma • Pneumonia • Lung abscess
Neoplasm	• Primary lung cancer • Metastasis

Etiologies of Hemoptysis (*Continued*)

Cardiovascular	• Pulmonary embolism • Heart failure • Mitral stenosis
Other	• Vasculitis (e.g., granulomatosis with polyangiitis, eosinophilic granulomatosis with polyangiitis, anti-glomerular basement membrane diseases (anti-GBM disease) • Arteriovenous malformation

Diagnostic workup of hemoptysis includes first ruling out etiologies of pseudohemoptysis (blood from the upper gastrointestinal tract or nasopharynx mimicking a lower respiratory tract source), via history and physical exam. Imaging studies such as a CXR or chest CT as well as bronchoscopy may help localize the source of bleeding. Laboratory studies such as PT, PTT, or CBC may be ordered to assess for coagulopathies. Infection is a common cause of hemoptysis (due to mucosal inflammation that causes rupture of superficial blood vessels) and can be evaluated using sputum Gram stain/culture; sputum cytology is useful to examine for malignant cells.

For management of massive hemoptysis, it is crucial to secure the airway (through intubation) to prevent death from asphyxiation. In the case of a unilateral source of bleeding, the patient should be placed bleeding side down (e.g., if source of bleeding is within the right lung, have patient lay on their right side) to prevent blood spilling over to the healthy lung. Possible next steps for diagnosis and treatment include angiography, bronchoscopy, or surgical resection. Management of hemoptysis that is not life-threatening involves identification and treatment of the underlying etiology.

CASE 14 | Bronchiectasis

An 18-year-old man with cystic fibrosis presents with a worsening productive cough, dyspnea, and fever for the past 5 days. He has had multiple similar episodes in the past, each of which eventually resolved with antibiotics. He has copious yellow-green sputum most prominent in the mornings; on occasion, the sputum has been tinged with blood. He has chronic generalized fatigue and weight loss and reports no smoking, sick contacts, chest pain, or recent travel. Temperature is 38.2°C, pulse is 104/min, respirations are 22/min, blood pressure is 124/76 mmHg, and SpO$_2$ 94% on room air. Pulmonary auscultation reveals diffuse coarse crackles; the cardiac and abdominal examinations are normal.

Conditions with Similar Presentations	**Pneumonia:** Presents with fever, productive cough, pulmonary crackles, and an infiltrate on chest imaging. **Acute bronchitis:** May have fever and cough. Most cases are viral and do not require antibiotics. The recurrent nature of this patient's symptoms suggests an underlying diagnosis beyond just pneumonia or acute bronchitis. **COPD** (including chronic bronchitis): Can also present with chronic cough, sputum production, and intermittent exacerbations but would be seen in an older patient with a smoking history.
Initial Diagnostic Tests	• Confirm diagnosis with CT chest • Check sputum for Gram stain/culture
Management	Antibiotics based on susceptibilities from previous and current cultures
Discussion	Bronchiectasis is due to chronic or recurrent airway inflammation that leads to destruction of epithelium and elastin which is replaced by collagen, resulting in abnormal bronchial dilation, stiff airways, and mucus plugs/sputum production. **History:** • History of chronic productive cough with foul-smelling sputum, occasionally with hemoptysis and intermittent exacerbations, which are usually bacterial in etiology. • May be predisposed by ↓ mucociliary escalator function (e.g., cystic fibrosis, primary ciliary dyskinesia, smoking, pulmonary malignancy). • Any condition that causes chronic/recurrent airway inflammation (e.g., TB, allergic bronchopulmonary aspergillosis, alpha-1 antitrypsin deficiency, rheumatoid arthritis, Severe Combined Immunodeficiency [SCID]). **Physical exam:** • During acute exacerbations, patients may be febrile and/or tachypneic (+/- accompanying tachycardia). • Pulmonary auscultation may reveal abnormalities such as crackles and rhonchi.

CASE 14 | Bronchiectasis *(continued)*

Discussion	**Diagnostics:**
	• Chest radiograph is a first-line study but is not diagnostic of bronchiectasis.
	• Diagnosed with CT chest showing dilated and thick-walled airways.

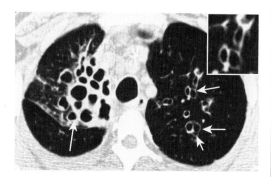

Chest computed tomography. (Left chest) Cylindrical bronchiectasis: dilated and thickened airways (arrows and insert). (Right chest) Saccular or cystic bronchiectasis: very dilated airways clustered into saccules, cysts, or grapelike clusters (arrow). (Reproduced with permission from Grippi MA, Elias JA, Fishman JA, Kotloff RM, Pack AI, Senior RM, Siegel MD. Fishman's Pulmonary Diseases and Disorders, 5e; Copyright © 2015 McGraw-Hill Education. All rights reserved.)

	• Additional evaluation includes sputum Gram stain/culture, CBC with differential.
	• If not already diagnosed, test for immunoglobulin levels and cystic fibrosis.
	Management:
	• Acute exacerbations: Antibiotics based on sputum Gram stain and culture. Resistant organisms (MRSA and *P. aeruginosa*) become more common with time.
	• Chronic management: Airway clearance techniques (chest physiotherapy) + manage underlying etiology if present (e.g., cystic fibrosis in this patient).
Additional Considerations	Antibiotic prophylaxis may be warranted for patients with frequent exacerbations.

CASE 15 | Rhinosinusitis

A 19-year-old woman presents with 4 days of cough, nasal congestion, purulent nasal discharge, and facial fullness. She has no fever, shortness of breath, or chest pain. She has been self-medicating with over-the-counter cold and allergy medications with partial symptom relief. On physical examination, her vital signs are normal and cardiopulmonary exam is unremarkable. Oropharyngeal exam reveals no erythema or exudates. There is mild facial tenderness. Anterior rhinoscopy shows mucosal edema and rhinorrhea.

Conditions with Similar Presentations	**Allergic rhinitis:** Also presents with nasal congestion and rhinorrhea but would not cause facial fullness or purulent nasal drainage. History may include personal or family history of atopy, allergic conjunctivitis. Exam findings include edematous nasal turbinates, allergic shiners (darkening under the eye), and allergic salute (transverse nasal crease, common in children). Allergic rhinitis is a type I hypersensitivity reaction to environmental triggers (e.g., pollen, dust, mold, animal hair), often in a seasonal pattern.
	Vasomotor rhinitis: Is triggered by cold exposure and resolves with removal of the offending cause. Symptoms are intermittent and are usually limited to nasal congestion and rhinorrhea.
	Acute bronchitis: Can also cause fever and cough but would not have purulent nasal discharge or facial pain tenderness.
Initial Diagnostic Tests	• Clinical diagnosis.
	• During outbreaks of influenza or COVID-19, consider performing rapid testing for these pathogens.
Next Steps in Management	• Acute viral rhinosinusitis (AVRS) is managed with acetaminophen or ibuprofen and nasal irrigation.
	• Acute bacterial rhinosinusitis (ABRS) warrants antibiotics (see discussion below).

CASE 15 | Rhinosinusitis (continued)

Discussion	Rhinosinusitis is inflammation of the nasal cavity and sinuses that is infectious or allergic in etiology, which leads to rhinorrhea and fluid buildup in the sinuses.
	• Acute infectious rhinosinusitis is most commonly viral; bacteria are responsible for a minority of cases.
	• AVRS may damage innate immune defenses and impede normal sinus drainage, predisposing to a secondary bacterial superinfection.
	Common viral pathogens are rhinovirus, parainfluenza, influenza, respiratory syncytial virus, and coronavirus. Bacterial causes are less common and include *S. pneumoniae*, *H. influenzae*, and *Moraxella catarrhalis*.
	History:
	• Rhinorrhea and facial pain/pressure/fullness are common symptoms. Location of pain indicates which sinuses are involved.
	• Cheeks: Ethmoid and or maxillary
	• Upper teeth: Maxillary
	• Around ear: Mastoid
	• Apex of head: Sphenoid
	• May report fevers, cough, congestion, fatigue, and/or myalgias.
	• May have exposure to sick contacts (e.g., family members) or work in higher-risk settings (e.g., daycare worker).
	• Symptoms are usually <4 weeks and are more common during winter.
	Physical exam:
	• May have sinus tenderness.
	• Rhinoscopy shows rhinorrhea and nasal edema.
	• +/− Fever.
	Diagnostics:
	Acute rhinosinusitis is a clinical diagnosis of:
	• ≤4 weeks of purulent nasal discharge *plus*
	• Nasal obstruction *or* facial pain/pressure/fullness.
	The vast majority of cases are viral in etiology (acute viral rhinosinusitis, AVRS).
	A *bacterial* etiology (ABRS) is suggested by:
	• Duration >10 days without improvement.
	• Biphasic pattern ("double-sickening"): Initial improvement but the after ≥3 days there is a new headache or discharge.
	• Severe manifestations for ≥3 days:
	• T >39°C
	• Purulent drainage
	• Facial pain
	Cultures of drainage should *not* be performed because they will be contaminated with normal flora. Sinus x-rays and CT are *not* indicated.
	For recurrent and/or cases unresponsive to treatment, endoscopic sinus cultures can be obtained to guide antibiotic therapy.
	Management:
	• AVRS is managed with acetaminophen, ibuprofen, nasal irrigation.
	• ABRS in immunocompetent patients with good follow-up can be managed with observation.
	• Antibiotics should be given for ABRS in immunocompromised patients, patients without assured follow-up, or patients who worsen during observation off antibiotics. Treatment is with amoxicillin-clavulanate. Second line if penicillin-allergic is doxycycline or fluoroquinolones.

CASE 15 | Rhinosinusitis (continued)

Additional Considerations	**Prevention:** Hand washing and personal protective equipment (PPE) help to limit spread of viral rhinosinusitis.
	Chronic sinusitis is diagnosed by meeting all three criteria below:
	• Sinusitis symptoms for >12 weeks.
	• Two of the following: nasal congestion/obstruction; mucopurulent drainage; facial pain/pressure/fullness; decreased sense of smell.
	• Signs of inflammation on physical exam or imaging (e.g., CT scan of sinuses).
	Surgical considerations: Sinus surgery may be indicated for chronic sinusitis that is severe or refractory to medical management.

Less common etiologies for cough include select eosinophilic pulmonary syndromes. These are relevant for Step 2.

Select Eosinophilic Pulmonary Syndromes

	Clinical Presentation	Comments
Acute eosinophilic pneumonia (PNA)	Acute onset cough, dyspnea, acute respiratory failure (70% need mechanical ventilation), pleural effusions Mostly in men and patients who smoke	BAL eosinophil count >25% *without* significant peripheral eosinophilia Pleural fluid is eosinophil-rich and exudative Tx: Steroids
Chronic eosinophilic PNA	Months of dyspnea, cough, or chest pain Mostly in women and non-smokers Associated with asthma and atopy	BAL eosinophil count >40% with peripheral eosinophilia Tx: Steroids
Eosinophilic granulomatosis with polyangiitis (EGPA)	History of severe corticosteroid-dependent asthma, rhinitis, and sinusitis May have multisystem vasculitis, arthralgias/myalgias, heart failure, renal failure, neuropathy, and/or palpable purpura	If active pneumonitis: eosinophilia on BAL and serum MPO-ANCA only positive in 40% Need four of six diagnostic criteria: asthma, peripheral eosinophilia >10%, neuropathy, pulmonary opacities, paranasal sinus abnormality, and a biopsy showing tissue eosinophilia Tx: Steroids, cyclophosphamide
Allergic bronchopulmonary aspergillosis (ABPA)	History of poorly controlled asthma or cystic fibrosis with a chronic productive cough or bronchiectasis	Peripheral blood eosinophilia, ↑ serum IgE, an immediate skin reaction and/or specific IgE/IgG antibodies to *Aspergillus fumigatus* due to type I and III hypersensitivity reactions, predisposing condition (asthma or cystic fibrosis) Radiographic findings: pulmonary opacities, central bronchiectasis, and mucus plugs Tx: Steroids; some may benefit from voriconazole
Parasites	Loffler syndrome: Coughing and wheezing with fever, coming from endemic areas; seen with Ascaris, strongyloides, toxocara, hookworm Tropical eosinophilia: Cough worse at night, splenomegaly, peripheral eosinophilia, coming from area endemic for *Wuchureria bancrofti*	Symptoms caused by the transpulmonary passage of helminth larvae causing transient pulmonary opacities and peripheral eosinophilia Stool and sputum evaluation for ova and parasites and ELISA for *Strongyloides* are helpful tests Tx: Antiparasitics (e.g., diethylcarbamazine); systemic glucocorticoids may be used for symptom control
Medications	Various presentations: Asymptomatic with pulmonary infiltrates, ±chronic cough, ±dyspnea, ±fever	Associated with NSAIDs, sulfasalazine, mesalamine, daptomycin, nitrofurantoin

Hemoptysis Mini-Cases

Cases	Key Finding
Epistaxis	**Hx:** Higher risk in patients who smoke or use intranasal drugs (cocaine), or are on anticoagulation or antiplatelet therapy for atrial fibrillation, stroke, or peripheral arterial disease (PAD) May occur due to nose picking, foreign body **PE:** Epistaxis, pseudohemoptysis **Diagnostics:** • Rhinoscopy may show bleeding, ulceration, clots • If significant bleeding, check CBC, type and screen, INR **Management:** • If anterior (more common and self-limited), perform cautery or nasal packing. • If anterior nasal packing unsuccessful, source likely posterior; consult ENT, and management includes use of posterior nasal packing (e.g., posterior balloon catheter or Foley catheter) or embolization of the bleeding vessel. • If life-threatening: Hold anticoagulation or antiplatelet therapy, consider correcting coagulopathy with blood products and consider arterial embolization. **Discussion:** Epistaxis can present as pseudohemoptysis (expectoration of blood from outside of the bronchial or pulmonary circulation). If concern for posterior epistaxis, ENT consult is needed.
Diffuse Alveolar Hemorrhage (DAH)	**Hx:** Risk factors: rheumatologic or connective tissue disease (SLE, anti-GBM disease, granulomatosis with polyangiitis, eosinophilic granulomatosis with polyangiitis). Symptoms: Abrupt onset of cough, fever, hemoptysis, shortness of breath. **PE:** Tachypnea and/or signs of autoimmune disease (e.g., skin changes, arthritis). **Diagnostics:** • CXR or CT chest may show patchy/diffuse opacities • Autoimmune studies if no known history • Bronchoscopy with bronchoalveolar lavage (BAL) will show increasingly bloody fluid to confirm diagnosis of DAH **Management:** • Supportive care including ventilatory support as needed (supplemental oxygen, mechanical ventilation) • Systemic steroids (methylprednisone) and additional immunosuppressive therapy (cyclophosphamide, rituximab) if rheumatologic cause known/suspected • Broad-spectrum antibiotics if underlying cause is unclear **Discussion:** DAH should be suspected in patients with hemoptysis and diffuse opacities on imaging. Once the diagnosis is of DAH is confirmed, underlying etiology should be identified and treated.

LUNG MALIGNANCIES

Lung cancer is the leading cause of cancer-related deaths in both men and women worldwide. High-risk exposures include tobacco use, asbestos, prior extrathoracic malignancy, radon, polycyclic aromatic hydrocarbons (produced when coal, wood, and other substances are burned), and various metals (e.g., nickel, chromium).

Lung cancer can be identified by lung cancer screening (50–80 years old, 20-pack-year or more smoking history, current tobacco use or quit in past 15 years), incidentally on chest imaging, or based on clinical signs and symptoms. Most patients who present with symptoms from their lung cancer have advanced disease. Symptoms include cough, hemoptysis, dyspnea, chest pain, and weight loss. On physical exam, wheezing and rhonchi are sometimes heard, and decreased breath sounds may be noted on the affected side due to a large lung mass or effusion. Less commonly, patients may have symptoms related to paraneoplastic syndromes. Although some paraneoplastic syndromes have classic associations with specific lung cancers (e.g., SIADH with small cell cancer), others, such as dermatomyositis and polymyositis, may also occur.

Schema for evaluation of patients with suspected lung cancer

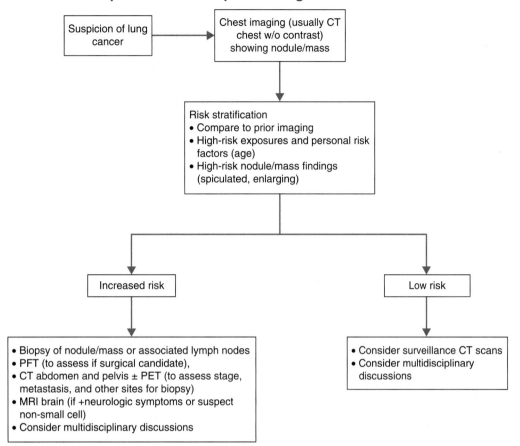

The diagnostic evaluation should be guided by shared decision making with the patient. Multidisciplinary discussions with pulmonologists, radiation oncologists, surgeons, interventional radiologists, and other specialists may be helpful in planning the evaluation. This schema does not include the workup of paraneoplastic syndromes.

Types of Lung Cancer

	Non-Small Cell			Small Cell
	Squamous	**Adenocarcinoma**	**Large Cell**	**Aka Oat Cell**
Key points		Most common 1° lung CA Most common lung CA in women and non-smokers		15% of lung CA
Associated with tobacco	Yes	No	Yes	Yes
Location	Central If peripheral, associated with cavitation	Peripheral	Peripheral	Central
Metastasis		Common to have distant mets		Early mets to brain, liver, bone
Histopathology	Nests of polygonal cells with eosinophilic cytoplasm and obvious nucleoli; intracellular bridges; Keratin pearls	Several subtypes exist; lepidic subtype has best prognosis +Mucin stain	Poorly differentiated, diagnosis of exclusion requiring surgical resection	Arise from neuroendocrine (Kulchitsky cells) in the basal bronchial epithelium Neuroendocrine markers (stains): Neuron-specific enolase, chromogranin A, synaptophysin, and CD56

Types of Lung Cancer (*Continued*)

	Non-Small Cell			Small Cell
	Squamous	**Adenocarcinoma**	**Large Cell**	**Aka Oat Cell**
Associated mutations	TP53 and P-450	Genetic mutations are *EGFR*, *KRAS*, and *ALK*, and are therapeutic targets		+ *myc* oncogene mutation
Paraneoplastic phenomena and other associations	Hypercalcemia due to PTHrP	Hypertrophic pulmonary osteoarthropathy (clubbing) Non-bacterial verrucous endocarditis (marantic endocarditis)	Gynecomastia	SVC syndrome, SIADH, Cushing syndrome, Lambert-Eaton syndrome
Treatment options	Surgery (if early stage and good lung function) Chemotherapy Immunotherapy (PDL1 and PD1 inhibitors) Targeted therapy (EGFR inhibitors, KRAS inhibitors) Radiation			Chemotherapy Immunotherapy Radiation

CASE 16 | Solitary Solid Pulmonary Nodule (SPN)

A 59-year-old man with a 30-pack-year smoking history presents to the ED with a dry cough, low-grade fevers, rhinorrhea, and mild dyspnea on exertion for the past week. Temperature is 36.8°C, pulse is 90/min, respirations are 18/min, blood pressure is 122/84 mmHg, and SpO_2 97% on room air. Physical exam shows nasal congestion and pharyngeal erythema without exudate. Cardiac examination is unremarkable, and the lungs are clear to auscultation bilaterally. There is no jugular venous distension, peripheral edema, or palpable lymphadenopathy. Rapid influenza and COVID-19 testing are negative. A chest radiograph shows no evidence of pneumonia, but there is an incidental finding of a single, round opacity in the lung parenchyma. There is no prior pulmonary imaging on file for the patient, who states he is generally healthy and has no chronic conditions.

Conditions with Similar Presentations	**Lung cancer:** Can present as a solid solitary nodule. **Metastatic cancer:** Probability increases with known non-pulmonary malignancy. Metastatic "cannonball" lesions are classically bilateral and multifocal. **Tuberculosis:** Has a predilection for mid-lung fields during primary infection, and upper lung fields during reactivation. May show early signs of cavitation. **Granulomatous diseases (non-TB)** (e.g., sarcoid, endemic fungi, granulomatosis with polyangiitis, and eosinophilic granulomatosis with polyangitis: May present as a pulmonary nodule but more commonly are multiple lesions. Fungi may have early signs of cavitation.
Initial Diagnostic Tests	• Check CT chest without contrast • Biopsy indicated based on size and irregular borders on CT
Management	Depends on size/appearance on imaging and clinical lung cancer risk factors (see following discussion)
Discussion	There are multiple possible etiologies of an incidental lung mass. In most cases, excluding malignancy is necessary. A SPN is defined by: • Rounded opacity on imaging surrounded by normal lung • ≤30 mm diameter • Surrounded by pulmonary parenchyma • No associated lymphadenopathy **History:** May be an incidental finding (as in this patient), detected on routine lung cancer screening, or discovered as part of cancer staging. **Factors increasing the suspicion for malignancy include:** • Large size (≥3 cm) • Spiculated/irregular borders or non-solid components • Smoking history • Emphysema • Advanced patient age 70 • Family history of lung cancer **Physical exam:** No specific findings.

CASE 16 | Solitary Solid Pulmonary Nodule (SPN) *(continued)*

Discussion	**Diagnostics:** • If nodule was NOT originally found on CT (e.g., in a chest radiograph as in this patient), obtain a CT chest without contrast to further characterize the lesion. • FDP-PET scanning assists in determining benign (low activity) and malignant (high activity) nodules. • If indicated, options for biopsy include bronchoscopy (ideal for central lesions) or surgery (better for peripheral lesions). Consider other studies: • Depending on the location and appearance of the lesion and clinical presentation, testing for infectious etiologies (e.g., tuberculosis) may be warranted. **Management:** Depends on size/appearance on imaging and clinical lung cancer risk factors. Most clinicians follow the Fleischner Society guidelines: • ≤0.6 cm: No follow-up required. Consider CT in 1 year if patient has a high-risk factor as listed earlier. • 0.6–0.8 cm: Repeat CT chest in 6–12 months, then consider every 18–24 months. If larger on repeat imaging, then biopsy/excision. • >0.8 cm: Biopsy/excision *or* PET/CT in 3 months, depending on risk of malignancy. • If there are multiple nodules, use the most suspicious nodule.
Additional Considerations	**Screening:** Patients who satisfy all three criteria below should have annual low-dose chest CT for lung cancer screening: • Age 50–80 • ≥20-pack-year smoking history • Currently smoking or quit within the past 15 years

Additional Clinical Syndromes Based on Tumor Location

CASE 17 | Superior Vena Cava (SVC) Syndrome

A 68-year-old woman with COPD and 50-pack-year tobacco use is brought to the ED for confusion. Her family reports that she has a worsening chronic cough as well as recent facial flushing and weight loss. Temperature is 37.5°C, pulse 110/min, respirations 30/min, blood pressure 120/80 mmHg, and pulse oximetry 93% on room air. She is oriented to self only. Her face is flushed, with blanching after applying gentle pressure (facial plethora), and she has engorged neck veins and bilateral pitting edema of her arms. On auscultation, breath sounds are diminished bilaterally but no wheezing is heard.

Conditions with Similar Presentations	**Thoracic outlet syndrome (TOS):** Presents with arm swelling and paresthesia and weakness in the ulnar distribution. Causes include trauma, tumors, or an extraneous cervical rib that may compress the nerves, arteries, or veins in the area from the neck to the axilla. TOS would not cause facial swelling, engorged neck veins, or confusion. **Upper extremity DVT:** Can present with swelling, redness, and pain in the arm and is usually found in patients with malignancy, trauma, or central venous catheters. This would not cause facial swelling, engorged neck veins, or confusion.
Initial Diagnostic Tests	• Chest CT with IV contrast. • Consider upper extremity venous duplex to rule out DVT.
Next Steps in Management	• Elevation of head of bed to decrease venous pressure • Consider mediastinal radiation if due to tumor • Intravascular stent to relieve obstruction • Consider anticoagulation if due to thrombus and no contraindication (brain metastases, coagulopathies)
Discussion	SVC syndrome is caused by compression or invasion of a tumor (usually a mediastinal mass) into the superior vena cava, preventing the return of blood to the heart. It is more commonly associated with centrally located tumors. **History/physical exam:** Signs and symptoms include facial swelling/plethora, formation of collateral blood vessels, distended neck veins on the side of the obstruction, and edema of the face, neck, arms, and upper thorax, and severe cases can present with stridor due to compromise of larynx or pharynx.

CASE 17 | Superior Vena Cava (SVC) Syndrome *(continued)*

Discussion	**Diagnostics:**
	• CT with IV contrast to identify obstructing lesion
	• Ultrasound of neck veins, venography in patients with severe presentation alongside endovascular intervention
	• Consider upper extremity venous duplex to rule out DVT
	Management:
	• Endovenous stenting in patients with life-threatening symptoms (stridor, airway compromise)
	• Investigate and treat obstructing lesion
Additional Considerations	**Complications:** Complications of SVC syndrome include edema in multiple locations including cerebral edema and laryngeal edema.
	Like SVC syndrome, another locoregional cancer syndrome is the **pancoast tumor**, also known as superior sulcus tumor. Compression of regional structures may cause an array of findings.
	Superior sulcus tumors (aka Pancoast tumor) can give rise to **Horner syndrome** (aka oculosympathetic syndrome, due to involvement of the paravertebral sympathetic chain and inferior cervical stellate ganglion causing unilateral ptosis, meiosis, anhidrosis, and enophthalmos), shoulder and arm pain (in the distribution of C8, T1, and T2 dermatomes), and weakness of the muscles of the hand. Superior sulcus tumors can also cause spinal cord compression and paraplegia due to invasion of the intervertebral foramina.
	• Recurrent laryngeal nerve → hoarseness
	• Superior vena cava → SVC syndrome
	• Brachiocephalic vein → brachiocephalic syndrome (unilateral symptoms)
	• Brachial plexus → sensorimotor deficits
	• Phrenic nerve → hemidiaphragm paralysis (hemidiaphragm elevation on CXR)
	Paraneoplastic syndromes associated with lung cancer are as follows:
	• **Hypercalcemia of malignancy** usually seen in non–small squamous cell carcinoma. The most common mechanism is tumor release of PTH-related protein (PTHrP). Other non-lung tumors may synthesize 1,25-dihydroxy vitamin D (calcitriol) or induce bone destruction through osteolytic metastases or local extension into bone.
	• **Cushing syndrome**, due to ACTH secretion by tumors, is seen in small cell CA.
	• **SIADH**, due to ADH secretion by tumors, is seen in small cell CA.
	• **Lambert-Eaton myasthenic syndrome.** Antibodies against presynaptic volume gated Ca^{2+} channels at neuromuscular junction, seen in small cell CA. It is characterized by proximal muscle weakness that improves with exercise (vs. myasthenia gravis, wherein weakness will worsen with exercise).
	• **Paraneoplastic encephalomyelitis.** Antibodies against Hu antigens in neurons are seen in small-cell CA.

CASE 18 | Malignant Mesothelioma

A 78-year-old man presents with right-sided dull chest pain and progressive shortness of breath over a 4-month period. He has a chronic cough and unintentional weight loss. He retired from being a pipefitter 13 years ago. He has no substance use. His vitals are temperature 37.2°C, blood pressure 114/74 mmHg, pulse 65/min, respirations 20/min, and oxygen saturation of 94% on room air. There is asymmetric chest wall expansion, dullness to percussion on the right hemithorax up to the midlung field, and diminished breath sounds on the right up to the midlung. A CXR shows fluid in the right pleural space and widespread dense opacities projecting over both lungs in a nonanatomic distribution (calcified pleural plaques).

Conditions with Similar Presentations	**Asbestosis:** Is a pneumoconiosis associated with shipbuilding, roofing, and plumbing and is a significant risk factor for bronchogenic carcinoma, which is more common than malignant mesothelioma. Asbestos bodies can be collected in bronchoalveolar lavage of sputum.
	Caplan syndrome: Is rheumatoid arthritis plus a pneumoconiosis (e.g., asbestosis, silicosis, anthracosis).
Initial Diagnostic Tests	• CT scan of the chest.
	• Video-assisted thoracoscopic surgery (VATS) and biopsy of pleural tissue.
Next Steps in Management	Multidisciplinary care and referral to surgery and oncology for treatment.

CASE 18 | Malignant Mesothelioma *(continued)*

Discussion	Mesothelioma is the most common primary tumor of the pleura. Approximately 70% of cases are associated with asbestos exposure. There is a long latency between asbestos exposure and disease development. There is not a clear dose–response relationship. Cigarette smoking, in the absence of asbestos exposure, is not a risk factor for developing malignant mesothelioma.
	Pleural plaques themselves do not become mesothelioma but are a marker for asbestos exposure.
	History:
	• Age ≥60 years.
	• Unilateral dull chest pain (non-pleuritic).
	• Progressive dyspnea and chronic cough.
	• History of exposure to asbestos (plumbing, shipbuilding trades, asbestos mining and milling, insulation work in construction).
	Physical exam:
	• Asymmetric chest wall expansion.
	• Unilateral dullness to percussion and decreased breath sounds.
	• Palpable unilateral chest nodules if disease has invaded the chest wall.
	Diagnostics:
	• CT chest: Unilateral diffuse pleural thickening and effusion with areas of calcification.
	• VATS performed to obtain biopsy.
	• Diagnosis is made by histologic evidence of mesothelioma on biopsy. The majority of tumors are the **epithelioid** variant with several subtypes (tubulopapillary, glandular, adenomatoid, and solid epithelioid). Stains are positive for **calretinin** and **cytokeratin 5/6**. Less common are **sarcomatoid** mesotheliomas.
	Management: Treatment is dictated by stage. Rarely is the tumor fully resectable. Systemic therapy with immune checkpoint inhibitors (nivolumab and ipilimumab) or pemetrexed and platinum are initial therapies, depending on histology (non-epithelioid or epithelioid, respectively).
	Complications: Prognosis is poor, with rare survival for >2 years. Patients develop respiratory failure due to tumor invasion of the ribs and intercostal structures. Disease can spread through the diaphragm, encasing the intraperitoneal organs and causing bowel obstruction.

6

Gastroenterology

Lead Authors: Asim Shuja, MD; Adam Mikolajczyk, MD; Euna Chi, MD
Contributors: Seoyeon (Sara) Kim, MD; Hwa-Pyung (David) Lim, MD; Aashutos Patel, MD

DYSPHAGIA AND ODYNOPHAGIA

Globus sensation is a functional esophageal disorder that is characterized by a nonpainful sensation of a lump or foreign body in the throat without any underlying structural abnormality, gastroesophageal reflux disease (GERD), or esophageal motility disorder.

Dysphagia is a subjective sensation of difficulty swallowing, while **odynophagia** is pain with swallowing, which is most often found in infectious and medication-induced esophagitis. Dysphagia can be further divided into oropharyngeal and esophageal dysphagia.

- Oropharyngeal dysphagia refers to difficulty initiating a swallow and can be accompanied by drooling, coughing, choking, nasal regurgitation, aspiration, or a sensation of food remaining in pharynx. This type of dysphagia is more prevalent in older populations.

- Esophageal dysphagia refers to difficulty swallowing several seconds after initiation and is often associated with a sensation of food getting stuck. Esophageal dysphagia can occur simultaneously with oropharyngeal dysphagia.

  Diagnostic Tests:

- Barium contrast swallow study (Esophagram): can detect the size, and location of any obstruction (*e.g.*, mass, stricture) or diverticula, and also assesses motility

- Upper endoscopy or esophagogastroduodenoscopy (EGD): to diagnose esophagitis, Barrett's esophagus, cancer

- Manometry: to identify motility disorders, *e.g.*, achalasia

- 24-hour pH testing: to quantify gastroesophageal reflux episodes

Causes of Oropharyngeal Dysphagia

Neurological	Structural	Myopathic	Infectious	Iatrogenic
• Stroke • Multiple sclerosis • Guillain-Barre syndrome (Miller Fisher syndrome variant) • Amyotrophic lateral sclerosis • Dementia • Parkinson disease	• Zenker diverticulum • Cervical webs and rings • Oropharyngeal tumors	• Connective tissue disease • Dermatomyositis • Polymyositis • Myasthenia gravis • Myotonic dystrophy • Sarcoidosis	• CMV* • Candida* • HSV* • Botulism • Tick paralysis	• Corrosive (pill, intentional) • Radiation • Medication (chemotherapy, neuroleptics) • Postsurgical

*Can also cause odynophagia

Causes of Esophageal Dysphagia

Mechanical		Motility
Intrinsic	**Extrinsic**	• Achalasia • Chagas disease • Primary motility disorders • Secondary motility disorders (systemic sclerosis, diabetes)
• Caustic esophagitis • Eosinophilic esophagitis • Infectious esophagitis (see above list) • Pill or radiation esophagitis • Strictures, rings, or webs • Diverticulum • Benign or malignant tumors • Hiatal hernia	• Enlarged aorta • Enlarged left atrium • Mediastinal mass (lung mass, lymphadenopathy)	

Approach to Dysphagia

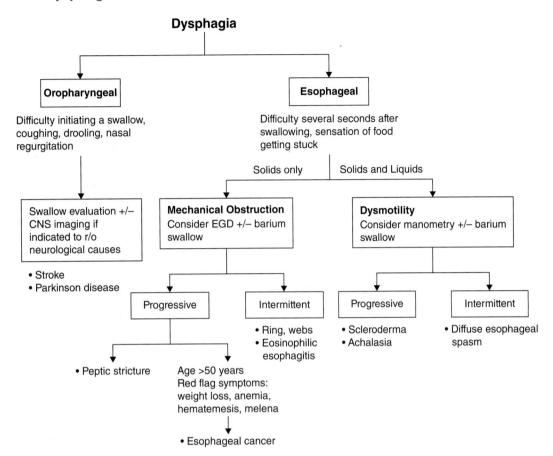

Dysphagia

→ **Oropharyngeal**
Difficulty initiating a swallow, coughing, drooling, nasal regurgitation

→ **Esophageal**
Difficulty several seconds after swallowing, sensation of food getting stuck

Oropharyngeal:
→ Swallow evaluation +/– CNS imaging if indicated to r/o neurological causes
- Stroke
- Parkinson disease

Esophageal:
- Solids only → **Mechanical Obstruction** Consider EGD +/– barium swallow
- Solids and Liquids → **Dysmotility** Consider manometry +/– barium swallow

Mechanical Obstruction:
- Progressive
- Intermittent
  - Ring, webs
  - Eosinophilic esophagitis

Progressive:
- Peptic stricture
- Age >50 years
  Red flag symptoms: weight loss, anemia, hematemesis, melena
  → Esophageal cancer

Dysmotility:
- Progressive
  - Scleroderma
  - Achalasia
- Intermittent
  - Diffuse esophageal spasm

CASE 1 | Achalasia

A 45-year-old man presents with progressive difficulty swallowing over the past 3 years. He is now having trouble swallowing both liquids and solids. Sometimes he notes regurgitation of undigested food but has had no weight loss. He tried proton pump inhibitors (PPIs) which did not help his symptoms. Physical exam is unremarkable.

Conditions with Similar Presentations	**Esophageal strictures:** May also present with solid foods getting stuck, but less difficulty with liquids. Fixed defects caused by chronic GERD, caustic ingestions, or radiation and treated with endoscopy, balloon dilation, and PPIs.
	Schatzki rings: Often asymptomatic but can present with dysphagia to solids and can be associated with hiatal hernia. Rings are circular membranes of mucosa and submucosa that form at the squamocolumnar junction of the distal esophagus.
	Eosinophilic esophagitis: Found in patients with food allergies, asthma, and atopy and presents with food impaction. It is a chronic, allergic inflammatory disease of the esophagus.
	Plummer-Vinson syndrome: Triad of dysphagia, esophageal web, and iron deficiency anemia and increased risk of squamous cell carcinoma (SCC) of the esophagus. Typically found in older women and confirmed with imaging or endoscopic visualization of the upper esophageal web.
	Diffuse esophageal spasm: Causes intermittent dysphagia to solids and liquids and retrosternal pain experienced seconds after initiating a swallow. Esophageal manometry is diagnostic, showing increased or premature contractions in the distal esophagus in at least 20% of swallows, and barium esophagram may show "corkscrew esophagus."

CASE 1 | Achalasia *(continued)*

Conditions with Similar Presentations	**Pseudoachalasia or Secondary achalasias:** May be caused by Chagas disease (*Trypanosoma cruzi*), scleroderma, or malignancies due to mass effect. Manometric findings of pseudoachalasia may be similar to those of achalasia. Esophagogastroduodenoscopy (EGD) should be done to rule out malignancies. Diffuse esophageal spasm. (Reproduced, with permission, from Loscalzo J, Fauci AS, Kasper DL, Hauser SL, Longo DL, Jameson JL, eds: Harrison's Principles of Internal Medicine. 21st ed. New York, NY: McGraw Hill; 2022.)
Initial Diagnostic Testing	• Confirm diagnosis with Barium esophagram and esophageal manometry. • Consider EGD to rule out other causes.
Next Steps in Management	• Pneumatic dilation, surgical myotomy. • Botulinum toxin injections or oral medications such as calcium channel blockers, nitrates, or sildenafil.

Discussion	Achalasia is an uncommon disorder that results from loss of normal peristalsis in the esophagus and failure of the lower esophageal sphincter (LES) to relax, due to a decrease in inhibitory neurotransmitters in the myenteric (Auerbach) plexus.
	
	History/Physical Exam:
	• Characterized by progressive dysphagia to solids and liquids over years and/or regurgitation unresponsive to PPIs.
	• Other symptoms include heartburn, regurgitation or vomiting, chest pain, epigastric pain, cough, wheezing, hoarseness, aspiration, unintentional weight loss.
	
	Diagnostics:
	• Confirm with esophagram and manometry.
	  • Barium esophagram: Dilated esophagus with narrow gastroesophageal junction (**"bird's beak" sign**).
	  • Manometry: Aperistalsis in the distal two-thirds of the esophagus with associated incomplete LES relaxation.
	• EGD to rule out other causes such as GERD, malignancy, or structural obstruction such as strictures or rings.
	
	Management: Goal is to decrease pressure of lower esophageal sphincter
	• Endoscopic pneumatic dilation or surgical myotomy is preferred.
	• If endoscopic/surgical options are contraindicated, other treatments include endoscopic botulinum toxin injections or oral medications (calcium channel blockers or nitrates).
	
	Dilated esophagus
	
	Achalasia. (Reproduced, with permission, from Farrokhi F, Vaezi MF: Idiopathic (primary) achalasia. Orphanet J Rare Dis. 2007;2:38.)

Additional Considerations	**Complications:** Achalasia is associated with increased risk of esophageal cancer. **Surgical considerations:** If medical treatment fails, refer for Heller myotomy If Heller myotomy fails and patient develops megaesophagus, refer for esophagectomy

CASE 2 | Zenker's Diverticulum

An 80-year-old woman presents with dysphagia and foul-smelling breath for several weeks. She regurgitates food into her mouth hours after eating, and now has a fever, cough, and shortness of breath. The patient's temperature is 38.7°C, heart rate is 90/min, respiratory rate is 22/min, blood pressure is 140/84 mmHg, and oxygen saturation is 93% on room air. She has normal dentition and no cervical lymphadenopathy. Audible crackles are noted in the right lower lung. There is no abdominal tenderness or masses, and her neurological exam is normal.

Conditions with Similar Presentations	**Strokes:** Can cause oropharyngeal (not esophageal) dysphagia and aspiration, and would have focal neurologic findings (e.g., focal weakness, facial droop). Dysphagia affects 50% of stroke patients and most recover function within 1–2 weeks. **Esophageal strictures and cancers:** Present with progressive dysphagia (solids more than liquids) and may cause aspiration. If suspected, EGD should be performed.
Initial Diagnostic Testing	• Confirm diagnosis with Barium esophagram (swallow). • Check CXR and consider EGD.

CASE 2 | Zenker's Diverticulum *(continued)*

Next Steps in Management	• Diverticulotomy is the definitive treatment of the diverticulum. • Treat aspiration pneumonia (if present) with antibiotics.
Discussion	Zenker's diverticulum results from altered pressure gradient inside the esophageal lumen, causing herniation of mucosal tissue at Killian's triangle (between thyropharyngeal and cricopharyngeal parts of inferior pharyngeal constrictor). It is more prevalent in middle-aged or older adults. **History/Physical Exam:** • Progressive dysphagia (usually to solids), regurgitation of undigested food, aspiration, foul breath (halitosis), noisy swallowing, cough, and weight loss. • May present with recurrent pneumonia due to aspiration. **Diagnostics:** • Barium esophagram shows a sac or pharyngoesophageal false diverticulum (Zenker's) • CXR to evaluate for aspiration pneumonia • Consider EGD to rule out cancer **Management:** • Surgical or endoscopic diverticulotomy is the main treatment for symptomatic patients. • Conservative management may be considered for patients with minimal or no symptoms. Esophagus Zenker diverticulum. (Reproduced, with permission, from Le T, et al: First Aid for the USMLE Step 1. 2022. New York, NY: McGraw Hill; 2022.)
Additional Considerations	**Complications:** Respiratory complications such as hoarseness, bronchospasm, pneumonia, lung abscess.

CASE 3 | Gastroesophageal Reflux Disease (GERD)

A 52-year-old man presents with globus sensation, dysphagia, chronic intermittent cough, and chest burning for several months. His symptoms are worse after large meals or lying down. Over-the-counter antacids are no longer helping with his symptoms. He has had no weight loss, nausea, vomiting, or change in his bowel movements. On exam he has mild tenderness to palpation in the epigastric region.

Conditions with Similar Presentations	**Esophageal strictures:** Sensation of food getting stuck, as strictures are due to a fixed defect. **Esophagitis:** Can also present with dysphagia but is often accompanied by odynophagia. • Causes include acid reflux, candida, CMV, and HSV (especially in immunocompromised patients), DM, chronic steroid use. • **Pill-induced esophagitis** may present with heartburn, odynophagia, or dysphagia but will have a history of ingestion of medications known to cause esophageal injury (e.g., doxycycline, aspirin, bisphosphonates, potassium chloride, NSAIDs, and iron compounds). **Angina pectoris:** Exertional chest pain relieved by rest, while GERD chest pain usually occurs after meals or when lying down to rest.
Initial Diagnostic Tests	• Clinical diagnosis, can confirm with empiric trial of PPI and/or pH monitoring (rarely done). • Obtain EGD if alarm/red flag symptoms (e.g., food getting stuck, weight loss, bleeding, anemia, vomiting).
Next Steps in Treatment/ Management	PPI and lifestyle modifications.
Discussion	GERD occurs when there is an impaired and transient decrease in the LES tone. GERD is more prevalent in Western countries. **History:** • Symptoms: Burning in the throat or chest (typically postprandially), hoarseness, chronic cough, sour taste in mouth, globus sensation, dysphagia, and new or worsening asthma symptoms. • Risk factors: Obesity, pregnancy, alcohol use, disordered/delayed esophageal motility (neuropathy, scleroderma), hiatal hernia, and Zollinger-Ellison syndrome (gastric acid hypersecretion caused by gastrinomas) or medications that affect the LES tone (e.g., calcium channel blockers).

CASE 3 | Gastroesophageal Reflux Disease (GERD) *(continued)*

Discussion	**Physical exam:** Normal or mild epigastric tenderness.
	Diagnostics: GERD is usually diagnosed clinically and does not require further testing.
	• Diagnosis confirmed by successful treatment with PPI or pH monitoring if diagnostic uncertainty.
	• EGD may show normal mucosa or erosion in mucosa (erosive esophagitis).
	• EGD is indicated for patients with alarm symptoms (weight loss, dysphagia, bleeding, anemia, recurrent vomiting) or unresponsiveness to PPI to rule out esophageal adenocarcinoma and Barrett esophagus.
	• **Barrett esophagus** (intestinal metaplasia) is associated with an increased risk of **esophageal adenocarcinoma** and requires chronic PPI therapy.
	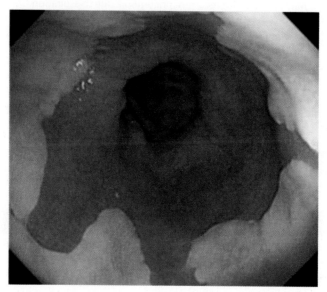
	Endoscopy shows irregular gastroesophageal junction. White/light pink mucosa is normal esophagus; salmon-colored mucosal tongues is Barrett esophagus.
	Management:
	• Trial of PPI (at least 30 minutes before breakfast) and lifestyle modifications (avoiding alcohol, caffeine, acidic foods/beverages, not lying down for several hours after a meal, sleeping with the head of the bed elevated, and weight loss).
	• Certain medications (such as calcium channel blockers, nitrates, albuterol, and anticholinergic drugs) should be avoided because they may aggravate symptoms by decreasing LES tone.
Additional Considerations	**Complications:** Chronic laryngitis, new or exacerbation of asthma, erosive esophagitis, stricture, Barrett esophagus, and esophageal adenocarcinoma.
	Surgical considerations: Anti-reflux surgery (e.g., Nissen fundoplication) can be offered to those with GERD unresponsive to high doses of PPIs or who cannot tolerate the medication.

CASE 4 | Esophageal Cancer

A 74-year-old woman with alcohol use disorder presents with progressive dysphagia to solids for the past 4 months, and difficulty swallowing liquids for the past 3 weeks. She has unintentionally lost 20 pounds since her last appointment 6 months ago. On exam, she has temporal wasting, conjunctival pallor, and poor dentition. The rest of the exam, including abdominal, is normal.

Conditions with Similar Presentations	**Neuromuscular causes of dysphagia** (e.g., **achalasia, diffuse esophageal spasm):** Typically present with simultaneous solid and liquid dysphagia, while dysphagia related to carcinoma usually starts with solid foods and progresses to liquids over time. **Esophageal rings, webs, strictures**, and **Zenker's diverticulum:** May all present with progressive dysphagia and weight loss. Diagnosis made with EGD.
Initial Diagnostic Testing	• Confirm diagnosis: EGD with biopsy. • Check CT neck/chest/abdomen with IV contrast, endoscopic US for staging.
Next Steps in Management	Depending on the tumor stage, chemotherapy and/or surgical resection.
Discussion	Esophageal cancer has two common types: squamous cell and adenocarcinoma. Squamous cell carcinoma is found in the upper two-thirds of the esophagus and is more prevalent in Eastern Europe and Asia, while adenocarcinoma is found in the lower one-third and is more prevalent in North America and Western Europe. By the time symptoms develop, esophageal cancer is usually advanced. Esophageal cancer spreads to adjacent and supraclavicular lymph nodes, liver, lungs, and bone. **History/Physical Exam:** • Risk factors for both types include men >50 years of age, smoking, achalasia. 　• Squamous cell carcinoma: Alcohol use disorder, nitrate consumption, ingestion of hot liquids, caustic strictures, and opiate use. 　• Adenocarcinoma: Chronic GERD, history of Barrett esophagus, obesity. • Symptoms: Progressive dysphagia (solids and liquids), odynophagia, persistent heartburn resistant to PPI (adenocarcinoma), chest pain, unintended weight loss, symptoms of anemia, bleeding/obstruction. **Diagnostics:** • Diagnosis with EGD and biopsy. • Locoregional staging by endoscopic US. • Distant metastases evaluated by neck, chest, and abdomen CT with contrast. If not detected on CT, PET-CT scans are done to look for occult metastases. **Management:** Esophageal cancer is treated with a combination of surgical resection, neoadjuvant chemoradiation, and adjuvant chemoradiation, depending on the staging.
Additional Considerations	**Screening:** Barrett esophagus is a premalignant finding. In Barrett esophagus, stratified squamous epithelium that normally lines the esophagus is replaced by intestinal columnar epithelium due to chronic inflammation caused by GERD. As metaplasia advances, it can eventually lead to esophageal adenocarcinoma, and endoscopic surveillance is recommended.

ABDOMINAL PAIN

Abdominal pain can be defined as either acute (≤7 days) or chronic. The clinical presentation may vary by the underlying etiology and may range from a self-limited condition to a serious condition requiring urgent intervention. Patients presenting with unstable vital signs, peritoneal signs on exam (rebound, voluntary guarding), or concerns for life-threatening causes (e.g., acute bowel obstruction, acute mesenteric ischemia, bowel perforation, myocardial infarction, ectopic pregnancy) require emergent evaluation. History and physical exam are important in creating a differential and often imaging and other diagnostic testing will be used to confirm the diagnosis. See *Surgery Chapter* for additional information and cases.

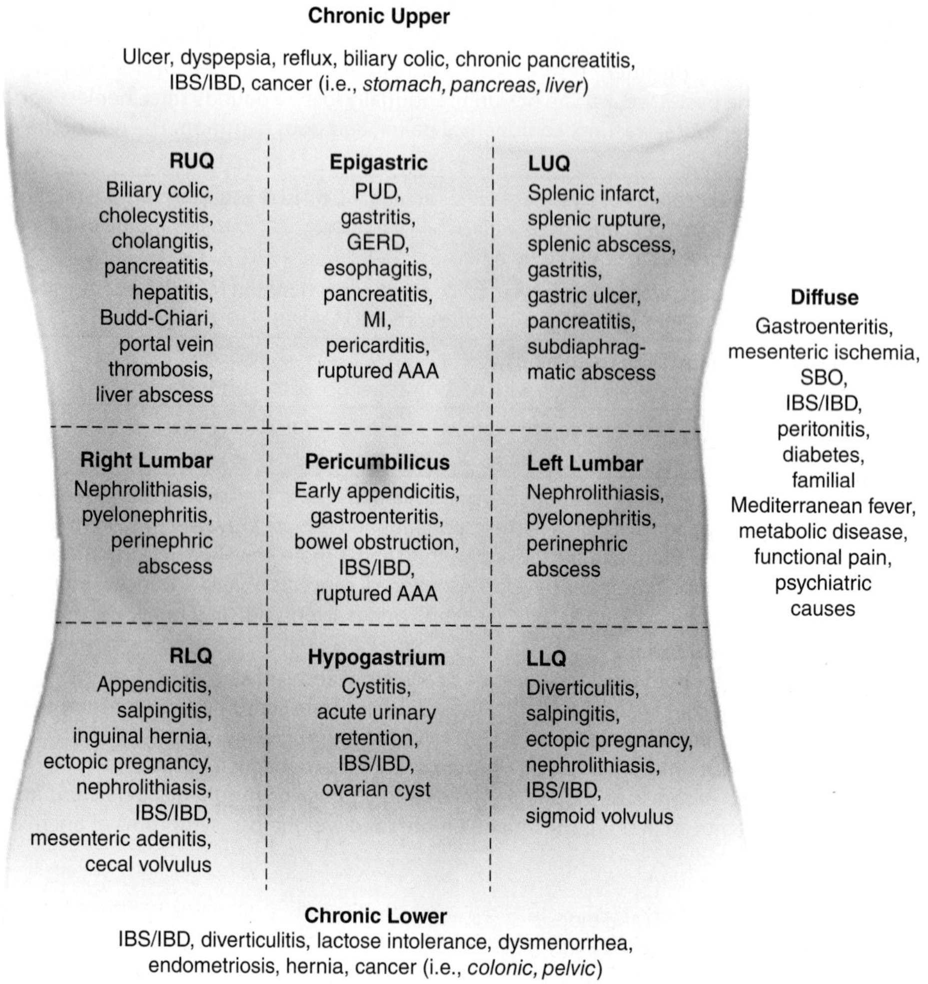

Chronic Upper

Ulcer, dyspepsia, reflux, biliary colic, chronic pancreatitis,
IBS/IBD, cancer (i.e., *stomach, pancreas, liver*)

RUQ
Biliary colic,
cholecystitis,
cholangitis,
pancreatitis,
hepatitis,
Budd-Chiari,
portal vein
thrombosis,
liver abscess

Epigastric
PUD,
gastritis,
GERD,
esophagitis,
pancreatitis,
MI,
pericarditis,
ruptured AAA

LUQ
Splenic infarct,
splenic rupture,
splenic abscess,
gastritis,
gastric ulcer,
pancreatitis,
subdiaphrag-
matic abscess

Diffuse
Gastroenteritis,
mesenteric ischemia,
SBO,
IBS/IBD,
peritonitis,
diabetes,
familial
Mediterranean fever,
metabolic disease,
functional pain,
psychiatric
causes

Right Lumbar
Nephrolithiasis,
pyelonephritis,
perinephric
abscess

Pericumbilicus
Early appendicitis,
gastroenteritis,
bowel obstruction,
IBS/IBD,
ruptured AAA

Left Lumbar
Nephrolithiasis,
pyelonephritis,
perinephric
abscess

RLQ
Appendicitis,
salpingitis,
inguinal hernia,
ectopic pregnancy,
nephrolithiasis,
IBS/IBD,
mesenteric adenitis,
cecal volvulus

Hypogastrium
Cystitis,
acute urinary
retention,
IBS/IBD,
ovarian cyst

LLQ
Diverticulitis,
salpingitis,
ectopic pregnancy,
nephrolithiasis,
IBS/IBD,
sigmoid volvulus

Chronic Lower

IBS/IBD, diverticulitis, lactose intolerance, dysmenorrhea,
endometriosis, hernia, cancer (i.e., *colonic, pelvic*)

Etiologies of pain by location. (Reproduced, with permission, from Huppert LA, Dyster TG: Huppert's Notes: Pathophysiology and Clinical Pearls for Internal Medicine. New York, NY: McGraw Hill; 2021.)

Etiologies that Cause Referred Pain

Cause	Site of Referred Pain
Myocardial infarction	Left chest wall, left neck or jaw, shoulders or arms
Cholecystitis	Right shoulder
Ruptured spleen	Left shoulder
Gastric ulcer or cancer	Epigastrium, midback between the scapula
Lower lobe pneumonia	Ipsilateral upper quadrant abdominal pain
Appendicitis	Periumbilical region
Kidney stone	Flank radiating to groin

Common Causes of Abdominal Pain and Diagnostic Tests

Diagnosis	Diagnostic test
Acute appendicitis, diverticulitis, bowel perforation, sigmoid volvulus	CT scan
Acute cholecystitis	Ultrasound
Acute pancreatitis	Serum lipase, CT scan
Peptic ulcer disease	EGD
Acute mesenteric ischemia	CT angiogram
Ischemic colitis	Colonoscopy
Intestinal obstruction	X-ray

CASE 5 | Diverticulitis

A 74-year-old woman with a history of diverticulosis presents with left lower quadrant (LLQ) abdominal pain, mild nausea, and low-grade fever for the past day. She also reports chronic constipation. Her temperature is 38.2°C, blood pressure is 110/80 mmHg, and pulse is 88/min. She has LLQ tenderness to palpation with no rebound tenderness or involuntary guarding.

Conditions with Similar Presentations	**Appendicitis:** Presents with initial periumbilical followed by right lower quadrant (RLQ) abdominal pain, fever, nausea/vomiting. Abdominal CT confirms diagnosis. **Inflammatory bowel disease (IBD):** May present with abdominal pain but is often accompanied by diarrhea and/or bloody stool. Patients have GI symptoms for several months before the presentation. **Colorectal cancer:** May present with abdominal discomfort and colonic wall thickening on abdominal CT, but symptoms of weight loss and anemia are usually present. **Gastroenteritis:** May present with abdominal pain; however, vomiting and/or diarrhea are usually the predominant symptoms and patients may have a history of recent travel. **Irritable bowel syndrome (IBS):** May present with abdominal pain and change in bowel habits. However, patients usually have symptoms of constipation and/or diarrhea several months prior to presentation and would not have fever.
Initial Diagnostic Tests	Abdominal CT with oral and intravenous contrast.
Next Steps in Management	NPO, IV fluids, IV antibiotics, pain control.
Discussion	**Diverticulosis** refers to presence of outpouchings of mucosa and submucosa herniating through a focal weakness in the colonic wall (false diverticula). They can occur anywhere but are typically seen in the sigmoid colon. When these diverticula become inflamed it is called **diverticulitis.** **History:** • Symptoms: Abdominal pain usually located in the LLQ (sigmoid colon), but RLQ may also be involved, and may have nausea, vomiting, constipation, or diarrhea. • Risk factors: Diverticulosis, older age, constipation, low fiber intake, obesity, and physical inactivity. **Physical exam:** • Abdominal distention, tenderness to palpation in LLQ, and low-grade fever. • Peritoneal signs (rebound tenderness, rigidity, and lack of bowel sounds) and hemodynamic instability (tachycardia, hypotension) suggest complicated diverticulitis including perforation. **Diagnostics:** • Confirm diagnosis with abdominal CT. Findings include pericolic fat infiltration or fat stranding, localized colonic wall thickening, and presence of diverticula. • CBC may show leukocytosis.

CASE 5 | Diverticulitis *(continued)*

Discussion	**Management:** Management depends on the level of severity. • Mild symptoms without complications (e.g., perforations, peritonitis, abscess, obstruction, fistulas) may be managed as outpatient: clear liquid diet, oral antibiotics, and follow-up in 2–3 days. • Moderate to severe diverticulitis or complicated diverticulitis should be managed as inpatients: NPO, IV fluids, pain control, and IV antibiotics. • Antibiotics with gram-negative and anaerobe coverage are used (e.g., ciprofloxacin and metronidazole or amoxicillin-clavulanate or ampicillin-sulbactam). • Most patients with acute diverticulitis are managed medically, but surgery may be indicated in complicated diverticulitis. • Colonoscopy 6–8 weeks after symptoms resolve to exclude colorectal cancer or inflammatory bowel disease.	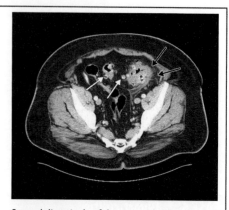 Several diverticula of the sigmoid colon as small round outpouchings *(white arrows)*. Extensive pericolonic fat stranding and wall thickening of that segment of colon *(black arrows)* consistent with acute diverticulitis. (Reproduced, with permission, from Elsayes KM, Oldham SAA, eds: Introduction to Diagnostic Radiology. New York, NY: McGraw Hill; 2014.)
Additional Considerations	**Surgical considerations:** Surgery should be considered for patients who have the following complicated forms of diverticulitis: abscesses, obstruction, perforation, or fistula formation. **Abscess:** Suspect if no improvement in abdominal pain or persistent fever despite antibiotics. If the fluid collection is <3 cm, treat with IV antibiotics and reserve surgery for patients with worsening symptoms. If the fluid collection is ≥3 cm, in addition to IV antibiotics, consider CT-guided percutaneous drainage. If symptoms are not controlled, surgical drainage and debridement is the next step. In complicated cases of obstruction, perforation, or fistula formation, management is via sigmoid resection of the affected portion of colon. Depending on the degree of affected bowel, patients may have to use a colostomy bag temporarily or permanently. **Perforation:** Acute diverticulitis with perforation is a surgical emergency. Rupture of inflamed diverticula or diverticular abscess may result in perforation with purulent or feculent peritonitis. Abdominal CT will show free air with or without extravasation of contrast. **Obstruction:** Both acute diverticulitis and colon cancer may present with obstruction. Colonic resection usually performed to relieve the symptoms and exclude malignancy.	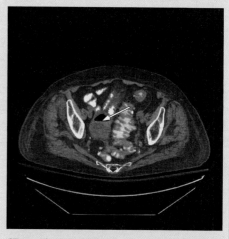 CT scan diagnostic of a localized intra-abdominal abscess. The patient has a rim-enhancing collection with an air-fluid level *(arrow)* secondary to acute diverticulitis. The sigmoid in the area is thick walled and has many diverticula. (Reproduced, with permission, from Hall JB, Schmidt GA, Kress JP, eds: Hall, Schmidt, and Wood's Principles of Critical Care. 4th ed. New York, NY: McGraw Hill; 2015.)

CASE 5 | Diverticulitis *(continued)*

Additional Considerations	**Fistula:** Inflammation from diverticula may lead to formation of a fistula between colon and adjacent viscera. Fistulas may involve bladder (most common), vagina, small bowel, uterus, or other pelvic structures. Fistulas are usually surgically corrected.

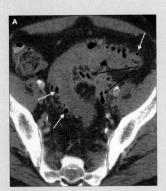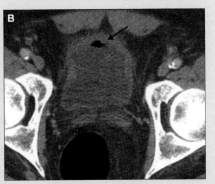

(A) Multiple sigmoid diverticuli (*white arrows*) with linear tract containing air outside the bowel lumen consistent with a fistula (*black arrow*) as a complication of diverticulitis. (B) Same patient showing air within the bladder (*black arrow*) consistent with a colovesical fistula from diverticulitis. (Reproduced, with permission, from Elsayes KM, Oldham SAA, eds: Introduction to Diagnostic Radiology. New York, NY: McGraw Hill; 2014.)

CASE 6 | Acute Pancreatitis

A 63-year-old woman with alcohol use disorder presents with severe abdominal pain. The pain is in the upper abdomen and radiates to the back. She has associated nausea, vomiting, and abdominal bloating. She is in acute distress secondary to pain and her vital signs are temperature 38.1°C, respiration rate is 24/min, heart rate is 104/min, and blood pressure 100/60 mmHg, and she has epigastric tenderness.

Conditions with Similar Presentations	**Acute cholecystitis:** May also have epigastric pain associated with fatty foods but is usually localized to RUQ with associated inspiratory arrest on deep palpation (Murphy sign). Abdominal US will show gallstones, bile sludge, pericholecystic fluid, and a thickened gallbladder.
	Choledocholithiasis: Presents with RUQ abdominal pain and may be concomitant with pancreatitis (gallstone pancreatitis). Patients may have a history of gallstones or biliary colic with normal lipase levels.
	Ascending cholangitis: Presents as a triad of jaundice, fever, and RUQ pain (Charcot triad) or as a pentad with additional altered mental status + shock (Reynolds pentad). May show elevations in ALT, AST, bilirubin, and/or ALP, but lipase levels will be normal.
	Peptic ulcer disease: Presents with epigastric pain which may be improved or worsened by food intake. May be accompanied by history of NSAID use or *Helicobacter pylori*.
	Perforated viscus: Presents with sudden-onset abdominal pain and will have peritoneal signs such as involuntary guarding, rigidity, and rebound tenderness. Upright chest and abdominal x-rays will show free air.
Initial Diagnostic Tests	• Check lipase to confirm diagnosis • Also check AST, ALT, ALP, bilirubin, lipid panel, and abdominal US • Consider CT abdomen with contrast
Next Steps in Management	NPO and supportive care including IV fluids and pain management

CASE 6 | Acute Pancreatitis *(continued)*

Discussion	Acute pancreatitis is a rapid-onset inflammatory process of the pancreas which can affect multiple organ systems due to systemic cytokine release. Pathophysiology involves injury to pancreatic acinar cells, leading to autodigestion by released trypsin and subsequent inflammatory response localized to pancreas (or systemic in severe disease). The most common causes are gallstones and alcohol use. 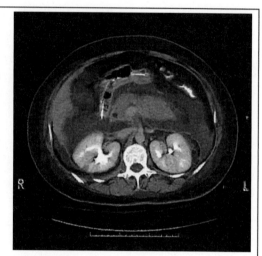 Acute pancreatitis. CT showing enlarged head and body of pancreas and surrounding fluid. (Reproduced, with permission, from Papadakis MA, McPhee SJ, Rabow MW, eds: Current Medical Diagnosis & Treatment 2023. 62nd ed. New York, NY: McGraw Hill; 2023.)

History:
- Risk factors mnemonic "I GET SMASHED": **I**diopathic, **G**allstones, **E**thanol, **T**rauma, **S**teroids, **M**umps, **M**alignancy (pancreatic cancer), **A**utoimmune, **S**corpion sting (outside of North America), **H**ypercalcemia, **H**ypertriglyceridemia, **E**RCP, **D**rugs (protease inhibitors, sulfonamide, 6-mercaptopurine, azathioprine, mesalamine, ACE inhibitors, nucleoside reverse transcriptase inhibitors)
- Symptoms: Severe epigastric or periumbilical pain radiating to the back, nausea and/or vomiting.

Physical exam:
- Epigastric tenderness to palpation.
- Although rare, there may be ecchymosis around umbilicus (Cullen sign) and flanks (Grey-Turner sign).

Diagnostics:
- Two out of three criteria required for diagnosis: epigastric pain ± radiation to the back, serum lipase >3× upper limit of normal, or radiological evidence of pancreatitis (US or CT scan). Contrast-enhanced CT typically shows enlarged pancreas surrounded by edema.
- Abdominal US to look for gallstones.
- If no clear common cause (gallstones, ethanol use) lipid panel to rule out hypertriglyceridemia (>1000 mg/dL) as cause.

Management:
- Initial management consists of NPO, aggressive fluid resuscitation with isotonic crystalloid solution (lactated ringers preferred over normal saline) and pain control (opioids).
- Early feeding as tolerated by the patient.

Additional Considerations	**Complications and surgical considerations:** Patients with pancreatitis usually recover without complications.
	- **Hypocalcemia** (precipitation of calcium soaps)
	- **Multiorgan Dysfunction**
	  - Shock
	  - Acute respiratory distress syndrome (**ARDS**)
	  - Renal failure
	- **Acute peripancreatic fluid collection:** Fluid collection without encapsulation.
	- **Pancreatic pseudocyst:** Well-circumscribed fluid collection without necrosis, surrounded by granulation tissue rather than epithelial lining. Typically develop 4–6 weeks after an episode of pancreatitis but can also develop after pancreatic injury and leakage following blunt abdominal trauma. Pseudocysts can become infected, obstruct the biliary tree or duodenum, and digestion by pancreatic enzymes can lead to pseudoaneurysm or pleural effusion. Diagnosis is confirmed by abdominal CT. If symptomatic, pseudocysts can be managed with endoscopic or percutaneous drainage. Patients undergoing ERCP can have mechanical injury from manipulation of ducts, injection of contrast media, or difficulty with cannulation that can result in **iatrogenic pancreatitis**. Patients with Sphincter of Oddi dysfunction are particularly at risk.

CASE 6 | **Acute Pancreatitis** *(continued)*

Additional Considerations	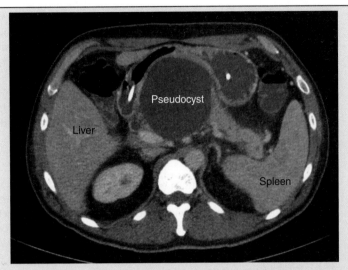 Abdominal CT scan reveals a large pancreatic pseudocyst compressing the stomach which can be treated with endoscopic cyst-gastrostomy with stent placement. (Reproduced, with permission, from Hall JB, Schmidt GA, Kress JP, eds: Hall, Schmidt, and Wood's Principles of Critical Care. 4th ed. New York, NY: McGraw Hill; 2015.) • **Necrotizing pancreatitis:** Pancreatic or peripancreatic necrosis, lack of pancreatic parenchymal enhancement on CT with IV contrast. May require percutaneous aspiration to rule out infected pancreatic necrosis, and if present, resection of affected tissue (necrosectomy).

CASE 7 | Ascending Cholangitis

A 55-year-old man presents with abdominal pain, fever, and yellow eyes. He reports intermittent RUQ abdominal pain for the past 2 weeks. For the past 2 days, the pain has been constant, and he had three episodes of vomiting. He is lethargic and diaphoretic and vital signs are temperature 102.5°F, blood pressure 85/55, and heart rate 115. On exam, he has conjunctival icterus and tenderness to palpation in the RUQ with associated inspiratory arrest (Murphy sign).

Conditions with Similar Presentations	**Acute cholecystitis:** Also presents with RUQ abdominal pain, fever, nausea, and vomiting. However, jaundice or increased alkaline phosphatase (ALP) are less likely due to the location of the obstruction in the biliary tree (blockage in cystic duct and not common bile duct, so flow of bile not impeded). **Choledocholithiasis:** Presents with episodic, postprandial RUQ pain, sometimes accompanied by nausea/vomiting. Abdominal exam is benign and patients lack systemic signs of inflammation including fever. ALP is elevated. **Acute pancreatitis:** Also presents with abdominal pain, nausea, and vomiting. However, the pain is epigastric and radiates to the back. Can present with jaundice if it is due to obstructing gallstones (gallstone pancreatitis). **Acute viral hepatitis:** Can present with RUQ abdominal pain, fever, and jaundice. However, patients also present with hepatomegaly and will have elevated transaminases without significant elevation in ALP. Patients may have risk factors (e.g., known outbreak, injection drug use, sexual contacts, travel history).
Initial Diagnostic Tests	• Obtain transaminases (ALT, AST), bilirubin (bili) and ALP, RUQ ultrasound and endoscopic retrograde cholangiopancreatography (ERCP) • Also check: CBC, BMP, blood cultures
Next Steps in Management	Empiric broad-spectrum IV antibiotics, aggressive IV fluid resuscitation

CASE 7 | Ascending Cholangitis (continued)

Discussion	Ascending cholangitis is an infection of the biliary tree which occurs when there is biliary stasis or obstruction. Many patients have symptomatic gallstone disease (biliary colic) which can progress to choledocholithiasis if a gallstone migrates to the common bile duct. If this obstruction persists, it predisposes to bacterial infection of the bile ducts (ascending cholangitis). **History/Physical Exam:** • Appear ill and typically present with jaundice, fever, and RUQ pain (**Charcot triad**). • If progression to sepsis, or in older patients, can also present with hypotension and altered mental status in addition to Charcot triad, which is known as **Reynolds pentad**. This can progress to multiorgan failure if obstruction is not removed. • Primary sclerosing cholangitis (PSC) is a risk factor for obstruction in the biliary tree secondary to strictures. **Diagnostics:** Confirm diagnosis with signs or labs consistent with a systemic illness (e.g., fevers, chills) or inflammatory response (e.g., ↑WBC or ↑CRP) and evidence of cholestasis and abnormal imaging. • ERCP: showing biliary dilation or potential cause (e.g., stone, stricture) • MRCP and endoscopic ultrasound (EUS) may also detect choledocholithiasis. • Elevated ALP, T bili, D bili (cholestatic pattern); AST and ALT may be elevated. • Abdominal US may show dilated common bile duct. • CBC with leukocytosis. **Management:** • Empiric IV antibiotics (piperacillin-tazobactam or ceftriaxone plus metronidazole or ampicillin-sulbactam) and IV fluids should be started promptly as many patients are bacteremic on presentation. • Urgent ERCP to remove the obstruction and provide source control of the infection, as antibiotics do not penetrate well into an obstructed biliary tree.
Additional Considerations	**Surgical considerations:** If ERCP unsuccessful, further intervention to remove the obstruction is indicated. If the obstruction is due to a stricture, endoscopic sphincterotomy and possible stent placement are performed. Open surgical intervention is reserved if this fails. Percutaneous biliary drainage is an alternative interventional radiological technique that can be used in scenarios where general sedation or anesthesia are to be avoided. Eventual cholecystectomy is indicated for patients due to risk of recurrent disease.

Upper Abdominal Pain Mini Cases

Cases	Key Findings
Peptic ulcer disease (PUD)	**Hx:** • Epigastric pain that may be worse or relieved after eating with possible associated weight loss, nausea, vomiting. May also present with complications including hematemesis or melena from bleeding (most common), early satiety and nausea/vomiting from gastric outlet obstruction, or severe diffuse abdominal pain from perforation. • **Gastric ulcers:** eating may exacerbate pain • **Pyloric channel ulcers:** often associated with signs of obstruction including bloating, nausea, vomiting • **Duodenal ulcers:** pain may occur mid-morning, relieved by food but recurs 2–3 hours after a meal. Pain may awaken the patient at night. • **Associated risk factors:** NSAID use, H. pylori infection, smoking history, alcohol history. **PE:** Epigastric tenderness. **Diagnostics:** • EGD ± biopsy to confirm diagnosis • Patients ≥50 years with new-onset dyspepsia or alarm features (unintended weight loss, early satiety, GI bleeding, iron deficiency anemia, dysphagia/odynophagia) require EGD and biopsy to rule out gastric cancer. • *H. pylori* testing (stool antigen or urea breath test) alone may be appropriate for younger patients without alarm features

Upper Abdominal Pain Mini Cases (continued)

Peptic ulcer disease (PUD)	**Management:** • Treat *H. pylori* with triple therapy (clarithromycin, amoxicillin, and PPI for 14 days) *or* quadruple therapy (bismuth subsalicylate, metronidazole, tetracycline, and PPI for 14 days). • Stool antigen or urea breath test to confirm eradication. • For uncomplicated peptic ulcer with history of NSAID use, stop NSAID and initiate PPI therapy. • Surgery is recommended for patients with ulcers refractory to medical management or with bleeding, perforation, and gastric outlet obstruction. **Discussion:** Peptic ulcers are defects in the gastric or duodenal wall that extend through muscularis mucosa into submucosa or muscularis propria. The two main risk factors are *H. pylori* infection and NSAID use. • Duodenal ulcers are more common and associated with *H. pylori* infection and acid hypersecretion. • *H. pylori*–associated ulcers have a 3- to 6-fold increased risk of gastric adenocarcinoma • **Zollinger-Ellison syndrome (ZES)** is a rare cause of peptic ulcers and is characterized by hypersecretion of gastric acid by duodenal or pancreatic neuroendocrine tumors (NETs; **gastrinomas**). ZES should be suspected with multiple or refractory peptic ulcers, ulcers distal to the duodenum, or diarrhea associated with PUD.
Chronic gastritis	**Hx:** Epigastric pain worse with meals, nausea, vomiting **PE:** May have epigastric tenderness **Diagnostics:** • EGD with biopsy for gastritis: Mucosal atrophy ± intestinal metaplasia, erosions due to chronic mucosal inflammation (gastritis); for gastric ulcers would see ulcerations. • *H. pylori* testing **Management:** • PPI and treat underlying cause **Discussion:** • Gastritis is an inflammatory process of the gastric mucosa and is most commonly caused by *H. pylori*, with other causes including drugs (NSAIDs, alcohol), autoimmune disease. • Increased risk of gastric cancer
Chronic pancreatitis	**Hx:** • Postprandial abdominal pain, nausea, vomiting, anorexia, weight loss, steatorrhea • Recurrent acute pancreatitis or alcohol use disorder **PE:** Epigastric tenderness **Diagnostics:** • Imaging (CT, MRI, US) may show pancreatic atrophy or calcifications • Lipase may not be elevated because of loss of acinar cells. • Pancreatic function tests (fecal elastase) may be used to document pancreatic insufficiency. **Management:** • Risk factor modification (smoking and alcohol cessation) • Multimodal pain control (acetaminophen and NSAIDs preferred but opioids often required) • Low-fat meals and pancreatic enzyme supplementation if exocrine pancreatic insufficiency (fecal elastase) along with PPI (to neutralize gastric acid and allow enzymes to function). **Discussion:** Chronic pancreatitis is due to repeated pancreatic injury. Patients are at risk for diabetes due to pancreatic destruction of islet cells and experience weight loss due to malnutrition and steatorrhea from pancreatic insufficiency.

CASE 8 | Gastric Adenocarcinoma

A 67-year-old woman with tobacco use and prior treatment for *H. pylori* infection presents with abdominal pain and 15-pound weight loss over 5 months. She has some nausea and occasional vomiting, but no hematemesis, melena, or blood in stool. On exam, she has a palpable left supraclavicular lymph node (Virchow node) and mild epigastric tenderness.

Conditions with Similar Presentations	**Chronic gastritis:** Can present with epigastric pain, nausea, vomiting, but would not expect alarm symptoms. **Gastrointestinal stromal tumor (GIST)** and **MALT lymphoma:** Rare gastric tumors that can be distinguished from gastric adenocarcinomas by biopsy. Should eradicate *H. pylori* infection in patients with MALT prior to surgical resection to reduce risks of second cancer. Eradication may cause remission of cancer.
Diagnostics	EGD with biopsy

CASE 8 | **Gastric Adenocarcinoma** *(continued)*

Treatment/ Management	Surgery and/or chemotherapy
Discussion	Gastric adenocarcinoma incidence is highest in Eastern Asia, Eastern Europe, and South America, and the diagnosis should be suspected in patients with alarm symptoms (new dyspepsia in patients >55 years, weight loss, GI bleed, iron deficiency anemia, palpable mass/lymph nodes). **History:** • Nonspecific symptoms such as anorexia, abdominal pain, weight loss, dyspepsia, or early satiety • Risk factors: Tobacco use, alcohol use, prior *H. pylori* infection, and high intake of nitrosamines, salt, or processed meat. Genetic risk factors include Lynch syndrome, Peutz-Jeghers syndrome, and familial adenomatous polyposis (FAP) **Physical exam:** • May have palpable left supraclavicular node (Virchow node), subcutaneous periumbilical node (Sister Mary Joseph nodule), and in females, metastatic bilateral ovarian masses (Krukenberg tumor) **Diagnostics:** • Upper endoscopy with biopsy confirms diagnosis • CT scan of chest, abdomen, and pelvis to evaluate for distant metastases **Management:** • Local disease (stage I–III) treated with combination of surgical resection and chemotherapy • Unresectable/stage IV disease treated with chemoradiation and referred to palliative therapy (5-year survival <10%)
Additional Considerations	**Complications:** Gastric obstruction, acute or chronic gastrointestinal bleeding.

Rare Gastric Tumors

Tumor	Association	Treatment
Mucosa-associated lymphoid tissue (MALT) lymphoma	*H. pylori*, autoimmune disorders (Sjogren syndrome, Hashimoto thyroiditis)	*H. pylori* triple therapy
Gastrointestinal stromal tumor (GIST)	KIT mutation	• Surgical or endoscopic resection • Imatinib (tyrosine kinase inhibitor) for recurrent/unresectable disease

CASE 9 | **Chronic Mesenteric Ischemia**

A 70-year-old man with diabetes, hypertension, smoking, and hyperlipidemia presents with generalized dull, cramping abdominal pain for the past several months. The pain occurs after meals, is associated with nausea and vomiting, and lasts about 30 minutes. He reports anorexia and has lost 15 pounds over the past year. On physical exam, he appears to be in moderate distress, but vital signs are normal and abdomen is soft and nontender.

Conditions with Similar Presentations	**Colonic ischemia or ischemic colitis:** Presents with crampy abdominal pain; however, it is more acute and is accompanied by loose stools or hematochezia. Patients usually have a history of hypoperfusion (septic shock, heart failure), recent cardiac or vascular surgery (coronary artery bypass or aortic dissection and repair), or atrial fibrillation.
	PUD: May also present with postprandial pain with associated nausea and vomiting. Patients usually have history of NSAID use or *H. pylori* infection.
	Biliary colic: Also associated with postprandial pain but is localized to the RUQ and sometimes radiating to the right shoulder or back. Weight loss is uncommon.
	Chronic pancreatitis: Also presents with postprandial abdominal pain and weight loss due to malnutrition and steatorrhea from pancreatic insufficiency. Patients usually have history of recurrent acute pancreatitis and/or alcohol use disorder.
	Abdominal aortic aneurysm (AAA): May present with chronic abdominal discomfort radiating to the back or buttocks, but is not associated with postprandial pain or weight loss. A pulsatile nontender abdominal mass may be palpated. An abdominal US should be performed to exclude AAA.

CASE 9 | Chronic Mesenteric Ischemia *(continued)*

Initial Diagnostic Tests	• CT angiogram (CTA) or magnetic resonance angiogram (MRA) of abdomen
Next Steps in Management	• Endovascular or surgical revascularization • Risk factor modification
Discussion	Chronic mesenteric ischemia (aka intestinal angina), is a rare condition seen more commonly in patients >60 and females. It is caused by atherosclerosis and involves arterial stenosis or occlusion of multiple vessels such as celiac, superior mesenteric, and inferior mesenteric arteries. Symptoms result from inadequate intestinal blood flow, especially during increased demand for blood flow after eating. **History:** • Risk factors: Cardiovascular risk factors such as smoking, hypertension, hyperlipidemia, diabetes. • Other evidence of atherosclerosis: Angina, myocardial infarction, stroke, or peripheral artery disease. • Symptoms: Dull, crampy postprandial abdominal pain which may lead to weight loss due to food aversion. Pain may be difficult to localize and often described as radiating to the back **Physical exam:** Physical exam is usually unremarkable. May auscultate abdominal bruit **Diagnostics:** • CT angiography or MRA of the abdomen and pelvis to evaluate for areas of vascular stenosis or obstruction. Mesenteric ischemia. Axial MDCT image shows lack of enhancement of the small bowel wall (arrow) and presence of pneumatosis (arrowhead). (From Blumberg R, Greenberger N, eds: Greenberger's Current Diagnosis & Treatment Gastroenterology, Hepatology, & Endoscopy. 3rd ed. New York, NY: McGraw Hill; 2016.) **Management:** • Revascularization (endovascular or surgical) indicated in patients with symptoms including abdominal pain and weight loss. • Address and treat risk factors such as smoking and secondary prevention of cardiovascular disease (statin therapy, blood pressure control, antiplatelet agents).
Additional Considerations	**Complications:** Chronic mesenteric ischemia may progress to acute mesenteric ischemia if not treated

Types of Mesenteric Ischemia

	Location	Onset	Cause	Symptoms/Signs
Acute mesenteric ischemia	Small intestine, superior mesenteric artery (SMA) occlusion most common	Acute	Acute arterial embolism (40–50%, from atrial fibrillation, valvular disease, or cardiovascular aneurysms), arterial thrombosis (25–30%)	Crampy abdominal pain out of proportion to physical exam If ischemia is prolonged, hematochezia and peritoneal signs (rebound tenderness, involuntary guarding)
Chronic mesenteric ischemia	Small intestine, celiac, SMA, or inferior mesenteric artery (IMA)	Chronic	Atherosclerosis of multiple intestinal vessels	Chronic postprandial pain Unremarkable physical exam
Colonic ischemia or ischemic colitis	Splenic flexure or rectosigmoid junction (watershed areas)	Acute	Low perfusion state due to recent coronary artery bypass or aortic repair, or medical history of heart failure	Abdominal pain Hematochezia Abdominal distention with vomiting due to ileus

NAUSEA AND VOMITING

- Controlled by pathways and neurotransmitters involving the brainstem chemoreceptor trigger zone, gut neurons, and smooth muscle cells.
- Medications, toxins, mechanical blockages, increased intracranial pressure, and even behavioral disorders can initiate this reflex.
- The list of causes is extensive, but initial focus should be on associated gastrointestinal (GI) symptoms, neurologic/vestibular symptoms, and medications to help narrow the differential.
- Regardless of the varying causes of nausea and vomiting, the medications that treat these symptoms focus on blocking receptors in the chemoreceptor trigger zone, e.g., 5HT3 (ondansetron), dopamine (metoclopramide), or act as prokinetic agents (erythromycin).

This section will focus on causes related to the GI system.

Key History and Exam Findings and Associated Diagnoses

Nausea/Vomiting with Key Associated Findings	Diagnoses
Diarrhea, recent travel or common meal outbreak	Gastroenteritis or food poisoning (*Bacillus cereus, Staphylococcus aureus, Clostridium perfringens*)
Cruise ship–associated diarrhea	Gastroenteritis—specifically norovirus
Uncontrolled diabetes mellitus, postprandial fullness	Gastroparesis, diabetic ketoacidosis (DKA)
Chemotherapy, new prescriptions	Medication-induced
Vertigo, worse with movement	Benign paroxysmal positional vertigo
Abdominal distension; high-pitched, tinkling bowel sounds	Small bowel obstruction
Hypoactive bowel sounds	Ileus, opioids
Calluses on fingers, dental caries/enamel erosion	Bulimia
Children, recent aspirin use, hepatomegaly, hypoglycemia	Reye syndrome
Infancy, projectile vomiting, palpable "olive-like mass"	Pyloric stenosis
Failure to pass meconium within the first 48 hours after birth	Hirschsprung disease, cystic fibrosis
Within first 2 days of life, "double bubble" sign on x-ray	Duodenal atresia
Poor feeding, smells like maple syrup	Maple syrup urine disease

CASE 10 | Diabetic Gastroparesis

A 73-year-old man with poorly controlled diabetes presents to the clinic with worsening nausea and vomiting over the past month. Patient reports decreased appetite, early satiety, and emesis after meals. The emesis is nonbilious and non-bloody. He was diagnosed with diabetes >20 years ago and his most recent A1C was 9.7. On exam, temperature is 98.5°F, blood pressure 125/75, heart rate 80, and he has abdominal distension. When the abdomen is shaken by moving the hips side to side, splashing sounds are heard (succussion splash).

Conditions with Similar Presentations	**Cyclic vomiting syndrome (CVS):** Presents with recurrent episodes of nausea and vomiting but is associated with migraine headaches. Diagnosis is made by the Rome IV criteria and treatment is with supportive care (IV fluids, antiemetics) and abortive therapy for migraines (sumatriptan).
	Cannabinoid hyperemesis syndrome (CHS): Presents with nausea and vomiting but is strongly linked to excessive and prolonged use of cannabis. Diagnosis made by history and treatment is cessation of cannabinoids.
	GERD: May present with nausea and vomiting; however, other symptoms include heartburn, regurgitation of sour liquid, postprandial substernal chest or epigastric pain, chronic cough, or dysphagia, which improve with PPI
	Bulimia nervosa: May present with nausea and vomiting and concomitant hoarseness, dental caries, or Russell sign (calluses on knuckles). Diagnosis made clinically, and treatment includes cognitive behavioral therapy, nutritional education/support, and SSRIs.
	Small bowel obstruction (SBO): Presents acutely with nausea and vomiting and causes include hernias, adhesions, strictures from prior surgeries, or tumors. Upright x-ray with presence of air–fluid levels.
Initial Diagnostic Tests	• Check Gastric emptying study (scintigraphy) • Consider: BMP, upper endoscopy, CT abdomen
Next Steps in Management	• Correct electrolyte abnormalities • Control diabetes • Antiemetics agents and pro-kinetic agents • Small meals with low fiber and low lipid content
Discussion	Gastroparesis is a condition of delayed gastric emptying in the absence of gastric obstruction, that presents with nausea, vomiting, and abdominal distension and may be idiopathic or develop secondary to various causes including medication, post-surgery or diabetes. Long-standing poorly controlled diabetes results in neuropathy over time and compromises gut sensorimotor function, resulting in diabetic gastroparesis. **History:** • Risk factors: Uncontrolled diabetes, pancreatic disease (chronic pancreatitis, pancreatic carcinoma), medications (e.g., opioids), mesenteric vascular insufficiency, scleroderma, and amyloidosis. • Symptoms: Early satiety, nausea, vomiting, and postprandial bloating/distension **Physical exam:** Abdominal distension, possible succussion splash **Diagnostics:** • Gold standard for diagnosis of gastroparesis is a **gastric emptying study** (**scintigraphy**); retention of 60% of the meal after 2 hours or >10% after 4 hours is abnormal. • If acute presentation of nausea and vomiting, an **upper endoscopy** is the first step to evaluate and rule out upper GI obstruction such as a mass or foreign body. • Non-contrast CT abdomen may be used to evaluate and rule out a lower GI obstruction. • Electrolyte abnormalities (hypochloremic metabolic alkalosis) if the vomiting is frequent and severe. **Management:** Initial treatment focuses on management of the vomiting and correcting electrolyte abnormalities. • For vomiting: Antiemetic agents such as ondansetron, diphenhydramine, prochlorperazine. • To increase gastric emptying: Prokinetic agents such as metoclopramide or erythromycin. These agents are used for short term only due to movement disorder adverse reactions (metoclopramide) or tachyphylaxis (erythromycin) leading to loss of efficacy. • Long-term management includes optimization of blood glucose to prevent further neurological damage, as well as eating small meals which are low in fiber/low residue and low in fat content.

GI BLEEDING (HEMATEMESIS, MELENA, HEMATOCHEZIA)

Patients with acute gastrointestinal bleeding can present with hematemesis or melena (signs of upper GI bleeding) or hematochezia (sign of lower GI bleeding). The first step is always to evaluate for hemodynamic instability and to resuscitate as needed. Once stabilized, diagnostic study with either upper or lower endoscopy is performed, during which sources of bleeding are identified and treated.

Approach to GI Bleeding

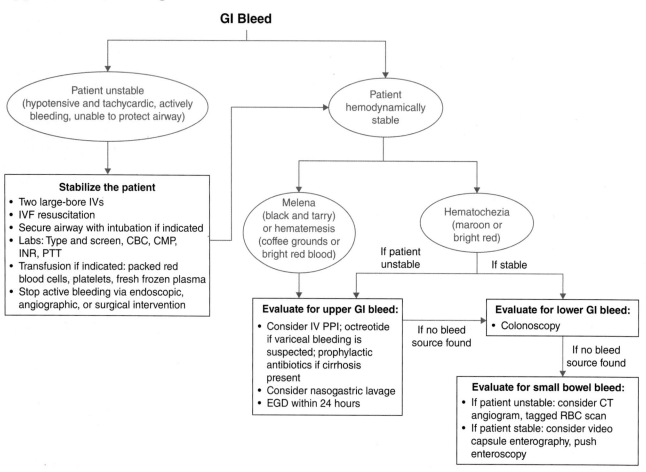

Differential Diagnoses GI Bleed

Upper GI Sources	Lower GI Sources
Esophageal or gastric varices	Arteriovenous malformations (AVM) or angiodysplasia
Boerhaave syndrome	Meckel diverticulum
Mallory-Weiss tear	Inflammatory bowel disease (IBD)
Esophagitis, gastritis, duodenitis	Ischemic colitis
Peptic ulcer disease (gastric, duodenal) (NSAID-induced or *H. pylori*–associated)	Infectious colitis
	• *Escherichia coli* O157:H7
Dieulafoy vascular malformation	• *Salmonella*
Esophageal or gastric cancer	• *Shigella*
	• *Campylobacter*
	• *Entamoeba histolytica*
	Colorectal cancer
	Diverticulosis
	Hemorrhoids/fissures

Key Associated Findings and GI Bleed Differential Diagnosis

GI Bleed with Key Associated Findings	Diagnoses
Male and <2 yo	Meckel diverticulum
NSAID use, epigastric pain, history of *H. pylori*	Peptic ulcer disease (PUD), gastritis
Improved with PPI/H2-blockers or antacids	GERD, PUD, gastritis
Hematemesis or large Hgb drop in a patient with stigmata of liver disease: ascites, scleral icterus, splenomegaly, spider angioma, telangiectasias, palmar erythema, gynecomastia, testicular atrophy, fluid wave, and shifting dullness	Esophageal varices
Hematemesis, retching, chest pain in setting of recurrent vomiting, ≥2:1 AST:ALT elevation (alcohol use disorder) or finger calluses and eroded tooth enamel (bulimia)	Mallory-Weiss tear
Weight loss, early satiety, history of tobacco, EtOH	Gastric cancer
Fever, diarrhea, recent travel or restaurant/picnic food, sick contacts	Infectious gastroenteritis
Weight loss, diarrhea, rash, arthralgias, eye irritation/redness	Inflammatory bowel disease (IBD)
Endoscopy revealing cobblestone mucosa and transmural inflammation with skip lesions and rectal sparing, noncaseating granulomas. String sign on barium swallow x-ray, fistulas	Crohn disease
Continuous colonic inflammation with rectal involvement, crypt abscesses on colonoscopy	Ulcerative colitis
Left-sided abdominal pain	Ischemic colitis
Abdominal pain, currant jelly stools	Intussusception (child), acute mesenteric ischemia (adult)
Abdominal pain after eating, food fear	Chronic mesenteric ischemia
Tenesmus, rectal pain after bowel movement	Anal fissure, or IBD with rectal involvement
Painless bright red blood per rectum (BRBPR), constipation	Diverticulosis, internal hemorrhoid
Weight loss, conjunctival pallor (iron deficiency anemia), abdominal pain, older age, strong family history of colon cancer, or not up-to-date on screening, change in stool caliber, ulcerative colitis, apple core lesion on barium enema; *Streptococcus bovis* bacteremia (rare)	Colorectal cancer
Immunocompromised, fever, abdominal pain, diarrhea with hematochezia	CMV colitis

---

CASE 11 | Esophageal Varices

A 64-year-old woman with alcoholic cirrhosis presents to the ED with hematemesis, dark, tarry, foul-smelling stools, and lightheadedness. Her clothes are covered in bright red blood. She looks weak and is tachycardic, hypotensive, and has cold/clammy extremities. She has palmar erythema, a distended abdomen with fluid wave, spider angiomas, and telangiectasias on her torso.

Conditions with Similar Presentations	**PUD:** May present with upper GI bleed; however, it is usually accompanied by epigastric pain that is associated with eating and history of NSAID use or *H. pylori* infection.
	Mallory-Weiss syndrome: May present with hematemesis following an increase in intra-abdominal pressure and a history of vomiting or retching.
	Esophagitis: May present with hematemesis, melena, or occult blood loss; however, it is usually associated with dysphagia/odynophagia or retrosternal pain. Patients may report a history of GERD, certain medication use (tetracyclines, trimethoprim-sulfamethoxazole, NSAIDs, bisphosphonates, potassium chloride, iron supplements), or infections (HSV, CMV, candida, HIV).
	Angiodysplasia: Mostly occult blood loss, but may present with hematemesis, hematochezia, melena. Patients may have a history of end-stage kidney disease (ESRD), aortic stenosis, von Willebrand disease, or hereditary hemorrhagic telangiectasia.

CASE 11 | Esophageal Varices *(continued)*

Initial Diagnostic Tests	Emergent EGD.
Next Steps in Management	• Hemodynamic stabilization: Airway protection, oxygen supplementation • Two large-bore IV access, fluid resuscitation • Blood transfusion if hemoglobin <7 g /dL • IV ceftriaxone and octreotide
Discussion	Variceal bleeding is a GI emergency and is associated with significant morbidity/mortality in patients with cirrhosis. Esophageal varices are dilated portosystemic collaterals that develop due to portal hypertension. Portal hypertension is most commonly found in cirrhosis and is known to result from combination of increased portal inflow from splanchnic vasodilation and increased resistance to outflow due to distorted hepatic sinusoids. Approximately half of cirrhotic patients develop varices, while one-third of patients with varices develop variceal bleeding. Risk of varices increases with the severity of liver disease. **History:** • Usually asymptomatic until rupture • Presentations include hematemesis, coffee-grounds emesis, melena, and hematochezia **Physical exam:** • No specific findings associated with esophageal varices • Exam findings associated with cirrhosis: Jaundice, spider angiomas, gynecomastia, ascites, splenomegaly, caput medusae, palmar erythema, testicular atrophy, and asterixis. **Diagnostics:** • EGD gold standard for diagnosis and recommended to be done within 12 hours in hemodynamically stable patients. • Type and cross, serial CBC • Coagulation studies (PT/INR, PTT), thromboelastography (TEG) = a functional measurement of coagulation **Management:** For all major GI bleeds, first steps are NPO, hemodynamic stabilization: airway protection, oxygen supplementation, two large-bore IV access, fluid resuscitation, and blood transfusion if hemoglobin <7 g /dL. • EGD within 12 hours with **endoscopic variceal ligation** (small elastic bands placed around varices) and/or **endoscopic sclerotherapy** (an injectable solution that causes inflammation and fibrosis is applied to obliterate the lumen of the bleeding vessel) • Balloon tamponade can be an effective way to stop the bleeding until the patient gets to the endoscopy suite • Continue octreotide for 2–5 days and bridge to nonselective beta blockers • Antibiotic prophylaxis (IV ceftriaxone) × 7 days to prevent primary spontaneous bacterial peritonitis (SBP) and decrease mortality • Vasoactive therapy (IV octreotide) to decrease splanchnic blood flow • Repeat EGD in 2–6 weeks for repeat endoscopic variceal ligation and continue until varices are eradicated • Consider rescue transjugular intrahepatic portosystemic shunt (TIPS) if refractory or recurrent bleeding
Additional Considerations	**Screening:** Patients with cirrhosis should undergo screening for varices. If no varices: Repeat EGD every 2–3 years in patients with compensated cirrhosis, or annually if hepatic decompensation occurs. **Prevention:** Treat medium-large varices with nonselective beta blockers (carvedilol, propranolol, or nadolol) or endoscopic ligation until eradication occurs for primary prophylaxis. **Surgical considerations:** In failed endoscopic cases or those with severe bleeding, placement of **TIPS** is the preferred therapy over open surgery. TIPS placement involves passing a catheter through the hepatic vein, advancing through the liver parenchyma into the portal vein where a stent is deployed. TIPS can be done without general anesthesia and is much less invasive than open surgery. Open emergency surgery to place a shunt is associated with significant complication and mortality rate and is therefore reserved for special, limited circumstances.

CASE 12 | Colorectal Cancer (CRC)

A 71-year-old man with a 30 pack-year history of tobacco use presents with fatigue and abdominal pain. He has no past medical history but has not seen a doctor in decades. He reports abdominal cramping, generalized malaise, and unintentional weight loss. His father had colon cancer at age 57. Physical exam is notable for conjunctival pallor and mild abdominal tenderness but no guarding. There is no palpable mass on digital rectal exam (DRE), but stool is positive for occult blood.

Conditions with Similar Presentations	**Diverticular bleed:** Presents with bright red blood but not weight loss. **Hemorrhoids:** Presents as painless bright red blood per rectum with bowel movements and other symptoms such as perianal irritation or itching. **IBD:** Also associated with GI bleeding, especially **ulcerative colitis**. However, IBD typically presents in younger patients and is associated with a history of intermittent episodes of bloody diarrhea. **Anal fissures:** Tears occur posteriorly where there is less perfusion, are generally painful and associated with constipation and low-fiber diets. Lateral fissures are associated with Crohn disease, anal cancer, or lymphoma. If a patient presents with associated rectal bleeding, endoscopy should be performed to evaluate for underlying malignancy.
Initial Diagnostic Testing	• Confirm diagnosis with colonoscopy and biopsy. • Consider checking CBC, baseline CEA, CT chest/abdomen/pelvis.
Next Steps in Management	Surgical resection of the primary colon tumor followed by chemotherapy
Discussion	CRC is the third most common cancer in men and women worldwide. It is more prevalent in ages >60 and more men are affected than women. Approximately 70% of all CRCs occur sporadically, while fewer than 10% are due to genetic predisposition. • The most well-known model for pathogenesis of CRC is the adenoma–carcinoma sequence, in which a series of mutations in genes such as APC and TP53 leads to development of adenoma to invasive carcinoma. • Another less common pathway (associated with Lynch syndrome) involves mutations in mismatch repair genes leading to microsatellite instability. **History:** • Risk factors: Red/processed meat, obesity, sedentary lifestyle, smoking, Lynch syndrome, FAP, hamartomatous polyposis syndromes (Peutz-Jeghers, juvenile polyposis). • Suspect in men and post-menopausal women presenting with iron deficiency anemia. • Symptoms: Rectal bleeding, change in bowel habits, fatigue, weight loss, abdominal pain, or anemia. • Cancers involving the ascending (right) colon present insidiously with iron deficiency anemia, while cancers affecting the descending (left) colon often present with change in bowel habits, hematochezia, and colicky pain (due to intermittent obstruction of lumen). **Physical exam:** Usually unremarkable but may have abdominal mass or pain. Rectal blood or mass may be noted on DRE (rectal cancer). **Diagnostics:** • Colonoscopy with biopsy confirms diagnosis. Tumors involving distal or left colon are commonly encircling (apple-core appearance on barium enema) and may narrow/occlude the bowel lumen, while tumors on the right colon are typically exophytic. • CT of chest, abdomen, and pelvis for metastases and pretreatment staging • CBC and iron studies may show iron deficiency anemia. • Obtain baseline serum CEA level to monitor for recurrence.

CASE 12 | Colorectal Cancer (CRC) *(continued)*

Discussion	**Management:** • Surgical resection and adjuvant chemotherapy depending on stage • Unresectable metastatic disease is treated with systemic chemotherapy, possibly in combination with targeted therapy Annular, constricting adenocarcinoma of the descending colon. This radiographic appearance is referred to as an "apple-core" lesion and is always highly suggestive of malignancy. (Reproduced with permission Loscalzo J, Fauci A, Kasper D, Hauser S, Longo D, Jameson J. Harrison's Principles of Internal Medicine, 21e; 2022.)
Additional Considerations	**Preventative:** Protective factors include fruits and vegetables, increased physical activity, and regular use of aspirin and NSAIDs. **Screening:** For average risk patients, start screening at age 45. Consider any of the following methods: • Colonoscopy every 10 years • Flexible sigmoidoscopy every 5–10 years • Fecal immunochemical test (FIT) annually or every 3 years in combination with sigmoidoscopy every 5 years • Guaiac occult blood test annually • CT colonography every 5 years • For patients at higher risk, see below table **Surgical considerations:** The sigmoid colon is the most common site of primary colon cancer. **Total colectomy** refers to removing the entire colon, **hemicolectomy** refers to removing the left or right portion of the colon, **proctocolectomy** involves removing the colon and rectum. During surgery, regional lymph node dissection is performed to inform prognosis and post-op management with chemo or radiation. Although it is ideal to restore bowel flow by primary anastomosis, some patients may require a temporary or permanent colostomy bag.

Colorectal Screening in Higher-Risk Populations

Risk	Key Points	Screening Interval/Test
Family history of colorectal cancer (CRC)	• In first-degree relative before age 60 or in two first-degree relatives at any age	• Colonoscopy every 5 years at age 40 or 10 years before the youngest age of CRC in the family (whichever comes first)
IBD	• Ulcerative colitis for >8–10 years • Crohn disease for >8 years	• Colonoscopy every 1–2 years
Familial cancer syndromes		
Familial adenomatous polyposis (FAP)	• Autosomal dominant mutation of the APC tumor suppressor gene • Risk of CRC is 100% • Associated with other cancers • Prophylactic total colectomy recommended	• Colonoscopy or flexible sigmoidoscopy annually beginning at age 10–15
Hereditary nonpolyposis colorectal cancer (HNPCC) syndrome (also known as Lynch syndrome)	• Autosomal dominant disorder of DNA mismatch repair genes • Consider diagnosis if family history is notable for three cases of (CRC), one case diagnosed before age 50, one is a first-degree relative of the other two, and at least two generations are affected • Increased risk for endometrial, gastric, ovarian, and skin cancers among others • Total colectomy only way to prevent disease recurrence	• Colonoscopy every 1–2 years beginning at age 20–25 or 2–5 years prior to the earliest age of CRC diagnosis in the family (whichever comes first)
Juvenile polyposis syndrome	• Affects children (<5 years of age) but may also affect adults • "Juvenile" refers to the polyps, and this autosomal dominant syndrome is characterized by numerous hamartomatous polyps in the colon, stomach, and small bowel • Initially benign but may become malignant in the future	• Colonoscopy every 1–3 years beginning at age 12 years
Peutz-Jeghers syndrome	• Autosomal dominant • Presents with numerous hamartomas in the GI tract and hyperpigmented mouth, lips, and hands • Associated with increased risk of breast and other GI cancers	• Baseline screening with upper endoscopy and colonoscopy at 8 years • Subsequent screening depends on whether polyps found

GI Bleed Mini Cases

Cases	Key Findings
Mallory-Weiss tear	**Hx/PE:** • Hematemesis or coffee-ground emesis, preceded by multiple episodes of non-bloody emesis, retching, or coughing. • Patients with severe bleeding may have signs of hemodynamic instability such as tachycardia or hypotension. **Diagnostics:** • Upper endoscopy confirms diagnosis (longitudinal mucosal tear in the esophagogastric junction). • CBC (Hgb) to assess blood loss. • Type and screen, coagulation studies (PT/INR, PTT) **Management:** • Resuscitate with IV fluid and/or blood products • Initiate IV PPI and give antiemetics as needed • Endoscopic therapy (e.g., clips, band ligation, thermal coagulation) for actively bleeding tears **Discussion:** • Mallory-Weiss tears are partial-thickness, longitudinal mucosal lacerations in the submucosa of the distal esophagus and proximal stomach resulting from behaviors that increase intra-abdominal pressure such as retching, coughing, or straining/lifting. • Classic presentation is someone with alcohol use disorder or patient with bulimia with a history of retching/vomiting, or pregnant patients with hyperemesis gravidarum.
Angiodysplasia	**Hx/PE:** • Usually occult blood loss, but can present as melena or hematochezia depending on if upper or lower source • Symptoms of anemia (fatigue, weakness, or exertional dyspnea) **Diagnostics:** • Upper (EGD) and/or lower (colonoscopy) endoscopy confirms diagnosis • Video capsule endoscopy considered if EGD negative. Angiodysplasias appear as small, dilated blood vessels radiating from a central vessel • CBC, type and screen, coagulation studies (PT/INR, PTT) **Management:** • Endoscopic treatment **Discussion:** • Angiodysplasia is dilated thin-walled vessels in veins, venules, and capillaries and can occur at any site in the stomach, small intestine, and colon • Colonic lesions are commonly found in the right colon (cecum) • Frequently detected in patients older than 60 years and associated with end-stage kidney disease (ESRD), von Willebrand disease, and aortic stenosis (**Heyde syndrome**)
Diverticular bleed	**Hx:** • Painless hematochezia • May have history of diverticulosis (bleeding occurs in 15% of patients with diverticulosis) **PE:** • DRE with blood and/or occult blood • May have signs of blood loss (anemia, pallor) **Diagnostics:** • Colonoscopy • CT angiography if bleeding not identified by colonoscopy • CBC, type and screen, coagulation studies (PT/INR, PTT) **Management:** • Volume resuscitation with isotonic fluid/blood, transfuse Hgb <7 or massive bleed • Colonoscopy both diagnostic and therapeutic (bleeding vessel treated with endoscopic therapy) **Discussion:** Diverticular bleeding is the most common cause of hematochezia. If bleeding cannot be stopped by endoscopic or angiographic intervention, surgery is required

GI Bleed Mini Cases (*continued*)

Anal cancer	**Hx:** • Initially rectal bleeding, itching, rectal pressure, followed by anorectal pain. • Risk factors: High-risk sexual behavior, HIV, immunosuppression, IV drug use, history of genital warts, cigarette smoking, history of cervical or vulvar or vulvar intraepithelial neoplasia or cancers. **PE:** DRE with palpable mass, inguinal adenopathy **Diagnostics:** • Anoscopy and rigid proctoscopy with biopsy • Biopsy with keratinized squamous cell hyperplasia with central necrosis, indicative of anal SCC **Management:** • Chemotherapy (combined fluorouracil or capecitabine plus mitomycin) and radiation therapy offers a potential for cure with preservation of anal sphincter function • For recurrent or unresponsive cases, resection of affected portions is an option. **Discussion:** Cancers of the anal canal include adenocarcinoma and squamous cell carcinoma. Squamous cell carcinoma is much more common and is associated with Human papillomavirus (HPV). **HPV-16** is closely linked to malignancies of the oropharynx, genital tract, anus, and rectum. • The proximal portion of the anal canal (above the dentate line) contains the squamo-columnar junction where columnar cells are gradually replaced by squamous cell types more distally. The anal transformation zone is the area where squamous metaplasia commonly occurs. • A third cancer that can arise in the region is squamous cell carcinoma that affects perianal skin instead of the canal itself. This category can be thought of similarly to other dermatologic cancers and are managed via wide local excision.

DIARRHEA

Diarrhea can be classified as acute (≤14 days), persistent (>14 to < 30 days), or chronic (>30 days). History, including risk factors and physical exam, will be helpful to narrow your differential and guide diagnostic investigations.

Acute diarrhea:

- Usually due to an infectious cause (most commonly viral) and self-limited.

- Diagnostic testing not recommended for uncomplicated traveler's diarrhea.

- Alarm symptoms include bloody diarrhea, signs of severe illness (fever, sepsis, severe abdominal pain, hospitalized, ≥6 bowel movements/24 hours), age >70, weight loss, immunocompromised host.

- Consider stool testing (stool PCR) for bacterial causes including *Salmonella*, *Shigella*, *Campylobacter*, *Yersinia*, *C. difficile*, and Shiga-toxin producing *E. coli* (STEC) in immunosuppressed hosts and those presenting with bloody diarrhea.

Chronic diarrhea can be due to:

- Malabsorption (celiac, lactose intolerance, pancreatic insufficiency)

- Inflammatory bowel disease (Crohn disease, ulcerative colitis)

- Irritable bowel syndrome (IBS)

- Chronic infections (*Cryptosporidium*, *Giardia*, Whipple disease)

- Secretory excess: secretagogues (vasoactive intestinal peptide, calcitonin, gastrin, glucagon, serotonin), bacterial overgrowth

Differential Diagnosis for Diarrhea

Infectious	Non-infectious	
Gastroenteritis Viral: Norovirus, Rotavirus Bacterial: *E. coli, Shigella, Salmonella, Yersinia, Campylobacter, Vibrio* Toxin producing: *B. cereus, C. perfringens, Staphylococcus aureus, C. difficile* **Colitis** *C. difficile, Klebsiella, E. coli, Shigella, Salmonella, Yersinia, Campylobacter* **Other** Parasites: *Giardia, Cryptosporidium, Entamoeba histolytica*; small bowel bacterial overgrowth	**Inflammatory** IBD: UC, Crohn's **Endocrine** Hyperthyroid Diabetes Gastrinoma VIPoma Carcinoid **Medication/substances** Metformin Antibiotics Laxatives Sorbitol, fructose	**Malabsorption** Lactose intolerance Laxative overuse Chronic pancreatitis Bile salt disorder Celiac disease Tropical sprue Short gut syndrome **Other** IBS Colon cancer

CASE 13 | Crohn's Disease

A 23-year-old man presents to clinic with diarrhea and intermittent abdominal cramping for the past 7 months. He reports up to six watery stools per day and sometimes during the night, with occasional mucus and blood. His abdominal pain is intermittent, and he reports feeling feverish at times and has lost about 10 pounds. Exam reveals pallor, aphthous oral ulcers, generalized abdominal tenderness to palpation, erythematous nodules on his anterior shins bilaterally (erythema nodosum), and perianal skin tags.

Conditions with Similar Presentations	**Ulcerative colitis:** Can also present similarly. *See comparison table.* **Chronic ischemic colitis:** Postprandial pain, and patients have other atherosclerotic disease (e.g., stroke, MI, peripheral vascular disease) or risk factors (e.g., HTN, smoking, DM, hypercholesterolemia). Patients may also have abdominal bruit on physical examination. **Infectious diarrhea:** Acute onset, and there is usually a travel/exposure history. Most infectious causes of diarrhea are self-limited and are treated primarily with supportive care (hydration). **Diverticulitis:** Pain is acute and localized to the LLQ. **Celiac disease:** Also presents with intermittent abdominal pain, weight loss, and malabsorption. However, symptoms will be related to gluten consumption and do not occur at night when fasting. Initial testing includes tissue transglutaminase antibody and confirmation of diagnosis by small bowel biopsy. Treatment is with a gluten-free diet. **IBS:** Can also present with intermittent abdominal pain and diarrhea but patients will not have signs of malabsorption, anemia, or weight loss. This is a diagnosis of exclusion and is treated with lifestyle modification (dietary changes, exercise, stress management). **Lactose intolerance:** Due to lactase deficiency, symptoms occur after dairy consumption and include flatulence/bloating. Diarrhea not present at night. There will be a high stool osmotic gap. If performed, endoscopy and biopsy are normal. **Tropical sprue:** Affects the small bowel and is seen in patients who visit or reside in the tropics, and responds to antibiotics. **Whipple disease:** More common in men, and is an infection due to *Tropheryma whipplei*. Patients also have migratory large joint arthralgia, dementia, and rarely endocarditis. Foamy macrophages are seen in the lamina propria on biopsy and the organism can be detected by PCR.
Initial Diagnostic Tests	• Confirm diagnosis with colonoscopy +/− upper endoscopy with biopsy • Consider: Rule out infection with stool culture, stool ova/parasites, and *C. difficile* toxin gene assay and tissue transglutaminase antibody to rule out celiac disease.
Next Steps in Management	• Steroids, immunosuppression • Nutritional supplementation depending on extent of malabsorption and nutritional deficiencies

CASE 13 | Crohn's Disease (continued)

Discussion	Crohn's disease is an inflammatory bowel disease which presents with chronic abdominal pain and diarrhea. Crohn's disease can involve any portion of the GI tract but typically spares the rectum. The mucosal inflammation is discontiguous ("skip lesions" involving various noncontinuous portions throughout the GI tract). The transmural inflammation specific to Crohn's disease can result in fistula and stricture formation. **History:** • Presents in the second to fourth decades of life, and risk factors include family history of IBD • Symptoms: Low-grade fevers, malaise, diarrhea, crampy abdominal pain, hematochezia, weight loss • Extraintestinal manifestations include rashes, joint pains (see below) **Physical exam:** • May have localized (RLQ if ileocecal involvement) or diffuse abdominal tenderness • May present with small bowel or colonic obstruction (from stricture formation due to transmural inflammation) • May have perianal disease **Diagnostics:** • Diagnosis with colonoscopy and biopsy showing noncaseating granulomas with lymphoid aggregates. • Visualization of GI tract may reveal a segmental pattern of involvement (skip lesions), erythema, and cobblestone sign (inflamed areas of bowel with deep ulcerations at the margins) Consider checking: • Markers of inflammation: CRP, ESR, fecal calprotectin • CBC: ↓Hgb secondary to GI bleed or anemia of chronic disease • B12 level (if there is ileal involvement) **Management:** • Treat acute flare with corticosteroids • Antibiotics (metronidazole, ciprofloxacin) may be used for acute flare • Chronic disease managed with 5-ASA agents (i.e., sulfasalazine, mesalamine), immunomodulating agents (i.e., azathioprine, methotrexate), or biologics (infliximab, adalimumab)
Additional Considerations	**Screening:** Colorectal cancer screening: 8 years after diagnosis and up to every 1–2 years onward **Complications:** *Strictures:* Sometimes seen on imaging as a "string sign," may occur in any portion of the GI tract due to chronic inflammation and stenosis of the intestinal lumen *Fistula:* May occur in any portion of the GI tract due to severe transmural inflammation; a common site is fistula formation between the ileocecal region and urinary bladder, known as an **enterovesical fistula.** This will typically present as dysuria and recurrent polymicrobial urinary tract infections *Small/Large Bowel Obstruction:* Presence of significant inflammation in a specific region of the bowel (i.e., ileitis, jejunitis, colitis) increases risk for acute complications such as a small or large bowel obstruction *Abscess:* May occur when the transmural inflammation results in a loss of integrity of the GI mucosa which can progress to transmural invasion by GI flora *Perforation:* May occur due to the transmural inflammatory nature of CD which results in loss of integrity of the GI tract; it typically occurs in the ileum or jejunum and requires emergent surgical intervention for treatment. *Malabsorption:* If there is involvement of specific regions of the small bowel or extensive disease, malabsorption of specific nutrients (i.e., iron, B12, vitamin D, niacin) may occur. **Extraintestinal manifestations of Crohn's disease:** Rashes such as pyoderma gangrenosum, erythema nodosum (red painful nodules on the patient's shins), ocular involvement including episcleritis and uveitis, oral ulcerations, kidney/gallstones, and spondyloarthropathy. **Surgical considerations:** Indications for surgical intervention include stricture/obstruction, massive hemorrhage, refractory fistula, abscess, or disease unresponsive to medical therapy. Surgery may alleviate symptoms; however, it is not curative as the disease process may recur in a different region of the GI tract.

Classic Distinguishing Characteristics of Crohn's Disease and Ulcerative Colitis

	Crohn's Disease	Ulcerative Colitis
Location of disease	Can affect any and multiple parts of the GI tract from the oropharynx to the anus, most commonly ileum and proximal colon	Starts distally in the rectum; extension is continuous proximally. Does not involve upper GI tract or small bowel (exception of rare involvement of the ileum ["backwash ileitis"])
Complications	Malabsorption (anemia, B12 deficiency, vitamin D deficiency). Intraabdominal and perianal fistulas, abscesses	Bleeding, fulminant colitis
Endoscopic findings	Skip lesions, cobblestoning Rectal sparing	Pseudopolyps Rectal involvement
Histologic findings	Transmural involvement Granulomas	Mucosal and submucosal involvement Crypt abscesses
Risk factors	Smoking, family history	Family history
Colon cancer screening	• Start 8 years after diagnosis of colon involvement, followed by surveillance colonoscopies every 1–2 years • If also with Primary sclerosing cholangitis (PSC), start at time of diagnosis, with annual surveillance	
Extraintestinal manifestations	• Ankylosing spondylitis, sacroiliitis, peripheral arthritis • Pyoderma gangrenosum, erythema nodosum • Uveitis, scleritis, episcleritis • PSC much more common with ulcerative colitis • Thromboembolism	

Malabsorption/Diarrhea Mini Cases

Cases	Key Findings
Celiac disease	**Hx:** • Chronic or recurrent GI symptoms such as diarrhea/steatorrhea, flatulence, abdominal pain, and bloating, and signs of malabsorption, or nutrient or vitamin deficiency. • Less commonly, may present with extraintestinal signs and symptoms (e.g., iron deficiency anemia, dermatitis herpetiformis, osteoporosis, arthritis, neurologic symptoms (peripheral neuropathy, ataxia), psychiatric disorders [anxiety, depression], amenorrhea, infertility, other autoimmune diseases). • Risk factors: Family history of celiac disease, type 1 diabetes, autoimmune thyroiditis, selective IgA deficiency, Down and Turner syndromes, and pulmonary hemosiderosis. **PE:** • Children and adolescents may have short stature and delayed puberty. • **Dermatitis herpetiformis**, characterized by erythematous, urticarial plaques, papules, and grouped vesicles, may be found on extensor surfaces of elbows and knees, scalp, posterior neck, and buttocks. • Signs of vitamin deficiency such as mucositis or ecchymosis may be seen. **Diagnostics:** • Diagnosis with both serologic evaluation with tissue transglutaminase (tTG) IgA antibody and upper endoscopy with small bowel biopsy. • Histologic findings of celiac disease include increased intraepithelial lymphocytes, atrophic mucosa with complete loss of villi.

Dermatitis herpetiformis. Papules, vesicles, and crusts on knees. (Reproduced, with permission, from Kang S, Amagai M, Bruckner AL, Enk AH, Margolis DJ, McMichael AJ, Orringer JS, eds: Fitzpatrick's Dermatology. 9th ed. New York, NY: McGraw Hill; 2019.)

Malabsorption/Diarrhea Mini Cases (*continued*)

Celiac disease	**Management:** • Lifelong gluten-free diet (avoid wheat, barley, and rye) • Dapsone for dermatitis herpetiformis **Discussion:** • Celiac disease is a chronic, multi-organ autoimmune disease caused by inappropriate immune response to dietary gluten in genetically predisposed individuals. It can occur in all ages from infancy to elderly. • Approximately 1% of Western population has celiac disease. • DEXA scan with osteopenia/osteoporosis is common in patients with celiac disease due to calcium and vitamin D deficiency. • Test for vitamin and mineral deficiencies such as copper, zinc, folic acid, and iron.
Infectious diarrhea	See Infectious Diseases Chapter
Irritable bowel syndrome (IBS)	**Hx:** • Abdominal pain/cramping related to defecation, constipation, diarrhea, or changes in consistency of stool. • No signs of weight loss, malabsorption, or anemia. **PE:** Unremarkable **Diagnostics:** Rome IV Criteria: Presence of intermittent abdominal pain at least once a week for 3 months with two of the following: 1. Pain related to defecation 2. Associated with change in stool frequency 3. Associated with change in stool appearance **Additional considerations:** • Normal CBC, CRP, TSH, BMP, tissue transglutaminase antibody and fecal calprotectin. • Investigate further if red flag symptoms (weight loss, anemia). **Management:** • Lifestyle changes (diet, exercise, trial of fiber [psyllium]). • Avoid gas-producing foods/recommend low FODMAP (Fermentable Oligo-, Di-, Monosaccharides, And Polyols) diet. These short-chain carbohydrates are poorly absorbed and can aggravate gut symptoms. • Medications based on predominant symptoms: Dicyclomine for cramping, other options depend on if diarrhea (loperamide) or constipation (psyllium, polyethylene glycol, lubiprostone, linaclotide, plecanatide) predominant symptoms. **Discussion:** IBS is the most common GI disorder and there does not seem to be one unifying pathophysiology that fits all patients (various contributions of altered GI motility, visceral hypersensitivity, intestinal inflammation, and alterations of bowel flora).
Carcinoid tumor	**Hx:** • Flushing (most common), watery diarrhea, bronchospasm, hypotension, symptoms of right-sided heart failure (ascites, edema, dyspnea), symptoms of niacin (B3) deficiency = pellagra (diarrhea, dermatitis, dementia). **PE:** • Cutaneous flushing • Tachycardia, hypotension, wheezing, dyspnea **Diagnostics:** • ↑ 24-hour urinary excretion of 5-HIAA (end product of serotonin metabolism) • CT with contrast or MRI of abdomen and pelvis to identify the primary tumor **Management:** • For nonmetastatic disease, surgical resection • Somatostatin analogs (octreotide, lanreotide) for carcinoid syndrome

Malabsorption/Diarrhea Mini Cases (*continued*)

Carcinoid tumor	Discussion:
	• Carcinoid tumors are rare, slow-growing neuroendocrine tumors (NETs). Most NETs are sporadic but some may be associated with genetic syndromes such as multiple endocrine neoplasia type 1 (MEN1) or von Hippel-Lindau disease (VHL) • Primary tumors are most commonly found in GI tract, followed by lungs and bronchi • Most are asymptomatic but may present with carcinoid syndrome • Carcinoid syndrome results from hypersecretion of amines and peptides (serotonins). Liver inactivates bioactive products secreted by the tumor, so carcinoid syndrome occurs when there are hepatic metastases or when the origin is outside of the GI tract • Carcinoid crisis (excessive flushing, diarrhea, bronchospasm, hypotension, hemodynamic instability) is a life-threatening condition and is treated with IV octreotide • Tryptophan depletion from excessive serotonin production can lead to niacin deficiency and pellagra

HEPATOCELLULAR INJURY

The liver plays an important role in detoxification, metabolism, digestion, storage of glycogen, minerals and vitamins, enzyme activation, and synthesizing plasma proteins. These essential functions may be compromised when the liver is injured due to various causes.

System	History, Physical Exam, and Lab Findings
Skin	Pruritis, jaundice, palmar erythema, spider angiomas, caput medusa, purpura, petechiae
HEENT	Conjunctival icterus, fetor hepaticus
Lungs	Dyspnea, decreased basilar breath sounds or dullness to percussion from ascites
CV	Peripheral edema
GI	Nausea/vomiting, anorexia, abdominal distension/pain, hematemesis, melena, hematochezia, ascites, hepatosplenomegaly
GU/renal	Amenorrhea, erectile dysfunction, gynecomastia, testicular atrophy, kidney injury
Neuro	Altered mental status (encephalopathy), asterixis
Hematologic	Pale conjunctiva, skin bruising, anemia, thrombocytopenia, coagulation disorders
Metabolic	Jaundice, hyperbilirubinemia, hyponatremia

History:

- Assess for possible exposures (e.g., alcohol, drug, medication usage, contaminated foods, blood transfusions)
- Elicit a sexual history, relevant family history, and history of diabetes or obesity.
- Inquire about jaundice, pruritus, abdominal pain, swelling, changes in bowels, changes in weight, nausea/vomiting, fevers, joint aches, pains or rashes, urine color, and stool color.

Physical exam: Look for stigmata of chronic liver disease (e.g., conjunctival icterus, splenomegaly, spider angioma, telangiectasias, palmar erythema, gynecomastia, testicular atrophy, ascites).

Diagnostics: When a patient presents with abnormal liver chemistries, one should first attempt to define the pattern of elevation:

- A hepatocellular pattern = $\uparrow$aspartate aminotransferase (AST) and alanine aminotransferase (ALT)
- A cholestatic pattern = $\uparrow$ALP ± bilirubin
- A mixed pattern will include both

Approach to Elevated AST/ALT

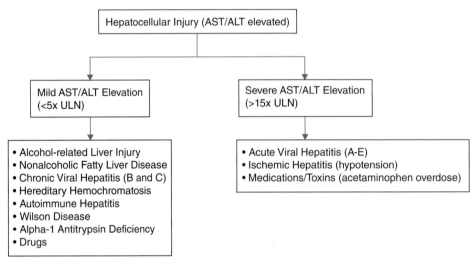

Acute liver injury (ALI): Elevated AST/ALT in a patient without preexisting liver disease or encephalopathy.

Acute liver failure (ALF): Significant liver dysfunction with a coagulopathy (INR ≥1.5) and hepatic encephalopathy in a patient without preexisting liver disease.

- Should be managed in an ICU at a liver transplantation center due to its poor prognosis when untreated.
- Acetaminophen toxicity most common cause of ALF in the United States and other developed countries, while viral hepatitis is more common cause in Asia and Africa.

Chronic liver disease: Progressive liver dysfunction for >6 months, marked histologically by fibrosis and eventually cirrhosis from continuous inflammatory damage and parenchymal regeneration.

- Chronic liver disease is more common than acute failure and increasing in prevalence.
- Alcohol and non-alcoholic fatty liver disease are the most common causes in the United States, while chronic infections with hepatitis viruses C or B ± D are more common in Asia and Africa.

Progression, Complications, and Treatment of Liver Injury

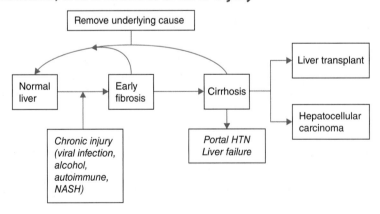

Serologic Profiles of Different HBV Statuses

	Anti-HBc Ab (Exposure)	HBsAg (Infection)	Anti-HBs Ab (Immunity)
HBV-Naive	−	−	−
Acute infection	+	+	−
Window period	+	−	−
Chronic infection	+	+	−
Resolved infection	+	−	+/−
Immunization	−	−	+

Positive anti-HBc IgM may indicate acute infection; anti-HBs typically persists for life but may disappear over time in some patients and allow for possible reinfection.

Relative Titers of HBV Serologic Markers Over Time

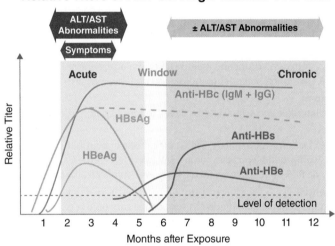

Relative titers of HBV serologic markers over time.

CASE 14 | Acute Hepatitis A

A 31-year-old woman presents to clinic with new-onset jaundice. She recently came back from a trip to Bangladesh. She initially had abdominal pain with nausea, vomiting, and generalized malaise followed by dark urine and yellowing of her eyes. She has not had any prescription or herbal medications, recent sexual activity, or alcohol. She is hemodynamically stable with a temperature of 38°C. Physical exam is notable for scleral icterus and jaundice, mild RUQ tenderness to palpation, and hepatomegaly. No asterixis is present.

Conditions with Similar Presentations	**Other viral hepatitis:** Hepatitis viruses B-E, CMV, EBV, HSV, yellow fever virus, and HIV may also present with elevated transaminases (ALT/AST) and nonspecific symptoms such as fever, fatigue, and lymphadenopathy. Hepatitis E should be considered in pregnant patients presenting with fulminant liver failure following fecal-oral exposure.
	Drug-induced liver injury (DILI): Many prescription and OTC drugs (e.g., acetaminophen, isoniazid, amoxicillin-clavulanate) are hepatotoxic and may present with jaundice and hepatomegaly. History and timing of exposure should be considered to rule out DILI.
	Autoimmune hepatitis: May be asymptomatic or present with liver failure, anorexia, fatigue, weight loss, and other extrahepatic manifestations from autoimmune diseases such as SLE, rheumatoid arthritis. More common in women and diagnosed with serologic markers (ANA, ASMA, LKM1, pANCA).
	Secondary syphilis: May present with elevated AST/ALT, lymphadenopathy, and constitutional symptoms, but will have other findings such as maculopapular rash.
Initial Diagnostic Tests	• Confirm diagnosis: Serum HAV IgM • Consider: B-HCG, LFTs, HBV, HCV, and HEV serologies, ANA, ASMA, ceruloplasmin, abdominal US to rule out other causes

CASE 14 | Acute Hepatitis A (continued)

Next Steps in Management	• Supportive care (bed rest, adequate nutrition and hydration) • Emergent liver transplantation for fulminant liver failure
Discussion	Hepatitis A virus (HAV) is one of the most common viral infections worldwide with an estimated 1.4 million cases each year. HAV is a picornavirus that is primarily transmitted via fecal-oral route via person-to-person contact or consumption of contaminated food or water. HAV reaches the liver through portal blood from the intestine where the virus replicates and assembles in hepatocytes for weeks before any evidence of liver injury. • Symptoms of liver inflammation and injury appear 15–50 days after infection (average 25–30 days). • IgM is the initial antibody that eliminates HAV, with IgG appearing shortly after symptom onset and conferring lifelong immunity. • Patients are infectious during the incubation period (average 28 days) until a week after jaundice appears. • Acute hepatitis A is usually self-limited and <1% of patients will develop fulminant liver failure requiring liver transplantation. **History:** • Risk factors: Highly endemic in parts of Africa and South Asia, but seen in high-risk populations (e.g., IV drug use, homeless individuals, health care workers, men who have sex with men) and from contaminated food • Children <6 years are typically asymptomatic, but >70% of adults have symptoms that persist for 2–8 weeks • Initial symptoms are abrupt and include fever, malaise, anorexia, nausea/vomiting, abdominal pain, and headache. Dark urine precedes jaundice, and patients may also have pale stools and pruritus **Physical exam:** • May have jaundice and scleral icterus, fever, tender hepatomegaly **Diagnostics:** • ALT and AST often >1000 units/L, Milder elevations of bilirubin, ALP are also seen • Diagnosis confirmed by positive serum HAV IgM (detectable 5–10 days after symptoms arise) • HAV RNA via PCR or genotyping (not widely available) can also confirm diagnosis but are rarely needed **Management:** • Symptomatic patients managed with supportive care only (e.g., rest, hydration, antiemetics) • Hospitalization may be required for complications such as hypovolemia from vomiting, coagulopathy, encephalopathy • Fulminant liver failure should be transferred to an ICU at a transplant center • Most important public health intervention is prevention through vaccination: all children ≥12 months and adults at risk of disease or complications from disease (men who have sex with men, chronic liver disease, clotting disorders, or travel to high-risk areas) • **Pre-exposure prophylaxis** with vaccination is recommended for patients planning travel to endemic countries • **Post-exposure prophylaxis** is vaccination within 2 weeks of exposure to HAV. IVIG prophylaxis should be used for children <12 months and individuals with contraindications to vaccination. It should be added to vaccination in those at high risk of exposure who are immunocompromised or have chronic liver disease
Additional Considerations	**Preventative:** Hepatitis A vaccine confers lifelong immunity to >90% of those receiving it. All children ≥12 months should receive two doses of the HAV vaccine 6 months apart **Complications:** Rare, but include fulminant liver failure (<1%), cholestatic hepatitis (5%), relapsing hepatitis (within 6 months of initial presentation in up to 10% of patients), and new-onset autoimmune hepatitis

CASE 15 | Chronic Hepatitis C

A 57-year-old woman presents to establish care with a primary care physician and is noted to have an AST 45 and ALT 62 on routine lab work. She does not drink alcohol but used intravenous heroin 30 years ago. On exam, she is well appearing, her BMI is 23, temperature 98.7°F, blood pressure 125/80 mmHg, heart rate 88/min, and respiratory rate 18/min. She has spider angiomas on her chest and palmar erythema.

Conditions with Similar Presentations	**Chronic hepatitis B** (see below), **alcohol-associated liver disease**, **non-alcoholic steatohepatitis**, **hemochromatosis**, **autoimmune hepatitis**, **Wilson disease**, and **medication side-effects** can present with asymptomatic chronic elevations in AST and ALT.
Initial Diagnostic Tests	• Confirm diagnosis: HCV antibody and RNA PCR. • Consider: Platelet count, serologies for HBV and HIV, US abdomen, and/or elastography for noninvasive fibrosis assessment.

CASE 15 | Chronic Hepatitis C *(continued)*

Next Steps in Management	• If detectable HCV RNA, treat with direct-acting antiviral therapy. • Assess for and manage extrahepatic manifestations of hepatitis C.
Discussion	Hepatitis C remains one of the major causes of cirrhosis in the United States, though this is slowly changing with the advent of the new highly effective antiviral therapies and increased screening efforts. Modes of transmission of HCV involve contact with contaminated blood through needlestick injuries, sharing needles among injection drug users, long-term dialysis use, or blood transfusions received prior to 1990. HCV is very rarely transmitted sexually or vertically. **History:** • Acute infection is rarely symptomatic and accounts for only 15% of all symptomatic acute hepatitis cases • Chronic HCV is usually asymptomatic and silently progresses to cirrhosis in 10–20% over 20–40 years **Physical exam:** • Initially normal, but signs of cirrhosis and portal hypertension if disease progresses (e.g., spider angiomas, palmar erythema, ascites) **Diagnostics:** • Positive Hep C antibody and subsequent detection of HCV RNA on a PCR test • HCV genotype should be assessed to inform antiviral selection but is becoming less utilized now that therapies are becoming effective for all genotypes. • Elastography studies (e.g., transient elastography) can be considered to noninvasively screen for advanced fibrosis **Management:** • Antiviral regimen and duration depend on extent of liver fibrosis, HCV genotype, and prior treatment history • Counsel the patient to avoid alcohol and other hepatotoxins • Counsel the patient on preventing transmission to others (blood donation, sharing needles, sexual transmission) • For intermittent or ongoing injection drug use, recommend counseling ± medication-assisted therapy • Vaccination for HAV and HBV
Additional Considerations	**Screening:** The USPSTF recommends one-time screening for HCV infection in adults 18–79 years old (Grade B). Consider repeat screening for those with ongoing risk factors **Complications:** Cirrhosis, HCC, and extraintestinal manifestations (e.g., mixed cryoglobulinemia, lymphoma, membranoproliferative glomerulonephritis, porphyria cutanea tarda, lichen planus, diabetes).

CASE 16 | Hemochromatosis

A 54-year-old woman with hypertension, congestive heart failure, and newly diagnosed type 2 diabetes mellitus presents for evaluation of abnormal liver chemistries. She does not drink alcohol or use any other substances, and is not taking supplements or herbal preparations. Review of symptoms is notable for chronic knee pain, bilateral wrist pain and paresthesias of the first three digits of her hands. She is afebrile with normal vital signs. Physical exam is notable for icteric sclera, diffuse bronze hyperpigmentation of the skin, jugular venous distension, S3, hepatomegaly, and bilateral lower extremity pitting edema and positive Tinel sign bilaterally. ALT is 120, AST is 99, albumin is 2.1. Electrolytes are normal.

Conditions with Similar Presentations	**Other causes of hepatitis:** Can also cause cirrhosis and its sequelae, including peripheral edema and jaundice. However, other causes of hepatitis would not cause bronze skin, arthralgia, or carpal tunnel syndrome. **Pancreatic cancer:** Can also present with new-onset diabetes and jaundice but would also have epigastric pain and weight loss. **Addison disease:** Can also present with weakness, arthralgia, and hyperpigmentation, but would also have fatigue, weight loss, postural hypotension, salt craving, hyponatremia, and hyperkalemia. **Wilson disease:** Can present with similar symptoms of systemic heavy metal deposition (copper instead of iron), including hepatomegaly, jaundice, cardiomyopathy, arthropathy, impotence, and may see Kayser-Fleischer rings.

CASE 16 | Hemochromatosis *(continued)*

Initial Diagnostic Tests	Iron studies; confirm with genetic testing
Next Steps in Management	• Phlebotomy (up to weekly if tolerated) • Iron chelation (e.g., deferoxamine) if phlebotomy is contraindicated due to anemia
Discussion	Hemochromatosis is a disease of iron overload due to abnormal deposition in body tissues over several decades. It is almost always hereditary. The most common form of hereditary hemochromatosis (HH) is seen in patients with European ancestry and is due to autosomal recessive mutations (most common C282Y) of the HFE gene. Other secondary causes of iron overload include excessive dietary iron consumption, multiple transfusions (≥10–20), and chronic liver disease. **History:** • Risk factors: Family history of HH. • Iron overload becomes symptomatic when total body accumulation reaches 20 g, which typically occurs after 40 years of age in males and after menopause in females. • May be asymptomatic or present with nonspecific symptoms such as weakness and lethargy, sequelae of cirrhosis, arthralgias, carpal tunnel syndrome, loss of libido, and impotence in men. **Physical exam:** • May have hepatosplenomegaly, skin hyperpigmentation ("bronze diabetes"), osteoarthritis (especially of the second and third metacarpophalangeal joints), testicular atrophy, gynecomastia, and/or signs of cirrhosis such as jaundice, spider angiomas, and palmar erythema. **Diagnostics:** • HH should be suspected in patients with elevated transaminases and/or cirrhosis, skin hyperpigmentation, arthritis, and new-onset diabetes mellitus. • Iron studies will show high ferritin and high % saturation of transferrin (Fe ÷ transferrin × 100) (>45%). • For HH associated with the HFE gene, genetic testing will show C282Y homozygosity or C282Y/H63D heterozygosity to confirm the diagnosis. • MRI can assess liver iron content noninvasively if iron studies not diagnostic. • Liver biopsy is not needed to confirm a diagnosis but may be helpful to rule out other liver diseases, quantify iron deposition, and evaluate the degree of fibrosis. • Consider genetic testing in individuals with a family history of HH in first- or second-degree relatives. **Management:** • Therapeutic phlebotomy to maintain ferritin levels of 50–100 mcg/L. • Iron chelators if unable to tolerate phlebotomy. • Avoid multivitamins that contain iron or vitamin C (increases iron absorption from gut). • Decrease or eliminate alcohol intake and take precautions against viral hepatitis and other causes of cirrhosis. • Liver transplant for decompensated cirrhosis or resectable HCC.
Additional Considerations	**Screening:** No screening unless family history of HH **Complications:** Complications occur due to Fe deposition in other organ systems and include diabetes mellitus, hypopituitarism, hypogonadism, hypothyroidism, arthropathy/arthritis, cardiomyopathy, conduction disturbances. Also increased risk of hepatocellular carcinoma (HCC). Patients are at risk of infections from siderophilic bacteria (e.g., *Vibrio vulnificus, Yersinia enterocolitica*), and thus should be counseled to avoid undercooked seafood. **Pediatric considerations:** Consider secondary hemochromatosis in pediatric patients with a history of multiple transfusions.

Hepatocellular Disease Mini Cases

Cases	Key Findings
Hepatitis B infection	**Hx:** • Most acute infections are asymptomatic, but common symptoms are fever, fatigue, loss of appetite, nausea, vomiting, RUQ pain, and jaundice • May have history of injection drug use, high-risk sexual behavior, and/or immigration from high-prevalence areas **PE:** • In symptomatic patients, exam may reveal fever, jaundice, hepatomegaly, splenomegaly, ascites, and RUQ tenderness • May have extrahepatic manifestations such as rash, arthralgias, and arthritis **Diagnostics:** • Suspect in patients with elevated hepatic transaminases ± signs and symptoms consistent with viral hepatitis • Diagnosis confirmed by hepatitis B virus (HBV) serology (*see figures below*), which should be accompanied by HIV testing and screening for HCV and HDV • Chronic HBV infection is defined as HBsAg positivity >6 months after initial exposure **Management:** • Treatment generally not necessary for acute HBV infection, as >95% of immunocompetent patients recover spontaneously. • For chronic infection, the timing and duration of antiviral therapy (e.g., nucleoside/nucleotide analogs) is contingent on the patient's serologic status and aimed at suppressing HBV replication and preventing cirrhosis **Discussion:** • The clinical manifestations of acute or chronic HBV infection range from asymptomatic to fulminant hepatitis • Both the likelihood of symptomatic illness and the risk of progression to chronic sequala are inversely related to age at time of initial infection. Fulminant liver failure is rare (0.1–0.5%) but is the leading cause of death from HBV infection • Acquisition of HBV varies geographically, with perinatal transmission and horizontal transmission in early childhood being most common in high-prevalence areas of southeast Asia and China, and sexual contact and percutaneous transmission (e.g., injection drug use) being most common in North America and Western Europe • Vaccination is recommended for all children and unvaccinated adults if at increased risk (e.g., health care workers, chronic liver disease, HIV, injection drug use, men having sex with men)
Wilson Disease	**Hx:** Unexplained combination of hepatic, neurologic, psychiatric, ocular, and other systemic findings (e.g., hemolytic anemia, Fanconi syndrome, arthropathy, cardiomyopathy, pancreatitis, impotence/infertility), typically in patients 5–35 years of age. **PE:** Kayser-Fleischer ring, hepatomegaly, splenomegaly, ascites/edema, and/or neurologic abnormalities (tremor, bradykinesia, chorea, dystonia, cognitive impairment). 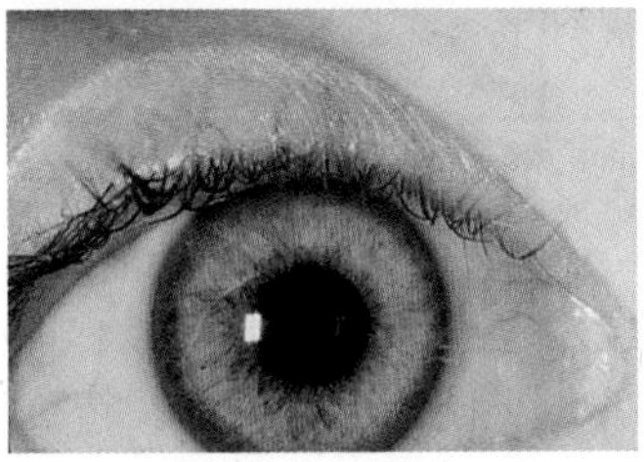 Kayser-Fleischer ring around the cornea in a patient with Wilson disease. (Reproduced, with permission Usatine RP, Smith MA, Mayeaux, Jr. EJ, Chumley HS. The Color Atlas and Synopsis of Family Medicine, 3e; McGraw-Hill 2019. FIGURE 63-9. Reproduced with permission from Marc Solioz, University of Berne.)

Hepatocellular Disease Mini Cases (*continued*)

Wilson Disease	**Diagnostics:** • Diagnosis confirmed by: 1) low serum ceruloplasmin, 2) high 24-hour-urinary copper excretion, and 3) Kayser-Fleischer rings on slit-lamp exam. • If all three criteria are not met, then liver biopsy to assess for elevated hepatic parenchymal copper concentration and/or testing for *ATP7B* gene mutations. **Management:** • Chelating agents (penicillamine or trientine) and oral zinc (interferes with copper absorption). • Lifelong treatment unless liver transplant performed for acute liver failure or refractory decompensated cirrhosis. • First-degree relatives should be screened for *ATP7B* gene mutations. **Discussion:** Wilson disease is an autosomal recessive genetic disorder of the *ATP7B* gene that encodes an ATPase that facilitates binding of copper to apoceruloplasmin to create ceruloplasmin, and also facilitates copper excretion in the bile. These defects lead to copper overload and subsequent deposition in various tissues. Most patients have liver disease that progresses silently into adolescence or adulthood, when they develop acute liver failure or cirrhosis. The spectrum of liver disease includes acute hepatitis, acute liver failure, chronic hepatitis, cirrhosis, and HCC.
Non-alcoholic fatty liver disease (NAFLD)	**Hx:** Most asymptomatic, but symptoms may include fatigue, RUQ fullness/pain, and jaundice. • Risk factors include obesity, diabetes and/or insulin resistance, and certain medications including steroids, antiretrovirals for HIV, methotrexate, and amiodarone. **PE:** Often obese with increased waist circumference; exam may reveal hepatomegaly and signs of cirrhosis (e.g., jaundice, ascites, spider angiomas, gynecomastia) **Diagnostics:** • Often incidental finding of elevated AST and ALT (2–5 × ULN) on blood tests or steatosis on imaging. • Rule out other etiologies of chronic liver disease (e.g., alcohol use, alpha-1 antitrypsin deficiency, Wilson disease, hemochromatosis). • Liver biopsy considered for patients at high risk of advanced fibrosis and/or with indeterminate initial testing **Management:** • Exercise, restrict caloric intake, lose ≥3–10% weight. • Counsel on reducing risk of developing cirrhosis from other etiologies, including avoidance of alcohol and treatment of concomitant viral hepatitis. • Pioglitazone, vitamin E, and GLP-1 agonists considered in certain patients after weighing individual risks vs. benefits. **Discussion:** NAFLD is the most common cause of elevated liver tests in United States adults, with a reported prevalence of 24–45%, which continues to increase with time given the obesity epidemic. Some patients with NAFLD can progress from steatosis to steatohepatitis to fibrosis and eventually cirrhosis and HCC.

Jaundice

Jaundice occurs with increased serum total bilirubin (>2.5 mg/dL). Clinically, patients present with yellowing of the skin and/or eyes (conjunctival icterus). Normally, when red cells break down, heme is converted to bilirubin and sent to the liver to be conjugated prior to its excretion. Therefore, hyperbilirubinemia can consist of either unconjugated (indirect) or conjugated (direct) bilirubin. Also, see Hematology and Oncology Chapter.

- Direct hyperbilirubinemia occurs when there is damage to the hepatocytes leading to inability to excrete conjugated bilirubin into the bile or obstruction of bile ducts after conjugated bilirubin has entered.

- Indirect hyperbilirubinemia occurs when there is overproduction of bilirubin (e.g., hemolysis) or problems with uptake and conjugation of indirect bilirubin (e.g., Gilbert, Crigler-Najjar syndromes).

- Patients can present with an isolated hyperbilirubinemia (no significant elevation of ALP or transaminases) which can be further separated into conjugated and unconjugated. The approach to this presentation is summarized below.

Approach to Isolated Hyperbilirubinemia

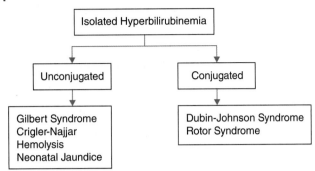

- Cholestatic liver injury pattern is when ALP and bilirubin are elevated more than serum aminotransferases. The first step in the evaluation of these patients is usually a right upper quadrant abdominal US which may show biliary ductal dilation. If isolated ALP elevation with normal bilirubin, an elevated GGT can confirm hepatobiliary source and distinguish it from a bone source.

Approach to Cholestatic Liver Injury

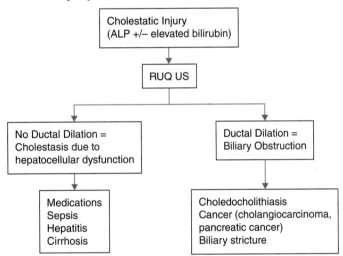

Key Associated Findings and Jaundice Differential Diagnoses

Jaundice with Key Associated Findings	Diagnoses
Travel to endemic country, contaminated water, fever	Hepatitis A or E
Obesity, T2DM	Nonalcoholic fatty liver disease/nonalcoholic steatohepatitis (NAFLD)
Injection drug use, multiple tattoos, or remote blood transfusions (pre-1992)	Hepatitis C
Hypercoagulable states	Hepatic vein thrombosis (Budd-Chiari syndrome)
Painless jaundice, weight loss	Pancreatic cancer, cholangiocarcinoma
Female, history of autoimmune disorders, ALP elevation	Primary biliary cholangitis (PBC)
PSC with worsening jaundice, weight loss	Cholangiocarcinoma
Skin hyperpigmentation, diabetes, cardiomyopathy, joint pains, elevated ferritin	Hemochromatosis
Conjunctival pallor, anemia, low haptoglobin, elevated indirect bilirubin, dark urine	Hemolysis

Key Associated Findings and Jaundice Differential Diagnoses (*Continued*)

Jaundice with Key Associated Findings	Diagnoses
Keyser-Fleischer rings, low ceruloplasmin, neuropsychiatric symptoms	Wilson disease
"Beads on a string" on cholangiogram; ulcerative colitis, ALP elevation	Primary sclerosing cholangitis (PSC)
Children, adolescents, and young adults	Congenital causes of hyperbilirubinemia: Gilbert, Crigler-Najjar, Dubin-Johnson, Rotor syndromes Breast-feeding jaundice and breast milk jaundice are causes of neonatal jaundice
Adolescents and young adults	Consider drug or toxin ingestions or viral hepatitis
Women	Fulminant hepatic failure in pregnant female—hepatitis E PBC is much more common in female patients
Pregnancy	Hepatitis E, HELLP, acute fatty liver of pregnancy, intrahepatic cholestasis of pregnancy (IHCP), are all causes of abnormal liver tests and jaundice in pregnancy

Additional Useful Labs

Condition	Useful Labs
Wilson disease	Low ceruloplasmin
Hemochromatosis	High ferritin and transferrin saturation (high iron, low TIBC)
PSC	+ pANCA;
PBC	+ antimitochondrial Ab (AMA); IgM: high
HAV	Anti-HAV IgM Ab+ (acute); anti-HAV IgG Ab+ (prior infection)
HBV	HBsAg+ (infection/carrier); HBsAb+ (immunity due to vaccine or previous infection); anti-HBcAg Ab+ (IgM: current infection/IgG: prior exposure or chronic infection)
HCV	HCV Ab+ (prior or current infection), HCV PCR
Autoimmune hepatitis	Numerous autoantibodies: ANA, anti-smooth muscle (ASMA) Ab, anti-liver-kidney microsomal-1 (LKM1) Ab, anti-soluble liver antigen (SLA) Ab, high IgG

Key Differences Between PBC and PSC

Features	Primary Biliary Cholangitis (PBC)	Primary Sclerosing Cholangitis (PSC)
Site of disease	• Intrahepatic • Small and medium bile ducts	• Intrahepatic and extrahepatic • Usually medium and large ducts*
Key demographic	• Middle-aged females	• Young males with ulcerative colitis (UC)
Histology	• Bile ducts disappear entirely • Florid duct lesion	• Scarring of bile ducts remains • Onion-skinning of bile ducts
Role of ursodiol	• Cornerstone of management	• Not helpful
Transplant curative?	• No	• No

*Can have small-duct PSC.

CASE 17 | Gilbert Syndrome

A 20-year-old woman presents to the clinic for evaluation of yellow eyes over the past 2 days. The patient also reports fever, malaise, rhinorrhea, and sore throat, all which started 4 days ago. The patient reports taking acetaminophen for fever. Her temperature is 38.5°C, blood pressure is 100/70 mmHg, and pulse is 96. On exam, her eyes have conjunctival icterus, there is nasal congestion, the posterior oropharynx is erythematous. Capillary refill is <2 seconds and there is no conjunctival pallor. There is no hepatosplenomegaly. Labs show normal ALT, AST, LDH, and ALP. Total bilirubin is 2.9 mg/dL and direct bilirubin is 0.3 mg/dL. Hgb, reticulocyte count, and haptoglobin are normal.

Conditions with Similar Presentations	**Crigler Najjar syndrome:** Also presents with jaundice and unconjugated hyperbilirubinemia but occurs in neonates. There is absent (Type 1) or markedly reduced (Type 2) hepatic UDP-glucuronsyltransferase which results in marked unconjugated hyperbilirubinemia (>10 mg/dL) and can cause bilirubin-induced neurologic dysfunction (BIND), also known as kernicterus (abundance of unconjugated bilirubin deposits in the CNS [basal ganglia/brainstem nuclei] resulting in neurological deficits [weakness, lethargy, audio/visual deficits, hypotonia, cerebral palsy]). **Hemolysis:** May also present with jaundice due to unconjugated hyperbilirubinemia; however, haptoglobin will be low and LDH and reticulocyte count are elevated. Medical history may include a known hemolytic disease (sickle cell disease, spherocytosis) or a new hemolytic process (autoimmune hemolytic anemia). **Large resolving hematomas:** May cause jaundice and an unconjugated hyperbilirubinemia from the breakdown of large amounts of blood. **Cirrhosis:** May also present with jaundice and an unconjugated hyperbilirubinemia. However, patients with cirrhosis have other stigmata of liver disease including fetor hepaticus, spider angiomas, gynecomastia, esophageal varices, caput medusae, and asterixis.
Initial Diagnostic Tests	• Confirm diagnosis: Unconjugated hyperbilirubinemia (high total and indirect, normal direct). • Consider: CBC with blood smear, reticulocyte count, haptoglobin, LDH to rule out hemolysis.
Next Steps in Management	Manage inciting stressor
Discussion	Gilbert syndrome is a benign inherited disorder of bilirubin metabolism present in ~5–10% of people. Patients have reduced activity of hepatic UDP-glucuronosyltransferase that results in a mildly increased unconjugated bilirubin following a stressful event (infection, fasting, exercise, hypovolemia, surgery). **History:** • Occurs in males more often than females and is often first diagnosed when a pubescent patient undergoes a stressful event • Triggered by an inciting stressful event **Physical exam:** Yellow discoloration of the conjunctiva, skin, and mucous membranes **Diagnostics:** • Elevated total and indirect bilirubin and normal direct bilirubin • Normal ALP, AST, and ALT • CBC, blood smear, reticulocyte count, haptoglobin, and LDH will be normal, which rules out hemolysis **Management:** • Address underlying cause, minimizing inciting events. Avoid any further testing.

CASE 18 | Primary Biliary Cholangitis (PBC)

A 45-year-old woman with celiac disease presents with new-onset jaundice and pruritis. She has not had alcohol or taken any new medications or supplements. Family history includes hypothyroidism and autoimmune hepatitis on her father's side. She is hemodynamically stable and afebrile. Physical exam is notable for scleral icterus, yellow skin, and hepatomegaly. The abdomen is soft and nontender to palpation, and there are several xanthomas along her neck and back. ALP is 490 and antimitochondrial antibody (AMA) is positive.

Conditions with Similar Presentations	**Autoimmune hepatitis:** May present similarly to or overlap with PBC in middle-aged women, but is characterized by presence of autoantibodies (antinuclear antibody [ANA] and anti-smooth muscle antibody [ASMA]) with elevated total IgG. **PSC:** May present similarly, but patients are typically younger men with IBD (especially ulcerative colitis). pANCA and ANA antibodies positive.

CASE 18 | Primary Biliary Cholangitis (PBC) *(continued)*

Conditions with Similar Presentations	**Cirrhosis:** Jaundice, fatigue, and pruritis can be nonspecific symptoms of cirrhosis due to any cause. **Pancreatic cancer:** May present with jaundice, fatigue, and upper abdominal pain, but would also expect weight loss and anorexia. Pruritus is uncommon.
Initial Diagnostic Tests	Check: ALP, AMA, and/or liver biopsy
Next Steps in Management	• Ursodeoxycholic acid (UDCA). • Cholestyramine for pruritis. • Liver transplantation for advanced liver disease.
Discussion	PBC is an autoimmune disease of the intrahepatic bile ducts caused by a combination of genetic and environmental factors and characterized by positive AMA (95% of cases). T cell–mediated damage to intrahepatic bile ducts leads to cholestasis, which triggers inflammatory processes leading to progressive fibrosis and cirrhosis. Disease progression may extend over several decades. **History:** • Women account for 90–95% of PBC cases, and most are 30–65 years of age. • Prevalence is highest in northern Europe and North America. • >50% asymptomatic, but common symptoms include fatigue, pruritus, and RUQ pain. • Risk factors include family history, exposure to infections or environmental toxins, and other autoimmune diseases (Sjögren syndrome, scleroderma, rheumatoid arthritis, autoimmune hepatitis, and celiac disease). **Physical exam:** • Exam may reveal jaundice, hepatomegaly, splenomegaly, abdominal distension, and RUQ tenderness. • Skin findings may include hyperpigmentation, xanthomas, xerosis or excoriations, and/or fungal infections. **Diagnostics:** Confirm diagnosis with ≥ two of: • Unexplained ALP ≥1.5 × upper limit of normal (ULN). • Serum AMA ≥1:40 or PBC-specific autoantibodies (e.g., gp210, sp100). • If AMA is positive, testing for other causes of liver/biliary injury usually not indicated because AMA is ~95% sensitive and ~98% specific for the diagnosis of PBC. • Liver biopsy: Destruction of small and medium bile ducts (granulomas may be seen); once destroyed, the bile ducts disappear completely. **Other tests:** • Ultrasound may reveal hepatomegaly. • Patients may also have elevations in GGT, AST (<5 × ULN), cholesterol and HDL, IgM, and/or bile acids. • ~70% are also ANA positive. • Biopsy is not required but may be useful in supporting the diagnosis and ruling out other etiologies of injury, including overlapping conditions like autoimmune hepatitis, as well as staging and prognosis. **Management:** • Start ursodiol as early as possible to slow disease progression. • Consider adding obeticholic acid if no response. • Cholestyramine for pruritus.
Additional Considerations	**Screening:** Routine screening is not indicated. **Complications:** Complications include portal hypertension (unlike other etiologies of cirrhosis, PBC may present with portal hypertension and esophageal varices before cirrhosis), cirrhosis, HCC, osteopenia, fat-soluble vitamin deficiencies, hypercholesterolemia ± xanthomas/xanthelasmas. **Surgical considerations:** PBC can recur after liver transplantation.

Cholestatic Liver Disease Mini Case

Case	Key Findings
Primary sclerosing cholangitis (PSC)	**History:** • Men account for 70% of cases, with a median age of diagnosis at 40 years. • Strong association with inflammatory bowel disease (80–90% of patients with PSC have IBD, mostly ulcerative colitis). • Common symptoms include pruritus, RUQ pain, fatigue, weight loss, and jaundice. • Development of a dominant stricture (60% of cases) may present with worsening jaundice/pruritus, ascending cholangitis, and malabsorption. **Physical exam:** Exam may be normal or reveal jaundice, hepatomegaly, splenomegaly, and RUQ tenderness. **Diagnostics:** • PSC should be suspected in patients with an elevation in ALP and GGT, particularly those with underlying IBD. • Diagnosis is established by demonstration of multifocal strictures and segmental dilation of intrahepatic and extrahepatic bile ducts on MRCP or ERCP ("beads on a string" appearance). • May be p-ANCA (+) and have elevated AST/ALT (usually not >300), IgG, and/or IgM. • Biopsy not required; it may be supportive of the diagnosis but is rarely diagnostic. Scarring ("onion-skinning") of the bile ducts may be seen. **Management:** • Like PBC, management of PSC consists of treating complications of portal hypertension and cirrhosis. • No drugs are known to alter progression of PSC, though cholestyramine may be used for pruritus. • ERCP can be used for dilation ± stenting of a dominant large duct stricture and to evaluate for cholangiocarcinoma. • Monitor for fat-soluble vitamin deficiencies and metabolic bone disease. • Monitor for development of cholangiocarcinoma, gallbladder adenocarcinoma, HCC (if cirrhotic), and colon cancer (especially with underlying IBD). • Liver transplantation is recommended for advanced disease, but similar to PBC, PSC can also recur after transplantation. **Discussion:** • PSC is a rare, progressive cholestatic liver disease most often found in young men with inflammatory bowel disease. • Many will have abnormal liver tests but are asymptomatic on initial presentation. • Pathophysiology of bile duct injury is unknown but thought to be due to an autoimmune process.

CASE 19 | Pancreatic Cancer

A 58-year-old woman with recently diagnosed diabetes mellitus presents with anorexia, malaise, and mid-epigastric pain for several weeks. The pain is dull, constant, and worsened by eating. She also reports unintentional 12-pound weight loss over the last month, and has noticed dark brown urine, pale stools, and generalized pruritus. She was diagnosed with superficial thrombophlebitis 4 weeks ago. She has no fevers, chills, vomiting, or dysphagia. Physical exam is notable for jaundice and scleral icterus with mild abdominal tenderness to deep palpation in the epigastrium.

Conditions with Similar Presentations	**Hepatitis/cirrhosis:** Liver disease of any etiology may also present with jaundice, abdominal pain, and generalized pruritus. History, labs, and imaging will help narrow the differential for above conditions. **Biliary obstruction:** (Choledocholithiasis, cholangiocarcinoma, primary sclerosing cholangitis, primary biliary cholangitis) may present similarly with jaundice, epigastric pain, pruritus, and weight loss. Imaging will help elucidate etiology. **Pancreatic NETs:** 50–85% of pancreatic NETs are nonfunctioning and thus indistinguishable from pancreatic adenocarcinomas on presentation. Functional tumors include insulinomas (episodic hypoglycemia), gastrinomas (Zollinger-Ellison syndrome; peptic ulcer disease and diarrhea), and less commonly, VIPomas, glucagonomas, somatostatinomas.
Initial Diagnostic Tests	• Confirm diagnosis: CT abdomen with IV contrast, US-guided biopsy • Consider: AST, ALT, ALP, lipase

CASE 19 | **Pancreatic Cancer** *(continued)*

Next Steps in Management	• Curative treatment is surgical resection with pancreaticoduodenectomy (Whipple procedure). • Consider neoadjuvant chemotherapy +/– radiation therapy for borderline resectable disease. • Palliative care referral if not resectable.
Discussion	Ductal adenocarcinomas account for ~90% of all pancreatic neoplasms and are aggressive tumors that have poor long-term prognosis (5-year survival <10%) when diagnosed at an advanced stage. Approximately 60–70% are in the pancreatic head, 20–25% in the body/tail, and the remainder involve the whole organ. Greater than 90% of tumors have *KRAS* oncogene activation and *CDKN2A* tumor suppressor gene inactivation. **History:** • Over 90% of cases occur in patients >55 years old, with peak incidence between 60–80 years. • Major risk factors include tobacco use, obesity, heavy alcohol use, chronic pancreatitis, diabetes mellitus, genetic predisposition, and family history. • Suspect in patients with **painless** jaundice, weight loss, and new-onset diabetes mellitus (up to 25% of cases). • May be asymptomatic or present with nonspecific symptoms such as subacute epigastric pain (often worse after eating and/or at night), weight loss, weakness, loss of appetite, dark urine, pale stools, jaundice, and nausea. • Less common symptoms include pruritus, back pain, diarrhea, vomiting, steatorrhea, superficial thrombophlebitis (Trousseau sign if migratory), and signs of metastatic disease. **Physical exam:** • May have scleral icterus/jaundice and hepatomegaly. • Less common findings include palpable RUQ/epigastric mass, cachexia, nontender palpable gallbladder at right costal margin (Courvoisier sign), and ascites. **Diagnostics:** • Preferred initial imaging is transabdominal US, followed by CT or MRI of pancreas and confirmed with endoscopic US-guided biopsy or open biopsy/resection. • Nonspecific findings are elevated transaminases, ALP, total and direct bilirubin and lipase. • CA 19-9 may help narrow the differential. • Carbohydrate antigen 19-9 (CA 19-9) is not a diagnostic tool because it is not always elevated in pancreatic cancer. However, if elevated, it can be used prognostically and to monitor for recurrence after surgical resection. **Management:** • If completely resectable, surgery can be curative and should be followed up with surveillance with imaging and CA 19-9. • Consider neoadjuvant chemotherapy ± radiation for potentially resectable disease. • The majority of patients will not have resectable disease. For locally advanced/metastatic disease, consider systemic chemotherapy and palliative care given poor prognosis. • Supportive care may include insulin, pancreatic enzymes, fat-soluble vitamins, and/or biliary stenting or bypass.
Additional Considerations	**Screening:** The USPSTF recommends against screening for pancreatic cancer in asymptomatic patients. Patients with strong family history of pancreatic cancer may consider germline genetic testing. **Complications:** Complications include biliary obstruction and GI complications (bowel obstruction, malabsorption due to decreased pancreatic enzymes entering the duodenum), superficial thrombophlebitis, and SIADH. **Surgical considerations:** If disease is deemed surgically unresectable, celiac plexus neurolysis for pain management, and/or biliary bypass or stent in patients with jaundice.

Cirrhosis/Complications and Liver Lesions

Cirrhosis is defined anatomically as diffuse fibrosis of the liver with nodule formation (both have to be present); it is the end result of fibrogenesis due to chronic liver disease. In patients diagnosed with liver disease, progression to cirrhosis may occur up to 30 years later. Patients with cirrhosis are classified as either compensated or decompensated.

- **Compensated** cirrhosis = liver able to perform vital functions. Asymptomatic with a median survival >12 years.
- **Decompensated** cirrhosis = inability to perform vital functions. Rapid clinical declines and median survival <2 years.

Decompensation:

- Defined by one or more of the following events: ascites, bleeding varices, hepatic encephalopathy, or jaundice (see figure below).
- Hepatorenal syndrome (HRS), hyponatremia, and spontaneous bacterial peritonitis (SBP) are also features of decompensation but are almost always preceded by ascites.
- Development of **portal hypertension** (defined as a pathologic increase in the portal venous pressure) is a hallmark in the clinical course of cirrhosis because it underlies the decompensating events described above.
- **Modified End-Stage Liver Disease (MELD) score** is the most commonly used prognostic score that incorporates sodium, bilirubin, creatinine, and INR and is utilized to prioritize patients for liver transplant. Liver transplantation should be considered for patients with decompensated cirrhosis and early-stage HCC.

Portal hypertension and subsequent complications occur as the result of increased intrahepatic resistance to blood flow and subsequent splanchnic vasodilation, which causes a decrease in effective arterial volume, hyperdynamic circulation, and central underfilling, including renal blood flow. Cirrhosis and both its portal hypertension-related complications and non-portal hypertension-related complications (e.g., HCC) are resource intensive.

Decompensated Cirrhosis

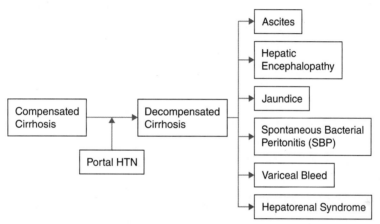

Ascites

Key Findings and Ascites Differential Diagnosis

Ascites with:	Diagnoses
Chronic liver disease of any type	Cirrhosis
Right-sided congestive heart failure	Cardiac ascites
Foamy urine, chronic kidney disease	Nephrotic syndrome → hypoalbuminemia → low oncotic pressure → ascites
Cachexia, severely low BMI, malnourished	Protein malnutrition → inability of liver to synthesize albumin → hypoalbuminemia → low oncotic pressure → ascites
Primary or metastatic intra-abdominal/gynecologic malignancy	Malignant ascites
Abdominal pain, fever with pre-existent ascites	Spontaneous bacterial peritonitis (SBP)
Endemic area of tuberculosis (TB) (e.g., Mexico, Southeast Asia) or known pulmonary TB	TB ascites

Diagnostics:

- Ultrasound or cross-sectional imaging to confirm and assess for liver disease and/or malignancy
- Paracentesis to assess total protein, albumin, serum-ascites albumin gradient (SAAG), Gram stain and culture, cell count with differential, and cytology.

- Useful initial tests on ascitic fluid are the total protein and SAAG (serum albumin minus ascitic fluid albumin)
  - SAAG >1.1 g/dL indicative of portal hypertension
  - SAAG <1.1 g/dL not indicative of portal hypertension as the primary cause of ascites
  - Total ascitic protein >2.5 g/dL suggests appropriate synthetic function of protein by the liver and cause of ascites is due to increased right heart hydrostatic pressure (right heart failure, tamponade, constrictive pericarditis) or non-cirrhotic intraabdominal processes (venous thrombosis, schistosomiasis)
  - Total ascitic protein <2.5 g/dL suggests either poor synthetic function by the liver, loss of albumin (nephropathy, enteropathy) or insufficient protein stores to make albumin (malnutrition)

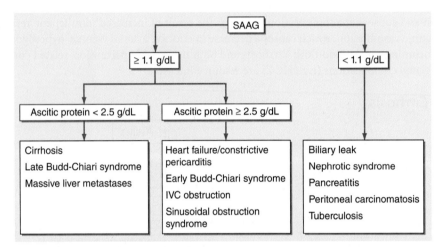

Algorithm for the diagnosis of ascites according to the serum-ascites albumin gradient (SAAG). IVC, inferior vena cava. (Reproduced, with permission, from Loscalzo J, Fauci AS, Kasper DL, Hauser SL, Longo DL, Jameson JL, eds: Harrison's Principles of Internal Medicine. 21st ed. New York, NY: McGraw Hill; 2022.)

CASE 20 | Alcohol-Associated Cirrhosis

A 55-year-old woman with alcohol use disorder presents with worsening abdominal distension and lower extremity edema for the past 3 weeks. She has been drinking about 10 beers daily for the past 18 years. She has no other drug use. Patient's temperature is 37°C (98.6°F), pulse is 90/min, respirations are 20/min, and BP is 100/64 mmHg. BMI is 21. On exam, she is cachectic, has slow speech, icteric conjunctiva, multiple spider angiomas, asterixis, and decreased breath sounds and dullness to percussion at bilateral lung bases. Abdomen is distended, caput medusae is present, there is a positive fluid wave. She has bilateral lower extremity pitting edema.

Conditions with Similar Presentations	**Heart failure exacerbation:** Presents with signs of hypervolemia but would not see jaundice, asterixis, or cutaneous signs of liver disease.
	Nephrotic syndrome: Presents with signs of hypervolemia but would not see jaundice, asterixis, or spider angiomas.
Initial Diagnostic Tests	• Suspect in patients with liver disease and prolonged history of alcohol use • Check US abdomen with Doppler, transaminases and albumin, platelet count, PT/INR • Consider checking HBV and HCV serologies • If suspect a less common etiology of cirrhosis, consider checking alpha-1 antitrypsin level and phenotype/genotype, ANA, ASMA, AMA, iron studies, serum copper, and ceruloplasmin.
Next Steps in Management	Diagnostic and therapeutic paracentesis with ascites fluid protein, albumin, and neutrophil count
Discussion	Alcohol-associated cirrhosis is the culmination of progressive liver injury from sustained alcohol use. Heavy alcohol use results in accumulation of fat in the liver, which can then trigger steatohepatitis and fibrosis. Alcohol-associated cirrhosis comprises a substantial portion of the overall cirrhosis burden, both in the United States and worldwide. Other causes of chronic liver disease, mainly chronic viral hepatitis B and C, should be ruled out because their presence may accelerate the development of cirrhosis.

CASE 20 | Alcohol-Associated Cirrhosis *(continued)*

Discussion	**History:** • Prolonged history of daily alcohol use (~1 standard drink) for a woman and (~2 standard drinks) for a man. • Nonspecific symptoms (weakness, fatigue), altered mental status, pruritis **Physical exam:** • Jaundice, peripheral edema, spider angiomas, palmar erythema, gynecomastia, nail changes, Dupuytren contractures, or testicular atrophy • Signs of decompensated cirrhosis include abdominal distension, GI bleed, confusion, asterixis, renal failure, and hypoxemia. **Diagnostics:** The following can help establish a diagnosis of cirrhosis in general: • Low platelet count, low albumin, and elevated PT/INR • US or cross-sectional imaging revealing nodular contour to the liver or evidence of portal hypertension (e.g., splenomegaly, recanalized periumbilical vein) • Elastography studies (a noninvasive radiographic assessment of the stiffness of the liver) show high liver stiffness • Ascitic fluid with SAAG >1.1 • Liver biopsy not needed if clinical picture, labs, and imaging strongly suggest cirrhosis The following can be suggestive of a diagnosis of *alcohol-associated* cirrhosis: • Elevated AST and ALT levels with AST:ALT ratio >2 and macrocytosis • Detectable biomarkers for alcohol use (e.g., phosphatidylethanol) • Biopsy demonstrating steatohepatitis **Management:** Primarily focused on symptom relief but should also include measures to treat and prevent complications. • Alcohol cessation and avoidance of other hepatotoxins; offer pharmacotherapy for those with alcohol use disorder • **Vaccinations:** HAV, HBV, and 23-valent pneumococcal vaccines • **Ascites:** Low-salt diet, diuretics (spironolactone and/or furosemide), prophylactic antibiotics to prevent SBP • **Varices:** Upper endoscopy to evaluate esophageal varices; nonselective beta blockers and/or endoscopic variceal ligation (banding) for prophylaxis • **Hepatic encephalopathy:** If present, treat with lactulose +/− rifaximin • **HCC:** Screen with liver US and alpha fetoprotein (AFP) every 6 months • **Nutrition:** Vitamin and micronutrient repletion, especially folate, thiamine, and pyridoxine in setting of alcohol use disorder; high-protein diet • Definitive treatment for eligible patients is liver transplantation
Additional Considerations	**Screening:** USPSTF recommends screening for unhealthy alcohol use in adults ≥18 years old, with brief behavioral counseling interventions for those engaged in risky or hazardous drinking (Grade B).

CASE 21 | Primary Peritonitis

A 64-year-old man with hepatitis C cirrhosis complicated by ascites and esophageal varices is brought for evaluation of diffuse abdominal pain and confusion. Vitals are notable for a temperature of 38.7°C, heart rate 104/min, and blood pressure of 97/58 mmHg. Physical exam is notable for scleral icterus and a tense, protuberant abdomen with a fluid wave but no rebound tenderness. There is no jugular vein distention (JVD) or peripheral edema.

Conditions with Similar Presentations	**Secondary bacterial peritonitis:** Occurs as a result of another intraabdominal infection (e.g., perforation, appendicitis, diverticulitis, cholecystitis, infected peritoneal dialysis catheter). **Peritoneal carcinomatosis:** Can also present with abdominal pain and distension from malignancy-related ascites. Ascitic fluid will have lymphocyte predominance, may be hemorrhagic, culture will be negative, and cytology may be positive for malignant cells. **Right heart failure:** May also cause ascites, fatigue, and anorexia, but would likely have dyspnea on exertion, and orthopnea. Exam would show peripheral edema and JVD. **Nephrotic syndrome:** Can also cause ascites from severe hypoalbuminemia secondary to urinary protein loss but would also be accompanied by peripheral edema and would not have jaundice.

CASE 21 | Primary Peritonitis *(continued)*

Initial Diagnostic Tests	• Confirm diagnosis: Diagnostic paracentesis with ascitic fluid analysis and culture. • Consider: CBC, CMP, PT/PTT, blood culture, imaging.
Next Steps in Management	• Empiric IV antibiotics with gram-negative and *Streptococcus pneumoniae* coverage (third-generation cephalosporins) • IV albumin
Discussion	Primary peritonitis or spontaneous bacterial peritonitis (SBP) is a common and potentially fatal infection in patients with advanced cirrhosis and ascites, accounting for 10–30% of bacterial infections in hospitalized patients with cirrhosis. Common causative agents in order of decreasing prevalence are *E. coli*, *Klebsiella pneumoniae*, and *Streptococcus pneumoniae*, *Staphylococcus* species, *Enterococcus* species, and *Streptococcus virida*. It develops when enteric bacteria organisms (or fungi) translocate across the edematous bowel wall and enter ascitic fluid. Decreased ability of the liver to create opsonins (specifically complement) predisposes to this and also explains why inflammatory manifestations (e.g., abdominal pain, tenderness, rebound) may be absent. **History:** • May be asymptomatic or present with diffuse abdominal pain/tenderness, vomiting, diarrhea, ileus, fever/chills, shock, and/or altered mental status secondary to precipitating hepatic encephalopathy. • Seen in cirrhotic patients with ascites. Risk factors include advanced age, more severe cirrhosis, GI bleeding, use of PPIs, and impaired renal function. **Physical exam:** • May have signs of advanced cirrhosis (e.g., palmar erythema, gynecomastia, spider angiomas) along with fever, tachycardia, tachypnea, hypotension, abdominal tenderness with rebound, encephalopathy, and asterixis. **Diagnostics:** • Diagnostic paracentesis with ascitic fluid ANC ≥250 cells/mm³ and positive ascitic fluid culture. **Management:** • Empiric broad-spectrum antibiotics with gram-negative and *S. pneumoniae* coverage (e.g., ceftriaxone, cefotaxime). • If nosocomial SBP suspected, consider carbapenem + daptomycin. • Decrease risk of hepatorenal syndrome with IV albumin. • Secondary prophylactic ciprofloxacin or TMP-SMX is recommended for patients with history of SBP treatment failure.
Additional Considerations	**Complications:** Complications may include AKI, acute on chronic liver failure, hepatorenal syndrome, and sepsis.

CASE 22 | Hepatocellular Carcinoma (HCC)

A 72-year-old man with alcohol use disorder presents with poor appetite, unintentional weight loss, abdominal distension, and jaundice. His physical exam is notable for conjunctival icterus, abdominal distension, anasarca, and a palpable RUQ mass.

| Conditions with Similar Presentations | **Decompensated cirrhosis:** May also present with jaundice or other complications of cirrhosis, including ascites, spontaneous bacterial peritonitis, variceal bleeding, hepatorenal syndrome, hepatopulmonary syndrome. HCC can be a cause of decompensated cirrhosis. However, unintentional weight loss, loss of appetite, and a palpable RUQ mass would not be expected for decompensated cirrhosis in the absence of HCC.

Cholangiocarcinoma: May also present with jaundice, weight loss, and palpable RUQ mass. However, patients will have signs/symptoms of biliary obstruction, including pruritus, clay-colored stools, and dark urine. Abdominal imaging will differentiate.

Liver metastases: May also present with fatigue, loss of appetite, fever, abdominal pain/distension, and jaundice. However, patients may have a recent or remote history of cancer (particularly GI, breast, lung, or melanoma), or symptoms of a primary malignancy.

Polycystic liver disease: May also present with abdominal pain and weight loss but is commonly associated with autosomal dominant polycystic kidney disease (ADPKD). Patients would have hypertension, hematuria, renal impairment, flank pain, cerebral aneurysms, and/or cardiac valvulopathies. More than one mass would be detectable. |

CASE 22 | Hepatocellular Carcinoma (HCC) *(continued)*

Initial Diagnostic Testing	• Confirm diagnosis: Triple-phase CT or MRI of the abdomen • Consider: Liver biopsy if imaging is not diagnostic for HCC (but avoid if suspect hepatic adenoma because of bleeding risk), CEA and CA 19-9 if suspect cholangiocarcinoma, chromogranin if suspect neuroendocrine tumor.
Next Steps in Treatment/ Management	• Surgical resection if possible • Liver transplant if available and patient meets eligibility criteria. • Nonsurgical: Radiofrequency ablation, transarterial embolization (TACE), transarterial radioembolization (TARE), stereotactic beam radiation therapy • Systemic therapy for refractory or metastatic disease
Discussion	HCC is the most common malignant tumor of the liver. Ninety percent of patients with HCC in Western countries have cirrhosis. HCC is twice as common in men and has a mean age at diagnosis of 60 years old. **History:** • Risk factors in the United States are cirrhosis (HBV, HCV, alcohol abuse, and nonalcoholic steatosis) and HBV (without cirrhosis) and in developing countries are HBV and aflatoxins. • Asymptomatic or nonspecific symptoms (e.g., mild to moderate upper abdominal pain, weight loss, early satiety, palpable mass). **Physical exam:** Patients with underlying cirrhosis may present with decompensated cirrhosis (e.g., ascites, jaundice/hyperbilirubinemia). **Diagnostics:** • Unlike other malignancies, HCC diagnosis does not require biopsy and can be made based on imaging alone. • Triple-phase abdominal CT or MRI findings will reveal a mass with late arterial phase enhancement and portal venous phase washout. • AFP not recommended as a diagnostic test due to its low sensitivity and specificity, but can be used to guide response to treatment and surveillance when combined with imaging. • If imaging is nondiagnostic, biopsy should be obtained. **Management:** Despite the existence of numerous treatment options, prognosis is poor, with a median survival of 6–20 months and 5-year survival rate of 18%. • Treatment involves multidisciplinary care with options including surgical resection, liver transplant, local treatment (ablation or transarterial chemoembolization/radioembolization), or systemic therapy for more advanced disease. • Given the poor prognosis of HCC, palliative care should be involved early in management for those with decompensated liver disease.
Additional Considerations	**Screening:** It is recommended to screen patients with cirrhosis for developing HCC with imaging +/– serum AFP every 6 months. **Complications:** Decompensation of cirrhosis. **Surgical considerations:** While the preferred therapy for hepatocellular carcinoma is surgical resection, tumor extent and cirrhosis severity may remove it as an option. Extent of cirrhosis is assessed by the Child-Pugh classification which assigns points based on the presence of ascites, encephalopathy, serum bilirubin, serum albumin, and PT/INR. Class A is considered well compensated disease, while class B and C indicate significant compromise and decompensated disease respectively. Class B and C classify the tumor as unresectable. In these cases, liver transplantation is the only curative option.

Other Benign and Malignant Liver Lesions

Cavernous hemangiomas	• Account for up to 73% of benign liver tumors and are most commonly diagnosed in women 30–50 years of age (W > M up to 5:1 ratio) but can occur in any age group • Etiology unknown but hemangiomas are not associated with oral contraceptive pill (OCP) use • Discovered incidentally in asymptomatic patients as solitary lesions <3 cm in diameter, though nearly 10% of patients have multiple localized lesions • Diagnosis is confirmed with further imaging and is based on features such as well-defined homogenous hyperintensity on T2 MRI and peripheral nodular enhancement on MRI or CT. • Avoid biopsy due to high risk of bleeding

Other Benign and Malignant Liver Lesions (*continued*)

Cavernous hemangiomas	• No treatment or follow-up are required in asymptomatic patients regardless of tumor size due to benign course and rarity of complications • Surgery is considered curative but is generally reserved for very large hemangiomas or those marked by symptomatic organ/vessel compression, complications (e.g., malignant transformation, rupture), and/or worsening or recurrent pain
Focal nodular hyperplasia (FNH)	• Second most common type of benign liver tumor and can be found in males and females of all ages • Discovered incidentally as a solitary lesion in women 35–50 years of age, though it is not associated with OCP use • 20–40% of patients are symptomatic with abdominal pain, and up to 20% of patients have concomitant hemangiomas • Key features for confirming the diagnosis on imaging include a hypo/isodense lesion with central scar and homogenous arterial enhancement on CT or hyperintense scar on T2-weighted MRI • Biopsy is not indicated • FNH has no risk of bleeding or malignant transformation, and no treatment or follow-up are required for asymptomatic patients with confirmed diagnoses who are not using OCPs • Surgical resection can be considered if lesions are symptomatic
Hepatic adenomas	• Rare (3–4 per 100,000 women), benign liver tumors that are most frequently associated with **oral contraceptive** or androgen use • Diagnosed incidentally in patients undergoing imaging studies for other reasons. Diagnosis can be made by features on MRI • No associated laboratory abnormalities • Biopsies for the evaluation of suspected hepatic adenomas are not performed due to the high risk of bleeding and lack of diagnostic benefit • Surgical resection is the definitive treatment of hepatic adenomas and is recommended for patients with large, symptomatic adenomas or those that have ruptured • Hormonal therapy should be stopped at the time of diagnosis
Intrahepatic cholangiocarcinoma	• Account for <10% of cholangiocarcinomas and constitute the second most common primary liver malignancy (up to 15%) • Risk factors include PSC, hepatolithiasis, and liver fluke infection, but nearly half of the cases have no identifiable risk factors • Triple-phase CT or MR shows minor peripheral enhancement as opposed to the homogenous enhancement seen with HCC • CEA and CA 19-9 for baseline assessment, but not to confirm diagnosis
Combined hepatocellular cholangiocarcinoma	• Rare, diagnosed by pathology
Metastases from other malignancies	Colon, breast, esophageal, stomach, pancreatic, lung, kidney, melanoma, and neuroendocrine tumors.

7

Infectious Diseases

Lead Authors: Sarah Messmer, MD; Mahesh C. Patel, MD; Fred A. Zar, MD
Contributors: Kimberly Orozco, MD; Artemis Gogos, MD, PhD; Helen Zhang, MD; Pooja Nayak, MD; Nikita Pillai, MD

INTRODUCTION

The general approach to patients with suspected infectious diseases is to obtain a full history, and explore activities that may have exposed the patient to a pathogen. Social history, dietary habits, animal exposures, and travel history may all hold clues to the etiology. It is important to identify the comorbidities that may affect the ability of the patient to defend against organisms including immunocompromised states, medications used, prior history of splenectomy, and immunization status. The physical exam including the skin, lymph nodes, and serial exams helps localize the anatomical compartment. Testing should be directed at likely sources identified by the history and physical exam findings. Further investigations include site-directed cultures, site-directed imaging, and lab tests that may include a WBC, Urinalysis (UA), ESR, CRP, and CMP. A careful history, exam, confirmatory tests, and cultures will help narrow the differential diagnosis, determine the etiology, and guide treatment and management. Most of the information in this chapter was obtained and/or confirmed from the following sources: CDC, DynaMed, Infectious Disease Society of America (IDSA) guidelines, and UpToDate.

Fever

- *Normal temperature:* This is regulated by input from the skin, core, and central nervous system to the hypothalamus, which maintains body temperature within the normal range by alterations in the autonomic nervous system and behavior. In a large diverse cohort of ambulatory patients, the mean temperature was 36.6°C (97.9°F) with a 99% range of 35.3–37.7°C (95.5°F–99.9°F).

- *Fever:* An elevated body temperature due to cytokine-mediated increased production of PGE2, which signals the hypothalamus to reset the temperature set point. The stimulus for this cytokine release may be infectious or noninfectious causes.

- *Hyperthermia:* An elevated body temperature (unlike fever) is not mediated by cytokine release resetting the hypothalamic temperature set point. It can be due to increased heat production by the body (heat stroke, malignant hyperthermia, neuroleptic malignant syndrome), injury to the hypothalamus (hypothalamic fever), or medications that inhibit heat loss (anticholinergics, sympathomimetics).

- *Pulse:* Assess the patient's pulse in the context of the fever. It generally increases by 10 bpm for each 1°F increase in temperature. If temperature ≥ 102°F, assess for relative bradycardia (pulse does not increase appropriately with the elevation in temperature). Relative bradycardia occurs in several infectious diseases, including Q fever, some viral diseases (dengue, yellow fever, Ebola), Mycoplasma, psittacosis, typhoid fever, Legionella, malaria, babesiosis, and Rocky Mountain spotted fever (RMSF). It may also be seen in drug fever and hypothalamic fever.

FEVER AND HEADACHE

Fever and headache in combination are concerning for infections involving the central nervous system (CNS) and should prompt immediate evaluation, diagnosis, and treatment. A variety of pathogens can cause infection of the brain, the meninges, or the spinal cord.

Brain abscesses are space-occupying infections that can also present with fever and headache and likewise can be due to a host of pathogens. Meningitis and encephalitis represent a spectrum of disease of the CNS involving the brain and/or spinal cord.

There is significant crossover in the presentation of these syndromes; fever, headache, and neck pain may be present in both. Classically, encephalitis patients also have altered mental status, because of involvement of the brain parenchyma. A thorough evaluation of risk factors for pathogens, as well as CNS imaging and cerebrospinal fluid (CSF) sampling, are paramount to making an accurate diagnosis.

There is some overlap between the CSF studies among these syndromes, but the basic patterns are very important to be familiar with to help narrow the differential diagnosis. CSF is secreted by the choroid plexus in the third and fourth ventricles. It is remarkably different from blood in that there normally are <5 WBCs/μL (none of which are neutrophils), it has protein of <50 mg/dL and glucose that is at least two-thirds of the blood glucose. Glucose is actively secreted into the CSF by the choroid plexus. Inflammation of the CNS causes WBCs and protein to cross into the CSF. Bacteria and fungi may consume glucose, and sufficient inflammation of the choroid plexus may impair its ability to secrete glucose.

Patterns of CSF Findings in Various Infections

Pathogen	White Cell Count (cells/uL)	Protein (mg/dL)	Glucose (mg/dL)
Normal	<5 (no neutrophils)	≤50	≥2/3 of serum glucose
Bacterial	>1000 (>80% PMNs/neutrophils)	100–500	<40 (can even be <10)
Fungal/TB	100–500 (mostly lymphocytes)	>50	<40 (in TB especially)
Viral	25–500 (mostly lymphocytes)	>50	Normal

The differential diagnosis for patients presenting with fever and headache is given below.

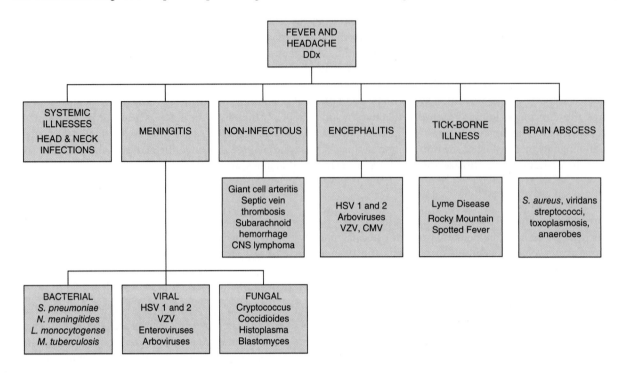

Key Differentials for Fever and Headache (HA)

Key Features-Associated Symptom(s) and Sign(s)	Diagnosis
Tick exposure Upper midwest and northeastern US	Lyme disease
Tick exposure; petechial rash Appalachian states or southeastern US	Rocky Mountain spotted fever (RMSF)
College student, living in dormitory; petechial rash Spread through close contact (via respiratory droplets)	*N. meningitidis*
Associated vesicular rash	HSV, VZV
Mosquito exposure in summer months; flaccid paralysis	West Nile virus
>50 years old; immunocompromised status; contaminated milk products; pregnancy	*Listeria* meningitis
Recent dental infection or oral abscess; history of bacterial endocarditis, Injection drug use, or new heart murmur; focal neurologic deficit	Pyogenic brain abscess
Altered mental status; focal neurologic deficit	Encephalitis
Housing instability, incarcerated, or travel to endemic area; cranial nerve deficits (if involving basilar brain structures)	TB meningitis
HIV/AIDS (CD4 <50–100); focal, ring-enhancing lesions on imaging	CNS toxoplasmosis or CNS lymphoma, cryptococcoma
HIV/AIDS (CD4 <50–100); meningitis or encephalitis	Cryptococcal meningitis or progressive multifocal leukoencephalopathy (from JC virus)
Southwestern US; eosinophilic meningitis	Coccidioidomycosis
Mississippi and Ohio River Valley	Histoplasmosis and blastomycosis
Latin America	Paracoccidioidomycosis
Eastern and central US: Great Lakes region	Blastomycosis

The diagnostic approach for patients with fever and headache is as below.

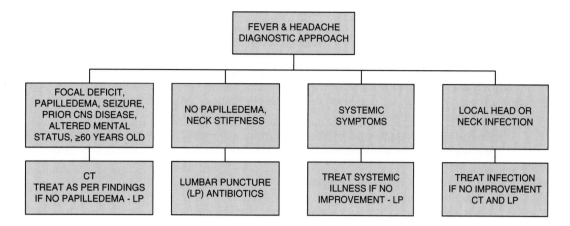

Headache and Fever Management

- Diagnostic lumbar puncture (LP)
- CSF analysis for CSF cell count, glucose, protein, Gram stain, pathogen cultures (bacterial, and when suspected, fungal)
- Tests for HSV PCR when suspected
- Blood cultures
- Glucocorticoids (dexamethasone) if bacterial meningitis suspected
- Empiric antibiotics without delay as shown in the algorithm below

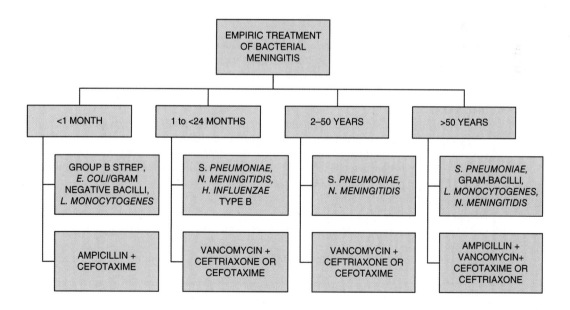

CASE 1 | *Neisseria meningitidis* Meningitis

A 19-year-old man is brought to the emergency department (ED) by his roommate for evaluation of severe headache and fever. He started with cold-like symptoms and a sore throat the day before, then reported a severe headache, sensitivity to light, body aches, and fever 12 hours ago. This was followed by the onset of nausea/vomiting and rash 8 hours ago. He lives in a college dormitory and is not sexually active. His exam is significant for a temperature of 39°C, pulse 120/min, respirations 24/min, and blood pressure 90/64 mmHg. He appears ill, is oriented only to person and place. He has a stiff neck and flexes his hips and knees when his neck is passively flexed (positive Brudzinski sign). When hip and knee are flexed to 90 degrees and then extension of the knee is attempted, there is restriction and pain in the neck beyond 135 degrees (positive Kernig sign). There is a petechial, maculopapular rash on his lower extremities.

Conditions with Similar Presentations	**Rocky Mountain spotted fever (RMSF):** Rash starts at the distal extremities and then spreads proximally and would have risk of tick exposure (caused by *Rickettsia rickettsii* and transmitted by *Dermacentor* dog tick). The following do not present with rash: • ***Streptococcus pneumoniae*** • **Bacterial encephalitis:** May have altered mental status and/or focal neurologic deficits • **Viral (aseptic) meningitis:** Often accompanied by inflammation of the brain parenchyma and therefore may involve mental status or subtle personality changes • **Brain abscess:** Typically has focal neurologic deficits and can be ruled out with a normal CT scan
Initial Diagnostic Tests	• Obtain Lumbar Puncture (LP) for CSF analysis (WBC count with differential, protein, glucose), Gram-stain and culture of CSF and PCR if available • Consider a CT scan prior to LP (see indications below) • Also check: Blood cultures, CBC, BMP, PT, PTT
Next Steps in Management	• Immediate empiric antibiotics: Vancomycin and ceftriaxone • Steroids (dexamethasone) to reduce inflammation-associated neurologic deficits
Discussion	*N. meningitidis* is an encapsulated, gram-negative diplococcus. The meningitis caused by it is also known as meningococcal meningitis. *N. meningitidis* has several virulence factors, including an antiphagocytic polysaccharide capsule and the presence of lipooligosaccharide, which can induce significant cytokine production and sepsis. It is spread by respiratory droplets and causes outbreaks in compressed living spaces, such as dormitories, military barracks, and prisons. Infants, adolescents, and young adults are most affected. **History:** Presents with fever, severe, abrupt-onset headache, stiff neck, photophobia, agitation, and petechial rash in individuals living in crowded quarters such as dormitories, military barracks, prisons. **Physical Exam:** Fever, agitation/confusion, or signs of shock (hypotension, tachycardia). Petechial rash, neck stiffness, positive Brudzinski, and Kernig signs (these signs have low sensitivity but high specificity). **Diagnostics:** • CSF analysis, shows high opening pressure, high WBCs >1000/mL (majority neutrophils), high protein >50 mg/dL, low glucose—less than two-thirds of blood glucose • If over age 60, focal neurologic deficits, altered mental status, immunodeficiency, prior CNS disease, new seizures or papilledema: obtain CT head before LP to rule out space-occupying lesion, which increases risk of herniation if LP is performed **Management:** • Empiric IV vancomycin and ceftriaxone • Steroids (dexamethasone) are given prior to antibiotics to reduce inflammation-associated neurologic deficits • Cultures should confirm the diagnosis and if *S. pneumoniae* is not found, vancomycin and steroids should be stopped
Additional Considerations	**Preventative:** Vaccination recommended between ages 11 and 18. Post-exposure prophylaxis: • For close contacts (e.g., household members, health care workers) directly exposed to secretions • Ciprofloxacin × 1 preferred; rifampin × 48 hours or ceftriaxone IM × 1 **Complications:** Bilateral adrenal cortical hemorrhage, known as **Waterhouse-Friderichsen syndrome,** results in shock due to acute adrenal insufficiency. **Pediatric Considerations:** Young children may have more nonspecific and subtle presentations with fever, poor feeding, seizures, high-pitched crying, and tachypnea

CASE 2 | Herpes Simplex Virus (HSV-1) Encephalitis

A 32-year-old man with no significant past medical history is brought by his wife to the ED for evaluation of 4 days of fever, headache, nausea, confusion, and a seizure 1 hour ago. There is no history of recent travel or sick contacts. Temperature is 38.5°C. He does not follow commands and a full neurological exam could not be completed.

Conditions with Similar Presentations	**HSV-2:** Is spread by direct contact and establishes latency in the sacral ganglia. It is a more common cause of viral meningitis than HSV-1, but a much less common cause of encephalitis.
	Arboviral encephalitis: Due to other causes can only be ruled out with testing. These include West Nile, Western equine encephalitis, cytomegalovirus (CMV), Epstein-Barr virus (EBV), varicella zoster virus (VZV).
	Bacterial meningitis, neurosyphilis, paraneoplastic and autoimmune encephalitis: Can be distinguished by further history and testing.
	Brain abscess, subdural hematoma (secondary or primary): Could present similarly but imaging would be diagnostic.
Initial Diagnostic Tests	• Obtain: PCR for HSV-1 in the CSF • Also check: CSF analysis, RPR, CBC, CMP, blood cultures
Next Steps in Management	Rapid initiation of empiric therapy with vancomycin, ceftriaxone, and acyclovir until CSF results return
Discussion	HSV encephalitis is an infection of the brain parenchyma and results in headache, altered mental status, focal neurologic deficits, seizures, and/or personality changes. Viral infections of the CNS often result in combined infection of the meninges and brain parenchyma, resulting in meningoencephalitis. The most common cause of sporadic encephalitis is herpes simplex virus-1 (HSV-1). HSV-1 is an enveloped, linear, double-stranded DNA virus. CSF findings are like other viral meningitis presentations—elevated protein, elevated lymphocytes, normal glucose—but a unique feature of HSV-1 encephalitis is that it is often hemorrhagic, and therefore the presence of numerous RBCs in the CSF is a common manifestation. HSV-1 infection results from an initial oropharyngeal infection that travels via the olfactory nerves and tracts to the brain, or from reactivation of latent virus within the trigeminal ganglion of cranial nerve V. This results in hemorrhagic necrosis of the temporal lobes, which can be unilateral or bilateral and may result in symptoms such as **temporal lobe seizures**, Wernicke's (receptive) aphasia, and olfactory hallucinations. Other causes of viral encephalitis may present similarly, so diagnosis is based on CNS imaging and CSF studies.

History:

Risk factors: Immunocompromised state, prior HSV-1 infections, prior neurosurgery or CNS radiation

Symptoms: Fever, headache, altered mental status, memory impairment, personality changes or seizures

Physical Exam: Fever, aphasia, focal neurologic deficits

Diagnostics:
• Polymerase chain reaction (PCR) for HSV-1 is the gold standard.
• CSF analysis would show elevated protein, elevated WBC with predominance of lymphocytes, elevated RBCs, and normal glucose.
• MRI brain reveals numerous hyperintense lesions on the temporal lobes with evidence of edema and hemorrhage.
• EEG shows numerous periodic lateralizing epileptiform discharges (PLEDS) originating from a temporal lobe. Not useful for diagnosis but predictive of future seizures.

Management:
• IV acyclovir
• Until diagnoses is confirmed, continue empiric IV antibiotics, vancomycin, and ceftriaxone and steroids (dexamethasone) to reduce inflammation-associated neurologic deficits
• Supportive care and seizure medications may be required

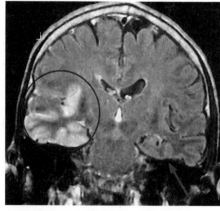

HSV encephalitis. Coronal FLAIR image of a young man with HSV encephalitis shows the characteristic MRI pattern within the cortex of the right temporal lobe (*circle*). The left temporal lobe is also involved (*arrow*), but to a lesser extent. (Reproduced with permission from Fauci AS, et al. *Harrison's Principles of Internal Medicine*, 17th ed. New York, NY: McGraw Hill, 2008.)

CASE 2 | Herpes Simplex Virus (HSV-1) Encephalitis *(continued)*

Additional Considerations	**Screening:** • HSV-1 can be transferred vertically to the neonate during delivery through the vaginal canal. Often the mother is asymptomatic and without genital lesions. • HSV screening is done routinely for pregnant patients to prevent vertical transmission and, if positive, the mother will be treated with acyclovir. **Pediatric Considerations:** • Infants can present with an encephalitis-like picture with lethargy, unusual behavior, seizures, fever (>100.4°F), poor feeding, headache, nausea, and vomiting. • An LP should be done for all infants with suspected encephalitis, and the diagnosis is clinical.

CASE 3 | Brain Abscess

A 27-year-old man is brought to the ED by his partner for worsening alteration of mental status (AMS) over the last few days. The partner notes that they both had a cold recently, though the patient developed more severe symptoms, including facial pain and worsening headache. Additionally, prior to arrival, the patient had an episode of projectile vomiting and became more confused. On exam, the patient is hemodynamically stable and febrile to 38.5°C. He is lethargic and oriented only to self. There is no evidence of head trauma. His neck is supple. He has left-sided paranasal and periorbital tenderness.

Conditions with Similar Presentations	**Meningitis:** Presents with headache and fever but also a stiff neck. **Encephalitis:** Presents with headache, fever, and altered mental status but would not have tenderness on facial exam. AMS and loss of consciousness could also suggest **toxic metabolic encephalopathy, subdural hematoma,** and **subarachnoid hemorrhage,** but these do not cause fever or facial tenderness. **Space-occupying lesions or malignancy:** Can also present similarly with focal neuro deficits, though these are more chronic in their presentation.
Initial Diagnostic Tests	Imaging is diagnostic
Next Steps in Management	• Drainage—needle aspiration to drain or surgical excision • Antibiotics

Discussion	Brain abscesses are purulent, focal collections in the brain parenchyma and arise as a complication of infection, head trauma, or surgical procedure. The most common causes are due to *Streptococcus* and *Staphylococcus*. Pathogens that enter through the lungs and seed the cerebral cortex include *Nocardia asteroides*, *Aspergillus* species, *Cryptococcus neoformans*, and *Coccidioides immitis*. *Listeria monocytogenes*, especially in patients on corticosteroids, can seed to the brain and brainstem. Other fungal infections that can invade the brain include *Candida* species and mucormycosis. Abscesses typically form along the middle cerebral artery distribution, along the grey–white matter junction. The integrity of the blood-brain barrier is damaged by micro-infarctions. There are several etiologies for how brain abscesses spread:
	• Direct inoculation by trauma or neurosurgical procedure
	• Contiguous or direct spread (20–60% of cases) of a primary infection, typically leading to a singular lesion
	  • Subacute/chronic otitis media or mastoiditis—inferior temporal lobes and/or cerebellum
	  • Frontal/ethmoid sinusitis—frontal lobes
	  • Dental infection—frontal lobes
	• Hematogenous seeding due to bacteremia/fungemia, leading to multiple lesions
	Symptoms arise from the immune response to the infective agent. The early stage (1–2 weeks) is cerebritis, which is characterized by a poorly demarcated lesion with associated edema and inflammation but no tissue necrosis. The later stage (2–3 weeks) is characterized by necrosis and liquefaction of parenchyma surrounded by a fibrotic capsule, and this clear demarcation leads to the ring-enhancing lesion.
		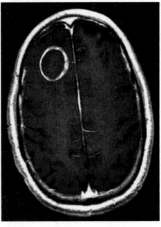
		MRI showing a right frontal brain abscesses associated with bacterial endocarditis (*S. aureus*) in a 55-year-old man. There is characteristic rim enhancement with gadolinium. (Reproduced with permission from Ropper AH, Samuels MA, Klein JP, Prasad S. Adams and Victor's Principles of Neurology, 11e; New York, McGraw-Hill 2019.)

CASE 3 | Brain Abscess *(continued)*

Discussion	**History:**
	Risk factors: Head trauma or neurosurgery, presence of infection in contiguous areas—sinusitis, otitis or dental abscess/infection or cyanotic heart disease. Immunocompromised hosts: *Toxoplasma gondii* can reactivate and cause multiple, ring-enhancing brain abscesses seen on imaging.
	Symptoms: The traditional triad (headache, fever, focal neural deficit) only occurs 20% of the time.
	• Severe headache, not relieved by analgesics, localizing to the side or region of the abscess
	• Change in mental status (confusion, lethargy, stupor, coma) due to cerebral edema
	• Vomiting due to increased intracranial pressure
	• Focal neurologic deficits (up to 50%) develop days to weeks after the headache
	• Seizure—grand mal, especially in frontal abscesses
	Physical Exam: Common signs on exam include focal neurologic deficits and signs of foci of contiguous infection or endocarditis.
	• Fever (50%)
	• Papilledema (25%)
	• Nuchal rigidity
	• Focal neurologic deficits (up to 50%)
	• CN III or CN VI deficits from increased ICP
	Diagnostics:
	• CT or MRI are the first steps
	• LP is contraindicated in patients with focal/unilateral symptoms because it may lead to brain herniation
	Management:
	• Initiate empiric antimicrobial therapy, with regimen depending on the suspected pathogen, which is dependent on the suspected origin
	• A common regimen for community-acquired infections is ceftriaxone and metronidazole (with vancomycin if MRSA is suspected)
	• If the microbiologic cause of the infection can be identified, the antimicrobial regimen should be narrowed
	• The course should last 4–8 weeks, with follow-up imaging to assess recovery
	• Surgical drainage or aspiration
Additional Considerations	**Complications:** Focal neurologic deficits, seizures, increased intracranial pressure, herniation.
	Surgical Considerations:
	• Surgical drainage or aspiration is performed, and removed contents aid in both treatment and diagnosis.
	• Surgical excision is indicated if the abscess was due to trauma, fungal abscesses, multiloculated abscesses, no clinical improvement following initial drainage/aspiration, or increased size of lesion.
	Pediatric Considerations:
	Children with congenital heart disease with right-to-left shunts and intrapulmonary right-to-left shunting with pulmonary arteriovenous malformations have a higher risk of brain abscesses.

Fever and Headache Mini-Cases

Cases	Key Findings
***Streptococcus pneumoniae* meningitis**	**Hx:** Classic features including rapid onset of fever, headache, and neck pain or stiffness. Consider underlying immunocompromising conditions (e.g., sickle cell disease, HIV, immunoglobulin deficiency).
	PE: Fever, neck stiffness. Brudzinski, and Kernig sign (sensitivity 10%, specificity 90%).
	Diagnostics:
	• Lumbar puncture for CSF analysis: Gram stain and culture: increased opening pressure, elevated neutrophils and protein with low CSF glucose (<40 mg/dL)
	• CT head is to be done before LP if indicated (see Case 1)
	Management:
	• Rapid initiation of dexamethasone and empiric antibiotics.
	• For adults, IV vancomycin and ceftriaxone.
	• If >50 years old or immunocompromised, add ampicillin to treat *Listeria*.
	Discussion: The most common pathogen causing bacterial meningitis across adults of all ages is *Streptococcus pneumoniae*, followed by *N. meningitidis*. In adults >50 or immunocompromised patients: *Listeria monocytogenes* becomes more common, causing 5–10% of cases. Bacterial or fungal meningitis is more severe than aseptic meningitis caused by viral pathogens.

Fever and Headache Mini-Cases (*continued*)

Viral Meningitis	**Hx:** Symptoms are like other forms of meningitis (fever, headache, neck pain) but are milder. May have a preceding upper respiratory infection. **PE:** Fever, neck stiffness. May see maculopapular or vesicular rash if coxsackievirus or echovirus. **Diagnostics:** LP for CSF analysis: increased WBCs (>5/mL) with a lymphocytic predominance, protein normal or mildly increased, glucose usually normal **Management:** • There are no effective antivirals against coxsackieviruses or echoviruses, and disease resolves without them in 1–2 weeks. • HSV meningitis should be treated with IV acyclovir followed by PO valacyclovir or famiciclovir. **Discussion: Enterovirus** is the leading cause of viral meningitis and is a member of the picornavirus family along with echovirus and coxsackie virus. These are positive-sense, single-stranded, icosahedral RNA viruses. Recovery is within 1–2 weeks for most.
CNS Toxoplasmosis	**Hx:** Fever, headache, lethargy, seizure Risk factors: • Eating undercooked meat • Exposure to cat feces, changing the litter box • Immunocompromised patients (HIV with CD4 <100) **PE:** Fever, white focal lesions on fundoscopy (toxoplasmosis chorioretinitis), focal neurologic deficits **Diagnostics:** • Brain MRI with and without contrast shows multiple ring-enhancing lesions and is diagnostic • IgG serology for anti-toxoplasma IgG antibodies only if imaging is not diagnostic **Management:** • First-line treatment is sulfadiazine and pyrimethamine, supplemented with leucovorin (folinic acid) to reduce hematologic side effects. If sulfa allergic, use clindamycin. • If patient fails to respond, consider brain biopsy to evaluate for CNS lymphoma **Discussion:** Toxoplasmosis is caused by ***Toxoplasma gondii***, that during acute infection may cause a mononucleosis-like syndrome in immunocompetent patients. In immunocompromised patients it can reactivate in the CNS to form brain abscesses and encephalitis. *T. gondii* is transmitted most commonly from cysts in undercooked meat but can be transmitted via food or water contaminated with oocysts in cat feces, because felines are the definitive host for the protozoan. An image showing bilateral ring-enhancing lesions in an immunocompromised host is sufficient to begin treatment. **Pediatric considerations:** *T. gondii* can also infect developing fetuses, resulting in **congenital toxoplasmosis**, presenting with a classic triad of chorioretinitis, hydrocephalus, and intracranial calcifications.	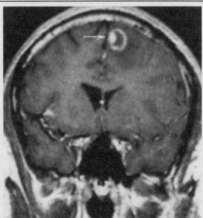 Central nervous system toxoplasmosis. A coronal postcontrast T1-weighted MRI scan demonstrates a peripheral enhancing lesion in the left frontal lobe, associated with an eccentric nodular area of enhancement (arrow); this so-called eccentric target sign is typical of toxoplasmosis. (Reproduced with permission from Loscalzo J, Fauci A, Kasper D, Hauser S, Longo D, Jameson J. Harrison's Principles of Internal Medicine, 21e; New York, McGraw Hill 2022.)

Conditions with Similar Presentations to Toxoplasmosis

Clinical Situation	Imaging	Diagnosis
Failure to respond to sulfadiazine and pyrimethamine therapy for toxoplasmosis	Ring-enhancing lesions in brain Uptake positive on PET scan	**Primary CNS lymphoma**
Immunosuppression, altered mental status, and decreased visual acuity	Non-enhancing areas of demyelination on MRI	**Progressive multifocal leukoencephalopathy** due to reactivation of JC virus which infects oligodendroglia and prevents myelin production
Immunosuppression, new onset of progressive headache	Soap-bubble lesions on brain MRI	***Cryptococcus* neoformans infection** Cryptococcal antigen in blood or CSF (+) CSF Gram stain shows encapsulated round yeast and grows *Cryptococcus neoformans*

FEVER AND COUGH

Fever and cough make up a clinical syndrome that generally is associated with infections of the lower respiratory tract, which consists of the trachea, bronchi (bronchitis), and alveoli (pneumonia). Cough is less common with infection of the upper respiratory tract (nose, mouth, sinuses, pharynx, and larynx). The differential diagnosis for acute infections of the respiratory tract is broad and ranges from common, mild infections that almost all humans have experienced (viral infections) to rare, life-threatening etiologies (e.g., *S. pneumoniae*, *Pneumocystis*, *Aspergillus*). As the clinical consequences of lower respiratory tract infections are much more severe, we will focus on pneumonia here. In general, the diagnosis of pneumonia is based on symptoms (fever, cough, sputum production, dyspnea, chest pain) and signs (fever, tachypnea, hypoxemia, rales, egophony, dullness to percussion, bronchial breath sounds, increased fremitus) in combination with a new pulmonary infiltrate on CXR or chest CT.

History

Consider patient's epidemiology and risk factors (immune-competent vs. compromised, health care exposure, prior antibiotic exposure, structural lung disease) and local geographic epidemiology (e.g., endemic mycoses, areas where TB is endemic). The first distinction to be made is between immunocompetent and immunocompromised (e.g., HIV/AIDS, transplant patients) hosts, as the latter group can be infected with opportunistic pathogens in addition to the usual common causes. A second important differentiation is between community-acquired infection and health care–associated/hospital-acquired infection, because the microbiologic epidemiology is quite different. Community-acquired pneumonia is most likely due to *Streptococcus pneumoniae*, atypical pathogens such as *Mycoplasma*, and common viruses (RSV, influenza). Health care–associated or hospital-acquired infections are more likely to be due to resistant bacterial pathogens such as methicillin-resistant *Staphylococcus aureus* (MRSA), *Pseudomonas aeruginosa*, and other drug-resistant gram-negatives. Following are some of the key differential diagnoses based on patient's risk profile.

The various etiologies for fever and cough among immunocompetent adults living in the community are as given below.

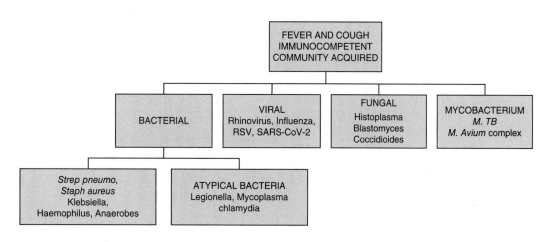

The various etiologies for fever and cough among immunocompetent hospitalized adults and immunocompromised adults are given below.

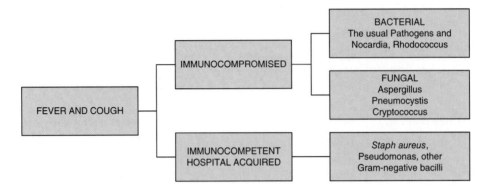

The common causes of pneumonia by age are as given below.

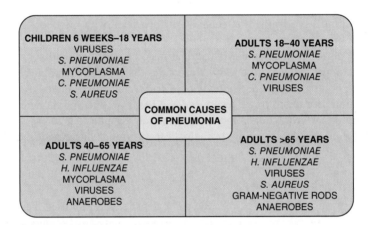

Key Differentials for Fever and Cough

Key Features and Associated Symptom(s) and Sign(s)	Diagnoses
Alcohol use disorder	Anaerobes (aspiration pneumonia)
	Klebsiella pneumoniae
Recent influenza infection	*Staphylococcus aureus, Streptococcus pneumoniae*
COPD	*Hemophilus influenzae, Moraxella catarrhalis, S. pneumoniae*
Hospitalized or ventilated patient develops pneumonia	Typical bacterial pneumonia
	Resistant bacterial pathogens (e.g., MRSA, *Pseudomonas*, and other drug-resistant gram negatives)
Cystic fibrosis, bronchiectasis	*Pseudomonas aeruginosa*
	Staphylococcus aureus
	Non-tuberculous *Mycobacteria* spp.
Exposure to water source (air conditioner, etc.) Hyponatremia, diarrhea, and pneumonia	*Legionella pneumophila*
Rash and pneumonia	*Mycoplasma pneumoniae*
	Blastomycosis, histoplasmosis, coccidioidomycosis
Erythema multiforme, bullous myringitis (inflammation of tympanic membrane)	*Mycoplasma pneumoniae*

Key Differentials for Fever and Cough

Key Features and Associated Symptom(s) and Sign(s)	Diagnoses
Pulse-temperature dissociation (high fever without much change in pulse)	Atypical pathogens (Mycoplasma, Legionella, Chlamydia)
Subacute (prolonged) symptoms	Atypical pathogens, fungal or Mycobacteria
HIV/AIDS (CD4 <200)	Typical bacterial pneumonia *Pneumocystis jirovecii* pneumonia (PJP) Mycobacteria
Stem cell or organ transplant recipients Leukemia/lymphoma	Typical bacterial pneumonia, fungal infections (e.g., *Aspergillus fumigatus*), rare bacterial pathogens (e.g., *Nocardia*)
Southwestern US, California, Northern Mexico	Coccidioidomycosis
Latin America	Paracoccidioidomycosis
Mississippi or Ohio River valley	Histoplasmosis or blastomycosis
Central and Eastern US; squamous cell carcinoma–type skin lesion	Blastomycosis
Bird exposure	Psittacosis, histoplasmosis, or *Cryptococcus neoformans*
New regurgitant heart murmur	Septic pulmonary emboli from endocarditis (*S. aureus* most common)

CASE 4 | Community-Acquired Pneumonia: *Streptococcus pneumoniae*

A 67-year-old man presents for evaluation of fever, shortness of breath, and productive cough with pleuritic chest pain for the last 3 days. Temperature is 39.7°C, pulse 115/min, respirations 29/min, blood pressure 87/62 mmHg, and SPO_2 89% on room air. On exam, crackles are auscultated posteriorly over the lower right lung field, along with dullness to percussion and egophony in the same location.

Conditions with Similar Presentations	**Aspiration pneumonia:** Fever, malaise, and a characteristic foul-smelling sputum due to presence of anaerobic organisms from the upper GI tract. The location of the infiltrate is gravity dependent. Risk factors include poor dentition, substance use disorders, intubation, GERD, impaired consciousness. **Recurrent pneumonia:** Multiple bouts of pneumonia with imaging showing consolidation in the same part of the lung raises the concern for a potential obstruction in that area, such as a tumor, or immunoglobulin deficiency (IgA deficiency, common variable immunodeficiency). **SARS-CoV-2 pneumonia (COVID-19):** This infection can result in a severe pneumonia and acute respiratory distress syndrome (ARDS).
Initial Diagnostic Tests	• Check chest x-ray • Also check: Gram stain and sputum culture, blood cultures, CBC, BMP
Next Steps in Management	• Antibiotics • Hospitalization and supportive care based on PSI or CURB-65 criteria
Discussion	Community-acquired pneumonia (CAP) results from an inflammatory response of the lung parenchyma triggered by a microbial agent. White cells move from capillaries into alveolar spaces due to cytokine release by alveolar macrophages. These cytokines trigger a systemic response when they reach the systemic circulation causing fever, tachycardia, and generalized symptoms (e.g., myalgias, fatigue, headache). The natural history of lobar pneumonia involves congestion, red hepatization, gray hepatization, and resolution of the infection, which occurs on average about 8 or more days. *Streptococcus pneumoniae* is a gram-positive lancet-shaped, encapsulated diplococcus. It can cause CAP (most common cause, lobar pneumonia), meningitis, otitis media in children, and sinusitis.

CASE 4 | Community-Acquired Pneumonia: *Streptococcus pneumoniae* (continued)

Discussion	Other common etiologies of pneumonia:

Other common etiologies of pneumonia:

- *Haemophilus influenzae, Moraxella catarrhalis* (Hib unvaccinated)
- *Legionella pneumophila* (hospitalized, travel to hotel/cruise)
- *Klebsiella pneumoniae* (hospitalized patients, aspiration)
- *Staphylococcus aureus*, including MRSA (CF, post-viral secondary bacterial pneumonia)
- *Pseudomonas aeruginosa* (CF, immunocompromised)
- Respiratory viruses (e.g., influenza, SARS-CoV-2, RSV, human metapneumovirus)

Should consider MRSA or *Pseudomonas* in patients with the following risk factors: Previous documented infection, recent hospitalization, or recent antibiotics

History:

Risk factors include: >65 years old, smokers, immunocompromised state, and reduced mucociliary clearance

Symptoms: Productive cough, fever, pleuritic pain, malaise

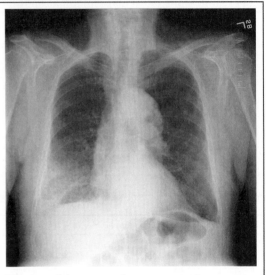

Right lower lobe pneumonia. (Reproduced with permission from Sylvia C. McKean, John J. Ross, Daniel D. Dressler, Danielle B. Scheurer: Principles and Practice of Hospital medicine, 2e, McGraw Hill, 2012.)

Our patient has CAP secondary to *S. pneumoniae* and presents with relatively rapid onset, severe symptoms (hypotension, toxic appearing). Pneumococcal pneumonia is associated with a productive "rusty" sputum (from minor bleeding), and patients with sickle cell disease, asplenia, or immunoglobulin deficiency are at increased risk of sepsis.

Physical Exam:

Lung exam: Crackles, dullness to percussion, egophony, tactile fremitus, bronchial breath sounds

Diagnostics:

- Obtain chest x-ray and/or CT scan to confirm diagnosis
- Consolidation typically occurs in one lobe but may involve all five lobes
- Additional tests: Gram stain sputum and obtain sputum/blood cultures for hospitalized patients with severe CAP, risk of antibiotic resistance, or MRSA colonization

Our patient has gram-positive, lancet-shaped diplococci and blood cultures grow *Streptococcus pneumoniae*. (This occurs ~10% of the time with pneumococcal pneumonia.)

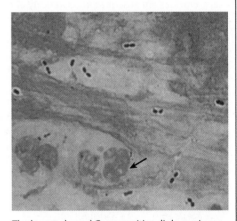

The lancet-shaped Gram-positive diplococci seen in the sputum specimen above are *Streptococcus pneumoniae*. The large, darker, irregular red shapes (*arrow*) are the degenerating nuclei of polymorphonuclear cells. The background shows mucus and amorphous debris. (Reproduced with permission from Stefan Riedel, Jeffery A. Hobden, Steve Miller, Stephen A. Morse, Timothy A. Mietzner, Barbara Detrick, Thomas G. Mitchell, Judy A. Sakanari, Peter Hotez, Rojelio Mejia, Medical Microbiology, 28e, McGraw Hill, 2019.).

Management:

Determine severity: **CURB-65 criteria** (see table) or the **Pneumonia Severity Index (PSI)** help you decide where the patient should be treated (based on mortality risk) and this determines what antibiotics are given. This patient has a CURB-65 score of 3 (age >65, BP <90/60 mmHg, respirations 31/min) and should be treated in the inpatient setting with possible ICU admission.

CASE 4 | Community-Acquired Pneumonia: *Streptococcus pneumoniae* (continued)

Discussion	If this patient had a higher BP and a lower respiratory rate (CURB-65 score of 1), he could be treated with antibiotics as an outpatient.
	• Low 30-day mortality risk (CURB-65 = 0 or 1)
	  • Outpatient management
	  • **Amoxicillin** or **doxycycline**
	  • If comorbid diseases (lung, heart, liver, kidney), give a fluoroquinolone or β-lactam + macrolide
	• Moderate 30-day mortality risk (CURB-65 = 2 or 3)
	  • Hospital admission—most likely to floor
	  • **B-lactam + macrolide** or **fluoroquinolone**
	• High 30-day mortality risk (CURB-65 = 4 or 5)
	  • Hospital admission—most likely to ICU
	  • **B-lactam + macrolide** or **β-lactam + fluoroquinolone**
	• MRSA or pseudomonal risk factors:
	  • Vancomycin (MRSA) or piperacillin-tazobactam (*Pseudomonas aeruginosa*).

Additional Considerations	**Immunizations:** PPSV and PCV vaccines against *S. pneumoniae* recommended for patients ≥65 years, or younger with comorbid conditions. **Complications:** Sepsis, acute respiratory distress syndrome (ARDS), pleural effusion, or empyema. **Pediatric Considerations:** School-aged children can present with bacterial pneumonia most commonly caused by *S. pneumoniae*. • Newborns and infants more often get viral pneumonia • Routine childhood immunizations protect against pneumonia by *H. influenza* type b and *S. pneumoniae*

CURB-65 Criteria for the Determination of CAP Severity on Presentation to Hospital

C	Confusion
U	BUN ≥20
R	Respiratory rate ≥30
B	Systolic BP <90 mmHg or diastolic BP ≤60 mmHg
65	Age ≥65 years old

One point applied for each item present:

0–1—Low mortality (0.7–2.1%). Possible outpatient treatment.

2—Intermediate mortality (9.2%). Consider hospital treatment.

3—High mortality (14.5%). Hospital admission.

4—Mortality of >40%. Admission. Consider intensive care unit.

Source: Data from Lim WS, van der Eerden MM, Laing R, et al. Defining community acquired pneumonia severity on presentation to hospital: an international derivation and validation study. Thorax. 2003;58:377-382.

CASE 5 | Pulmonary Tuberculosis

A 62-year-old woman presents with fever, night sweats, and a productive cough for the past 2 months. She recently emigrated from Indonesia. Her vitals are temperature 38.7°C, pulse 90/min, respirations 24/min, and blood pressure 110/84 mmHg, with SpO$_2$ 92% on room air. On exam, auscultation reveals coarse crackles in the right upper lobe posteriorly with increased tactile fremitus.

Conditions with Similar Presentations	**Histoplasmosis:** Is more commonly seen in Ohio and Mississippi River valley regions. Can be transmitted in bird and bat droppings, so it is important to ask about the patient's hobbies, such as spelunking. On microscopy, *Histoplasma* can be found within macrophages. **Blastomycosis:** Is more commonly seen in eastern and central United States (US) and can form granulomas and verrucous skin lesions when spread. On microscopy, broad-based buds can be seen. **Anaerobic lung infections:** Are subacute as well, but patients would have risk factors such as poor dentition, seizure history, substance abuse, or gag reflex abnormalities. **Pulmonary sarcoidosis:** Is often asymptomatic but may present with cough, hilar adenopathy, erythema nodosum, and noncaseating granulomas. It has similarities in presentation to TB and the above endemic fungi. Because the treatment of sarcoidosis is corticosteroids, endemic fungi and TB should be ruled out before steroid treatment is initiated.

CASE 5 | Pulmonary Tuberculosis (continued)

Initial Diagnostic Tests	• Confirm with chest x-ray and sputum culture for acid-fast bacilli (AFB) • Consider interferon gamma-release assay (IGRA) or tuberculin skin test (TST), but these only confirm past exposure, not active infection
Next Steps in Management	Rifampin, isoniazid, pyrazinamide and ethambutol

Discussion	Pulmonary tuberculosis is caused by lower respiratory tract infection with *Mycobacterium tuberculosis* spread via airborne droplets. Although there is low incidence of tuberculosis (TB) in the US, the disease burden of TB is very high worldwide, with ~25% of the population infected. Pulmonary tuberculosis can present in several ways.
	• Initial infection (**primary tuberculosis**) presents with classic TB symptoms (cough, fever, night sweats, weight loss) in addition to development of ipsilateral hilar adenopathy and a middle lung lesion with hilar adenopathy known as a **Ghon complex**.
	• Most patients, if untreated, will develop **latent TB**, during which the patient is asymptomatic and no longer contagious. Latent TB is diagnosed if an asymptomatic individual has a positive result on TST or an interferon-γ release assay. Chest x-ray should be ordered to rule out active infection.
	• **Reactivation of TB** can occur and results in formation of a fibrocaseous cavitary lesion often within the upper lobes, as is seen in this patient. Reactivation TB can lead to localized destruction with caseation and scar formation.
	• Rarely, primary or secondary tuberculosis can cause progressive lung disease or bacteremia, which can lead to **miliary TB** with extrapulmonary manifestations. 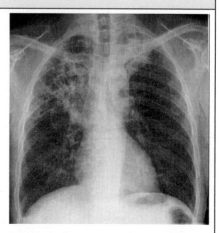
	Postprimary (reactivation) tuberculosis. (A) Frontal chest radiograph demonstrates patchy airspace opacities in the right upper lung, and to a much lesser extent in the left apex as well. In the appropriate clinical setting, opacities that demonstrate an apical predominance should raise suspicion for reactivation tuberculosis. (Reproduced with permission from Khaled M. Elsayes , Sandra A.A. Oldham . Introduction to Diagnostic Radiology; New York, NY: McGraw Hill: 2015.)
	
	History:
	Risk factors: Endemic area, close contact with someone who has TB, high TB transmission settings (e.g., undomiciled, incarceration, health care work), HIV/AIDS
	Subacute presentation (6 weeks of symptoms) of cough, hemoptysis, night sweats, and constitutional symptoms (fever, weight loss)
	Physical Exam: Fever, low SpO$_2$, localized crackles on pulmonary exam
	Diagnostics:
	For active symptoms:
	• Obtain CXR (may show a cavitary lesion in upper lobes and hilar lymphadenopathy)
	• Our patient: Right hilar and mediastinal and right hilar lymphadenopathy and consolidation in the right upper lobe consolidation.
	• Induce sputum for AFB
	Additional tests:
	TST
	• A subcutaneous injection of tuberculin, a mycobacterial protein. Positive results vary by risk factors and include an induration of:
	  • >5 mm: immunosuppressed, HIV/AIDS, TB contact
	  • >10 mm: health care, endemic area, intravenous drug use (IVDU)
	  • >15 mm in the general population
	• Patients may have a false negative TST test in conditions with decreased cell-mediated immunity, such as HIV/AIDS and chronic kidney disease

CASE 5 | Pulmonary Tuberculosis (*continued*)

Discussion	Interferon gamma release assay (IGRA)
	• Measures the amount of interferon-γ released by a patient's CD4 T-cells after stimulation with a TB-specific antigen
	• BCG vaccine can cause a false-positive TST, so IGRA is preferred in individuals who had BCG vaccine
	Management:
	• RIPE therapy: First-line treatment for TB involves four drugs: **R**ifampin, **I**soniazid, **P**yrimethamine, **E**thambutol.
	  • Patients take all four drugs daily for 2 months, then two drugs (isoniazid and rifampin) daily for 4 additional months.
	  • If susceptibility testing reveals sensitivity to RIP, the ethambutol can be discontinued sooner than 2 months.
	• Reportable disease to Department of Public Health.
	• Testing of close contacts and family members.
		
		Acid-fast stain and culture of sputum: induced sputum culture with acid-fast stain is positive for acid-fast bacilli of *Mycobacterium tuberculosis* seen at 100 × power with oil immersion microscopy. (Reproduced with permission from Richard P. Usatine, Mindy A. Smith, E.J. Mayeaux, Jr., Heidi S. Chumley. The Color Atlas and Synopsis of Family Medicine, 3e, McGraw Hill, 2019. Figure 56-2, ISBN 9781259862045. Reproduced with permission from Richard P. Usatine, MD.)

Additional Considerations	**Pediatric Considerations:** Children <2 years should be tested using TST over IGRA. **Complications and other Infectious Syndromes caused by *Mycobacterium tuberculosis*:** **Latent TB:** Patients will present with a positive TST or IGRA but clear chest x-ray. Treatment to prevent reactivation is rifampin for 4 months or isoniazid for 9 months. **Reactivation TB:** Results in formation of a fibrocaseous cavitary lesion often within the upper lobes of the lungs which are more highly oxygenated. **Miliary TB:** Primary or secondary TB can cause progressive lung disease or bacteremia, which can lead to miliary TB with extrapulmonary manifestations. This progressive form of TB is more common in immunocompromised patients with HIV/AIDS or malnutrition. **Tuberculous adrenalitis** can cause primary adrenal insufficiency. **Tuberculous spondylitis (Pott disease)** **Tuberculosis meningitis** can lead to hypopituitarism (secondary adrenal insufficiency, hypothyroidism, hypogonadotropic hypogonadism). CT scan of the head will show basilar meningeal enhancement and mild hydrocephalus.	

Common Side Effects and Toxicities Associated with TB Drugs

Drug	Side Effects and Toxicities
Rifampin	Red-orange body fluids, interstitial nephritis, induction of P450 enzyme causing effects such as: • Increased degradation of vitamin D (vitamin D deficiency) • Increased dose requirement of levothyroxine, warfarin, phenytoin • Decreases effectiveness of oral contraceptives • Decreased hepatic uptake of bilirubin (hyperbilirubinemia)
Isoniazid	Sideroblastic anemia, hepatotoxicity, peripheral neuropathy, which are all caused by depletion of pyridoxine (B6). **Pyridoxine supplementation** is indicated in patients who are at an increased risk for neurotoxicity, such as those who are pregnant, malnourished, have alcohol use disorder, or have diabetes.
Pyrazinamide	Hyperuricemia.
Ethambutol	Decreased visual acuity, optic neuritis, red-green colorblindness. Very rare at low doses.

CASE 6 | *Pneumocystis jirovecii* Pneumonia (PJP)

A 29-year-old woman with HIV infection presents with fever, dyspnea, and dry cough for 3 weeks. She has been inconsistent with taking her HIV medications. She denies night sweats, weight loss, and has never used IV drugs. She lives alone in her own apartment. On exam, the patient has a temperature of 38.7°C, pulse 105/min, respirations 22/min, blood pressure 110/74 mmHg, and SpO_2 89% on room air. Faint crackles are appreciated bilaterally on lung auscultation.

Conditions with Similar Presentations	**Community-acquired pneumonia:** Presents more acutely and usually unilateral. **Tuberculosis** and other **fungal infections:** From endemic fungi, have a more prolonged clinical course and present with cavitary lung disease rather than interstitial infiltrates. **CMV pneumonitis:** Would present with ground-glass opacities and pleural effusion on chest x-ray, and is seen in patients with CD4 <100.
Initial Diagnostic Tests	• Check Chest x-ray • Confirm with induced sputum for PJP • If negative, do BAL • Also check CD4 count and ABG
Next Steps in Management	• First line: Trimethoprim-sulfamethoxazole (discussed below) • Corticosteroids with moderate to severe disease
Discussion	PJP pneumonia, formerly known as *Pneumocystis carinii* (hence the commonly used acronym PCP) is caused by the opportunistic fungus *Pneumocystis jirovecii* and is the most common opportunistic infection in patients with immunocompromised states. **History:** Risk factors: HIV/AIDS (especially if CD4 <200 or high viral load), transplant patients (risk is usually greatest in the 6 months following transplantation). Common symptoms: Cough, fever, and dyspnea. **Physical Exam:** Crackles on auscultation, often a low SpO_2 on room air. **Diagnostics:** • Chest x-ray: shows bilateral diffuse interstitial pulmonary infiltrates and ground-glass opacities extending from the hilar areas in a "bat-wing" pattern. • Induced sputum or bronchoscopy with bronchoalveolar lavage (BAL): Reveals a disc-shaped yeast on silver stain. 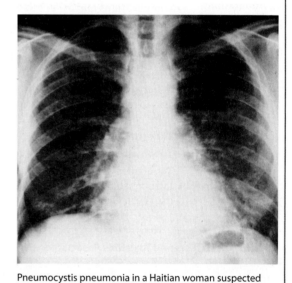 Pneumocystis pneumonia in a Haitian woman suspected of having underlying HIV/AIDS. Typical chest radiograph showing bilateral diffuse interstitial infiltrates extending out from the hilar areas. (Reproduced with permission from Maxine A. Papadakis, Stephen J. McPhee, Michael W. Rabow, CMDT, 16e, McGraw Hill 2021, Figure 31-2, ISBN 9781260469868.) Additional tests: • CD4+ count for patients with HIV/AIDS. • ABG to assess severity with a PaO_2 >70 considered mild and <70 considered as moderate to severe disease. This identifies who should receive steroids. • CT scan, if obtained, would show ground-glass opacities. **Management:** • Trimethoprim-sulfamethoxazole (TMP-SMX) for 21 days • Patients with sulfa allergy can receive clindamycin and primaquine (check for G-6-PD deficiency if this regimen is used) • Steroids if patient has SpO_2 <92%, PaO_2 ≤70 mmHg, or alveolar-arterial gradient ≥35 mmHg on room air
Additional Considerations	**Prevention:** Prophylactic therapy with TMP-SMX is indicated in patients with CD4 counts <200 or those on chronic glucocorticoid therapy.

Fever and Cough Mini-Cases

Cases	Key Findings
Legionella Pneumonia	**Hx:** Risk factors: Age >50, immunocompromised status, diabetes, smoking, chronic lung disease, and exposure to aerosols from contaminated water or soil (e.g., hot tubs, swimming pools, domestic plumbing systems, respiratory devices and nebulizers). Symptoms: Fever, fatigue, nonproductive cough, and shortness of breath 2–10 days after exposure. May also have gastrointestinal symptoms (nausea, vomiting, diarrhea), headaches, neurologic abnormalities, delirium, myalgias, or chest pain. **PE:** High fever (>39°C). Relative bradycardia may be seen. Crackles or other signs of consolidation on pulmonary exam. **Diagnostics:** • Chest x-ray: May show patchy infiltrates or lobar consolidation but varies greatly and are not specific to Legionella. • Confirm with: Legionella-specific testing with urinary antigen testing or culture of lower respiratory tract secretions (sputum or bronchoalveolar lavage). • Testing indicated in adults with severe CAP or for those in whom clinical suspicion for Legionella is high (recent travel, association with recent outbreak). Additional tests: • Gram stain: Shows leukocytes but no bacteria because Legionella's cell wall does not stain well. • Leukocytosis, hyponatremia, hypophosphatemia, and elevated transaminases may be present on laboratory studies. **Management:** • Fluoroquinolone or azithromycin are preferred therapies for Legionella. • Doxycycline may be used as alternative therapy. • Patients should be empirically treated for community- or hospital-acquired pneumonia until diagnosis is confirmed. **Discussion:** **Legionnaire's disease** is another name for *Legionella* pneumonia and is a cause of atypical CAP among elderly and immunocompromised patients. **Pontiac fever** refers to a self-limited febrile illness without pneumonia caused by *Legionella* and usually occurs in outbreaks.
Influenza	**Hx:** Risk Factors: Exposure to a sick contact within incubation period of 1–4 days Symptoms: Acute onset of fever, upper tract symptoms (sneezing, sore throat), cough, headache, myalgia, malaise, weakness. **PE:** Fever (37.8–40.0°C, can reach 41.1°C) and cervical lymphadenopathy. Unremarkable pulmonary exam unless influenza pneumonia has occurred. **Diagnostics:** • Molecular assay is preferred (RT-PCR, rapid molecular) • Rapid antigen testing is less preferred due to lower sensitivity • Serologic testing and viral culture are not indicated because they take too long to turn positive **Management:** • Supportive care for any symptomatic patient • Within 48 hours of symptom onset: Antiviral therapy with a neuraminidase inhibitor (zanamivir, oseltamivir, peramivir) or endoculease inhibitor (baloxavir) • The goal of antiviral therapy is to reduce the length of symptoms and prevent complications, especially morbidity and mortality in high-risk groups. Prevention: • Yearly immunization for everyone over 6 months of age • Live vaccine contraindicated in immunocompromised • High-dose vaccine indicated for those ≥65 **Discussion:** The average duration of symptoms is 3 days. Some patients with certain risk factors are more likely to have more severe and a longer duration of symptoms (>50 years, obesity, young children, pregnant women, and patients with other chronic medical diseases).

Fever and Cough Mini-Cases (*continued*)

SARS-CoV-2 (COVID-19)	**Hx:** Risk factors: Exposure, travel history or residence in area with community transmission. Incubation period of 2–14 days (mean ~5 days) and estimated 33% of infections are asymptomatic.
	Symptoms: Fever and acute respiratory symptoms (cough, sore throat, rhinorrhea) are the most common. Systemic symptoms (myalgia, malaise, fatigue); taste/smell changes (anosmia, ageusia); gastrointestinal (diarrhea, nausea, vomiting) may also occur. New or worsening dyspnea tends to develop a week after onset of initial symptoms
	PE: Fever, hypoxia without increased work of breathing or dyspnea.
	Diagnostics:
	• RT-PCR assay (for detecting COVID-19 RNA in an upper respiratory tract sample) is the preferred initial diagnostic test.
	• Antigen testing is less sensitive but can be used in serial testing
	• Chest imaging may show pneumonia, characterized by bilateral infiltrates, including characteristic ground-glass opacities
	Management:
	Asymptomatic or mild cases (no dyspnea or oxygen requirement):
	• Manage at home with supportive care, with distancing precautions for 5-10 days. Can discontinue after that time if >24 hours afebrile and symptoms improving.
	• Monoclonal antibody spike protein inhibitors, or nirmatrelvir + ritonavir is indicated if risk of clinical progression is high (e.g., COPD, heart failure, age ≥65).
	Hospitalized patients:
	• Management of hypoxia, with treatment including oxygen supplementation, mechanical ventilation, and extracorporeal membrane oxygenation (ECMO).
	• Remdesivir is recommended for all hypoxic patients, while adding dexamethasone is reserved for those requiring supplemental oxygen or higher levels of oxygenation support. Tocilizumab should be added if patient requires ventilation or ECMO.
	• Thromboprophylaxis is indicated for all patients.
	Discussion: SARS-CoV-2 is a novel Coronavirus that was first reported in the US in 2020 and causes COVID-19.
	• Infection control is by cleaning hands with alcohol-based sanitizers, maintaining social distancing and use of masks.
	• All vaccines with boosters are helpful in reducing hospitalization and death.
Lung Abscess	**Hx:** Risk factors include advanced age, gingival disease, alcohol use disorder, bronchial obstruction due to underlying tumor/foreign body, and other risk factors for aspiration pneumonia.
	Symptoms: Present sub-acutely with fever, cough, and purulent sputum (foul smelling in 50% of patients), arising over several weeks.
	PE: Potential findings include fever, cavernous breath sounds on lung exam, and poor dentition.
	Diagnostics:
	• Chest x-ray may reveal a cavity with a thick-wall and air-fluid level.
	• Computed tomography is indicated for patients with pneumonia unresponsive to antibiotic treatment as it has better detection of small abscesses and/or malignancy.
	Management:
	• Preferred regimen is ampicillin-sulbactam IV or amoxicillin clavulanate PO for ~6–8 weeks based on the patient's clinical and radiographic response.
	• If penicillin-allergic, clindamycin or a fluoroquinolone +/– metronidazole.
	• If there is no improvement, abscess may require surgery or percutaneous or endoscopic drainage.
	Discussion: Lung abscess is a circumscribed collection of pus in the lung caused by necrosis of lung due to infection. Aspiration-related abscesses are polymicrobial. The majority (85–90%) of patients improve with antibiotics. Fever may persist for 4–8 days after initiation, and radiographic infiltrates may initially progress.

Fever and Cough Mini-Cases (*continued*)

Invasive Pulmonary Aspergillosis (*Aspergillus fumigatus*)	**Hx:** Classic triad of fever, pleuritic chest pain, and hemoptysis in an immunocompromised patient (neutropenia or HIV with CD4 <50).

PE: Rales on lung exam, also can have sinus tenderness, nasal discharge if sinuses involved.

Diagnostics:
- Chest x-ray shows "halo sign"—nodules with surrounding ground-glass infiltrates.
- CT with dense, well-circumscribed dense lesions which may or may not have the halo sign or air-crescent sign (seen in a cavitating lesion)
- Serum biomarkers for fungal cell wall components (galactomannan, beta-D-glucan)
- Confirm with sputum or tissue biopsy demonstrating septated hyphae with acute angle (45°) branching.
- Biopsy demonstrating tissue invasion with *Aspergillus* is the gold standard for diagnosis but is often difficult to obtain.

Management:
- Treat with voriconazole
- Liposomal amphotericin B, if diagnosis is uncertain and patient is not improving

Discussion: Invasive pulmonary aspergillosis (IPA) is caused by *Aspergillus sp.* such as A. *fumigatus*, A. *flavus*, A. *niger* and A. *terreus*. These are ubiquitous environmental fungi transmitted via the airborne route. It occurs in immunocompromised patients, especially in those with prolonged neutropenia or individuals with chronic granulomatous disease and neutrophil dysfunction. *Aspergillus* tends to invade vasculature, which can lead to widespread disease and to manifestations such as hemoptysis from pulmonary blood vessel invasion. Even with treatment, mortality rates are >50%.

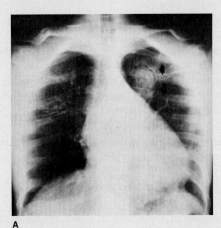

A

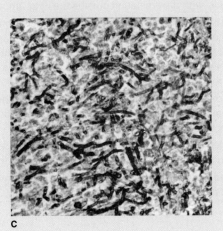

C

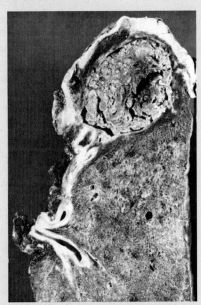

B

Pulmonary aspergilloma. A. Monad's sign: The arrows show a solid mass within a cavity surrounded by a rim of air between the mass and cavity wall. B. Specimen showing "fungus ball" occupying an old, fibrotic cavity. C. Histologic stain showing *Aspergillus hyphae* which invades the wall of the cavity. (Reproduced with permission from F. Charles Brunicardi, Dana K. Andersen, Timothy R. Billiar, David L. Dunn, Lillian S. Kao, John G. Hunter, Jeffrey B. Matthews, Raphael E. Pollock, CMDT, 16e, McGraw Hill 2021.)

Fever and Cough Mini-Cases (*continued*)

Invasive Pulmonary Aspergillosis (*Aspergillus fumigatus*)	Additional Considerations: **Allergic bronchopulmonary aspergillosis (ABPA)**, a hypersensitivity response to *Aspergillus*, presents with wheezing, fever, eosinophilia, and bronchiectasis, classically in patients with asthma or cystic fibrosis. Susceptible individuals develop an abnormal T-lymphocyte cellular immune response to *A. fumigatus*, which results in activation of the complement cascade that leads to inflammation. Damage can progress to bronchiectasis, pulmonary cavities, focal emphysema, and fibrosis. Patients will usually have peripheral eosinophilia, elevated *Aspergillus*-specific IgG antibodies, high total serum IgE, and positive immediate and delayed skin reactions to *Aspergillus* antigens. On CXR, fleeting parenchymal opacities that respond to corticosteroids are seen. End-stage ABPA will manifest with cavitation and fibrosis. **Aspergillomas:** Form in cavity formed by aspergillus or in a preexisting lung cavity such as from a prior tuberculosis infection.
Histoplasmosis	**Hx:** Risk factors: Living in or traveled to the midwest region of the US (Mississippi and Ohio River valleys). Occupational and recreational activities that expose patients to contaminated soil (e.g., spelunking, moving soil, building demolition). Symptoms: Most patients (>99%) are asymptomatic and most cases are self-limiting. Symptomatic infection typically occurs 7–21 days after exposure and is more likely in immunocompromised patients. Symptoms include malaise, fever, chills, headaches, anorexia, and weight loss. Additional features vary by type: • **Pulmonary histoplasmosis:** Dyspnea, chest pain, cough, and hemoptysis may be present. • **Progressive disseminated histoplasmosis:** Painful mucocutaneous lesions, diarrhea, liver and spleen infection, and rarely CNS infection. **PE:** Fever and lymphadenopathy may be present in both pulmonary and disseminated forms. Additional findings vary by type and may include: • **Pulmonary histoplasmosis:** Rales on lung exam, erythema nodosum or multiforme on skin exam and/or hepatosplenomegaly on abdominal exam • **Disseminated histoplasmosis:** Petechiae, skin ulcers, nodules, or molluscum-like papules on skin exam, ulcerations on oropharyngeal exam, hepatosplenomegaly and, if the brain is involved, focal neurologic deficits and/or altered mental status **Diagnostics:** • Antigen testing of the blood or urine is positive in the majority of patients • Sputum Gram stain may reveal the organism and is diagnostic because endemic fungi are never normal flora • Culture is gold standard, but results take days to weeks **Management:** • No treatment recommended for asymptomatic or mild to moderate disease of < 4 weeks duration. • For mild to moderate infection > 4 weeks, treat with itraconazole. • For severe cases, especially with dissemination outside the lung, amphotericin B is indicated. **Discussion:** Histoplasmosis is a mycotic infection caused by *Histoplasma capsulatum*. *H. capsulatum* is found in soil contaminated with bird feces or bat droppings. Spores are inhaled into lower airways, where they are phagocytized by alveolar macrophages and multiply throughout the reticuloendothelial system. In immunocompetent patients, cellular immunity develops in a few weeks and the yeast is destroyed within the macrophages. In patients with deficient cell-mediated immunity, the fungus can proliferate and spread throughout the body, leading to disseminated disease. Any histoplasma infection outside of the lung is an AIDS-defining illness in HIV-infected individuals. **Pulmonary histoplasmosis:** In the acute form, symptoms are usually self-limiting. The chronic form presents as a chronic pneumonia, unresponsive to antibacterials used to treat CAP. **Progressive disseminated histoplasmosis:** Seen in immunocompromised patients and causes painful mucocutaneous lesions, diarrhea, liver and spleen infection, and rarely CNS infection.

Fever and Cough Mini-Cases (*continued*)

Blastomycosis	**Hx:** Risk factors: Individuals who spend time outdoors and live in the Ohio and Mississippi River areas. Symptoms: Months of fever, night sweats, productive cough, weight loss, and skin lesions. **PE:** Fever; well-circumscribed, verrucous ulcers with crusted irregular borders on nose or face. **Diagnostics:** • Chest x-ray may show lytic bone lesions or lobar consolidation with or without cavities. • Antigen testing of the blood or urine is positive in the majority of cases. • Microscopy showing broad-based budding yeast with a double-layered cell wall and culture of sputum or body tissues. Endemic fungi are never normal flora. **Management:** • All patients should be assessed for underlying immunocompromised state and treated regardless of severity. • Oral itraconazole for mild to moderate disease, not involving the CNS. • For severe disease, treatment starts with amphotericin B, then transitions to itraconazole. **Discussion:** Blastomycosis is seen in states surrounding the Great Lakes as well as the Mississippi and Ohio River valleys. The most common form of infection is pneumonia, but disseminated disease (with or without concomitant pulmonary involvement) may occur, including skin lesions, osteomyelitis, prostatitis, meningitis, or brain abscesses. Although the fungus can cause more severe disease in immunocompromised patients, disseminated disease may occur even in immunocompetent patients. **Cutaneous blastomycosis** is the most common extrapulmonary manifestation of systemic blastomycosis.
Coccidioidomycosis	**Hx:** Associated with southwestern region of the US and northern Mexico. Symptoms of primary pulmonary infection can occur 1–3 weeks after exposure and resemble acute pneumonia: Cough, dyspnea, arthralgias, night sweats, fever lasting 3 weeks. **PE:** In addition to signs of pneumonia, erythema nodosum may be seen. **Diagnostics:** • Gram stain is diagnostic but low yield. • Culture is the gold standard but may take weeks to grow. • Serial serology tests. Initially, test for IgM (1–3 weeks—acute infection) and IgG (rising titer after 2–3 weeks) with enzyme-linked immunoassay (EIA), then immunodiffusion tests. • Chest x-ray: Normal or with infiltrates, nodules, cavities, mediastinal hilar adenopathy, pleural effusions. **Management:** • Many cases are subacute, mild, and resolve without treatment. • If symptomatic but not severe, treat with triazoles (fluconazole, itraconazole). • Severe or disseminated disease, treat with amphotericin B. **Discussion:** Initial infection may be asymptomatic but may reactivate, warranting treatment, especially in immunocompromised patients (HIV; after transplant). Signs of primary pulmonary infection resemble acute pneumonia and this is known as **Valley Fever** (named after the San Joaquin Valley in California).
Nocardiosis	**Hx:** Risk factors: Immunocompromised patients. Symptoms: Cough, dyspnea, chest pain, night sweats, fever, and weight loss. May also have headache, altered mental status, and/or focal deficits if CNS involvement. **PE:** Fever, abnormal lung sounds, cutaneous findings include ulcers or purulent lesions at site of inoculation. **Diagnostics:** • Chest x-ray with consolidations or cavitary lesions. • Modified acid-fast staining and Gram staining from multiple sites (e.g., skin biopsy, abscess drainage) showing branching gram-positive rods. Takes weeks to grow. **Management:** • TMX-SMP for mild/moderate pulmonary disease or cutaneous infection alone. • Use TMX-SMP with amikacin for disseminated disease, and add imipenem for CNS involvement. • Drain abscesses surgically. **Discussion:** Nocardia can disseminate to any organ, most frequently the brain (brain abscesses). The infection is prone to relapse or further progression despite appropriate therapy. Nocardia is endemic in soil and routes of infection include trauma (skin lesions) and inhalation (pulmonary symptoms in *immunosuppressed* patients (HIV, chronic steroids, history of transplant))

Fever and Cough Mini-Cases (*continued*)

Anthrax	**Hx/PE:** Risk factors: Exposure or inhalation of spores (handling animal wool, hair, or other products) or from bioterrorism.
	• *Inhalation* (most deadly form). Biphasic symptoms begin 4-6 days after exposure.
	• Prodromal phase: Lasts about 4-5 days and is characterized by flu-like symptoms (fever, cough, malaise), hemoptysis and odynophagia.
	• Fulminant phase: Quickly follows prodromal phase and is characterized by pulmonary hemorrhage and shock, and if untreated, leads to death. Meningitis may also occur.
	• *Cutaneous* (most common form). Develops 1–7 days after exposure, starting as a pruritic papule, enlarges into a bulla (later an ulcer), ultimately forming a black eschar by day 7–10.
	• *Gastrointestinal* (secondary to ingestion of undercooked or contaminated meat). Symptoms develop in 3–6 days and include nausea, vomiting, abdominal pain, dysphagia, and bloody diarrhea.
	Diagnostics:
	• Diagnose with a positive culture isolation (e.g., blood, pleural fluid, sub-eschar swab, stool) or two nonculture tests (PCR, IHC, ELISA).
	• Chest x-ray in inhalation anthrax does not show infiltrates, but rather widened mediastinum and pleural effusions.
	Management:
	• Systemic disease (inhalation, gastrointestinal, cutaneous disease of face/head/neck): 1 of each of the following 3 groups:
	• Fluoroquinolone, ß-lactam (carbapenem, or penicillin/ampicillin), and other (linezolid, clindamycin, rifampin, chloramphenicol).
	• In addition two monoclonal antibodies are available (obiltoxaximab, raxibacumab).
	• Cutaneous disease only: ciprofloxacin, doxycycline.
	• Post-inhalation exposure prophylaxis: ciprofloxacin or doxycycline + anthrax vaccine.
	Discussion: Anthrax infection is caused by contact with spores of the *Bacillus anthracis* bacterium, as seen when exposed to or handling animal wool, hair, or other products or bioterrorism. There is no person-to-person spread. Complications of systemic disease include meningitis (which can lead to hemorrhagic meningitis) and should be treated with ciprofloxacin, meropenem, and linezolid.

Common Side Effects and Toxicities Associated with Antifungal Drugs

Antifungal Agent	Indication	Adverse Effects
Nystatin	Mostly used for treatment of Candidiasis. Swish and swallow for oral thrush.	Diarrhea, nausea, vomiting, and abdominal pain.
Clotrimazole	Topical use for tinea pedis, tinea corporis.	
Terbinafine	Topical use for tinea pedis, cruris, and corporis. Oral use for onychomycosis and tinea capitis.	Hepatotoxicity, headache, diarrhea, dyspepsia.
Griseofulvin	Oral agent used mainly for treatment of tinea capitis.	Rash, urticaria, CYP-450 inducer.
Itraconazole	Oral drug that treats aspergillosis, blastomycosis, and histoplasmosis as well as dermatophytes.	Hepatotoxicity, nausea, vomiting, diarrhea, abdominal pain, hypertension, peripheral edema, and hypokalemia.
Amphotericin B	Reserved for life-threatening fungal infections. Used in combination with flucytosine to treat cryptococcus neoformans.	Hypotension, hypokalemia, hypomagnesemia, fevers, and chills (shake and bake), anemia, renal tubular acidosis type 1, phlebitis. Many side effects, hence, the moniker "amphoTERRIBLE."
Micafungin, Caspofungin or Anidulafungin	Candidemia, disseminated candidiasis, candidal endocarditis, febrile neutropenia.	Anaphylaxis, hypersensitivity reaction, GI side effects, hepatotoxicity, hemolysis, thrombocytopenia, neutropenia.

ENDOCARDITIS

Infective endocarditis (IE) is an infection of the endocardium due to various organisms. Suspect infective endocarditis in patients with:

- Bacteremia and risk factors: prosthetic valve, intravascular devices, hemodialysis, IV drug use, structural heart disease, previous endocarditis
- Bacteremia with fever and new murmur
- Bacteremia with no clear source
- Fever in illnesses that do not normally have fever (e.g., stroke, myocardial infarction, congestive heart failure, vascular aneurysm)
- Staphylococcal bacteremia

The common etiologic agents of infective endocarditis are as below.

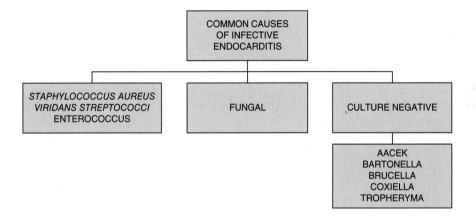

Clues to Potential Etiology of Endocarditis

History of:	Potential Organism(s)
Dental procedures	Viridans group *Streptococcus*
Colon cancer	*S. gallolyticus* (*S. bovis* biotype)
GI/GU procedure	*Enterococcus*
Prosthetic valves	*S. epidermidis*
IV drug use	*S. aureus, Pseudomonas aeruginosa, Candida albicans*
Negative cultures	*Coxiella burnetti*, Bartonella, AACEK (**A**ggregatibacter aphrophilus, **A**ggregatibacter actinomycetemcomitans, **C**ardiobacterium hominis, **E**ikenella corrodens, **K**ingella kingae)
SLE, metastatic cancer, hypercoagulable states	Consider nonbacterial thrombotic endocarditis

The diagnostic approach for patients presenting with fever, new murmur, and a positive blood culture is as below.

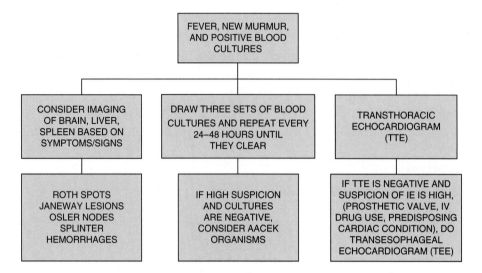

Modified Duke Criteria for Diagnosing Endocarditis

Endocarditis diagnosis: two major criteria, 1 major + 3 minor, or all 5 minor criteria
Possible endocarditis: 1 major, 1 minor OR 3 minor
Major criteria
1. Multiple positive blood cultures with an organism that commonly causes endocarditis
2. Echocardiogram with a vegetation, or abscess, or new prosthetic valve dehiscence OR a new valvular regurgitation murmur on exam
Minor criteria
1. History of IV drug use or predisposing valvular disease
2. Fever ≥38°C
3. Vascular phenomena: major arterial embolus, septic PE, mycoctic aneurysm, intracranial bleed, conjunctival hemorrhages, Janeway lesions.
4. Immunologic phenomena: Glomerulonephritis, Osler nodes, Roth spots or rheumatoid factor (+)
5. Blood culture suggestive of endocarditis, but not meeting major criteria

Approach to Therapy

- Empiric parenteral therapy is based on valve type (see below chart)
- Narrow antibiotic spectrum once cultures confirm organism
- Surgical indications (see below chart)

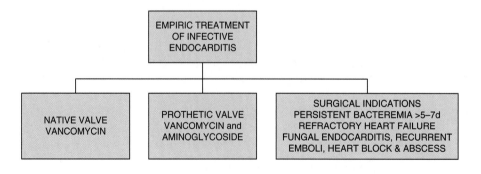

CASE 7 | Subacute Bacterial Endocarditis

A 47-year-old man with rheumatic heart disease and mitral stenosis presents with new dyspnea and cough for the past few days. He also reports fevers, night sweats, decreased appetite, weight loss, malaise, and arthralgias for the last 3 weeks. Over a month ago, he had an infected dental implant repaired. He has a temperature of 38.4°C, pulse 115/min, blood pressure 90/62 mmHg, RR 23, and SpO$_2$ 98% on room air. Fundoscopic exam shows flame hemorrhages with white centers (Roth spots). A pan systolic murmur is heard at the cardiac apex radiating to the axilla. There are several tender, raised lesions on his finger and toe pads (Osler nodes); small nontender, black lesions on palms and soles (Janeway lesions); and the nail beds have linear reddish-brown lesions (splinter hemorrhages).

Conditions with Similar Presentations	**Nonbacterial endocarditis:** Also called marantic or thrombotic endocarditis, can be seen secondary to underlying malignancy (marantic endocarditis), hypercoagulable states, or lupus (Libman-Sachs endocarditis). High-grade **bacteremia** or **fungemia:** May also have similar features without valve involvement.
Initial Diagnostic Tests	• Obtain at least three blood cultures prior to initiation of any antibiotic therapy and a transthoracic echocardiography. • Consider: Chest x-ray, CBC, BMP
Next Steps in Management	• Prolonged bactericidal, parenteral antibiotic treatment, initially empiric (e.g., vancomycin) • Remove any implanted devices • Consider valve repair or replacement if hemodynamic compromise

Discussion	Infective endocarditis (IE) is the infection of the innermost layer of the heart, which can damage the valvular endothelium, chordae tendineae, and mural endocardium. Initial endocardial injury in the process of healing leads to the development of a platelet-fibrin nidus. Nidus becomes infected by a microbe already circulating in the blood, due to a concurrent infection (e.g., skin infection, dental abscess, minor trauma from procedures) or transient bacteremia. Microbial growth activates the coagulation cascade and leads to increased deposition of fibronectin, ultimately developing into a vegetation. The vegetation encases a bacterial center with an outer layer of platelets, fibrin, and other tissue, allowing for the persistence of the mass.
	• Most cases of native valve endocarditis are left-sided.
	• IVDU and indwelling vascular catheters increase the risk for endocarditis (caused by *S. aureus*) on a right-sided valve because the tricuspid valve is the first valve encountered in the heart by bacteria traveling in the bloodstream as well as particulate material injected directly injuring the tricuspid valve.
	History: Symptoms: Low-grade, intermittent fever (90%), chills, anorexia, weight loss, night sweats, malaise.
	Risk factors:
	Cardiac risk factors: Congenital heart disease, especially cyanotic heart disease that has not been surgically repaired; prosthetic valves, especially within the first 12 months following surgery, cardiac devices, prior endocarditis.
	Noncardiac risk factors: IVDU, prolonged bacteremia, mild trauma from procedures in the following areas: gastrointestinal (GI), genitourinary (GU), and dental (poor dental hygiene, dental abscess).
	Physical Exam:
	• Fever (95%)
	• Murmur (85%)
	• New murmur (50%)
	• Splenomegaly (10%)
	• Rare (<10%) but highly specific
	  • Conjunctival hemorrhages
	  • Janeway lesions
	  • Osler nodes
	  • Roth spots
	Diagnostics:
	• Obtain three sets of blood cultures from different sites drawn at least 1 hour apart
	• Transthoracic echocardiogram (TTE) showing a vegetation
	• Transesophageal echocardiogram (TEE) if suspicion is high despite negative TTE
	• Duke criteria—see above table
	Management:
	• IV antibiotics should be bactericidal: beta-lactams, glycopeptides, aminoglycosides, cyclic lipopeptides (daptomycin)
	• Native valve endocarditis: Vancomycin and (ceftriaxone or gentamicin)
	• Prosthetic valve endocarditis: Vancomycin and gentamicin and rifampin
	• Any potential implanted nidus, such as a central venous catheter or an implanted cardiac device, should be removed during treatment.
	• Consider valve repair or replacement (see Surgical considerations below)
	• If the infectious agent is a *Streptococcus bovis* biotype (e.g., *S. gallolyticus* or *S. infantarius*), the patient needs to be evaluated for colon cancer.

CASE 7 | Subacute Bacterial Endocarditis *(continued)*

Discussion	**Prophylaxis:** Antimicrobial prophylaxis (amoxicillin) for patients who have a high-risk cardiac condition (prosthetic material or prior endocarditis) and a planned high-risk procedure for transient bacteremia (dental procedure leading to bleeding, infected skin/SQ tissue procedure, or respiratory procedure with biopsy or surgery all of which can cause transient bacteremia).
Additional Considerations	**Complications:** Six-month mortality is 27%. Eventual need for valve surgery is ~50% • Cardiac complications include: CHF (most common cause of mortality and most common indication for surgery), perivalvular abscess (can progress to heart block), pericarditis, and intracardiac fistula • Septic emboli: Can occur in any part of the circulatory system and can cause metastatic abscesses • Neurologic: Brain abscess, stroke, meningitis • Musculoskeletal: Vertebral osteomyelitis, septic arthritis **Surgical Considerations:** A valve repair or replacement may be needed if the damage is causing significant complications such as: Refractory CHF due to valve dysfunction, multiple emboli, annular or aortic abscess, heart block and left-sided endocarditis due to *S. aureus* or infection that is difficult to treat due to resistance to cidal antibiotics or persistent bacteremia ≥5 days **Pediatric Considerations:** Highest risk factor for IE in pediatric cases is congenital heart disease, especially cyanotic heart disease

FEVER AND BONE/JOINT INFECTIONS

Fever and arthritis:

- Can be infectious or noninfectious
- Can involve one joint (monoarticular) or multiple joints (polyarticular)
- Can be acute or chronic
- Arthrocentesis and synovial fluid analysis are needed to determine etiology

The most urgent and important monoarticular diagnosis to make is septic arthritis (acute bacterial arthritis). Bacterial septic arthritis is both joint threatening and potentially life-threatening, and can be mimicked by noninfectious causes such as gout. Of note, up to 40% of patients with septic arthritis lack fever. Arthrocentesis and synovial fluid analysis are the primary means of discerning the etiology of a joint with arthritis.

The following are some of the key diagnoses.

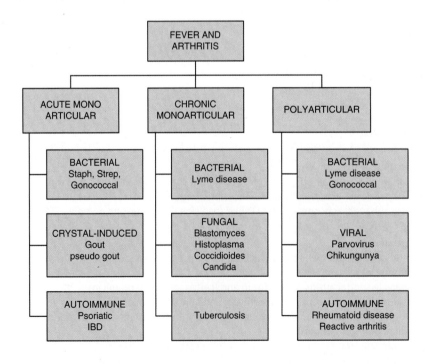

Differential Diagnosis for Arthritis Based on Arthrocentesis and Synovial Fluid Analysis

Measure	Normal	Inflammatory (e.g., Gout)	Septic (Bacterial)
Color	Clear/Transparent	Yellow/Opaque	Yellow/Opaque
WBC	<200	>2000	>50,000
PMNs (%)	<25%	>50%	>75%
Culture	Negative	Negative	Positive
Crystals	Negative	Positive (uric acid, calcium pyrophosphate)	Negative

Key Differential Diagnoses for Fever and Arthritis

Key Features and Associated Symptom(s) and Sign(s)	Diagnoses
Multiple, symmetric small joint arthritis	Rheumatoid arthritis
Metabolic syndrome, obesity, alcohol use Arthritis of the first metatarsophalangeal (MTP) joint	Gout
Young, sexually active, monoarticular arthritis	Gonorrhea
Triad of tenosynovitis, rash (pustular/necrotic), polyarthralgia	Disseminated gonococcal infection
Recent diarrheal illness or STI	Reactive arthritis (e.g., *Campylobacter* or *Chlamydia*)
Exposure to sick child Lacy, reticular rash New onset of anemia	Parvovirus
Undomiciled, incarcerated, travel to endemic area	Tuberculosis
IVDU New regurgitant heart murmur	Septic arthritis secondary to endocarditis (*Staphylococcus aureus* most common), *Candida albicans*, *Pseudomonas*
Prosthetic joint	*S. aureus*, other gram positives (e.g., *Propionibacterium acnes*, coagulase-negative staphylococci such as *S. epidermidis*) as well as gram negatives if the infection occurs postoperatively
History of erythema migrans ("bulls-eye" rash) Northeast US, Wisconsin, California and tick exposure	Lyme disease (*Borrelia burgdorferi*)
Southwestern US, Northern Mexico	Coccidioidomycosis
Mississippi or Ohio River valley	Histoplasmosis or Blastomycosis
Caribbean countries, mosquito bite	Tropical diseases such as chikungunya, dengue virus, Zika virus

CASE 8 | Septic Arthritis (*Staphylococcus aureus*)

A 62-year-old man with gouty arthritis and type 2 diabetes presents with right knee pain, swelling, redness, and difficulty walking for 2 days. His previous episodes of gout were localized to his left big toe. He is sexually active with his wife and has no history of IVDU. On exam, he has a temperature of 38.5°C, pulse 110/min, respiratory rate of 18/min, and blood pressure 128/78 mmHg. His right knee is edematous, warm, erythematous, and he has restricted active and passive range of motion.

Conditions with Similar Presentations	Acute monoarticular arthritis can be due to infection (bacterial, fungal), crystal deposition (gout, CPPD), immune mediated (psoriatic arthritis, SLE, reactive arthritis) or trauma.
Initial Diagnostic Test	Obtain synovial fluid for evaluation
Next Steps in Management	Initiate empiric antibiotics if synovial fluid consistent with infection

CASE 8 | Septic Arthritis (*Staphylococcus aureus*) *(continued)*

Discussion	Septic arthritis is defined as infection of one or more joints. Infection of the joint is most commonly due to hematogenous spread but also can occur from direct inoculation or contiguous spread of nearby skin infection. *S. aureus* is most common. Gram-negative infection (e.g., gonococcus), fungi, and atypical organisms are less common.
	History: Risk factors include older age, IV drug use, immunosuppression, prosthetic joint, underlying joint damage, and diabetes.
	Symptoms: Warm, painful, and erythematous joint.
	Physical Exam:
	• Fever usually is present. Evaluate range of motion and for signs of inflammation in affected joint.
	• Assess for cellulitis, abscesses, or signs of infective endocarditis as potential sources of hematogenous or contiguous spread to the affected joint.
	Diagnostics:
	• Obtain synovial fluid for evaluation (cell count and differential, Gram stain and culture, and polarizing microscopy) to confirm diagnosis and help rule out other causes.
	• For our patient, fluid showed gram-positive cocci in clusters on initial Gram stain consistent with **S. aureus**.
	Other studies to obtain:
	• Blood cultures (×2).
	• Complete blood count (CBC) with differential (WBC may be elevated).
	• C-reactive protein (CRP), and erythrocyte sedimentation rate (ESR) to monitor therapy (initially elevated).
	• Comprehensive metabolic panel (CMP) to assess for end-organ damage and assist with choice of antibiotics/dosing.
	• Imaging: X-ray can be obtained as baseline assessment of joint damage. Magnetic resonance imaging (MRI) used only if osteomyelitis suspected. Imaging does not differentiate septic arthritis from other causes of inflammatory arthritis.
	• Consider: PCR of synovial fluid and serology for suspected Lyme disease, PCR for tuberculosis, gonococcus, or chlamydia if standard culture is unrevealing.
	Management:
	• The affected joint should be aspirated until dry, and repeat aspirations should occur if effusion recurs.
	• Vancomycin is commonly used for empiric therapy in those with gram-positive cocci on Gram stain, then de-escalated if organism is MSSA.

Fever and Joint Pain Mini-Cases

Cases	Key Findings
Disseminated Gonococcal Infection	**Hx:** Fever, tenosynovitis, dermatitis, polyarthralgia, sexually active.
	Over 90% are women, and it has a predilection to occur during menses.
	PE: Warmth and erythema of affected joint(s).
	• Pustules on the hands and feet
	• Pain with flexion of fingers, tenderness over flexor tendons
	Diagnostics:
	• Positive blood culture or synovial fluid culture confirms the diagnosis and urine nucleic acid amplification test (NAAT) supports it.
	• Arthrocentesis: neutrophilia of synovial fluid, gram-negative intracellular diplococci
	• Blood cultures or synovial fluid cultures growing *Neisseria gonorrhoeae* confirm the diagnosis
	• Pustule culture (<30% yield)
	Management: Ceftriaxone and drainage of the septic joint.

Fever and Joint Pain Mini-Cases (*continued*)

Disseminated Gonococcal Infection	**Discussion:** Disseminated gonococcal infection (DGI) presents as either a monoarticular purulent arthritis or with the triad of tenosynovitis (pain/inflammation at insertion sites), dermatitis, and polyarthralgia in a sexually active patient. The causative pathogen is *N. gonorrhoeae*, a gram-negative diplococcus that is often found intracellularly inside neutrophils. In addition to disseminated gonococcal infection and septic arthritis, infection with *N. gonorrhoeae* can cause urethritis, neonatal conjunctivitis, pelvic inflammatory disease, and Fitz-Hugh-Curtis syndrome.
Osteomyelitis	**Hx:** Risk factors: Diabetes, IVDU, surgery, peripheral vascular disease. **PE:** Tenderness in affected site, erythema, possible ulcer or sinus tract. **Diagnostics:** • X-ray (may not show anything for first 7–14 days) • MRI can show elevation of the periosteum ("Codman's triangle") and bone edema • Elevated CRP/ESR and leukocytosis • Bone biopsy will provide definitive diagnosis • Bone culture is necessary to identify specific pathogens and guide therapy **Management:** • Antibiotics directed at bone culture results. Do not rely on superficial cultures. • Surgical debridement required to remove necrotic tissue. **Discussion:** *S. aureus* is the most common organism causing osteomyelitis. Consider *S. aureus* or *Pseudomonas aeruginosa* if there is a history of IV drug use, Salmonella if the person has sickle cell disease, *Pseudomonas* if there is a puncture wound involving the foot, and polymicrobial infection if the patient has diabetes. In adults, osteomyelitis usually develops from contiguous seeding of the bone by nearby tissue, while in children it more often develops from hematogenous seeding of the bone. In all age groups, penetrative trauma or contact with surgical tools are also leading causes of osteomyelitis. Osteomyelitis can be acute or chronic. • Acute osteomyelitis is usually seen in children and has been present about 2 weeks. • Chronic osteomyelitis is seen in adults and involves symptoms that persist for months or years after initial infection, such as draining sinus tracts or ulcers. It is often caused by *S. aureus*, *P. aeruginosa*, and Enterobacteriaceae.

FEVER AND SORE THROAT

Fever with acute-onset sore throat most commonly is viral in etiology but can also be caused by bacterial pathogens.

The viruses commonly causing pharyngitis and their characteristics are given below.

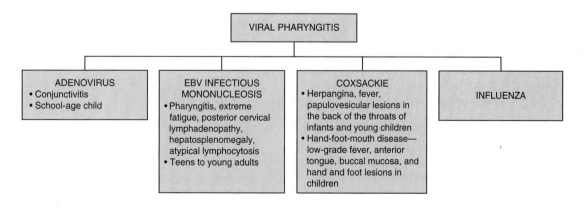

The various bacteria commonly causing pharyngitis and their characteristics are given below.

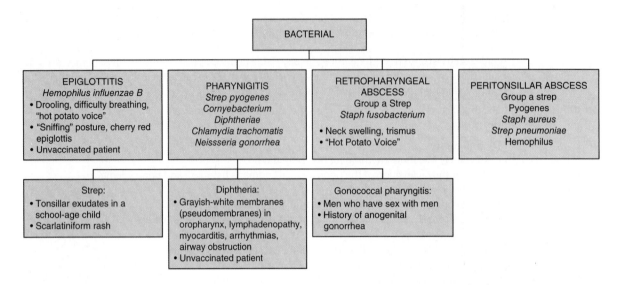

CASE 9	Streptococcal Pharyngitis

A 29-year-old school teacher presents to clinic for evaluation of fever and sore throat for 2 days. He has no cough, rhinorrhea, or nasal congestion. His temperature is 38.7°C, blood pressure is 110/70 mmHg, pulse is 90 bpm, and respiratory rate is 18/min. On physical exam, there are erythematous and swollen tonsils covered in exudates.

Conditions with Similar Presentations	**Adenovirus:** Can cause fever and sore throat. Conjunctivitis is common and does not occur with strep. **Diphtheria:** Would be uncommon in someone who is up to date on their immunizations, and grayish-white exudates would be visible in the posterior oropharynx. **Peritonsillar abscess:** Is a deeper infection of the head and neck and would present with a "hot potato" voice along with swelling noted in lateral wall of the oropharynx on the affected side. Usually, the pain is more severe on one side of the neck than the other, often with referred pain to the ipsilateral ear. The most common causal organism isolated from the abscesses is *Streptococcus pyogenes*.
Initial Diagnostic Tests	• Rapid streptococcal antigen test if Centor score >2 • Confirm negative rapid test with a throat culture
Next Steps in Management	Penicillin or amoxicillin

Discussion	Streptococcal pharyngitis presents as rapid onset of throat pain and a high fever (often greater than 38.3°C). Antibiotic treatment is instituted to prevent noninfectious sequelae, principally rheumatic heart disease and glomerulonephritis. *S. pyogenes* bacteria infect the tonsils and forms pyogenic exudates.
	
	History: Most common in children ages 6–12. Fever, sore throat with lack of cough, rhinorrhea, or nasal congestion.
	
	Physical Exam: Tonsillar exudates, tender anterior lymphadenopathy
	
	Diagnostics:
	• Rapid streptococcal antigen test
	  • If positive treat
	  • If negative obtain culture because antigen testing is only 80% sensitive
	• **Centor criteria** (presence of tonsillar exudates, fever, and tender anterior cervical lymphadenopathy along with the absence of cough) are used to determine the likelihood of streptococcal pharyngitis and whether testing is indicated
	
	Management:
	• Penicillin (PCN) or amoxicillin
	• If PCN allergy, use clindamycin

CASE 9 | Streptococcal Pharyngitis *(continued)*

Additional Considerations	**Pediatric Considerations:** Centor criteria were developed for use in adults; however, there are modified Centor criteria that can be used in children that take patient age into consideration. **Surgical Considerations:** • Recurrent streptococcal pharyngitis may be an indication for removal of the tonsils, which can harbor Group A Streptococcus (GAS). • Recurrent infection can also lead to the formation of crypts which can harbor malodorous tonsil stones—patient may desire tonsillectomy **Complications:** See table below.

Complications of Strep Pharyngitis

Exam and Findings	Complications
Fever, chills and desquamating, sandpaper-like rash overlying the flexural areas	**Scarlet Fever:** Seen after pharyngitis with strains of *S. pyogenes* expressing erythrogenic toxin.
Migratory arthritis, erythema marginatum, subcutaneous nodules, carditis, and Sydenham chorea	**Acute rheumatic fever (ARF):** Carditis due to host antibody production to the streptococcal M protein, which shows molecular mimicry with proteins on heart valves. Incidence dramatically reduced after adequate antibiotic treatment of streptococcal pharyngitis.
Symptoms related to damage of the mitral valve (regurgitation, stenosis) due to repeated episodes of ARF	**Rheumatic heart disease (RHD):** Patients with existing valvular damage are at increased risk of progression of RHD with repeated episodes of ARF and require penicillin prophylaxis (monthly injections until the age of 40).
Edema, hypertension, and hematuria several weeks after an incident of streptococcal pharyngitis or streptococcal skin infection (impetigo)	**Post-streptococcal glomerulonephritis (PSGN):** C3 levels will be low due to activation of the complement system and formation of immune complex deposits in the glomerulus. Unlike rheumatic fever, the incidence of PSGN is *not* reduced after adequate antibiotic treatment.

Throat Pain Mini-Cases

Cases	Key Findings
Peritonsillar Abscess	**Hx:** Most common in young adults. • Fever, malaise, severe sore throat, dysphagia, odynophagia, and muffled ("hot potato") voice • Sore throat more severe on one side of the neck, sometimes with ipsilateral referred otalgia • May be associated with recurrent infectious pharyngitis, previous peritonsillar abscess **PE:** • Trismus (difficulty opening mouth), drooling, rancid breath • Unilateral swelling of the affected lateral wall of oropharynx → medially displaced tonsil + uvula displaced to the contralateral side • Cervical lymphadenopathy **Diagnostics:** • Clinical diagnosis in patient with deviated uvula + medial displacement of tonsil. • Confirmed (and differentiated from cellulitis) with pus at time of drainage • CT neck is for patients in whom there is a suspicion of extension of infection outside the peritonsillar space **Management:** • Drainage of abscess and antibiotics. • Empiric antibiotic therapy, commonly ampicillin-sulbactam, amoxicillin-clavulanate, or clindamycin. Patients with a toxic appearance should have IV vancomycin added to the regimen. • Supportive therapy (hydration, pain control) **Discussion:** Peritonsillar abscesses are the most common deep-space infections of the neck. They are polymicrobial infections and should be treated with empiric antibiotics, covering group A streptococcus, *S. aureus*, and oral/respiratory anaerobes. Complications include airway compromise due to extension of infection into deep neck, internal jugular vein thrombosis, and aspiration.

Throat Pain Mini-Cases (*continued*)

Infectious Mononucleosis (Epstein-Barr Virus)	**Hx:** Sore throat, fever, and fatigue lasting a few weeks making it difficult to keep up with daily activities. Suspect in children with three Ds—dysphagia, drooling, and distress (respiratory). **PE:** Bilateral enlarged tonsils and pharyngeal exudates, posterior cervical lymphadenopathy, splenomegaly. **Diagnostics:** • A heterophile antibody test is positive in 80% IgM capsid Ab is present in > 95% of cases caused by EBV. Additional tests: • CBC shows lymphocytosis • Peripheral blood smear will show atypical lymphocytes (CD8+ cytotoxic T lymphocytes) • Consider streptococcal antigen and HIV tests to rule out those causes **Management:** • Symptomatic and supportive care. • Avoid contact sports for one month to avoid splenic rupture • Steroids considered only if impending airway obstruction **Discussion:** Infectious mononucleosis presents with fever, exudative pharyngitis, posterior cervical lymphadenopathy, and fatigue. It is spread by saliva or respiratory secretions. Mononucleosis is most commonly caused by the Ebstein-Barr virus (EBV). Less commonly, mononucleosis can be caused by CMV, in which case the heterophile antibody test will be negative and exudates are rare. EBV is also associated with other conditions, including Burkitt lymphoma, nasopharyngeal carcinoma, and lymphoproliferative disease in transplant patients.
Epiglottitis	See Pediatrics Chapter

FEVER AND LYMPHADENOPATHY

History

In patients with fever and palpable lymphadenopathy, consider risk factors and signs and symptoms of malignancy and review infectious exposures, medications, and travel history.

Physical Exam

Enlarged lymph nodes are at least 1 cm. Painful lymphadenopathy with fever points to an infectious etiology, while painless lymphadenopathy suggests lymphoma or autoimmune causes (with the exception of tuberculosis). The texture of the lymph nodes can also suggest different etiologies:

• Firm and rubbery: may indicate lymphoma

• Fluctuance with suppuration: bacterial infection

• "Shotty" (like buckshot): viral illness

• Matted lymphadenopathy, or the feeling that the lymph nodes move together with palpation, may suggest infectious (tuberculosis) and/or malignant (lymphoma) causes.

It is useful to categorize the distribution as regional (limited to one group) or generalized (involving two or more, noncontiguous). Regional lymphadenopathy and fever often point to an obvious, infectious cause in the area of drainage but should still warrant careful exam to search for additional sites of lymphadenopathy. Generalized lymphadenopathy and fever should always initiate a workup for systemic or disseminated infections or malignancy.

Regional Lymphadenopathy and Fever

Location	Drains from	Associated Diagnoses
Submandibular	Lips and mouth, tongue, submaxillary gland	Local infection (including pharyngitis, as well as head, neck, sinuses, ears, eyes, scalp, pharynx)
Submental	Lower lip, floor of mouth, tip of tongue, buccal skin	Mononucleosis—EBV, CMV
Anterior cervical (jugular)	Tongue, tonsil, pinna, parotid	Pharyngitis

Regional Lymphadenopathy and Fever

Location	Drains from	Associated Diagnoses
Posterior cervical	Cervical and axillary nodes Scalp, neck, skin of arms/pectorals, thorax	Mononucleosis—EBV, CMV Kikuchi disease Rubella
Suboccipital	Head, scalp	Local infection
Postauricular	External auditory meatus, pinna, scalp	Rubella
Preauricular	Eyelids/conjunctiva, pinna, temporal region scalp	External otitis (no fever)
Supraclavicular node	Right: Mediastinum, lungs, esophagus Left: Thorax, abdomen	Malignancy most likely Possible infection
Axillary	Arm, thoracic wall, breast	Cat-scratch disease Brucellosis
Epitrochlear	Ulnar aspect of forearm and hand	Tularemia Secondary syphilis Sarcoidosis
Inguinal	Pelvis, genitals, lower abdominal canal, anal canal (inferior to pectinate line)	Leg/foot infections Sexually transmitted infections
Periumbilical	Intraabdominal	Malignancy

Key Differential Diagnoses for Fever and Lymphadenopathy

Fever and Lymphadenopathy with Key Associated Findings	Diagnoses
Hypercalcemia (increased vitamin D 1,25)	Lymphoma
IVDU	HIV
High-risk sexual behavior	HIV, syphilis, HSV, CMV
Night sweats	Lymphoma, TB
New medication, itching, arthralgias, malaise	Serum sickness
Chronic lung disease, bronchiectasis	Non-tuberculosis mycobacteria (e.g., *M. avium-intracellulare* [MAI])
High fever, sore throat	Infectious mononucleosis (EBV, CMV) Streptococcal pharyngitis
Ulcer at inoculation site; hunters, trappers	Tularemia, anthrax
Cat scratch or bite	Bartonella
Exposure to cats, flu-like illness, myalgia OR asymptomatic	Toxoplasmosis
Animal exposure (sheep, cattle, goats) Unpasteurized milk and cheese consumption	Brucellosis
Travel to endemic area Undomiciled, incarceration, health care worker	Tuberculosis
Eastern and Central US, Great Lakes region	Blastomycosis
Mississippi and Ohio River valleys (overlap with blastomycosis)	Histoplasmosis
Southwestern US, California and Northern Mexico	Coccidioidomycosis
Central and South America	Paracoccidioidomycosis

Fever and Lymphadenopathy with Key Associated Exam Findings	Diagnoses
Rales (crackles), especially upper lobe	TB, blastomycosis, histoplasmosis
Splenomegaly	EBV, CMV, lymphoma, disseminated TB or fungal disease
Rash	HIV, secondary syphilis, Rubella
Rash, conjunctivitis, mucositis	Kawasaki disease
Rash, conjunctivitis, cough	Measles
Skin lesion near lymphadenopathy	Cutaneous infection, skin neoplasm

HIV/AIDS AND OPPORTUNISTIC INFECTIONS

Though the differential diagnosis for fever in a patient with HIV/AIDS is broad, infection due to common pathogens is often the cause. This section, however, will focus on pathogens that are mostly seen in immunocompromised patients, known as opportunists. Given the variety of infections causing fever in patients with HIV/AIDS, it can be helpful to categorize them by type of pathogen. Alternatively, one can categorize them by body system (e.g., skin, CNS, pulmonary, disseminated).

Key Differential Diagnoses for Fever and HIV/AIDS

Fever and HIV/AIDS with Key Associated Findings	Diagnosis
Fever, diffuse lymphadenopathy, sore throat, +/- rash ("mono-like" syndrome)	Acute retroviral (HIV) infection
Demyelination, multiple white matter changes, loss of visual acuity	Progressive multifocal leukoencephalopathy (PML) due to JC virus
Headache, meningoencephalitis, increased intracranial pressure (ICP)	Cryptococcal meningitis
Focal neurological deficit, multiple well-circumscribed lesions (basal ganglia)	Central nervous system (CNS) toxoplasmosis
Cotton wool spots on fundoscopy, intraretinal hemorrhage, "ketchup-and-mustard" retina	Cytomegalovirus (CMV) retinitis
Odynophagia, oral thrush	Candida esophagitis
Cavitary lung lesion, positive TST or IGRA	Pulmonary tuberculosis
Cough, fever, hypoxemia, diffuse bilateral infiltrates on CXR or "ground glass" opacities on chest CT	Pneumocystis jirovecii pneumonia (PJP)
Hemoptysis, pleuritic chest pain, pulmonary nodules, acute angle branching septate hyphae	Invasive aspergillosis
Systemic illness, elevated transaminases, hepatosplenomegaly, residence/travel to Mississippi or Ohio River valley	Disseminated histoplasmosis
Systemic illness, skin lesions (similar appearance to squamous cell cancer), CNS disease, residence/travel to Mississippi or Ohio River valley	Disseminated blastomycosis
Systemic illness, skin lesions, CNS disease, residence/travel to southwestern US	Disseminated coccidioidomycosis
Linear ulcers on GI endoscopy, bloody stools	CMV colitis
Diarrhea, severe anemia (<10 g/dL), and fever without localizing symptoms	Disseminated *Mycobacterium avium* complex (MAC)
Diarrhea, "acid-fast" oocysts	Cryptosporidiosis, *Cystoisospora*, Cyclospora
Skin lesions and cat scratch	Bacillary angiomatosis
Rash on palms and soles, sexually active	Secondary syphilis
Painful genital ulcers, inguinal lymphadenopathy	Herpes simplex virus (HSV)
Vesicular, painful rash in different stages in a dermatomal distribution	Varicella zoster

CASE 10 | Acute HIV Infection

A 36-year-old man presents with 3 weeks of diarrhea, nausea, abdominal cramps, night sweats, and a 10-pound weight loss. He reports unprotected intercourse during the last 2 months. During the past week, he noticed a macular rash on the upper torso, and oral lesions have developed that are painful when he eats. He currently has a temperature of 100.9°F. On physical exam, he has nontender lymphadenopathy of his cervical and inguinal lymph nodes.

Conditions with Similar Presentations	**Infectious mononucleosis:** Presents with fever, exudative pharyngitis, posterior cervical lymphadenopathy, fatigue, and splenomegaly. **Secondary syphilis:** Presents with fever, lymphadenopathy, malaise, skin rash on the palms of the hands and soles of the feet, and mucous patches, condyloma lata, alopecia, and multi-organ injury.
Initial Diagnostic Tests	• HIV screening test • Viral load (HIV RNA PCR)—usually >100,000 copies/mL
Next Steps in Management	Start antiretroviral therapy (ART)
Discussion	Acute HIV infection presents 2–4 weeks following infection. HIV virus enters the body and starts to multiply rapidly, leading to viremia. Eventually, virus-specific CD8+ T lymphocytes emerge, and patients during this transient period of high viral loads are very contagious to others. Ninety percent of patients in this acute phase of HIV infection present with a vague mononucleosis-like illness that lasts from a few days to a few months. HIV screening test may still be negative as patient may not yet have seroconverted so if acute HIV infection is suspected, viral load will be the most useful test to order. **History:** Risk factors: IVDU, incarceration, unprotected intercourse, multiple sexual partners. Symptoms: Fever, lymphadenopathy, sore throat, arthralgias, headache, diarrhea, weight loss, rash. **Physical Exam:** Macular rash and oral ulcers (both lasting 1 week). **Diagnostics:** • The key is detection of HIV in plasma in patients whose symptoms precede seroconversion by either the P24 antigen assay or the HIV RNA nucleic acid amplification test (if the P24 antigen test is negative and acute HIV syndrome is suspected). • Viral load in the blood and resistance testing CD4+ T cell count **Management:** • All HIV-infected patients should be treated with lifelong ART regardless of CD4 count • Patients should be monitored for ART-associated toxicity such as dyslipidemia, glucose intolerance, cardiovascular disease, and hypertension • Immunizations (avoid live vaccines) are particularly important in patients with HIV (see table below) • Partner notification and prophylaxis such as pre-exposure prophylaxis (PrEP)
Additional Considerations	**Complications:** Opportunistic infections and malignancies (see below) **Screening:** All people over 18 should be offered screening with HIV test that looks for antibodies against HIV as well as p24 antigen and is reliable within 1 week of infection. **Prevention:** • Ensure routine immunizations are up to date in addition to below • Partner notification and prophylaxis such as PrEP • PrEP consists of antiretroviral agents designed to be used in uninfected individuals who are at high risk for HIV transmission **Obstetric considerations:** Pregnant patients should continue taking ART during pregnancy to decrease the rate of perinatal transmission **Pediatric Considerations:** Neonates born to mothers with HIV should be treated based on the mother's viral load during delivery

Antibiotic Prophylaxis against Opportunistic Infections in Patients with HIV

Opportunistic Infection	Indications	Prophylaxis
MAC	CD4 <50/mm³	If on ART, no prophylaxis If not on ART, initiate prophylaxis with macrolide
TB	Close contact with person with TB, or positive IGRA or PPD without active disease	*Isoniazid + pyridoxine 9 months or alternative regimens*
PJP	CD4 <200/mm³	Daily TMP-SMX
Toxoplasma	CD4 <100/mm³	Daily TMP-SMX

Opportunistic Infections in Patients with HIV/AIDS Mini-Cases

Cases	Key Findings
Disseminated *Mycobacterium avium* Complex (MAC)	**Hx:** Risk factors: Immunocompromised state—HIV/AIDS, not on antiretroviral medications (CD4 <50), organ transplant or neutropenic patients, patients on chronic steroids, chemotherapy, or other immunosuppressants. Symptoms: Fever, fatigue, weight loss, night sweats, watery diarrhea, crampy abdominal pain. **PE:** Febrile, lymphadenopathy, hepatosplenomegaly, abdominal tenderness. **Diagnostics:** • Sputum, stool or tissue demonstration of AFB, and isolation of the organism confirms the diagnosis. • Must rule out TB • Pancytopenia (from marrow invasion) and ↑LDH and ↑alkaline phosphatase (from liver infection) can be seen **Management:** Patients are often treated presumptively prior to culture results • Macrolides (azithromycin or clarithromycin), combined with rifampin and ethambutol, is the treatment regimen of choice, based on sensitivity • Treat underlying/precipitating immunocompromised state **Discussion:** Disseminated *Mycobacterium avium-intracellulare* complex (MAC) is an infection caused by one of two nontuberculous mycobacteria (*M. avium* or *M. intracellulare*). Mycobacteria can infect both immunocompetent and immunocompromised patients; however, disseminated disease is most seen in HIV+ patients with a CD4 count <50. In addition to disseminated disease, MAC can also cause a focal lymphadenitis. Prophylactic antibiotics were previously recommended for individuals with CD4 counts <50; however, prophylaxis is no longer recommended for those on ART because the CD4 count will rapidly rise above 50.
Secondary Syphilis	**Hx:** Risk factors: Immunocompromised patients with untreated primary syphilis. Symptoms: Fever, fatigue, headache, sore throat, rash on palms and soles. **PE:** Polymorphic rash on trunk and the palms and soles, generalized nontender lymphadenopathy, condyloma lata (painless, wart-like lesions on genitals), patchy alopecia, mucous patches (oral shallow ulcerations). **Diagnostics:** • Positive VDRL or RPR (nonspecific serologic testing) in 99% of cases. • Confirm with FTA-ABS (fluorescent treponemal antibody-absorption) (specific serologic testing) **Management:** • Penicillin G benzathine IM × 1 • If allergic, pregnant patients should be desensitized to penicillin and treated • If patients are highly allergic to penicillin, doxycycline or ceftriaxone are alternative treatments **Discussion:** Syphilis is sexually transmitted and caused by the spirochete *Treponema pallidum*. Patients may or may not recall the preceding painless chancre of primary syphilis. Secondary syphilis manifests several weeks after primary syphilis and occurs due to the systemic spread of spirochetes, inducing an immunologic reaction in the body. Manifestations of secondary syphilis include wart-like condyloma lata on the genitals, patchy hair loss, and mucosal ulcers in the mouth.

Opportunistic Infections in Patients with HIV/AIDS Mini-Cases (*continued*)

Secondary Syphilis	After starting treatment (2–24 hours) for secondary syphilis, some patients develop the **Jarisch-Herxheimer reaction**, a self-limiting immune-mediated response characterized by flu-like syndrome (fever, headache, and myalgias) caused by antigens released by the killed spirochetes. This reaction can be symptomatically treated with NSAIDs or acetaminophen.
Candidiasis (*Candida esophagitis*)	**Hx:** Risk factors: Diabetes, immunocompromised state -HIV/AIDS, not on ART (CD4 <100), organ transplant or neutropenic patients, patients on chronic steroids, chemotherapy, or other immunosuppressants. Symptoms: Dysphagia, odynophagia, retrosternal pain. **PE:** White, scrapeable plaques/pseudomembranes with a red base in the mouth or throat, extending to the esophagus (visualized on endoscopy). **Diagnostics:** Clinical diagnosis • Confirm with KOH stain (characteristic filamentous yeast with pseudohyphae) **Management:** • Fluconazole for 14–21 days. • Systemic therapy with an azole is required for esophagitis. • Mild oral *Candida* infections can be treated with topical medications like clotrimazole and nystatin. **Discussion:** *Candida* esophagitis is an AIDS-defining illness and is caused by the opportunistic fungus *Candida albicans*. *Candida* is a dimorphic fungus that forms pseudohyphae and budding yeasts and is present normally in low numbers on the skin, in the oral cavity, and in gastrointestinal and genitourinary tracts. It causes only minor infections in immunocompetent patients, such as diaper rash or, vulvovaginitis. In immunocompromised patients, *Candida* can cause oral thrush (mouth and throat), esophagitis, or disseminated disease that may affect any organ system and can lead to sepsis. It is also a common cause of fungemia in the blood of patients with intravascular catheters and can cause endocarditis in a person who injects drugs.
Cryptococcal Meningitis	**Hx:** Subacute onset of headache, altered mental status, seizures, neurological deficits due to increased intracranial pressure as disease progresses. **PE:** Fever, altered mental status, focal neurological deficits, fundoscopic exam with papilledema (sign of increased intracranial pressure). In disseminated disease, may have skin findings (abscess or skin nodules) and/or exam consistent with pneumonia. **Diagnostics:** • LP with CSF analysis (<50 WBCs, high protein, low to normal glucose, high opening pressure) • Positive India Ink preparation of the CSF (stains round encapsulated yeast, but low sensitivity) • Positive CSF cryptococcal antigen test (very sensitive and specific) **Management:** • Amphotericin B in combination with 5-flucytosine. • Treat underlying immunosuppression • Address elevated intracranial pressure by repeated LPs **Discussion:** Cryptococcal meningoencephalitis is an opportunistic infection of the CNS caused by *Cryptococcus neoformans*. *Cryptococcus* is found in soil and pigeon droppings and can be acquired via inhalation. After inhalation, it can enter the bloodstream and spread to the meninges and brain. Individuals with cryptococcus meningitis who receive antifungal treatment still have a high mortality. In addition to meningoencephalitis, immunocompromised patients may also present with **pulmonary cryptococcosis**. **Cutaneous cryptococcus** presents as a single, chronic, non-healing ulcer or abscess without signs of infection. Skin biopsy is needed given generalized appearance of lesion. Cutaneous cryptococcus can appear like acne, cutaneous syphilis, molluscum contagiosum, or basal cell carcinoma. Ruling out disseminated disease is most important before treating.

Opportunistic Infections in Patients with HIV/AIDS Mini-Cases (*continued*)

Cytomegalovirus (CMV)	**Hx/PE:** Patient with HIV and CD4 <50 cells/mm³, can have reactivation of CMV. Infection can be severe, disseminated disease and often can affect the gastrointestinal tract, retina, liver, lung, and brain. *Gastrointestinal*—most common • Colitis (diarrhea, hematochezia, abdominal pain, weight loss) • Esophagitis (odynophagia with linear ulcerations) *CMV retinitis*—most concerning due to possible blindness • Floaters and photopsia (flashing lights) high predictor of CMV retinitis, blurring/loss of central vision • Painless (unlike HSV), initially unilateral but can progress to bilateral involvement • Can progress to retinal detachment and blindness *Other manifestations*—pulmonary (pneumonitis, interstitial pneumonia) and/or neurologic (encephalitis, myelitis, radiculomyelopathy, peripheral neuropathy) involvement. **Diagnostics:** • GI involvement—endoscopy/colonoscopy would reveal linear ulcerations; biopsy and histopathology would confirm diagnosis ("owl's eye" inclusions) • Retinitis—fundoscopy showing retinal hemorrhage (cotton wool spots, "pizza pie" retinopathy) • PCR of plasma or whole blood or vitreous/aqueous fluid can be done • Serology is not useful for diagnosis because this is a reactivation, not an initial infection **Management:** • Ganciclovir, foscarnet, or cidofovir • Management of underlying HIV **Discussion:** Seroprevalence of CMV is approximately 80% of the world's population. In immunocompetent patients, most are asymptomatic infections or have mononucleosis-type symptoms. Other patients at risk for the above serious complications of disseminated CMV disease include organ transplant recipients (especially within the first 100 days).

FEVER AND NIGHT SWEATS

- Night sweats are significant if they are drenching sweats requiring changing of clothes
- History and exam should guide the laboratory and imaging evaluation

Generally, hold antipyretics to monitor the fever curve except if high fevers, cardiopulmonary conditions, pregnant patients, or if the patient desires symptomatic relief.

Key Differential Diagnoses for Fever and Night Sweats

Fever and Night Sweats with Key Associated Findings	Diagnoses
Travel to an endemic region Undomiciled, incarceration, health care worker Lung exam with rales (crackles), especially upper lobe	Tuberculosis
Sexually active, IVDU	Acute HIV infection
Lymphadenopathy	Lymphoma, TB, acute HIV
Valvular heart disease, history of rheumatic fever Poor dentition, new or changing heart murmur, Janeway lesions, Osler nodes, splinter hemorrhages, Roth spots, conjunctival petechiae	Subacute bacterial endocarditis
Chronic lung disease, bronchiectasis	Non-tuberculosis mycobacteria such as *M. avium-intracellulare* (MAI)
HIV/AIDS and other immunocompromised hosts	TB, disseminated MAI, disseminated histoplasmosis, or non-Hodgkin lymphoma
Hypercalcemia (increased vitamin D 1,25)	Lymphoma

Key Differential Diagnoses for Fever and Night Sweats

Fever and Night Sweats with Key Associated Findings	Diagnoses
Animal exposure (sheep, cattle, goats) Unpasteurized milk and cheese consumption	Brucellosis Brucella (rare cause of endocarditis)
Eastern and central US, Great Lakes region Rales (crackles), especially upper lobe	Blastomycosis
Mississippi and Ohio River valleys	Histoplasmosis and blastomycosis
Southwestern US, California and Northern Mexico	Coccidioidomycosis
Central and South America	Paracoccidioidomycosis
Wheezing, skin flushing	Carcinoid syndrome
Severe hypertension	Pheochromocytoma
Exophthalmos, hair thinning, tremor, pretibial myxedema	Hyperthyroidism (Graves' disease)
Splenomegaly	Lymphoma, disseminated TB or fungal disease

CASE 11 | Fever of Unknown Origin (FUO)

A 37-year-old man with no significant past medical history presents for follow-up of intermittent fevers to ~38.6°C for the past 2 months. He does not endorse any symptoms other than generalized malaise and night sweats. He does not take any medications and reports no recent travel, sick contacts, known tick bites or animal exposures, or consumption of raw or unpasteurized meats. Physical exam is unremarkable except for fever of 38.4°C.

Conditions with Similar Presentations	Differential diagnosis of FUO includes: Infections, inflammatory conditions, malignancy, drugs, subacute thyroiditis, serum sickness, and hemolytic anemia.
Initial Diagnostic Tests	• Clinical diagnosis: See definition below • Perform detailed and thorough history and physical exam • Initial tests to check: CBC, CMP, TSH, ESR/CRP, HIV, UA, CXR • Ensure routine screening tests are up to date
Next Steps in Management	• Avoid empiric antibiotics unless hemodynamically unstable • Discontinue medications that can cause drug fever
Discussion	FUO is defined as fever >38.3°C (101°F) >3 weeks with unknown diagnosis after ≥3 visits or 3 days of hospitalization. FUO can be caused by infections, noninfectious inflammatory diseases, malignancy, drug fever, and other miscellaneous causes (subacute thyroiditis, familial fever syndromes, factitious fever). **History:** Review fever pattern and explore past medical history, surgical history, family history, thorough review of systems. • Social history should assess for sick contacts, travel history, occupational exposures, tick or animal exposures, consumption of contaminated food or water, sexual history, intravenous drug use, and incarceration • Review all medications to assess for conditions such as drug fever • Enquire about risk factors for malignancy, HIV, autoimmunity, or foreign body infection which may cause fever **Physical Exam:** General evaluation of any mental status changes, cachexia, wasting, skin changes, or local or general lymphadenopathy. • Thorough examination of oropharyngeal cavity (sinuses, eyes, nose, oral cavity), thyroid, and carotids • Note any relative bradycardia and carefully assess for signs of endocarditis • Assess lungs for consolidation or effusion • Assess for hepatomegaly, splenomegaly, or signs of abdominal tenderness • Assess all joints for erythema, warmth, tenderness, and range of motion • Assess extremities for clubbing, rashes, or signs of endocarditis or DVT • Examine rectum for perirectal fluctuance or a boggy prostate • Assess via GU/pelvic presence of genital lesions

CASE 11 | Fever of Unknown Origin (FUO) (continued)

Discussion	**Diagnostics:**
	Diagnostic workup should be broad: check initial/baseline tests as above
	If initial tests are nondiagnostic, consider:
	• Blood and urine cultures, drug screen
	• Computer tomography (CT) of chest and abdomen, echocardiography, and positron emission tomography
	• Can also consider checking: Cryoglobulins, complement studies, thyroid function tests, antinuclear antibodies, immunoglobulins, and lymphocyte phenotyping for immunodeficiencies, antibody titers to known vaccinations, neutrophil function testing
	Management:
	• Empiric therapy should be avoided if possible, as antibiotics and corticosteroids may mask fever patterns.
	• Empiric therapy with glucocorticoids should be considered if there is a high suspicion of temporal arteritis, and with antibiotics if there is a high suspicion of leptospirosis, CNS tuberculosis or endocarditis.
	• Management is based on etiology once it is detected.

CASE 12 | Febrile Neutropenia

A 67-year-old woman with recently diagnosed acute myeloid leukemia presents with new-onset fever, chills, and night sweats. She received her first cycle of chemotherapy 8 days ago. On physical exam, she appears ill, and has a temperature 38.9°C, pulse of 110/min, respiratory rate of 14/min, blood pressure of 100/65 mmHg, and SpO_2 98% on room air. The rest of the exam is unremarkable. Labs 2 days ago were significant for an absolute neutrophil count (ANC) of 400 cells/mm³.

Conditions with Similar Presentations	Fever in a neutropenic patient should always be assumed to be from an infectious disease even though it less commonly is due to drug fever, cytolosis from chemotherapy, or the malignancy being treated.
Initial Diagnostic Tests	• Clinical diagnosis: See definition below • Obtain CBC, CMP, UA and urine culture, two sets of blood cultures and CXR
Next Steps in Management	Start immediate empiric broad-spectrum antibiotics directed at gram-negative aerobic bacilli including *Pseudomonas aeruginosa* (within 1 hour of presentation)
Discussion	Febrile neutropenia is defined as a single fever >38.3°C (101°F) or a sustained elevated temperature >38°C (100.4°F) in a patient with a current or anticipated **ANC <500 cells/mm³**. Febrile neutropenia most commonly presents in patients receiving cytotoxic chemotherapy. Lack of WBCs contributes to lack of an inflammatory response at sites of infection, so patients with febrile neutropenia may not have any localizing symptoms.
	History: History should thoroughly evaluate type and timing of chemotherapy, other immunosuppressive medications, comorbidities, prior latent infections that may reactivate, new exposures, sick contacts, and recent blood transfusions.
	Physical Exam: A thorough physical exam should be performed, including careful assessment of the skin, vascular access sites, oropharynx, lungs, and the GI tract.
	Diagnostics:
	• All patients should be evaluated with CBC with differential, serum creatinine and blood urea nitrogen, electrolytes, liver transaminases, and total bilirubin
	• Two sets of blood cultures should be collected, including culture from peripheral line and any indwelling catheter
	• Urinalysis and urine culture
	• Chest x-ray should be performed
	Management: Patients are classified as either high risk or low risk, which determines empiric antibiotic regimen, treatment setting, and antibiotic duration.
	Low-risk patients—Those with anticipated brief neutropenic periods (≤7 days) and few comorbidities.
	• Oral ciprofloxacin AND oral amoxicillin clavulanate.
	• Can be managed in the outpatient setting if patient is stable after receiving first dose of antibiotics and can easily return to clinic.

CASE 12 | Febrile Neutropenia *(continued)*

Discussion	*High-risk patients*—Those with anticipated prolonged (>7 days) and severe neutropenia (ANC ≤100 cells/mm³) OR significant medical comorbid conditions (hypotension, pneumonia, new abdominal pain, or neurologic changes). • Should be managed inpatient with IV cefepime OR piperacillin/tazobactam OR antipseudomonal carbapenem (imipenem, meropenem). • Vancomycin added to regimen if patient is hemodynamically unstable or has multiorgan failure, pneumonia, suspected line sepsis, skin or soft tissue infection, mucositis, or known colonization with MRSA. • Should add empiric antifungal therapy with caspofungin if patient has a persistent fever with 4–7 days of broad-spectrum antibiotics with no identified source or high suspicion of fungal infection. • Modify initial empiric regimen based on clinical and microbiologic evidence.
Additional Considerations	**Prophylaxis:** In patients deemed to have ≥ 20% risk of febrile neutropenia, should give fluoroquinolone and colony-stimlulating factor prophylaxis.

DYSURIA

Dysuria (broadly defined as burning, tingling, pain, and/or discomfort associated with voiding) is a very common presenting symptom, particularly in the outpatient setting. Refer to Chapters 12 (Nephrology) and 14 (Obstetrics and Gynecology) for additional cases.

Dysuria can be due to infectious or noninfectious causes, as listed below.

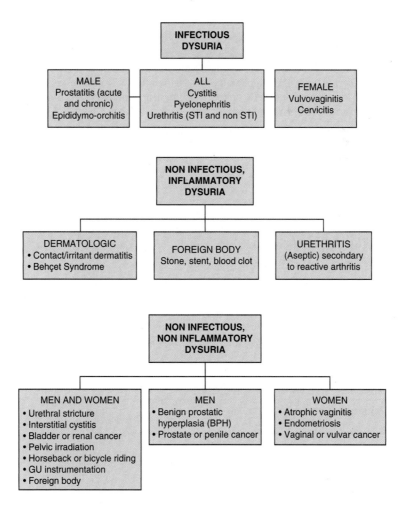

Key Differential Diagnoses for Dysuria

Dysuria with Key Associated Findings	Diagnosis
Urinary urgency, increased frequency, possible suprapubic pain and tenderness on exam	Cystitis
Urinary urgency, increased frequency, fever and flank pain and costovertebral angle (CVAT) tenderness	Pyelonephritis
Fever, myalgias, "tip of penis" pain and an enlarged, tender prostate	Acute prostatitis
Dribbling, decreased stream, hesitancy, urinary incontinence and an enlarged, nontender prostate	Benign prostatic hyperplasia (BPH)
Testicular pain, possible scrotal swelling and tenderness	Epididymo-orchitis
Vulvovaginal dryness, dyspareunia (pain with sexual intercourse) and vaginal atrophy	Atrophic vaginitis, UTI
Vaginal discharge	Vulvovaginitis
Purulent discharge from cervix	Cervicitis
Urethral discharge	Urethritis (associated with STI)
Urethritis (aseptic), arthritis and enthesitis, following an enteric infection	Urethritis secondary to reactive arthritis
Prior treatment with cyclophosphamide	Interstitial cystitis
Oral and genital ulcers, uveitis	Behçet syndrome
Perineal rash or irritation	Contact/irritant dermatitis

CASE 13 | Lower Urinary Tract Infection (Acute Cystitis)

A 25-year-old woman presents with dysuria and urinary frequency for the past 2 days. No fevers, chills, nausea, vomiting, flank pain, vaginal discharge, or irritation are reported. The patient has a temperature is 37.3°C, pulse of 86/min, respiratory rate of 14/min, blood pressure is 109/70 mmHg, and SpO_2 99% on room air. Physical exam is remarkable for mild suprapubic tenderness without rebound or guarding. No costovertebral tenderness.

Conditions with Similar Presentations	**Female:** **Acute urethritis:** Due to an STI presenting with dysuria and urinary frequency. Will have pyuria without bacteriuria. **Vulvovaginitis:** May present with dysuria but without urinary frequency. Presence of discharge, odor, pruritus, and dyspareunia. **Pelvic inflammatory disease:** May have dysuria with fever and lower abdominal/pelvic pain but exam findings include mucopurulent endocervical discharge and/or cervical motion tenderness. **Painful bladder syndrome:** Diagnosis of exclusion in a patient with dysuria and frequency after infection or other causes have been ruled out. **Male:** **Acute urethritis:** Must consider in sexually active men presenting with dysuria and urinary frequency. Exam may show penile ulcerations and/or urethral discharge. **Acute prostatitis:** May present with dysuria, urinary frequency, urgency but also have fever, chills, malaise, myalgias, pelvic or perianal pain, or obstructive symptoms (hesitancy, dribbling) and exquisitely tender prostate.
Initial Diagnostic Tests	• Clinical diagnosis • Can confirm with urinalysis/urine culture
Next Steps in Management	• Empiric treatment with antibiotics (see below)

CASE 13 | Lower Urinary Tract Infection (Acute Cystitis) *(continued)*

Discussion	Urinary tract infection (UTI) is an infection of the lower (cystitis) or upper (pyelonephritis) urinary tract. Lower urinary tract infections are further categorized as uncomplicated or complicated. A complicated UTI is defined as an infection in a patient with increased risk for failing treatment or for complications. This includes a UTI in patients with functional and structural abnormalities of the urinary tract. It also includes patients with diabetes, immunosuppression, prior resistant organism infection, and all males. *E. coli* is the most common cause of cystitis. Other microbial causes include other *Enterobacteriaceae* (*Klebsiella pneumoniae, Proteus mirabilis*) and *Staphylococcus saprophyticus*. UTIs are more common among females due to the shorter length of the urethra.
	History: Risk factors include sexual intercourse, spermicide use, new sexual partner, and history of UTIs.
	Symptoms: Dysuria, urgency and frequency, without vaginal discharge or irritation are highly suggestive of acute cystitis.
	• Except for children, patients with uncomplicated cystitis tend to present without fever or other systemic symptoms
	• Symptoms in patients with complicated UTI vary greatly in severity, but they are more likely to develop systemic symptoms
	• Presentation may be subtle or atypical in elderly, immunocompromised, catheterized, obstructed, or neurologically impaired patients
	Physical Exam:
	• Patients with uncomplicated cystitis may exhibit suprapubic or pelvic tenderness on physical exam.
	• Fever, signs of sepsis or systemic toxicity are more likely to be present in complicated UTI (complicated cystitis or pyelonephritis)
	• Flank pain and costovertebral(CVA) tenderness indicates infection of the upper urinary tract (pyelonephritis)
	Diagnostics:
	• Acute uncomplicated cystitis: Clinical diagnosis in patients with characteristic symptoms (dysuria, frequency, urgency) and no vaginal discharge or irritation.
	• Can confirm diagnosis with a positive UA or urine dipstick. Urine culture is sent if antibiotic resistance is suspected.
	• If there is a chance that patient may be pregnant, send a urine pregnancy test, as management of UTI is different in the pregnant patient
	Management:
	• Patients with acute uncomplicated cystitis and normal renal function may receive empiric treatment with either oral nitrofurantoin for 5 days OR trimethoprim/sulfamethoxazole for 3 days OR fosfomycin for a single dose.
	• Treatment with trimethoprim/sulfamethoxazole should not be used if resistance of *E. coli* is >20% in the community.
Additional Considerations	**Complications:** Complications of UTI include bacteremia or sepsis, renal and perinephric abscess (complication of pyelonephritis), acute kidney injury, and emphysematous pyelonephritis or emphysematous cystitis.
	Screening: Pregnant women should be screened for **asymptomatic bacteriuria** in early pregnancy with urine culture and treated if positive, as treatment may reduce the risk of pyelonephritis, preterm labor, and low birth weight. Patients having endoscopic urologic procedures with mucosal trauma should also be screened, and if positive, treated for bacteriuria.
	Asymptomatic bacteriuria is diagnosed when culture demonstrates $\geq 10^5$ colony-forming (CF) units/mL of single bacterial species from two consecutive voided urine specimens in asymptomatic women, one specimen in men, or $\geq 10^2$ CF units/mL of a single bacterial species from any single catheterized specimen.
	Complicated urinary tract infection (UTI): Defined as an infection of the upper or lower urinary tract in a patient who is at an increased risk of failing treatment or developing complications. Diagnosed when culture demonstrates $\geq 10^5$ CF units/mL of single bacterial species. Mild to moderately ill patients may receive fluoroquinolones (ciprofloxacin, levofloxacin) if resistance is <10% and no complications. Severely ill patients or those at risk for fluoroquinolone-resistant organisms should receive IV cefepime OR IV ceftazidime OR IV piperacillin-tazobactam OR meropenem IV.
	Catheter-associated urinary tract infection (CAUTI): The approach to antibiotic treatment is the same as for complicated UTI. Prior to antibiotic therapy, catheter should be removed or replaced and urine culture should be obtained to guide therapy.

242   CHAPTER 7   INFECTIOUS DISEASES

CASE 13 | Lower Urinary Tract Infection (Acute Cystitis) (continued)

Additional Considerations	**Pediatric Considerations:**
	Children <2 weeks old: Presents with temperature instability, hypothermia, and tachypnea.
	Patients <3 months old: First presenting sign of UTI may be fever. Should be evaluated for other serious occult bacterial infection including UTI, if temperature is ≥38°C.
	Children >3 years old present with classic symptoms of dysuria, urinary frequency, and urgency.
	Children 3–36 months with an unexplained temperature ≥39°C should be evaluated for a UTI.
	• Urinalysis and culture should be performed in all children presenting with symptoms of a UTI or unexplained fever.
	• Imaging in Pediatrics: Perform renal and bladder ultrasound (RBUS) to rule out obstruction of the urinary tract in infants <24 months with a febrile UTI or in children with a complicated UTI. Voiding cystourethrography (VCUG) should be performed following first febrile UTI if there are abnormal findings on RBUS, findings suggestive of high-grade vesicoureteral reflux or obstructive uropathy, or other complex clinical circumstances. VCUG should be performed in all children <2 years following a second febrile UTI.

CASE 14 | Acute Pyelonephritis

A 35-year-old woman presents with a 1-day history of fever, flank pain, nausea, and several episodes of vomiting. Three days prior to the above symptoms, she began to have dysuria, increased urinary frequency, and urgency. On exam, the patient is acutely ill and has chills. Her vitals are temperature 39.0°C, pulse 104/min, respirations 14/min, and blood pressure 108/72 mmHg. Her abdominal exam is notable for suprapubic tenderness and she has left CVA tenderness. Her pelvic exam is normal.

Conditions with Similar Presentations	**Cystitis:** Symptoms of dysuria, frequency, and urgency are consistent with lower tract UTI, but the presence of flank pain, back pain, CVA tenderness, high fever (≥39.0°C), chills, and nausea make pyelonephritis (an upper tract UTI) more likely.
	Pelvic inflammatory disease (PID): Usually also have vaginal discharge and cervical motion tenderness on exam.
	Kidney stones: Potential diagnosis if antecedent colicky pain radiating to the groin, hematuria, or history of stones are present.
	For men, consider **prostatitis** if recurrent UTI or pelvic/perineal pain in the setting of pyelonephritis.
Initial Diagnostic Tests	• Obtain urinalysis, urine culture and sensitivity • CBC, BMP and blood cultures in hospitalized patients
Next Steps in Management	• Patients with severe symptoms and signs should be hospitalized and treated with IV antibiotics and supportive care • Milder cases can be treated with a fluoroquinolone as an outpatient
Discussion	Acute pyelonephritis is a bacterial infection of the renal parenchyma. Bacteria usually ascend from the lower urinary tract but may also reach the kidney via the bloodstream. Common pathogens include *Escherichia coli* followed by *Klebsiella pneumoniae*, *Enterococcus* spp. and other gram-negative rods. Hematogenous pyelonephritis may be due to *S. aureus*. Acute pyelonephritis is much more common in females than in males because the shorter urethra in women facilitates colonization by fecal flora such as *E. coli*. Uncomplicated pyelonephritis occurs in healthy people and women who are not pregnant; otherwise, the infection is considered complicated and will have a more severe course.
	History: Dysuria, frequency and urgency, fever, chills, nausea/vomiting.
	Physical Exam: High temperatures (>100.4°F/38°C), CVA tenderness, suprapubic tenderness.
	Diagnostics: • Evaluation includes a urinalysis, urine culture, and sensitivity. • Urinalysis consistent for UTI may be cloudy, leukocyte esterase and nitrite positive, and have numerous WBCs and/or WBC casts • CBC will often show an elevated WBC count • BMP and blood cultures should be obtained in hospitalized patients Additional tests: • Consider urethral/cervical swab for gonorrhea and chlamydia; NAAT tests to rule out STI if patient is at risk.

CASE 14 | Acute Pyelonephritis *(continued)*

Discussion	**Management:** • For complicated pyelonephritis that requires hospitalization, ceftriaxone or piperacillin-tazobactam is indicated. • For uncomplicated pyelonephritis that does not require hospitalization, oral fluoroquinolones if *E. coli* resistance is <10% in the community • Imaging with ultrasound or CT to rule out renal or perinephric abscess should be considered if there is no clinical improvement after 48 hours of appropriate treatment
Additional Considerations	**Complications:** Complications include bacteremia, sepsis, renal abscess, renal papillary necrosis, or chronic pyelonephritis causing scarring and chronic kidney disease. **Obstetric considerations:** Screening for a UTI is indicated at least once early in pregnancy. The incidence of pyelonephritis is higher than in the general population, likely because of physiologic changes in the urinary tract during pregnancy. Progesterone causes relaxation of the ureteral smooth muscle, which increases the risk of bacteria from the bladder ascending to the kidney. **Pediatric Considerations:** Children usually can be treated as outpatients; however, if children are <2 months of age, are septic, vomiting, immunocompromised, or fail to respond to prior treatments as outpatients, they should be treated as inpatients.

CASE 15 | Gonococcal Urethritis

A 28-year-old man presents with severe dysuria and a whitish discharge from his penis for the past 2 days. He tested positive for chlamydia and was treated last year. He is currently sexually active with men and women and has had three partners in the last 6 months. He has inconsistent condom use. He reports no testicular pain. On exam, he is afebrile and his vital signs are normal. There are no areas of fluctuance upon palpating the urethra, but mild tenderness is noted on the most distal aspect, and a purulent discharge is milked from the urethra.

Conditions with Similar Presentations	**Nongonococcal urethritis (NGU):** Presents as a nonpurulent urethritis and is often due to *Chlamydia trachomatis*. Gonococcal urethritis is typically more purulent and painful than Chlamydia urethritis in men. **HSV:** Should be considered as a rare cause of NGU, but a history of vesicles, recurrent HSV, and/or ulceration will be clues to the diagnosis. **Acute prostatitis:** Usually seen in older men from *E. coli* infections. Younger individuals with acute bacterial prostatitis are typically infected with *N. gonorrhoeae* or *C. trachomatis*. Patients with acute bacterial prostatitis will present with pelvic pain, fever, and a tender prostate along with dysuria and increased frequency. **UTI** (in males): Would not have discharge.
Initial Diagnostic Tests	• NAAT of first-void urine sample or urethral swab • Consider urinalysis
Next Steps in Management	• Treatment with ceftriaxone • Add doxycycline if rapid testing for Chlamydia not available
Discussion	Urethritis is inflammation of the urethra, which classically presents with urethral discharge and dysuria. In clinical practice, the term often implies infection-induced urethral inflammation, though noninfectious etiologies exist. Urethral infections are usually sexually transmitted and are categorized as gonococcal (*Neisseria gonorrhoeae*) and nongonococcal (most commonly *Chlamydia trachomatis*). Other causes of NGU include *Mycoplasma genitalium*, *Trichomonas vaginalis*, herpes simplex virus, and adenovirus. **History:** • Males present with urethral discharge and severe dysuria 2–7 days after exposure. • Asymptomatic infections in males are rare. • The primary site of *N. gonorrhoeae* infection in females is the cervix, which is often asymptomatic unless it spreads to the vagina, urethra, or rectum. **Physical Exam:** • Purulent urethral discharge, erythema of the meatus, or testicular or epididymal tenderness.

CASE 15 | Gonococcal Urethritis *(continued)*

Discussion	**Diagnostics:**
	• Use NAAT of the first-void urine sample or urethral swab to diagnose *N. gonorrhoeae* or *Chlamydia trachomatis* urethritis.
	• Culture with urethral swab is the gold standard for diagnosis but is not immediately available, and treatment decisions should be made as soon as possible.
	• Gram stain will show gram-negative diplococci with ~90% sensitivity and close to 100% specificity.
	• Additional evaluation should include testing for other sexually transmitted infections (HIV, syphilis, HSV, and chlamydia).
	
	Management:
	• Treat patients empirically for both *N. gonorrhea* and *C. trachomatis* if chlamydia has not been ruled out with rapid testing
	  • First line for *N. gonorrhoeae* is a single dose of ceftriaxone
	  • Chlamydial urethritis: Doxycycline for 7 days or azithromycin for pregnant individuals
	
	Sexual partners should be referred for testing and treatment. If sexual partner may not be able to access a health care provider, can give treatment to patient to give to their sexual partner(s).

Additional Considerations	**Complications:** Disseminated gonococcal infection, seen in less than 3% of infected patients, 90% of which are females. Causes skin pustules and septic arthritis that is oligoarticular and distal (digits). *N. gonorrhoeae* also causes neonatal conjunctivitis and pelvic inflammatory disease (PID). Perihepatic inflammation due to ascending infection can be seen in PID and is known as the **Fitz-Hugh-Curtis syndrome.** "Violin-string" adhesions of the peritoneum to the liver are seen if laparoscopy is performed. **Screening:** Women should be screened annually through age 25 and then if at high risk or living with HIV. Men should be screened for gonorrhea annually if they have sex with men or high risk behavior with women.

GENITAL LESIONS AND SEXUALLY TRANSMITTED INFECTIONS

Most genital lesions, particularly ulcerative lesions, can be attributed to sexually transmitted infections (STIs). Despite this, lesions that do not respond appropriately to treatment should always prompt further evaluation, often including biopsy. See Obstetrics and Gynecology Chapter for additional cases.

Genital Lesions

History/Physical Exam	Other Findings	Diagnosis
Painful papules that evolve into pustules then painful well demarcated necrotic ulcers with a friable/exudative base. From Le, Tao and Bhushan, Vikas. First Aid for the USMLE Step 2 CK, Tenth Edition ISBN 9780071793025. pg 256(B)., (Reproduced with permission from Wolff K, Johnson RA, Saavedra AP. Fitzpatrick's Color Atlas & Synopsis of Clinical Dermatology, 7th ed. New York, NY: McGraw-Hill; 2013.)	Inguinal adenopathy	Chancroid due to *Hemophilus ducreyi*
Multiple small painful vesicles that leave behind a shallow ulcer 3–7 days after exposure From Le, Tao and Bhushan, Vikas. First Aid for the USMLE Step 2 CK, Tenth Edition ISBN 9780071793025. pg 256 (C)., (Reproduced with permission from Wolff K, Johnson RA, Saavedra AP. Fitzpatrick's Color Atlas & Synopsis of Clinical Dermatology, 7th ed. New York, NY: McGraw-Hill; 2013.)	Malaise, myalgias, and fever with burning and pruritus in initial outbreak	Herpes simplex virus (HSV) HSV 1 or HSV 2

Genital Lesions

History/Physical Exam	Other Findings	Diagnosis
Multiple warts Painless irregular pink or white papules. (Condyloma acuminata) From Le, Tao and Bhushan, Vikas. First Aid for the USMLE Step 2 CK, Tenth Edition ISBN 9780071793025. pg 256(D). (Reproduced courtesy of Dr. Wiesner, Public Health Image Library, Centers for Disease Control and Prevention, Atlanta, GA.)	Pruritus	HPV
Painless papule Single painless ulcer (chancre) with a clear/clean base and raised border 1 cm in size From Le, Tao and Bhushan, Vikas. First Aid for the USMLE Step 2 CK, Tenth Edition, Page 256 (E) ISBN 9780071793025. (Reproduced courtesy of Public Health Image Library, Centers for Disease Control and Prevention, Atlanta, GA.)	Regional adenopathy	Primary syphilis *Treponema pallidum*
Painless initial vesicle → papule → ulcer that resolves followed by inguinal adenopathy flanking the inguinal ligament (groove sign) Reproduced with permission from Sewon Kang, Masayuki Amagai, Anna L. Bruckner, Alexander H. Enk, David J. Margolis, Amy J. McMichael, Jeffrey S. Orringer Fitzpatrick's Dermatology, 9e, McGraw Hill, 2019.	Lymph nodes may erode into cutaneous fistulae	Lymphogranuloma venereum due to *Chlamydia trachomatis* (L1 through L3 serovars)
Painless hypertrophic papule changing to an ulcer Raised red lesions with rolled white borders 0.5–1 cm in size From Le, Tao and Bhushan, Vikas. First Aid for the USMLE Step 2 CK, Tenth Edition. New York: McGraw-Hill Education, 2018, page 250. (Image reproduced with permission from Longo DL, et al. Harrison's Principles of Internal Medicine, 18th ed. New York, NY: McGraw-Hill; 2012.)	No lymphadenopathy but can have nodular cutaneous lesions in the groin known as pseudo-buboes	Granuloma Inguinale due to *Klebsiella granulomatis*—also known as Donovanosis

Sexually Transmitted Infection Mini-Cases

Cases	Key Findings
Herpes Simplex Virus (HSV)	**Hx/PE:** Multiple small, painful vesicular lesions with a shallow ulcerative base (see above table). May have malaise, fever, lymphadenopathy with primary outbreak **Diagnostics:** • Genital swab of vesicle with PCR for HSV–1 and HSV–2 DNA • Multinucleated giant cells seen on Tzanck smear as shown **Management:** • Antivirals: acyclovir, famciclovir, valacyclovir • Antiviral drugs for suppression should be considered in patients with frequent recurrences, or complications of recurrences including erythema multiforme, eczema herpeticum, or aseptic meningitis **Discussion:** HSV-1 and HSV-2 can both cause genital herpes, with HSV-2 being more common and more likely to recur than HSV-1. HSV-1 also causes gingivostomatitis, keratoconjunctivitis, herpes labialis, and herpes encephalitis. Both types remain latent in the sensory ganglia and can cause disease when they reactivate. Arrows show the multinucleated giant cells in this positive Tzanck smear in a patient with genital herpes (HSV-2). (From Le, Tao and Bhushan, Vikas. First Aid for the USMLE Step 2 CK, Tenth Edition, ISBN 9781260440300, page 239. Image modified with permission from Yale Rosen.)
Syphilis	**Hx/PE:** • In primary syphilis, patients present with a single painless ulcer (chancre) with a clean, raised base • May have associated mild, tender lymphadenopathy **Diagnostics:** • Combination of nontreponemal (RPR, VDRL) and treponemal (FTA-ABS, TPPA) testing to diagnose syphilis; can order one or the other, with reflex to the other test if positive. • Nontreponemal tests can be used to monitor therapy, while treponemal tests remain positive for life and are not helpful for monitoring. Effective treatment should result in a reduction of titers to positive at 1:1 or undetectable one year after treatment. • Note that nontreponemal tests are nonspecific and may be positive in pregnancy, autoimmune disorders, bacterial endocarditis, and other chronic conditions. **Management:** • Penicillin G benzathine is the drug of choice for all forms except neurosyphilis. • Primary and secondary and early latent syphilis: 2.4 million units intramuscularly as a single dose. • Late latent non-neurologic tertiary syphilis (aortitis, gummatous): 2.4 million units IM weekly for 3 weeks. • Neurosyphilis (as well as ocular and otic syphilis) should be treated with 3–4 million units penicillin G intravenously every 4 hours for 14 days. Recent data supports the use of ceftriaxone as an alternative. • Patients with PCN allergy can be treated with doxycycline or tetracycline unless it is neurosyphilis or during pregnancy, in which case PCN desensitization should be done.

Sexually Transmitted Infection Mini-Cases (*continued*)

Syphilis	**Discussion:**
	• *Primary syphilis:* Presents 1 week to 3 months after exposure with a painless chancre at the site of infection.

• *Secondary syphilis:* Presents 2–8 weeks after chancre resolution and can present with fever, local or diffuse mucocutaneous lesions (maculopapular rash including palms and soles), condyloma lata, generalized lymphadenopathy, mucous patches (oral mucosa ulcers), alopecia, and neurologic disease.

• *Tertiary disease:* Occurs years later and has three forms:
  • Cardiovascular syphilis: Proximal aortitis leading to aneurysm and aortic valve insufficiency
  • Gummatous syphilis: Painless necrotic lesions that can occur anywhere in the body
  • Neurosyphilis: Also has three major forms: aseptic meningitis, tabes dorsalis (posterior column destruction with gait disturbance and Romberg sign), and general paresis. Symptoms of general PARESIS are:
    • **P**ersonality changes
    • **A**ffect changes
    • **R**eflexes increased
    • **E**ye findings: Argyll-Robertson Pupil (reacts to accommodation but not light- Accommodation Reflex Present- Pupillary Reflex Absent)
    • **S**ensorium changes
    • **I**ntellectual deterioration
    • **S**peech defect

Ophthalmic and otic neurosyphilis may also occur

• *Latent syphilis* is defined as serologic evidence of syphilis with no current signs or symptoms. It is considered early if it is within 1 year of signs or symptoms of syphilis, or late if it is > 1 year of signs or symptoms of syphilis or there never were any signs or symptoms.

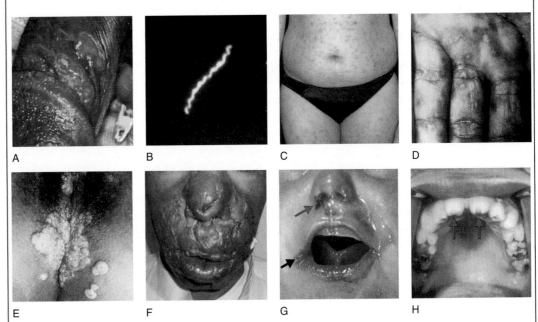

Syphilis. (A) Localized disease presenting with painless chancre and (B) dark-field microscopy visualizing treponemes in fluid from chancre in 1° syphilis. (C) Maculopapular rash ([D] including palms and soles) and (E) condylomata lata in 2° syphilis. (F) Gummas (chronic granulomas) in 3° syphilis. (G) Rhagades (linear scars at angle of mouth), snuffles (nasal discharge), saddle nose, and (H) notched (Hutchinson) teeth in congenital syphilis. (A, Reproduced courtesy of Public Health Image Library, Centers for Disease Control and Prevention, M. Rein; B, Reproduced courtesy of Public Health Image Library, Centers for Disease Control and Prevention, W.F. Schwartz; C, From Le, Tao and Bhushan, Vikas. First Aid for the USMLE Step 2 CK, Tenth Edition. New York: McGraw-Hill Education, 2018, Fig.2.8-25. ISBN 9781260440300. Reproduced with permission from Dr. Richard Usatine.; D, Reproduced courtesy of Public Health Image Library, Centers for Disease Control and Prevention, Robert Sumpter; E, Reproduced courtesy of Public Health Image Library, Centers for Disease Control and Prevention, Richard Deitrick; F, From Le, Tao and Bhushan, Vikas. First Aid for the USMLE Step 2 CK, Tenth Edition. New York: McGraw-Hill Education, 2018, Fig.2.8-25. ISBN 9781260440300. Modified with permission from Chakir K, Benchikhi H. Centro-facial granuloma revealing a tertiary syphilis. Pan Afr Med J. 2013;15:82; G, Reproduced courtesy of Public Health Image Library, Centers for Disease Control and Prevention, Dr. Norman Cole; H, Reproduced courtesy of Public Health Image Library, Centers for Disease Control and Prevention, Susan Lindsley)

Sexually Transmitted Infections Mini-Cases (*continued*)

Chancroid (*Haemophilus ducreyi*)	**Hx/PE:** • Single painful ulcer with friable/exudative base (see table) • Often with suppurative and tender lymphadenopathy **Diagnostics:** • Clinical diagnosis and exclusion of syphilis and HSV infection by serology and PCR testing, respectively • Culture available but requires special media and is not sensitive **Management:** • Azithromycin OR ceftriaxone as a single dose • Alternatives are ciprofloxacin or erythromycin • Buboes should be aspirated and drained
Condyloma Acuminata	**Hx/PE:** • Variable appearance of lesions • Can be flat, cerebriform, or verrucous • Can be dome-shaped, cauliflower-shaped, or pedunculated (see table) **Diagnostics:** Clinical diagnosis **Management:** • Can perform watchful waiting or use a variety of wart removal treatments • Topical destructive therapies (imiquimod, trichloroacetic acid) or if large, wide local excision or laser resection, although recurrence is high. • Consider biopsy if concern for squamous cell lesions **Discussion:** • Condyloma acuminatum (anogenital warts) is a proliferation of anogenital skin and mucosa due to HPV infection • HPV 6 and 11 are the cause of 90% of genital warts and confer a low risk of malignancy
Lymphogranuloma Venereum (LGV)	**Hx/PE:** • Painless genital ulcer • Followed by tender, inguinal lymphadenopathy above and below the inguinal canal (grove sign) weeks later (see table) • Constitutional symptoms may be present **Diagnostics:** • Swab or aspiration of lesion for NAAT testing • Culture or serology **Management:** Doxycycline for 21 days **Discussion:** LGV is an ulcerative genital disease caused by the L1, L2, and L3 biovars of *Chlamydia trachomatis* and is mostly seen in tropical areas, though in recent years there have been outbreaks in temperate climates among men who have sex with men (MSM). Primary infection is characterized by an ulcer at the site of inoculation. Secondary infection is characterized by extension into reginal lymph nodes and late LGV by strictures and fibrosis that may cause genital elephantiasis and other complications.

INFECTIOUS DIARRHEA

Diarrhea is the passage of unusually soft or liquid stools more than three times in 24 hours OR >250 g of unformed stool/day.

- Categorized by duration of symptoms
  - Acute ≤14 days
  - Persistent >14–30 days
  - Chronic >30 days

History

Inquire about food exposures, travel, animal exposures, sick contacts, antibiotic use, immunocompromised state. Fever and/or bloody diarrhea suggests invasive organisms.

Exam

Check for orthostatic hypotension, frank hypotension, rash, abdominal tenderness. Any diarrhea if severe can cause hypovolemia and hypotension.

Diagnosis/Management

Ultimately, most causes of acute diarrhea are self-limited and managed with supportive care, so identifying causes that require antimicrobial therapy, such as *Clostridioides difficile*, is important.

The following are some of the key differential diagnoses for various types of diarrhea.

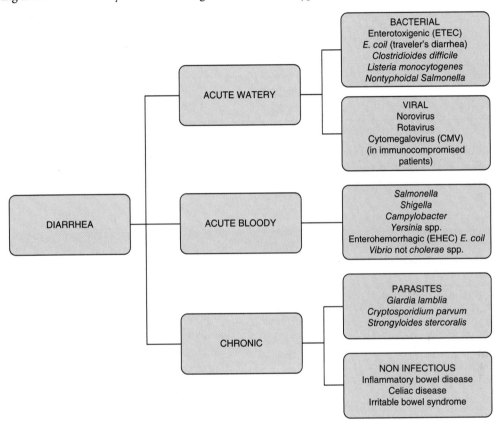

Key Differential Diagnoses for Infectious Diarrhea

Diarrheas with Key Associated Findings	Diagnoses
Recent antibiotic exposure, recent hospitalization Pseudomembranous colitis appearance on endoscopy	*C. difficile*
Hemolytic uremic syndrome (HUS), hemolysis, thrombocytopenia, and acute kidney injury	EHEC (O157:H7)
Cruise ship outbreak	Norovirus
Freshwater exposure, time in the woods/hiking Common variable immune deficiency (CVID), IgA deficiency	*Giardia lamblia*
Daycare center exposure	*G. lamblia*, rotavirus
Unpasteurized milk Pregnancy	*Listeria monocytogenes*
Undercooked poultry, fever	*Campylobacter, Shigella, Salmonella*
Reptile/turtle exposure	*Salmonella*

Key Differential Diagnoses for Infectious Diarrhea (*Continued*)

Diarrheas with Key Associated Findings	Diagnoses
"Rose spot" rash on abdomen	*Salmonella enterica* serotype *typhi*—typhoid fever
Diarrhea followed by polyarticular arthritis, conjunctivitis	Reactive arthritis, which is associated with *Campylobacter, Shigella, Salmonella, Yersinia*
Hemochromatosis on iron-chelating therapy Severe RLQ pain: "pseudo-appendicitis" due to severe ileocolitis and regional adenopathy	*Yersinia* spp.
Diarrhea followed by flaccid, ascending weakness on exam	*Campylobacter* (the most associated diarrheal cause with Guillain-Barre syndrome)
Men who have sex with men (MSM) Diarrhea and liver abscess	*Entamoeba histolytica*
Eosinophilia	*Strongyloides stercoralis*
Cirrhosis and salt water exposure	*Vibrio vulnificus* and *parahemolyticus*

Immunocompromising conditions such as HIV/AIDS and organ transplantation broaden the differential to include opportunistic causes of diarrhea. The primary diagnostic tool is stool examination, which can help to identify organisms through PCR, culture, and staining.

Causes of Diarrhea in Immunocompromised Patients

Symptoms	Labs	Organism/Treatment
Frequent bloody diarrhea, abdominal pain, low-grade fever	CD4 <50/mm^3	*Cytomegalovirus* Treatment with ganciclovir
Watery diarrhea, cramping abdominal pain, RUQ pain (acalculous cholecystitis)	CD4 <100/mm^3	*Cryptosporidium, Microsporidium, Cystoisospora, Cyclospora* Antiretroviral therapy to increase CD4 count Specific antimicrobials: *Cryptosporidium*: nitazoxanide *Microsporidium*: albendazole *Cystoisospora*: TMP/SMX *Cyclospora*: TMP/SMX
Watery diarrhea, high-grade fever (>39˚C), weight loss	Elevated alkaline phosphatase, anemia	*Mycobacterium avium* complex Treatment with macrolide + ethambutol

Considerations in Travelers

The differential diagnosis of infectious diarrhea is expanded for patients who recently have traveled and consumed contaminated food or water. Treatment is supportive unless the diarrhea is incapacitating or persists, in which case antibiotics are administered.

Bismuth subsalicylate has been shown to prevent the incidence of diarrhea and can be utilized as a short-term (<3 weeks) preventative measure. However, it is very inconvenient (two tablets four times a day), causes side effects such as black tongue and dark stools, and can cause salicylate toxicity in adults taking aspirin, and Reye syndrome in children.

Symptoms	Cause/Treatment
Acute watery diarrhea	Enterotoxigenic *E. coli* (ETEC) Antibiotics not recommended, supportive measures only

Symptoms	Cause/Treatment
Progressive presentation: • First week: fever • Second week: abdominal pain, bloody diarrhea, faint red macules (Rose spots) • Third week: intestinal bleeding and perforation	Typhoid fever (*Salmonella enterica*, serotype Typhi) Typhoid vaccine given before travel to endemic areas Treatment with ceftriaxone is crucial, as typhoid fever can be fatal
Bloody diarrhea, often with RUQ pain and fever if liver abscess has developed Characteristic, *flask-shaped amoebic ulcers* on colonoscopy	*Entamoeba histolytica* Treatment with metronidazole and paromomycin
Profuse watery diarrhea, self-limiting (10–14 days) in healthy patients, low-grade fever	*Cryptosporidium* No treatment unless immunocompromised
Person in tropical/subtropical area with intermittent watery diarrhea over the course of years, often accompanied by pruritus and urticaria	Strongyloidiasis (*Strongyloides stercoralis*) Treat with ivermectin
Steatorrhea, abdominal cramps, flatulence Associated with freshwater streams in US	Giardiasis (*Giardia lamblia*) Treat with tinidazole

Infectious Diarrhea Mini-Cases

Cases	Key Findings
Viral Gastroenteritis	**Hx:** Watery diarrhea, abdominal pain, emesis, fever. **PE:** Signs of dehydration such as orthostatic hypotension, dry mucous membranes. **Diagnostics:** • Clinical diagnosis. • Stool PCR if indicated (immunocompromised, not improving) **Management:** • Volume resuscitation with oral or IV fluids. • Symptoms resolve within a few days. **Discussion:** In the US, viral gastroenteritis is most often caused by **norovirus** (50% of all acute diarrhea). Many outbreaks are associated with schools and cruise ships. **Rotavirus** also causes viral gastroenteritis and is particularly seen in unvaccinated individuals and children 2 years of age and younger. A live rotavirus vaccine is part of the routine childhood immunization schedule.

***Clostridioides difficile* Infection**	**Hx:** Watery stools, abdominal pain, recent hospitalization, or antibiotic exposure.
	PE: Fever, signs of dehydration such as orthostatic hypotension.
	Diagnostics: Stool PCR for *C. diff* toxin B gene.
	Management:
	• First episode: PO vancomycin or fidaxomicin
	• First recurrence:
	  • Fidaxomicin or tapering doses of vancomycin
	  • Bezlotoxumab, a monoclonal antibody against toxin B, should be added with comorbidities or age > 65.
	• Subsequent recurrences: Fidaxomicin or tapering doses of vancomycin or vancomycin and rifaximin, or fecal microbiota transplantation
	• In **fulminant *C. diff*** (hypotension, shock, ileus, megacolon), use IV metronidazole + PO vancomycin and consider colectomy
	• IV fluids and electrolyte repletion as needed
	Discussion:
	Clostridioides is a gram-positive, spore-forming, obligate anaerobic rod that produces exotoxins: Toxin A enterotoxin damages intestinal enterocytes driving watery diarrhea and toxin B is a cytotoxin that drives epithelial necrosis and pseudomembrane formation. Despite appropriate treatment, recurrence is common, and patients may need prolonged antibiotic therapy or a fecal microbiota transplant.

VECTOR-BORNE DISEASES

CASE 16	Malaria	
A 40-year-old man with no past medical history presents with intermittent fevers, shaking chills, sweats, and diffuse myalgias. He returned from Somalia 1 week ago and was not taking any medications while traveling. His symptoms last a few hours and recur every 48–72 hours. On exam, he has a fever of 41.5°C and is tachycardic. There is conjunctival icterus, pallor, and hepatosplenomegaly.		
Conditions with Similar Presentations	**West Nile virus (WNV) encephalitis:** Is a form of viral meningoencephalitis that can present with fever, altered mental status, and flaccid paralysis. However, infections in immunocompetent, healthy adults are mostly asymptomatic. WNV is an arbovirus spread by the female *Culex* mosquito and is seen in the summer months. There is no specific therapy for WNV, but supportive care can help improve outcomes. Those at highest risk of severe disease include immunocompromised, elderly, or very young patients.	
	Dengue fever: Caused by another flavivirus (dengue virus), it is spread by the *Aedes* mosquito. It is prevalent in tropical and subtropical regions. It presents with flu-like symptoms, headache, fever, myalgias, arthralgias, and retro-orbital pain. If severe it can cause thrombocytopenia and capillary leak syndrome.	
Initial Diagnostic Tests	• Confirm with parasitological testing of peripheral blood smear with PCR testing or Giemsa stain to detect intraerythrocytic *Plasmodium* • Also check CBC, CMP and PT, PTT	
Next Steps in Management	• Uncomplicated infection: chloroquine (if sensitive) or mefloquine or atovaquone/proguanil (if resistant) or oral artemisinin combination therapy (ACT) • Treat severe cases with intravenous artesunate	
Discussion	Malaria is transmitted by infected Anopheles mosquitos and is caused by **Plasmodium species.** The five malaria species that infect humans are *P. falciparum*, *P. vivax*, *P. malariae*, *P. ovale*, and *P. knowlesi*. *P. falciparum*: Is the most common and deadliest and complications include cerebral malaria, hemolytic anemia, hypoglycemia, lactic acidosis, and cardiopulmonary, renal, and liver damage. *P. malariae*: Can have a delayed onset presentation, even >2 months after the traveler has returned and even if the traveler has had adequate prophylaxis. *P. vivax* and *P. ovale*: Can be dormant in the liver as a hypnozoite and reactivate after years. This can be eradicated by using primaquine. **History:** Risk factors: Travel to endemic areas include Africa, Central and South America, Caribbean, Asia, and Eastern Europe, and South Pacific Islands. Not using antimalarial prophylaxis. Symptoms: Tertian (every 48 hours) or quartan (every 72 hours) pattern of fever. Headache, shaking chills, sweats **Diagnostics:** • Microscopic examination of Giemsa-stained thick and thin smears of peripheral blood smear is the gold standard lab test. The parasite can be in the ring stage (purple spot in a ring), trophozoite stage (small spot in a larger spot), schizont stage, or gametocyte stage (banana shaped in *P. falciparum*). • PCR is useful for low-level parasitemia. • CBC notable for mild normocytic anemia and thrombocytopenia. **Management:** • Consult CDC website to assess whether chloroquine resistance is present in country of origin of infection. 　• If species is *P. falciparum*, treat with artemisinin combination therapy. 　　• If not *P. falciparum*, if chloroquine sensitive, use chloroquine. • If resistant use atovaquone-proguanil or any two of: quinine, doxycycline, or clindamycin. • If pregnant use chloroquine if sensitive, quinine plus clindamycin or mefloquine if resistant in all trimesters.	
Additional Considerations	**Preventative:** Prophylaxis for travelers to endemic areas is recommended with chloroquine, atovaquone-proguanil, mefloquine, doxycycline, or primaquine. Travelers are also advised on steps to take to avoid mosquitoes, including protective clothing and netted and enclosed sleeping sacks.	

Tick-Borne Illnesses

Many tick-borne diseases present with similar early symptoms of fatigue, fever, and myalgias. However, the presence and type of rash can help differentiate between them.

CASE 17 | Lyme Disease

A 38-year-old man with no previous medical history presents with fever, malaise, and myalgias for 48 hours. He has had no sick contacts, and no one else in the family is sick. He just returned from camping in upstate New York earlier this week. On exam, his vitals are temperature 38.5°C, pulse 85/min, respirations 16/min, and blood pressure 121/79. On his left leg, he has a targetoid, erythematous macule measuring 6 cm.

Conditions with Similar Presentations	Differential diagnosis includes other tick-borne illnesses (RMSF, babesiosis, ehrlichiosis), influenza and Juvenile idiopathic arthritis. However, none of these would cause the skin lesion described.
Initial Diagnostic Tests	• Clinical diagnosis • Serologies not recommended for early disease because they may be negative early on, and erythema migrans is diagnostic
Next Steps in Management	Start treatment for early disease with doxycycline, amoxicillin, or cefuroxime
Discussion	Lyme disease is a tick-borne illness carried by the spirochete *Borrelia burgdorferi. Ixodes scapularis* ticks that carry it are endemic to the Pacific coast, northeast, and northern midwest. Infection usually occurs after a tick attaches to the skin and feeds for >48 hours. For patients with a known tick bite, be wary of potential Lyme disease transmission if the tick is found to be *Ixodes scapularis* and there are high local transmission rates of Lyme disease. 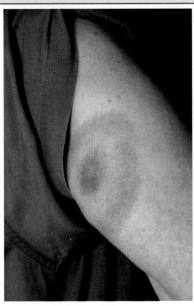 Erythema chronicum migrans seen in Lyme disease. Note the classic "bull's eye" lesion, which consists of an outer ring where the spirochetes are found, an inner ring of clearing, and central erythema caused by an allergic response at the site of the tick bite. (Reproduced courtesy of Public Health Image Library, Centers for Disease Control and Prevention) **History/Physical Exam:** Risk factors: Travel to an endemic area, tick attached for 48–72 hours. Systemic symptoms of early disease are vague (fever, headache, myalgias, fatigue, and/or arthralgias). • *Early localized disease:* Erythema migrans presents as a small, erythematous macule or papule that gradually enlarges over the course of days to weeks. There is often central clearing, commonly referred to as a targetoid or "bull's-eye" rash. Fever may also be present. • *Early disseminated disease:* Migratory polyarthropathy, bilateral facial nerve palsy, lymphocytic meningitis, conduction abnormalities (second- or third-degree heart block) and myocarditis. • *Late disease:* Arthritis and subacute encephalitis **Diagnostics:** *Early Lyme disease:* • A clinical diagnosis made on basis of erythema migrans and travel to endemic area. • For early Lyme disease, serology is not recommended as antibodies only become present 1–6 weeks after onset of erythema migrans and the skin lesion is diagnostic. *Late Lyme disease:* • Diagnose via serology. If ELISA IgM and IgG are (+) or equivocal, order Western blot to confirm. • For late or disseminated Lyme disease, do not use Western blots for screening or without high degree of suspicion. Western blots sent without ELISA have high false (+) rates. **Management:** • Early Lyme disease should be treated with doxycycline, amoxicillin, or cefuroxime. • For pregnant patients and children <8 years old, use amoxicillin. • Give empiric treatment for any patient with erythema migrans, arthralgias, or known tick bite in endemic area. • For late Lyme disease, oral therapy with the same drugs can be given • More severe manifestations (meningitis, carditis) can be treated with ceftriaxone
Additional Considerations	**Prophylaxis:** Give one dose of doxycycline if *Ixodes scapularis* tick has been attached for ≥36 hours, local infection rate is >20% AND prophylaxis can be started within <72 hours of removal

Tick-Borne Illness Mini-Cases

Cases	Key Findings
Rocky Mountain Spotted Fever (RMSF)	**Hx:** Risk factors: Dog tick (*Dermacentor*) bite transmitting *Rickettsia rickettsia* anywhere in the continental US, but commonly in the south and southeast. Symptoms: Fever >38.9°C, malaise, severe headache, and rash. **PE:** • Rash arises 2–4 days after fever onset and is initially macular and begins on wrists and ankles • Later it turns petechial and begins to spread centrally • Altered mental status and disseminated intravascular coagulation (DIC) can occur in severe cases 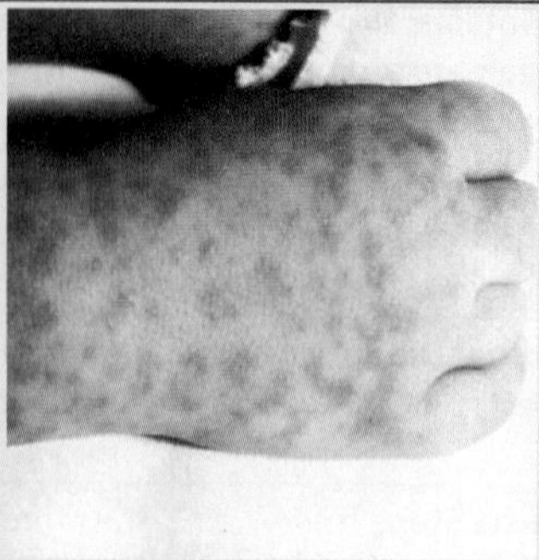 Involvement of the foot with Rocky Mountain spotted fever. (Reproduced with permission from Le, Tao; Bhushan, Vikas; and Sochat, Matthew. First Aid for the USMLE Step 1 2021. New York: McGraw-Hill , 2021. Pg 150.). **Diagnostics:** • Skin biopsy and indirect immunofluorescence. Serologies turn positive but treatment should be given prior to that. • Characteristic lab findings include thrombocytopenia, hyponatremia, and elevated transaminases **Management:** • Doxycycline **Discussion:** • High rate of fatality if left untreated • Where the clinical suspicion is high, doxycycline is started while awaiting biopsy results 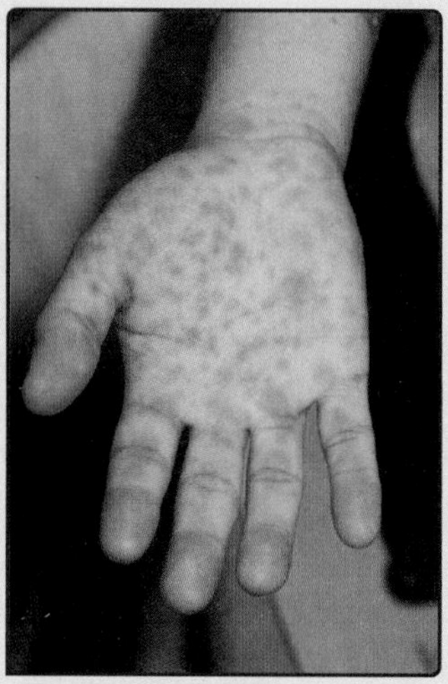 Erythematous macular lesions on palm in Rocky Mountain spotted fever.: (From Kang S, Amagai M, Bruckner AL, Enk AH, Margolis DJ, McMichael AJ, Orringer JS. Fitzpatrick's Dermatology, 9e; 2019. Figure180-2, ISBN 9780071837798., Used with permission from Daniel Noltkamper, MD. Reprinted from Hardin JM. Cutaneous conditions. In: Knoop KJ, Stack LB, Storrow AB, et al, eds. The Atlas of Emergency Medicine, 4th ed. New York, NY: McGraw-Hill, 2016.)
Babesiosis	**Hx:** May be asymptomatic or symptoms (flulike symptoms and easy bruising/bleeding (from intravascular hemolysis)) can occur several weeks after tick bite **PE:** Fever, may have pallor and tachycardia (from anemia), jaundice, bruising/bleeding. **Diagnostics:** • Ring-shaped or "Maltese cross" organisms can be seen on thin smear of blood inside RBCs. • If smear is negative, can order PCR • Above tests may be negative with low levels of parasitemia. A four-fold rise in serology is then diagnostic Additional tests: Labs may show thrombocytopenia, leukopenia, elevated transaminases, and hematuria/proteinuria. **Management:** • Azithromycin and atovaquone • Azithromycin should be IV if ≥4% parasitemia • Transfusions if severe anemia **Discussion:** *Babesia* is a protozoa that can invade and lyse RBCs. *Ixodes* tick vector may transmit *Babesia*, *B. burgdorferi* or *Anaplasma*. Tick avoidance and precautions should be taken in endemic areas. Symptoms resolve in 1 week, but immunocompromised patients are more likely to have severe symptoms and longer duration of symptoms.

Tick-Borne Illness Mini-Cases (*continued*)

Ehrlichiosis and Anaplasmosis	**Hx:** Risk factors: Travel to south and southeastern US (ehrlichiosis) or northeastern and north central US (anaplasmosis), tick bite (see Discussion).
	
	Symptoms: May present with rapid-onset fever, chills, headache, myalgias, and altered mental status. Symptoms are usually more severe in ehrlichiosis.
	
	PE: Fever
	
	Rash is seen in 30% of ehrlichiosis, but <5% of anaplasmosis
	
	Diagnostics:
	• PCR is most sensitive during acute infection
	• Peripheral smear shows intracytoplasmic organisms (morulae)
	  • In polymorphonuclear cells if *Anaplasma*
	  • In lymphocytes if *Ehrlichia*
	• Serology and culture less used
	
	Additional tests: Labs show thrombocytopenia, leukopenia (neutropenia if *Anaplasma* and lymphopenia if *Ehrlichia*), and elevated transaminases.
	
	Management:
	• Doxycycline
	• Severe illness can rapidly progress to CNS involvement and sepsis with or without organ dysfunction; empiric treatment should be started immediately if clinical suspicion is high.
	
	Discussion:
	• Ehrlichiosis is transmitted by Lone Star tick (*Amblyomma americanum*) after travel to south and southeastern US.
	• Anaplasmosis is transmitted by the deer tick (*Ixodes scapularis*) in northeastern and north central US.
		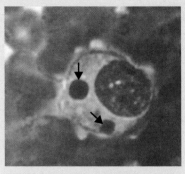
		Monocytes forming morulae in cytoplasm in ehrlichiosis. (Reproduced with permission from Le, Tao; Bhushan, Vikas; and Sochat, Matthew. First Aid for the USMLE Step 1 2021. New York: McGraw-Hill, 2021.)
		
		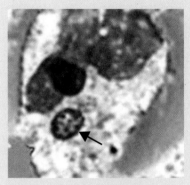
		Granulocytes forming morulae in cytoplasm in anaplasmosis. (Reproduced with permission from Le, Tao; Bhushan, Vikas; and Sochat, Matthew. First Aid for the USMLE Step 1 2021. New York: McGraw-Hill, 2021.).)

Zoonotic Diseases Transmitted Between Animals and Humans

Disease/ Species/ Transmission	Presentation	Diagnosis	Treatment
Transmitted by Ticks			
• Anaplasmosis (e.g., human granulocytic anaplasmosis) • *Anaplasma phagocytophilum* • *Ixodes scapularis* tick (on deer and mice)	Endemic in NE and Midwestern U.S. in spring/summer; may see co-infection with other *Ixodes*-transmitted diseases (Lyme disease, babesiosis); fever, chills, malaise, myalgia, headache, nausea/vomiting, cough, arthralgias; infects PMNs and causes neutropenia	PCR, serology, and/ or blood smear demonstrating morulae in PMNs (do not delay treatment); evaluate for co-infections	Doxycycline (PO or IV)
• Babesiosis • *Babesia microti* • *Ixodes scapularis* tick (on deer and mice)	Same geographic distribution as anaplasmosis and Lyme disease and may see co-infection with them; fever, fatigue, myalgia, headache; infects RBCs and causes hemolytic anemia and jaundice. Severe if immunocompromised or asplenic; can lead to ARDS, heart failure, DIC	Pancytopenia; elevated bilirubin, LDH, and ALT/AST; thin blood smear with Wright-Giemsa stain showing "Maltese cross" in RBCs	Atovaquone and azithromycin; in severe cases, consider quinine with clindamycin

Zoonotic Diseases Transmitted Between Animals and Humans (*Continued*)

Disease/ Species/ Transmission	Presentation	Diagnosis	Treatment
• Ehrlichiosis (human monocytic ehrlichiosis) • *Ehrlichia chaffeensis* • *Amblyomma americanum* or Lone Star tick (on white-tail deer)	Endemic in SE and Mid-Atlantic U.S. during spring/summer; fever, chills, malaise, myalgia, headache, nausea/vomiting, cough, arthralgias, rash in ~1/3. Infects lymphocytes and causes lymphocytopenia.	PCR, serology, and/ or blood smear demonstrating morula in lymphocytes (do not delay treatment)	Doxycycline (PO or IV)
• Lyme disease • *Borrelia burgdorferi* • *Ixodes scapularis* tick (on deer and mice)	Same geographic distribution as anaplasmosis and babesiosis and may see co-infection with them. Erythema migrans in majority of cases; minority of patients will develop disseminated disease with flu-like symptoms, lymphadenopathy, carditis (AV conduction block), facial nerve palsy, meningitis, arthritis	Erythema migrans is diagnostic. For later stages, perform serology	Oral doxycycline, amoxicillin, or cefuroxime Severe neurologic or cardiac disease: IV ceftriaxone
• Rocky Mountain spotted fever • *Rickettsia rickettsia* • *Dermacentor* (dog) tick	Endemic in Southeastern and South-Central U.S.; early symptoms include fever, headache, malaise, myalgias, arthralgias, nausea; erythematous macules beginning on ankles and wrists that becomes petechial	Clinical, confirm with PCR or DFA of skin biopsy (do not delay treatment)	Early empiric treatment with PO or IV doxycycline
**Transmitted by Pets, Farm Animals, or Other Animals**			
• Cat scratch disease; bacillary angiomatosis • *Bartonella henselae* • Cat scratch or bite, cat fleas	Cat scratch disease – Initial macule then papule then pustule at site of scratch/bite; tender regional lymphadenopathy (commonly axillary) Bacillary angiomatosis – immunocompromised patient with violaceous, papular skin lesions; may have internal organ involvement (respiratory or GI tract); can be fatal	Cat scratch disease – clinical, confirm with PCR of blood or biopsy, or serology Bacillary angiomatosis – PCR of blood or biopsy	Cat scratch disease – azithromycin Bacillary angiomatosis – doxycycline or erythromycin; add rifampin if severe. Antiretroviral therapy if HIV+
• Cellulitis, osteomyelitis • *Pasteurella multocida* • Animal bite (cats, dogs), cat scratch	Rapidly progressing soft tissue infection including cellulitis, abscesses, necrotizing infections; septic arthritis; osteomyelitis; respiratory tract infection; may have characteristic mouse-like odor	Gram stain and cultures from wound	Empiric amoxicillin-clavulanate; narrow based on culture results; wound care (including debridement if needed)
• Leptospirosis • *Leptospira* spp. • Animal urine in water; recreational water use	Prevalent in tropical regions. Abrupt fever, rigors, myalgias, headache, conjunctival suffusion without purulent discharge; can lead to aseptic meningitis, uveitis; minority of patients can develop icteric form (Weil's disease) with jaundice, conjunctival icterus, renal failure, pulmonary disease	Can be made clinically, definitive diagnosis via PCR, serology, and/or urine cultures (do not delay treatment)	PO doxycycline or azithromycin If severe, IV penicillin, doxycycline, ceftriaxone, or cefotaxime; renal replacement therapy if renal failure
• Plague • *Yersinia pestis* • Rodent fleas or bites. Pneumonic form transmissible person-to-person	Most commonly presents as bubonic plague, with sudden onset of fever, chills, weakness, headache, lymphadenopathy followed by intense pain and swelling in a lymph node area (bubo);other forms are septicemic (sepsis with no cutaneous lesions) and pneumonic (acute pneumonia).; can be fatal	Clinical, confirm with culture and Wright-Giemsa stain or serology (do not delay treatment)	Bubonic plague – aminoglycoside, fluoroquinolone, and doxycycline Septicemic or pneumonic plague – aminoglycoside or fluoroquinolone
• Psittacosis • *Chlamydia psittaci* • Parrots or other birds	Abrupt fever, headache, photophobia, dry cough, rigors, sweats, myalgias; pneumonia	Serology (do not delay treatment)	Doxycycline PO
• Q fever • *Coxiella burnetiid* • Aerosols from amniotic fluid or waste of cattle, goats, or sheep	Fever fatigue, myalgia, severe (retro-orbital) headache, photophobia, pneumonia, hepatitis; endocarditis in those with valvular disease	Elevated liver enzymes, thrombocytopenia; serology or PCR (do not delay treatment)	Doxycycline PO If chronic or endocarditis, add hydroxychloroquine

Zoonotic Diseases Transmitted Between Animals and Humans

Disease/ Species/ Transmission	Presentation	Diagnosis	Treatment
• Tularemia • *Francisella tularensis* • Rabbits, ticks, deer flies	Multiple subtypes; abrupt onset of fever, chills, anorexia, malaise; ulcerative skin lesions, regional tender lymphadenopathy; pneumonia with hilar adenopathy; can be fatal	Serology (do not delay treatment)	Mild or moderate infection – ciprofloxacin or doxycycline PO Severe infection – IM or IV gentamicin, IM streptomycin
Less Commonly Transmitted by Animals			
• *Campylobacter* gastroenteritis • *Campylobacter* • Contaminated food (poultry, milk); poor hand-hygiene; feces from infected pets or farm animals	Acute, inflammatory, bloody diarrhea (may be watery initially), abdominal pain (often periumbilical) and cramping, tenesmus; may precede Guillain-Barré syndrome or reactive arthritis	Stool culture or molecular testing	Usually a mild, self-limited infection. If severe treat with azithromycin or a fluoroquinolone
• Leprosy (Hansen's disease) • *Mycobacterium leprae, Mycobacterium lepromatis* • Respiratory transmission or skin-to-skin contact from other infected patients; (rarely) armadillo in Southern U.S.	Typically occurs in resource-limited settings with chronic skin lesions Tuberculoid leprosy – few hypopigmented, well-defined skin plaques, loss of hair follicles, decreased sensation or paresthesias along cutaneous nerves Lepromatous leprosy – diffuse skin thickening and erythematous lesions, hair loss, leonine facies, paresis, loss of sensation, blindness	Clinical with confirmation by skin biopsy, PCR, and/or serology	Multi-drug therapy: Tuberculoid leprosy – dapsone and rifampicin Lepromatous leprosy – dapsone, rifampicin, and clofazimine
• *Salmonella* (nontyphoidal) gastroenteritis • *Salmonella* enterica (except *S. enterica* serotype typhi) • Reptiles; poultry, eggs, and milk products	Usually self-limited diarrhea (may be bloody), nausea/vomiting, fever, abdominal cramps, other constitutional symptoms (fatigue, malaise), weight loss	Stool culture or molecular testing	Usually a mild self-limited infection. If severe illness, or high risk of invasive disease treat based on susceptibilities trying to avoid fluoroquinolones (resistance increasing)

INFECTIONS OF THE EYES AND EARS

CASE 18	Bacterial Conjunctivitis
A 7-year-old girl with no previous medical history presents with right eye irritation for 2 days. She reports feeling itching and like something is "stuck" in her eye but denies pain. Her mother notes crusting on her eyelashes. On exam, she has unilateral inflamed, erythematous conjunctiva with thick, whitish-yellow mucopurulent discharge. Her visual acuity is preserved.	
Conditions with Similar Presentations	Other conditions can present with red eye such as mechanical or toxic irritation or dry eye disease. **Allergic conjunctivitis:** Symptoms bilateral; may have asthma or other allergies. **Viral conjunctivitis:** Serous discharge vs. purulent in bacterial. **Blepharitis:** Chronic inflammatory disorder of skin, lashes, and eyelid glands. **Angle-closure glaucoma:** Narrowing or closure of anterior chamber angle causes sudden eye pain and/or vision loss.
Initial Diagnostic Tests	• Clinical diagnosis • For severe infections, Gram stain and culture is indicated

CASE 18 | Bacterial Conjunctivitis (continued)

Next Steps in Management	Treat with antibiotic drops/ointment for nongonococcal, bacterial conjunctivitis.
Discussion	Inflammation of the conjunctiva can be found in both children and adults. It is most commonly bacterial (*S. aureus, S. pneumoniae, H. influenzae, M.catarrhalis*) or viral (adenovirus) in etiology. However, it is important to exclude allergic, fungal, and chemical conjunctivitis before initiating treatment. Viral is most common overall and prevalent in summer. **History:** Risk factors: Overcrowding, exposure to infected persons, or contaminated multidose vials of eye drops. Symptoms: Serous discharge if viral, purulent if bacterial, sticky eyelids, itching and foreign body sensation in eye. There is no pain or loss of visual acuity **Physical Exam:** Conjunctival injection, ocular discharge (mucopurulent discharge—suggestive of bacterial infection), sticky lids, and normal acuity. • Look for red flags that suggest intraocular infection (pain with eye movements and visual acuity loss), acuity should be normal, lid margins and lashes show crusting, conjunctival injection • Cornea—epithelial defects and keratitis suggest HSV **Diagnosis:** Clinical diagnosis • However, it is important to determine the cause behind infectious conjunctivitis (gonococcal, nongonococcal, chlamydial, viral) based on history and physical exam. • Gram stain and culture is indicated for severe infection, neonatal conjunctivitis, chronic or recurrent conjunctivitis, or suspected gonococcal conjunctivitis **Management:** • Refer to ophthalmologist if there are features like pain, blurred vision, or hyper-purulent discharge • If viral, use artificial tears and cold compresses • If bacterial with more than mild symptoms, use topical antibiotics like ciprofloxacin or erythromycin
Additional Considerations	***N. gonorrhoeae:*** Medical emergency, as corneal involvement can lead to blindness. Hyper-purulent discharge. Gram stain shows Gram-negative intracellular diplococci. Treat with IM or IV ceftriaxone and consult ophthalmology. ***C. trachomatis:*** Mucopurulent infection in newborns. Diagnose with NAATs. Treat with erythromycin or azithromycin ointment for 3–4 weeks. *C. trachomatis* also causes **trachoma**, leading worldwide cause of preventable blindness. **Adenovirus:** Copious watery discharge and redness, often bilateral. Also presents with severe irritation and preauricular lymphadenopathy. Contagious and common in children attending daycare. Self-limiting.

Eye Infection Mini-Cases

Cases	Key Findings
Orbital Cellulitis	**Hx/PE:** Occurs in children and adults due to trauma or sinusitis. Risk factors include immunocompromised states and diabetes. Symptoms and Signs: Acute-onset fever, pain with eye movement and tenderness around eye area, proptosis, decreased extraocular movement, and diplopia (due to injury to extraocular muscles). **Diagnostics:** Clinical diagnosis • Obtain blood and tissue fluid culture. • Obtain imaging (CT or MRI) to confirm diagnosis, assess for drainable focus, and rule out cavernous sinus thrombosis. **Management:** • Admit for IV antibiotics and ophthalmology/ENT consult. • Treat empirically until culture results. • Drain abscesses if present. **Discussion:** **Preseptal cellulitis** should be distinguished from orbital cellulitis. Preseptal cellulitis presents with eyelid edema that may extend to the brow, but there is no pain with eye movements or diplopia. **Orbital cellulitis** has eyelid edema limited to superior orbital boundary, pain with eye movements, limited extraocular eye movements and possible diplopia.

Eye Infection Mini-Cases (continued)

Orbital Cellulitis	Cavernous sinus thrombosis is a medical emergency if orbital cellulitis spreads to the cavernous sinus behind the orbit causing thrombosis. The cavernous sinus contains cranial nerves III, IV, and the first two divisions of V, along with the carotid artery. Cranial nerve VI lies adjacent to it. Thus, thrombosis can cause complete ophthalmoplegia, which can extend to the contralateral side because the cavernous sinuses are connected. Most common pathogens causing cellulitis include streptococci and staphylococci (including MRSA), and *H. influenzae* in children. Suspect **mucormycosis** in patients with diabetic ketoacidosis or immunocompromised patients with palatal or nasal mucosal ulceration. Mucormycosis is often associated with cavernous sinus thrombosis and should be treated with amphotericin B and surgical debridement.
Acute Dacryocystitis	**Hx:** Pain and redness at inner corner of eye. **PE:** Tenderness and erythema in medial canthus. Possible fever. **Diagnostics:** Clinical diagnosis. **Management:** Empiric antibiotics to prevent orbital cellulitis.
Herpes Simplex Keratitis	**Hx:** Risk factors: Prior history of HSV, immunocompromised states. Symptoms: Pain, blurred vision, tearing, and redness. **PE:** Corneal vesicles and dendritic ulcers. **Diagnostics:** Clinical diagnosis • Epithelial scrapings reveal multinucleated giant cells. **Management:** • Treat with oral antivirals (acyclovir, famciclovir) or topical antivirals (acyclovir, trifluridine, ganciclovir). • Episodes generally self-limited. **Discussion:** Reactivation of latent herpes simplex causes corneal infection and is the leading cause of corneal blindness in developed countries. It can be recurrent in immunocompromised patients.
Contact Lens Keratitis	**Hx:** Pain and redness of eye and history of contact lens use. **PE:** Opacification and ulceration of cornea. **Diagnostics:** Clinical diagnosis. **Management:** Immediately remove contact lens and treat with topical broad-spectrum antibiotics such as fluoroquinolones. **Discussion:** Emergent infection in contact lens wearers, commonly caused by *Pseudomonas*. Other contact lens–associated adverse events, such as papillary conjunctivitis and corneal hypoxia, are not bacterial infections and are inflammatory reactions caused by mechanical irritation.

Ear Infection Mini-Case

Cases	Key Findings
Otitis Media	See Pediatric Chapter
Otitis Externa	**Hx:** Pain and pruritus of outer ear. Often in children and adults who spend a lot of time in water (called "swimmer's ear") **PE:** • Tenderness with movement of tragus/pinna • Ear canal is erythematous and edematous • Purulent discharge is possible **Diagnostics:** Clinical diagnosis **Management:** • Topical agents (fluoroquinolone drops, steroid drops, or combination agents) • Keep ear clean, dry, and avoid submerging in water • If case is severe or refractory, can culture ear • If patient appears toxic, order CT to assess for deeper involvement **Discussion:** Patients with diabetes are at risk for **malignant (necrotizing) otitis externa** which is almost always caused by *Pseudomonas aeruginosa*. This is an invasive infection that can lead to osteomyelitis, meningitis, and brain abscess. Patients should be admitted for IV anti-pseudomonal beta-lactams and a CT scan to rule out cartilage and/or bone involvement.

NEUROTOXIC CLOSTRIDIAL INFECTIONS

CASE 20 | Tetanus

A 34-year-old man presents with new onset of facial spasms and jaw stiffness. Ten days ago, he stepped on a nail in his backyard which pierced his foot. He has no other medical problems and is not taking any medications or drugs. He has not seen a health care provider in over 15 years and does not recall when he last received his tetanus vaccine. On exam, the wound contains a lot of debris and dirt.

Conditions with Similar Presentations	**Drug-induced spasms:** Certain drugs can cause dystonia, like phenothiazine antipsychotics, but this can be differentiated from a tetanus reaction because eye deviations will be present, while no eye deviations are seen with tetanus.
	Neuroleptic malignant syndrome (NMS): Patient will present with muscle rigidity, which may mimic tetanus; however, fever, altered mental status, and recently taking an antipsychotic or antiemetic distinguishes NMS from tetanus.
	Trismus due to dental infection: Deep space neck infections can inflame muscles of mastication causing jaw stiffness. Fascial spasms would be absent and a dental source seen on exam and/or imaging.
Initial Diagnostic Tests	Clinical diagnosis (see Discussion for clinical features)
Next Steps in Management	Tetanus toxoid vaccine and tetanus immune globulin
Discussion	Tetanus results in a neurologic syndrome caused by the *Clostridium tetani* toxin, tetanospasmin. Tetanospasmin ascends into the spinal cord and brain stem where it enters inhibitory neurons and blocks release of their neurotransmitters. This results in uninhibited firing of lower motor neurons and sympathetic neurons. This causes facial spasms resulting in a "sardonic smile" (risus sardonicus), inability to open the jaw (lockjaw), extreme back extension (opisthotonus) and sympathetic lability with hypertension, tachycardia, and other arrhythmias, and fever from peripheral vasoconstriction. Consciousness is not altered. The organism is ubiquitous in soil. Wounds prone to tetanus are punctures or crush injuries (produce an anaerobic environment) or contaminated with dirt/feces (high inoculum of organism).
	History: Risk factors: Unvaccinated and tetanus-prone wound
	Symptoms: Fever, elevated blood pressure, muscle spasms, lockjaw
	Physical Exam: Trismus, lockjaw, spasms, hypertension, fever
	Diagnostics: Clinical diagnosis
	Management:
	• Patients with tetanus by definition have not received adequate immunization, which includes a primary series of three tetanus toxoid injections and boosters every 10 years. Therefore, they must be given passive immunity using tetanus immune globulin (TIG), which contains high levels of antibody to tetanus toxin.
	• Tetanus toxoid is also given to produce active immunity toward prevention of future episodes.
	• Cases are reportable to the local health authorities.
	• Hospitalization is required, and the wound must be debrided.
	• Benzodiazepines are used to address muscle spasms and sedate the patient.
	• Ventilator use may be indicated if spasms of the diaphragm inhibit respirations.

CASE 20 | Tetanus *(continued)*

Discussion	**Algorithm for Tetanus Prophylaxis**

Algorithm for Tetanus Prophylaxis

Tetanus Prophylaxis

- **>3 or equal - lifetime tetanus doses**
  - **Clean/Mild Wound** Tetanus, toxoid vaccine only if last dose was greater than or equal to 10 years ago — NO TIG
  - **Dirty/Major Wound** Tetanus toxoid vaccine only if last booster was over greater than or equal to 5 years ago — NO TIG
- **<3 lifetime tetanus doses or unsure or none**
  - **Clean/Mild Wound** Tetanus toxoid vaccine only — NO TIG
  - **Dirty/Major Wound** Tetanus toxoid vaccine — YES TIG

Additional Considerations	**Pediatric Considerations:** Neonates (<28 days old) without passive immunity from their mother are at increased risk for tetanus and may have more nonspecific physical exam findings, such as inability to feed, muscle spasms, or stiffness.
	Prevention: The number of cases of tetanus in the US have been dramatically reduced by immunization, now <40 cases a year.
	The DTap (diphtheria toxoid, tetanus toxoid, and acellular pertussis vaccine) vaccine five-dose series should be given at 2, 4, 6, 15–18 months, and 4–6 years.
	The Tdap vaccine should be given to adolescents 11–12 years of age, with booster every 10 years. All adults should get Tdap one time.
	Pregnant women should receive the Tdap vaccine (at 27–36 weeks' gestational age) for every pregnancy; time of prior Tdap vaccine does not change this recommendation.

Mini-Case

Botulism	**Hx/PE:** Risk factors: Ingestion of honey or home-canned goods contaminated with *Clostridium botulinum*, which makes a preformed botulinum toxin. Symptoms start 12–36 hours after toxin ingestion.
	• Gastrointestinal symptoms present initially, if foodborne.
	• Dry mouth and eyes.
	• Symmetric descending paralysis.
	• Cranial nerve motor palsies (III, IV, VI, VII). Mydriasis.
	• No fever or altered mental status.
	Diagnostics: Clinical diagnosis
	Management: Equine antitoxin
	Discussion: *C. botulinum* is ubiquitous in the soil and can contaminate foods, especially if they are placed in an anaerobic environment (such as home canning). It produces botulinum toxin which prevents acetylcholine release from neurons of the motor system and parasympathetic system. This results in cranial nerve palsies, mydriasis, and dry mouth and eyes. In infants, botulism presents as peripheral nerve weakness ("floppy baby") or dysphagia, poor feeding, unable to cry, respiratory distress. Honey should be avoided in infants until 1 year of age to prevent this possibility.

8

Hematology and Oncology

Lead Authors: Eshana E. Shah, MD; Shikha Jain, MD
Contributors: Sofia Ahmed, MD; Minji Seok, MD; Analisa Taylor, MD; Anthony Carrera, MD

ANEMIA

Anemia is defined as a hemoglobin (Hb) or hematocrit (Hct) below the lower limit of normal. It varies by lab assay, but generally is Hb <13 in males and <12 in females, or Hct <42 in males and <37 in females. Anemia is usually categorized by size of red blood cells (RBCs) using mean corpuscular volume (MCV).

Mean corpuscular hemoglobin concentration (MCHC) is an indicator of hemoglobin levels. Erythrocytes or RBCs containing the normal amount of hemoglobin (normal MCHC) are called normochromic. When the MCHC is abnormally low they are called hypochromic (e.g., iron deficiency anemia), and when the MCHC is abnormally high, hyperchromic (e.g., B12 and folate deficiency).

Red cell distribution width (RDW) measures difference in the volume and size of the RBCs. High RDW means increased variation in RBC size (e.g., early iron deficiency anemia, sickle cell, sideroblastic anemia, and dimorphic anemia [e.g., mixed iron and folate deficiency]).

Mean corpuscular volume (MCV) is more commonly used as an indicator of RBC size. Normal MCV is approximately 80–100 fL, with smaller cells being referred to as "microcytic," larger cells being referred to as "macrocytic," and cells within the range referred to as "normocytic."

- **Microcytic anemia:** MCV<80 fL
  - Iron deficiency, thalassemia, sideroblastic anemia
  - Borderline low MCV may be seen in anemia of chronic disease.
- **Macrocytic anemias:** MCV >100 fL.
  - **Megaloblastic:** Presence of hypersegmented neutrophils (DNA synthesis is impaired usually from folate or B12 deficiency)
  - **Nonmegaloblastic:** Neutrophils normal (DNA synthesis is unimpaired—e.g., liver disease, hypothyroidism, alcohol, drugs [methotrexate, hydroxyurea, certain chemotherapies], myelodysplastic syndrome)
- **Normocytic anemia:** MCV 80–100 fL
  - **Underproduction (reticulocyte count <2%)**
    - Anemia of chronic disease: mildly low MCV or normocytic; total body iron is normal but sequestered and unable to be used by RBC precursors.
    - Chronic kidney disease (CKD): ↓ erythropoietin
    - Bone marrow failure: caused by failure or the destruction of myeloid stem cells (e.g., radiation, medications, viral infections [HIV, parvovirus B19], idiopathic, and genetic disorders). Findings include: ↓ reticulocyte count, ↑ erythropoietin, pancytopenia.
  - **Destruction/Loss (reticulocyte count >2%)**
    - **Bleeding**
    - **Hemolytic anemias:** Erythrocytes may be destroyed intravascularly or extravascularly and due to intrinsic or extrinsic problems.
      - Hemolysis may be classified by site of destruction:
        - Intravascular (hemolysis within blood vessels): ↑ total/indirect bilirubin, ↑ LDH, ↑ reticulocyte count, ↓ haptoglobin (binds to Hb and destroyed by macrophages), ↑ urine hemosiderin
        - Extravascular (hemolysis within the spleen): e.g., hereditary spherocytosis
        - Both intravascular and extravascular hemolysis occur in:
          - Sickle cell disease
          - Glucose-6-phosphate dehydrogenase (G6PD) deficiency (hemolysis occurs after oxidative stress)
      - Hemolysis may also be classified if abnormality is intrinsic or extrinsic to erythrocyte:
        - Intrinsic (a problem with the erythrocyte itself leading to hemolysis): membrane defects (hereditary spherocytosis, paroxysmal nocturnal hemoglobinuria), enzyme defects (G6PD deficiency, pyruvate kinase deficiency), hemoglobinopathies (sickle cell disease).
        - Extrinsic (erythrocytes normal but another process causes hemolysis):
          - Microangiopathic: arteriole and capillary obstructed or narrowed, causing passing RBCs to be sheared (e.g., DIC, TTP/HUS, HELLP syndrome, malignant hypertension). These are medical emergencies. **Schistocytes** seen on peripheral smear.

- Macroangiopathic (e.g., mechanical heart valves).
- Infections (e.g., malaria, babesiosis).
- Immune: alloimmune (transfusion reactions) vs. autoimmune (AIHA)—see below.
  - **Autoimmune hemolytic anemia (AIHA):** Autoantibodies (Ab) are formed against normally present erythrocyte membrane antigens(s), resulting in hemolysis. These immunoglobulins can be identified using a direct and indirect **Coombs test (direct antibody test [DAT] positive).**

Warm AIHA	Cold AIHA
• IgG-mediated chronic process • Ab most active at "warm" body temperature • May see spherocytes on smear	• IgM mediated acute process • Ab most active at "cold" room temperature
Causes: • Autoimmune diseases (e.g., SLE) • Neoplasms (lymphoma, CLL) • Drugs (α-methyldopa) • Idiopathic	Causes: • Infections (e.g., *Mycoplasma pneumoniae*, infectious mononucleosis) • Neoplasms (lymphoma, CLL) • Idiopathic

MCV Approach to Anemia

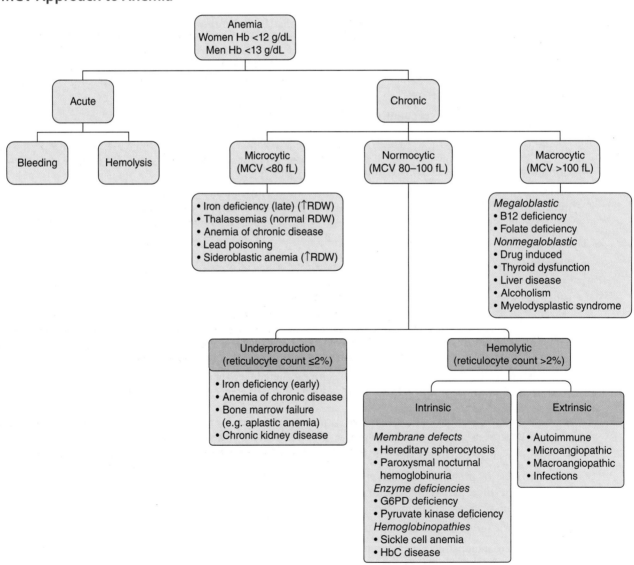

Key Associated Findings and Anemia Differential Diagnoses

Anemia with Key Associated Findings	Diagnoses
History of heavy menses, GI bleed, pica, esophageal webs (Plummer-Vinson syndrome) Spoon nails (koilonychia), or cheilosis Lab findings: ↓ Hb, ↓ ferritin (<30 ng/mL), ↓ iron, ↑ TIBC, ↓ transferrin saturation (<16%)	Iron deficiency anemia (IDA)
Chipped paint exposure, encephalopathy, abdominal colic Foot/wrist drop, gingival lines Lab findings: ↓ MCV, erythrocyte basophilic stippling, sideroblastic anemia, ↑ blood lead levels	Lead poisoning
Hereditary or acquired (alcohol, lead poisoning, vitamin B6 deficiency, malignancy, isoniazid) Lab findings: ↓ MCV, ↓ Hb, ↑ iron, Prussian blue staining with ringed sideroblasts on blood smear Reproduced with permission from Lichtman MA, Shafer MS, Felgar RE, Wang N, Lichtman's Atlas of Hematology 2016. New York, NY: McGraw-Hill 2017.	Sideroblastic Anemia (defect in heme metabolism)
Asian, African, or Mediterranean descent Family history of anemia Lab findings: ↓ MCV, normal iron studies, normal RDW	Thalassemia
History of autoimmune or inflammatory disease Lab findings: ↑ ferritin and ↓ TIBC, mildly ↓ or normal MCV	Anemia of chronic disease
Travel to endemic regions	Malaria
Family history sickle cell disease Priapism, dactylitis Asplenia, avascular necrosis (AVN), or pulmonary HTN	Sickle cell disease
Drug exposure (sulfas, antimalarial), infection, food (fava beans) African or Middle Eastern decent Lab findings: Heinz bodies, bite cells	G6PD Deficiency
Lab findings: ↑ indirect/total bilirubin, LDH, reticulocyte count, ↓ haptoglobin	Hemolytic anemia (intravascular)
Lab findings: pancytopenia, ↓ reticulocyte count, ↑ erythropoietin	Aplastic anemia
If Hb <7.0 consider the following five etiologies:	• Chronic kidney disease • Acute or chronic bleed • Acute or chronic hemolysis • Megaloblastic anemia • Aplastic anemia

CASE 1 | Iron Deficiency Anemia (IDA)

A 34-year-old woman with uterine fibroids and heavy menses presents with several months of progressive fatigue. She has recently been craving ice chips and has had difficulty sleeping due to an urge to move her legs at night. On exam, she has conjunctival pallor and spoon-shaped nails (koilonychia). Labs show Hb 8 g/dL and MCV 71 fL.

Conditions with Similar Presentations	**Sideroblastic anemia:** Also causes microcytic anemia with a high RDW but has a normal or ↑ iron level. Causes are hereditary or acquired (e.g., lead poisoning, alcohol, vitamin B6 deficiency). Ringed sideroblasts on peripheral smear or bone marrow are diagnostic.
	Thalassemias: Also cause microcytic anemia, but the RDW and iron level is normal. These are hereditary disorders and typically present at a younger age.
	Anemia of chronic disease: May cause a borderline microcytic anemia but not as low as in this patient. Unlike IDA, serum ferritin would be ↑. It is seen in chronic infectious/inflammatory conditions.
Initial Diagnostic Tests	Confirm diagnosis with CBC and iron studies (iron, ferritin, TIBC, transferrin saturation).
Next Steps in Management	• Iron replacement therapy • Evaluate and treat source of anemia (inadequate nutritional intake, blood loss)
Discussion	IDA is the most common cause of anemia and occurs because decreased body iron stores are inadequate for heme synthesis. IDA is a microcytic, hypochromic anemia that can be caused by nutritional deficiency, poor absorption (malabsorption syndromes), or chronic blood loss (e.g., colon cancer). **History:** • Fatigue, dyspnea on exertion, dizziness, pica symptoms (cravings for ice, dirt, clay, or other nonfood substances that contain iron) • More common in children and women of childbearing age **Physical Exam:** • Conjunctival pallor (if Hb <9), palmar pallor (if Hb <7), cheilosis, koilonychia (spoon nails) **Diagnostics:** • Iron studies: ↓ ferritin, ↓ iron, ↑ TIBC, ↓ transferrin saturation • CBC with microcytic (MCV <80), hypochromic (central pallor) anemia **Management:** • Iron repletion with either oral (preferred) or IV therapy (if severe and symptomatic or patient cannot tolerate oral iron) • Evaluate for underlying source of iron deficiency: inadequate intake vs. malabsorption vs. blood loss (chronic menorrhagia, GI bleed) • GI evaluation is warranted in males or postmenopausal females presenting with iron deficiency anemia • Blood transfusion if Hb <7 or if severe cardiovascular symptoms secondary to anemia (e.g., chest pain)	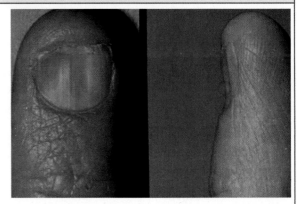 Koilonychia. (Reproduced with permission from Lichtman MA, Shafer MS, Felgar RE, Wang N, Lichtman's Atlas of Hematology 2016. New York, NY: McGraw-Hill 2017.) 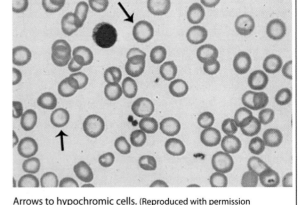 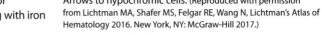 Arrows to hypochromic cells. (Reproduced with permission from Lichtman MA, Shafer MS, Felgar RE, Wang N, Lichtman's Atlas of Hematology 2016. New York, NY: McGraw-Hill 2017.)
Additional Considerations	**Pediatric Considerations:** • IDA can occur in exclusively breastfed infants if not supplemented with iron • Can occur in children who begin consuming high amounts of cow's milk or nonfortified formulas as part of their diet prior to 12 months of age • Screening for IDA with Hb level is done in all infants 9–12 months per CDC recommendations **Obstetric Considerations:** • Pregnant women have physiologic anemia secondary to volume expansion of plasma during pregnancy and increased iron requirements for increased RBC production. • Most pregnancy supplements will contain iron to ensure adequate fetal growth and development.

CASE 2 | Macrocytic Anemia (Vitamin B12 [Cobalamin] Deficiency)

A 37-year-old previously healthy woman presents with chronic fatigue and worsening forgetfulness that is starting to affect her job. She also reports numbness and tingling of her bilateral lower extremities. She has no past medical or surgical history. She gets regular exercise and has followed a strict vegan diet for 8 years. She is a nonsmoker and has one to two alcoholic drinks per week. Physical exam is notable for conjunctival pallor, a swollen, beefy red tongue with absence of papillae, hyperreflexia, decreased sensation of her bilateral lower extremities, and an ataxic gait. There is a positive Romberg sign. Notable labs include hemoglobin 8 g/dL, hematocrit 24%, MCV 115 fL, and decreased absolute reticulocyte count.

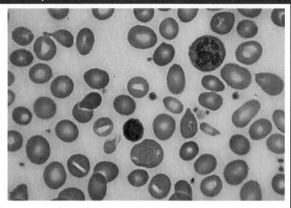

Peripheral blood smear with sickle cells. (Reproduced with permission from Lichtman MA, Shafer MS, Felgar RE, Wang N, Lichtman's Atlas of Hematology 2016. New York, NY: McGraw-Hill Education 2017.)

Conditions with Similar Presentations	**Folate deficiency:** Is also a megaloblastic, macrocytic anemia; however, neurologic impairment will not be present, and labs will show low folic acid levels and normal methylmalonic acid. Folate deficiency can develop in weeks, whereas B12 deficiency develops over years. **Alcoholism/liver disease:** Can cause macrocytic, non-megaloblastic anemia. Patient will have a history of significant alcohol intake and/or signs of chronic liver disease (ascites, jaundice). **Myelodysplastic syndrome (MDS):** Can present with macrocytic, non-megaloblastic anemia, bleeding, or infection depending on the cell lines primarily affected. Labs can show thrombocytopenia and lymphopenia. The peripheral smear shows dysplastic cells and nucleated RBCs. **Drugs:** Can cause isolated macrocytic, non-megaloblastic anemia. Common offending drugs include hydroxyurea, chemotherapy (methotrexate, purine or pyrimidine analogs), antiretrovirals (zidovudine), anti-epileptics (phenytoin, valproic acid), and antibiotics (TMP-SMX). **Reticulocytosis:** As a robust response to acute hemorrhage or hemolysis, will increase the MCV. The macrocytosis is due to the larger size of reticulocytes compared to RBCs. There will be no megaloblastic changes.
Initial Diagnostic Testing	• Confirm diagnosis: CBC showing macrocytic anemia (MCV often >115), peripheral smear showing hypersegmented neutrophils, and low serum B12 level. • Consider: Methylmalonic acid, homocysteine levels, anti-intrinsic factor antibody (IF-Ab).
Next Steps in Management	Oral (unless due to malabsorption) or parenteral supplementation with vitamin B12 (cyanocobalamin)

Discussion	Vitamin B12 deficiency is a nutritional deficiency caused by inadequate oral intake or malabsorption that causes macrocytic anemia and/or neuropsychiatric deficits. Megaloblastic anemia is exclusive to B12 and folate deficiencies due to impaired DNA synthesis. A peripheral smear will show hypersegmented neutrophils. Non-megaloblastic macrocytic anemias will have normal neutrophils.
	• B12 is important in the synthesis of myelin, and deficiency leads to demyelination of the peripheral and central nervous system (dorsal/posterior and lateral columns of the spinal cord, and neurocognitive changes). It is marked by morphologic abnormalities seen in the bone marrow called megaloblastic changes.
	• Vitamin B12 deficiency affects up to 5% of younger patients but is more frequent in older adults >60 years old. There are several causes of vitamin B12 deficiency:
	  • Inadequate oral intake: B12 is found in animal products (meat, eggs, dairy), thus strict vegans are at risk for deficiency. B12 deficiency can develop within 2–3 years once body stores are depleted.
	  • **Pernicious anemia:** Gastric parietal cells secrete intrinsic factor (IF) which binds vitamin B12 for absorption. Pernicious anemia is characterized by autoantibodies against IF or gastric parietal cells so B12 is not absorbed.
	  • Gastrectomy or bariatric surgery: similar to pernicious anemia, these patients are unable to produce IF.
	  • Intestinal malabsorption: the B12-IF complex is absorbed in the ileum. Malabsorption can occur due to small bowel intestinal overgrowth (SIBO), inflammatory bowel disease, or small bowel resection. Malabsorption due to GI infections such as tapeworms is common in developing areas.
	  • Pancreatic insufficiency: insufficient protease production results in inability to unbind ingested B12 resulting in impaired B12-IF binding and decreased absorption in terminal ileum.
	  • Medications: acid blockers (PPI, H2-blockers, or antacids) which increase the gastric pH and impair B12-IF binding. Metformin affects ileal absorption of B12.

CASE 2 | Macrocytic Anemia (Vitamin B12 [Cobalamin] Deficiency) *(continued)*

Discussion	**History:** • May be asymptomatic, or present with symptomatic anemia (fatigue, dyspnea on exertion), or neurologic symptoms (sensory deficits notably peripheral neuropathy, ataxic gait, or cognitive impairment). • Review history (e.g., vegan diet, bariatric surgery, IBD) and medications (metformin, PPI) for cause of macrocytosis and B12 deficiency **Physical Exam:** • Depending on severity of anemia, patients may present with conjunctival pallor and/or a flow murmur. • Beefy red swollen tongue (**glossitis**) with a smooth surface (e.g., absent papillae) can be seen. • Neurologic exam can demonstrate various deficits including mood changes or irritability, memory issues, impaired position/vibration sensation, gait ataxia. **Diagnostics:** • CBC with anemia and ↑ MCV >115 is suggestive of a megaloblastic disorder such as vitamin B12 or folate deficiency • Peripheral smear with hypersegmented neutrophils. • ↓ Serum B12 level • If marginally low B12, check: ↑ homocysteine, ↑ methylmalonic acid • Check for presence of IF-Ab to evaluate for pernicious anemia in susceptible populations (patients with other autoimmune conditions or elderly) to assess utility of oral B12 administration **Management:** • Intramuscular (IM) vitamin B12 injections initially if symptoms of neuropathy or evidence of malabsorption (e.g., pernicious anemia) • Oral supplementation when B12 deficiency is caused by poor dietary intake and those without absorption issues • Patients can present with multiple nutritional deficiencies, with most common being concurrent folate or iron deficiency
Additional Considerations	**Complications:** Prolonged B12 deficiency can result in irreversible CNS and peripheral nervous system injury.

CASE 3 | Autoimmune Hemolytic Anemia

A 33-year-old woman presents to clinic with generalized weakness and fatigue for the past month. She also reported that she has had pain in her elbows, hands, and knees for the past 6 months. The patient's vitals are temperature of 38.0°C, pulse 97/min, respirations 17/min, blood pressure 105/62 mmHg, and SpO$_2$ 95% on room air exam. Physical exam is notable for conjunctival pallor, splenomegaly, and a malar rash sparing the nasolabial fold. Labs notable for Hb 7.4, reticulocytes >2%, ↑ total and indirect bilirubin, ↑ LDH, ↓ haptoglobin, peripheral blood smear with spherocytes, no schistocytes, and urinalysis with hemoglobin but no RBCs.

Conditions with Similar Presentations	**HIV:** Can cause hemolytic anemia but would not have malar rash. **Hypersplenism:** Would have splenomegaly and anemia, but would also have leukopenia and thrombocytopenia. Causes include cirrhosis (alcohol, viral hepatitis), infections (EBV, CMV, malaria) hematologic malignancies (lymphomas, leukemias, myeloma). **Hereditary spherocytosis (HS):** May see spherocytes, but Coombs would be negative. It is a genetic defect of spectrin so would not present in adulthood. **Mechanical (macroangiopathic) hemolysis** (associated with heart valves) and **microangiopathic hemolytic anemias (DIC/TTP/HUS):** Also cause a hemolytic anemia, but peripheral smear will have schistocytes due to mechanical shearing (intravascular hemolysis) and thrombocytopenia.
Initial Diagnostic Tests	• Confirm with direct antiglobulin test (DAT) or Coombs test • Also check CBC with differential, peripheral smear, LDH, haptoglobin, bilirubin
Next Steps in Management	Treat warm AIHA with corticosteroids
Discussion	AIHA occurs secondary to development of autoantibodies against the patient's own normal RBCs. RBCs are coated with autoantibodies which are subsequently cleared by the liver and spleen. When the RBCs lyse, they release hemoglobin and LDH. AIHA can be primary/idiopathic (about 50% of cases) or secondary to another underlying condition (e.g., systemic lupus erythematosus [SLE]). • Warm hemolytic anemia is more common and is an IgG-mediated chronic process caused by autoimmune diseases (e.g., SLE). • Cold hemolytic anemia: IgM autoantibodies can lead to symptoms when the patient is exposed to cold. (IgM is a potent activator of the classical complement pathway which leads to complemented-mediated lysis of RBCs).

CASE 3 | Autoimmune Hemolytic Anemia *(continued)*

Discussion	**History and Physical Exam:**
	• Signs and symptoms of anemia like pallor, fatigue, dyspnea on exertion
	• **Warm AIHA:**
	  • May be associated with leukemia, lymphoma, SLE, rheumatoid arthritis, and inflammatory bowel disease
	  • Splenomegaly
	• **Cold AIHA:**
	  • May be associated with infections with pathogens such as mycoplasma, Epstein-Barr virus
	  • May see acrocyanosis in distal extremities
	Diagnostics:
	• CBC: usually normocytic anemia (MCV may be higher if reticulocytes very high), smear with spherocytes (warm type), high RDW
	• Reticulocytes >2%
	• Hemolysis labs: ↑ LDH, ↓ haptoglobin, ↑ total and indirect bilirubin
	• Direct antiglobulin test (DAT) or Coombs test positive for IgG autoantibodies (warm AIHA) or an IgM-directed antibody against the I/i carbohydrate on the RBC surface complement antibodies (cold AIHA)
	• Should evaluate for underlying cause of hemolysis (e.g., G6PD, sickle cell disease, infections, SLE, malignancy)
	Management:
	• Warm AIHA: corticosteroids are first-line, splenectomy considered for recurrent disease, can consider other immunosuppressants (e.g., azathioprine, rituximab)
	• Cold AIHA: avoidance of cold exposures, rituximab for more severe disease, splenectomy less effective
	• Folic acid
	• Treat underlying cause
	• RBC transfusion if severe or symptomatic anemia

Additional Considerations	**Pediatric Considerations:** AIHA has a better prognosis in children and is generally self-limiting. **Paroxysmal cold hemoglobinuria** (aka Donath-Landsteiner syndrome) is a rare form of AIHA, though more common in children. Binding of autoantibodies occurs in the cold but intravascular hemolysis occurs when warmed. Causes include viral upper respiratory infections.

Anemia Mini Cases

Anemia of Chronic Disease (ACD)	**Hx/PE:** If symptomatic may present with symptoms or signs of anemia. It is associated with autoimmune and inflammatory disorders (IBD, SLE, vasculitis), chronic infections (HIV and HCV), and malignancies. Exam often unremarkable or findings related to underlying cause. Often found incidentally on CBC. **Diagnostics:** • Normocytic or borderline microcytic anemia with a low reticulocyte count • ↑ Ferritin level due to chronic inflammation • ↓ TIBC because the iron stores are elevated so liver downregulates production of transferrin **Management:** • Identify and treat underlying inflammatory process **Discussion:** Anemia of chronic disease (ACD), also known as anemia of chronic inflammation, is seen in conditions causing chronic inflammation such as autoimmune diseases, chronic liver or kidney disease, infections, or cancers. • Systemic, chronic inflammation causes elevated acute phase reactants such as interleukin-6 (IL-6) and ferritin • IL-6 can promote increased synthesis and release of hepcidin from the liver, which decreases iron absorption from the gut and prevents release of intracellular iron from macrophages resulting in low serum iron levels • Elevated ferritin promotes increased intracellular storage of iron, further contributing to low serum iron levels
Hereditary Spherocytosis (HS)	**Hx/PE:** • Symptoms and signs of chronic hemolysis (e.g., pallor, jaundice, splenomegaly, dark urine) • Family history of hemolytic anemia

Anemia Mini Cases *(continued)*

Hereditary Spherocytosis (HS)	**Diagnostics:** • CBC showing anemia with elevated MCHC (often >36), and ↑ reticulocyte count • Hemolysis labs: ↑ total and indirect bilirubin, ↑ LDH, ↓ haptoglobin, negative Coombs test • Peripheral blood smear showing spherocytes (small RBCs without central pallor) • Confirmation with osmotic fragility testing and low eosin-5'-maleimide (EMA) staining of RBCs **Management:** • RBC transfusion if severe or symptomatic anemia • Folate supplementation • Splenectomy if transfusion-dependent	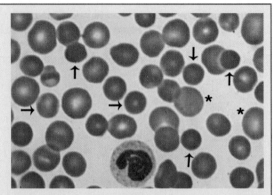 Spherocytes. (Reproduced with permission from Lichtman MA, Shafer MS, Felgar RE, Wang N, Lichtman's Atlas of Hematology 2016. New York, NY: McGraw-Hill 2017.)
	Discussion: • An intrinsic cause of hemolysis, due to defects in red cell membrane skeleton proteins (e.g., ankyrin, spectrin, band 3, or band 4.2 proteins) that decrease deformability of RBCs and shorten their life span	
Glucose-6-Phosphate Dehydrogenase (G6PD) Deficiency	**Hx/PE:** • Infants: neonatal hyperbilirubinemia and kernicterus (lethargy, poor muscle tone, apneic episodes, seizure) • Adults: hemolytic episodes triggered by oxidative stress from specific foods, medications, or infection. • Signs of anemia (fatigue, pallor) and hemolysis (jaundice, dark urine). • Jaundice, splenomegaly **Diagnostics:** • ↓ G6PD blood level • CBC showing anemia and ↑ reticulocyte count • Hemolysis labs: ↑ total and indirect bilirubin, ↑ LDH, ↓ haptoglobin • Peripheral blood smear: bite cells (arrows) and Heinz bodies (hemoglobin precipitates)	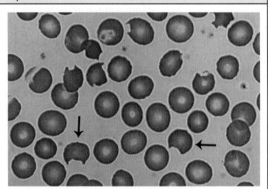 Bite cells. (Reproduced with permission from Lichtman MA, Shafer MS, Felgar RE, Wang N, Lichtman's Atlas of Hematology 2016. New York, NY: McGraw-Hill 2017.)
	Management: • Supportive care (hydration) • RBC transfusion if symptomatic • Phototherapy or exchange transfusion in neonates with severe hyperbilirubinemia • Education on avoidance of triggers such as food (fava beans), medications (nitrofurantoin, dapsone, quinolones, sulfa-containing drugs, sulfonylurea) **Discussion:** Most prevalent in endemic malaria regions and found in people of Mediterranean, African, or Asian descent. X-linked inheritance pattern, affects males > female.	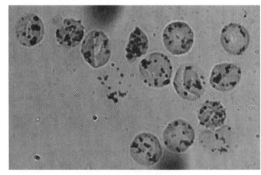 Heinz bodies. (Reproduced with permission from Lichtman MA, Shafer MS, Felgar RE, Wang N, Lichtman's Atlas of Hematology 2016. New York, NY: McGraw-Hill 2017.)

CASE 4 | Sickle Cell Disease (SCD): Vaso-occlusive Crisis (Acute Chest Syndrome)

A 25-year-old man with SCD who initially presented for generalized bony pain develops new-onset shortness of breath 3 days after admission. Vitals show 38.5°C, pulse 118/min, respirations 32/min, blood pressure 102/53 mmHg, and O_2 saturation 91%. Labs show WBC 16,500/mm³ with neutrophil predominance, hemoglobin 5.7 g/dL with MCV 74, LDH 1273 U/L and elevated reticulocytes. He has conjunctival icterus, crackles on lung exam, and CXR shows a new focal infiltrate.

Conditions with Similar Presentations	Hemoglobin electrophoresis will differentiate between below two conditions. **Hemoglobin C disease:** Is a hemoglobinopathy caused by a different mutation in the beta globin. Homozygous patients (HbCC phenotype) present with mild chronic hemolysis, splenomegaly (as opposed to asplenia seen in HbSS), and jaundice. CBC shows a microcytic anemia with an increased MCHC. Smear will show target cells and Hb C crystals. Patients with combination sickle cell and hemoglobin C disease (HbSC) are more symptomatic than HbCC but have less severe sickling and VOC than HbSS. **Alpha- and beta-thalassemia:** May also present with anemia and hemolysis due to mutations in either alpha or beta globin genes but patients do not have sickling. **AIHA:** Can also present with acute anemia and features of hemolysis (jaundice, ↑ total and indirect bilirubin, ↓ haptoglobin) but are Coombs-positive, often occur in setting of underlying autoimmunity or malignancy, and will not have vaso-occulsive complications.
Initial Diagnostic Tests	• Acute chest syndrome is a clinical diagnosis in a patient with SCD • Check CXR +/− CT to evaluate for infiltrate • Consider: arterial blood gas (ABG) and evaluate for precipitating cause
Next Steps in Management	• Supportive care (fluids, pain control, oxygen, incentive spirometry) • Empiric antibiotics • Exchange transfusion

Discussion	Sickle cell anemia occurs due to a single nucleotide mutation leading to an amino acid substitution (E6V) in the beta globin gene. It is inherited in an autosomal codominant pattern. Homozygous inheritance produces SCD, and heterozygotes (carriers) have sickle cell trait. The geographic distribution of SCD parallels malaria, as shorter-lived RBCs are thought to provide a survival advantage against malaria. SCD causes both intravascular and extravascular hemolysis. Severely painful vaso-occlusive crises are experienced by patients with sickle cell anemia and can be accompanied by medical emergencies such as stroke, acute chest syndrome, priapism, as well as dactylitis and avascular necrosis.
	
	History:
	Acute chest syndrome can present with chest pain, dyspnea or fever, and often occurs several days after a vaso-occlusive pain crisis. Must assess for precipitating causes.
	
	Physical Exam: Pulmonary crackles, tachycardia, tachypnea
	
	Diagnostics:
	SCD: Diagnosis confirmed with hemoglobin electrophoresis (measure HbS concentration)
	
	Vaso-occlusive crisis (VOC):
	• Confirmed by patient's history (no labs to determine presence of pain)
	• CBC: ↓ Hb, smear with sickle and target cells
	• ↑ reticulocyte count, ↑ indirect bilirubin, ↑ LDH
	
	Acute chest syndrome:
	• Check CXR +/− CT to evaluate for infiltrate
	• Consider ABG to evaluate for hypoxia
	• Evaluate for precipitant: infection (blood culture, urine culture), CT to evaluate for pulmonary embolus
	
	Management:
	• Painful vaso-occlusive crisis: supportive care (fluids, pain control with NSAIDs/opioids, oxygen, incentive spirometry, hydroxyurea)
	• Acute chest syndrome
	  • Treat underlying cause (e.g., empiric antibiotics for pneumonia)
	  • Consider exchange transfusion in patients not responding to the above measures
	• Indications for exchange transfusion include acute chest syndrome, acute stroke, multiorgan failure, and severe priapism.
	
	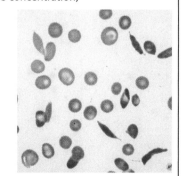
	Peripheral blood smear with sickle cells. (Reproduced with permission from Laposata M. Laposata's Laboratory Medicine Diagnosis of Disease in Clinical Laboratory, 3rd ed. New York, NY: McGraw Hill; 2019.)

CASE 4 | Sickle Cell Disease (SCD): Vaso-occlusive Crisis (Acute Chest Syndrome) *(continued)*

Additional Considerations	**Screening:** Screening usually done as part of neonatal screen with hemoglobin electrophoresis. **Complications:** Patients with SCD can develop complications from vaso-occlusion and hemolysis. **Painful bone crisis:** • Most common vaso-occlusive crisis, which is due to bone marrow ischemia or infarction. • Can be precipitated by dehydration, stress, infection, asthma, acidosis, sleep apnea, high altitude, pregnancy, and menstruation. • Presents with sudden onset of pain in the extremities, chest, and back in adults. In children it can present as dactylitis with pain and swelling in the hands and feet. • It may precede other complications like acute chest syndrome or multiorgan system failure. **Acute chest syndrome:** • Defined as the presence of new pulmonary infiltrates with respiratory complaints and hypoxia, with or without fever • Increased adhesion of sickled red cells to pulmonary vasculature causing vaso-occlusion, V/Q mismatch and hypoxia • Can be precipitated by pneumonia, asthma, pulmonary embolus, or non-pulmonary infections • It has a high mortality and potential for developing into chronic lung disease **Splenic sequestration crisis:** • Result of RBCs accumulating in splenic sinuses leading to rapid enlargement of the spleen. • Usually occurs in children <5 years before auto-splenectomy. • May present with severe abdominal pain and distention, signs of hypovolemia, decreased Hb with elevated reticulocyte count. • Consider splenectomy if recurrent acute splenic sequestration and/or symptomatic hypersplenism. **Aplastic crisis:** • Temporary cessation of RBC production that is typically caused by infection with parvovirus B19, but may also be caused by other infections. • Symptoms of anemia and labs with markedly ↓ Hb and ↓ reticulocytes. • Supportive care (transfusion) while awaiting resolution. **Hepatic sequestration:** • Self-limiting condition that occurs due to vaso-occlusion in hepatic sinusoids and consequent ischemia. • Presents with RUQ pain, hepatomegaly, elevated liver enzymes (AST, ALT), elevated bilirubin, and fever. • Supportive care (hydration, pain control). **Chronic complications:** Include functional asplenia due to chronic splenic vaso-occlusion and auto-splenectomy (increased infection risk with encapsulated organisms), avascular necrosis (AVN), pulmonary hypertension, renal papillary necrosis resulting in chronic kidney disease, and retinopathy. 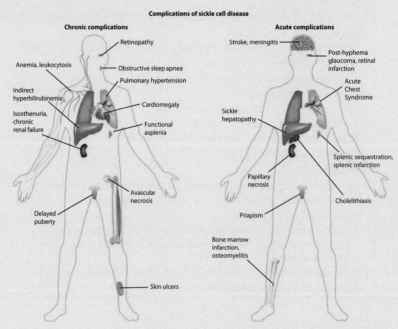 Complications of sickle cell disease Reproduced with permission from Jesse B. Hall, Gregory A. Schmidt, John P. Kress: Principles of Critical Care, 4th ed, New York: McGraw Hill, 2015.

PORPHYRIA

Porphyrias are a group of hereditary or acquired conditions that cause accumulation of heme precursors due to defective heme synthesis. Affected individuals may present with a constellation of intermittent symptoms; it's important to identify triggers.

Porphyrias Mini-Cases

Condition	Key Findings
Acute Intermittent Porphyria (AIP)	**Hx:** Symptoms include intermittent moderate to severe, colicky lower abdomen pain lasting hours to days. Nausea, vomiting, weakness, constipation, and mood changes (depression or anxiety) are other commonly reported symptoms of an acute attack. **PE:** Can reveal peripheral neuropathy. It is important to note that AIP does *not* have cutaneous manifestations. **Diagnostics:** ↑ urine porphobilinogen (PBG) to confirm diagnosis **Management:** • Administer glucose and IV hemin • Discontinue known drug triggers **Discussion:** • AIP is an autosomal dominant disorder with low penetrance caused by a mutation of porphobilinogen deaminase, causing a buildup of porphobilinogen • Difficult to diagnose due to vague and nonspecific symptoms • Symptoms include the 5 P's: **p**ainful abdomen, **p**ort wine–colored urine, **p**eripheral neuropathy, **p**sychological disturbances (anxiety, confusion, psychosis, dementia), and **p**recipitation by starvation and drugs (sulfa drugs, barbiturates, cytochrome P-450 inducers antipsychotics, alcohol) • Goals of treatment are to avoid precipitants and treat with glucose and hemin infusion for severe attacks that will inhibit ALA synthase, thereby inhibiting the accumulation of PBG
Porphyria Cutanea Tarda (PCT)	**Hx/PE:** Erosions and bullae on sun exposed areas (face, neck, forearms, back of hands), which resolve to blisters and vesicles after a few days **Diagnostics:** ↑ urine or fecal porphyrins confirms diagnosis. **Management:** • Avoidance of sun exposure, alcohol consumption, smoking, estrogen, and iron supplements • Phlebotomy or hydroxychloroquine can usually produce remission • Iron chelation if these are not tolerated **Discussion:** • Porphyria cutanea tarda (PCT) is the most common porphyria and is usually seen in adult males. • It is an autosomal dominant disorder caused by deficiency of uroporphyrinogen decarboxylase, resulting in the accumulation of uroporphyrin and resulting in blistering cutaneous lesions and hyperpigmentation in sun-exposed areas. • Attacks often exacerbated by alcohol consumption, smoking, and estrogen treatments, including hormonal contraception. • Association with hepatitis C and HIV • Chronic blistering of skin can lead to severe thickening and calcification of skin.

BLEEDING DISORDERS, PLATELET DISORDERS, AND COAGULOPATHIES

Conditions that cause bleeding due to abnormal hemostasis are broadly categorized as either platelet disorders or coagulopathies:

- **Platelet disorders** are divided into decreased platelets or platelet dysfunction (see table). Patients with platelet disorders usually have mucosal bleeding (e.g., from mouth, nose, gastrointestinal or genitourinary tracts) and petechiae. Consider ITP or acute leukemia in patients with new-onset spontaneous bruising/bleeding.

- **Coagulopathies** arise from either factor deficiencies or inhibitors. Patients with coagulopathies present with deep tissue bleeding, often into soft tissue, muscles, and joints. After procedures, they can present with delayed bleeding.

- These disorders are either congenital (inherited) or acquired. Patients with a congenital disorder will present earlier, often in childhood. Adults will usually have acquired etiologies, such as in the setting of a new hematologic malignancy, renal or liver disease, nutritional deficiency, or medication use. See Pediatric Chapter for additional cases.

Platelet Disorder			Coagulopathy	
Decreased Platelets		Platelet Dysfunction	Congenital	Acquired
Increased destruction	• DIC, TTP, ITP • Drug induced (heparin)	• von Willebrand disease • Uremia • NSAID use • Congenital platelet disorders (Bernard-Soulier, Glanzmann)	• Hemophilia A/B/C • Rare other factor deficiencies	• Drug induced • DIC • Acquired factor deficiencies • Liver disease • Renal disease • Vitamin K deficiency
Decreased production	• Viral • Bone marrow disorders			
Sequestration	• Splenomegaly			

Approach to Thrombocytopenia

Thrombocytopenia is defined as a platelet count <150,000/mm^3. Mechanisms of thrombocytopenia are:

- ↓ platelet production
- ↑ platelet destruction
- Platelet sequestration
- Hemodilution

First, ensure the patient is clinically stable and then rule out life-threatening causes.

- Mild to moderate thrombocytopenia may be asymptomatic, and clinically significant spontaneous bleeding usually does not occur until platelets are below 10–20/mm^3.
- Evidence of bleeding on history includes epistaxis, menorrhagia, hematuria, and gastrointestinal bleeding. Often, the history (current illness, comorbidities, and medications) will provide clues to the etiology.
- Evidence of bleeding on exam include petechiae, purpura, and ecchymosis.

		Potential Etiology	Additional Workup	Mechanism/Clinical Course
History	Critical Illness	• DIC • Sepsis-induced myelosuppression	Coagulation studies (rule out DIC)	Platelet activation and consumption via thrombin or cytokines
	Medications	Heparin-induced thrombocytopenia (HIT)	HIT ELISA, Serotonin release assay	Type 1: non-immune, platelets normalize despite continued heparin therapy Type 2: heparin-PF4 antibodies
		Drug-induced ITP: • antibiotics (Piperacillin/tazobactam, TMP-SMX, rifampin) • H2 blockers (famotidine, cimetidine) • antiplatelet (GPIIb/IIIa blockers) • antipsychotics (haloperidol)	In vitro detection of drug-dependent platelet antibodies	Onset: 5–10 days after medication start. Plt nadir often <20 K. Plt normalize in 2–4 weeks after drug discontinuation
		Non-immune mechanisms: ethanol, chemotherapy, linezolid, thiazides	–	Direct toxicity on platelets and/or megakaryocytes
	Thrombosis	HIT, TTP, DIC, DITMA, antiphospholipid syndrome	Blood smear, coags	Thrombotic microangiopathy
	Transfusion	Post-transfusion purpura	Platelet antibody assays (serum antibodies to HPA-1a)	Delayed transfusion reaction, occurs 5–10 days after transfusion. Plt nadir <20 K Treatment: steroids, IVIG

		Potential Etiology	Additional Workup	Mechanism/Clinical Course
History	Hematologic malignancy	• Malignancy-associated ITP • Evans syndrome (ITP + autoimmune hemolytic anemia)	Coombs if associated with AIHA	Commonly seen with Hodgkin lymphoma, non-Hodgkin lymphoma, low-grade lymphoproliferative disorders
	Autoimmune disorder	SLE, RA	• ANA, anti-dsDNA, anti-Smith • RF	Autoimmune secondary to anti-platelet glycoprotein antibodies
		Antiphospholipid syndrome	Lupus anticoagulant, β2-glycoprotein and/or anti-cardiolipin antibodies	Associated with recurrent arterial and/or venous thromboses and miscarriages
	Cardiac conditions	CABG	–	Platelet loss on artificial surface (bypass circuit)
		Valvular disorders	TTE	Increased platelet turnover
	Pregnancy	HELLP	LFTs, LDH, haptoglobin, blood smear	Seen in third trimester or postpartum
		Gestational thrombocytopenia	–	Plt >50 Self-limiting, benign condition
	Family History	VWD type 2B	VWF:Ag, VWF:RCo, Factor VIII	Increased clearance of platelets
		Hereditary thrombocytopenia	Platelet function assay	Associated with Bernard-Soulier syndrome, May-Heggelin anomaly, Gray platelet syndrome
Exam	Lymphadenopathy	Malignancy	Lymph node biopsy	Associated with lymphomas with marrow involvement or autoimmune ITP
		Viral infection	EBV, HIV	HIV infection impairs platelet production
	Splenomegaly	Malignancy	Biopsy	Commonly seen in CML, lymphoma
		Liver disease	RUQ US	Decreased thrombopoietin (TPO) synthesis
		Portal hypertension	RUQ US with Doppler	Splenic sequestration
Smear	Platelet Clumping	Pseudothrombocytopenia	Repeat test with sodium citrate tube	EDTA-dependent in vitro platelet agglutination
	Schistocytes	Microangiopathic hemolytic anemia (TTP/HUS/DIC)	ADAMTS13, coagulation studies (PTT, INR)	schistocytes >5/hpf
	Blasts	MDS Leukemia	Flow cytometry, bone marrow biopsy	Multiple lineage cytopenias (isolated thrombocytopenia rare)
	Parasitic Inclusions	Malaria, babesiosis, ehrlichiosis	PCR or thick/thin blood smear	Platelet destruction +/– hypersplenism
	Large Platelets	ITP Hereditary thrombocytopenia	—	—
	Atypical Lymphocytes	Viral infection	EBV	Hemophagocytosis

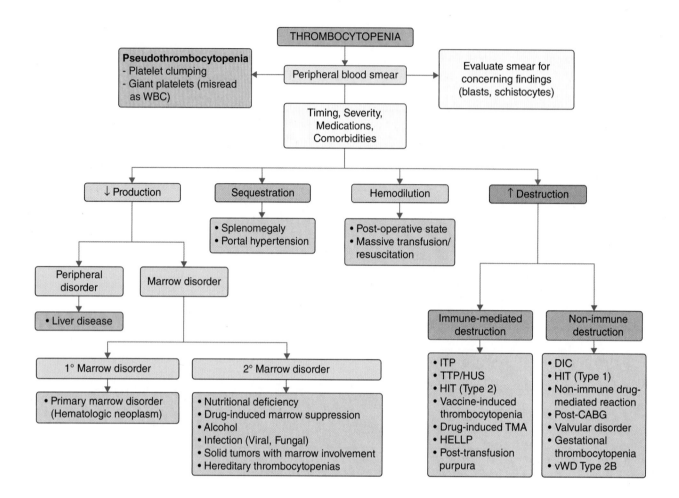

COAGULOPATHIES

Disorders of coagulation can cause arterial or venous thrombosis or bleeding disorders. The risk of developing a thrombus can increase due to the presence of elements of Virchow's triad (endothelial injury, blood stasis, and hypercoagulable state), such as long airplane flights or immobility due to hospitalization. In the absence of any of the components of Virchow's triad, an undiagnosed hypercoagulable state should be suspected. See Pediatrics Chapter for additional cases.

Approach to Coagulopathy

As with thrombocytopenia, the clinical history is important in providing information on the underlying condition.

Clinical Condition	Is patient acutely ill?
Personal History	Comorbid conditions
Bleeding History	Type of bleeding events (spontaneous, dental extraction, trauma-related, menstruation)
	Frequency of bleeding
	Severity of bleeding
	Need for transfusion support
	Response to procedures/surgeries (i.e., hemostatic challenges)
Family History	First-degree relatives with bleeding events
	Inheritance pattern can be X-linked (hemophilia A and B), autosomal dominant or autosomal recessive

Physical Exam Findings

Signs and Conditions Associated with Bleeding

- Pallor, oral blood blisters, telangiectasias
- Petechiae, purpura, perifollicular hemorrhages
- Skin pigmentation changes from recurrent bleeds, ecchymoses, hematomas
- Signs of underlying hematologic disorder (e.g., splenomegaly, lymphadenopathy)
- Signs of acute or chronic liver disease (hepatomegaly, jaundice, palmar erythema, spider nevi)
- Signs of collagen vascular disorder (hyperextensibility)
- Signs suggestive of syndromic bleeding disorder (albinism, hearing impairment)

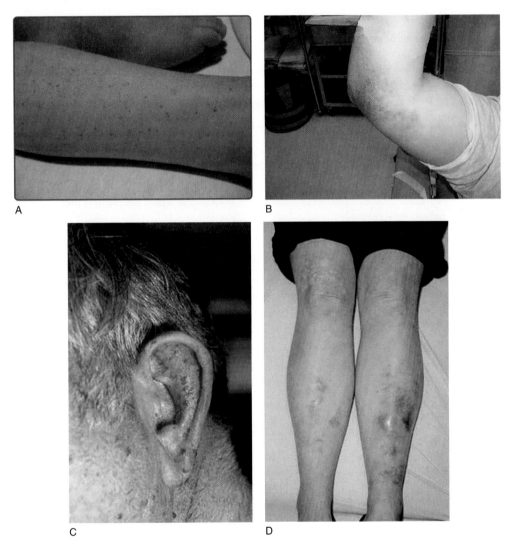

a) Petechiae (Reproduced with permission from Sewon Kang, Masayuki Amagai, Anna L. Bruckner, Alexander H. Enk, David J. Margolis, Amy J. McMichael, Jeffrey S. Orringer, Fitzpatrick's Dermatology, 9e. New York, NY: McGraw-Hill 2019.); b) hemarthroses with overlying ecchymoses (Reproduced with permission from Lichtman MA, Shafer MS, Felgar RE, Wang N, Lichtman's Atlas of Hematology 2016. New York, NY: McGraw-Hill 2017.); c) hereditary hemorrhagic telangiectasia (Reproduced with permission from Lichtman MA, Shafer MS, Felgar RE, Wang N, Lichtman's Atlas of Hematology 2016. New York, NY: McGraw-Hill 2017.); d) Ehler Danlos syndrome. Purpura on lower extremities (Reproduced with permission from Lichtman MA, Shafer MS, Felgar RE, Wang N, Lichtman's Atlas of Hematology 2016. New York, NY: McGraw-Hill 2017.)

CASE 5 | Immune (Idiopathic) Thrombocytopenic Purpura (ITP)

A 54-year-old man presents with new-onset easy bruising and small red spots underneath his skin. He has no personal or family history of a bleeding disorder, has no recent infections, and takes no medications. Physical exam is normal, without lymphadenopathy or hepatosplenomegaly. Labs include WBC 7000/mm³ with normal differential, hemoglobin 14.8 g/dL, and platelets 17,000/mm³. Peripheral blood smear confirms thrombocytopenia with occasional large platelets. No schistocytes are seen.

Conditions with Similar Presentations	**Drug-induced Immune Thrombocytopenia:** Also presents with thrombocytopenia but in a patient taking medications. Commonly implicated medications include heparin, antibiotics (penicillin, sulfa, linezolid), GPIIb/IIIa inhibitors, and H2-blockers. After drug discontinuation, platelets will normalize within several weeks.
	Secondary ITP: Is also an immune-mediated thrombocytopenia, but is seen in patients with an underlying condition such as autoimmune disorders (e.g., SLE, RA, IBD), malignancies (e.g., CLL, lymphoma), or infection (e.g., CMV, EBV, HIV, HBV, HCV). Treatment of the underlying condition will improve thrombocytopenia.
	HIT: Presents with gradually decreasing platelet count in a hospitalized patient 5–10 days after heparin exposure (may occur earlier if previously exposed).
	TTP, HUS: Also present with thrombocytopenia but would also see a hemolytic anemia with schistocytes on peripheral smear.
Initial Diagnostic Testing	• Diagnosis of exclusion • Check: CBC, peripheral smear, and rule out other causes • Consider: PT/ INR, PTT (especially in patients with active bleeding), testing for HIV and hepatitis C, LFTs
Next Steps in Management	Treatment indicated if platelets <30,000/mm³, bleeding, or a planned invasive procedure. Otherwise observation is reasonable. • Steroids • IVIG (if immediate need to increase platelet count) • Platelet transfusions (if critical bleeding [e.g., intracranial bleed, hemodynamically unstable bleed])
Discussion	ITP is a common bleeding disorder seen in children and adults, characterized by isolated thrombocytopenia and bleeding/petechiae, though patients with mild ITP can be asymptomatic. • Often an incidental finding in patients and is a diagnosis of exclusion after more serious etiologies have been ruled out. • Anti-platelet antibodies form against the GPIIb/IIIa fibrinogen receptor on platelets, creating platelet-antibody complex which is then cleared by the spleen. Given the low sensitivity of antiplatelet antibodies (negative in up to 50% of patients), this is not routinely used in diagnosis. • ITP can be idiopathic (primary) or secondary to drugs, autoimmune disease, viral infections, or malignancies. **History:** • May be an incidental finding on routine labs, or patients present with new unprovoked mucocutaneous bleeding • Significant bleeding usually occurs with severe thrombocytopenia (<30,000/mm³) • Often preceded by a viral infection (anti-virus antibodies cross-react with the platelet surface leading to ITP) • Inquire about recent infections, medications, underlying medical conditions (liver disease, autoimmune conditions), or signs/symptoms of hematologic malignancy to identify secondary causes of thrombocytopenia. **Physical Exam:** • Unremarkable in mild-moderate thrombocytopenia • If severe, thrombocytopenia can have petechiae, easy bruising, or mucocutaneous bleeding (epistaxis, gingival bleeding) **Diagnostics:** • Diagnosis of exclusion after other etiologies have been ruled out. CBC will show platelet count <100,000/mm³, PT/ INR, PTT will be normal. • Consider tests looking for underlying medical conditions (ANA, RF, HIV, hepatitis C, B12, folate) to rule out secondary ITP.

CASE 5 | Immune (Idiopathic) Thrombocytopenic Purpura (ITP) *(continued)*

Discussion	**Management:** Treatment is based on the platelet count and bleeding events • Platelet count >30,000/mm³: close observation • Platelet count <30,000/mm³ and asymptomatic: steroids (methylprednisolone or dexamethasone pulse, or prednisone taper) • Active bleeding: steroids and IVIG; platelet transfusions can be given if active bleeding • In refractory settings, consider splenectomy • Secondary ITP: treat underlying condition

CASE 6 | Heparin-Induced Thrombocytopenia (HIT)

A 62-year-old woman hospitalized 1 week ago for pneumonia develops left calf swelling and pain while on prophylactic subcutaneous heparin. Labs are notable for platelets 60,000/mm³ (210,000/mm³ on admission). PT/INR, PTT, fibrinogen are normal. A peripheral smear is normal. A Doppler ultrasound of the left leg shows a popliteal deep vein thrombosis. The HIT ELISA optical density is 1.8 (normal <0.4) and a functional serotonin release assay is positive.

Conditions with Similar Presentations	**ITP:** Presents as an isolated thrombocytopenia with or without bleeding. **TTP:** Also presents with thrombocytopenia, but will also include microangiopathic hemolytic anemia, fever, neurologic symptoms, and elevated creatinine. **DIC:** Also presents with thrombocytopenia but coags (PT/PTT/INR) and D-dimer will be elevated, and fibrinogen will be decreased. It is usually found in a hospitalized patient with a critical illness or injury (sepsis, malignancy), and patients can have bleeding or thrombosis.
Initial Diagnostic Testing	Risk stratify with 4T score, if intermediate or high probability send HIT immunoassay (HIT ELISA) +/− functional assay (serotonin release assay)
Next Steps in Management	• Immediately stop heparin products if suspicion for HIT • Start alternative therapeutic anticoagulation with direct thrombin inhibitors or direct oral novel anticoagulants

Discussion	HIT is an immune-mediated drug reaction leading to thrombocytopenia and thrombosis in patients exposed to heparin products. HIT is caused by IgG autoantibodies that recognize and bind to the heparin-platelet factor 4 (PF4) complex. Thrombocytopenia occurs from widespread clumping of IgG-coated platelets that can cause catastrophic venous and arterial clotting.
	
	HIT affects up to 1 in 5000 hospitalized patients. The risk is higher for patients receiving unfractionated heparin than low molecular weight heparin. Surgical patients, especially those undergoing cardiac surgery, are more likely to develop HIT.
	
	History/Physical Exam:
	• Suspect if >50% platelet drop 5–10 days after heparin exposure, or within 1 day if exposed to heparin in the preceding 30 days
	• Up to 50% will also have arterial or venous thrombosis
	• Bleeding is not seen
	• Patients can either be asymptomatic or have signs and symptoms associated with thrombosis (extremity swelling for DVT, shortness of breath (SOB)/tachycardia for PE, headache for sinus venous thrombosis, or stroke-like symptoms, or evidence of limb ischemia)
	
	Diagnostics:
	• Risk stratification based on the **4T score** (**t**hrombocytopenia, **t**iming relative to heparin exposure, **t**hrombosis, likelihood of other causes of **t**hrombocytopenia), which assigns points to the presence and/or severity of these phenomena.
	  • Low probability 4T score → unlikely to have HIT, and laboratory testing is not recommended
	  • Intermediate or high 4T score → screen with HIT ELISA immunoassay for heparin-PF4 antibodies
	    • HIT ELISA with low optical density rules out HIT and high optical density is suggestive of HIT
	    • An intermediate HIT antibody test (ELISA) result should be confirmed with functional testing such as a serotonin release assay (SRA)
	• Monitor platelets and consider duplex ultrasound of extremities if new swelling or pain to evaluate for thrombosis

CASE 6 | Heparin-Induced Thrombocytopenia (HIT) *(continued)*

Discussion	**Management:** • Stop heparin products when HIT suspected • Start alternative therapeutic anticoagulation, such as direct thrombin inhibitors (argatroban, bivalirudin, fondaparinux) or direct oral anticoagulants (apixaban, rivaroxaban)
Additional Considerations	There are two types of HIT: • **Type 1 HIT:** Due to a nonimmune direct effect of heparin on platelets and results in mild thrombocytopenia with a platelet nadir >100,000/mm³. Heparin does not need to be discontinued and the platelet count normalizes despite continued use. • **Type 2 HIT:** Clinically relevant and is described in this case.

CASE 7 | Thrombotic Thrombocytopenic Purpura (TTP)

A 51-year-old man presents with 2 weeks of malaise and increasing confusion. On examination, he has a temperature of 102°F, mild conjunctival icterus, and petechiae on his lower legs. Notable labs show hemoglobin 9 g/dL, platelets 11,000/mm³, serum creatinine 1.8 mg/dL, haptoglobin is undetectable, indirect bilirubin 3.5 mg/dL, and reticulocyte count is elevated. Schistocytes are present on the peripheral blood smear.

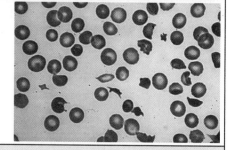

Schistocytes on peripheral smear. (Reproduced with permission from Lichtman MA, Shafer MS, Felgar RE, Wang N, Lichtman's Atlas of Hematology 2016. New York, NY: McGraw-Hill 2017.)

Conditions with Similar Presentations	**Hemolytic uremic syndrome (HUS):** Can also present with thrombocytopenia, anemia, and acute kidney injury but is usually in a child with a history of bloody diarrhea and ADAMTS13 >10%. **DIC:** Also presents with signs of bleeding but is usually in a hospitalized patient with an underlying illness (sepsis, malignancy) or injury. PTT/INR and D-dimer will be elevated, fibrinogen will be low. **HELLP:** Also presents with hemolytic anemia and thrombocytopenia; however, occurs only in pregnancy and is also marked by elevated liver enzymes. **Drug-induced thrombotic microangiopathy (DITMA):** Also presents with thrombocytopenia, hemolytic anemia, and signs/symptoms of organ damage (especially the kidney), from microvascular thrombi due to offending medications (e.g., chemotherapy [gemcitabine, VEGF inhibitors], calcineurin inhibitors [tacrolimus], opioids [oxymorphone, oxycodone], quinine, interleukin). **ITP:** Presents with isolated thrombocytopenia and is often an incidental finding.
Initial Diagnostic Testing	• Confirm diagnosis: CBC, peripheral blood smear, ADAMTS13 activity level <10%, and anti-ADAMTS13 antibodies • Consider: CMP, LDH, haptoglobin, PTT and INR, fibrinogen, Coombs test
Next Steps in Management	TTP is a medical emergency. • Urgent plasmapheresis if strong clinical suspicion • High-dose steroids
Discussion	TTP is an acquired thrombotic microangiopathy that causes small vessel microthrombi leading to **microangiopathic hemolytic anemia (MAHA)** and organ damage (e.g., renal dysfunction, altered mental status). It is a life-threatening condition and prompt recognition and treatment are essential to reduce mortality. • Classic pentad of symptoms: fever, anemia with fragmented RBCs (schistocytes), thrombocytopenia, kidney injury, and neurologic symptoms. • Acquired TTP is due to autoantibodies against von Willebrand factor (VWF) metalloproteinase ADAMTS13. ADAMTS13 normally cleaves VWF multimers immediately after their release from vascular endothelium, and its absence results in ultra-large VWF multimers that aggregate platelets to form platelet-rich microthrombi in capillaries, shearing RBCs as they pass through, leading to a MAHA. • Acquired TTP usually presents in adulthood and is more common in women. Episodes of TTP can be precipitated by underlying conditions such as infection or pregnancy.

CASE 7 | Thrombotic Thrombocytopenic Purpura (TTP) *(continued)*

Discussion	**History:**
	• Symptoms related to anemia (fatigue, malaise) and thrombocytopenia (bleeding, bruising)
	• Neurologic symptoms if CNS involved
	
	Physical Exam:
	• Fever, altered mental status
	• May have conjunctival icterus/jaundice from hemolysis, and mucosal bleeding or petechiae/purpura from thrombocytopenia
	
	Diagnostics:
	• Hallmark is classic pentad of symptoms, though all symptoms are present in <10% of cases:
	  • MAHA with schistocytes on peripheral smear ($\uparrow$ indirect bilirubin, $\uparrow$ LDH, $\uparrow$ reticulocyte count, $\downarrow$ haptoglobin). Coagulation studies will be normal.
	  • Severe thrombocytopenia (platelets $<30 \times 10^9$/L)
	  • Acute kidney injury.
	  • Neurologic symptoms most commonly include altered mental status, headache, or focal deficits (motor/sensory or speech problems).
	  • Fever
	• Decreased ADAMTS13 activity level and anti-ADAMTS13 antibodies are specific for TTP
	• Consider testing for secondary causes of TTP (e.g., HIV, hepatitis B and C, pregnancy)
	
	Management:
	• Initiate plasmapheresis while waiting for ADAMTS13 level if there is strong clinical suspicion
	• Pulse-dose methylprednisolone or high-dose oral prednisone followed by taper
	• Rituximab decreases relapses and is usually added to initial therapy
	• Supportive care with RBC transfusions and platelets if significant bleeding

Thrombocytopenia Mini-Cases

Cases	Key Findings
Disseminated Intravascular Coagulation (DIC)	**Hx:** Presents in patients with critical conditions such as sepsis (most commonly from gram-negative bacteria), trauma, burns, acute promyelocytic leukemia (APL), pancreatitis, nephrotic syndrome, transfusions, and obstetric complications. **PE:** • Usually have bleeding, ranging from cutaneous findings (ecchymoses, bleeding from venipuncture sites or other indwelling devices, mucosal membranes), to life-threatening bleeding • Manifestations of microvascular thrombosis include thrombophlebitis, skin infarcts or necrosis, discoloration of distal extremities **Diagnostics:** • $\downarrow$ platelets, $\uparrow$ PT/PTT, $\uparrow$ D-dimer, $\downarrow$ fibrinogen • Peripheral blood smear may show schistocytes • No single lab test to confirm DIC; diagnosis established with above constellation of lab findings in the appropriate clinical setting **Management:** • Treat underlying illness (e.g., infection, malignancy) • Transfusion of platelets (goal platelets >20–50,000/mm³), FFP or vitamin K, and/or cryoprecipitate (goal fibrinogen >150 mg/dL) to decrease bleeding **Discussion:** • DIC is characterized by over activation of the coagulation cascade leading to widespread clotting resulting in consumption of coagulation factors and platelets that can result in bleeding • Organ failure (renal, pulmonary, CNS) can be seen
Hemolytic Uremic Syndrome (HUS)	**Hx:** Macroangiopathic hemolytic anemia (MAHA) similar to TTP with main differences: • Children more commonly affected than adults • Neurologic dysfunction less common than in TTP but are more likely to present with acute kidney injury than TTP • History of bloody diarrhea; classic etiology is Shiga-like toxin from *E. coli* (EHEC, e.g. O157:H7 strain)

Thrombocytopenia Mini-Cases *(continued)*

Hemolytic Uremic Syndrome (HUS)	**PE:** • May be febrile; can have conjunctival icterus and jaundice from hemolysis and mucosal bleeding or petechiae/purpura from thrombocytopenia • Signs of dehydration from diarrhea (decreased skin turgor, decreased capillary refill time, and dry mucus membranes) **Diagnostics:** • CBC: ↓ Hb, ↓ platelets, peripheral smear with schistocytes • ↑ Creatinine, ↑ indirect bilirubin, ↑ LDH • Stool positive for Shiga toxin; ADAMTS13 level >10% **Management:** • Supportive care with fluids and electrolyte replacement • People infected with a Shiga-/Shiga-like toxin–producing bacteria should *not* be treated with antibiotics, as this can increase the risk of developing HUS • Avoid antimotility medications • Dialysis if acute renal failure • Plasmapheresis or anti-complement therapy (eculizumab) can be considered for severe neurologic symptoms

Hypercoagulable States

Antithrombin III deficiency	Antithrombin inhibits the action of factors IIa, IXa, and Xa; deficiency of this protein results in a hypercoagulable state. Antithrombin III may be decreased as an inherited deficiency or it can be lost in the urine of patients with nephrotic syndrome.
Factor V Leiden	Due to an autosomal dominant point mutation (Arg506Gln) with incomplete penetrance that results in factor V being resistant to cleavage by protein C, causing a hypercoagulable state. Factor V Leiden is the most common cause of hypercoagulability in individuals of European descent.
Prothrombin gene mutation	DNA mutation results in increased production of prothrombin, a procoagulant, resulting in a hypercoagulable state.
Protein C and S deficiency	Proteins C and S are involved in inhibiting the actions of factor Va and factor VIIIa; deficiency of these proteins results in less cleavage of these factors, leading to thrombosis.
Antiphospholipid syndrome (APS)	An autoimmune condition involving the development of antiphospholipid antibodies that cause activation of the complement system and coagulation cascade. This process also inhibits the action of proteins C and S.

Inherited or Acquired Causes of Bleeding

Rare inherited factor deficiencies	• Severity of disease is associated with the factor level • Include fibrinogen, factor II, V, X, and XIII deficiency • Treatment: Replace the missing coagulation factor
Hemophilia A	• X-linked inherited bleeding disorder • ↓ factor VIII level and ↑PTT • Treat with factor VIII replacement therapy or desmopressin, which promotes release of vWF to elevate factor VIII concentration
Hemophilia B	• X-linked inherited bleeding disorder • ↓ factor IX • Treat with factor IX
Hemophilia C	• Autosomal recessive disorder • ↓ factor XI • Treat with factor XI
Acquired factor deficiencies	• Immune causes (such as acquired factor VIII inhibitor) or nonimmune due to reductions in factors from vitamin K deficiency, liver disease, hemodilution, snakebites
von Willebrand disease	• ↓ factor VIII, ↓ VWF antigen and abnormal VWF activity (ristocetin cofactor assay) • Treat with desmopressin (DDAVP) for mild to moderate bleeding and VWF concentrates for more severe bleeding

Inherited or Acquired Causes of Bleeding

Acquired von Willebrand disease	• Nonimmune acquired von Willebrand disease seen in severe valvular disease or aortic stenosis. The turbulent flow unfolds the VWF multimer making it more susceptible to ADAMTS13 degradation. Immune type seen with IgG paraprotein. • ↓ factor VIII and ↓ VWF levels • Treatment: DDAVP
Renal disease/ Uremia	• Uremia impairs platelet adhesion and aggregation. • ↑ Bleeding time • Treatment: Platelet transfusion in patients with active bleeding • DDAVP can help restore platelet activity and be used as adjunct therapy in bleeding patients.
Liver disease	• Thrombocytopenia due to decreased synthesis of thrombopoietin and/or decreased production of coagulation factors.
Vitamin K deficiency	• Factors II, VII, IX, and X are dependent on vitamin K for γ-glutamyl carboxylation. • Liver disease can cause an acquired vitamin K deficiency • GI malabsorptive conditions and/or broad spectrum antibiotics that reduce gut bacteria can lead to vitamin K and other fat-soluble vitamin deficiencies • Treatment: Vitamin K and correct the underlying disorder
Acquired hemophilia	• Acquired hemophilia is the result of development of autoantibodies, usually against factor VIII. It can be associated with pregnancy, malignancies, or autoimmune conditions. • Unlike congenital hemophilia, incidence of hemarthrosis is low but there is increased soft tissue, abdominal, and retroperitoneal bleeding. • Treatment: Recombinant VIII
Drug induced	• Aspirin, NSAIDs, platelet function inhibitors, anticoagulants
DIC	• Widespread consumption of coagulation factors including fibrinogen, thrombocytopenia • Causes include infection, postpartum consumptive states, prostate or other cancers, snakebites

LEUKEMIA

Leukemias are a malignancy of hematopoietic stem cells and are characterized by the type of cell involved (myeloid or lymphoid) and the level of differentiation (blasts = acute, mature cells = chronic). An unregulated proliferation of one cell line in the bone marrow leads to marrow failure, a reduction in other cell lines, and dysfunctional circulating cell types.

Acute leukemia can present with signs and symptoms related to cytopenias: ↓ RBC (signs and symptoms of anemia), ↓ WBC (infections), and ↓ platelets (bleeding). Initial diagnostic workup includes CBC with differential, comprehensive metabolic panel, and coagulation studies. Bone marrow biopsy is essential for confirmation of diagnosis. See Pediatric Chapter for additional cases.

Leukemia Classification

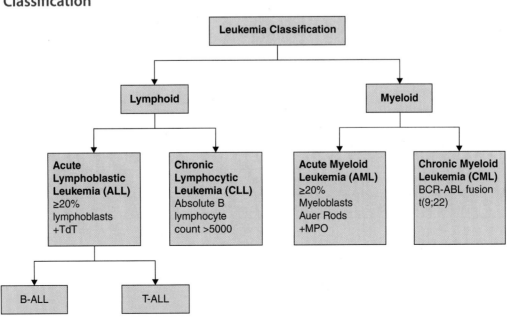

Acute Leukemias

	AML	APL	ALL
Etiology	Proliferation of undifferentiated myeloid blasts Eight subtypes (M0–M7)	Subtype of AML (M3) with t(15:17) translocation	Proliferation of undifferentiated lymphoid blasts
Epidemiology	Adults: Increasing incidence with age (median 68 years)	Seen in younger adults (median 40 years)	B-ALL: Bimodal distribution in children/young adults and older adults T-ALL: Most common in young children (<5 years old) and adolescents
Presentation	Fatigue, DOE, infection, bleeding, pancytopenia, or hyperleukocytosis	Fatigue or DOE, pallor, infection, bleeding Commonly presents with DIC	Fatigue, DOE, infection, bleeding, pancytopenia or hyperleukocytosis More likely to have lymphadenopathy, organomegaly, bone pain
Diagnosis	Myeloblasts (immature granulocytic precursor) with Auer rods +MPO	Promyelocyte with Auer rods and t(15;17) translocation +MPO	≥20% Lymphoblast (immature lymphoid precursor) +TdT
Management	Cytarabine + anthracycline, stem cell transplant (SCT) for cure	All-trans retinoic acid + arsenic trioxide	Multi-agent chemotherapy +/– SCT

CASE 8 | Acute Myelogenous Leukemia (AML)

A 75-year-old man with no significant past medical history presents with bleeding gums, fatigue, and shortness of breath for a few weeks. On examination he has a low-grade fever, tachycardia, tachypnea, erythematous papules and nodules on his chest and back, and scattered ecchymosis on the extremities. Labs show hemoglobin 9.0 g/dL; WBC 80,000/mm³ with numerous large granulocytic cells; platelets 28,000/mm³. Bone marrow biopsy shows a hypercellular marrow with 70% myeloblasts.

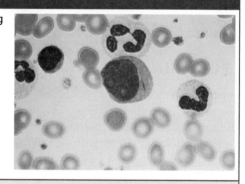

Leukemic myeloblast with an Auer rod. Note the large, prominent nucleoli in each cell. (Reproduced with permission from Joseph Loscalzo, Anthony Fauci, Dennis Kasper, Stephen Hauser, Dan Longo, J. Larry Jameson, Harrison's Principles of Internal Medicine, 21e. New York, NY: McGraw Hill LLC 2022.)

Conditions with Similar Presentations	**CML blast crisis:** Also has ≥20% myeloblasts in peripheral blood or bone marrow but can be distinguished by the detection of the Philadelphia chromosome [BCR-ABL fusion protein t(9;22)]. **MDS:** Is also seen in older adults with a median age of 70 years and can present similarly to AML with fatigue and cytopenias. However, bone marrow aspirate and biopsy will have <20% blasts and show abnormal features (dysplasia) in all cell lines. **ALL:** Will demonstrate lymphoblasts (+TdT) as opposed to myeloblasts (+MPO). The cell types are differentiated using immunohistochemistry and flow cytometry techniques. **Acute promyelocytic leukemia (APL):** Is a subtype of AML, characterized by t(15;17) which produces the PML-RARA fusion protein. **Leukemoid reaction:** Presents with elevated WBC count (often >50,000/mm³) but cells are mature and are positive for leukocyte alkaline phosphatase (LAP). This is a reactive process seen in infection.
Initial Diagnostic Testing	Check peripheral blood smear or bone marrow (≥20% Myeloblasts)
Next Steps in Management	• Hydration and allopurinol to prevent tumor lysis syndrome • Chemotherapy with cytarabine and an anthracycline • For patients with APL, use all-trans retinoic acid (ATRA)

CASE 8 | Acute Myelogenous Leukemia (AML) *(continued)*

Discussion	AML is a hematologic malignancy arising from aggressive, unchecked clonal proliferation of immature myeloid precursors (blasts). As blasts accumulate in the bone marrow, normal hematopoiesis is disturbed leading to cytopenias. There are eight subtypes (M0–M7). AML can occur at any age but is most often seen in older adults (≥65) and can arise de novo or occur secondarily (in setting of prior chemotherapy, underlying MDS, or myeloproliferative neoplastic [MPN] syndromes).
	History:
	• Risk factors include ionizing radiation, or exposure to drugs known to cause DNA damage (alkylators and topoisomerase inhibitors). There is also an association with Down syndrome and bone marrow failure syndromes
	• May present with fever, infection or signs/symptoms of:
	• Pancytopenia: fatigue, dyspnea, infection, bleeding (epistaxis, gingival, menorrhagia, GI bleed)
	• Leukostasis: vision changes, headache, AMS, chest pain, SOB/dyspnea on exertion (DOE), cranial nerve palsies
	Physical Exam:
	• Fever, pallor, petechiae, bleeding
	• Swollen/bleeding gums/gingival hyperplasia (M5 subtype)
	• Leukemic infiltration seen in skin presents as violaceous papules, plaques, or nodules (leukemia cutis)
	Diagnostics:
	• Blood smear and/or bone marrow with ≥20% myeloblasts
	• Myeloblasts with Auer rods are characteristically seen in the peripheral smear and stain positive for myeloperoxidase (MPO).
	• May also have pancytopenia (due to blasts overcrowding marrow space) or marked leukocytosis (spillage of blasts into blood)
	• Consider rule out underlying infection
	Management:
	• Hyperleukocytosis can cause leukostasis as blasts (which are "sticky") cause vascular congestion leading to pulmonary (SOB, DOE), cardiac (chest pain, ACS), and neurologic (TIA, stroke) symptoms
	• Monitoring and prevention of tumor lysis syndrome
	• Chemotherapy with cytarabine + anthracycline
	• Allogeneic stem cell transplant in fit patients
	• APL (subtype of AML (M3)) often presents with disseminated intravascular coagulation (DIC) and requires urgent treatment with ATRA and arsenic trioxide
Additional Considerations	**Complications:**
	Tumor lysis syndrome: Seen in patients with leukemias and lymphomas in which massive tumor destruction causes ↑ K+, ↑ phos, ↑ uric acid, and ↓ Ca+ (due to precipitation with phosphate) and resulting AKI, arrhythmias, and death. Prevention and treatment involve aggressive IV hydration, allopurinol or rasburicase, and/or dialysis.
	Infections: Antibiotic prophylaxis indicated in patients with neutropenia.

Oncologic Emergency Mini-Cases

Cases	Key Findings
Tumor Lysis Syndrome (TLS)	**Hx/PE:**
	Risk factors: Induction chemotherapy for leukemias and lymphomas
	Symptoms, signs, presentation: Gastrointestinal (nausea, vomiting, diarrhea, anorexia), cramps/tetany (from hypocalcemia), seizures, cardiac arrhythmias, and sudden death.
	Diagnostics:
	• ↑Potassium, ↑phosphate, ↓calcium, ↑uric acid, and ↑creatinine
	• Suspect tumor lysis syndrome in patients who develop acute renal failure with hyperuricemia and hyperphosphatemia after chemotherapy.
	Management:
	• IV fluids and correction of electrolyte abnormalities
	• Prevention is key and includes IV fluids and the use of allopurinol or rasburicase.

Oncologic Emergency Mini-Cases *(continued)*

Tumor Lysis Syndrome (TLS)	**Discussion:** Rapid lysis of malignant cells usually after chemotherapy leads to a rapid release of intracellular contents. This directly increases serum potassium and phosphate. Phosphate combines with calcium and causes hypocalcemia. Nucleic acids released are metabolized to uric acid leading to hyperuricemia. Precipitation of uric acid and calcium phosphate in the renal tubules can cause renal failure.
Leukostasis	**Hx/PE:** Risk factors: Hematologic malignancies; seen in AML and ALL in the setting of hyperleukocytosis (WBC >50–100,000/mm^3) Symptoms, signs, presentation: Dyspnea, hypoxia, chest pain, altered mental status, visual abnormalities, and headache or AMS **Diagnostics:** Clinical diagnosis in the appropriate setting (elevated blasts, respiratory or neurologic compromise) **Management:** Rapid lowering of WBC count with induction chemotherapy, leukapheresis, hydroxyurea **Discussion:** High numbers of blasts (which are "sticky") occlude microvasculature and lead to decreased tissue perfusion and ischemia. (Elevated numbers of normal white blood cells do not cause leukostasis.)
Febrile Neutropenia	**Hx/PE:** Risk factors: Can be a complication of myelosuppressive chemotherapy or in patients with neutropenia due to malignancy. Symptoms, signs, presentation: Neutropenia (ANC <500 cells/mm^3) + fever (101°F [or 38.3°C]). **Diagnostics:** • Clinical diagnosis: Fever in a neutropenic patient • Determine source with a targeted history and physical exam, blood cultures, chest imaging, UA **Management:** Start urgent empiric antibiotics with pseudomonal coverage (cefepime, meropenem, imipenem, or piperacillin-tazobactam). **Discussion:** Caused by bacterial or fungal infection in the setting of neutropenia. See Febrile Neutropenia case in Infectious Disease Chapter.

MYELOPROLIFERATIVE NEOPLASMS

Myeloproliferative neoplasms (MPNs) encompass a heterogenous group of chronic myeloid conditions characterized by clonal overproduction of differentiated cells. Chronic myeloid leukemia (CML) is an MPN defined by the BCR-ABL mutation. The classic BCR-ABL negative MPNs include polycythemia vera (PV), essential thrombocytosis (ET), and primary myelofibrosis (PMF). Less common conditions include chronic neutrophilic leukemia, chronic eosinophilic leukemia, and mast cell disorders. MPNs have certain molecular, laboratory, and clinical features in common:

- Mutations in the genes JAK2, CALR, and MPL define these conditions.
- Patients are at risk of clotting, leading to morbidity from stroke or other thrombosis.
- Patients may have constitutional symptoms (fatigue, fevers, night sweats) and/or complications from extramedullary hematopoiesis (splenomegaly, bone pain).
- MPNs should be considered in patients with unusual sites of thrombosis, such as splenic thrombosis, portal or hepatic vein thrombosis (in absence of liver disease), or cerebral sinus vein thrombosis.
- Over time, PV and ET can progress to a secondary myelofibrosis (also termed post-PV or post-ET MF) and all conditions (PV, ET, and both primary and secondary myelofibrosis) can progress to an acute leukemia.

		PV	ET	PMF
Molecular Mutations	JAK2	++++	+++	+++
	CALR	None	++	++
	MPL	None	+	+
Exam Findings	Erythromelalgia	+	++	None
	Plethora	++	None	None
	Pallor	None	None	Variable
	Splenomegaly	+	+	+++
	Hepatomegaly	None	None	+
Laboratory Findings	Erythrocytosis	+++	None	None
	Thrombocytosis	Variable	+++	Variable
	Leukocytosis	Variable	Variable	Variable
	↓ Serum EPO	+++	None	None

Natural History of MPNs

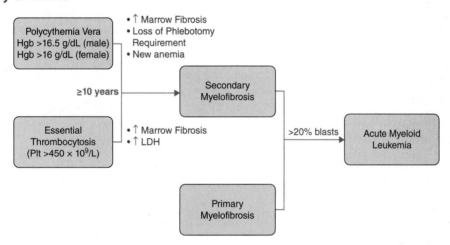

Causes of Secondary Erythrocytosis

	Etiology	Cause	Notes
Relative erythrocytosis	Hypovolemia	Dehydration, vomiting/diarrhea, diuretics, burns	Normal red cell mass with ↑ Hb due to contracted plasma volume. Normal or ↑EPO
Secondary erythrocytosis (congenital)	Oxygen-sensing pathway	Familial erythrocytosis (mutations in VHL, HIF2a)	May have normal or ↓ EPO but exhibit persistent erythrocytosis
	Hemoglobin variants with high oxygen affinity	High oxygen-affinity hemoglobin, 2,3-BPG deficiency (rare)	↑EPO to compensate for ineffective oxygen transport and release
Secondary erythrocytosis (acquired)	Relative hypoxia	Pulmonary disease, smoking, obstructive sleep apnea, high altitude, cyanotic heart conditions	↓SaO_2 (<92%)
	Drug-induced	Androgens, erythropoietin-stimulating agents (i.e., epoetin)	↑EPO levels
	Impaired tissue oxygen delivery	Carbon monoxide poisoning, methemoglobinemia	CO displaces O_2 on Hb molecules; methemoglobin cannot bind O_2
	EPO-producing tumors	Renal cell carcinoma (RCC), hepatocellular carcinoma (HCC), ovarian and uterine tumors, pheochromocytoma, cerebellar hemangioblastoma	Tumors may be benign or malignant

CASE 9 | Chronic Myelogenous Leukemia (CML)

A 58-year-old woman presents for a routine exam. Review of systems is positive for mild fatigue, night sweats, and weight loss. Physical exam is notable for splenomegaly. Labs show hemoglobin 11 g/dL; WBC 175,000/mm^3; platelets 100,000/mm^3. Peripheral blood smear reveals predominantly mature neutrophils. Leukocyte alkaline phosphatase (LAP) activity is low. Bone marrow biopsy reveals granulocyte hyperplasia. Cytogenetic testing shows the presence of a *BCR-ABL1* fusion protein resulting from a t(9;22), Philadelphia chromosome.

Conditions with Similar Presentations	**Leukemoid reaction:** Refers to hyperleukocytosis >50,000/mm^3, most often due to infection. LAP activity will be high in leukemoid reaction and low in CML due to the low activity of malignant neutrophils. **Chronic lymphocytic leukemia (CLL):** Is also mostly seen in older adults, and patients may be asymptomatic or present with fatigue, lymphadenopathy, and splenomegaly. However, CLL has a predominance of lymphocytes on the WBC differential instead of neutrophils. **AML:** Also presents with hyperleukocytosis, but it is differentiated by the presence of increased blasts (immature) as opposed to the mature neutrophils seen in CML. AML is also less likely due to the lack of acuity of the presentation which is more suggestive of chronic leukemia.
Initial Diagnostic Tests	Check cytogenetic testing (t(9;22) translocation confirms diagnosis)
Next Steps in Management	Tyrosine kinase inhibitors (TKIs)
Discussion	CML is a neoplastic proliferation of myeloid cells, resulting in the production of the full spectrum of mature granulocytes such as neutrophils, basophils, and eosinophils. Median age of onset is 50–60 years old. CML has three phases: 1. Chronic phase (about 90% of cases on presentation): <15% blasts 2. Accelerated phase: 15–20% blasts and ≥20% basophils 3. Blast crisis phase: ≥20% blasts on bone marrow Without intervention, patients will advance through the accelerated phase and ultimately transform into a blast crisis. **History/Physical Exam:** • Commonly presents in adults aged 50–60. • ~40% of cases diagnosed incidentally (leukocytosis on routine CBC) • Symptoms may include fatigue, night sweats, malaise or weight loss, LUQ pain (from splenomegaly), and weakness • Patients in accelerated or blast crises may present with lymphadenopathy, extramedullary masses, and bone pain **Diagnostics:** • Cytogenetic testing (chromosomal analysis or FISH) demonstrating t(9;22) translocation (Philadelphia chromosome) confirms the diagnosis • CBC with leukocytosis (median ~100,000) showing a normal range of neutrophilic cells, basophilia, eosinophilia • Consider checking LDH (↑) and leukocyte alkaline phosphatase activity (LAP↓) • Bone marrow biopsy reveals granulocyte hyperplasia **Management:** • TKIs such as imatinib, dasatinib, or nilotinib bind to and inhibit BCR-ABL tyrosine kinase, preventing unregulated cell proliferation.
Additional considerations	**Complications:** Patients are at an increased risk of infections, bleeding, and leukostasis. Massive splenomegaly can result in splenic infarctions. **CML blast crisis:** Transformation to acute leukemia (either AML or ALL).

CASE 10 | Polycythemia Vera (PV)

A 67-year-old woman with a history of splenic vein thrombosis presents with burning of the extremities. She notes that her feet intermittently turn red, warm, and burn (erythromelalgia) (see image). She also has intermittent headaches and generalized pruritis, which is worse after hot showers (aquagenic pruritis). She does not smoke. On exam, she has a ruddy complexion (facial plethora), a blood pressure of 158/94 mmHg, an enlarged liver, skin excoriations, and erythematous extremities with hypersensitivity to touch. CBC shows WBC 11×10^9/L, hemoglobin 18 g/dL, RBC 6×10^{12}/L, platelets 425×10^9/L.

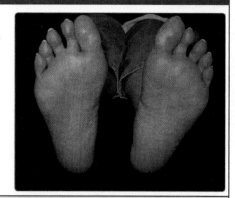

Intense erythema of the feet with associated burning pain typical of erythromelalgia. (Reproduced with permission from Sewon Kang, Masayuki Amagai, Anna L. Bruckner, Alexander H. Enk, David J. Margolis, Amy J. McMichael, Jeffrey S. Orringer, Fitzpatrick's Dermatology, 9e. New York, NY: McGraw-Hill 2019.)

Conditions with Similar Presentations	**Relative polycythemia (erythrocytosis):** Is caused by volume contraction and leads to an apparent increase in hemoglobin and hematocrit (e.g., dehydration, GI losses, burns, diuretic use). Though ↑ Hb, would have normal or ↑ epoetin alfa (EPO). **Secondary polycythemia:** Is caused by non-hematologic conditions that alter hemoglobin production, including conditions causing tissue hypoxia, hemoglobin mutations leading to abnormal oxygen dissociation, or EPO-producing tumors. See table for secondary causes.
Initial Diagnostic Testing	Check CBC, EPO level, JAK2 mutation analysis, and bone marrow biopsy.
Next Steps in Management	• Aspirin and therapeutic phlebotomy • High-risk patients should receive hydroxyurea

Discussion	PV is a myeloproliferative disorder marked by increased RBC mass due to mutations in JAK2 (95% of cases). PV is the most common MPN and the median age of onset is 60 years old. Patients with PV can also have concomitant secondary causes of erythrocytosis based on risk factors (e.g., from sleep apnea).
	
	History/Physical Exam:
	• Majority asymptomatic. Symptoms may include headaches, visual disturbances, Raynaud phenomenon (from hyperviscosity) pruritis especially after hot showers (**aquagenic pruritis**), neuropathy, hypertension, or constitutional symptoms.
	• Classic symptom is **erythromelalgia**, periodic attacks of burning pain with erythema and swelling that primarily affects the hands and feet.
	• On exam, patients may have **facial plethora** or a ruddy complexion. Splenomegaly may be present.
	
	Diagnostics:
	• Patients with the following meet criteria for PV:
	  • Hemoglobin >16.5 g/dL (males) or >16 g/dL (females)
	  • Bone marrow biopsy with trilineage hypercellularity
	  • JAK2 mutation and/or ↓serum EPO
	• It is important to rule out secondary causes of polycythemia (see table above).
	
	Management: Vascular complications due to hyperviscosity are a significant cause of morbidity, and treatment is targeted at reducing the risk of thrombosis.
	• Aspirin and phlebotomy to reduce hematocrit <45%
	• High-risk patients (age >60, prior thrombosis) should receive hydroxyurea
	• Alternative agents include ruxolitinib and interferon if not responsive or intolerant of hydroxyurea

Additional Considerations	**Complications:** PV can progress to **AML** or **myelofibrosis**. Anemia, no longer needing phlebotomy, worsening splenomegaly or new constitutional symptoms should raise suspicion of disease transformation. Patients with any MPN can present with **arterial or venous thrombosis** in unusual sites, such as splenic thrombosis, **Budd-Chiari syndrome** (in absence of liver disease), or cerebral sinus vein thrombosis.

CASE 11 | Primary Myelofibrosis

A 57-year-old woman presents with low-grade fevers, weight loss, fatigue. She also reports bone pain and early satiety from abdominal fullness. She denies cough or dysuria. On physical exam, she has conjunctival pallor and hepatosplenomegaly. CBC reveals a hemoglobin of 9.8 g/dL. A peripheral blood smear shows numerous teardrop-shaped RBCs (see image).

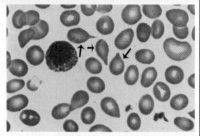

Peripheral smear with teardrop cells. (Reproduced with permission from Lichtman MA, Shafer MS, Felgar RE, Wang N, Lichtman's Atlas of Hematology 2016. New York, NY: McGraw-Hill 2017.)

Conditions with Similar Presentations	**Granulomatous disease (tuberculosis or histoplasmosis):** Can also present with constitutional symptoms (fatigue, fever, night sweats), but patients would have risk factors (e.g., TB: incarceration, housing instability, health care worker, injection drug use; histoplasmosis: endemic area) and biopsy/culture of affected organs confirming diagnosis and/or positive histoplasma urine Ag testing.
	Metastatic carcinoma: Including solid tumors (e.g., lung cancer, prostate cancer, breast cancer) and lymphomas that infiltrate the marrow can cause **secondary myelofibrosis** but clinical history and bone marrow biopsy will differentiate from primary myelofibrosis.
	Chronic myeloid leukemia (CML): Presents with splenomegaly, leukocytosis, and thrombocytosis, but teardrop cells and a fibrotic bone marrow are not seen.
Initial Diagnostic Testing	• Confirm diagnosis with bone marrow biopsy • Consider: Abdominal ultrasound to evaluate for hepatosplenomegaly; molecular mutation testing
Next Steps in Management	• JAK1/2 inhibitor (ruxolitinib or fedratinib) • Hydroxyurea • Stem cell transplant
Discussion	Myelofibrosis (MF) is a clonal hematologic malignancy marked by proliferation of atypical megakaryocytes, which secrete cytokines and growth factors that increase fibroblast activity leading to increased deposition of reticulin and collagen in the bone marrow leading to marrow fibrosis. Median age of onset is 65 years old. Patients develop extramedullary hematopoiesis, especially in the bones, liver, lungs, or spleen leading to massive splenomegaly. • Myelofibrosis can be diagnosed de novo "**primary**" or be the terminal manifestation of other myeloproliferative conditions such as polycythemia vera (PV) or essential thrombocytosis (ET) "**secondary**." • It is the least common of the MPNs. The natural history of MF is variable, with some patients progressing to acute leukemia within 10 years of diagnosis. **History/Physical Exam:** • May have history of PV or ET • Most common symptom is fatigue but can have other constitutional symptoms (fever, weight loss) or pruritis • Splenomegaly found in most patients, and can present as abdominal fullness, early satiety, and/or LUQ pain • Hepatomegaly also common and can cause ascites, variceal complications, or portal vein thrombosis • Bone and joint involvement can cause significant pain

CASE 11 | Primary Myelofibrosis *(continued)*

Discussion	**Diagnostics:** • CBC with differential shows anemia with variable WBC and platelet counts (either increased or decreased) • Peripheral smear often shows "teardrop" cells, nucleated RBCs, and immature forms of WBCs (**leukoerythroblastosis**), which are signs of the replacement of normal bone marrow with fibrosis • Bone marrow biopsy is required for diagnosis which shows abnormal megakaryocytes and advanced reticulin/collagen deposition Reticulin stain of marrow myelofibrosis. Silver stain of a myelofibrotic marrow showing an increase in reticulin fibers (black-staining threads). (Reproduced with permission from J. Larry Jameson, Anthony S. Fauci, Dennis L. Kasper, Stephen L. Hauser, Dan L. Longo, Joseph Loscalzo, Harrison's Principles of Internal Medicine, 20e. New York, NY: McGraw-Hill 2018.) • Molecular testing will show specific clonal mutations associated with myelofibrosis • JAK2 mutations in 50% **Management:** Treatment is stratified according to risk and symptom burden. • Observation is an option in patients with asymptomatic, low risk disease • Patients with symptomatic MPN (splenomegaly, pain, constitutional symptoms) should be treated with JAK inhibitors (ruxolitinib or fedratinib) or hydroxyurea • Stem cell transplant is the treatment of choice for high-risk or refractory disease if the patient has good functional status (usually young and medically fit patients)
Additional Considerations	**Complications:** • Transformation to acute leukemia (AML) is a major cause of mortality. • Higher risk for infections. • Similar to other MPNs, patients at risk of thrombosis. They can also have splenic infarcts from splenomegaly.

Myeloproliferative Disorder Mini-Cases

Cases	Key Findings
Myelodysplastic Syndrome (MDS)	**Hx:** Risk factors: There may be a past history of chemotherapy, ionizing radiation, exposure to benzene, or hereditary conditions such as Down syndrome, or ataxia telangiectasia. A history of autoimmune disease (e.g., rheumatic heart disease, rheumatoid arthritis, pernicious anemia) is seen in ~20%. Symptoms: Often asymptomatic and found incidentally in a CBC. If present, symptoms related to the specific cytopenia(s). Fatigue, DOE, SOB from anemia, neutropenia predisposing to an infection easy bruising or bleeding due to thrombocytopenia. **PE:** Findings depend on the cell line(s) affected; there may be tachycardia, pallor, or cutaneous signs of bleeding. Some patients have splenomegaly. **Diagnostics:** • At least one cytopenia on CBC • Dysplasia of one or more cell lines is seen on peripheral smear • Bone marrow with ≥10% dysplasia in at least one cell line but <20% blasts. There may be ringed sideroblasts, pseudo-Pelger Huet cells, and hypogranulation of myelocytes.

Myeloproliferative Disorder Mini-Cases *(continued)*

Myelodysplastic Syndrome (MDS)	**Management:** • Treat symptomatic anemia or thrombocytopenia with transfusions. • Persistent symptoms may also be treated with "low-intensity" regimens (epoetin, thrombopoietin receptor agonists), azacitidine, lenalidomide. • Cytotoxic chemotherapy is not routinely effective. • Allogeneic hematopoietic stem cell transplant in selected individuals **Discussion:** MDS are a group of hematologic malignancies that have in common abnormal clonal proliferation, at least one cytopenia, and increased blood cell apoptosis. Median age of onset is 70 years old with a male predominance and symptoms depend on which cell line(s) are most greatly affected. MDS can transform into AML in ~40% of cases.
Essential Thrombocythemia (ET)	**Hx/PE:** • Median age at diagnosis of 60 years. Females are more likely to be affected than males. Family history of myeloproliferative neoplasms may be present. • ~50% are asymptomatic; incidental finding on CBC. • Some have constitutional symptoms (fatigue, night sweats, weight loss, fever) or vasomotor symptoms (headaches, pruritis) from microvascular thrombi. • Patients with extreme thrombocytosis (platelet count >1 million) may present with bleeding-related issues such as epistaxis or hematomas. • Erythromelalgia (pain or erythema in hands or feet from microvascular thrombi) or cutaneous bruising is more common in ET than other MPNs. • Splenomegaly in 20–35%. • Exam may also reveal manifestations of arterial or venous thrombotic events such as stroke, DVT. **Diagnostics:** • Suspect in patients with thrombocytosis (platelet ≥450 × 10⁹/L). • Evaluate for secondary causes of thrombocytosis (reactive thrombocytosis in setting of infection or trauma, post-splenectomy state, iron-deficiency anemia). • Mutational analysis for Jak2/CALR/MPL. • Absence of other MPNs (CML, PV). **Management:** The goal is to reduce thrombotic complications. • Lower risk (<60 years and no history of thrombosis): observation or aspirin • Higher risk (>60 years and/or have history of thrombosis): hydroxyurea + aspirin • Interferon alpha can be considered in high-risk pregnant patients where hydroxyurea is contraindicated. **Discussion:** ET is a chronic MPN characterized by elevated platelet count. Thrombotic complications are a source of morbidity. ET is a clonal process driven by mutations including Jak2 V617F (50–65%), CALR (20–25%) or MPL (5%). Most patients will have a normal life expectancy, though the risk of progression to myelofibrosis or acute leukemia increases over time. • ET can have overlapping clinical and laboratory features with other MPNs, notably leukocytosis or erythrocytosis. • Patients with extreme thrombocytosis (platelet count >1 million) are at risk of having acquired von Willebrand disease (vWD). • Surgical Consideration: There is increased risk for thrombosis or bleeding in patients with ET undergoing surgery.

LYMPHOMAS

Lymphomas are malignancies arising from lymphoid cells, most commonly the lymph nodes. Presentation is classically associated with "B symptoms" including fevers, night sweats, and weight loss. They are primarily categorized as Hodgkin lymphoma (HL) or non-Hodgkin lymphoma (NHL):

• HL has a bimodal age distribution and is characterized by Reed-Sternberg, or "owl-eye nuclei," cells. HL originates in lymph nodes, spreads contiguously within them, and has rare extranodal involvement.

• NHL may originate outside of lymph nodes and has noncontiguous spread. It has a peak incidence 65–75 years of age.

Non-Hodgkin Lymphoma

Type	Presentation	Epidemiology	Genetics	Prognosis/Treatment
Follicular lymphoma	Lymphadenopathy and B symptoms	Adults, median age 65 years	t(14;18) (BCL-2 rearrangement)	Indolent malignancy, treatable but not curable
Diffuse large B cell lymphoma (DLBCL)	Lymphadenopathy and B symptoms. Indolent lymphomas (CLL, FL) can transform to DLBCL May present as extranodal mass (head and neck or GI tract)	Adults (most common NHL)	No pathognomonic alteration May see Bcl-2, Bcl-6 alterations	Aggressive malignancy but curable Treat with chemotherapy with R-CHOP (**R**ituximab-**C**yclophosphamide, Doxorubicin (**H**ydroxydaunomycin), Vincristine (**O**ncovin), **P**rednisone)
Mantle cell lymphoma	B symptoms, GI symptoms, lymphadenopathy, hepatosplenomegaly	Adult, men > women	t(11;14) (cyclin D1 rearrangement) Bone marrow with tiny cells	Aggressive and usually presents at a high stage.
Burkitt lymphoma	1. Endemic form seen in Africa presents as jaw mass (associated with EBV) 2. Sporadic form presents with diffuse lymphadenopathy (associated with HIV)	More common in children than adults	t(8;14) (c-*myc* gene rearrangement) Bone marrow: starry sky appearance, phagohistiocytosis	Aggressive malignancy Treat with multi-agent chemotherapy Good prognosis in children

CASE 12 | Hodgkin Lymphoma (HL)

A 27-year-old woman presents for evaluation of recurrent fevers. She has a 1-month history of low-grade fevers, as well as a 14-lb weight loss and night sweats. She has no past medical history and takes no medications. Physical exam reveals nontender lymphadenopathy in the anterior cervical and axillary regions, and a large supraclavicular node. The lymph nodes are firm and immobile; biopsy shows cells with bilobed "owl-eyes" nuclei (Reed-Sternberg cells). HIV test is negative.

Conditions with Similar Presentations	**Infectious mononucleosis:** Is due to EBV infection, which may also play a role in the pathogenesis of HL. Patients usually present with sore throat and positive heterophile antibody test. **Tuberculosis:** Can also cause night sweats and weight loss. Other symptoms include hemoptysis and chronic cough. Biopsy shows caseating granulomas, and patients typically have risk factors of traveling or living in endemic areas or working in healthcare or prison systems. **Sarcoidosis:** May present with fevers and weight loss but also commonly includes respiratory symptoms (cough, dyspnea), and biopsy would show noncaseating granulomas.
Initial Diagnostic Tests	• Excisional lymph node biopsy • PET/CT scan
Next Steps in Management	Chemotherapy
Discussion	HL is a B-cell malignancy, and patients present with lymphadenopathy and may have constitutional "B" symptoms (fever, night sweats, weight loss). **History/Physical Exam:** • Presents in a bimodal age distribution, affecting young adults approximately 20 years of age and older adults with average age of 65 years. • May see B-symptoms and can have severe pruritis unresponsive to topical agents and oral medication. • Risk factors include a history of infectious mononucleosis caused by EBV, immunosuppression, or autoimmune disease such as rheumatoid arthritis, SLE, or sarcoidosis. • Painless lymphadenopathy in cervical, supraclavicular, and mediastinal regions. "Rubbery," fixed, nontender lymphadenopathy (often cervical or supraclavicular).

CASE 12 | Hodgkin Lymphoma (HL) *(continued)*

Discussion	**Diagnostics:**
	• Diagnosis is confirmed via excisional lymph node (LN) biopsy showing Reed-Sternberg cells (bilobed nuclei, "owl eyes" appearance) and immunohistochemistry (see image).
	• PET/CT scan to determine stage which determines treatment:
	• I: Single enlarged LN
	• II: >1 LN, same side of diaphragm
	• III: LN both sides of diaphragm
	• IV: Extranodal involvement (i.e., bone marrow)
	• *If presence of B symptoms, add "B" to the stage*
	Management:
	• Chemotherapy with ABVD (**A**driamycin, **B**leomycin, **V**inblastine, and **D**acarbazine).
	• Consider post-chemotherapy radiation for limited stage; however, may avoid due to long-term radiation side effects.
	• Survival is excellent; >75% of patients are cured of their disease, but some may require stem cell transplant to achieve remission.
Additional Considerations	**Complications: SVC syndrome** can occur secondary to mediastinal lymphadenopathy.

Reed-Sternberg cells. (Reproduced with permission from Kenneth Kaushansky, Marshall A. Lichtman, Josef T. Prchal, Marcel M. Levi, Oliver W. Press, Linda J. Burns, Michael Caligiuri, Williams Hematology, 9e. New York, NY: McGraw-Hill 2016.)

PLASMA CELL DYSCRASIAS

Plasma cell dyscrasias (PCDs) are disorders caused by a malignant proliferation of a monoclonal plasma cells, producing excess immunoglobulins and/or fragments (heavy and light chains). The two most common conditions are multiple myeloma (MM) and monoclonal gammopathy of undetermined significance (MGUS). Other disorders that also fall into this category include Waldenström macroglobulinemia and amyloidosis.

CASE 13 | Multiple Myeloma

A 68-year-old woman presents with low back pain, fatigue, and 20-lb weight loss over the last 5 months. She attributes weight loss to two separate episodes of pneumonia in the last year. She has numbness and tingling in her upper and lower extremities but denies incontinence of bowel or bladder, or lower extremity weakness. Physical exam reveals bony tenderness over the spine. Labs with hemoglobin 7.9 g/dL, MCV 88 fL, creatinine 2.3 mg/dL, calcium 12.2 mg/dL. Imaging reveals multiple lytic lesions in the skull and other bones, along with compression fracture of L3 vertebra. Serum protein electrophoresis (SPEP) reveals presence of a monoclonal IgG protein measuring 3.5 g/dL. Bone marrow biopsy reveals 15% plasma cells.

Conditions with Similar Presentations	**Monoclonal gammopathy of undetermined significance (MGUS):** Also has an elevated monoclonal protein but is quantified as <3 g/dL, bone marrow has <10% plasma cells, and end-organ damage would be absent.
	Waldenstrom macroglobulinemia: Is a lymphoplasmocytic lymphoma that causes a monoclonal IgM gammopathy. Patients present with fatigue, B symptoms, GI symptoms, and hyperviscosity syndrome. Exam may be notable for lymphadenopathy, rash, decreased visual acuity, hepatosplenomegaly, and neuropathy but do not present with lytic lesions or renal insufficiency.
	Primary bone cancer or metastatic cancer to the spine: Could also cause bone pain and vertebral compression fracture; however, would not produce a monoclonal protein on SPEP.
Initial Diagnostic Tests	Confirm diagnosis with serum and urine protein electrophoresis (SPEP), serum and urine light chains, bone marrow biopsy with >10% plasma cells.
Next Steps in Management	• Management of end-organ damage (hypercalcemia, bone pain or fractures, anemia) • Chemotherapy, stem cell transplant

CASE 13 | Multiple Myeloma *(continued)*

Discussion	Multiple myeloma (MM) is a plasma cell malignancy where unregulated proliferation of a clonal plasma cell population produces excess immunoglobulins (monoclonal protein, also known as M protein). MM can arise from MGUS, which is an asymptomatic and premalignant condition, or smoldering MM (SMM). Progression to MM is dependent on signs of end-organ dysfunction (CRAB findings—see below).
	
	History/Physical Exam:
	• Median age 60–70s. Risk factors include MGUS (progresses to MM ~1% per year) and SMM (progresses to MM ~10% a year).
	• Anemia is present in the majority of patients and may present with symptoms of fatigue, SOB, DOE, and signs of pallor.
	• Approximately half present with bony pain in axial skeleton (vertebra, pelvis/femur, shoulder) due to lytic lesions causing fractures. Vertebral compression fractures can cause radiculopathy.
	• Approximately half of patients have kidney disease which may be symptomatic.
	• Hypercalcemia is seen in ~25% and may present as altered mental status, kidney stones, or abdominal pain.
	
	Diagnostics:
	• ≥10% clonal plasma cells on bone marrow biopsy or extramedullary plasmacytoma and any one of the following CRAB or biomarkers of malignancy.
	• CRAB
	  • hyper**C**alcemia
	  • **R**enal insufficiency
	  • **A**nemia
	  • **B**one lesions (osteolytic)
	• Biomarkers of malignancy
	  • Clonal bone marrow plasma cells ≥60%
	  • Involved:uninvolved serum free light chain ratio ≥100
	  • >1 focal lesion on MRI
	
	Additional findings:
	• Elevated total protein
	• Peripheral smear: Rouleaux formation of RBC, which resembles stacked poker chips (see image)
	
	Management:
	• Fluorescent in situ hybridization (FISH) to assess for translocations that are used for risk stratification
	• Hematopoietic cell transplantation recommended for all eligible patients
	• If not eligible, patients should receive chemotherapy
	• Bisphosphonates help ↓ hypercalcemia and treat lytic lesions
	• Radiation can also treat lytic lesions
	
	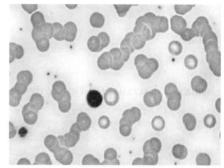
	Rouleaux formation on peripheral smear. (Reproduced with permission from J. Larry Jameson, Anthony S. Fauci, Dennis L. Kasper, Stephen L. Hauser, Dan L. Longo, Joseph Loscalzo, Harrison's Principles of Internal Medicine, 20e. New York, NY: McGraw-Hill 2018.)

Additional Considerations	**Complications: Hyperviscosity syndrome** can be caused by elevated immunoglobulins (most common with IgM) and presents as stroke-like symptoms, ocular abnormalities, and respiratory distress.

ONCOLOGY

For specific solid organ tumor cases, please refer to the appropriate chapters (i.e., hepatocellular carcinoma and colon cancer in Gastroenterology Chapter, ovarian and cervical cancer cases in Obstetrics and Gynecology Chapter, brain tumors in Neurology Chapter, breast cancer in Surgery Chapter, and thyroid and other endocrine tumors in Endocrinology Chapter. General information regarding staging and treatment is provided below.

Tumor Grading and Staging Nomenclature

Tumor Grade: Describes how closely the cancerous cells resemble their cells of origin.

- Well-differentiated cells have similar resemblance to the cells of origin, and thus replicate more slowly and are associated with a better prognosis.
- As the tumor grade increases (i.e., intermediate- and poorly differentiated), cancer cells have greater histopathologic differences and usually replicate more quickly and are associated with a worse prognosis.
  - *Tumor grading spectrum: Well-differentiated → intermediate-differentiated → poorly differentiated → undifferentiated*
- While tumor grade is an indicator of aggressiveness, the extent of tumor spread (staging) most closely predicts prognosis.

Tumor Stage: Describes the degree of tumor spread.

- Staging is based on the TNM system for solid tumors. (*T = primary tumor; N = lymph node involvement; M = presence of metastases*)
- The presence of metastases correlates with worse prognosis

Tumor Stage

T (Tumor)	N (Lymph Nodes)	M (Metastasis)
T0: no evidence of tumor	N0: no lymph node involvement	M0: no distant tumor spread
T1-4: degree of local/direct tumor invasion	N1-3: number and sites of lymph nodes involved	M1: distant tumor spread
Tx: unable to assess	Nx: unable to assess	Mx: unable to assess

Hereditary Cancer Syndromes

Syndrome	Gene	Inheritance	Associated Cancers	Screening
MEN 1 **MEN 2A** **MEN 2B**	MEN1 RET	Autosomal Dominant (AD)	MEN1: Pituitary, pancreatic neuroendocrine tumors, parathyroid adenoma MEN 2A/2B: Medullary thyroid cancer, pheochromocytoma, mucosal neuromas (2B only)	MEN1: Annual biochemical monitoring for parathyroid and neuroendocrine tumor MEN 2A/2B: Annual biochemical monitoring for pheochromocytoma
Lynch syndrome	MLH1, MSH2, MSH6, PMS2	AD	Colorectal, endometrial, ovarian, stomach	Annual colonoscopy starting at age 25 or 5–10 years before earliest onset in age in family Consider risk-reducing hysterectomy and oopherectomy in women, or annual endometrial sampling at age 30–25 or 5–10 years before earliest onset in age in family
FAP (Familial adenomatous polyposis)	APC	AD	Gastric polyps, colorectal polyps and cancer, desmoid tumor	Classic FAP: Annual colonoscopy starting at age 12–14; annual EGD starting at age 25–30
Hereditary breast and ovarian cancer syndrome	BRCA1, BRCA2	AD	BRCA1: Breast, ovarian, pancreatic BRCA2: Breast, ovarian, stomach, pancreatic, prostate, melanoma	Annual breast MRI +/– mammogram starting at age 25–29
Li-Fraumeni	TP53	AD	Soft tissue and bone sarcomas, leukemia, breast, brain, adrenocortical cancers	Annual breast MRI +/– mammogram starting at age 20–25
von Hippel Lindau	VHL	AD	Renal cell cancer, pheochromocytoma, hemangioblastoma	Annual biochemical monitoring for pheochromocytoma starting age 5–10; biennial MRI brain and total spine starting at age 11

Hereditary Cancer Syndromes

Syndrome	Gene	Inheritance	Associated Cancers	Screening
Neurofibromatosis type 1 and 2	NF1, NF2	AD	NF type 1: Optic gliomas, neurofibromas, malignant peripheral nerve sheath tumor, breast, pheochromocytoma NF type 2: Meningioma, schwannoma	NF1: Annual breast MRI +/− mammogram starting at age 30 NF2: Brain and spine MRI starting at age 10

Paraneoplastic Syndromes and Associated Cancers

Organ System	Paraneoplastic Syndrome	Associated Cancers	Etiology
Neuromuscular	Lambert-Eaton	Small-cell lung cancer	Antibody to presynaptic calcium channels
	Myasthenia gravis	Thymoma	Anti-acetylcholine receptor antibody or anti-muscle-specific tyrosine kinase
	Opsoclonus-myoclonus ataxia syndrome	Neuroblastoma (children), small cell lung cancer (adults)	Antibody to Purkinje cells
Endocrine	Cushing syndrome	Small-cell lung cancer Bronchial carcinoid	ACTH
	Hypercalcemia	Squamous-cell lung cancer Lymphoma Multiple myeloma	PTHrP, calcitriol, or osteoclast activation
	SIADH	Small-cell lung cancer	ADH
Rheumatologic	Dermatomyositis	Breast, ovarian, lung, prostate	Cross-reactivity with tumor antigens
	Hypertrophic osteoarthropathy	Thoracic tumors Rhabdomyosarcoma	VEGF, PDGF, prostaglandin
Dermatologic	Sweet syndrome	AML	Unknown
	Leukocytoclastic vasculitis	Leukemia/MDS Lymphoma	Small vessel immune complex formation from circulating tumor antigens
	Paraneoplastic pemphigus	Non-Hodgkin lymphoma CLL	Antibodies to epidermal proteins
Hematologic	Polycythemia	Renal cell cancer, HCC	EPO production
	Pure red cell aplasia	Thymoma	Antibodies to RBCs

Hypercalcemia of Malignancy Mini-Case

Hypercalcemia of Malignancy	**Hx/PE:** • May have known malignancy or may be the initial presentation, especially in patients with multiple myeloma • Depending on the calcium level, may be asymptomatic or have symptomatic hypercalcemia • Symptoms: "stones" (renal calcium-based stones), "bones" (bone pain), "groans" (abdominal pain, constipation), and "psychiatric overtones" (altered mental status, confusion, lethargy) • Signs and symptoms of dehydration from polyuria (dry mucous membranes, reduced skin turgor, orthostasis, low blood pressure) **Diagnostics:** • Elevated serum calcium (confirm with ionized calcium) • Low serum PTH (rule out primary hyperparathyroidism) • 1,25-hydroxyvitamin D and/or, PTHrP elevated depending on the mechanism of hypercalcemia of malignancy.

Hypercalcemia of Malignancy Mini-Case *(continued)*

| Hypercalcemia of Malignancy | **Management:**
• *Mild* hypercalcemia (corrected calcium <12 mg/dL) and asymptomatic: Monitor; acute treatment not required
• *Moderate* hypercalcemia (corrected calcium level 12–14 mg/dL), or symptoms, treat with isotonic saline infusion
• *Severe* hypercalcemia (corrected calcium ≥14 mg/dL) and/or significant symptoms (i.e., neurologic), treat with isotonic saline infusion and additional therapy including **calcitonin** to quickly decrease calcium levels and **bisphosphonates** which have a slower onset (>24 hours) but have a longer-lasting effect on hypercalcemia

Discussion: Primary hyperparathyroidism and malignancy account for 90% of the cases of hypercalcemia. Malignancy is the most common cause of hypercalcemia in the inpatient setting. There are three common mechanisms by which malignancy causes hypercalcemia:
1. Ectopic production of PTHrP (solid tumor malignancies)
2. Ectopic production of 1,25-dihydroxyvitamin D (lymphomas and granulomas)
3. Osteolytic bone metastases through RANKL activation and local cytokine release (myeloma and solid tumors with osteolytic bone lesions)

Additional Considerations:
• Calcitonin has tachyphylaxis and loses effectiveness after 24–48 hours
• Long-term use of bisphosphonates can be associated with osteonecrosis of the jaw and atypical femur fractures
• Bisphosphonates are contraindicated if CrCl <30 or in dialysis-dependent patients
• Denosumab can be given in patients with renal insufficiency |

CHEMOTHERAPY AND IMMUNOTHERAPY

Chemotherapy

• Cytotoxic medications that usually target different phases of the cell cycle (mitosis) which cause DNA damage or impair DNA synthesis or repair.

• These include alkylating agents which cause abnormal cross-linking and DNA strand breaks, purine and pyrimidine antagonists that affect DNA replication, and microtubule inhibitors that inhibit mitosis.

• Some chemotherapy agents are not cell-cycle specific and can directly damage DNA and lead to irreversible cell death.

• Healthy cells undergoing normal cell division are also affected. Hair, the GI tract, and blood cells are some of the faster dividing cells and are disproportionately affected. This leads to common toxicities of many chemotherapy drugs: alopecia, nausea/vomiting/diarrhea, and cytopenias.

Monoclonal Antibody

• Monoclonal antibodies (mAb) are lab-derived antibodies produced against a specific epitope/target, usually a cell surface marker that is commonly expressed in certain cancers.

• Administration of these agents will target only cells displaying the marker.

• Cells "flagged" by the mAb will be recognized by the immune system (macrophages, NK cells) or complement and undergo cell death by phagocytosis or cell lysis.

Immunotherapy

• Cancer cells have developed mechanisms to evade surveillance and killing by the immune system, specifically by cytotoxic T-cells.

• Immunotherapy agents (PD-L1, PD-1, and CTLA-4 inhibitors) disrupt this evasion and allow recognition and destruction of cancer cells.

• Unfortunately, the activated immune system may attack normal organs, leading to autoimmune complications (e.g., hypothyroidism, diabetes, pneumonitis, hepatitis, colitis).

Radiotherapy

- Ionizing radiation therapy (photon or proton beams) damage DNA and cause cell death.
- Radiation therapy can be used in many different ways:
  - Given concurrently with chemotherapy to synergize efficacy
  - Used alone in cases where a tumor is inoperable (brain or spine tumors) or if the patient is not able to undergo surgery
  - Given as adjuvant treatment after other treatments to reduce the risk of recurrence
- Adverse side effects depend on which organs are involved in the radiation field.

Chemotherapy and Side Effects

Chemotherapeutic Agent	Side Effects	Notes
Platinum agents (cisplatin, carboplatin)	Neurotoxicity, peripheral neuropathy, ototoxicity nephrotoxicity	• Testicular, bladder, ovarian, and lung cancers • Nephrotoxicity minimized with adequate hydration
Bleomycin	Pulmonary fibrosis	• Testicular cancer, Hodgkin lymphoma
Anthracyclines (doxorubicin, daunorubicin)	Cardiomyopathy	• Breast cancer, leukemia • Risk of toxicity increases with greater cumulative doses • Can decrease risk of cardiomyopathy with dexrazoxane
Cyclophosphamide	Hemorrhagic cystitis, SIADH	• Leukemia, lymphoma, and many solid tumors • Hemorrhagic cystitis prevented with Mesna and hydration • Used in autoimmune disorders (lupus nephritis)
Anti-HER2 mAb (trastuzumab)	Cardiomyopathy	• HER-2+ breast cancer • Cardiomyopathy reversible with discontinuation of drug
Anti-estrogen (tamoxifen)	Endometrial carcinoma, thromboembolism (DVT, PE), osteoporosis	• Treat and prevent breast cancer
Taxanes (docetaxel, paclitaxel)	Neurotoxicity, peripheral neuropathy	• Ovarian and breast cancers
Vinca alkaloids (vincristine)	Neurotoxicity, peripheral neuropathy, paralytic ileus	• Acute lymphoblastic leukemia (ALL), lymphoma, sarcoma
Methotrexate	Myelosuppression, hepatotoxicity, folate deficiency, mucositis	• Leukemia, lymphoma, other solid tumors • Also used to treat ectopic pregnancy and autoimmune conditions • Leucovorin administration minimizes mucositis and cytopenias
Hydroxyurea	Myelosuppression	• Myeloproliferative disorders • Sickle cell disease to prevent vaso-occlusive crises (increases fetal hemoglobin)

TRANSFUSION MEDICINE

Transfusion Reactions

Blood transfusion reactions are potentially serious complications occurring after transfusion of platelets, plasma products, or RBCs.

- Mediated by **immunologic** or **non-immunologic** factors.
- Can occur within minutes to hours of a transfusion but can be delayed for weeks. Timing of reaction and clinical manifestations are useful in determining the etiology of the reaction.
- Regardless of the etiology, the first step in management is always to stop the transfusion.

	Immediate	0–6 hours	0–24 hours	Delayed
Immunologic	• Allergic—urticaria	• Febrile non-hemolytic transfusion reaction (FNHTR) • Transfusion-related lung injury (TRALI)	• Acute hemolytic transfusion reaction (ABO incompatibility)	• Delayed hemolytic transfusion reaction • TA-GVHD • Post-transfusion purpura
Non-immunologic		• Bacterial contamination • Transfusion-associated circulatory overload (TACO)		• Viral transmission (e.g., HBV, HCV, HIV)

Blood Product	Product Components	Use
Red blood cells	Red blood cells, prepared by removing plasma from whole blood	Acute blood loss, symptomatic anemia or Hb <7.0
Fresh frozen plasma (FFP)	All coagulation factors, fibrinolytic proteins, immunoglobulins, albumin, plasma proteins	Correct coagulopathy in patients with coagulation defects (i.e., warfarin use, liver disease)
Cryoprecipitate	Fibrinogen, factor VIII, factor XIII, VWF, and fibronectin	Increase fibrinogen levels in patients with fibrinogen consumption (i.e., DIC) or dysfunction
Platelets	Pooled or single donor platelets, collected by apheresis or from whole blood	Prevent or control bleeding in patients with thrombocytopenia or platelet dysfunction
Whole blood	Blood that has not been separated into blood components	Severe hemorrhage; may be used if apheresis platelets not available

Transfusion Reaction Mini-Cases

Cases	Key Findings
Allergic and Anaphylactic Transfusion Reaction	**Hx/PE:** Symptoms occur within minutes of transfusion • Allergic reactions: Mild symptoms (e.g., urticaria, pruritis, flushing) • Anaphylactic reactions: Can be severe and life-threatening (e.g., angioedema, lip/tongue swelling, bronchospasm, wheezing, respiratory distress) and have hemodynamic instability (hypotension) **Diagnostics:** Clinical diagnosis made in setting of transfusion • Rule out other types of acute transfusion reactions and anaphylaxis • Consider other causes (e.g., food or drug allergy) • Consider evaluation for IgA deficiency **Management:** • Stop transfusion • Treat allergic reactions with antihistamines • Treat anaphylactic reactions with epinephrine and antihistamines • Monitor airway and oxygen status • IVF and vasopressors if hypotensive **Discussion:** Allergic and anaphylactic transfusion reactions are uncommon type I hypersensitivity reactions against proteins in the plasma of administered blood products. Anaphylactic reactions are a severe form of allergic reactions and occur due to massive histamine and tryptase release from mast cells. Anaphylactic transfusion reactions are more common in patients with IgA deficiency. Patients with IgA deficiency should receive washed (hence IgA-deficient) blood products.
Febrile Nonhemolytic Transfusion Reaction	**Hx/PE:** Presents within 6 hours of a transfusion • More common to occur after either pRBC or platelet transfusion, less common after plasma transfusion • Fever; no evidence of hemolysis or hemodynamic instability **Diagnostics:** Clinical diagnosis, exclude other acute transfusion reactions and work up other causes of fever/infection **Management:** • Stop transfusion • Ask blood bank to recheck for ABO compatibility • Supportive care (antipyretics for fever, meperidine for rigors if bothersome)

Transfusion Reaction Mini-Cases *(continued)*

Febrile Nonhemolytic Transfusion Reaction	**Discussion:** Febrile nonhemolytic transfusion reactions (FNHTR) occur due to cytokines (IL-1, IL-6, TNF-a), which are created by and accumulate from residual white blood cells during storage. Cytokine release during transfusion causes an inflammatory response. It is the most common of the transfusion reactions, occurring in up to 1% of transfusions, but is not life-threatening. Leukocyte reduction prior to storage can decrease incidence.
Acute and Delayed Hemolytic Transfusion Reaction (HTR)	**Hx/PE:** • Acute hemolytic transfusion reaction (AHTR): Usually occurs within minutes of a transfusion but can be as late as 24 hours • Delayed hemolytic transfusion reaction (DHTR): Can occur days to weeks after transfusion, is clinically silent, and diagnosed on repeat type and screen • Classic triad of AHTR: Fever, flank pain, and hematuria/dark urine. • Severe cases can lead to DIC and/or renal failure • Severity of the reaction is dependent on the type of recipient mismatch and the volume of blood product transfused **Diagnostics:** • Recheck for ABO compatibility and CBC, coags • Positive direct Coombs test • Positive hemolysis studies ($\uparrow$ LDH, $\downarrow$ haptoglobin, $\uparrow$ indirect bilirubin) • Positive serum free hemoglobin **Management:** Medical emergency that requires prompt management. • Stop transfusion • Administer IVF to maintain renal blood flow and minimize renal injury • Monitor serial Hb • Monitor potassium, as hemolysis can cause hyperkalemia • Monitor for and treat DIC (PT, PTT, fibrinogen, d-dimer, Plt). **Discussion:** Acute and delayed hemolytic transfusion reactions are immune-mediated hemolytic responses to unrecognized antigens on RBCs. AHTR usually occurs because of ABO incompatibility, and DHTR is an amnestic response to minor RBC antigens. For instance, when a patient with blood type O (and therefore has anti-A and anti-B antibodies) receives type A RBCs, the patient's anti-A antibodies will cause hemolysis. Hemolysis can be either intravascular or extravascular.
Transfusion-Related Lung Injury (TRALI)	**Hx/PE:** Symptoms present within 1–2 hours after transfusion but can be delayed up to 6 hours • Patients will have sudden hypoxemia and/or dyspnea • Other findings include fever and/or hypotension • If severe, cyanosis from hypoxia can be present; pink-tinged frothy secretions may be visualized in the ET tube of intubated patients **Diagnostics:** • Chest x-ray: Bilateral pulmonary infiltrates; ABG to determine severity of hypoxemia • Rule out other causes of acute transfusion reactions **Management:** • Stop transfusion • Supplemental oxygenation as needed (nasal cannula, CPAP, BiPAP, mechanical ventilation) • Support hemodynamics with IVF or vasopressors • Diuretics **Discussion:** TRALI is a life-threatening condition characterized by non-cardiogenic pulmonary edema. TRALI occurs when donor anti-leukocyte antibodies attack recipient pulmonary endothelium, causing endothelial damage, capillary leak, and pulmonary edema. TRALI can have an insidious onset and no apparent risk factors. Like TACO, it presents with predominantly respiratory distress, hypoxia, and pulmonary infiltrates, but is a form of acute respiratory distress syndrome (ARDS) rather than circulatory overload.

Transfusion Reaction Mini-Cases *(continued)*

Transfusion-Associated Circulatory Overload (TACO)	**Hx/PE:** Symptoms usually present within 12 hours • Risk factors include age <3 or >60 years, preexisting cardiac disease, or high volume of blood product administration • Patients may present with cough, dyspnea, or orthopnea • Patients may have hypoxia, tachycardia, new S3 or jugular venous distension, rales, or wheezing **Diagnostics:** Clinical diagnosis • Elevated BNP and chest x-ray demonstrating pulmonary edema in the clinical context of recent high-volume transfusions • Rule out other causes of heart failure and acute transfusion reactions **Management:** • Stop transfusion • Support oxygenation as needed • Diuretics **Discussion:** TACO is acute pulmonary edema from transfusion volume overload. TACO should be differentiated from other similarly presenting conditions such as TRALI or heart failure. Elevated BNP after transfusion is suggestive of TACO.
Transfusion-Associated Graft-versus-Host Disease (TA-GVHD)	**Hx/PE:** Occurs from 4–30 days after transfusion. • Risk factors include immunosuppression and partial HLA matching of the donor. • The most common symptom is rash (initial maculopapular rash followed by generalized erythroderma). • The majority of patients will have fever. Abdominal pain and diarrhea are seen in about 50%. • Pancytopenia may cause fatigue, easy bruising/bleeding, or infection. **Diagnostics:** • Biopsy of affected organs showing lymphocytic infiltrate • Rule out other possible causes (drug reaction, viral infection, hematologic malignancy, hemophagocytic lymphohistiocytosis) **Management:** Immunosuppression can decrease activity of donor T cells, but patients with TA-GVHD have irreversible bone marrow aplasia and require hematopoietic stem cell transplantation. **Discussion:** TA-GVHD occurs when leukocytes from the transfusion product engraft and attack the recipient. Normally transfused leukocytes are recognized and eliminated by the recipient, but this may not occur when the patient is immunocompromised or there is partial HLA matching. In TA-GVHD, alloreactive T-cells attack recipient organs, most commonly the GI tract, liver, skin, and bone marrow. TA-GVHD has high mortality, reaching >90%, and the only successful treatment is hematopoietic stem cell transplantation. TA-GVHD can be prevented with irradiation of blood products, which inactivates T-cells. Irradiated blood products are recommended before giving to susceptible recipients (patients with immunodeficiency or stem cell transplant).

9

Endocrinology

Lead author: Daniel Joseph Toft, MD, PhD
Contributors: Jorge W. Rivera, MD; Tessa Eckley, MD

INTRODUCTION

The endocrine system consists of multiple organs throughout the body that are connected through hormonal pathways.

Disorder of the endocrine system generally fall into two categories:

- Hormone excess
- Hormone deficiency

Etiologies include, but are not limited to genetic mutations, medication effects, malignant and benign tumors, environmental factors, autoimmune disorders, and trauma.

Each of the endocrine pathways is closely related, resulting in clinical presentations that may be vague and non-specific. Therefore, it is important to obtain a complete history and physical exam.

Some common abnormal findings on physical exam are demonstrated in the following table.

System	Key Features/Findings
Vitals	Alterations in heart rate, blood pressure, weight/BMI/abdominal circumference
Volume status	Dry mucous membranes, abnormal skin turgor, orthostatic hypotension
Eyes	Papilledema, visual field defects (e.g., bitemporal hemianopsia), proptosis
Thyroid	Goiter, nodules
Abdomen	Masses (pancreatic, adrenal)
Skin	Hyperpigmentation, acanthosis nigricans, striae
Genitourinary	Alterations in pubic hair, testicular volume, other secondary sex characteristics
Neuromuscular	Weakness, abnormal sensation, hypo or hyper reflexes

The information in this chapter is based on the authors experience in this field and was confirmed using online resources and references such as Dynamed, Greenspan's Basic & Clinical Endocrinology, Harrison's Principles of Internal Medicine, Endocrine Society Guideline, American Thyroid Association Guidelines, AACE/ACE 2020 Clinical Practice Guidelines, ADA: Standards of Medical Care in Diabetes and Gene Reviews.

HYPOTHALAMIC-PITUITARY-HORMONE AXIS

The hypothalamus and the pituitary start each axis of hormonal regulation. Hormones then act on various endocrine organs throughout the body. Examples of these axes and their associated feedback regulation are demonstrated in the figure.

The hypothalamus releases hormones including:

- Corticotropin-releasing hormone (CRH)
- Thyrotropin-releasing hormone (TRH)
- Growth hormone-releasing hormone (GHRH)
- Gonadotropin-releasing hormone (GnRH)
- Prolactin inhibitory factor (PIF), which is dopamine

These hypothalamic hormones act on the pituitary gland, divided into two lobes based on embryologic development, which secretes hormones that then act on glands and organs throughout the body.

Anterior lobe (adenohypophysis):

- Adrenocorticotrophic hormone (ACTH, corticotropin)
- Thyroid-stimulating hormone (TSH, thyrotropin)
- Growth hormone (GH, somatotropin)
- Follicle-stimulating hormone (FSH)

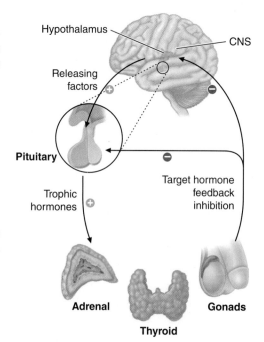

Feedback regulation of endocrine axes. (Reproduced, with permission, from Jameson JL, Fauci AS, Kasper DL, Hauser SL, Longo DL, Loscalzo J, eds. Harrison's Principles of Internal Medicine. 20th ed. New York, NY: McGraw-Hill; 2019.)

- Luteinizing hormone (LH)
- Prolactin
- Melanocyte-stimulating hormone (MSH)

Posterior lobe (neurohypophysis):

- Antidiuretic hormone (ADH; vasopressin, arginine vasopressin [AVP])
- Oxytocin

Disorders of the hypothalamus will affect the function of the pituitary and downstream end-organs, but it is often difficult clinically to distinguish dysfunction of the hypothalamus from dysfunction of the pituitary. Disorders can be categorized into primary, secondary, or tertiary based on where the disease process begins.

	Location of Pathology	Examples
Primary	Secreting gland (e.g., thyroid, adrenal gland)	Hypothyroidism due to Hashimoto thyroiditis Adrenal insufficiency due to lack of cortisol production (Addison disease)
Secondary	Pituitary	Hypothyroidism due to TSH deficiency Adrenal insufficiency due to ACTH deficiency (e.g., in the setting of cessation of chronic corticosteroid use)
Tertiary	Hypothalamus	Hypothyroidism due to TRH deficiency Adrenal insufficiency due to CRH deficiency

Dysfunction in the hypothalamus and pituitary gland can impact the function of multiple glands and organs downstream, leading to an even wider variety of symptoms than can be attributed to a single axis.

Pituitary disorders cause symptoms related to:

- Hormone excess (from functional tumors that release hormones like prolactin or cortisol)
- Hormone deficiency (due to tumors compressing hormone-releasing cells, preventing them from functioning normally)
- Mass effect—headache, diminished vision in the outer visual fields (**bitemporal hemianopsia**) due to compression of the optic chiasm

MRI of the brain is often helpful for diagnosing hypothalamic and pituitary pathology. Specific findings associated with pituitary hormone abnormalities are listed below.

Prolactin

Prolactin is a hormone secreted by the anterior pituitary. Secretion of prolactin is physiologic during pregnancy to support milk production for breastfeeding. Common causes of elevated prolactin include:

- **Pregnancy**—physiologic increase in prolactin; most common cause
- **Hypothyroidism**—lack of feedback inhibition leads to elevation in TSH and TRH, with TRH directly stimulating prolactin secretion
- **Medications:**
  - **Dopamine antagonists** including antipsychotics (e.g., haloperidol, risperidone) and metoclopramide
    - Dopamine is also known as prolactin-inhibiting factor, normally released by hypothalamus to regulate secretion of prolactin
  - Other medications that increase prolactin levels include verapamil, estrogens, H2-receptor antagonists
- **Renal failure**—decreased clearance of prolactin by the kidney

Symptoms/Signs	Hormone Abnormality	Differential Diagnosis
Galactorrhea Menstrual irregularities Infertility Decreased libido	Prolactin excess	Prolactinoma (most common) Drug-induced hyperprolactinemia (e.g., antipsychotics) Breastfeeding (delayed postpartum ovulation to prevent pregnancy) Chronic diseases (e.g., hypothyroidism, liver disease, kidney disease)
Impaired lactation	Prolactin deficiency	Hypopituitarism (craniopharyngioma, pituitary adenoma, infection, Sheehan syndrome, traumatic brain injury, primary or metastatic cancer)

Growth Hormone (GH), Somatotropin

GH promotes growth of the skeleton and organs. It stimulates production of insulin-like growth factor 1 (IGF-1), mainly in the liver, which is the primary effector of GH signaling.

Symptoms/Signs	Hormone Abnormality	Differential Diagnosis
Large tongue Jaw prognathism Frontal bossing Large hands and feet Diaphoresis Hyperglycemia Rapid growth in children Peripheral neuropathy Hyperglycemia	Growth hormone excess	GH-secreting pituitary adenoma Gigantism (GH excess occurs before the growth plate closes) Acromegaly (GH excess occurs after the growth plate closes)
Short stature Hypoglycemia Micropenis in male infants	Growth hormone deficiency	Hypopituitarism (craniopharyngioma, pituitary adenoma, infection, Sheehan syndrome, traumatic brain injury, primary or metastatic cancer)

Antidiuretic Hormone (ADH)

ADH (also called vasopressin) is a hormone that causes the kidney to retain free water, resulting in increased concentration of the urine.

- It is synthesized in the paraventricular and supraoptic nuclei of the hypothalamus and then transported for storage to the posterior pituitary.
- ADH **decreases serum osmolality by increasing urine osmolality**
- Acts on renal collecting duct, promoting insertion of aquaporin channels to facilitate **water reabsorption**, thus regulating blood volume and pressure

Symptoms/Signs	Hormone Abnormality	Differential Diagnosis
Nausea Headache Altered mental status (All due to hyponatremia)	ADH excess	Syndrome of inappropriate antidiuretic hormone secretion (SIADH) Paraneoplastic ADH secretion (e.g., small cell lung cancer)
Polydipsia Polyuria Nocturia	ADH deficiency	Central diabetes insipidus (DI) (can be seen with hypopituitarism) Nephrogenic DI

There are two forms of diabetes insipidus (DI):

- **Central DI:** Lack of ADH production by the posterior pituitary
- **Nephrogenic DI:** Kidney unable to appropriately respond to ADH

They are differentiated by a water deprivation test. In central DI, several hours without water intake will cause a rise in both serum sodium and plasma osmolality, with no change in urine osmolality.

When the ADH analog desmopressin is subsequently given, the urine osmolality will rise >50%. This step helps to differentiate central from nephrogenic DI.

In nephrogenic DI, the plasma osmolality and urine osmolality will not change in response to desmopressin.

CASE 1 | Cushing Disease (ACTH-Secreting Pituitary Adenoma)

A 42-year-old woman with hypertension and obesity presents with difficulty losing weight. Despite calorie restriction and increased activity, she has had a 10-pound weight gain over the last 6 months. She also reports polyuria, polydipsia, several vaginal yeast infections, easy skin bruising, and increased facial hair and acne. On exam, her blood pressure is 160/100 mmHg and she has central obesity with thin extremities and a rounded plethoric face. Posterior cervical and supraclavicular fat pads are enlarged, and wide violaceous striae are visible along the abdomen and axilla. Proximal muscle strength is decreased.

CASE 1 | Cushing Disease (ACTH-Secreting Pituitary Adenoma) *(continued)*

Conditions with Similar Presentations	**Obesity, hypothyroidism, polycystic ovarian syndrome (PCOS):** Would not have plethora and violaceous striae. Menstrual irregularities would be seen in PCOS.
Initial Diagnostic Tests	• Check 24-hour urinary cortisol ($\uparrow$), late night salivary cortisol ($\uparrow$), or dexamethasone suppression test. • Consider: A1c or other tests to confirm diagnosis of diabetes and TSH to rule out thyroid disorders. • MRI brain to confirm adenoma.
Next Steps in Management	Surgical removal of pituitary tumor via transsphenoidal approach.
Discussion	Cortisol is secreted by the adrenal cortex, and cortisol secretion is regulated by ACTH from the anterior pituitary, which is in turn regulated by CRH secreted from the hypothalamus. **Cushing disease** is cortisol excess resulting specifically from an ACTH-producing pituitary adenoma, and most commonly affects women of reproductive age. **Cushing syndrome** is a state of excess cortisol from any cause such as adrenal gland (adenoma, bilateral hyperplasia, carcinoma), exogenous glucocorticoids, and paraneoplastic ACTH secretion. **History:** • Weight gain • New or worsening of diabetes, hypertension, and hyperlipidemia • Proximal muscle weakness • Menstrual irregularities • Psychiatric manifestations—depression, anxiety **Physical Exam:** • Central obesity and thin extremities • Facial plethora (due to erythrocytosis and thin skin), "moon facies" (rounded face) due to preauricular fat pad deposition, "buffalo hump" (supraclavicular and dorsocervical fat pads) • Hypertension, abdominal striae • Skin thinning, bruising, and red abdominal striae due to cortisol inhibition of fibroblast function combined with central fat deposition stretching the skin and bleeding into the skin. • Skin hyperpigmentation due to ACTH binding to MSH receptors Reproduced, with permission, from Hammer GD, McPhee SJ. Pathophysiology of Disease: An Introduction to Clinical Medicine. 8th ed. New York, NY: McGraw Hill; 2019.

Psychiatric effects ("steroid encephalopathy," depression) (50–80%)

Growth retardation (in child) (85%)

Androgen excess (in female)
• Virilization (in adrenal carcinoma) (20%)
• Acne (50%)
• Menstrual irregularity (70%)
• Infertility (70%)
Increased mineralocorticoid effect
• Hypertension (80%)
• Hypokalemic alkalosis (in ectopic ACTH) (85%)

Diabetes mellitus (80%)
• Increased gluconeogenesis

Redistribution of body fat
• Central obesity (80%)
Moon facies (80%)
Thick neck (80%)
Fat trunk or abdomen (80%)
Thin extremities (80%)
Atrophy of skin and dermal connective tissue (striae) (70%)
Thinning of bones (osteoporosis) (50%)
Muscle wasting and weakness (steroid myopathy) (70%)
Easy bruising (50%), delayed healing (40%)

CASE 1 | Cushing Disease (ACTH-Secreting Pituitary Adenoma) *(continued)*

Discussion	**Diagnostics:**
	1. Initial tests (any 2 of the following) that confirm the presence of **Cushing syndrome:**

- 24-hour urinary cortisol (↑)
- Late-night salivary cortisol (↑)
- Low-dose dexamethasone suppression test (cortisol levels remain (↑), after low-dose steroid given)

2. Next, check **plasma ACTH levels** to determine the source of excess cortisol:
   - (↑) with either pituitary ACTH or ectopic ACTH secretion
   - (↓) with adrenal hypersecretion or exogenous steroids
3. To differentiate between pituitary ACTH or ectopic ACTH production:
   - Perform **high-dose dexamethasone suppression test.** Cells in a pituitary adenoma have ACTH receptors that when stimulated with a high dose of dexamethasone will decrease ACTH secretion and therefore decrease cortisol. Ectopic cells do not have these receptors, so cortisol will remain elevated.
   - **CRH stimulation test**—alternative to dexamethasone suppression test, will cause (↑) cortisol in Cushing disease because pituitary adenoma has CRH receptors but ectopic cells do not.
4. Obtain MRI brain if tests consistent with **Cushing disease** (pituitary adenoma) to confirm presence and assess resectability.

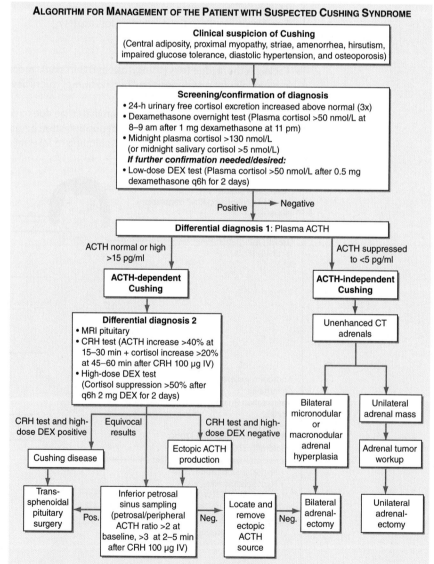

Management of patient with suspected Cushing syndrome. (Reproduced, with permission, from Jameson JL, Fauci AS, Kasper DL, Hauser SL, Longo DL, Loscalzo J, eds. Harrison's Principles of Internal Medicine. 20th ed. New York, NY: McGraw Hill; 2019.)

CASE 1 | Cushing Disease (ACTH-Secreting Pituitary Adenoma) *(continued)*

Discussion	**Management:** • First-line for Cushing disease: Surgery to remove the ACTH-secreting pituitary adenoma (transsphenoidal hypophysectomy). • Refractory cases may require bilateral adrenalectomy with lifelong glucocorticoid and mineralocorticoid replacement therapy.
Additional Considerations	**Complications:** • Increased susceptibility to infections (due to the effects of cortisol on the immune response) • Osteoporosis—increased risk of fractures • Diabetes mellitus • Cardiovascular disease

Cushing Syndrome Mini-Cases

Cases	Key Findings
Exogenous Corticosteroid Use	**Hx:** Weight gain, metabolic abnormalities (e.g., DM, HTN, dyslipidemia), easy bruising, or fractures in the setting of long-term or high-dose steroids use for inflammatory conditions (e.g., SLE or RA) **PE:** Same as Cushing disease but no hyperpigmentation. **Diagnostics:** Cortisol levels ($\uparrow$) and ACTH ($\downarrow$) **Management:** • Taper off steroids. • Switch to steroid-sparing therapy if possible. **Discussion:** • Chronic use of exogenous corticosteroids is the commonest cause of Cushing syndrome. • Low ACTH due to exogenous cortisol causes negative feedback on hypothalamus and anterior pituitary. • Important to taper steroid dose over weeks to months to avoid adrenal crisis or acute adrenal insufficiency in the setting of HPA axis suppression due to long-term glucocorticoid therapy.
Adrenal Hypersecretion of Cortisol (Adenoma or Carcinoma)	**Hx:** Weight gain, metabolic abnormalities (e.g., DM, HTN, dyslipidemia), easy bruising, or fractures. No exogenous steroid use. **PE:** Same as Cushing disease but no hyperpigmentation. **Diagnostics:** Cortisol levels ($\uparrow$) and ACTH ($\downarrow$) • CT abdomen may show adrenal mass or bilateral hyperplasia. **Management:** Adrenalectomy (surgical removal of tumor) **Discussion:** • Uncommon cause of Cushing syndrome. • Occurs in setting of adrenal adenoma, carcinoma, or bilateral hyperplasia. • High cortisol from adrenal exerts negative feedback on HPA axis, causing low ACTH. • With adenoma or carcinoma, increased pituitary ACTH causes atrophy of contralateral adrenal gland.
Paraneoplastic ACTH Secretion	**Hx:** Metabolic abnormalities (e.g., DM, HTN, dyslipidemia), easy bruising, or fractures. No exogenous steroid use. Risk factors suggesting lung tumor (smoking history, weight loss, cough, shortness of breath). **PE:** Same as Cushing syndrome. In addition, may have findings consistent with cancer (temporal wasting, abnormalities on lung exam). **Diagnostics:** • Cortisol levels ($\uparrow$) and ACTH ($\uparrow$) • Dexamethasone suppression test (cortisol levels stay [$\uparrow$]). • CT chest and abdomen to localize the tumor. **Management:** • Treat the underlying cause (the ACTH-secreting tumor). • Consider bilateral adrenalectomy. **Discussion:** • Most commonly from small cell lung cancer. • Other causes: Bronchial carcinoid tumors, other neuroendocrine tumors, pheochromocytoma. • Tumor secretes ACTH, which increases cortisol secretion from adrenals. • Normal negative feedback loop absent because tumor cells do not have ACTH receptors. • Differentiate from Cushing disease by lack of cortisol suppression on high-dose dexamethasone suppression test.

CASE 2 | Hypopituitarism (Pituitary Adenoma)

A 48-year-old man presents with erectile dysfunction. He has reduced interest in sexual activity, and he has not been experiencing early morning erections for the last year. He also notes low energy, modest weight gain, constipation, cold intolerance, and headaches. He does not have any recent testicular trauma or symptoms of depression. On exam, his blood pressure is 98/56 mmHg and he has cool dry skin, central obesity, and a normal genitourinary exam. Visual acuity is normal, but visual field confrontation testing reveals bitemporal hemianopsia.

Conditions with Similar Presentations	**Primary hypogonadism** and **primary hypothyroidism:** Would not have visual field defects. Other presentations of hypopituitarism: **Sheehan syndrome:** Form of acute hypopituitarism due to ischemic infarction of the pituitary in the setting of postpartum hemorrhage. **Empty Sella syndrome:** More common in obese women, due to atrophy or compression of the pituitary gland. **Craniopharyngioma:** Suprasellar tumor, more common in children and the elderly. **Prolactinoma** (see the following Case 3): Prolactin levels >200.
Initial Diagnostic Tests	• Evaluate for pituitary hormone deficiency: TSH ($\downarrow$), free T4 ($\downarrow$), FSH ($\downarrow$), LH ($\downarrow$), ACTH ($\downarrow$), cortisol ($\downarrow$), IGF1 ($\downarrow$), testosterone ($\downarrow$), prolactin (normal) • Also check MRI given visual field defect
Next Steps in Management	• Hormone replacement therapy (see details below) • Dopamine agonists (cabergoline) if prolactinoma is the cause. • Transsphenoidal hypophysectomy.
Discussion	**Hypopituitarism** is insufficient production of multiple pituitary hormones, can result from injury to the normal gland and can cause: • GH deficiency • Prolactin deficiency • Secondary hypogonadism • Secondary hypothyroidism • Secondary hypoadrenalism • DI **Pituitary adenomas** arise from anterior pituitary cells. Most tumors are non-functional (non-secreting) and they may be clinically silent or cause insidious symptoms due to compression of surrounding structures. Functional tumors secrete hormones and cause clinical presentations such as **acromegaly** or **Cushing disease.** **History:** Patients will present with symptoms depending on which pituitary cells are affected by the adenoma. These include: • **Hypothyroidism:** Weight gain, constipation, dry skin, cold intolerance • **Hypogonadism:** $\downarrow$libido or erectile dysfunction in men, amenorrhea or infertility in women • **Hypoadrenalism:** Fatigue, weight loss, symptoms of hypoglycemia • **GH deficiency:** $\downarrow$ muscle mass in adults, delayed growth in children • **Mass effect:** Headaches, visual impairment, oculomotor nerve impairment **Physical Exam:** • Visual field testing—**bitemporal hemianopsia** due to **compression of the optic chiasm** • Hypotension and bradycardia may be seen in the setting of hypothyroidism or hypoadrenalism **Diagnostics:** • Diagnostic testing depends on specific symptomatology of the patient • Testing for end-organ abnormalities: free T4 ($\downarrow$), cortisol ($\downarrow$), testosterone ($\downarrow$) • Pituitary hormone levels: TSH ($\downarrow$), FSH ($\downarrow$), LH ($\downarrow$), ACTH ($\downarrow$), IGF1 ($\downarrow$), prolactin (normal) to differentiate primary vs. secondary cause. Pituitary hormone levels may be inappropriately normal with low peripheral hormones when pituitary tumors are present. • MRI pituitary to assess size of adenoma if present

CASE 2 | Hypopituitarism (Pituitary Adenoma) *(continued)*

Discussion		End-Organ Hormone	Pituitary Hormones
	Central hypothyroidism	Free T4 ↓	TSH ↓
	Central hypogonadism	Testosterone ↓ Estradiol ↓	FSH ↓ LH ↓
	Central adrenal insufficiency	Cortisol ↓	ACTH stimulation test, Insulin tolerance test
	Growth hormone deficiency	IGF-1 ↓	GH stimulation test, Insulin tolerance test

Management:
- Transsphenoidal hypophysectomy of pituitary adenoma, especially if tumor is large enough to cause symptoms such as visual field defects.
- Hormone replacement therapy to compensate for loss of pituitary function with hydrocortisone, thyroxine once hydrocortisone given, testosterone for men, estrogen-progestin for women. GH and prolactin do not need to be replaced in adults.
- Dopamine agonists (cabergoline) if prolactinoma is the cause

Additional Considerations	**Complications:** **Pituitary apoplexy:** • Enlarging pituitary adenoma with fragile blood vessels suddenly outgrows its blood supply. • Hemorrhage into the sella turcica may present with severe headache, visual disturbances, sudden loss of pituitary function • Can manifest as acute adrenal insufficiency with hypotension and shock

CASE 3 | Hyperprolactinemia (Prolactinoma)

A 27-year-old woman presents with irregular menses and milky nipple discharge. She has had only two periods in the last 6 months, and they have been lighter than usual. She is not sexually active and is not on any medications. Physical exam reveals bilateral milky nipple discharge with no breast masses. No visual fields defects are noted.

Conditions with Similar Presentations	**Pregnancy, hypothyroidism, medications** (e.g., dopamine antagonists), or **renal failure** can cause elevations in prolactin.
Initial Diagnostic Tests	• Check serum prolactin (↑) • Also check TSH, pregnancy test, and basic metabolic panel (BMP) (to rule out kidney disease) • MRI of the brain to assess size of prolactinoma
Next Steps in Management	• Treat with dopamine agonists—cabergoline, bromocriptine. • Consider transsphenoidal hypophysectomy surgery in refractory cases.
Discussion	Hyperprolactinemia may be due to physiologic, pathologic, or iatrogenic causes. • Physiologic causes include pregnancy, stimulation of the nipple/breast, and stress. • Pathologic causes include prolactinomas (most commonly in females aged 20–50) and any process that interferes with dopamine release or transfer from the hypothalamus to the anterior pituitary such as non-pituitary tumors and infiltrative diseases (e.g., sarcoidosis), trauma. • Iatrogenic causes are mainly from medications that antagonize dopamine receptors on the pituitary gland. Examples are antipsychotics (specifically risperidone and haloperidol) and gastric motility drugs (metoclopramide, domperidone). **History:** • Females: galactorrhea, oligomenorrhea, and/or infertility (due to low LH and FSH resulting in anovulation) • Males: present later than females with decreased libido, erectile dysfunction, headaches from pituitary mass effect **Physical Exam:** • Females: Bilateral milky nipple discharge • Males: Gynecomastia • Bitemporal hemianopsia if tumor is large enough to compress optic chiasm (more common in males due to larger tumor size because of later diagnosis)

CASE 3 | Hyperprolactinemia (Prolactinoma) *(continued)*

Discussion	**Diagnostics:** • Prolactin levels in prolactinoma are usually elevated >200 ng/mL; however, lower levels may be present with smaller prolactinomas or other pituitary growths that block inhibitory dopamine signaling ("stalk effect") • Pregnancy test and TSH should be checked to rule out these causes of hyperprolactinemia • MRI of the brain will identify a lesion in the pituitary • If large pituitary tumor, should be screened for hypopituitarism by checking other pituitary hormone levels **Management:** • Dopamine agonists: Cabergoline preferred over bromocriptine due to less adverse reactions • Consider transsphenoidal hypophysectomy if refractory to medical therapy • Do not treat asymptomatic medication-induced hyperprolactinemia.
Additional Considerations	May be seen as part of **MEN 1 syndrome**—consider with a family history or other manifestations of MEN 1 (pancreatic endocrine tumors, parathyroid hyperplasia).

CASE 4 | Acromegaly

A 42-year-old man with poorly controlled hypertension presents for a follow-up appointment after his blood pressure medications were recently increased. He is accompanied by his partner who reports that the patient snores and appears to stop breathing at night. The patient also notes morning headaches, polyuria, polydipsia, weight gain, and wrist/hand pain and weakness. He states he is taking his four blood pressure medications as prescribed. On exam, his blood pressure is 172/92 mmHg. He has coarse facial features, prominent jaw and brow, enlarged tongue, widely spaced teeth, and prominent protruding forehead with broad nasal bridge (frontal bossing). Finger and toe thickening is noted more prominently at his joints. When he flexes his wrists for one minute, he starts to feel tingling and numbness in his fingers (Phalen sign). Hepatomegaly is noted on abdominal exam.

Conditions with Similar Presentations	**Hemochromatosis:** Is a genetic condition marked by excess iron absorption and iron overload. It may present with joint pains and new onset or worsening diabetes, but not other findings such as coarse facial features and frontal bossing. **Diabetes mellitus and insipidus:** Can present with polyuria/polydipsia, **sleep apnea** (OSA), labored breathing during sleep, morning headaches, and resistant hypertension. However, other findings and facial characteristics would not be seen in isolated cases of DM, DI, or OSA.
Initial Diagnostic Tests	• Check serum IGF-1 level (markedly ($\uparrow$) is diagnostic) • If IGF-1 level is only mildly ($\uparrow$), obtain GH suppression test (failure of GH to suppress with oral glucose challenge confirms the diagnosis). • Check MRI brain to assess for mass • Consider checking serum glucose levels and/or A1C to rule out DM, serum ferritin to rule out hemochromatosis, and a sleep study to evaluate for sleep apnea
Next Steps in Management	Surgical resection of pituitary adenoma (transsphenoidal)
Discussion	Acromegaly is a disease caused by excess GH, most commonly caused by a GH-producing pituitary adenoma. **History:** • Joint pain, weight gain, fatigue • Carpal tunnel syndrome, arthropathy, arthritis • Shoes, hats, and rings no longer fitting due to bony enlargement • Features of related conditions such as heart failure and diabetes **Physical Exam:** • Frontal bossing, enlargement of the hands and feet • Coarse facial features, large tongue, deep voice, excessive sweating • Bitemporal hemianopsia may be present due to compression of the optic chiasm

CASE 4 | Acromegaly *(continued)*

Discussion	**Diagnostics:** GH works to stimulate production of IGF-1, mainly in the liver, which is the primary effector of GH signaling.
	• GH levels fluctuate considerably during the day so are not the initial screening test.
	• IGF-1 level is a highly sensitive screening test and is almost always elevated; normal results rule out acromegaly.
	• IGF-1 levels may be falsely elevated in various conditions (e.g., pregnancy).
	• Confirmatory test (GH suppression test with oral glucose challenge) should be performed if the IGF-1 level is equivocally elevated. Oral glucose challenge in a normal person causes suppression of the GH level.
	• Failure to suppress GH 2 hours after giving 75 g of glucose confirms the diagnosis of acromegaly.
	• MRI of the pituitary demonstrates the presence of a mass and aids in surgical planning.
	• Consider checking other pituitary hormone levels (TSH, ACTH, LH/FSH, prolactin) and visual field assessment.
	Management: Transsphenoidal surgical resection of the pituitary adenoma to remove the source of excess GH.
	Medical options (used if surgery is not possible or if surgery leaves residual tumor) include:
	• Pegvisomant—GH receptor antagonist that prevents production of IGF-1 by the liver.
	• Octreotide (somatostatin analog) and cabergoline (dopamine agonist)—suppress GH production by the pituitary.
	• Mild cases can be treated with cabergoline
	Also screen with:
	• **Colonoscopy**—as patients at increased risk for colorectal polyps and colorectal cancer
	• **Polysomnography**—to evaluate for obstructive sleep apnea
Additional Considerations	**Complications:**
	• Most common cause of death is congestive heart failure
	• Joint disease (carpal tunnel, arthropathy, arthritis)
	• T2DM, hypertension, sleep apnea
	• Jaw or dental problems
	Pediatric Considerations:
	• In children, excess GH manifests as **gigantism** due to promotion of longitudinal growth prior to the closure of epiphyseal growth plates.
	• Once the growth plates are closed, excess GH causes acromegaly, with growth mainly in the distal extremities.

CASE 5 | Central Diabetes Insipidus (DI)

A 39-year-old man presents with polyuria and polydipsia for few months after a motor vehicle accident that resulted in traumatic brain injury. Over the last 2 months, he has felt constant thirst and he has had five or six episodes of nocturia. He only has relief with consumption of large volumes of cold water. Physical exam is significant for dry mucous membranes.

Conditions with Similar Presentations	**Nephrogenic DI:** May have a similar presentation but occurs due to failure at the level of the kidney to respond to circulating ADH and would not occur from head trauma. Etiologies include:
	• Medication side effect (lithium, demeclocycline)
	• Hypercalcemia, hypokalemia, renal disease
	• Inherited genetic defects in ADH receptor or aquaporin channels
	Primary polydipsia: A disorder of pathologic water drinking.
	• Commonly seen in patients with psychiatric disturbances, and thirst is the primary factor driving the polyuria
	• Diagnosed with normalization of urine osmolality during the water deprivation test
	Diabetes mellitus (DM) and **diuretics:** Can cause polyuria.
Initial Diagnostic Tests	• Check serum sodium and plasma and urine osmolality before and after water deprivation test. (Confirm diagnosis if after water deprivation test: serum sodium ($\uparrow$), plasma osmolality ($\uparrow$), and urine osmolality (unchanged).
	• Consider checking A1C or blood glucose to rule out DM.

CASE 5 | Central Diabetes Insipidus (DI) *(continued)*

Next Step in Management	Desmopressin (DDAVP) and free access to liquids.

Discussion	DI is a disorder related to impaired activity of ADH. In central DI, there is deficient production of ADH by the hypothalamus and/or release by the posterior pituitary which results in free water loss, polyuria (production of large volumes of dilute urine), and high-normal or high plasma osmolality triggers thirst (polydipsia). Most cases are idiopathic and may be due to autoimmune attack on hypothalamus and/or pituitary stalk. Other known causes include:
	• Pituitary tumors (e.g., adenoma, craniopharyngioma), metastases
	• Traumatic brain injury, ischemia (e.g., Sheehan syndrome), consequence of neurosurgery
	
	History: Polyuria, polydipsia, nocturia
	
	Physical Exam: Possibly signs of dehydration due to insufficient water intake
	
	Diagnostics:
	• Initially mild hypernatremia, high-normal or slight increase in plasma osmolality and low urine osmolality (<300 mOsm/kg), low urine specific gravity (<1.006).
	• Diagnosis is confirmed with **water restriction test**. This will cause a rise in serum sodium to above 145 mEq/L and plasma osmolality >295 mOsm without changing urine osmolality. Next step is to administer the ADH analog desmopressin to distinguish central DI from nephrogenic DI:
	  • **Central DI**—the urine osmolality will rise >50%
	  • **Nephrogenic DI**—no change in urine osmolality
	• MRI brain, may reveal structural reason for central DI
	
	Urine osmolality interpretation in water deprivation test. (Reproduced, with permission, from Gardner DG, Shoback D. Greenspan's Basic & Clinical Endocrinology. 10th ed. New York, NY: McGraw Hill; 2018.)
	
	Management: Desmopressin (DDAVP), an ADH analog—given intranasally or orally

CASE 6 | Syndrome of Inappropriate Anti-Diuretic Hormone (SIADH)

A 64-year-old man with a 40-pack-year tobacco use history is brought for evaluation of altered mental status. His family notes the patient has been more confused in the last week and he recently started coughing up bloody sputum. On exam, he is afebrile, respirations are 10/min, pulse is 100/min, and blood pressure is 122/78 mmHg. He is lethargic, has moist mucous membranes and no signs of volume overload. Labs are notable for a serum sodium of 122 mEq/L.

| Conditions with Similar Presentations | **Psychogenic polydipsia:** Hyponatremia caused by excess consumption of free water. Patient would have polyuria and very low urine osmolality.

Tea and toast diet/beer potomania: Seen in patients who consume low protein, low solute, high water diets. Impaired ability to excrete free water causes hyponatremia.

Adrenal insufficiency and **hypothyroidism:** Are often associated with fatigue, hypotension, weight changes. |

CASE 6 | Syndrome of Inappropriate Anti-Diuretic Hormone (SIADH) (continued)

Initial Diagnostic Tests	• Check serum sodium (↓), serum osmolality (↓), urine osmolality (↑), and urine fractional excretion of sodium (↑). • Consider checking: TSH and cortisol to rule out thyroid and adrenal causes.
Next Steps in Management	• Mild/moderate hyponatremia: Fluid restriction • Severe and symptomatic hyponatremia (usually serum sodium <120 mEq/L): **Slowly** correct hyponatremia using hypertonic saline (3% NaCl).

Discussion	Syndrome of inappropriate antidiuretic hormone secretion (SIADH) is a disorder of water homeostasis. ADH is normally released when serum osmolality is high and causes free water retention. SIADH results from excess ADH secretion in the setting of low or normal serum osmolality; therefore, patients present with euvolemic hyponatremia due to impaired free water excretion.
	
	 History:
	 Risk Factors:
	 • Ectopic ADH production (small cell lung cancer)
	 • Intracranial tumors, elevated intracranial pressure
	 • Pulmonary disease (pneumonia)
	 • Medications: SSRIs, carbamazepine, cyclophosphamide
	 • SIADH is common in postoperative state in the setting of pain, nausea, stress, and narcotic administration
	
	 Patients may be asymptomatic or have the following symptoms due to hyponatremia:
	 • Lethargy, nausea, vomiting
	 • Possible coma, seizure, and death
	
	 Physical Exam: Euvolemic on exam, no signs of either fluid overload or dehydration.
	
	 Diagnostics:
	 1. Determine patient's volume status to rule out hyponatremia associated with hypervolemia (e.g., elevated JVP, S3, edema, crackles on lung exam) or hypovolemia (e.g., dry mucous membranes, orthostatic hypotension)
	 2. SIADH is characterized by:
	   • Hyponatremia
	   • ↓ serum osmolality (<280 mOsm/kg H2O)
	   • ↑ urine osmolality (>100 mOsm/kg H2O)
	   • ↑ urine sodium (>20 mEq/L)
	   • Urine osmolality > serum osmolality, due to kidneys concentrating urine inappropriately
	   • BUN, creatinine, uric acid will be low due to dilution
	 3. Check TSH to rule out hypothyroidism or early morning cortisol to rule out adrenal insufficiency.
	 4. Obtain CT chest if concerned for lung cancer-associated paraneoplastic syndrome.
	
	 Management: Goal of treatment is to correct hyponatremia and identify and treat the underlying cause.
	   • Treat mild hyponatremia with fluid restriction.
	   • Treat severe and symptomatic hyponatremia with careful administration of hypertonic saline (3%).
	   • Frequent sodium monitoring to ensure serum Na correction does not exceed 8–10 mEq/L in the first 24 hours.
	   • Add loop diuretic or sodium tablets as needed.
	   • ADH antagonists (conivaptan and tolvaptan)—bind to V2 vasopressin receptor in principal cells of renal collecting duct to prevent action of ADH, causing increased water excretion with loss of electrolytes, allowing serum sodium to increase.

Additional Considerations	**Complications:** If serum sodium concentration increases too rapidly, can result in **osmotic demyelination syndrome** (also called central pontine myelinolysis). This may lead to the **locked-in syndrome** (quadriplegia, complete loss of cranial nerve function except for blinking and vertical eye movements).

ADRENAL GLAND

The adrenal cortex secretes three main categories of steroids: mineralocorticoids, glucocorticoids, and androgens. The adrenal medulla is responsible for secreting catecholamines like norepinephrine and epinephrine.

Aldosterone

Aldosterone is a mineralocorticoid hormone secreted by the zona glomerulosa of the adrenal cortex. It plays an important role in **regulation of sodium levels and volume status.**

- Secreted in response to decreased blood volume (via angiotensin II in the RAAS system) and increased plasma potassium
- Acts on the late distal tubule and collecting ducts to stimulate reabsorption of sodium and secretion of potassium and H$^+$

Symptoms/Signs	Hormone Abnormality	Differential Diagnosis
Hypertension Hypokalemia	Aldosterone excess	Aldosterone-producing adrenal adenoma (Conn syndrome)
		Bilateral adrenal hyperplasia
		Congenital adrenal hyperplasia (17 α-hydroxylase or 11 β-hydroxylase deficiency)
		Syndrome of apparent mineralocorticoid excess (e.g., black licorice ingestion)
		Renovascular hypertension
		Juxtaglomerular cell tumors
		Edema (e.g., cirrhosis, heart failure, nephrotic syndrome)
Hypotension Hyperkalemia Hyponatremia Salt craving	Aldosterone deficiency	Primary adrenal insufficiency
		Renal tubular acidosis type IV
		Congenital adrenal hyperplasia (21-hydroxylase deficiency)

Cortisol

Cortisol is secreted by the zona fasciculata of the adrenal cortex and plays important roles in the regulation of appetite, blood pressure, insulin resistance, gluconeogenesis, lipolysis, wound healing, inflammatory responses, bone formation, and more. It is **regulated by ACTH,** released from the anterior pituitary, which is in turn regulated by CRH, released from the hypothalamus.

The secretion of excess cortisol is known as Cushing syndrome (**see Case 1**). There are multiple causes of Cushing syndrome, depending on the source of excess cortisol:

- ACTH-secreting pituitary adenoma (Cushing disease)
- Exogenous corticosteroid use
- Adrenal hypersecretion of cortisol
- Paraneoplastic ACTH secretion (e.g., small cell lung cancer, carcinoid)

Symptoms/Signs	Hormone Abnormality	Differential Diagnosis

Hypertension
Hyperglycemia
Excessive weight gain
Truncal obesity
Buffalo hump
Abdominal purple striae
Bruising
Proximal muscle weakness
Decreased linear growth in children
	Cortisol excess	Cushing disease (pituitary hypersecretion)
		Cushing syndrome
		   Exogenous steroids
		   Adrenal adenoma
		   Adrenal hyperplasia
		   Paraneoplastic ACTH secretion

Symptoms/Signs	Hormone Abnormality	Differential Diagnosis
Hypotension Hypoglycemia Anorexia Weight loss Abdominal pain Fatigue Decreased libido Hyperpigmentation	Cortisol deficiency	Hypopituitarism (craniopharyngioma, pituitary adenoma, infection, Sheehan syndrome, traumatic brain injury, primary or metastatic cancer) Addison disease Adrenoleukodystrophy Autoimmune polyglandular syndromes Waterhouse-Friderichsen syndrome Abrupt discontinuation of chronic exogenous steroid use

Catecholamines

Catecholamines (including norepinephrine, epinephrine, and dopamine) are secreted by the adrenal medulla, the innermost layer of the adrenal gland. They function throughout the body to activate the sympathetic nervous system. Catecholamine deficiency is rare and not associated with a specific clinical syndrome.

Symptoms/Signs	Hormone Abnormality	Differential Diagnosis
Hypertension Palpitations Headaches Sweating	Catecholamine excess	Pheochromocytoma Paraganglioma Aldosterone-producing adrenal adenoma (Conn syndrome) Bilateral adrenal hyperplasia Congenital adrenal hyperplasia (17 α-hydroxylase or 11 β-hydroxylase deficiency) Syndrome of apparent mineralocorticoid excess (e.g., black licorice ingestion) Renovascular hypertension Juxtaglomerular cell tumors Edema (e.g., heart failure, cirrhosis, nephrotic syndrome)

Androgens

Androgens are released by the zona reticularis of the adrenal cortex. Adrenal androgens include dehydroepiandrosterone (DHEA) and dehydroepiandrosterone sulfate (DHEAS) and serve as precursors to hormones including testosterone and estrogen.

Symptoms/Signs	Hormone Abnormality	Differential Diagnosis
Females: Increased male pattern body hair (chin, chest, back) Hair loss (central, temporal) Acne Early pubic/axillary hair development Clitoromegaly Irregular menses Deepened voice **Males:** Increased penile length Early pubic/axillary hair development in children	Androgen excess	Congenital adrenal hyperplasia (21-hydroxylase deficiency) Premature adrenarche Adrenal tumor Exogenous androgen exposure Polycystic ovarian syndrome FSH- or LH-secreting pituitary adenoma (rare)
Delayed puberty Menstrual irregularities Micropenis in male infants Decreased libido Infertility Decreased pubic/axillary hair	Androgen deficiency	Hypogonadotropic hypogonadism (e.g., Kallman syndrome) Congenital adrenal hyperplasia (17-α-hydroxylase deficiency)

CASE 7 | Primary Hyperaldosteronism (Conn Syndrome)

A 60-year-old man with hypertension returns to clinic for repeat blood pressure check. His current medications include once-daily hydrochlorothiazide 25 mg, amlodipine 10 mg, lisinopril 20 mg, and thrice-daily hydralazine. On his last visit, his hydralazine was increased from 50 mg to 100 mg TID. He takes his medications regularly, follows a low-salt diet, and exercises regularly. He lost 20 pounds intentionally. His blood pressure at home is also consistently elevated. On exam, he has a normal body mass index (BMI), blood pressure is 175/110 mmHg, heart rate is 80 bpm, and he has no signs of peripheral edema. Review of the patient's chart shows intermittent hypokalemia for the past 4 years.

Conditions with Similar Presentations	**Secondary hyperaldosteronism:** Increased renin secretion leads to increased aldosterone production. May occur with renal artery stenosis, renin-secreting tumors, or edema secondary to cirrhosis, heart failure, or nephrotic syndrome. The first two could cause refractory hypertension but the edematous disorders would not.
	Bartter syndrome: Renal tubular defect that presents with polyuria, polydipsia, metabolic alkalosis, hypokalemia, however, patients are usually normotensive.
	Liddle syndrome: Renal tubular defect that presents similarly to hyperaldosteronism, but with decreased aldosterone levels.
	The same presentation can also be caused by **syndrome of apparent mineralocorticoid excess**, often caused by **licorice ingestion.**
Initial Diagnostic Tests	• Check plasma renin and aldosterone (plasma aldosterone concentration/plasma renin activity [PAC/PRA] ratio >20) • Saline suppression test to confirm • Abdominal CT or MRI
Next Steps in Management	• For unilateral disease: Laparoscopic adrenalectomy • For bilateral disease: Mineralocorticoid receptor antagonists
Discussion	Primary hyperaldosteronism (Conn syndrome) is a syndrome of increased aldosterone secretion from the adrenal cortex due to aldosterone-secreting adrenal adenoma, bilateral adrenal hyperplasia, or adrenal carcinoma (very rare). The normal action of aldosterone is to stimulate sodium reabsorption, potassium secretion, and H^+ secretion by the kidney. Abnormal aldosterone secretion causes hypokalemia and metabolic alkalosis (due to loss of H^+), and high levels of aldosterone act in a negative feedback loop to decrease renin release.
	History: • Difficult-to-control hypertension despite multiple medications and confirmed adherence to treatment. • Symptoms associated with hypertension (e.g., headache), • Fatigue and muscle weakness due to hypokalemia,
	Physical Exam: • Hypertension and no peripheral edema on exam

	Diagnostics:
	• BMP consistent with hypokalemia, metabolic alkalosis
	• ↑ **plasma aldosterone, ↓ plasma renin, PAC/PRA ratio >20.**
	• Confirmatory testing:
	  • **Saline infusion test** (introduction of saline should suppress aldosterone <5 ng/dL); aldosterone remains elevated in primary hyperaldosteronism
	  • **Oral sodium loading:** Patient follows high-sodium diet for 2–3 days, which normally inhibits aldosterone secretion; urine aldosterone and sodium levels remain elevated in primary hyperaldosteronism
	• Abdominal CT/MRI and, if no localizing lesion, adrenal vein sampling to differentiate unilateral adrenal adenoma from bilateral adrenal hyperplasia.

	Management: • For unilateral adrenal adenoma, definitive treatment is laparoscopic adrenalectomy. If not a good surgical candidate, mineralocorticoid receptor antagonists (spironolactone, eplerenone). • For bilateral adrenal hyperplasia, treat medically with mineralocorticoid receptor antagonists (spironolactone, eplerenone).

CASE 8 | Primary Adrenal Insufficiency (Addison Disease)

A 47-year-old woman presents with fatigue, anorexia, and unintentional weight loss and cravings for salty/sweet foods. On exam, she is afebrile; respirations are 16/min, pulse is 94/min, blood pressure is 110/70 mmHg supine and 96/58 mmHg standing. She has hyperpigmentation of the face and palmar creases.

Conditions with Similar Presentations	**Secondary or tertiary adrenal insufficiency:** May present similarly but would not have skin and mucosal hyperpigmentation.
Initial Diagnostic Tests	• Check early morning cortisol level ($\downarrow$) and serum ACTH ($\uparrow$) • Confirm with ACTH stimulation test (cortisol remains low) • Also check BMP [NA ($\downarrow$), K ($\uparrow$), glucose ($\downarrow$)] and consider checking for chronic causes of primary adrenal insufficiency (e.g., HIV, TB, ferritin)
Next Steps in Management	Glucocorticoid (hydrocortisone) and mineralocorticoid (fludrocortisone) replacement therapy.
Discussion	Primary adrenal insufficiency is also known as Addison disease and most commonly occurs due to chronic autoimmune destruction of the adrenal cortex, resulting in low levels of mineralocorticoids, glucocorticoids, and androgens. Antibodies to the adrenal enzyme anti-21-hydroxylase are present in most cases. Non-immune causes include infection (TB, HIV, syphilis, endemic fungi), infiltrative diseases (hemochromatosis, sarcoidosis, tumors), and vascular (thrombosis, or hemorrhage [Waterhouse-Friderichsen syndrome]). In response to decreased cortisol levels, the anterior pituitary increases the release of ACTH. **History:** It is often associated with other autoimmune disorders (e.g., thyroid disease or type 1 diabetes mellitus) Symptoms include: • Fatigue, weakness, weight loss, salt craving • Nausea, vomiting, abdominal pain • Low androgen production in women causes decreased libido, loss of axillary and pubic hair (androgens are also produced by the testes in men) **Physical Exam:** • Orthostatic hypotension • Hyperpigmentation of the skin, due to increased production of α-melanocyte stimulating hormone (α-MSH). α-MSH is derived from the same precursor molecule as ACTH (proopiomelanocortin) **Diagnostics:** • **Morning cortisol ($\downarrow$) and ACTH levels ($\uparrow$).** • If morning cortisol levels are not diagnostic, cosyntropin stimulation test should be performed. Cosyntropin is made of the active 24 N terminal amino acids of ACTH. Low cortisol production following this test is diagnostic of primary adrenal insufficiency • May also see hyponatremia, hyperkalemia, hypoglycemia, eosinophilia, and antibodies against 21-hydroxylase **Management:** • If possible, treat the underlying cause • Treat with hydrocortisone and fludrocortisone to replace the glucocorticoids and mineralocorticoids that are no longer being produced by the adrenal glands
Additional Considerations	**Secondary Adrenal Insufficiency:** • Failure of adrenal hormone release secondary to decreased ACTH production by pituitary gland • Most common cause is **sudden cessation of long-term steroid use** or increased metabolic demand (e.g., infection, surgery) in a patient on long-term steroids • Chronic suppression of ACTH causes adrenal atrophy which inhibits ability to make adrenal hormones if steroids are stopped or during increased metabolic demand • No skin/mucosal hyperpigmentation (low ACTH) or hyperkalemia (RAAS intact) **Tertiary Adrenal Insufficiency:** • Decreased corticotropin-releasing hormone (CRH) from hypothalamus • Leads to decreased ACTH release by pituitary and decreased steroid release from adrenals • Very rare

CASE 8 | Primary Adrenal Insufficiency (Addison Disease) *(continued)*

Additional Considerations	**Complications:**
	Acute adrenal insufficiency can occur in a patient with chronic adrenal insufficiency
	• Generally, in the setting of an **acute stressor** (trauma, infection, surgery).
	• Manifests as **hypotension and shock.**
	• Immediate infusion of large volumes of normal saline.
	• Hydrocortisone immediately and every 6 hours. Dexamethasone is an alternative but has no mineralocorticoid activity.
	Waterhouse-Friderichsen syndrome
	• Acute primary adrenal insufficiency resulting from bilateral adrenal infarction and/or hemorrhage
	• Often in setting of bacteremia, *Neisseria meningitidis* is most common pathogen
	• Presents as acute illness characterized by fever, malaise, headaches, followed by sudden shock and abdominal/flank pain
	• Petechial rash, coagulopathy (DIC), and shock

CASE 9 | Pheochromocytoma

A 39-year-old man presents with palpitations and shortness of breath. For the past year he has been having progressively worsening bitemporal headaches and episodic blurry vision. He is not using any medications, supplements, or drugs. On exam his vitals are temperature 37.5°C, blood pressure 210/110 mmHg supine which drops to 180/90 when standing, respirations 17/min, and pulse 108/min. He is diaphoretic and appears anxious. Lungs are clear to auscultation. Cardiac exam notable for tachycardia with regular rhythm. On neurological exam, there is a fine anti-gravity action hand tremor bilaterally and arteriovenous nicking on fundoscopic exam.

Conditions with Similar Presentations	**Drug use** (e.g., stimulants, sympathomimetics)
	Panic attacks: Diagnosis of exclusion and would not have hypertension
	Other causes of **secondary hypertension** include:
	• Fibromuscular dysplasia (would not have tremor)
	• Primary hyperaldosteronism (would not have tremor and no orthostasis)
	• Hyperthyroidism (would not have orthostasis)
Initial Diagnostic Tests	• Check plasma free metanephrines (↑) or 24-hour urine metanephrines (↑), homovanillic acid (↑), and vanillylmandelic acid (↑)
	• Consider: TSH, plasma renin, and aldosterone to evaluate for thyroid and hyperaldosteronism
Next Steps in Management	• Check abdominal CT or MRI to detect tumor
	• Prior to adrenalectomy, treat with α-blocker (phenoxybenzamine) followed by β-blocker (e.g., propranolol, metoprolol)
Discussion	Pheochromocytoma is a catecholamine-secreting neuroendocrine tumor. The "10% rules" are helpful: 10% are malignant, 10% are bilateral, 10% are extra-adrenal (paraganglioma), 10% are associated with multiple endocrine neoplasia type 2 (MEN 2), 10% occur in childhood. Pheochromocytomas may secrete catecholamines in a pulsatile manner leading to intermittent symptoms in those patients.
	History: Risk factors include germline mutations including MEN 2, Von Hippel-Lindau disease, and neurofibromatosis
	Symptoms include:
	• Headache, palpitations, diaphoresis, flushing, anxiety, and tremor
	• The tremor is best brought out with anti-gravity action (arms out in front with fingers spread) and is due to an exaggerated physiologic tremor brought about by catecholamines
	Physical Exam:
	• Hypertension refractory to medications
	• May be present episodically, so patient may be normotensive during exam
	• May be associated with orthostasis because catecholamine secretion is already at maximum and cannot be increased by baroreceptor input

CASE 9 | Pheochromocytoma *(continued)*

Discussion	• Early onset of end organ injury from
	  • Fundoscopic changes
	  • Kidney injury
	  • Atherosclerotic disease
	Diagnostics: Hormone metabolites are generally two- to three-fold the upper limit of normal. Levels of epinephrine and norepinephrine are too variable to be useful because of their short half-lives measured in minutes.
	• **Plasma or urine metanephrines** ($\uparrow$)
	• May have elevated levels of urinary homovanillic acid or vanillylmandelic acid
	• Check abdominal CT or MRI to help localize the tumor(s)
	• Possible polycythemia (due to EPO-secreting tumors) and hyperglycemia (due to catecholamine inhibition of insulin secretion)
	Management:
	• Surgical resection if possible
	• To avoid intraoperative catecholamine surge and hypertensive crisis, treat first with an α-adrenergic antagonist (phenoxybenzamine) 7–14 days prior to surgery to normalize the blood pressure. Add β-blocker treatment 2–3 days prior to surgery. Do not administer β-blockers in the absence of α-blockers because this can precipitate a hypertensive crisis due to unopposed α-agonism.

Additional Considerations	**Paraganglioma:** • Extra-adrenal catecholamine-secreting tumor (represent about 10% of pheochromocytomas) • Locations include organ of Zuckerkandl at the bifurcation of the aorta, wall of the bladder, level of the carotid body in the neck

THYROID DISORDERS

The thyroid gland regulates metabolism, and various etiologies can cause thyroid deficiency or excess. It is also important to note that the same disease process may result in both hyper- and hypothyroidism. For example, thyroiditis (inflammation of the thyroid gland) can lead to hyperthyroidism initially due to the release of thyroid hormone following the destruction of thyroid follicles. However, over time, the thyroid loses ability to synthesize additional T3 and T4 as more follicles are destroyed, ultimately resulting in hypothyroidism.

Patients may also present with biochemical markers of thyroid dysfunction (e.g., elevated TSH), without any clinical symptoms. This phenomenon represents subclinical dysfunction and may resolve on its own or be the precursor to future symptoms.

Excess Thyroid Hormone

Symptoms related to excess thyroid hormone and heightened metabolism include weight loss, tachycardia, palpitations, hypertension, warm, dry skin, sweating, diarrhea, tremors, brisk reflexes, difficulty concentrating, insomnia, menstrual irregularity, or infertility.

Assess for the following on physical exam:

• Thyroid gland for enlargement, nodules, or bruit.

• **Proptosis** (bulging of the eyes) and **lid lag** (upper eyelid remains static with downgaze when it normally would close slightly)—seen in **Graves' disease**.

• Tremors, brisk reflexes.

Diagnostic testing involves thyroid function testing (TSH, free T4) and may include radioactive iodine uptake (RAIU) scan.

• Free T4 (fT4) and T3 (fT3) have negative feedback loop with pituitary, so high levels of thyroid hormones should cause compensatory decrease in TSH.

• **RAIU scan**—incorporation of radioiodine into thyroid hormone can differentiate "hot" (hormone-producing) nodules from "cold" (hypo-functioning) nodules, along with determining amount and location of thyroid tissue affected.

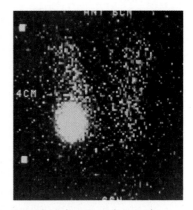

Exemplar radioactive iodine uptake (RAIU) and scan of functioning nodule in a patient with a palpable nodule in right lower thyroid gland. (Reproduced, with permission, from Gardner DG, Shoback D. Greenspan's Basic & Clinical Endocrinology. 10th ed. New York, NY: McGraw Hill; 2018.)

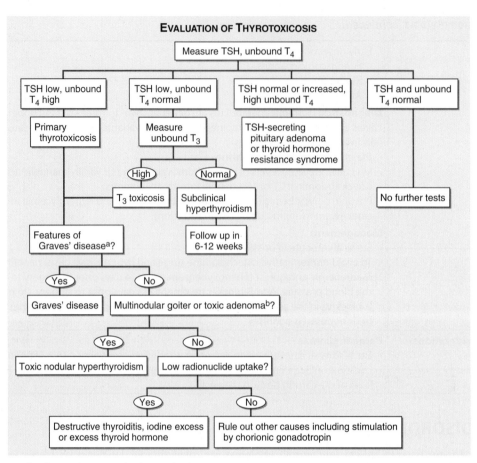

EVALUATION OF THYROTOXICOSIS

This algorithm presents the diagnostic process for thyrotoxicosis. (Reproduced, with permission, from Jameson JL, Fauci AS, Kasper DL, Hauser SL, Longo DL, Loscalzo J, eds. Harrison's Principles of Internal Medicine. 20th ed. New York, NY: McGraw Hill; 2019.)

Causes of Excess Thyroid Hormone and Associated Symptoms, Signs, and Studies

Diagnosis	Symptoms/Signs	TSH	Free T4, T3	Radioactive Iodine Uptake Scan	Thyrotropin Antibodies
Graves' disease	Proptosis Lid lag Goiter with bruit	↓	↑	Diffuse uptake	Present
Toxic adenoma, toxic multinodular goiter	Nodular or asymmetric goiter	↓	↑	Focal uptake	Absent
Thyroiditis (e.g., subacute (painful), infectious, radiation, trauma	Smooth goiter, may be painful or painless	Acutely ↓, followed by ↑ (hypothyroid phase)	↑ (hyperthyroid phase), then ↓ (hypothyroid phase)	↓	Absent
TSH-producing pituitary adenoma	Headache Visual field defects Pituitary adenoma on MRI brain	↑	↑	Diffuse uptake	Absent
Iodine-induced hyperthyroid (Jod-Basedow phenomenon)	Smooth goiter History of iodine exposure (e.g., IV contrast, amiodarone)	↓	↑	Variable, depending on preceding exogenous iodine load	Absent

It is important to note that **ophthalmopathy** is specific to **Graves' disease** and is not present in other forms of hyperthyroidism. Ophthalmopathy is characterized by lymphocyte infiltration into connective tissue the secretion of proinflammatory cytokines, and the stimulation of retro-orbital fibroblasts to produce excess glycosaminoglycans causing proptosis.

Other less common causes of hyperthyroidism include:

- **Factitious** or **iatrogenic thyrotoxicosis**—inappropriate use or excessive dose of levothyroxine.
- **Central hyperthyroidism**—pituitary dysfunction leading to inappropriately normal or ↑ TSH despite ↑ in T3 and T4.
- **Medications**—(e.g., amiodarone) given to someone who has subacute hyperthyroidism.
- **Choriocarcinoma**—hCG and TSH share a common subunit, so high levels of hCG can cause overstimulation of TSH receptors.

Pregnancy is an important cause of changes in thyroid function and can result in both hyper- and hypofunction of the thyroid gland. Also refer to Obstetrics and Gynecology Chapter for additional information.

- First trimester: High levels of hCG stimulate the thyroid to produce thyroid hormone causing transient gestational hyperthyroidism (which is usually asymptomatic).
- During pregnancy, T4 reference ranges set about 1.5 times the non-pregnant normal range.

CASE 10 | Graves' Disease

A 48-year-old woman presents with intermittent palpitations, frequent stools, heat intolerance, irregular menses, and trouble sleeping. On exam, she is afebrile; blood pressure is 160/95 mmHg, and pulse is 108/min. She appears anxious and her skin is warm. Exam notable for exophthalmos, thyromegaly, lid lag, brisk reflexes, and mild bilateral anti-gravity action tremor.

Conditions with Similar Presentations	Other causes of hyperthyroidism (**toxic multinodular goiter, thyroiditis**) would not cause ophthalmopathy. **Menopause, pheochromocytoma** (see the previous Case): No ophthalmopathy, brisk reflexes, or abnormal thyroid on physical exam.
Initial Diagnostic Tests	• Check TSH (↓), free T4 (↑), thyroid antibodies (↑) • Consider checking total T3, if free T4 normal
Next Steps in Management	• Symptom control with β-blocker • Antithyroid medications like propylthiouracil and methimazole
Discussion	Graves' disease is the most common cause of hyperthyroidism. It is an autoimmune disease in which stimulatory thyrotropin receptor antibodies activate the thyrotropin receptor mimicking the action of TSH and causing excess thyroid hormone synthesis and secretion. It is more common in females 30–60 years of age. **History:** Risk Factors: include genetic susceptibility, dietary iodine levels, radioactive iodine treatment, immune reconstitution, recent viral infection Symptoms include: • Weight loss, heat intolerance, palpitations • Insomnia, anxiety, tremor • Frequent stools of low volume • Menstrual changes **Physical Exam:** • Tachycardia, anti-gravity action tremor • Warm and moist skin • Thinning hair • Brisk reflexes • Ophthalmopathy—exophthalmos and periorbital edema with lid-lag • Pretibial myxedema due to stimulation of dermal fibroblasts resulting in swelling of anterior shins **Diagnostics:** • TSH (↓), free T4 (↑): confirm the diagnosis of hyperthyroidism • If TSH (↓), and free T4 normal, then check total T3, if T3↑ will diagnose T3 toxicosis • Thyrotropin receptor antibodies elevated • Check radioactive iodine uptake (RAIU) scan if thyroid nodules present

CASE 10 | Graves' Disease *(continued)*

Discussion	**Management:** • Symptomatic management with beta blockers. • Propylthiouracil (PTU) or methimazole (MMI) (preferred) to reduce thyroid hormone production. • MMI preferred because of more rapid onset, once daily dosing, and less adverse reaction • Definitive treatment with thyroidectomy or radioiodine therapy, generally results in need for lifelong thyroid hormone replacement • Glucocorticoids for active progressive Graves' ophthalmopathy
Additional Considerations	**Surgical Considerations:** • Risk of damaging surrounding structures, including parathyroids (creating hypoparathyroidism), recurrent laryngeal and/or superior laryngeal nerve (hoarseness, dysphagia, dysphonia). • Surgery on hyperthyroid patients may precipitate thyroid storm (see Case "Thyroid Storm"). **Pregnancy Considerations:** • PTU is preferred medication in first trimester due to lower risk of teratogenicity. • In second and third trimesters (once organogenesis is complete), methimazole is preferred. **Pediatric Considerations:** **Neonatal hyperthyroidism:** • TSH-R antibodies can cross placenta and stimulate fetal thyroid gland. • Transient condition that resolves within 4–5 months. • Treat with methimazole.

Medications Used in the Treatment of Hyperthyroidism

Drug Name	Mechanism of Action	Side Effects	Additional Considerations
Propylthiouracil (PTU)	Blocks thyroperoxidase (TPO) reducing the synthesis of new thyroid hormone; and decreases T4 → T3 conversion	Agranulocytosis especially in first 3 months Liver injury Rash	Avoid in children Interacts with warfarin
Methimazole	Blocks TPO reducing the synthesis of new thyroid hormone	**Agranulocytosis** Rash Arthritis Vasculitis Pancreatitis Hepatotoxicity	Contraindicated in hypersensitivity First-line except for first trimester of pregnancy Interacts with bupropion and warfarin

CASE 11 | Thyroid Storm

A 28-year-old man is brought to the emergency department (ED) with fever, sweats, palpitations, tremors, and confusion. According to family, for the past few months he has been complaining of palpitations, sweating, frequent stools, weight loss, and anxiety. One day ago, he had minor foot surgery for a bunion. Patient is not known to be on any other medications or substances/supplements. On exam, vitals are temperature 39.8, HR 130, BP 150/60 (widened pulse pressure) RR 20, SpO$_2$ 98% on room air. Patient appears anxious and confused, oriented to name only. He is diaphoretic with a notable stare and lid lag. Thyroid gland is symmetric and five times larger than normal with bruit present. Lungs are clear to auscultation and cardiac exam has an irregularly irregular tachycardic rhythm and a 2/6 systolic murmur at the cardiac apex. Symmetric non-pitting lower extremity edema is noted. Right foot surgical scar is clean dry and intact.

CASE 11 | Thyroid Storm *(continued)*

Conditions with Similar Presentations	**Pheochromocytoma, drug withdrawal, drug toxicity, or surgical site infection.** **Arrhythmia** alone would not cause other symptoms (e.g., loose stools, weight loss) **Serotonin syndrome:** May occur in patients on multiple serotonergic medications or with increasing dose of medications (SSRIs, SNRIs, migraine medications, bupropion, tramadol, linezolid) **Neuroleptic malignant syndrome:** May occur with dopaminergic medications (antipsychotics, metoclopramide, anti-Parkinson medications). Findings include lead-pipe rigidity, hyporeflexia, elevated CK **Malignant hyperthermia:** Present with muscle rigidity and increasing oxygen requirements and end-tidal CO_2 during anesthesia
Initial Diagnostic Tests	• Clinical diagnosis • Check: TSH ($\downarrow$), free T4 ($\uparrow$) and/or T3 ($\uparrow$) to confirm thyrotoxicosis • Consider: ECG to confirm diagnosis of atrial fibrillation • CBC, BMP, blood cultures, and toxicology screen to rule out other pathology
Next Steps in Management	• Antithyroid drugs (methimazole, propylthiouracil) • Beta-blockers (propranolol, esmolol) • Potassium iodide (once above given). This paradoxically prevents organification of iodine (Wolff-Chaikoff effect) • Glucocorticoids (block T4 to T3 conversion and treat any possible relative adrenal sufficiency due to hypermetabolic state) • Active cooling measures and acetaminophen
Discussion	Thyroid storm is a severe form of thyrotoxicosis leading to multi-organ dysfunction and is a medical emergency with mortality rate of 15–20%. It occurs in patients with underlying hyperthyroidism (which may or may not be symptomatic), who then have a trigger that results in excessive thyroid stimulation, and release of excess thyroid hormone. In addition, there is hyperactivity of the sympathetic nervous system and increased response to endogenous catecholamines. **History:** It is most commonly seen in individuals with underlying Graves' disease Triggers include: • Acute illnesses: Infection, heart attack, surgery, trauma, stroke, diabetic ketoacidosis • Medications: Thyroid hormone ingestion, amiodarone (contains two iodine molecules), salicylates, interferon alpha, interleukin 2, tyrosine kinase, anesthetics, radioactive iodine therapy • Abrupt discontinuation of antithyroid medication Symptoms: • Central nervous system: Altered mental status, agitation, delirium, eventual stupor and coma if not treated • Gastrointestinal: Nausea, vomiting, frequent stools, abdominal pain, jaundice • Cardiovascular system: Tachycardia, atrial fibrillation, arrhythmias, lower extremity edema, heart failure, cardiogenic shock **Physical Exam:** • High fever due to increased vasoconstriction and decreased heat loss • Jaundice • Signs of heart failure, arrhythmia • In addition to findings of Graves' disease if present

CASE 11 | Thyroid Storm *(continued)*

Discussion	**Diagnostics:** • Clinical manifestations are diagnostic, especially if there is a known hyperthyroid state • TSH ($\downarrow$), free T4 ($\uparrow$) • Check ECG to assess for arrhythmia and ischemia • Thyroid antibodies such as thyroid-stimulating immunoglobulin (TSI) and thyroid receptor antibody (TRab) are positive if hyperthyroidism is due to Graves' disease **Management:** Treat the underlying cause if possible. • Beta-blockade: To control symptoms and block T4 to T3 conversion • Methimazole: To block T4 synthesis • Potassium iodine: Only after above given to decrease thyroid hormone production (Wolff-Chaikoff effect) • Glucocorticoids: Block T4 to T3 conversion and treat any relative adrenal insufficiency brought on by hypermetabolic state • Cooling blankets: To treat hyperthermia • Once the patient is stable, treat underlying cause of hyperthyroidism.

Thyroid Hormone Deficiency

• Symptoms of hypothyroidism include weight gain, dry skin, brittle hair and nails, fatigue, constipation, dyspnea on exertion, menstrual irregularities, cold intolerance, and depression.

• Physical exam: Evaluate thyroid gland for presence of goiter. Other exam findings may include bradycardia, dry skin, brittle nails, hair loss.

• **In infants,** symptoms may include developmental delay, poor linear growth, and delayed puberty. Exam findings may include widened anterior fontanelle, jaundice, macroglossia, hypothermia, umbilical hernia/ abdominal distention.

   Common causes of thyroid hormone deficiency include:

• Thyroiditis (thyroid gland inflammation)—including Hashimoto thyroiditis (by far the most common), postpartum, post-viral

• Iodine deficiency

• Medications (e.g., lithium, amiodarone)

• Prior thyroid ablation or resection

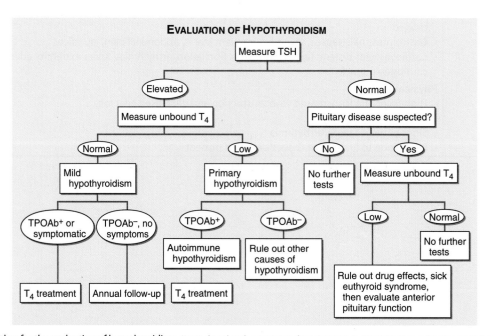

Diagnostic algorithm for the evaluation of hypothyroidism. (Reproduced, with permission, from Jameson JL, Fauci AS, Kasper DL, Hauser SL, Longo DL, Loscalzo J, eds. Harrison's Principles of Internal Medicine. 20th ed. New York, NY: McGraw Hill; 2019.)

CASE 12 | Hashimoto Thyroiditis

A previously well 44-year-old woman presents with weight gain, irregular menses, and fatigue for several months. Despite dieting and exercising she is unable to lose weight. She also reports constipation and cold intolerance. On exam, blood pressure is 130/92 mmHg, pulse is 60, and BMI is 30. She has dry skin and her reflexes have delayed relaxation. The thyroid gland is diffusely enlarged and non-tender.

Conditions with Similar Presentations	Other forms of thyroiditis resulting in an eventual hypothyroid state: **Postpartum thyroiditis, subacute granulomatous (deQuervain) thyroiditis** (painful thyroid gland following viral illness)**, Riedel (fibrous) thyroiditis** (very hard, painless goiter).
	Other conditions presenting with weight gain, irregular cycles, and fatigue:
	Central hypothyroidism: Can be caused by hypopituitarism (secondary), hypothalamic causes (tertiary), or severe illness (functional).
	Metabolic syndrome: Would not affect reflexes or cause enlarged thyroid.
	Polycystic ovarian syndrome: Hirsutism and other signs of increased androgens.
Initial Diagnostic Tests	• Check TSH ($\uparrow$), Free T4 ($\downarrow$) • Consider checking thyroid antibodies
Next Steps in Management	Levothyroxine (thyroid hormone replacement)
Discussion	Hashimoto thyroiditis (chronic lymphocytic thyroiditis) is the most common cause of hypothyroidism in iodine-sufficient regions. It is a chronic autoimmune process with infiltration of the thyroid by lymphocytes resulting in a painless goiter. Initially, patients may present with signs/symptoms of hyperthyroidism as thyroid follicles are destroyed and thyroid hormones are released resulting in higher levels of hormone. Over time, the thyroid is unable to synthesize additional T3 and T4, resulting in hypothyroidism. Most commonly affects women aged 30–50.
	History:
	Risk factors include genetic predisposition, dietary iodine intake, exposure to radioiodine, and immune-modulating medications
	Symptoms include:
	• Fatigue, dyspnea on exertion, weight gain, dry skin/hair • Menstrual irregularity • Cold intolerance, constipation • Depressed mood, sleep disturbance
	Physical Exam:
	• Bradycardia • Diastolic hypertension • Diffuse alopecia, brittle hair and nails, dry skin • Puffy facies, periorbital edema, generalized non-pitting edema (myxedema) • Proximal muscle weakness, carpal tunnel syndrome • Slow return phase of deep tendon reflexes • Thyroid gland may be small, normal, or large
	Diagnostics: • TSH ($\uparrow$), free T4 ($\downarrow$) • Antibodies present in autoimmune hypothyroidism include anti-thyroid peroxidase antibody, anti-thyroglobulin antibody • May see hyperlipidemia, hyponatremia, elevated CK
	Management: • Symptomatic patients should be treated with levothyroxine (thyroid hormone replacement) • TSH levels monitored every 6–8 weeks and medications accordingly adjusted until patient is euthyroid • Start with lower doses and increase more slowly if increased age, severe/long-standing hypothyroidism, coronary artery disease

CASE 12 | Thyroid Storm *(continued)*

Additional Considerations	**Complications:** Include myxedema coma, carpal tunnel syndrome, anemia
	Pregnancy complications:
	Increased risk of miscarriage, stillbirth, preterm birth, postpartum hemorrhage, and gestational hypertension
	Pediatric considerations:
	Congenital hypothyroidism occurs when there is decreased or absent action of thyroid hormone during development and early infancy
	• Most common cause is thyroid dysgenesis but other etiologies include inborn errors of thyroid hormone synthesis, iodine deficiency, antibody-mediated maternal hypothyroidism, dyshormonogenic goiter
	• Symptoms include increased head circumference, feeding difficulties, enlarged and protuberant tongue, constipation, umbilical hernia, pale puffy face, hyperbilirubinemia, poor brain development
	• Generally identified on newborn screening and early treatment is critical to prevent neurodevelopmental delay

Hypothyroidism Mini-Cases

Cases	Key Findings
Central Hypothyroidism	**Hx:** Hypopituitarism may lead to hypotension, salt wasting, fatigue, irregular menses.
	PE: Goiter, other signs of hypothyroidism.
	Diagnostics: TSH (↓), free T4 (↓)
	• Other pituitary hormones usually low (e.g., ACTH, estrogen/testosterone)
	Management:
	• Levothyroxine
	• Other hormone replacement as necessary
	Discussion: Due to pituitary dysfunction (secondary) or hypothalamic dysfunction (tertiary)
	• Distinguish from primary hypothyroidism with low TSH
Subacute (de Quervain) Thyroiditis	**Hx:** May present with anterior neck pain in setting of recent viral infection. Initially may have signs and symptoms of hyperthyroidism (thyrotoxic phase) followed by hypothyroid signs and symptoms (hypothyroid phase).
	PE: Very tender thyroid gland.
	Diagnostics: Initially TSH (↓), free T4 (↑), ESR (↑)
	Other abnormalities may include WBC (↑), Hg (↓)
	Management:
	• NSAIDs, beta-blockers for mild symptoms
	• Corticosteroids if moderate-severe thyroid pain or severe symptoms of thyrotoxicosis
	Discussion: Self-limited inflammatory disease. The initial hyperthyroid phase is followed by a hypothyroid phase and subsequent return to euthyroid state.
Riedel (Fibrous) Thyroiditis	**Hx:** May present with anterior neck discomfort, hoarseness, dyspnea, dysphagia, stridor.
	PE: Fixed firm thyroid mass
	Diagnostics: Open biopsy of thyroid mass or surgical resection required for definitive diagnosis. Histology shows inflammatory process of thyroid and surrounding tissue, presence of fibrous tissue, absence of giant cells, lymphoid follicles, without evidence of thyroid malignancy.
	Management:
	• Corticosteroids to decrease mass size and arrest progression
	• If refractory can use tamoxifen or rituximab
	• Consider surgery if blocking airway
	Discussion:
	• Rare, inflammatory process resulting in infiltrative fibrosclerosis and progressive destruction of thyroid gland
	• Can cause compressive symptoms and endocrine abnormalities
	• Most common in women aged 30–50
	• Thyroid manifestation of IgG4-related disease

CASE 13 | Myxedema Coma

A 63-year-old woman is brought to the ED by her family for evaluation of increased lethargy and confusion for the last 2 days. She has a past medical history of breast cancer treated with radical mastectomy, radiation, and chemotherapy 10 years ago. Her family notes that she has been complaining of constipation, cold intolerance, fatigue, insomnia, dry skin, and thinning hair for the past several years. Her vital signs are temperature 34.0 C, BP 85/50, HR 45, RR 8, SpO$_2$ 87% on room air. She is lethargic and does not answer questions appropriately. She is obese, has a puffy face, thin hair, and an enlarged tongue. She has thickened, non-pitting edematous skin over her legs. During the evaluation, her mental status declines and she is intubated for airway protection.

Conditions with Similar Presentations	**Metabolic encephalopathy**
	Substance overdose (e.g., benzodiazepines, barbiturates, opiates): May see pupillary changes (pinpoint for opiates, mydriasis for others), would not cause hypothermia and other exam findings.
	Adrenal insufficiency: History of weight loss rather than weight gain
	Other vital organ failures: Kidney, liver
Initial Diagnostic Tests	• Check TSH (↑), free T4 (↓) • Consider checking CBC, BMP, toxicology screen, ECG, CXR, serum cortisol, ACTH
Next Steps in Management	• IV glucocorticoids (to prevent relative adrenal insufficiency when metabolism increases after levothyroxine) • IV levothyroxine
Discussion	Myxedema coma is a rare form of extreme hypothyroidism and is a medical emergency with high mortality rate that leads to the dysfunction of multiple organs. There usually is a trigger that disrupts the neurovascular adaptations which maintain homeostasis in chronic hypothyroidism (such as chronic peripheral vasoconstriction) and can result in decreased hypoxic drive leading to respiratory failure. **History:** Usually seen in women over age 60 with incompletely treated hypothyroidism and triggers (e.g., cold weather, infection, myocardial infarction, stroke, trauma). Risk factors include hypothyroidism and medication nonadherence, therapeutic chest or neck radiation, positive anti-TPO antibodies, thyroidectomy, family history of hypothyroidism and/or other autoimmune processes. Symptoms: • Altered mental status/memory loss • Hypothyroid symptoms (e.g., cold intolerance, constipation, facial puffiness, tongue enlargement) **Physical Exam:** • Reduced respiratory drive leading to hypoxemia and hypercapnia • Hypothermia, hypotension, bradycardia • Fluid retention, facial puffiness, tongue enlargement • Skin thickening and discoloration (due to deposition of glycosaminoglycans in the dermis) in the setting of long-standing hypothyroidism **Diagnostics:** TSH (↑), free T4 (↓) **Management:** • Maintain airway (intubation if necessary) • IV hydrocortisone to prevent adrenal crisis • Then, IV levothyroxine to reestablish euthyroid state • Initiate treatment prior to receiving lab results • Patient requires ICU level of care

Thyroid Nodule/Malignancy

Thyroid nodules may be an incidental finding on physical exam, although large nodules may be noticed by the patient. Nodules may be asymptomatic if non-functioning, or they may cause hyperthyroidism if autonomously producing thyroid hormone.

Nodules may be benign or malignant. Examples of benign nodules include:

- **Thyroid adenoma**—majority are nonfunctional or "cold," may rarely be "hot" or "toxic" (meaning they secrete thyroid hormone). Hot nodules are almost never malignant. Cold nodules need to be assessed for malignancy.

- **Toxic multinodular goiter**—focal patches of hyperfunctioning follicular cells that release T3 and T4 independent of TSH regulation.

Thyroid malignancies, because they are usually nonfunctional, are most commonly asymptomatic until they are large enough to encroach on surrounding structures, such as the recurrent laryngeal nerve or the trachea. Common symptoms include hoarseness, dysphagia, and dysphonia.

Diagnostics:

- Thyroid function tests to assess if there is hypo or hyperthyroidism.
- TPO antibodies to assess for autoimmune thyroid disease.
- Thyroid ultrasound, radionuclide scanning, and FNA-guided biopsy as shown below.

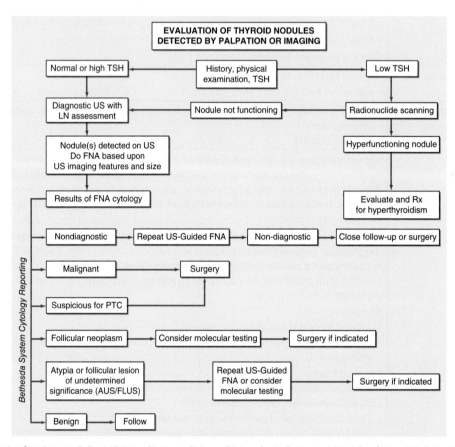

Reproduced, with permission, from Jameson JL, Fauci AS, Kasper DL, Hauser SL, Longo DL, Loscalzo J, eds. Harrison's Principles of Internal Medicine. 20th ed. New York, NY: McGraw Hill; 2019.

CASE 14 | Papillary Thyroid Cancer

A 39-year-old man who received radiation treatment as a child for Hodgkin lymphoma presents for a progressively enlarging neck mass. He reports worsening anterior neck discomfort for 6 months, difficulty swallowing solid food for the last 3 months with occasional regurgitation of food, and difficulty breathing when lying flat on his back. He has a visible mass in his right anterior neck that is mildly tender to palpation with associated enlarged cervical lymph nodes.

| Conditions with Similar Presentations | Other thyroid masses/cancers:
• **Benign adenoma**—may cause symptoms of hyperthyroidism; resect only if symptomatic
• **Follicular thyroid cancer**—known for hematogenous spread to other organs, including lungs and skeleton
• **Medullary thyroid cancer**—arises from **parafollicular "C cells"** of thyroid, produces calcitonin; patients should be tested for germline RET mutations to rule out MEN syndromes
• **Anaplastic thyroid cancer**—usually affects the elderly; aggressive tumor that presents with extensive invasion of nearby structures; poor prognosis with 1-year survival around 20% |

CASE 14 | Papillary Thyroid Cancer *(continued)*

Conditions with Similar Presentations	**Nontoxic/nonobstructive multinodular goiters:** Slow growing, and surgery indicated if suspicious for malignancy or causing compressive symptoms.
	Toxic multinodular goiter (Plummer disease): Occurs when two or more thyroid nodules secrete thyroid hormone autonomously. Patients may present with compressive symptoms and symptoms of hyperthyroidism. RAIU scan with increased radioiodine uptake corresponding to nodules. "Hot" nodules rarely malignant, treat with antithyroid medication, radioactive iodine, thyroidectomy.
	Thyroglossal duct cyst: Remnant of thyroglossal duct that does not fully close during development and is often diagnosed in childhood but more than one-third present in patients >20 years. Asymptomatic, midline mass above the hyoid bone, that elevates with protrusion of tongue and swallowing.
Initial Diagnostic Tests	• Check ultrasound, RAIU scan (if hyperthyroidism present), and fine needle aspiration/biopsy to confirm diagnosis • Also check thyroid function tests (often normal)
Next Steps in Management	Thyroidectomy potentially followed by radioiodine therapy depending on surgical pathology findings and levothyroxine treatment.
Discussion	Papillary thyroid cancer is the most common malignancy of the thyroid gland and occurs in thyroid follicular cells and can spread slowly through the lymphatic system. Genetic association include BRAF and RAS mutations. RET/PTC rearrangements seen more commonly after radiation exposure or in childhood papillary thyroid cancer.
	History: Patients often asymptomatic and mass found incidentally.
	Risk factors include exposure to radiation exposure and a history of thyroid cancer in the family.
	Physical Exam: Concerning features include: • Rapid, progressive growth of thyroid nodule • Nodule with partial mobility or fixed to underlying tissue • Hoarseness (indicates involvement of recurrent laryngeal nerve) • Cervical lymphadenopathy
	Diagnostics: • Ultrasound (features suggestive of malignancy include irregular borders, low echogenicity, taller than wide in transverse plane, increased vascularity, internal microcalcifications) • Fine needle aspiration with empty-appearing nuclei with central clearing, laminated calcium deposits (psammoma bodies), nuclear grooves • Because they are nonfunctional, TSH and T4 are normal • If TSH is low, RAIU scan should be done (hyper-functioning nodules do not need biopsy)
	Management: • Hemi- or total thyroidectomy • May need adjuvant radioiodine therapy postoperatively • Levothyroxine to replace thyroid hormone and to suppress TSH to prevent stimulation of any remaining cancer cells
Additional Considerations	**Complications:** Surgical complications include: • Hoarseness (damage to recurrent laryngeal nerve) • Hypocalcemia (damage or removal of parathyroids) • Dysphagia, dysphonia (damage to recurrent and/or superior laryngeal nerves)

PARATHYROID DISORDERS

The parathyroid glands are a group of two to six glands located along the posterior aspect of the thyroid gland. The chief cells in the gland secrete parathyroid hormone (PTH) which:

- ↑ serum calcium by
  - ↑ reabsorption of calcium from bone
  - ↑ reabsorption of calcium in the kidney
  - ↑ dihydroxylation of vitamin D which ↑calcium reabsorption in the bowel
- ↓ serum phosphorus by
  - ↑ renal excretion of phosphorus

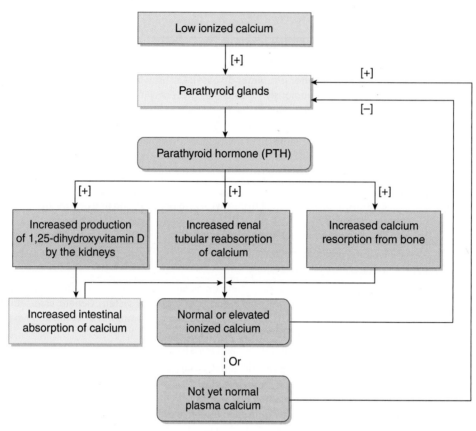

Disorders of the parathyroid glands result in excess or deficiency of PTH, resulting in an imbalance of calcium and phosphate levels. Loss of homeostasis of the calcium parathyroid axis can lead to increased secretion of PTH and the following conditions:

- **Primary hyperparathyroidism** occurs when PTH secretion is ↑ due to an adenoma, carcinoma, or hyperplasia of the gland resulting in elevated calcium and low phosphorus.
- **Secondary hyperparathyroidism** occurs when there is hypocalcemia that stimulates ↑PTH secretion. This can occur from chronic kidney disease (CKD), gut malabsorption, or vitamin D deficiency.
- **Tertiary hyperparathyroidism** occurs after long-standing secondary hyperparathyroidism seen in CKD. The parathyroid glands become autonomous, producing ↑PTH that can cause hypercalcemia.

In addition to assessing for signs and symptoms of hyper- and hypocalcemia, it is important to inquire about thyroid conditions, neck surgeries, and/or kidney disease.

Symptoms and signs of **hypercalcemia** include polyuria, polydipsia, abdominal pain, bone pain, constipation, weakness, and neuropsychiatric disturbances.

Symptoms and signs of **hypocalcemia** include:

- **Acute hypocalcemia** (e.g., anterior neck surgery with damage to the parathyroid glands)
  - Neuromuscular irritability: perioral numbness, numbness of fingers and toes, tetany, myalgias, cramps, seizures
  - Cardiovascular: cardiac arrhythmias secondary to prolonged QT intervals, hypotension, congestive heart failure
- **Chronic hypocalcemia**
  - Neurologic symptoms
  - Blurred vision
  - Constipation, abdominal cramping
  - Fatigue
  - Depression

- Exam findings of hypocalcemia include:
  - **Chvostek sign:** provider taps on patient's cheek below zygomatic arch, causes twitching of the face due to excitement of the facial nerve
  - **Trousseau sign:** patient develops spasm in outstretched hand when BP cuff inflated above systolic pressure for ≥3 minutes

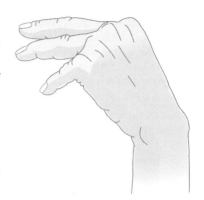

Trousseau sign. (Reproduced with permission from Ganong WF: Review of Medical Physiology, 17th ed. New York: McGraw Hill; 1995.)

Causes of Hyper- or Hypocalcemia and Associated Diagnostic Studies

Disorder	Manifestations	Calcium	Phosphorus	Vitamin D	Parathyroid hormone (PTH)
Primary hyperparathyroidism (parathyroid adenoma, parathyroid hyperplasia, parathyroid carcinoma)	Kidney stones, hypercalciuria, altered mental status, bone pain, osteitis fibrosa cystica	(↑)	(↓)	(↓) or normal	(↑)
Secondary hyperparathyroidism (CKD, hypocalcemia, vitamin D deficiency)	Renal osteodystrophy, osteomalacia	(↓) or normal	(↑) in renal failure (↓) in other causes	(↓)	(↑)
Tertiary hyperparathyroidism (CKD)	Kidney stones, hypercalciuria, altered mental status, bone pain, osteitis fibrosa cystica	(↑)	(↓) or normal	(↓) or normal	(↑)
Additional Causes of Hypercalcemia					
Ectopic secretion of PTH-related peptide (PTHrp) (tumors: squamous cell carcinoma of lung, head, neck; kidney, bladder, breast, ovarian carcinoma)	May have symptoms/signs of hypercalcemia and underlying malignancy	(↑)	(↓)	(↓) or normal	(↓)
Excess vitamin D, vitamin A, or calcium intake	May have symptoms/signs of hypercalcemia and underlying disorder	(↑)	(↓) or normal	(↓), normal, or (↑)	(↓)
Familial hypocalciuric hypercalcemia	Usually asymptomatic	(↑)	Normal	Normal	Normal-(↑)
Additional Causes of Hypocalcemia					
Hypoparathyroidism (surgical resection, autoimmune destruction, DiGeorge syndrome)	Tetany, Chvostek sign (see above), Trousseau sign (see above), fatigue, seizures, arrhythmia	(↓)	(↑)	Normal	(↓)
Vitamin D deficiency (rickets)	Muscle weakness, rachitic rosary, fractures	(↓)	(↓)	(↓)	(↑)
Pseudohypoparathyroidism (end-organ resistance to PTH, Albright hereditary dystrophy)	Shortened 4th/5th digits, short stature, obesity, developmental delay	(↓)	(↑)	Normal	(↑)
Pseudo-pseudohypoparathyroidism (defective G protein, but no PTH resistance—paternally inherited disorder)	Shortened 4th/5th digits, short stature, obesity, developmental delay	Normal	Normal		Normal

CASE 15 | Primary Hyperparathyroidism

A 44-year-old woman presents for evaluation of fatigue and muscle weakness for the last month. The weakness has worsened over the last couple of weeks and she fractured her arm in a recent fall. She has a history of recurrent kidney stones and on review of systems reports polyuria, polydipsia, and constipation. She does not take any vitamins or supplements. Routine labs show an elevated calcium level.

Conditions with Similar Presentations	**Thyroid dysfunction** (either hypo- or hyperthyroidism): Would not see hypercalcemia, recurrent kidney stones, polyuria.
	Sarcoidosis: Patients often present with respiratory symptoms, and hypercalcemia is due to ($\uparrow$) 1,25-OH vitamin D produced by giant cells in the granulomatous lesions.
	Familial hypocalciuric hypercalcemia (FHH): Asymptomatic and does not require treatment. Occurs due to an autosomal dominant mutation in G-protein-coupled calcium-sensing receptor (CASR) which increases threshold range of calcium required to trigger PTH release, resulting in normal or mildly ($\uparrow$) serum calcium and ($\uparrow$) PTH and ($\downarrow$) calcium in urine, due to retention of calcium by the kidney.
	Vitamin D toxicity: Vitamin D level ($\uparrow$) and PTH ($\downarrow$)
Initial Diagnostic Tests	• Check calcium ($\uparrow$), phosphorus ($\downarrow$), PTH level ($\uparrow$) • Also check BMP, 25-OH vitamin D level, serum albumin or ionized calcium
Next Steps in Management	Depends on severity of presentation • If symptomatic, manage hypercalcemic crisis with IV hydration and bisphosphonates. • If asymptomatic or after treating acute hypercalcemia, evaluate patient for parathyroidectomy. • If not a surgical candidate, medical therapy includes bisphosphonates or cinacalcet to reduce serum calcium.
Discussion	Parathyroid adenomas cause about 85% of cases of primary hyperparathyroidism. The excess PTH results in hypercalcemia and hypophosphatemia. Multi-gland parathyroid hyperplasia is seen in <15%, and parathyroid carcinoma is rare.
	History: Most commonly seen in women over age 50. It can also be seen in multiple endocrine neoplasia (MEN) type 1 or 2A. Risk factors include genetic predisposition, lithium, ionizing radiation exposure. Most patients are asymptomatic and diagnosis is often made incidentally when an elevated serum calcium is noted on labs.
	Symptoms/Presentations: Include kidney stones, osteoporosis, fragility fractures, bone pain, polyuria, abdominal pain, nausea, vomiting, fatigue, depression, neuromuscular manifestations.
	Physical Exam: Findings in severe cases may include muscular weakness, flat affect (due to depression).
	Diagnostics: ($\uparrow$) PTH with ($\uparrow$) calcium
	Calcium levels should be corrected based on serum albumin or an ionized calcium level obtained.
	Additional studies prior to surgery: • 24-hour urine calcium and creatinine to rule out FHH; patients with FHH will have fractional excretion of calcium <1% • 25-OH D levels because concurrent hypovitaminosis D is associated with more severe disease • Ultrasound to determine location of parathyroid adenomas, four-gland hyperplasia, or neoplastic appearance of a gland • Technetium 99m sestamibi scan to look for areas of increased uptake correlating to a parathyroid adenoma
	Radiographic findings may include: • Subperiosteal thinning and erosions within the phalanges • Osteitis fibrosa cystica caused by formation of cystic bone spaces that fill with brown fibrous tissue • "Salt and pepper" skull on imaging

CASE 15 | Primary Hyperparathyroidism *(continued)*

Discussion	Consider checking:
	• Dual energy x ray absorptiometry (DEXA) scan including views of the 1/3rd forearm (cortical bone is most affected by primary hyperparathyroidism)
	• Renal US to assess for kidney stones if symptomatic
	Management:
	• Manage hypercalcemic crisis with IV hydration and bisphosphonates
	• Loop diuretics assist in calcium excretion
	• Calcitonin may be added but has short-lived effect
	• Definitive treatment for symptomatic disease is parathyroidectomy (removal of hypersecreting parathyroid tissue while preserving the remaining glands)
	• Surgery recommended for asymptomatic patients if: serum calcium is ≥1 mg/dL above normal, osteoporosis (T score <2.5), fragility or vertebral fractures, renal manifestations (stones, GFR <60 mL/min), age <50, 24-hour urine calcium >400 mg/d
	• If surgery is not an option, medical therapy with bisphosphonates or cinacalcet to reduce serum calcium
Additional Considerations	**Surgical Complications:**
	• Risk of damage to recurrent laryngeal or superior laryngeal nerve
	• Permanent hypoparathyroidism may occur
	• "Hungry bone syndrome" if vitamin D deficiency also present

CASE 16 | Secondary Hyperparathyroidism

A 60-year-old man with end-stage renal disease awaiting a kidney transplant presents to the clinic for evaluation of bone pain, depressed mood, and numbness in his fingers and toes. He receives dialysis to treat renal failure secondary to hypertensive renal vascular disease first diagnosed 2 years ago. His dialysis labs have shown an elevated phosphorus and low calcium level, even when corrected for his albumin.

Conditions with Similar Presentations	Patients who do not take phosphorus binders with food can present with hyperphosphatemia.
	Hypomagnesemia: Can present with hypocalcemia and can be differentiated by checking magnesium levels.
Initial Diagnostic Tests	• Check calcium (↓), serum phosphorus (↑), PTH (↑), 25-OH vitamin D (↓)
	• Consider: BMP, CBC, TSH
Next Steps in Management	• Calcium and vitamin D supplementation
	• Low-phosphate diet
	• Phosphate binders (sevelamer) or calcimimetics (cinacalcet) to treat hyperphosphatemia
Discussion	Secondary hyperparathyroidism is commonly a result of CKD. The lack of calcitriol (activated vitamin D) decreases calcium absorption in GI tract. In addition, decreased phosphate excretion by the kidney leads to hyperphosphatemia, which binds to free calcium. The hypocalcemia triggers release of PTH, which results in further hyperphosphatemia (unable to excrete phosphorus) and hypovitaminosis D (unable to activate vitamin D).
	History: Risk factors include CKD, malabsorption syndromes (inflammatory bowel disease, celiac disease, lactose intolerance, history of gastric bypass), pancreatitis, and dietary restrictions. Symptoms include bone pain, fractures, muscle twitching/spasms, numbness, depression, lethargy, headaches, impaired vision.
	Physical Exam:
	• Chvostek sign (see above)
	• Trousseau sign (see above)
	• Dry skin and brittle hair due to hypocalcemia
	Diagnostics:
	• Calcium (↓), phosphorus (↑), PTH secretion (↑)
	• Low 25-OH vitamin D (↓) and 1,25-OH vitamin D (↓)
	• BMP (BUN and creatinine elevated in underlying renal disease)

CASE 16 | Secondary Hyperparathyroidism *(continued)*

Discussion	**Management:** • Dietary changes—limiting phosphorus, increasing calcium (supplementation if necessary) • Calcitriol may be given as oral supplement • Phosphate binders (sevelamer, aluminum hydroxide, calcium acetate) • Calcimimetic (cinacalcet) modulates the calcium sensing receptor in the parathyroid glands to lower PTH levels
Additional Considerations	**Screening:** In CKD patients, regularly check BMP, 25-OH vitamin D, PTH, and phosphorus levels. **Complications:** **Tertiary hyperparathyroidism:** • Develops in response to refractory or untreated secondary hyperparathyroidism • Chronic hypocalcemia results in compensatory hyperplasia of parathyroid cells that become autonomous • Significantly elevated PTH, elevated serum calcium • May require parathyroidectomy with advanced CKD and PTH levels >800 with no response to medical therapy

Medications Used in the Treatment of Secondary Hyperparathyroidism

Drug Name	Mechanism of Action	Side Effects	Additional Considerations
Sevelamer	Binds phosphate in dietary tract and decreases absorption	Abdominal pain, constipation, diarrhea, indigestion, nausea and vomiting	Contraindicated in bowel obstruction Interacts with ciprofloxacin, levothyroxine, mycophenolate mofetil, erdafitinib Minimal fetal risk
Cinacalcet	Causes an increase in the sensitivity of calcium sensing receptors on parathyroid glands thereby decreasing serum PTH and Ca	Hypocalcemia, adynamic bone disease, nausea, vomiting, diarrhea, myalgias, dizziness, hypertension, asthenia	Swallow tablets whole, with food Strong CYP2D6 inhibitor (other substrates include antidepressants, antipsychotics, beta-blockers, morphine, codeine, and tramadol), partially metabolized by CYP3A4

CASE 17 | Hypoparathyroidism

A 28-year-old man with primary hyperparathyroidism undergoes resection of a parathyroid adenoma. Immediately post-op, the patient reports leg pain, cramping in hands and legs, and perioral numbness. On exam, vital signs are stable, but twitching of the patient's lip, ala nasi, and orbicularis oculi is noted. When a blood pressure cuff is inflated for 3 minutes there is spastic flexion of wrist, metacarpophalangeal joints; abduction of thumb and extension of interphalangeal joints is observed (Trousseau sign).

Conditions with Similar Presentations	**CKD:** Symptoms related to hypocalcemia occur more gradually and are not so severe. **Hypomagnesemia:** Low magnesium levels may also cause neuromuscular excitability and cardiac arrhythmias in severe cases.
Initial Diagnostic Tests	• Check serum total and ionized calcium ($\downarrow$), PTH ($\downarrow$), serum albumin. • Consider: ECG, BMP, serum magnesium, vitamin D level.
Next Steps in Management	• Calcium supplementation (IV then PO) • Possible magnesium supplementation and vitamin D supplementation if needed

CASE 17 | Hypoparathyroidism *(continued)*

Discussion	There is a sudden drop in PTH that accompanies surgical removal of parathyroid tissue. Bones increase uptake of calcium, phosphate, magnesium, resulting in low serum levels. This is known as hungry bone syndrome. **History:** Risk factors include resection or damage to parathyroid glands, autoimmune destruction of parathyroid glands, infiltrative disease (amyloidosis, sarcoidosis), parathyroid aplasia (DiGeorge syndrome). Symptoms include: • Neuromuscular irritability (numbness around perioral region, fingertips and toes) • Myalgias, cramps, tetany • Palpitations (due to cardiac arrhythmias secondary to prolonged QT) • Seizures **Physical Exam:** • Chvostek and Trousseau signs • Dry skin, brittle hair • Decreased visual acuity • Dental abnormalities (enamel hypoplasia) **Diagnostics:** • Inappropriately (↓) PTH levels (<20 pg/mL) • (↓) serum calcium levels (<8.4 mg/dL) • Correct serum calcium based on albumin level or check ionized calcium • Serum magnesium to rule out hypomagnesemia • ECG to check for QT prolongation **Management:** • Acute severe and/or symptomatic hypocalcemia: IV calcium gluconate or calcium chloride • Chronic management with calcium and vitamin D supplements • May consider recombinant PTH replacement therapy (but risk of osteosarcoma)
Additional Considerations	**Complications:** Cardiomyopathy, heart failure, cataracts, papilledema, fractures. **Surgical Considerations:** Calcium and vitamin D supplementation given prior to removal of parathyroid adenoma to prevent hungry bone syndrome from developing. **Pediatric Considerations:** Calcitriol given to regulate calcium and phosphorus levels for hypoparathyroidism secondary to 22q11.2 deletion syndrome.

CASE 18 | Osteoporosis

A 63-year-old woman with COPD and type 2 diabetes presents with acute back pain after lifting a box. She says she felt like something cracked in her back and has been in severe pain since then. She has no loss of sensation in either leg or loss of urinary or bowel function. She has smoked one pack of cigarettes daily for 40 years, and her diabetes is currently controlled with metformin. Her last menstrual period was 8 years ago. She has focal spinal tenderness at T10 level.

Conditions with Similar Presentations	**Osteopenia:** Low bone mass that occurs with age and is defined as a T-score between −1.0 and −2.5 **Primary hyperparathyroidism:** Elevated PTH causing increased bone turnover. **Pathologic fracture:** Usually occurs in thoracic or lumbar spine in the setting of metastatic lesion or infection and patients may have other systemic or localized symptoms of infection, or known malignancy.
Initial Diagnostic Tests	• Check thoracic spine X-ray to confirm compression fracture at T10. • If no other etiology found, this is considered a fragility fracture and is diagnostic of osteoporosis. In the absence of a fracture, a DEXA scan with a T-score <2.5 is diagnostic. • Consider: 25-OH vitamin D, BMP, PTH, alkaline phosphatase, AST/ALT, 24-hour urinary calcium.
Next Steps in Management	• Pain control • Antiresorptive agents or anabolic medications (recombinant PTH) • Calcium and vitamin D supplementation

CASE 18 | Osteoporosis *(continued)*

Discussion	Osteoporosis is caused by an imbalance between osteoblastic and osteoclastic activity in bone remodeling. It is characterized by decreased bone strength, which predisposes to increased fracture risk. Primary osteoporosis is due to increasing age in men and women and post-menopausal status in women. Reduced estrogen production in the post-menopausal state results in excess production of RANK-L, which promotes osteoclastogenesis and bone resorption.

History:

Risk Factors: Include female sex, low calcium, and vitamin D intake or malabsorption, smoking, alcohol use, primary ovarian insufficiency, hyperparathyroidism, CKD, autoimmune diseases, medications (warfarin, glucocorticoids, vitamin A, loop diuretics, chemotherapy, anti-epileptic drugs, proton pump inhibitors, thiazolidinediones, aromatase inhibitors), parental history of fracture, porphyria, and osteogenesis imperfecta.

Symptoms: Often asymptomatic but may present with fragility fracture (extremity or back pain).

Physical Exam:

Possible kyphosis or focal tenderness at fracture site with associated limited mobility and pain with active/passive range of motion of affected site

Diagnostics:

Imaging:
- X-ray used to detect fracture in the affected bone
- DEXA used in outpatient setting to assess bone mineral density

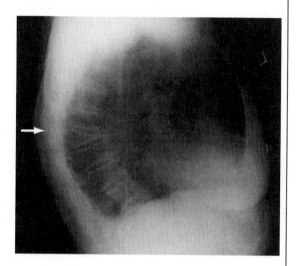

Lateral spine x-ray showing wedge-type deformity (severe anterior compression) and severe osteopenia. (Reproduced, with permission, from Jameson JL, Fauci AS, Kasper DL, Hauser SL, Longo DL, Loscalzo J, eds. Harrison's Principles of Internal Medicine. 20th ed. New York, NY: McGraw Hill; 2019.)

Diagnostic criteria for osteoporosis include:
- Presence of a fragility fracture without other metabolic bone disorders, independent of bone mineral density
- DEXA scan showing T score ≤2.5 in lumbar spine, total hip, femoral neck or 33% radius, even without prevalent fracture
- T-score between –1 and –2.5 and high fracture risk assessment fracture probability

T-scores are determined by DEXA scan and measure standard deviations of bone mineral density from a mean for age and gender.

Consider workup for secondary causes of osteoporosis in men and premenopausal women.

Management:
- Antiresorptive medications (e.g., bisphosphonates, denosumab, selective estrogen receptor modulators) or anabolic medications (e.g., teriparatide, romosozumab)
- Lifestyle modifications and increased dietary intake of calcium, vitamin D
- If fragility fracture, also treat pain

CASE 18 | Osteoporosis *(continued)*

Additional Considerations	**Preventative:** Lifestyle modifications (abstinence from alcohol and smoking, moderation of caffeine, increasing weight-bearing activities, exercise) and increased dietary intake of calcium, vitamin D, and protein. Bisphosphonates and selective estrogen receptor modulators can also prevent postmenopausal osteoporosis.
	Screening: USPSTF Grade B recommendation for screening in postmenopausal women at least 65 years of age (or younger than 65 years with increased risk of osteoporotic fracture).
	Complications: • Fractures result in loss of freedom and independence, often require long-term physical therapy to regain previous level of function • Women have 12–20% increased mortality for 2 years following hip fracture • Over 50% of patients with hip fracture do not return to independent living

Medications Used in the Management of Osteoporosis

Drug Class/Name	Mechanism of Action	Side Effects/Contraindications	Additional Considerations
Bisphosphonates Alendronate Ibandronate Zoledronate Risedronate	Binds hydroxyapatite at sites of active remodeling in bones and ↓ activity of osteoclasts	Side effects: Esophagitis, dysphagia, osteonecrosis of the jaw, atypical femoral fractures Contraindications include active esophageal disease, upper GI disease, GFR <30	Take in the morning on an empty stomach with full glass of water Wait 30 minutes before ingesting other medications, food, or water
Selective estrogen receptor modulator (SERM) Raloxifene	Binds to and activates estrogen receptors at bones to ↓resorption	Side effects: VTE, retinal vein thrombosis, stroke, hot flashes, myalgias, flu-like symptoms Contraindications: Hypersensitivity to drug/class, venous thromboembolism, pregnancy/breastfeeding	Does not require renal adjustments Also used for treatment of breast cancer SERMs lower the risk of vertebral fractures but do not lower hip fracture risk
Denosumab (Prolia)	Monoclonal antibody that prevents the binding of RANKL to receptors, causing a reduction in the differentiation of precursor cells into mature osteoclasts	Back pain, muscle pain, high cholesterol, bladder infection, osteonecrosis of the jaw and atypical femoral fractures Contraindications: Hypocalcemia (hypoparathyroidism and osteomalacia), pregnancy	Does not require renal adjustments Delivered by subcutaneous injection every 6 months
Calcitonin	Recombinant naturally occurring hormone that counteracts PTH	Nausea, local inflammatory reactions, vasomotor symptoms if injected;	Comes in either injectable or nasal spray Not useful for fracture reduction but can be used for the initial treatment of hypercalcemia
Recombinant PTH Teriparatide Abaloparatide	Recombinant form of PTH and PTHrp, intermittent use activates osteoblasts as opposed to osteoclasts to decrease bone resorption	Transient nausea, orthostatic hypotension, hypercalcemia, leg cramps Contraindicated in patients who are at increased risk of osteosarcoma, including patients with Paget disease of the bone, history of irradiation of the skeleton, open epiphyses, or unexplained elevation of alkaline phosphatase of skeletal origin	Delivered by daily subcutaneous injection Should measure PTH, serum calcium, alkaline phosphatase. and 25-OH vitamin D level prior to starting medication Teriparatide is also approved for treatment of steroid-induced osteoporosis and osteoporosis in men

Medications Used in the Management of Osteoporosis (*Continued*)

Drug Class/Name	Mechanism of Action	Side Effects/Contraindications	Additional Considerations
Romosozumab	Monoclonal antibody against sclerostin, a protein that ↑formation of bone and to a lesser extent ↓bone resorption	Joint pain, headaches, hypocalcemia Like other agents, osteonecrosis of the jaw is a rare potential side effect Possible ↑risk of heart attack and stroke	Considered a "rescue therapy" for patients at very high fracture risk who have failed other therapies; can be used in patients with previous radiation exposure and renal insufficiency

PANCREATIC ENDOCRINE DISORDERS

The endocrine pancreas is responsible for producing insulin, glucagon, and somatostatin.

Insulin and glucagon: Maintain glucose homeostasis

- Insulin: Promotes glucose uptake by cells and formation of glycogen
- Glucagon: Promotes glycogenolysis and release of glucose from cells into the bloodstream

Somatostatin:

- Inhibits the secretion of insulin, glucagon, and other GI hormones
- Decreases gastric and gallbladder contraction
- Decreases fluid secretion from the intestine and pancreas

Symptoms related to pancreatic dysfunction are often related to excess or deficiency of glucose.

- Hypoglycemia: Altered mental status, palpitations, diaphoresis
- Hyperglycemia: Polyuria, polydipsia, polyphagia
- Elevations in glucagon may cause DVT, skin changes (specifically migratory necrolytic erythema)

The most common example of pancreatic dysfunction is **diabetes mellitus**. Type 1 and type 2 diabetes are discussed in detail in the cases below. However, there are several complications that are common to both conditions that are described here.

Diabetes Mellitus

Microvascular Complications:

Retinopathy

- Annual screening with dilated fundoscopy
- Non-proliferative retinopathy: Dot and blot hemorrhages, hard exudates, microaneurysms
- Proliferative retinopathy: Neovascularization, vitreous hemorrhage; treat with anti-VEGF agents (bevacizumab), laser photocoagulation

Nephropathy

- Annual screening with urine albumin/creatinine ratio
- Glomerular hyperfiltration precedes microalbuminuria
- Prevent and treat with ACE inhibitors or ARBs

Neuropathy

- Annual screening with foot exam using monofilament
- Symmetric sensorimotor polyneuropathy; treat with TCAs, gabapentin, pregabalin, duloxetine
- Gastroparesis, neurogenic bladder, erectile dysfunction

<u>Macrovascular Complications:</u> Coronary artery disease (CAD), cerebrovascular accident (CVA), peripheral vascular disease (PVD)

<u>Other Complications:</u>

Diabetic ketoacidosis (DKA): See case below

- May be the initial presentation of type 1 diabetes
- Presents with nausea, vomiting, altered mental status, fruity odor to breath (signifying ketones), Kussmaul respirations (rapid purse lipped breathing).
- May progress to death if untreated

Hyperosmolar hyperglycemic state (HHS): See case below

- Presents with several days of polyuria, polydipsia, weight loss
- Lethargy, focal neurologic deficits, coma
- May progress to death if untreated
- Often precipitated by triggering event (e.g., infection, dehydration, discontinuation of insulin)

CASE 19 | Hypoglycemia

A 65-year-old man with type 1 diabetes is brought to the ED for decreased mental status. The patient reports having palpitations, feeling tremulous, and sweaty. He took lispro insulin in the morning but was in a hurry to get to work and did not finish eating breakfast. He is currently being treated with glargine 35 units at night and lispro 7 units with meals. On exam he is afebrile with a blood pressure of 128/86 mmHg, pulse of 102/min, respiratory rate of 12/min, and he is lethargic.

Conditions with Similar Presentations	**Sepsis:** Usually has fever and localizing signs of infection
	Substance misuse (e.g., narcotics): May present with mioisis, decreased deep tendon reflexes, bradycardia, hypoventilation
	Insulinoma or **surreptitious use of hypoglycemic medication:** Need history and laboratory data to differentiate
Initial Diagnostic Tests	• Check serum blood glucose ($\downarrow$) • Consider checking: CBC, drug screen, ECG, TSH
Next Steps in Management	• Oral glucose vs. IV dextrose, depending on level of consciousness • If no IV access, give IM glucagon
Discussion	Hypoglycemia is low plasma glucose causing autonomic or neuroglycopenic signs/symptoms. It is caused by a disruption in balance between glucose uptake and glucose release. Without glucose available to provide energy for the body, neuroglycopenic symptoms arise relating to loss of glucose and the activation of the sympathetic system. The term *hypoglycemia unawareness* refers to reduced sympathetic response, which results in lack of symptoms until glucose levels are dangerously low. It is more common in type 1 than type 2 diabetes. **History:** Risk Factors: In patients with diabetes include overtreatment with medications that cause hypoglycemia, skipping meals, poor oral intake, and reduced renal function. Causes of hypoglycemia in patients without diabetes include surreptitious or accidental use of medications causing hypoglycemia, insulinoma (tumor of insulin-secreting β cells), adrenal insufficiency (low cortisol production), post-gastric bypass. Symptoms of hypoglycemia include sweating, tremors, palpitations, lightheadedness, dizziness, anxiety, hunger, confusion. In patients without diabetes, may present with **Whipple triad:** • Presence of symptoms • Documentation of low glucose level (often <55 mg/dL) • Resolution of symptoms with proper treatment

CASE 19 | Hypoglycemia *(continued)*

	Sugar Level mg/dL (Approximation)	Severity
Discussion	80	Lower limit of physiologic euglycemia (endogenous insulin production is inhibited)
	65	Hypoglycemia (glucagon release, adrenaline and GH release)
	55	Symptomatic hypoglycemia (cortisol release)
	50 and below	Neurophysiologic dysfunction (autonomic symptom onset and cognitive dysfunction)
	25	Severe neuroglycopenia (coma, seizure)

Physical Exam: Altered mental status, loss of consciousness, tremors, diaphoresis, tachycardia.

Diagnostics:
- Low blood glucose confirms diagnosis.
- If considering other causes besides overtreatment with medications, check: Serum insulin and its precursors (proinsulin and C-peptide)
  - Elevations in proinsulin and C-peptide will only be seen with an endogenous insulin source (insulinoma, sulfonylurea use)
  - In exogenous insulin use, insulin levels will be high while proinsulin and C-peptide will be low

Management:
- Oral glucose, IV glucose, or IM glucagon (depending on patient's level of consciousness and ability to protect the airway).
- If patient continues to require glucose to maintain blood sugar, possible culprit medications include octreotide, diazoxide, nifedipine (all inhibit release of insulin from beta cells), acarbose (lowers glucose absorption).

Mangement of Symptomatic Hypoglycemia

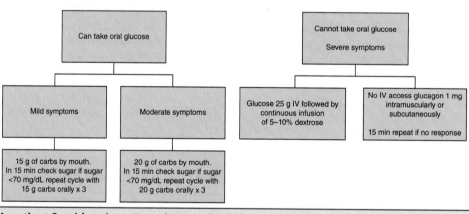

Additional Considerations | **Inpatient Considerations:** Hypoglycemia should be on the differential for any patient who has loss of consciousness or altered sensorium, especially if they are taking insulin.

CASE 20 | Type 2 Diabetes Mellitus (T2DM)

A 54-year-old woman with hypertension presents with blurred vision for the last couple of days and fatigue for the last several weeks. She thinks she is tired because she wakes up several times at night to urinate. She has no dysuria but has tingling in her feet. She has lost 10% of her weight over the last month. On exam, blood pressure is 128/80 mmHg and BMI is 33. There is a velvety hyperpigmentation on the back of neck (acanthosis nigricans), and monofilament testing of feet shows areas of decreased sensation. The rest of the exam is normal.

Conditions with Similar Presentations	**UTI, DI:** May have polyuria, but not have other symptoms associated with DM (blurry vision, unintentional weight loss, neuropathy)
	Glucagonoma: Presents clinically with hyperglycemia/DM and may have necrolytic migratory erythema, DVT, weight loss
Initial Diagnostic Tests	• Check blood glucose (↑) or A1C (↑) • Consider checking: BMP, Urinalysis
Next Steps in Management	• Diabetes education and lifestyle modification. • Metformin is preferred initial oral medication unless there is renal disease • Add insulin if blood glucose >300 mg/dL, A1C >10%, or symptoms of hyperglycemia
Discussion	T2DM is a common endocrine disorder with strong genetic predisposition. Hyperglycemia is caused by insulin resistance and relative insulin deficiency. Peripheral tissues are resistant to insulin, causing decreased glucose uptake by muscles and fat, and inappropriate hepatic gluconeogenesis. Hyperglycemia occurs gradually. It can progress to hyperosmolar hyperglycemic state, but DKA is rare.

History:

Risk factors: Obesity, family history, high-carbohydrate diet, sedentary lifestyle, advancing age. medications (e.g., glucocorticoids, atypical antipsychotics, thiazide diuretics, some HIV medications).

May be asymptomatic or present with symptoms of hyperglycemia mediated symptoms like polyuria, polydipsia, nocturia, polyphagia, blurred vision, and weight loss.

Physical Exam:

Patients may have increased BMI, retinopathy, neuropathy, and/or acanthosis nigricans on back of neck and other intertriginous folds

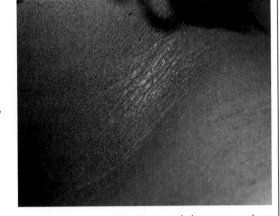

Acanthosis nigricans: Hyperpigmented plaques on a velvet-appearing verrucous surface on the neck. (Reproduced, with permission, from Jameson JL, Fauci AS, Kasper DL, Hauser SL, Longo DL, Loscalzo J, eds. Harrison's Principles of Internal Medicine. 20th ed. New York, NY: McGraw Hill; 2019.)

Diagnostics: Criteria for diagnosis include two consecutive positive tests of any of the following:

1. A1c ≥6.5%
2. Fasting plasma glucose ≥126 mg/dL
3. Two-hour oral glucose tolerance test ≥200 mg/dL
4. Random plasma glucose ≥200 mg/dL in a patient with hyperglycemic symptoms

(If checked, anti-islet cell and anti-GAD antibodies will be negative in T2DM.)

Test	Normal Glucose Tolerance	Pre-Diabetes	Diabetes
Fasting glucose	100 mg/dL	100–125 mg/dL	≥126 mg/dL
2-hour post-prandial glucose	140 mg/dL	140–199mg/dL	≥200 mg/dL
A1c	<5.6%	5.7–6.4%	≥6.5%

CASE 20 | Type 2 Diabetes Mellitus (T2DM) *(continued)*

Discussion	**Management:** • Diabetes education and lifestyle modification • Goals: A1C <7%, fasting blood glucose 80–130 mg/dL, 2-hour postprandial <180 mg/dL • First-line oral medication is metformin • Often combination treatment is needed; common medications include SGLT2 inhibitors and GLP-1 agonists (preferred in patients with known cardiovascular or renal disease), sulfonylureas, thiazolidinediones, DPP-4 inhibitors, insulin • Add insulin if blood glucose >300 mg/dL, A1C >10%, or symptoms of hyperglycemia (start basal insulin at 0.1–0.2 units/kg/day and titrate accordingly) • Monitor A1C every 3–6 months • Counsel patients about symptoms of hypoglycemia (shakiness, confusion, irritability, sweating, tachycardia, hunger; treat with glucose or glucagon) • Perform annual dilated eye exam and foot exam including monofilament. • Check urine albumin (spot urine albumin-to-creatinine ratio goal <30 mg/g Cr), estimated GFR, lipids. • Monitor blood pressure (goal <130/80 mmHg) • Treat hypertension and albuminuria with ACE inhibitor or ARB • Treat hyperlipidemia with lifestyle modifications and statins • Routine immunizations and Pneumovax starting at age 19 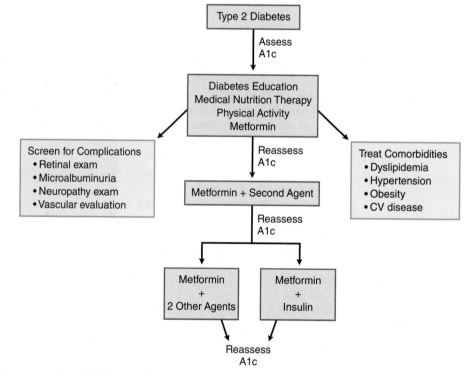 Management of type 2 diabetes mellitus. (Reproduced, with permission, from Brunton LL, Hilal-Dandan R, Knollmann BC, eds. Goodman & Gilman's the Pharmacological Basis of Therapeutics. 13th ed. New York, NY: McGraw Hill; 2018.)
Additional Considerations	**Screening:** USPSTF recommends screening asymptomatic overweight or obese adults aged 35–70 years. **Complications:** See introductory material for complications common to both type 1 and type 2 diabetes mellitus. **HHS:** Serious complication of T2DM. **DKA:** Uncommon in patients with T2DM and is characterized by anion gap acidosis. **Inpatient Considerations:** Hold oral hypoglycemic medications and metformin and manage hyperglycemia with insulin

CASE 20 | Type 2 Diabetes Mellitus (T2DM) *(continued)*

Additional Considerations	**Pediatric Considerations:** Not all the same oral hypoglycemic agents are used in treating children and adolescents as in adults. In patients with elevated A1c without evidence of acidosis or ketosis, can start metformin and if A1c is 2% above target, add another agent. If A1c is above target on dual or triple oral therapy or >10%, add insulin. If acidosis or ketosis is present, patients should be managed with insulin, but metformin can be initiated after acidosis has resolved. Presence of pancreatic autoantibodies warrants discontinuation of metformin and initiation of insulin monotherapy if not already started. For patients without pancreatic autoantibodies who have poor blood sugar control on metformin +/- insulin, liraglutide can be used if there are no contraindications. Please review Pediatric Chapter for more information.

Medications Used to Manage Type 2 Diabetes Mellitus

Drug Class and Examples	Mechanism of Action	Side Effects and Contraindications	Additional Considerations
Biguanide Metformin	Improves peripheral insulin sensitivity Inhibits hepatic gluconeogenesis	GI side effects: Nausea, diarrhea (usually resolves within a few weeks) Do not use in patients with renal insufficiency (eGFR <30 mL/min/1.73 m^2), advanced cirrhosis, or heart failure to avoid lactic acidosis	Used to treat PCOS Avoid excessive alcohol while taking metformin May cause B12 deficiency
Sulfonylureas Glimepiride Glipizide Glyburide	Increase endogenous insulin secretion	Hypoglycemia especially glyburide, weight gain, dizziness, heartburn, headache Contraindicated in DKA Use with caution in the elderly and those with liver or renal insufficiency	Glyburide is a pregnancy class B drug Interactions with many other medications including beta blockers, oral anticoagulants, diuretics, calcium channel blockers, and NSAIDs Glyburide can cause a disulfiram-like reaction with alcohol consumption
GLP-1 receptor agonists/ Incretins (-tides) Exenatide Liraglutide Dulaglutide Semaglutide	Delay food absorption Increase insulin secretion Decrease glucagon secretion	Nausea, vomiting, diarrhea, weight loss, pancreatitis (rarely) Risk medullary thyroid cancer (contraindicated in patients with history of MEN 2) Avoid in patients with CKD (stages 4–5)	Can be delivered SQ and oral (semaglutide) Preferred for patients with cardiovascular disease (ventricular function preservation and anti-inflammatory effect [Dulaglutide, Semaglutide, liraglutide]) Exenatide may decrease effect of oral agents due to slowing of gastric emptying Promote weight loss
SGLT-2 inhibitors (-flozins) Canagliflozin Dapagliflozin Empagliflozin	Inhibit SGLT2 in proximal tubule to decrease glucose reabsorption	Can cause weight loss, dehydration, hypotension glucosuria, UTI, vulvovaginal candidiasis, hypokalemia Rare risk euglycemic DKA, Fournier gangrene Contraindicated in dialysis, ESRD, severe renal impairment	Oral medications empagliflozin and canagliflozin have been shown to have a CV benefit and Reno protective effect Major drug interactions: Hydroxychloroquine, octreotide

Medications Used to Manage Type 2 Diabetes Mellitus (*Continued*)

Drug Class and Examples	Mechanism of Action	Side Effects and Contraindications	Additional Considerations
Thiazolidinedione Pioglitazone Rosiglitazone	Peroxisome proliferator-activated receptor gamma agonist Decrease insulin resistance at peripheral sites Decreased hepatic glucose production	Edema, weight gain, hepatotoxicity Avoid in heart failure Risk of bladder cancer (pioglitazone) Increased ischemic CV complications (rosiglitazone) Increased fracture risk (P>R)	Requires the body to be able to produce its own insulin to be effective Interacts with gemfibrozil and ketoconazole (inhibit metabolism)
DPP-4 inhibitors (-gliptins) Sitagliptin Saxagliptin Linagliptin Alogliptin	Inhibit degradation of GLP-1 Enhance incretin effects	Headaches, joint pain, upper respiratory infections Rare side effects: Angioedema, urticaria, SJS, pancreatitis	Oral medication Does not cause hypoglycemia when used as monotherapy Should reduce dose in CKD (except linagliptin which is mostly hepatically metabolized)
Alpha glucosidase inhibitors Acarbose Miglitol	Decrease brush border enzymes to decrease postprandial intestinal absorption of carbohydrates	Flatulence, loose stools Contraindications: Cirrhosis, colonic ulceration and IBD, intestinal obstruction, DKA	Oral medications Take with first bite of food at each main meal
Amylin analog Pramlintide	Inhibits inappropriately high glucagon post prandial Slows gastric emptying and rate of glucose absorption reduces food intake and increases satiety	Severe hypoglycemia, GI intolerance, and nausea Contraindicated in patients with confirmed gastroparesis, lack of self-awareness of hypoglycemia, poor compliance with insulin regimen	Injectable medication Only used as adjunct to insulin therapy in patients who have failed other agents When initiating, should cut mealtime insulin in half
Insulin Long acting: Glargine, detemir, degludec Intermediate: NPH Short acting: Regular Rapid acting: Lispro, aspart	Promotes glucose absorption into muscle, fat, and liver tissue and promotes glycogenesis and triglyceride formation	Hypoglycemia, weight gain	Delivered SQ or inhaled May be initiated in the hospital setting when oral hypoglycemic agents are discontinued. First-line agent in diabetes management in pregnancy, T1DM

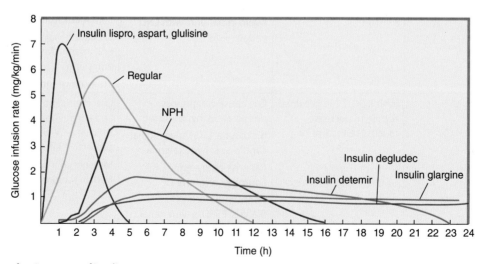

Duration of action of various types of insulin. (Reproduced, with permission, from Katzung BG, Vanderah TW, eds. Basic & Clinical Pharmacology. 15th ed. New York, NY: McGraw Hill; 2021.)

CASE 21 | Diabetic Ketoacidosis (DKA)

A 34-year-old man with T1DM is brought to the ED when he was found less responsive by his wife. She reported that he had been complaining of abdominal pain and vomiting for the last 2 days and noticed he was not easily arousable this morning. Review of systems is positive for increased thirst, increased urination, nocturia, fatigue, and weight loss. On exam, pulse is 145/min; blood pressure is 80/50 mmHg; and respirations are deep at 40/min with a fruity odor. Capillary refill is delayed, and he has dry mucous membranes.

Conditions with Similar Presentations	**Sepsis, or intoxication** **Hyperglycemic hyperosmolar state:** More common in type 2 diabetes and would not have fruity odor.
Initial Diagnostic Tests	• Check serum glucose, BMP, ABG, serum ketones • Consider checking: Urinalysis, CXR, ECG, toxicology screen, blood and urine cultures
Next Steps in Management	• IV fluids and IV insulin • Give potassium if serum level normal or low, because insulin will drive potassium intracellularly
Discussion	DKA is a life-threatening complication of diabetes mellitus resulting from a severe deficiency of insulin and is characterized by hyperglycemia, acidosis, and ketonemia. It is caused by an absolute insulin deficiency, triggered by infection, insufficient insulin injection, and/or increased counterregulatory hormones. This results in increased gluconeogenesis and glycogenolysis and hyperglycemia. The increased sugar causes osmotic diuresis, dehydration, increased thirst, and potassium loss in the urine, causing total body potassium depletion. Excess fat breakdown due to absence of insulin results in free fatty acids that are made into acidic ketone bodies (β-hydroxybutyrate > acetoacetate). Acetoacetate is metabolized into acetone, producing the fruity breath odor. Increased ketone bodies lead to increased anion gap metabolic acidosis. **History:** Ask about precipitating factors: poor metabolic control, missed insulin doses, illness/infection, medications (steroids). Symptoms include polyuria, polydipsia, fatigue, weight loss, altered mental status, lethargy, and coma due to decreased perfusion from dehydration. **Physical Exam:** • Decreased capillary refill, dry mucous membrane and decreased skin turgor, hypotension or orthostatic hypotension due to dehydration from osmotic diuresis • Tachypnea (Kussmaul breathing) to compensate for underlying acidemia by allowing the body to expel CO_2 and create more bicarbonate to buffer the rise in acidic serum ketones **Diagnostics:** • Hyperglycemia—serum glucose will be elevated • Ketonemia—serum ketones are present (β-hydroxybutyrate > acetoacetate) • Acidosis <table><thead><tr><th></th><th>Mild</th><th>Moderate</th><th>Severe</th></tr></thead><tbody><tr><td>Serum pH</td><td>7.2–7.3</td><td>7.1–7.2</td><td><7.1</td></tr><tr><td>Bicarbonate</td><td>10–15</td><td>5–10</td><td><5</td></tr></tbody></table> **Management:** • Goals are to hydrate and close anion gap and normalize blood sugar • Normal saline for rehydration and to increase intravascular volume and help kidneys excrete excess glucose • Potassium included in IV fluids due to total body deficit and to prevent hypokalemia as insulin is given • Once serum glucose lowered to 200 mg/dL, may need to add 5% dextrose to IV fluids • IV regular insulin to close anion gap and reduce production of ketones • Transition to subcutaneous insulin once serum bicarbonate >15 mEq/L and patient able to eat

CASE 21 | Diabetic Ketoacidosis (DKA) *(continued)*

Additional Considerations	**Complications:** Mucormycosis infection, cerebral edema, cardiac arrhythmias, heart failure.
	Higher risk of complications in younger patients, those with more severe DKA, and with administration of bicarbonate
	Pediatric Considerations: Children may initially present in DKA with abdominal pain, vomiting, dehydration, and fruity odor before being diagnosed with T1DM. DKA and its complications are the most common cause of hospitalization, mortality, and morbidity in children with T1DM. Fluids given in boluses to correct fluid status and then transitioned to maintenance fluids

CASE 22 | Hyperglycemic Hyperosmolar State (HHS)

A 75-year-old man with T2DM and chronic kidney disease is brought to the ED with lethargy, confusion, vomiting, and generalized weakness progressing over the course of a day. He is lethargic, disoriented, and is unable to follow simple commands. The exam is notable for a pulse of 128/min, blood pressure of 100/64 mmHg, dry mucous membranes, and decreased skin turgor. Capillary blood glucose is >600.

Conditions with Similar Presentations	**Acute delirium:** In the elderly may be due to infections (URI, UTI, pneumonia), medications, ACS, stroke, metabolic causes, hypoglycemia.
	Diabetic ketoacidosis (DKA): Usually type 1 rather than type 2 diabetes.
Initial Diagnostic Tests	• Check: Blood glucose, ABG, BMP, serum osmolality to confirm diagnosis • Also check: CBC, TSH, ECG, CXR, urinalysis, urine culture and blood cultures, toxicology screen.
Next Steps in Management	• IV fluids, insulin drip with regular monitoring of glucose. • Potassium, with goal >3.3.
Discussion	HHS is a serious complication associated with T2DM with a 5–20% mortality rate, which is higher than DKA. **History:** Occurs in patients with T2DM and often triggered by an insult such as infection and/or abrupt cessation of insulin. Symptoms include polyuria, polydipsia, weight loss, lethargy, delirium, coma. **Physical Exam:** May have signs of dehydration: Dry mucous membranes, sunken eyes, decreased skin turgor, and orthostatic hypotension May be febrile if infection is triggering event and may have neurologic symptoms due to neuronal dehydration **Diagnostics:** • Diagnostic criteria for HHS include plasma glucose >600 mg/dL, arterial pH >7.3, serum bicarbonate >18 mEq/L, serum osmolality >320 mOsm/kg, severe dehydration, altered mental status, small or no urine, and serum ketones • May have normal or low sodium levels (often pseudohyponatremia due to hyperglycemia; correct by adding 1.6 mg/dL sodium for every 100 mg/dL of glucose above 100 mg/dL). • Serum potassium may be elevated, but there is an overall deficit due to extracellular shift caused by insulin deficiency, and hypertonicity. • ECG may show prolonged PR intervals, ST depression or U-waves related to hypokalemia, flattened T-waves, and prolonged QT interval due to hypomagnesemia. **Management:** • IV fluids (normal saline) for rehydration and IV regular insulin to decrease blood sugar. • Give IV potassium to maintain K >3.3 to prevent cardiac arrhythmias • Once serum glucose lowered to 300 mg/dL, 5% dextrose added to IV fluids • Transition from IV to subcutaneous insulin when hyperosmolality resolves, mental status normalizes, and patient is able to eat. • IV insulin should be continued for a couple of hours after initiation of subcutaneous insulin to prevent recurrence of hyperglycemia while re-establishing basal insulin levels.
Additional Considerations	**Complications:** Overly rapid correction of serum osmolality may result in central pontine myelinolysis and/or seizures. **Pediatric Considerations:** • Fluid resuscitation with normal saline boluses of 20 mL/kg until peripheral perfusion restored. • Potassium replacement initiated if K <5 mEq/L. • Magnesium replacement in children with hypomagnesemia and hypocalcemia.

CASE 23 | Gestational Diabetes (GDM)

A G4P3 32-year-old woman at 22 weeks' gestation presents to her obstetrician's office for an ultrasound and routine lab work. She notes that she is having urinary frequency without dysuria and has been drinking more water to compensate. She did not have any of these symptoms prior to her pregnancy. Her last A1C from her primary physician's office was 5.4% a year ago. Prior to pregnancy her BMI was 31 kg/m².

Conditions with Similar Presentations	**T2DM:** Unlikely with normal A1C 1 year ago.
	Pregnancy: Increased urinary frequency due to pressure on bladder from growing uterus and inability for complete bladder distention.
	Urinary tract infection: Less likely given absence of dysuria
Initial Diagnostic Tests	• Check: glucose level and confirm with two-step glucose tolerance test (1-hour followed by 3-hour).
	• Consider: Urinalysis.
Next Steps in Management	Lifestyle modifications (diet, exercise with limitations) and insulin
Discussion	GDM is glucose intolerance that is diagnosed during pregnancy. In normal pregnancy, maternal insulin resistance increases due to placental secretion of diabetogenic hormones (GH, placental lactogen, corticotropin-releasing hormone, prolactin and progesterone). These increase blood glucose and facilitate glucose delivery to the fetus. However, if too much insulin resistance occurs, blood glucose becomes elevated and may cause vascular changes within the placenta. Maternal hyperglycemia leads to fetal hyperinsulinemia and increases fetal growth. Insulin resistance is greatest in the third trimester of pregnancy.
	History:
	Risk Factors: Severe obesity, advanced maternal age, strong family history of T2DM, a previous history of GDM.
	Usually asymptomatic but may have polyuria and polydipsia.
	Physical Exam: No specific findings
	Diagnostics:
	• First step is 1-hour glucose tolerance test with 50-g glucose load
	• If glucose level >130–140 mg/dL, this is followed by 3-hour glucose tolerance test with 100-g load
	• Diagnosis made if patient meets or exceeds ≥2 of the following on the 3-hour test: (1) fasting glucose ≥95 mg/dL; (2) 1-hour ≥180 mg/dL; (3) 2-hour ≥155 mg/dL; (4) 3-hour ≥140 mg/dL.
	Management:
	• Lifestyle modifications to reduce risk factors for developing further insulin resistance.
	• Insulin (initiated at time of diagnosis or after 1–2 weeks of lifestyle modification if glycemic targets not met).
	• Metformin and glyburide are considered second-line therapies.
	• Glycemic targets for maternal glucose: fasting ≤95 mg/dL, 1-hour post prandial ≤140 mg/dL, and/or 2-hour postprandial ≤ 120 mg/dL.
Additional Considerations	**Screening:** All pregnant women are screened for GDM at 24–28 weeks' gestation.
	Complications: Increased risk of developing type 2 diabetes, metabolic syndrome.
	Pediatric/Fetal Considerations:
	• Complications of uncontrolled maternal hyperglycemia for the fetus include hyperinsulinemia, macrosomia, polycythemia, cardiac septal hypertrophy.
	• Macrosomia (large for gestational age) causes increased risk of shoulder dystocia or clavicular fracture during delivery.
	• Polycythemia (develops due to placental vasculopathy and decreased oxygen delivery) can result in hemolysis or hyperbilirubinemia after birth.
	• Fetal hyperinsulinemia increases risk of stillbirth and neonatal hypoglycemia.
	• These complications are different from those of infants born to diabetic mothers (who tend to be small for gestational age, with increased risk of congenital abnormalities).

CASE 24 | Obesity/Metabolic Syndrome

A 32-year-old woman presents to clinic for an annual visit. She feels well and reports no medical problems. She has noticed progressive weight gain in recent years after she took a new job. She attributes this to her inability to find sufficient time for exercise and she is eating out more often. She has tried several diets on and off over the years without much long-term success. Physical exam is notable for BP 144/92 and a BMI of 38, as well as a waist circumference of 37 inches.

Conditions with Similar Presentations	**T2DM**
	Cushing syndrome: Would expect other findings (e.g., skin atrophy, purple striae, proximal muscle weakness, abnormal fat deposition in preauricular and upper back).
	Polycystic ovary syndrome: Often comorbid with metabolic syndrome and obesity in women of reproductive age but additional features include hyperandrogenism (acne, hirsutism) and menstrual abnormalities (oligomenorrhea, infertility).
Initial Diagnostic Tests	Consider: A1c, lipid panel, liver enzymes, TSH
Next Steps in Management	• Lifestyle modification with diet and exercise is first-line treatment. • Treat comorbidities and consider medications for weight loss: Orlistat, liraglutide, phentermine/topiramate. • Bariatric surgery.
Discussion	Obesity results from an imbalance between energy intake (determined by factors such as diet and appetite) and energy expenditure (determined by metabolic activity and physical activity) and results from both genetic and environmental influences. Obesity affects about one-third of the United States population and is defined as BMI ≥30 (calculated as weight in kg/height in m²). Metabolic syndrome is diagnosed when a set of criteria are met, including elevated blood pressure, dyslipidemia, and insulin resistance. Obesity and metabolic syndrome frequently occur together and increase the risk of conditions such as diabetes mellitus and cardiovascular disease. **History:** Risk factors for obesity include medical conditions (Cushing syndrome, hypothyroidism, PCOS), medications (glucocorticoids, antiepileptics, antipsychotics), sleep disturbances, and stress. **Physical Exam:** • May be normal other than elevated BMI and central adiposity • Hypertension • Acanthosis nigricans (due to insulin resistance) **Diagnostics:** • BMI is the first measure for determining obesity, with classification as follows: • Underweight: <18.5 • Normal weight: 18.5–25 • Overweight: 25–30 • Class I Obesity: 30–34.9 • Class II Obesity: 35–39.9 • Class III Obesity: >40 • Waist circumference ≥40 inches in men and ≥35 inches in women is an additional risk factor for cardiometabolic comorbidities • Evaluate for metabolic syndrome using lipid panel, glucose, blood pressure, and waist circumference. **Metabolic syndrome** (National Cholesterol Education Program) (≥three must be present): • Insulin resistance (fasting glucose ≥100 mg/dL) • Elevated blood pressure (≥130/85 mmHg) • Elevated triglycerides (≥150 mg/dL) • Low HDL (<40 mg/dL in men, <50 mg/dL in women) • Abdominal obesity (waist circumference ≥40 inches in men, ≥35 inches in women) **Management:** • First-line management of obesity and/or metabolic syndrome is with lifestyle modifications, including dietary changes and physical activity. • Medical management of comorbidities with antihypertensives, antihyperglycemics or insulin, and statins.

CASE 24 | Obesity/Metabolic Syndrome *(continued)*

Discussion	• Some medications are available to specifically aid with weight loss, such as liraglutide (GLP-1 agonist also used in the treatment of type 2 diabetes), phentermine, buproprion/naltrexone, and topiramate, and orlistat (inhibits pancreatic lipase) • Bariatric surgery is also a very effective option—available procedures include sleeve gastrectomy or Roux-en-Y gastric bypass. • Eligibility criteria for bariatric surgery include BMI ≥40 or BMI ≥35 with significant comorbidities related to obesity (e.g., hypertension, diabetes). Patients must demonstrate a history of failed attempts at management with diet and exercise prior to being considered for surgical options.
Additional Considerations	**Screening:** All patients should be screened annually for obesity with a BMI calculation. **Complications:** Associated with a wide range of conditions, including coronary artery disease, diabetes, hypertension, hyperlipidemia, nonalcoholic fatty liver disease (NAFLD), stroke, osteoarthritis, various cancers, and obstructive sleep apnea (OSA).

NEUROENDOCRINE TUMORS

Neuroendocrine tumors are a class of epithelial neoplasms that may secrete functional hormones. Four of the most important to recognize are carcinoid tumor, gastrinoma, insulinoma and glucagonoma. Please review *Surgery Chapter* for additional information. Rare genetic conditions such as MEN syndromes predispose to the development of multiple neuroendocrine tumors. Tumors may be treated medically and/or surgically.

Multiple Endocrine Neoplasia Syndromes

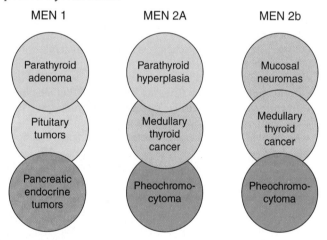

CASE 25 | Multiple Endocrine Neoplasia 1 (MEN 1) Syndrome

A 28-year-old woman presents with a year of intermittent bilateral milky breast discharge. She has had menstrual changes with cycles every other month, and persistent mid-abdominal pain. Medical history includes primary hyperparathyroidism with previous parathyroidectomy.

Conditions with Similar Presentations	Other causes of galactorrhea: **Pregnancy, antipsychotic medications** (dopamine antagonists), **hypothyroidism** (TRH stimulates release of prolactin, which can cause galactorrhea)
	Prolactinoma: May occur independently of MEN 1

CASE 25 | Multiple Endocrine Neoplasia 1 (MEN 1) Syndrome *(continued)*

Initial Diagnostic Tests	• Check PTH, calcium, phosphorus, serum glucose, prolactin, TSH, cortisol, gastrin levels • Consider: pregnancy test, CMP, CBC • Confirm with imaging
Next Steps in Management	• Dopamine agonists (bromocriptine, cabergoline) for prolactinoma • Surgical resection of gastrinoma or other pancreatic tumors • Consider parathyroidectomy for parathyroid hyperplasia/adenoma
Discussion	MEN 1 is a very rare autosomal dominant syndrome caused by germline mutations in the *MEN 1* tumor suppressor gene, encodes the protein menin. *MEN 1* mutation leads to endocrine tumors summarized by the "3 Ps" (Parathyroid, Pancreatic, Pituitary) • Parathryoid hyperplasia or adenoma: Primary hyperparathyroidism • Pancreatic endocrine tumors: Gastrinomas are most common, also insulinomas, glucagonomas, VIPomas • Pituitary tumors: Often functional, usually prolactin or GH-secreting • Other tumors include angiofibromas, meningiomas, lipomas • Tumors mostly benign, although malignancy can occur **History:** Risk Factors: Personal or family history of parathyroid, pancreatic, and pituitary tumors. Symptoms: • Hyperparathyroidism: Fatigue, constipation, renal stones, abdominal pain (due to hypercalcemia) • Prolactinoma: Vision changes, headache, galactorrhea and amenorrhea in women, decreased libido and infertility in men • Gastrinoma: Abdominal pain, GI bleed due to recurrent ulcers • VIPoma: Watery diarrhea • Glucagonoma: Diabetes symptoms **Physical Exam:** • Bilateral milky nipple discharge, visual field defects like bitemporal hemianopsia (prolactinoma) • Somatotropinoma—acromegaly • Corticotropinoma central obesity, moon facies, buffalo hump, easy bruising, purple striae • Thyrotropinimea—excessive sweating, tachycardia, muscle weakness, tremor • Glucagonoma—necrolytic migratory erythema • Abdominal tenderness (gastrinoma, other pancreatic tumors) **Diagnostics:** • Two or more tumor manifestations of MEN 1 listed above *or* one manifestation of MEN 1 + first degree relative with MEN 1 *or* genetic testing • For pituitary tumors: ↑ in prolactin, IGF-1, ACTH, cortisol, TSH depending on tumor type • For pancreatic tumors: ↑ in gastrin, insulin, glucagon, VIP depending on tumor type • For parathyroid: ↑ PTH, ↑ calcium, ↓ phosphorus • Brain MRI for pituitary tumors; abdominal CT or MRI for pancreatic tumors • Genetic testing for germline *MEN 1* mutation **Management:** • Surgical resection for most pancreatic tumors • Treat gastrinomas with PPIs, H2-receptor antagonists, or octreotide • Parathyroid adenoma requires resection • Parathyroid hyperplasia treated with parathyroidectomy • Prolactinomas are treated medically with dopamine agonists • Surgical removal of other pituitary tumors
Additional Considerations	**Screening:** Regular screening and monitoring is needed for future tumor development in patients and family members with MEN 1 beginning at age 5.

Neuroendocrine Mini-Cases

Cases	Key Findings
MEN 2A	Multiple endocrine neoplasia type 2A (MEN 2A) triad of: • Primary hyperparathyroidism (usually multiglandular) • Medullary thyroid cancer (MTC) with elevated calcitonin levels • Pheochromocytoma **Hx:** Neck pain, renal stones, constipation, abdominal pain (due to hypercalcemia), episodic headache, diaphoresis, palpitations (due to pheochromocytoma) **PE:** Enlarging neck mass (due to medullary thyroid carcinoma) and constant or intermittent severe hypertension (due to pheochromocytoma) **Diagnostics:** • Clinical diagnosis with ≥ two of: MTC, pheochromocytoma, or parathyroid adenoma in a single person or in close relatives • ↑ PTH, ↑ calcium, ↓ phosphorus • ↑ plasma and 24-hour urine metanephrines, abdominal CT for adrenals if positive • Calcitonin (↑ in MTC), thyroid ultrasound and biopsy • Genetic testing for *RET* mutation **Management:** Surgical resection of pheochromocytoma and parathyroid adenoma and total thyroidectomy. **Discussion:** • Germline mutations in the RET oncogene are associated with MEN 2. • Medullary thyroid cancer is treated with total thyroidectomy, dissection and removal of any local or regional metastases, followed by life-long thyroid hormone replacement and close monitoring for recurrence. • Surgical resection of pheochromocytoma, following pretreatment with α and β adrenergic blockade, prevent hypertensive crisis perioperatively, and prevent unopposed β stimulation. • Patients with asymptomatic hypercalcemia from primary hyperparathyroidism can be monitored; however, eventually parathyroid surgery is usually required for MEN 2 patients.
MEN 2B	Multiple endocrine neoplasia type 2B (MEN 2B) triad of: • Medullary thyroid cancer • Pheochromocytoma • Mucosal neuromas, intestinal ganglioneuromas, marfanoid habitus **Hx:** Neck pain and swelling (MTC), headache, palpitations (pheochromocytoma). **PE:** Marfanoid habitus (long limbs, wingspan greater than height, hyperlaxity) and mucosal neuromas. **Diagnostics:** • Plasma and urine metanephrines (↑ in pheochromocytoma) • Abdominal CT • Calcitonin (↑ in MTC) thyroid ultrasound and biopsy • Genetic testing for *RET* mutation **Management:** Total thyroidectomy and resection of pheochromocytoma. **Discussion:** • Also caused by germline mutations in the RET oncogene • Most aggressive form of MEN 2 • Differentiated from MEN 2A by absence of hyperparathyroidism and presence of mucosal neuromas (generally self-limited)
Carcinoid tumors	**HX/PE:** May be sporadic or associated with genetic syndromes like MEN1, von Hippel Lindau, tuberous sclerosis, neurofibromatosis type 1. Symptoms and signs vary depending on site of tumor and hormones secreted. Patients may have diarrhea, abdominal pain, wheezing, bronchospasm, altered mentation, facial flushing, rash, skin hyperpigmentation, edema or signs of right-sided valvular heart disease (e.g., tricuspid regurgitation, pulmonic stenosis)

Neuroendocrine Mini-Cases (*continued*)

Carcinoid tumors	**Diagnostics:** • 24-hour urine collection of 5-HIAA (breakdown product of serotonin) • Tumor localization and staging with CT, MRI, and somatostatin receptor nuclear scans using radiolabeled octreotide or Ga68-Dotatate (synthetic somatostatin analog) **Management:** • Somatostatin analogs (octreotide) • Surgical resection with regional lymph node dissection for non-metastatic disease • Peptide receptor radionuclide therapy with lutetium-177 dotatate, chemotherapy, radiation therapy • Hepatic arterial embolization for hepatic disease **Discussion:** Carcinoid tumors most commonly present in GI tract and lungs, but also may be in the liver, and pancreas. Within the GI tract, the most common location is in the small bowel. Symptoms are caused primarily by the secretion of serotonin (5-HT) as well as numerous other substances (histamine, kallikrein, and prostaglandins) by the tumor. The liver and lung metabolize serotonin so carcinoid tumors are usually asymptomatic until they metastasize past the liver or lungs.

Gastrinoma (Zollinger-Ellison Syndrome)	**Hx/PE:**
	• Abdominal pain/epigastric tenderness
	• Weight loss, nausea/vomiting, diarrhea
	• In severe cases, upper GI bleeding or history of distal peptic ulcers (duodenal or jejunal)
	
	Diagnostics: Diagnose with elevated fasting gastrin. If borderline, abnormal secretin stimulation test (normally secretin inhibits gastrin, but will see an increase in patients with gastrinoma)
	• Elevated fasting gastrin level (>1000 pg/mL)
	• Gastric pH ≤2
	• If fasting gastrin is elevated but <1000 pg/mL, perform a secretin stimulation test
	• CT/MRI abdomen to identify the tumor and blood tests for endocrinopathies related to MEN 1
	
	Management:
	• PPIs (e.g., omeprazole)
	• Octreotide (somatostatin analogue)
	• Surgical resection
	
	Discussion:
	• Neuroendocrine tumor arising from pancreas or duodenum
	• Produces high levels of gastrin, resulting in hypersecretion of gastric acid from parietal cells of stomach
	• Predisposes to multiple gastric and small bowel ulcers, possible GI bleeding or perforation
	• Diarrhea due to three mechanisms
	  • Gastric hypersecretion overwhelming ability of colon to reabsorb water
	  • High HCl concentration in the duodenum overwhelming pancreatic bicarbonate to create the alkaline environment necessary for pancreatic enzyme function resulting in malabsorption
	  • Exudation from multiple ulcers
	• 60% are malignant, often metastasize to liver

Insulinoma	**Hx/PE:** Episodes of hypoglycemia and catecholamine release in response to hypoglycemia can cause: palpitations, diaphoresis, lightheadedness, confusion, anxiety, tachycardia, tremor
	
	Diagnostics:
	• Significant hypoglycemia without appropriate suppression of insulin
	• ↑ serum fasting insulin level
	• ↑ C-peptide level which is part of proinsulin (the insulin precursor protein)
	  • Elevated C-peptide indicates endogenous insulin secretion, whereas elevated insulin with a low C-peptide level indicates exogenous insulin administration as a cause of the hypoglycemia
	  • Be aware that sulfonylurea drugs will also increase the C-peptide level
	• Imaging studies to localize tumor

Neuroendocrine Mini-Cases (*continued*)

Insulinoma	**Management:** • Dietary modifications to prevent hypoglycemia • Definitive treatment is surgical resection **Discussion:** • Tumors that arise from the pancreatic β cells • Overproduction of insulin leads to symptoms of hypoglycemia, which persists even with prolonged fasting • Diazoxide is often used to control glucose and symptoms of hypoglycemia • Most often are benign, and surgical resection is generally curative
Glucagonoma	**Hx:** • Mild diabetes mellitus, usually not requiring medication • Weight loss, diarrhea • Neuropsychiatric symptoms **PE:** Migratory necrolytic erythema (skin rash consisting of pruritic and erythematous patches with central areas of bronze induration and necrosis) **Diagnostics:** ↑ serum glucagon levels **Management:** Surgical resection **Discussion:** • Rare neuroendocrine tumors of the pancreas • Many tumors are already metastatic at the time of diagnosis
VIPoma	**Hx/PE:** Chronic watery odorless diarrhea and muscle weakness and cramping **Diagnostics:** • VIP >75 pg/mL • Hypokalemia • Abdominal CT or MRI to localize the tumor **Management:** Octreotide and surgical resection **Discussion:** • Rare tumor of the pancreas, resulting in increased secretion of vasoactive intestinal peptide (VIP) • Also referred to as WDHA syndrome (watery diarrhea, hypokalemia, achlorhydria)
Somatostatinoma	**Hx/PE:** Steatorrhea, gallstones (RUQ tenderness), new onset diabetes (polyuria and polydipsia) **Diagnostics:** CT abdomen revealing a tumor in the pancreas **Treatment:** Octreotide (somatostatin analog, allows for feedback inhibition) **Discussion:** • Tumors of the delta cells of the pancreas • Somatostatin inhibits the secretion of cholecystokinin, gastrin, glucagon and insulin, leading to derangements in blood sugar, gallstones and steatorrhea due to gallbladder stasis and reduced signaling to the gallbladder to release bile salts

10

Rheumatology and Musculoskeletal Disorders

Lead Author: Mina Al-Awqati, MD
Contributors: Benjamin Follman, MD; Laura Krivicich, MD; Zafar Siddiqui, MD

Musculoskeletal Overview
Upper Extremity (UE)
Hand, Wrist, and Elbow

1. Carpal Tunnel Syndrome
2. Lateral Epicondylitis (Tennis Elbow)
   UE Pain and/or Paresthesia Mini-Cases
   De Quervain Tenosynovitis
   Olecranon Bursitis

Shoulder and Neck

3. Rotator Cuff Tear
   Shoulder/Neck Pain Mini-Cases
   Adhesive Capsulitis ("Frozen Shoulder")
   Anterior Shoulder Dislocation

Posterior Shoulder Dislocation
Cervical Radiculopathy
Cervical Spinal Stenosis
Thoracic Outlet Syndrome
Pancoast Tumors
Winged Scapula
Erb's Palsy
Klumpke's Palsy

Lower Extremity
Foot and Ankle

4. Ankle Sprain (Anterior Talofibular Ligament Injury)
   Foot/Ankle Pain Mini-Cases
   Plantar Fasciitis
   Tarsal Tunnel Syndrome (Tibial Nerve Injury)

MUSCULOSKELETAL OVERVIEW

When approaching musculoskeletal concerns, even though the problematic pathology may be attributable to a single anatomic structure, you are more likely to be presented with symptoms relating to a group of structures. Your task as a test taker and clinician will often be to parse out what specific structures are affected from a more generalized local complaint, and then to choose the appropriate treatment plan. A good rule of thumb when choosing treatments is to err for the most conservative option first, with surgical solutions reserved for refractory cases.

The history and physical are critical pieces in diagnosing musculoskeletal concerns; imaging is often ancillary. When a patient presents with musculoskeletal symptoms, consider the time course. **Acute symptoms** should prompt a thorough history assessing for possible trauma (such as a fall broken by an outstretched arm) leading to a structural abnormality. The mechanism of injury will always point to the diagnosis. **Chronic symptoms** may indicate a lower threshold injury such as sprain or strain, presenting with ongoing swelling or irritation, especially with use. Repetitive use of the upper extremity in daily recreational or work-related activities may inform the diagnosis in the absence of acute trauma.

As with any non-rheumatoid musculoskeletal concerns, remember that the test question may often be simplified down to four main components: **bones, tendons, ligaments, and nerves**. A fifth component is possible—**vascular**—but is not commonly tested on Step 2, with rare exceptions (such as *avascular necrosis of the hip* and scaphoid fracture).

The information in this chapter was obtained and confirmed from the American College of Rheumatology, DynaMed, Harrisons Principles of Internal Medicine, Rheumatology Secrets, and UpToDate. Please see Surgery Chapter for additional orthopedic cases.

Definitions

Sprain: injury to ligaments

Strain: injury to muscles

Bursa: fluid-filled sac around joints prone to friction

Bursitis: inflammation of bursa usually due to repetitive movements

Enthesis: site where tendons or ligaments insert into the bone

Enthesitis: inflammation of the entheses

Tenosynovitis: infectious or noninfectious inflammation of the fluid-filled sheath (synovium) that surrounds a tendon resulting in joint pain, swelling, and/or stiffness

Dactylitis: inflammation of a digit (finger or toe) resulting in pain and swelling (sausage shaped)

Spondyloarthropathies: chronic arthritic conditions that share the following features: involve the spine and sacroiliac joints and present with asymmetric oligoarthritic, dactylitis and enthesitis.

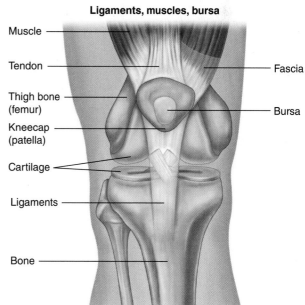

Ligaments, muscles, bursa

Muscle

Tendon

Thigh bone (femur)

Kneecap (patella)

Cartilage

Ligaments

Bone

Fascia

Bursa

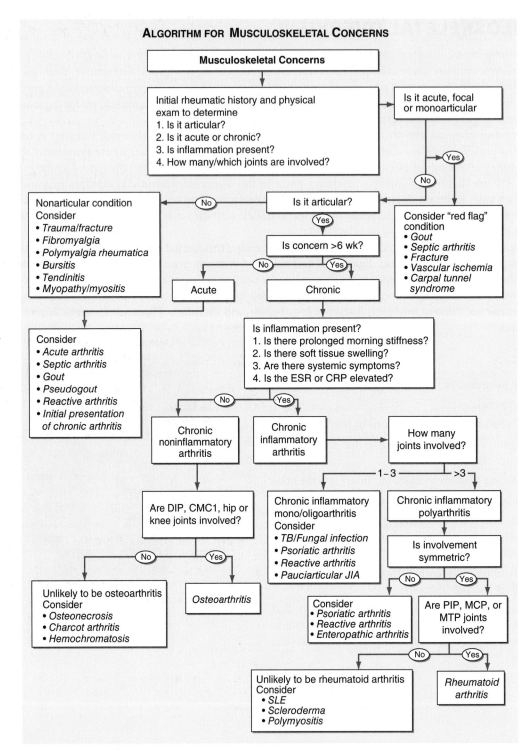

Reproduced with permission from J. L. Jameson, A.S. Fauci, D.L Kasper, et al., Harrison's Principles of Internal Medicine, 20th ed, New York: McGraw Hill, 2018.

UPPER EXTREMITY

- Upper extremity (UE) symptoms are often localized to a single joint (most tested: shoulder, elbow, wrist, and hand) but may be related to a systemic problem
- Assess nearby structures to isolate the concern (e.g., weakness or paresthesia of the hand may be attributable to pathology anywhere along UE all the way to the dorsal root ganglia of the spine)
- Attempt to localize neurologic symptoms to a specific nerve distribution

HAND, WRIST, AND ELBOW

The hand and wrist are particularly complex, but a few pathologies are commonly tested.

The elbow is a simple joint with two basic functions (flexion and contraction and supination and pronation), and the most common causes of pathology are medial and lateral epicondylitis.

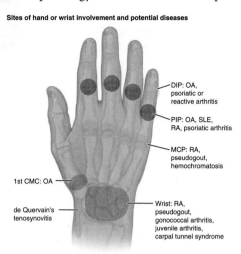

Sites of hand or wrist involvement and potential diseases

DIP: OA, psoriatic or reactive arthritis

PIP: OA, SLE, RA, psoriatic arthritis

MCP: RA, pseudogout, hemochromatosis

1st CMC: OA

de Quervain's tenosynovitis

Wrist: RA, pseudogout, gonococcal arthritis, juvenile arthritis, carpal tunnel syndrome

Reproduced with permission from J. L. Jameson, A.S. Fauci, D.L Kasper, et al., Harrison's Principles of Internal Medicine, 20th ed, New York : McGraw Hill, 2018 and From JJ Cush et al [eds], Evaluation of musculoskeletal complaints, in Rheumatology: Diagnosis and Therapeutics, 2nd ed. Philadelphia, Lippincott Williams & Wilkins, 2005. Reproduced with permission from Dr. John J Cush.

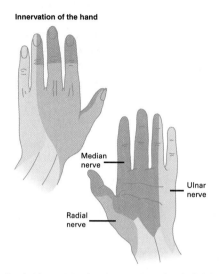

Innervation of the hand

Median nerve

Ulnar nerve

Radial nerve

Reproduced with permission from Raj Mitra: Principles of Rehabilitation Medicine, McGraw Hill, 2019 and Reproduced with permission from Young DM, Hansen SL. Hand Surgery. In: Doherty GM, eds. CURRENT Diagnosis & Treatment: Surgery, 14e; New York: McGraw-Hill; 2014.

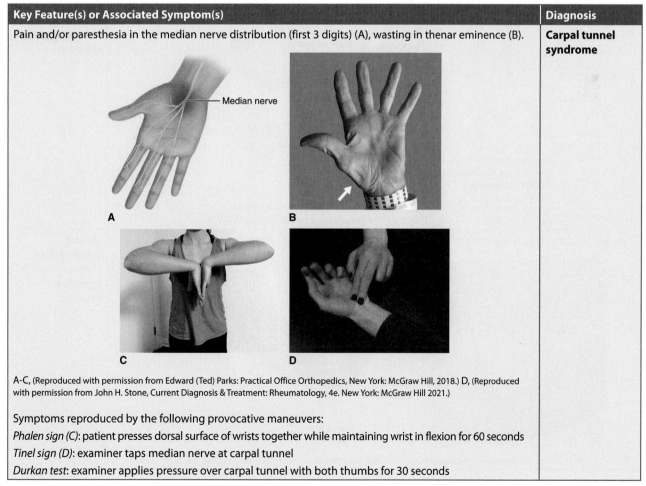

Key Feature(s) or Associated Symptom(s)	Diagnosis
Pain and/or paresthesia in the median nerve distribution (first 3 digits) (A), wasting in thenar eminence (B).	**Carpal tunnel syndrome**

Median nerve

A   B

C   D

A-C, (Reproduced with permission from Edward (Ted) Parks: Practical Office Orthopedics, New York: McGraw Hill, 2018.) D, (Reproduced with permission from John H. Stone, Current Diagnosis & Treatment: Rheumatology, 4e. New York: McGraw Hill 2021.)

Symptoms reproduced by the following provocative maneuvers:

Phalen sign (C): patient presses dorsal surface of wrists together while maintaining wrist in flexion for 60 seconds

Tinel sign (D): examiner taps median nerve at carpal tunnel

Durkan test: examiner applies pressure over carpal tunnel with both thumbs for 30 seconds

(Continued)

Key Feature(s) or Associated Symptom(s)	Diagnosis
Pain at the radial aspect of the wrist that is worse with gripping or rotating the wrist *Finkelstein test* (B): pain is elicited when patient grasps their thumb in their fist and ulnar deviates the wrist 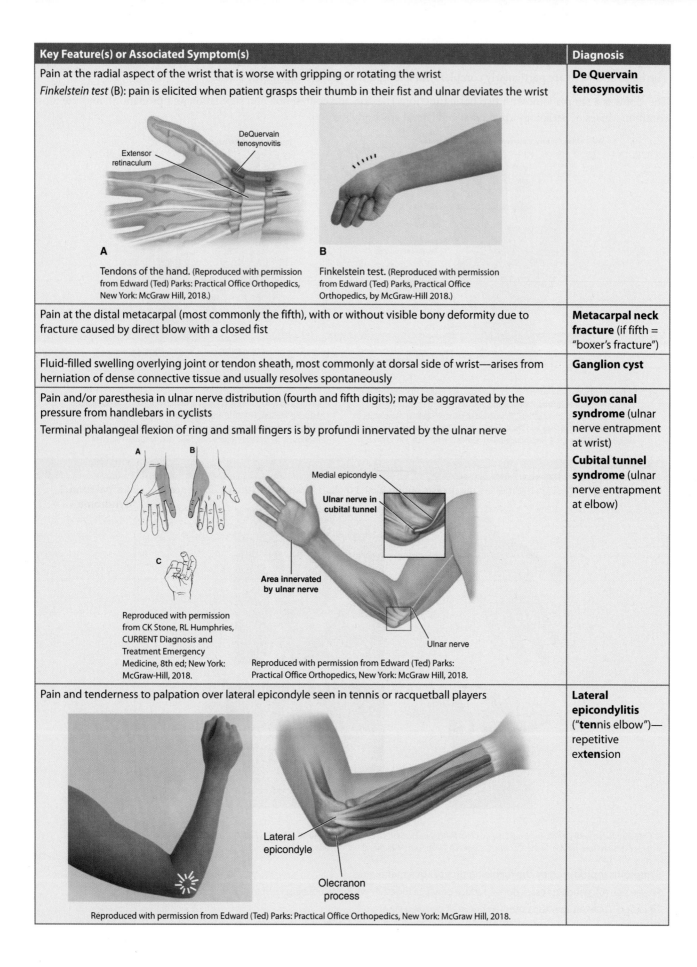 **A** Tendons of the hand. (Reproduced with permission from Edward (Ted) Parks: Practical Office Orthopedics, New York: McGraw Hill, 2018.) **B** Finkelstein test. (Reproduced with permission from Edward (Ted) Parks, Practical Office Orthopedics, by McGraw-Hill 2018.)	**De Quervain tenosynovitis**
Pain at the distal metacarpal (most commonly the fifth), with or without visible bony deformity due to fracture caused by direct blow with a closed fist	**Metacarpal neck fracture** (if fifth = "boxer's fracture")
Fluid-filled swelling overlying joint or tendon sheath, most commonly at dorsal side of wrist—arises from herniation of dense connective tissue and usually resolves spontaneously	**Ganglion cyst**
Pain and/or paresthesia in ulnar nerve distribution (fourth and fifth digits); may be aggravated by the pressure from handlebars in cyclists Terminal phalangeal flexion of ring and small fingers is by profundi innervated by the ulnar nerve Reproduced with permission from CK Stone, RL Humphries, CURRENT Diagnosis and Treatment Emergency Medicine, 8th ed; New York: McGraw-Hill, 2018. Reproduced with permission from Edward (Ted) Parks: Practical Office Orthopedics, New York: McGraw Hill, 2018.	**Guyon canal syndrome** (ulnar nerve entrapment at wrist) **Cubital tunnel syndrome** (ulnar nerve entrapment at elbow)
Pain and tenderness to palpation over lateral epicondyle seen in tennis or racquetball players Reproduced with permission from Edward (Ted) Parks: Practical Office Orthopedics, New York: McGraw Hill, 2018.	**Lateral epicondylitis** ("**ten**nis elbow")—repetitive ex**ten**sion

Key Feature(s) or Associated Symptom(s)		Diagnosis
Pain and tenderness to palpation over medial epicondyle		**Medial epicondylitis** ("golfer's elbow")— repetitive flexion
Pain and swelling over olecranon process; often someone resting their elbows on a hard surface for long periods of time ("student's elbow") 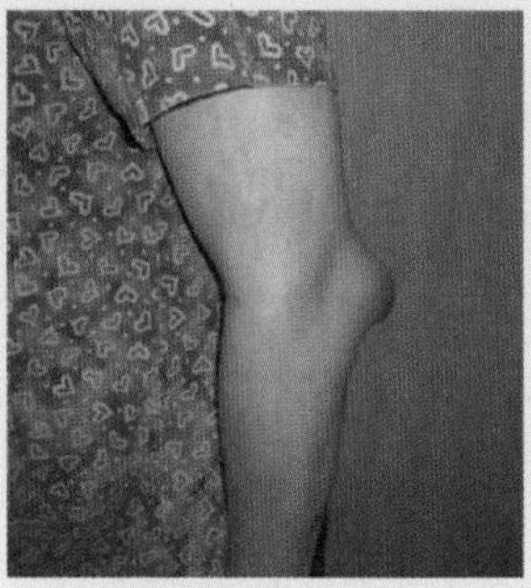 Reproduced with permission from Richard P. Usatine, Mindy A. Smith, E. J. Mayeaux, Jr.,Heidi S. Chumley The Color Atlas and Synopsis of Family Medicine, 3e, McGraw Hill, MD.2019, Figure 103-2, ISBN 9781259862045 From Raj Mitra, Principles of Rehabilitation Medicine, by McGraw-Hill 2019. FIGURE 30–48. ISBN: 9780071793339. Used with permission from Richard P. Usatine, MD.		**Olecranon bursitis**

Nerve distributions in the UE are extremely important, and compression of the median, ulnar, or radial nerve (in that order) is one of the most common concerns managed in orthopedics.

Symptoms and Signs	Nerve Involved	Cause(s)
Decreased sensation over deltoid Flattened deltoid Decreased abduction	Axillary (C5–C6)	• Humeral neck fracture • Anterior dislocation humerus
Decreased sensation of posterior forearm and dorsum of hand (radial) Weakness in hand and finger extension: **wrist drop**	Radial (C5–T1)	• Humeral mid-shaft fractures • Tumors compressing nerve • Compression of the radial nerve at the spiral groove ("Saturday night palsy"/prolonged use of crutches)
Decreased sensation in first three half-digits and thenar area Inability to make a fist Loss of thumb opposition **Pope's blessing** (damage of median nerve) **Ape hand** (damage of recurrent branch of median nerve) 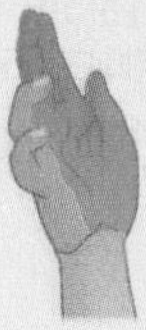	Median (C5–T1)	• Supracondylar humeral fracture • Carpal tunnel syndrome
Decreased sensation in fourth and fifth digits Medial elbow pain if injury is at the elbow Weak grip **Ulnar claw** (clawing of fourth and fifth fingers) 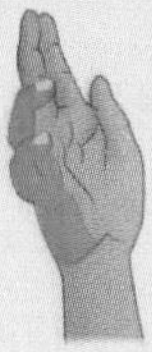	Ulnar (C8–T1)	• Compression of ulnar nerve due to prolonged elbow resting on desk, osteophytes, or other mass lesions • Ulnar nerve injury at the wrist due to constant use of hand tools, bicycling, or hook of hamate fracture

CASE 1 | Carpal Tunnel Syndrome

A 45-year-old man with diabetes presents with several months of numbness and tingling in the right thumb and index fingers which is now starting to wake him up at night. He is finding it difficult to use the keyboard and mouse at work because of this. On exam, there is subtle wasting of the thenar muscles. Tapping over the carpal tunnel (Tinel sign) and holding the wrist in a flexed position for a minute (Phalen sign) elicits pins-and-needles sensation in the thumb and index fingers.

Conditions with Similar Presentations	**Ulnar nerve entrapment:** Can occur at the elbow (cubital tunnel syndrome) or the wrist (Guyon canal syndrome); however, symptoms occur in the fourth and fifth digits. **De Quervain tenosynovitis:** Pain is typically at the base of the thumb and is due to swelling and thickening of the first dorsal compartment (may present as a painful bump over the wrist).
Initial Diagnostic Tests	Clinical diagnosis
Next Steps in Management	Wrist splinting
Discussion	Carpal tunnel syndrome (CTS) is the most common entrapment neuropathy, and characteristic symptoms occur when the median nerve is compressed within the carpal tunnel (roof: transverse carpal ligament; floor: proximal carpal row; medial/ulnar border: pisiform and hook of hamate; lateral/radial border: scaphoid and trapezium) either due to narrowing of the anatomic pathway or the presence of external pressure. **History:** CTS is more common in women, and risk factors include obesity, pregnancy, osteoarthritis (OA), rheumatoid arthritis(RA), and diabetes. • Some other conditions associated with CTS include gout, amyloidosis, long-term dialysis, hypothyroidism, acromegaly, and hemochromatosis • Pain over the distal forearm and thenar area and paresthesias in the median nerve distribution (first, second, third, and lateral/radial half of the fourth digit) • Symptoms can be worse with repetitive movements and flexion, are worse at night, and can be bilateral **Physical Exam:** • Objective sensory and motor deficits in the median nerve distribution may be present, especially in advanced disease • Assess for muscle weakness or atrophy of the thenar eminence • Tinel sign, Phalen sign, and Durkan test are all provocative maneuvers to diagnose CTS. See above table **Diagnostics:** • The diagnosis is often made by history and physical exam alone (positive Phalen and/or Tinel signs) • Electromyography (EMG) and nerve conduction velocity (NCV) may be used to confirm the diagnosis if it is in question or to quantify the severity of nerve compression • Consider evaluation for associated conditions (e.g., TSH, ferritin) **Management:** • Initial conservative approach is wrist splinting • Other options include corticosteroid injections into the carpal tunnel and surgery for refractory cases
Additional Considerations	**Complications:** Failure to treat CTS may lead to irreversible sensory loss in the median nerve distribution as well as significant wasting of the thenar muscles, which in turn can cause weak grasp and thumb opposition. **Surgical Considerations:** Surgical decompression is considered in the following cases: • Failure of conservative approach • Muscle atrophy or weakness • Symptoms interfering with quality of life Surgery can be open or done endoscopically and can decrease pressure on the median nerve by dividing the transverse carpal ligament and antebrachial fascia. **Other Considerations:** Pay attention to comorbid conditions when presented with potential CTS. Step 2 CK heavily emphasizes comorbid conditions such as pregnancy, hypothyroidism, and patients on dialysis as key history findings that implicate CTS.

CASE 2 | Lateral Epicondylitis (Tennis Elbow)

A 45-year-old woman presents with right elbow pain for the past few weeks. She started playing racquetball a few months ago and has worsening pain with backhand shots. The pain is over the lateral elbow and forearm and is worsened by gripping and resisted wrist extension. The pain improves with ibuprofen and rest. On exam, there is tenderness at the lateral epicondyle at the insertion of extensor carpi radialis brevis, and this is exacerbated by wrist and third digit extension.

Conditions with Similar Presentations	**Medial epicondylitis (golfer's elbow):** Pain near the medial epicondyle elicited with forearm pronation or wrist flexion. Results from repetitive flexion as seen in forehand shots. **Olecranon bursitis:** Pain associated with swelling over the olecranon process.
Initial Diagnostic Tests	Clinical diagnosis
Next Steps in Management	Conservative treatment with rest, NSAIDs, avoidance of aggravating activity
Discussion	Lateral epicondylitis (tennis elbow) is chronic tendinosis due to overuse of the common extensor tendon by repetitive wrist extension. The lateral epicondyle is the origin for several muscles that extend the wrist, which comprise the common extensor tendon. The extensor carpi radialis brevis (ECRB) is stressed during wrist extension and forearm pronation, like when hitting a backhand shot. The ECRB inserts at the base of the third metacarpal distally. Repetitive motions may lead to vascular hyperplasia, fibroblast hypertrophy, and disorganized collagen, resulting in tendinopathy or tendonitis. **History:** Risk increases with age, and risk factors include occupations and sports that require repetitive wrist movement such as in racquetball players or laborers. Symptoms include lateral elbow pain in the setting of work or recreational activity that requires repetitive use of the forearm extensors **Physical Exam:** Tenderness at the level of the elbow laterally and resisted extension of the third digit may reproduce the pain. See above table Resisted extension. (Reproduced with permission from Edward (Ted) Parks, Practical Office Orthopedics, by McGraw-Hill 2018.) **Diagnostics:** Clinical diagnosis **Management:** Conservative treatment with rest, oral analgesics, and avoidance of aggravating activity
Additional Considerations	**Surgical Considerations:** Surgical management may be considered in cases refractory to conservative management (such as with symptoms persisting greater than 6 months). Surgical approaches offer no clear benefit over nonoperative treatment. **Pediatric Considerations:** The classic mechanism of injury for **radial head subluxation** or **nursemaid's elbow** is sudden pulling or grabbing a child's arm to prevent an incident. • The annular ligament slips into the radiohumeral joint and becomes trapped between the two joint surfaces, where it remains stuck • Exam will reveal a pronated arm and partially flexed elbow that is held close to the body, as well as tenderness of the radial head

UE Pain and/or Paresthesia Mini-Cases

Cases	Key Findings
De Quervain Tenosynovitis	**Hx:** Pain at the radial aspect of the wrist which is increased with gripping or rotating the wrist and repetitive movements at the wrist. New mothers holding infants and texting with thumbs are common causes. **PE:** *Finkelstein test*—Pain upon ulnar deviation of the wrist after making a fist with thumb in full opposition. See above table. **Diagnostics:** Clinical diagnosis. Imaging can aid in ruling out fracture or other pathology. **Management:** NSAIDs, splinting. Consider steroid injections or surgery for refractory cases. **Discussion:** De Quervain tenosynovitis is a disease affecting the extensor pollicis brevis and abductor pollicis longus tendons. To confirm this diagnosis clinically, pain is elicited by stretching these tendons by adducting and flexing the thumb with ulnar deviation of the wrist.
Olecranon Bursitis	**Hx:** Follows overuse via prolonged pressure, often secondary to resting elbows on a hard surface for long periods of time (such as with students). **PE:** Often a sack-like swelling and tenderness in superficial bursae of elbow. Exam may demonstrate point tenderness over the olecranon. See above table. **Diagnostics:** Clinical diagnosis. Consider bursal fluid aspiration when there is a concern for infection or crystalline arthritis. **Management:** NSAIDs for symptomatic relief. Avoid aggravating maneuvers; cushion the bony prominence of the elbow when resting on surfaces or avoid this position altogether. **Discussion:** Inflammation of the olecranon bursa on the posterior facet of the elbow occurs from repeated trauma or pressure from excessive time spent leaning the elbow on hard surfaces. It is usually self-limited but can be complicated by infection, especially in superficial bursae. Distinguish from joint effusion.

SHOULDER AND NECK

Shoulder pain and other symptoms (paresthesias, weakness, decreased range of motion) can be caused by damage to the rotator cuff and/or referred from cervical pathology.

The four rotator cuff muscles (**SITS** mnemonic: supraspinatus, infraspinatus, teres minor, subscapularis) are the basis for most shoulder-related test questions.

Rotator Cuff Muscles

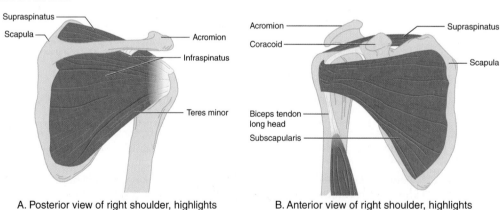

A. Posterior view of right shoulder, highlights infraspinatus and teres minor

B. Anterior view of right shoulder, highlights subscapularis, supraspinatus

Reproduced with permission from Edward (Ted) Parks: Practical Office Orthopedics, New York: McGraw Hill, 2018.

As with any musculoskeletal pathology, it is important to consider an injury "up the chain." While working up a rotator cuff pathology, be sure to rule out cervical pathology.

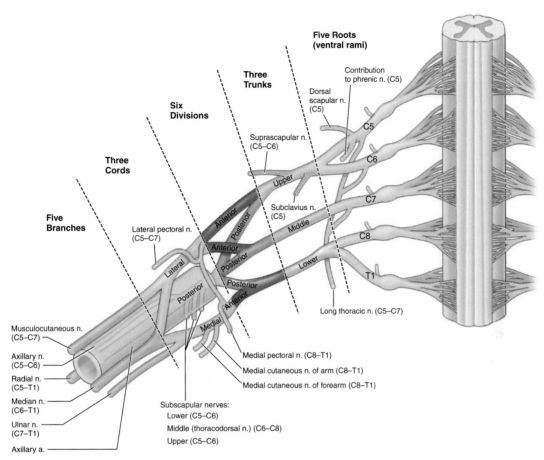

Schematic of the brachial plexus showing the branches, cords, divisions, trunks, and roots. (Reproduced with permission from Overview of the Upper Limb, Morton DA et al., In: DA Morton, K Bo Foreman et al, The Big Picture: Gross Anatomy, Medical Course & Step 1 Review, 2nd ed, NY: McGraw Hill, 2018.)

Muscle	Nerve	Action
Supraspinatus	Suprascapular nerve	Abduction
Infraspinatus and teres minor	Suprascapular nerve Axillary nerve	External rotation
Subscapularis	Upper and lower subscapular nerves	Internal rotation

Key Physical Exam Maneuvers and Findings and Shoulder and/or Neck Pain Differential Diagnosis

Key Associated Exam Findings		Diagnoses
Hawkins-Kennedy test: Patient flexes elbow and shoulder forward 90 degrees while examiner internally rotates arm, bringing forearm downward reproducing pain **Painful arc test:** Patient abducts arms (pain with abduction between 60 and 120 degrees is positive) **Neer test:** Raising internally rotated (thumb pointing down) and extended arm forward in scapular plane elicits pain Reproduced with permission from John H. Stone, Current Diagnosis & Treatment: Rheumatology, 4e by McGraw Hill 2021.		Subacromial impingement or rotator cuff tendonitis or tendinosis

(Continued)

Key Associated Exam Findings	Diagnoses
Jobe test/empty can test: Internally rotate fully extended arms with thumb pointing down and elevate while the examiner applies resistance reproducing weakness **Drop arm sign:** Examiner fully abducts patient's arm and then asks patient to slowly lower and attempt to hold at 90 degrees (inability to hold is positive for weakness or tear)	Rotator cuff injury, supraspinatus pathology
Elbow flexed to 90 degrees and rotated externally while the examiner applies resistance (pain and/or weakness with external rotation is positive) Reproduced with permission from S G.Waxman: Clinical Neuroanatomy, 29ed, NY: McGraw Hill, 2020.	Rotator cuff injury infraspinatus or teres minor pathology
Lift-off test: Patient places hand behind (midlumbar and slightly off back) and attempts to push away from the body while the examiner applies resistance (inability to hold extremity in position is positive) (figure B) **Belly press test:** Patient presses hand against their abdomen with elbow abducted away from the body while the examiner tries to pull hand away from belly (inability to hold extremity in position is positive) (figure A) Reproduced with permission from Edward (Ted) Parks: Practical Office Orthopedics, New York: McGraw Hill, 2018.	Rotator cuff injury, subscapularis pathology
Apprehension test: Patient lies supine, and examiner flexes elbow to 90 degrees, abducts shoulder to 90 degrees, and then maximally externally rotates (apprehension to this position can be positive for anterior shoulder dislocation) **Relocation test:** As with the apprehension test, but the examiner simultaneously applies pressure to the shoulder posteriorly (less apprehension or pain with posterior glide of humerus is positive)	Shoulder dislocation, subluxation, or glenohumeral instability
O'Brien test: Shoulder is flexed 90 degrees and slightly adducted and internally rotated (with thumb pointing down), and patient raises arm while the examiner applies resistance. Repeat with palm facing upward. Test is positive if pain or crepitus in internally rotated position and better with palm facing up.	Glenohumeral joint labral tears (superior labral tear from anterior to posterior [SLAP tear]) or impingement
Speed test: Patient extends elbow, supinates arm, and attempts to flex elbow while examiner resists. Test is positive if pain is reproduced in anterior shoulder/bicipital groove.	Biceps tendinopathy
Reproduces radicular symptoms (pain and/or paresthesia into upper extremity): **Axial loading or compression:** Pressing downward on the seated patient's head reproduces radicular symptoms (pain and/or paresthesia into upper extremity) **Spurling test:** Pressing downward on the patient's head (axial loading or axial compression) while the neck is extended and flexed to the affected side reproduces radicular symptoms	Cervical radiculopathy (cervical nerve root impingement)
Atrophy of intrinsic hand muscles (claw hand), diminished pulses and edema of hand	Thoracic outlet syndrome
Atrophy of intrinsic hand muscles (claw hand)	Klumpke's palsy
Arm hangs by side medially rotated; wrist is flexed and pronated (waiter's tip)	Erb's palsy
Protrusion of scapula when patient leans with arms against the wall (winged scapula)	Winged scapula (C5–C7 injury)

CASE 3 | Rotator Cuff Tear

A 35-year-old mail carrier presents with right shoulder pain for the past 2 weeks after he tripped and fell. Since then, he has difficulty reaching overhead and the pain often keeps him awake at night. When the patient's arm is passively abducted and then let go, patient is unable to hold the position in the horizontal plane, and reports pain and "drops" the arm (positive drop arm test). There is weakness and pain with resisted elevation in the plane of the scapula (supraspinatus test/empty can test). Lift-off test is negative. Tenderness is present over the lateral aspect of the right shoulder. Shoulder x-rays were negative for fracture.

Conditions with Similar Presentations	**Fracture** and/or **dislocation:** Can be excluded by imaging. **Adhesive capsulitis:** (frozen shoulder) Presents with insidious pain, progressive stiffness, and decreased range of motion. It usually affects women over 40 years with endocrine conditions such as diabetes and can occur after rotator cuff tear.
Initial Diagnostic Tests	• Clinical diagnosis • MRI can confirm rotator cuff tear
Next Steps in Management	Initial treatment includes NSAIDs and physical therapy
Discussion	This is a common presentation for a **rotator cuff injury**; specifically, a **supraspinatus tear**. The rotator cuff consists of four muscle groups: supraspinatus, infraspinatus, teres minor, and subscapularis, and it is innervated mostly by C5–C6. The primary function of the rotator cuff is to provide dynamic stability of the shoulder joint by keeping the humeral head against the glenoid. Supraspinatus pathology (tendinosis or tendonitis) is the most common cause of shoulder pain and can result from trauma, impingement, or degeneration. • **Supraspinatus** is innervated by the suprascapular nerve and abducts arm initially (0–30 degrees) • **Infraspinatus** is innervated by the suprascapular nerve and externally rotates the arm (pitching injury) • **Teres minor** is innervated by the axillary nerve adducts and externally rotates the arm • **Subscapularis** is innervated by the lower subscapular nerve and internally rotates and adducts arm. **History:** Risk factors for supraspinatus pathology include age, participation in sports, and occupations that require repetitive overhead activity. Symptoms include shoulder pain and weakness. Pain is located over the anterolateral shoulder and is exacerbated by overhead activities, and often presents with difficulty sleeping on the affected side. Weakness is noted, especially in large or full-thickness tears **Physical Exam:** Assess for swelling, deformity, focal tenderness, range of motion, sensation, strength, and pulses. See table for special shoulder maneuvers to help distinguish between the various pathologies. Jobe test (empty can test) and drop arm sign helpful in confirming supraspinatus pathology. **Diagnostics:** The diagnosis is often made clinically. • Plain radiographs are obtained to evaluate for alternative or concomitant bone/joint pathology such as fractures or dislocations. In the case of rotator cuff tear, a migrating humeral head in relation to the glenoid and acromion maybe seen. • MRI provides more accurate diagnosis, especially for full-thickness tear. **Management:** • The first line of treatment is physical therapy and pain control. • Rotator cuff surgical repair is offered to patients who have failed conservative treatment or have a full-thickness tear.
Additional Considerations	**Complications:** Failure to treat may lead to impairment of daily living activities and developing a frozen shoulder. **Surgical Considerations:** While conservative treatment (PT, rest, pain management) is first-line for partial-thickness tears, for acute full-thickness tears, surgery is the initial choice of treatment. Acute full-thickness tears are more associated with acute trauma and shoulder dislocation than with chronic overuse. Rotator cuff repair or reverse total shoulder arthroplasty are common surgical interventions used to treat a complete tear.

Shoulder/Neck Pain Mini-Cases

Cases	Key Findings
Adhesive Capsulitis ("Frozen Shoulder")	**Hx:** • Severe diffuse unilateral (less commonly bilateral) shoulder pain with progressive stiffness • More common in women; >40 years old (rarely seen before age 40) • Risk factors include endocrine conditions (e.g., diabetes, hypothyroidism) or any shoulder condition that causes shoulder pain that leads to limiting the motion of the shoulder (e.g., rotator cuff tear) **PE:** Reduced active and passive range of motion (unlike rotator cuff pathology in which only active range of motion is affected). **Diagnostics:** Clinical diagnosis Imaging (radiography, ultrasound, and MRI) helpful in excluding other etiologies **Management:** • Patient education and range of motion exercises • Physical therapy and pain control with acetaminophen, NSAIDs, and/or intra-articular steroids • Consider surgery for refractory cases **Discussion:** Adhesive capsulitis and rotator cuff pathology are two of the most common causes of shoulder pain. Both conditions can cause pain, stiffness, and limited range of motion. Frozen shoulder is often a self-limiting condition, although many patients may not experience complete resolution.
Anterior Shoulder Dislocation	**Hx:** Most common type of dislocation. Patient may report sudden pain and instability following a traumatic blow to the shoulder or following load-bearing exercise. **PE:** Loss of normal shoulder contour and prominence of acromion may be visible. Arm will be held abducted and externally rotated. **Diagnostics:** Clinical diagnosis; plain radiographs and ultrasound can aid diagnosis, assist in differentiation of frank dislocation from subluxation, and assess for concomitant pathology. **Management:** Reduce the dislocation; consider confirmation of reduction via plain radiograph or ultrasound. Consider orthopedic follow-up, especially if there is concern for concomitant pathology such as rotator cuff injury, and to assess risk of re-dislocation (risk decreases with increasing age of first dislocation). **Discussion:** Anterior shoulder dislocations occur because the rotator cuff is weakest at the anterior–inferior aspect, thus this area of the rotator cuff is most susceptible to insufficiency in the case of trauma or load bearing.
Posterior Shoulder Dislocation	**Hx:** Uncommon; typically occurs following trauma, seizure. **PE:** Loss of normal shoulder contour with flattening of the anterior facet and prominence of the coracoid process may be visible. Arm will be held adducted and internally rotated. **Diagnostics:** Clinical diagnosis; plain radiographs and ultrasound can aid diagnosis, assist in differentiation of frank dislocation from subluxation, and assess for concomitant pathology. **Management:** Reduce the dislocation; consider confirmation of reduction via plain radiograph or ultrasound. Consider orthopedic follow-up, especially if there is concern for concomitant pathology such as rotator cuff injury, and to assess risk of re-dislocation (risk decreases with increasing age of first dislocation). **Discussion:** Posterior shoulder dislocations occur when all muscles are activated simultaneously due to a form of overstimulation (such as a seizure or lightning strike). When this occurs, the internal rotators of shoulder are stronger than external rotators, so when all muscles fire at once, internal rotators win out and cause posterior shoulder dislocation.
Cervical Radiculopathy	**Hx:** Usually history of an underlying cervical spondylosis or disc herniation. More common in older adults. History of weakness and/or numbness that may radiate anywhere from the neck into the shoulder, arm, hand, or fingers. **PE:** Dermatomal sensory and motor deficits may be present; lower cervical nerve roots (C7) are more commonly impacted than upper cervical nerve roots. Diminished deep tendon reflexes, weakness, and/or paresthesias may be present. Spurling maneuver may be positive and is specific. **Diagnostics:** MRI and CT may confirm diagnosis but are generally reserved for cases of significant neurological deficits. EMG can also demonstrate dermatomal denervation. **Management:** In nonprogressive and mild cases, conservative treatment with NSAIDs and avoidance of provocative maneuvers is the first-line treatment. Steroid injections may be used for symptomatic relief in progressive or moderate cases. Surgical decompression is reserved for severe cases. **Discussion:** Cervical radiculopathy is a clinical condition that results from inflammation or damage of a nerve root in the cervical spine, resulting in a change in neurological function. Most individuals experiencing cervical radiculopathy improve without specific treatment; however, symptoms often recur.

Shoulder/Neck Pain Mini-Cases *(continued)*

Cervical Spinal Stenosis	**Hx:** Can be asymptomatic but can also present with neck pain, numbness, or paresthesia in the arm. Occurs in older individuals and often a complication of cervical spondylosis. **PE:** • Forward flexion of the neck causing shock-like sensation down the arms or back (Lhermitte sign) • Weakness in the upper extremities, and in more severe cases, atrophy of some muscles of the upper extremities may be observed • Weakness, spasticity, or gait abnormalities in the lower extremities can also be present in more severe cases. • Impaired proprioception **Diagnostics:** MRI of the cervical spine is the best diagnostic tool, although nerve conduction studies can sometimes be helpful in ruling out other etiologies. **Management:** • Pharmacologic measures include NSAIDs, acetaminophen, and muscle relaxants, along with medications such as gabapentin or amitriptyline for neuropathic pain • Nonpharmacologic nonsurgical measures include physical therapy and neck immobilization • Surgical options include laminectomy, laminoplasty, discectomy, and corpectomy **Discussion:** Cervical spinal cord myelopathy from cervical spinal stenosis is a common cause of neck pain, and symptoms are usually progressive in nature. In the setting of an acute spinal cord compression, immediate surgical intervention is required, and corticosteroids can help reduce spinal cord edema.
Thoracic Outlet Syndrome	**Hx:** Can present with pain and paresthesia if nerves are compressed, swelling and discoloration if veins are compressed, and the five P's (pain, pallor, pulselessness, poikilothermia [temperature changes], and paresthesias) if arteries are compressed. Patients will often have a history of genetic structural abnormalities, trauma, repetitive motion (especially of abduction + external rotation), or more rare causes, such as Pancoast tumors. **PE:** • Brachial plexus compression (most common): sensory loss most commonly in the ulnar distribution, atrophy of intrinsic hand muscles. • Subclavian vein compression: swelling, discoloration. • Subclavian artery compression: pulselessness, pallor, poikilothermia, decrease in BP in affected arm. **Diagnostics:** X-rays of shoulder may show structural abnormalities. CT/MRI can be useful to rule out other causes of symptoms such as rotator cuff tendinopathy, Pancoast tumors, or cervical disc pathologies. Nerve conduction studies, duplex ultrasonography, and MR angiography can all be obtained, depending on predominance of symptoms. **Management:** • Nonpharmacologic measures include physical therapy focusing on strengthening muscles around the shoulder, and practicing proper posture • Surgical involvement is required if there is venous or arterial involvement or if nerve compression symptoms do not respond to conservative management **Discussion:** Thoracic outlet syndrome is a term that encompasses many conditions that all involve neurovascular compression in the passageway from the lower neck to the axilla. Symptoms are based on whether compression is primarily of the nerves, veins, or arteries.
Pancoast Tumors	**Hx:** In addition to shoulder/chest pain, can present with symptoms typical of lung cancer: hemoptysis, dyspnea, weight loss, and fever. May also present with unique symptoms because of compression of important structures: swelling of head, neck, and upper extremities (SVC compression), hoarseness (recurrent laryngeal nerve compression), paralysis of hemidiaphragm (phrenic nerve), dysphagia (esophageal compression). **PE:** • SVC compression: swelling of head, neck, and upper extremities, dilated arm veins, jugular venous distension, papilledema • Compression of sympathetic chain: ptosis, miosis and anhidrosis **Diagnostics:** X-ray can show tumor as well as diaphragmatic elevation if there is phrenic nerve involvement. CT can show what structures are involved. **Management:** • Treatment will be largely guided by the type and classification of the lung tumor. • Involvement and compression of important structures by a Pancoast tumor may make surgery more difficult. Patients may require neoadjuvant or radiation therapy prior to surgery. **Discussion:** Pancoast tumors are lung tumors in the superior sulcus of the upper lobes. Symptoms are caused by compression of important neurovascular structures.

Shoulder/Neck Pain Mini-Cases *(continued)*

Winged Scapula	**Hx:** Patients will often have an inciting event (trauma, surgery). Can sometimes be painful, and often leads to difficulty lifting arm above the head and limitations with activities of daily life. **PE:** • Winged scapula: medial scapula protrudes from the ribcage, more pronounced when patient pushes against something • May complain of impaired abduction of the arm **Diagnostics:** Clinical diagnosis. X-ray, CT, and MRI can rule out other diagnoses. **Management:** • Strength training and physical therapy are initial interventions aimed at increasing strength of serratus anterior • Surgical intervention required if symptoms continue to be severe **Discussion:** Winged scapula is a condition caused by damage to the long thoracic nerve which innervates the serratus anterior muscle. This muscle acts to pull the scapula forward, and denervation causes protrusion or "winging" of the scapula. This can have iatrogenic causes such as complications of axillary node dissection or other causes such as trauma to the area. Physical therapy is often initiated but if symptoms are severe, surgery is required.
Erb's Palsy	**Hx:** Unilateral loss of feeling in affected upper extremity, partial or total paralysis, weakness, numbness, and limited motion of the affected upper extremity. **PE:** Lack of active shoulder abduction and elbow flexion with preserved hand function. **Diagnosis:** Clinical diagnosis based on history of injury and pattern of involvement. **Management:** Physical therapy and range-of-motion exercises to prevent contractures. Surgical procedures like nerve graft/nerve transfer if physical therapy does not lead to improvement. **Discussion:** Erb's palsy is a form of obstetric brachial plexus injury resulting from damage of superior trunk (C5/C6) of the plexus. It is often caused by shoulder dystocia. It can occur in adults following a traumatic force downward on the upper arm and shoulder.
Klumpke's Palsy	**Hx:** Lack of ability to use muscles of the hand, and C8/T1 dermatome distribution numbness. Involvement of T1 may result in drooping of eyelid(ptosis). **PE:** Weakness of intrinsic hand muscles and the wrist. with difficulty flexing the wrist and fingers. If C8/T1 is involved, Horner syndrome (ptosis, miosis, and anhidrosis on the ipsilateral side) can occur due to damage to the adjacent sympathetic chain. **Dx:** Clinical. EMG and nerve conduction studies can be used to determine location and severity of the injury. **Management:** • Physical and occupational therapy including passive ROM exercises and supportive splints to prevent contractures and help restore normal function • Surgery is reserved for cases of severe injury or when functional recovery is not achieved **Discussion:** Klumpke's palsy results from an injury to the brachial plexus involving C8 and T1. This causes paralysis affecting the interossei, thenar, and hypothenar muscles (intrinsic hand muscles) as well as the flexors of the fingers and wrists.

LOWER EXTREMITY

As with the upper extremity, identify the presenting concern as a local or systemic problem.

Traumatic lower extremity (LE) injuries often occur as part of a chain, e.g., a fall from a height onto one's feet is unlikely to affect only the feet, but there may be complaints of pain in the ankle, knees, hips, and back as well. Complex trauma is not commonly tested, but it is important to know about a few key LE trauma presentations.

FOOT AND ANKLE

• Foot and ankle parallel the hand and wrist in their complexity.
• For ankle or foot symptoms—consider trauma, sprains and strains, infection, neuropathy, arthritis, and crystalline disease in the differential diagnosis.
• Understanding ankle anatomy as well as the structures enables an informed history and physical.
• The anterior talofibular ligament is the most common ligament injured in ankle sprains and is often due to over inversion/supination of foot.

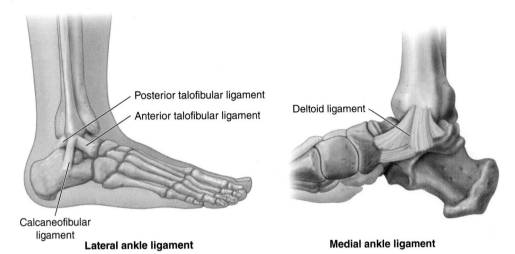

Ankle ligaments. (Reproduced with permission from Edward (Ted) Parks: Practical Office Orthopedics, New York: McGraw Hill, 2018.)

Ankle Sprains

- Common both in practice and on exams
- The physical exam for a sprain is guided by the mechanism of injury
- Plantar flexion with inversion injuries are the most common causes of sprain, as they stretch the lateral ankle structures

Key Exam Maneuvers and Findings	Diagnosis
Anterior drawer test: With the ankle in slight plantar flexion, downward pressure is applied to the lower leg, and the heel is lifted anteriorly; the test is positive if the talus moves more anteriorly compared to the contralateral side.	Anterior talofibular ligament laxity/injury Reproduced with permission from Ian B. Maitin, Ernesto Cruz, CURRENT Diagnosis & Treatment: Physical Medicine & Rehabilitation by McGraw-Hill 2015.
Talar tilt or inversion stress test: When the ankle is inverted or adducted, the test is positive if there is instability or inversion greater than the contralateral side.	Calcaneofibular ligament laxity/injury Reproduced with permission from Ian B. Maitin, Ernesto Cruz, CURRENT Diagnosis & Treatment: Physical Medicine & Rehabilitation by McGraw-Hill 2015.

(Continued)

Key Exam Maneuvers and Findings	Diagnosis
Pain in the plantar region of the midfoot near the heel, which is worse with the first steps in the morning. Tenderness over the medial tuberosity of the calcaneus. Dorsiflexion of the foot and extension of the toes increase patient's pain. Point of tenderness in plantar fasciitis. (Reproduced with permission from Edward (Ted) Parks: Practical Office Orthopedics, New York: McGraw Hill, 2018.)	Plantar fasciitis 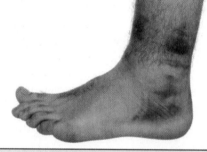 Plantar fascia Reproduced with permission from Edward (Ted) Parks: Practical Office Orthopedics, New York: McGraw Hill, 2018.
Painful, swollen big toe in a patient who has alcohol use disorder.	Podagra (gout)

CASE 4 | Ankle Sprain (Anterior Talofibular Ligament Injury)

A 21-year-old man presents with left ankle pain after a fall. He twisted the ankle while stepping off a curb. He has a limp when he walks and there is bruising and swelling over the lateral aspect of the ankle. There is tenderness just distal and anterior to the distal tip of the fibula. With the ankle in slight plantar flexion, the talus translates significantly more anteriorly with anterior pull on the foot when compared to the contralateral side (anterior drawer test). There is no instability or pain when varus stress is applied with the ankle in dorsiflexion (talar tilt test).

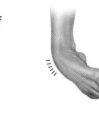

From Edward (Ted) Parks, Practical Office Orthopedics, by McGraw-Hill 2018. FIGURE 5-30. ISBN: 9781259642869. Licensed from Luis Santos/Shutterstock

Conditions with Similar Presentations	**Ankle fracture:** Usually presents in setting of a high-impact mechanism of injury, and risk of fracture is low when the patient can walk immediately after the injury. Fracture and sprains can be differentiated with the Ottawa ankle rules (see below). **Medial ankle sprain:** Occurs with sprain of the deltoid ligament, and results from a forced eversion of the foot. Medial ankle sprains are significantly less common than lateral ankle sprains because the deltoid ligament is a much stronger structure than the relatively weak anterior talofibular ligament of the lateral ankle.
Initial Diagnostic Tests	• Clinical diagnosis • Consider x-rays to rule out fracture
Next Steps in Management	Conservative treatment with rest, ice, compression, and elevation (RICE)
Discussion	The most injured ligament in a low ankle sprain is the anterior talofibular ligament (ATFL). The mechanism of injury is plantar flexion and inversion, which stresses the ATFL. The calcaneofibular ligament (CFL) is the second most sprained ligament in the ankle. The injury takes place during dorsiflexion and inversion. 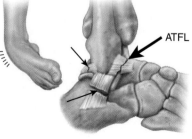 ATFL Anterior talofibular ligament. (Reproduced with permission from Edward (Ted) Parks: Practical Office Orthopedics, New York: McGraw Hill, 2018.)

CASE 4 | Ankle Sprain (Anterior Talofibular Ligament Injury) *(continued)*

Discussion	**History:** Risk factors include ligamentous laxity (e.g., Ehlers-Danlos syndrome, deconditioning (lack of muscular stabilization), footwear that lacks ankle support. The mechanism of injury guides the differential; ankle sprains are associated with low-impact injuries (such as "rolling" the ankle, stepping off the curb). Patients with sprains can usually walk after the injury and may have a history of ligamentous injuries, including previous ankle sprains **Physical Exam:** • Patients with ATFL injury show pain with weight bearing but are still able to walk • They often have focal tenderness and swelling over the ATFL or CFL • The anterior drawer test may show anterior translation of the talus • Increased foot inversion compared to the non-injured ankle may be seen with the tilt test • Grade 2 and grade 3 ankle sprains present with ecchymosis and difficulty bearing weight, and are differentiated by the fact that grade 3 sprains have a significant loss of function as opposed to some loss of function **Diagnostics:** Clinical diagnosis • X-rays, if obtained will be negative (can help rule out other causes, such as fracture or osteochondral lesions of the talus) **Management:** • Conservative treatment with RICE • A supportive ACE bandage, air cast brace, or walking boot may be used for support, depending on the severity of the sprain. • Functional rehabilitation is recommended for all patients

Additional Considerations	**Complications:** Chronic ankle instability may occur following a minority of ankle sprains and is characterized by ongoing pain or instability in the ankle more than 6 months after the initial injury.
	
	Surgical Considerations: Surgical management is considered when ankle ligaments rupture, rather than simply sprain.
	
	Ottawa Ankle Rules: Help dictate whether an ankle injury warrants imaging by plain radiographs as workup for a potential fracture. Consider x-rays when either criteria 1 or 2 below is met.
	1. There is pain in the malleolar zone AND
	  • There is bony tenderness of the lateral or medial malleolus at the posterior edge or tip OR
	  • The patient cannot bear weight immediately after the injury or cannot walk four steps in the clinical setting
	2. There is pain in the midfoot zone AND
	  • There is bony tenderness at the navicular bone or base of the fifth metatarsal OR
	  • The patient cannot bear weight immediately after the injury or cannot walk four steps in the clinical setting

Foot/Ankle Pain Mini-Cases

Cases	Key Findings
Plantar Fasciitis	**Hx:** Pain at the bottom of the foot/inferior heel, which is worse when initiating walking, especially the first steps in the morning or after a period of inactivity. Obesity is a risk factor, and dancing and running are common causes. **PE:** Tenderness is elicited by dorsiflexing the patient's toes and simultaneously palpating along the fascia from the heel to the forefoot. **Diagnostics:** Clinical diagnosis. Consider imaging to rule out other etiologies and in refractory cases (ultrasound or MRI would show thickening of the plantar fascia). **Management:** Conservative measures such as stretching exercises, ice, and avoiding flat shoes and triggering activities. • Short-term NSAIDs for symptomatic relief • Steroid injections can be considered if conservative measures fail • Surgery is reserved for severe refractory cases **Discussion:** Plantar fasciitis is one of the most common causes of self-limiting foot pain in adults. It can be caused by chronic overuse or stress on the plantar fascia, which causes microtears and recurrent inflammation. Heel spurs may coexist with plantar fasciitis; however, causality is unclear.

Foot/Ankle Pain Mini-Cases *(continued)*

Tarsal Tunnel Syndrome (Tibial Nerve Injury)	**Hx:** Sharp, shooting pain in the medial foot/ankle, worse with standing, walking, and at night. May radiate to the sole and/or associated numbness of sole. Risk factors include trauma, diabetes, hypothyroidism, space-occupying lesions (e.g., lipomas, ganglion cysts).
	PE: Tapping over the tarsal tunnel may reproduce pain (positive Tinel sign), and loss of sensation over plantar foot may be present.
	Diagnostics: Clinical diagnosis • Comparison with the contralateral, unaffected body part is helpful • Imaging such as foot and ankle x-ray can be used to ensure there are no bony abnormalities such as bone spurs or changes due to previous trauma • Ultrasound can be used to evaluate for soft tissue structures such as ganglion cysts • EMG/NCS would reveal decreased amplitude in the sensory/motor components of the medial and lateral plantar nerves
	Management: NSAIDs, physical therapy, and orthotic shoes. If there is a source of compression of the tibial nerve such as a ganglion cyst, operative decompression can be helpful.
	Discussion: The tibial nerve gets compressed/injured in the ankle area as it passes through the tarsal tunnel. This occurs due to trauma (ankle sprain/fracture). The tarsal tunnel also contains the medial and lateral plantar nerves.

KNEE

Commonly tested pathologies involve the bones and ligaments of the knee joint. Understanding the anatomy of the ligamentous structures and how they are tested by isolating and stretching them relative to other structures helps in making the correct diagnosis.

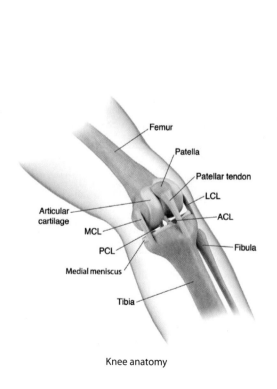

Knee anatomy

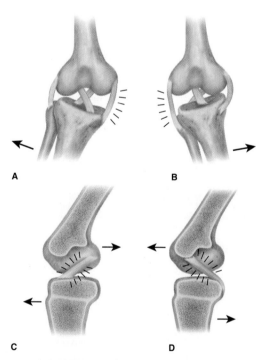

The medial collateral ligament (MCL) prevents valgus deformities (A). The lateral collateral ligament prevents varus deformities (B). Varus and valgus deformities are prevented by the collateral ligaments, while the anterior and posterior translation of the tibia are prevented by the cruciate ligaments. The anterior cruciate ligament prevents anterior tibial translation (C). The posterior cruciate ligament prevents posterior tibial translation (D). (Reproduced with permission from Edward (Ted) Parks: Practical Office Orthopedics, New York: McGraw Hill, 2018.)

Varus and **valgus** describe the angular deformities in the coronal plane. Deviation of the distal segment of the articulation (the tibia and fibula in the case of a knee joint) towards the midline is described as a varus deformity. Deviation of the distal segment away from the midline is described as a valgus deformity.

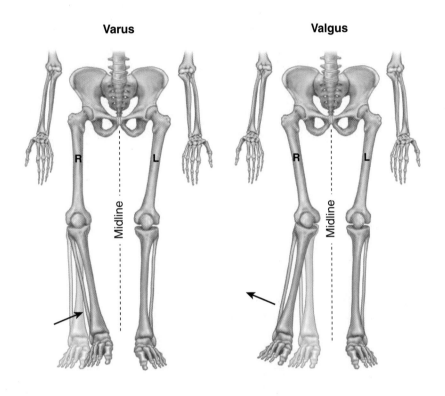

Key Exam Maneuvers and Findings	How to Perform the Maneuvers	Diagnosis
Increased anterior glide of tibia relative to femur is due to ACL injury: **Anterior drawer test:** Patient lying with feet flat on table and hips flexed and knee bent at 90 degrees while examiner pulls the tibia forward with both hands *or* **Lachman test** (more sensitive): Patient lying with knee bent 30 degrees and examiner places one hand on thigh and pulls the tibia forward with other hand	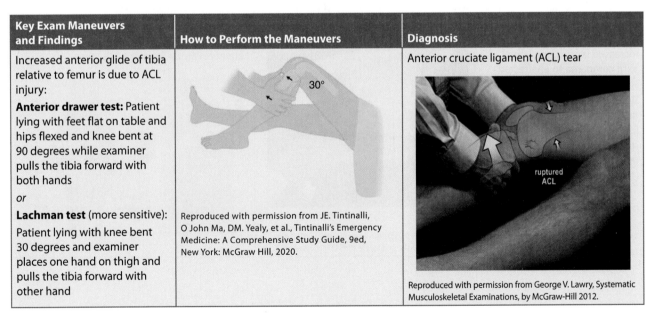 Reproduced with permission from JE. Tintinalli, O John Ma, DM. Yealy, et al., Tintinalli's Emergency Medicine: A Comprehensive Study Guide, 9ed, New York: McGraw Hill, 2020.	Anterior cruciate ligament (ACL) tear ruptured ACL Reproduced with permission from George V. Lawry, Systematic Musculoskeletal Examinations, by McGraw-Hill 2012.

(Continued)

Key Exam Maneuvers and Findings	How to Perform the Maneuvers	Diagnosis
Increased posterior translation of tibia relative to femur compared with unaffected side with the following test: **Posterior drawer sign:** Patient lying with feet flat on table and hips flexed and knee bent at 90 degrees while examiner pushes the tibia posteriorly with both hands. Increased posterior glide is due to PCL injury *or* **Posterior sag test:** Place patient's feet on elevated surface so knees and hips bent to 90 degrees and observe for excessive posterior positioning of tibia	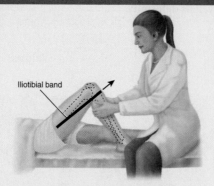 Reproduced with permission from Edward (Ted) Parks: Practical Office Orthopedics, New York: McGraw Hill, 2018.	Posterior cruciate ligament (PCL) tear 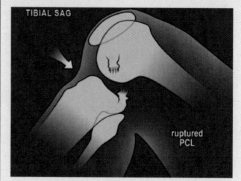 Reproduced with permission from Lawry GV: Systematic Muskuloskeletal Examinations, New York: McGraw Hill, 2012.
Increased laxity along medial joint compared to unaffected side with: **Valgus** (lateral force) **stress test** (abnormal passive abduction): Examiner places one hand laterally against knee and pushes laterally at the ankle	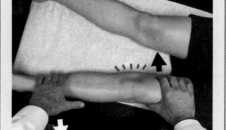 A Reproduced with permission from Edward (Ted) Parks, Practical Office Orthopedics, New York: McGraw-Hill 2018.	Medial collateral ligament (MCL) tear 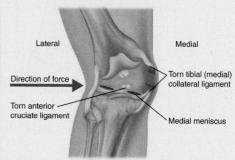
Increased laxity along lateral joint compared to unaffected side with: **Varus** (medial force) **stress test** (abnormal passive adduction): Examiner places one hand medially against knee and pushes medially at the ankle	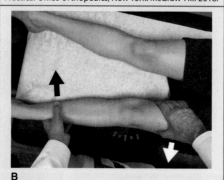 B Reproduced with permission from Edward (Ted) Parks, Practical Office Orthopedics, New York: McGraw-Hill 2018.	Lateral collateral ligament (LCL) tear 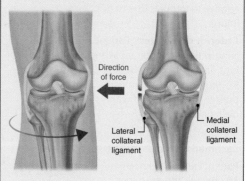

Key Exam Maneuvers and Findings	How to Perform the Maneuvers	Diagnosis
Pain and/or clicking or popping reproduced in knee with: **Thessaly test:** Patient stands on affected leg with knee bent 20 degrees and rotates knee internally and externally *or* **McMurray test:** Patient is placed in supine position and while grasping the ankle with one hand, the other hand is placed over the affected knee. The knee is flexed maximally, externally rotated and slowly extended to assess the medial meniscus. The knee is flexed maximally, internally rotated and slowly extended to assess the lateral meniscus. A painful "click" is a positive McMurray test.	 McMurray test. McMurray's test for a torn meniscus. (Reproduced with permission from The Knee In: Parks E. Practical Office Orthopedics, New York: McGraw-Hill, 2017.)	 External rotation — Medial tear Internal rotation — Lateral tear Meniscus injury/tear Reproduced with permission from Le Tao, Bhushan Vikas, Sochat Matthew, First Aid for the USMLE Step 1 2021, 31st ed. New York: McGraw-Hill Education, 2021.

CASE 5 | Anterior Cruciate Ligament (ACL) Tear

A 24-year-old man presents with acute left knee pain and swelling. He was playing football when he made a cutting move and felt a sudden "pop" in his left knee, followed by significant swelling. On physical exam, the left knee is swollen but there is no point tenderness. With the knee bent at 30 degrees, the tibia translates anteriorly approximately 0.5 cm without a firm endpoint (positive Lachman test). With the knee at 90 degrees, the tibia similarly translates anteriorly with stress, compared to the contralateral side (positive anterior drawer test); however, the tibia does not translate posteriorly (negative posterior drawer test) or medially.

Conditions with Similar Presentations	**Medial meniscus tear:** Often occurs due to twisting injury to the knee. Diagnosis is often made clinically with a positive McMurray or Thessaly test. **Lateral tears:** Often occur in the setting of an acute ACL injury. **PCL injuries:** Can be caused by several mechanisms: direct blow to the tibia with a posteriorly directed force (e.g., proximal tibia of a flexed knee slams into dashboard), hyperextension of the knee, or associated with other knee injuries. Most isolated PCL injuries are treated nonoperatively. **Patellofemoral pain syndrome:** Presents with dull, aching pain under or around patella of gradual onset, may be described as a locking sensation; however, true mechanical locking of the knee is not present. **Prepatellar bursitis:** Presents with pain and swelling of the patella with overlying erythema, warmth, and swelling that worsens with knee flexion. **Iliotibial (IT) band syndrome** presents with lateral knee pain due to friction of the IT band against the lateral femoral epicondyle secondary to overuse of the lateral knee (e.g., in runners). **Tibial plateau fracture:** Occurs due to trauma and will be apparent on x-ray.
Initial Diagnostic Tests	• Clinical diagnosis • MRI to confirm if considering surgery • Consider x-ray to rule out fracture or dislocation
Next Steps in Management	Conservative treatment with physical therapy

CASE 5 | Anterior Cruciate Ligament (ACL) Tear *(continued)*

Discussion	The ACL is the most frequently injured ligament in the knee. It is a single ligament comprised of two ligamentous bundles: an anteromedial and posterolateral bundle. Together, these bundles resist anterior translation of the tibia in reference to the distal femoral condyles, thus providing intra-articular stability to the knee. **History:** Common injury in sports requiring sudden twisting and pivot motions (e.g., "stop-and-go" athletics such as soccer, gymnastics, basketball). • Snapping sensation or "pop" followed by swelling due to a bloody effusion • May report instability while walking or pivoting • With chronic ACL tears, patients may report their knee unexpectedly "giving out" **Physical Exam:** Hemarthrosis may limit the sensitivity of exam maneuvers. • The anterior drawer test, Lachman test, and the pivot shift test are the three most sensitive and specific tests for ACL tear • When performing a knee examination for ACL tear, all other cruciate and collateral ligaments, as well as meniscal bodies, should be examined, as many structures may be damaged simultaneously **Diagnostics:** MRI is the gold standard for diagnosis. However, an MRI is often ordered only to inform surgical planning, if there is uncertainty in the diagnosis, or to determine if the ACL tear occurred in conjunction with other injuries in the knee, such as a meniscal tear. **Management:** • Initially, conservative management with physical therapy and activity modification—goals include strengthening exercises to maximize knee stability. • Physical therapy is also sometimes recommended as pre-habilitation prior to surgery and postoperatively to ensure the patient achieves full range of motion, proprioception, and strength.
Additional Considerations	**Complications:** ACL tears often occur as part of the "unhappy triad," in which the patient suffers an ACL tear, medial meniscal tear, and medial collateral ligament (MCL) tear simultaneously. The unhappy triad most commonly results from a lateral blow to the knee causing an acute valgus deformity. **Pediatric and Surgical Considerations:** ACL tears do not heal on their own. Therefore, in younger active patients, ACL repair surgery is the treatment of choice. MRI should be obtained to gather information regarding anatomy, measurements, and other injuries. A tendon graft from the patella, hamstring, quadriceps are commonly used for reconstruction. In addition to restoring full mobility and activity, surgery helps to prevent the development of longer-term complications of injury, namely osteoarthritis. For patients who lead a sedentary life or have contraindications to surgery, bracing and physical therapy can be effective to maintain some function without undergoing surgery.

Anterior view of left knee

Le T, Bhushan V, Sochat M. First Aid for the USMLE Step 1 2021. New York: McGraw-Hill Education, 2021. (Reproduced with permission from Le Tao,Bhushan Vikas, Sochat Matthew, First Aid for the USMLE Step 1 2021, New York: McGraw-Hill Education, 2021.)

Knee Pain Mini-Cases

Case	Key Findings
Meniscal Tear	**Hx:** Occurs in sports where pivoting is common, as well as onset of pain that occurs when there is a sudden adjustment in speed along with a directional change. Patients may report experiencing a tearing or popping sensation in the knee at the time of the event. Later, patients report their knee "catching" or "locking," along with pain and delayed effusion in the knee. In older patients, degenerative tears can result from minimal trauma.

Knee Pain Mini-Cases (continued)

Meniscal Tear	**Physical Exam:** Positive McMurray or Thessaly test. Joint line tenderness. **Diagnostics:** Clinical diagnosis. MRI can aid in diagnosis if surgery is contemplated. **Management:** Treatment depends on the location and size of the tear—most are treated conservatively with physical therapy; some may require partial meniscectomy or meniscal repair. **Discussion:** Medial tears are more common than lateral tears. Acute tears result from sudden adjustment of speed and change in direction while the knee is flexed, causing torsional stress on the trapped meniscus; these tears are more commonly seen in young, active individuals and are more commonly treated surgically. Degenerative tears occur due to reduced compliance of the menisci, which become stiffer with age, and are usually seen in patients over age 40; these tears are more commonly managed conservatively, if tolerable given the patient's lifestyle.
Baker/Popliteal Cyst	**Hx:** Occurs following trauma, overuse, prolonged pressure, direct injury, infection, or due to inflammatory arthritis. Usually occur in association with underlying joint disease. **PE:** Sometimes an obvious sack-like swelling and tenderness in posterolateral corner of knee. Patient may demonstrate tenderness to palpation or limited range of motion. **Diagnostics:** Clinical diagnosis. Consider bursal fluid aspiration when there is a concern for infection or crystalline arthritis. **Management:** NSAIDs for symptomatic relief. For severely symptomatic cases, consider combination of local anesthetic and glucocorticoid injections. **Discussion:** Inflammation of the popliteal bursa on the posterior facet of the knee occurs in association with underlying joint disease. When symptomatic, this condition must be differentiated from DVT. It is most commonly self-limited and resolves with treatment of the underlying joint condition but can be complicated by infection. 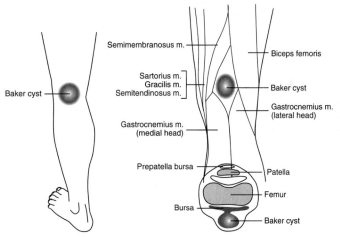 Baker cyst. (Reproduced with permission from Manish Suneja, Joseph F. Szot, et al, DeGowin's Diagnostic Examination, 11e; New York: McGraw-Hill Education, 2020.)
Medial Tibial Stress Syndrome (Shin Splints)	**Hx:** Shin pain and diffuse tenderness in runners. Occurs when bone resorption outpaces bone formation in tibial cortex. **PE:** Tenderness to palpation diffusely over anterior tibia. No palpable lesions. **Diagnostics:** Clinical diagnosis. Plain radiographs may be used to rule out tibial stress fracture, but shin splints demonstrate normal radiographic findings. **Management:** Conservative treatment via rest, ice, and use of NSAIDs as needed. **Discussion:** Differentiating shin splints from a tibial stress fracture can be challenging in cases of overuse. Shin splints generally demonstrate a more diffuse pattern over the anterior tibia, while stress fractures demonstrate more focal tenderness. Shin splints frequently recur due to overuse or inadequate treatment intervals; in cases of recurring shin splints, consider ruling out a stress fracture.

Knee Pain Mini-Cases *(continued)*

Posterior Cruciate Ligament (PCL) Tear	**Hx:** Pain that worsens over time, instability in the knee while walking or pivoting. Stiffness, difficulty walking, and a snapping sensation or "pop" followed by swelling due to a bloody effusion. With chronic PCL tears, patients may report their knee unexpectedly "giving out."
	PE: The posterior drawer test may be positive, and it correlates to the severity of the tear. Examine all other cruciate and collateral ligaments, as well as meniscal bodies due to high potential for concomitant injury.
	Diagnostics: Clinical diagnosis. MRI is the gold standard.
	Management: • Conservative management, physical therapy, and activity modification—goals include strengthening exercises to maximize knee stability • Crutches to limit weight bearing • Knee brace to help with instability • Surgery for severe cases (physical therapy is also recommended as pre-habilitation prior to surgery and postoperatively to ensure the patient achieves full range of motion, proprioception, and strength)
	Discussion: The PCL is the strongest ligament in the knee, and its injury is far less common than ACL. Injury occurs by knee hyperextension or direct trauma. Active patients whose lifestyles involve recreational activities or work duties dependent on knee stability are candidates for PCL repair. Younger patients are more likely to warrant surgical correction, as these patients are more active.
Prepatellar Bursitis	**Hx:** Follows trauma, overuse, prolonged pressure, direct injury, infection, or due to inflammatory arthritis. **Physical Exam:** Often an obvious sack-like swelling and tenderness in superficial bursae of knee; less obvious in deep bursae. Chronic bursitis has more swelling but less pain. **Diagnostics:** • Clinical diagnosis. Consider bursal fluid aspiration when there is a concern for infection or crystalline arthritis **Management:** • NSAIDs for symptomatic relief • For deeper bursae, consider combination of local anesthetic and glucocorticoid injections **Discussion:** Prepatellar bursal inflammation in front of the kneecap occurs from repeated trauma or pressure from excessive kneeling (also called "housemaid's knee"). It is usually self-limited but can be complicated by infection, especially in superficial bursae. Distinguish from joint effusion.	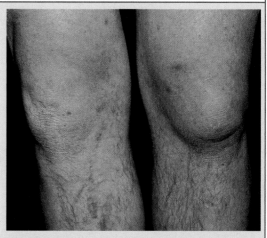 Prepatellar bursitis. (From Kevin J. Knoop, Lawrence B. Stack, Alan B. Storrow, R. Jason Thurman, The Atlas of Emergency Medicine, 5e, by McGraw Hill 2021. FIGURE 12.22. ISBN 9781260134940. Photo contributor: Kevin J. Knoop, MD, MS.)

HIP

The hip presents a unique challenge as a joint because it is particularly hard for patients to accurately describe the location of their pain for such a deep structure. The physical exam can help localize the pathology, and it is important to distinguish if pain is originating from the hip or spine. Pain and stiffness on passive internal and external hip rotation in 90 degrees flexion (windshield wiper test) suggests hip joint arthritis.

Approach to Hip Pain

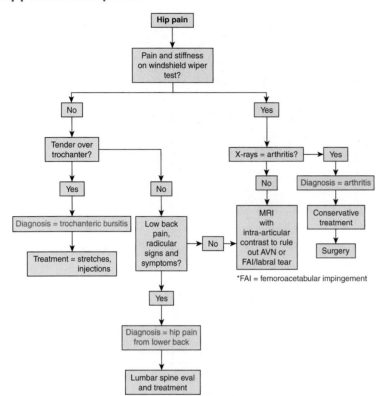

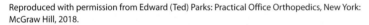

Reproduced with permission from Edward (Ted) Parks: Practical Office Orthopedics, New York: McGraw Hill, 2018.

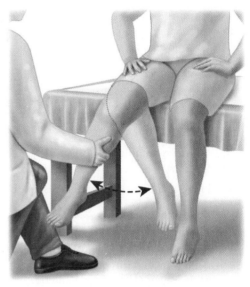

Windshield wiper test. (Reproduced with permission from Edward (Ted) Parks: Practical Office Orthopedics, New York: McGraw Hill, 2018.)

Key Exam Maneuvers and Findings	Diagnoses
Log roll test: Specific test to confirm hip pathology. While patient is supine, extended leg is internally and externally rotated. If pain, clicking, or increased or decreased range of motion is detected, it helps confirm hip pathology vs. pain from outside of the hip joint (i.e., referred from back). **Windshield wiper test:** Passive internal and external hip rotation in 90 degrees of flexion. Pain and stiffness suggest hip joint arthritis.	Hip pathology (e.g., arthritis, osteonecrosis, slipped capital femoral epiphysis [SCFE], piriformis syndrome)
FADIR test (flexion, adduction, internal rotation): Pain reproduced with flexing the hip of a supine patient to 90 degrees, and internally rotating and adducting the hip by placing one hand on bent knee and ankle. 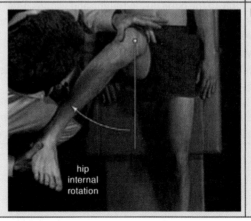 Reproduced with permission from George V. Lawry, Systematic Musculoskeletal Examinations, by McGraw-Hill 2012.	Intra-articular pathology

(Continued)

Key Exam Maneuvers and Findings		Diagnoses
FABER test (flexion, abduction, external rotation): Pain reproduced with flexing the hip of a supine patient to 45 degrees, and externally rotating and abducting the hip by placing one hand on bent knee and ankle. Reproduced with permission from George V. Lawry, Systematic Musculoskeletal Examinations, by McGraw-Hill 2012.		Posterior pain: SI joint, lumbar spine, or posterior hip Groin pain: Intra-articular pathology

- There are many pathologies of the hip, especially in the pediatric population (see Pediatrics Chapter), but there are relatively few commonly tested pathologies of the bones, tendons, ligaments, or nerves.
- However, as mentioned earlier, there is a fifth essential category: vascular.

CASE 6 | Avascular Necrosis (AVN) of the Hip

A 38-year-old woman status post(s/p) renal transplant, on chronic steroid therapy presents with 2 months of worsening right hip pain. Pain is worse with weight bearing, walking, climbing stairs, and prolonged standing. There is no history of falls or trauma. Physical exam reveals normal range of motion of the hip, but it elicits pain in the groin region with positive log roll test.

Conditions with Similar Presentations	**Fracture:** Occurs acutely in setting of trauma. **OA:** More common in older patients. **Septic arthritis:** Would have fever, erythema, and swelling of the joint.
Initial Diagnostic Tests	Confirm with plain radiography (maybe normal at early stages)
Next Steps in Management	• Analgesia and non-weight bearing of the affected side • Early surgical intervention has more promising results than medical management
Discussion	AVN (osteonecrosis) of the hip is a pathologic process that is poorly understood. It results from impaired blood supply to the bone due to trauma and various other causes. In cases of hip trauma, fractures of the femoral neck may interrupt the ascending branch of the medial femoral circumflex artery's blood supply to the head of the femur. **History:** The most common symptom is groin pain. Traumatic risk factors include fracture of the femoral neck and "the bends" (caisson/decompression disease). Other risk factors include chronic steroid use, alcoholism, sickle cell disease, Legg-Calve-Perthes, Gaucher disease, slipped capital femoral epiphysis (SCFE), and hypercoagulable states. **Physical Exam:** Groin pain may be exacerbated by abduction or internal rotation.

CASE 6 | Avascular Necrosis (AVN) of the Hip *(continued)*

Discussion	**Diagnostics:** X-ray showing an example of AVN of the femoral head. Note the "step-off" on the articular surface of the ball and fragmentation of the femoral head.
	
	 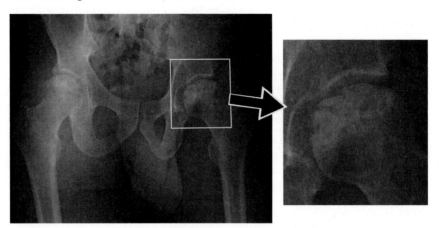
	
	 Reproduced with permission from Edward (Ted) Parks, Practical Office Orthopedics, by McGraw-Hill 2018.
	
	 • Initial plain radiographs may be normal.
	 • Late plain radiographs may show a mottled appearance of the affected area because of the presence of "cysts" (which represent areas of dead bone resorption) and contiguous sclerosis (which represent areas of bone repair). These changes develop as follows:
	    • Development of a region of generalized osteopenia
	    • Collapse of the cancellous bone beneath the subchondral plate
	    • The development of a radiolucent line is pathognomonic and referred to as the crescent sign.
	 • If the x-rays are not diagnostic, MRI is the radiologic method with most sensitivity and highest accuracy. MRI shows decreased signal on both T1 and T2 sequences.
	 • Bilateral hips are involved 50–80% of the time; therefore, bilateral imaging should be considered.
	
	 Management:
	 • Medical management: Tapering patients off glucocorticoids, discontinuing weight bearing and pain control.
	 • Surgical management: See below.

Additional Considerations	**Screening:** Routine screening for osteonecrosis is not recommended; attempts should be made to correct risk factors if possible. Glucocorticoids and alcohol represent the most common risk factors, and both are modifiable. **Complications:** • Articular surface collapse may occur in cases of AVN of the hip with extensive involvement. • AVN may also occur at the scaphoid following a fall on outstretched hands. • Bisphosphonate usage is a risk factor for osteonecrosis of the jaw, especially in patients with malignancy. **Surgical Considerations:** If caught early, it is possible to use conservative measures such as bracing, splinting, and rest to preserve the joint. However, given the progressive nature of the disease as well as the risk of joint collapse, surgical intervention to preserve or replace the joint entirely is often indicated. Options for surgery include bone grafting (to replace necrosed tissue), core decompression (to drill inside the bone and remove necrosed tissue), or total hip arthroplasty. **Pediatric Considerations:** Osteonecrosis of the hip in children is referred to as Legge-Calvé-Perthes disease (see Pediatrics Chapter).

Hip Pain Mini-Cases

Cases	Key Findings
Hip Fracture	**Hx:** Typically occurs after trauma and risk increases with osteoporosis. **PE:** Leg will be shortened and externally rotated. **Diagnostics:** Plain films may demonstrate fracture. If clinical suspicion is high and plain films are negative, evaluate further using CT or MRI. **Management:** Operative fixation via hemi or total arthroplasty. Unless there is active bleeding, anticoagulate to decrease likelihood of DVT. **Discussion:** Hip fracture surgery should be performed within 24 hours of admission. In hip fractures secondary to osteoporosis, bisphosphonate therapy is recommended following operative fixation.

Hip Pain Mini-Cases *(continued)*

Hip Dislocation	**Hx:** Following trauma ("dashboard injury").
	PE: Leg will be internally rotated, flexed, and adducted if posterior dislocation. Posterior dislocation may be associated with AVN and/or sciatic nerve deficits. Anterior dislocation may demonstrate obturator nerve deficits.
	Diagnostics: Plain films should demonstrate dislocation and indicate whether the dislocation was anterior or posterior.
	Management: Closed reduction, with affected leg kept in abduction using bracing following reduction.
	Discussion: In the event of significant trauma, advanced imaging of the pelvis with CT may be pursued; these images provide more utility in surgical planning. Significant pelvic trauma should be evaluated in the setting of the mechanism of injury. Red flag symptoms of severe pelvic trauma include hematuria, lower extremity weakness or decreased sensation, abnormal position of the lower extremities, and bony tenderness.
Greater Trochanteric Pain Syndrome	**Hx:** Lateral hip pain. More common in middle-aged female patients. Comorbid conditions include obesity, arthritis, plantar fasciitis. **PE:** Tenderness over the greater trochanter, associated gait abnormalities (e.g., waddling gait). **Diagnostics:** Clinical diagnosis • Ultrasound can be used to assess for an enlarged trochanteric bursa • X-rays of the hip can be helpful to rule out other pathology **Management:** • Often self-limited, but physical therapy and NSAIDs are helpful • Steroid injections can be used if still symptomatic • Surgery is used in refractory cases **Discussion:** Greater trochanteric pain syndrome (also known as trochanteric bursitis) is common and is due to inflammation of the gluteal tendon and trochanteric bursa of the femur (deep to the iliotibial band and superficial to the hip abductor muscles). During running, the iliotibial band repeatedly rubs over the bursa and can lead to irritation and inflammation. It can often present similarly to sacroiliitis, but sacroiliitis is worse at night and improves in the morning.	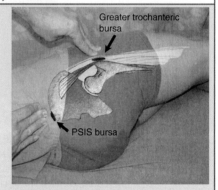 Reproduced with permission from John H. Stone, Current Diagnosis & Treatment: Rheumatology, 4e by McGraw Hill 2021.
Iliotibial (IT) Band Syndrome	**Hx:** Pain at lateral aspect of the knee that worsens with activity. Gradual onset, starting with mild pain after extended use and becoming more severe over time with an earlier onset. Primarily affects physically active people, especially runners and cyclists. **PE:** Tenderness at epicondyle. *Noble compression test*: patient lays on their side with the injured side facing up while a physician applies pressure to the distal IT band while flexing the patient's knee slowly from 0 to 90 degrees while applying pressure on the lateral epicondyle of the femur and palpating for crepitus with the thumb of the other hand. **Diagnostics:** Clinical diagnosis **Management:** Conservative approach such as rest, ice, NSAIDs and physical therapy **Discussion:** IT band syndrome is an overuse injury. Distinguish from patellofemoral pain by location based on tenderness at lateral knee rather than at the patellofemoral joint.

BACK PAIN

History

In addition to enquiring about onset, timing/duration, severity/intensity, location/radiation, quality/character, associated symptoms, exacerbating and alleviating factors, ask about alarm or red flag symptoms. Urgent identification and treatment of any etiologies that involve or put the spinal cord at risk are critical to avoid potential irreversible sequelae due to spinal cord injury.

Alarm or red flag symptoms warranting further imaging and investigation:

- Trauma history
- Previous history of cancer
- Extremes of age: <16 or >50 with new-onset pain
- Fevers/chills or history of significant infection or injection drug use
- Unintentional weight loss, malaise, or other systemic symptoms
- Additional pain in chest, abdomen, pelvis, or other joints

- Chronic steroid use or immunosuppression
- History of osteoporosis
- Severe night-time pain or rest pain
- Duration >1 month
- Saddle anesthesia
- Bowel or bladder incontinence or urinary retention
- New neurological deficit: weakness, tingling, numbness

Approach to Back Pain

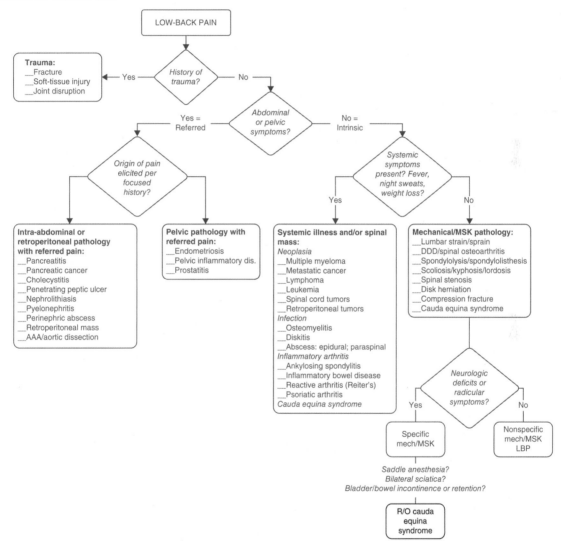

The following conditions cause **nonspecific** back pain, as there is not always a definitive relationship between the pain and anatomical findings:

- Lumbar strain/sprain: Musculotendinous (strain) or ligamentous (sprain) injuries secondary to over-stress of the structures
- Degenerative disease: Disk and facet-joint deterioration and arthritic changes (degenerative disk disease)
- Spondylolisthesis: Forward displacement of a vertebra
- Spondylolysis: Fracture or defect of the vertebral pars interarticularis
- Scoliosis: Sideways curvature of the spine
- Kyphosis: Exaggerated rounding of the upper back
- Lordosis: Inward curvature of lower back

The following conditions typically cause *specific* back pain since there is a definitive relationship between the pain and the anatomical findings. Neurologic signs and symptoms are often present, as well.

- Spinal stenosis: Abnormal narrowing of the spinal canal

- Disk herniation: Rupture and extrusion of the intervertebral disk with impingement on the spinal nerve root

- Vertebral compression fracture: Often caused by osteoporosis

- Cauda equina syndrome: Compression of the cauda equina nerve roots secondary to herniated disk (or other pathology), resulting in motor and sensory deficits that can lead to incontinence and/or possible paralysis

Diverse systemic processes may affect the structures of the spine:

- Neoplasia: Multiple myeloma, metastatic cancer, leukemia, lymphoma, retroperitoneal tumors, primary spinal-cord tumors, infection, osteomyelitis, diskitis, paraspinal or epidural abscess

- Inflammatory arthritis: Ankylosing spondylitis, Inflammatory bowel disease (IBD), associated arthritis, reactive arthritis (occurring after an infection), psoriatic arthritis

Sources of referred pain include the following: pancreatitis or pancreatic cancer, cholecystitis, penetrating peptic ulcer, nephrolithiasis, pyelonephritis, perinephric abscess, retroperitoneal lymphadenopathy or mass, abdominal aortic aneurysm or aortic dissection, endometriosis, pelvic inflammatory disease (PID), prostatitis.

Physical Examination

Pertinent exam maneuvers related to the back are listed below. Like the upper extremity, it is important to localize neuropathic symptoms of the lower extremity to dermatomes; any neuropathic concern should prompt an investigation of the nerve from the root at the spine to the tip.

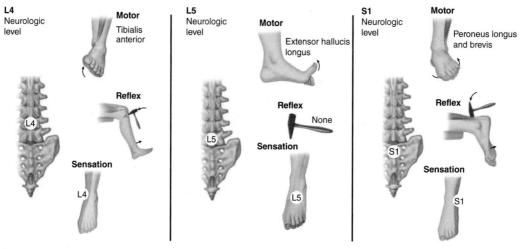

Distribution of nerves and nerve roots. (Reproduced with permission from Edward (Ted) Parks: Practical Office Orthopedics, New York: McGraw Hill, 2018.)

Physical Examination	Clinical Implications
Vital signs/general appearance	Elevated temperature may indicate infection or systemic illness
Inspection of the spine	Kyphosis or lordosis or disk herniation/muscular spasm
Range of motion/gait	Abnormal heel walking may indicate L5 pathology
	Abnormal toe walking may indicate S1 Pathology
Palpation of spine	Focal spinal tenderness may indicate infection tumor or compression fracture
	Costovertebral angle (CVA) may indicate kidney infection
	Sacroiliac joints tenderness may indicate inflammatory arthritis
Reflexes	Diminished patellar reflex may indicate L4 pathology
	Diminished Achilles tendon reflex may indicate S1 pathology
	Hyperreflexia or presence of Babinski when assessing plantar reflex indicates upper motor neuron disease and thus suggests myelopathy

Physical Examination	Clinical Implications
Sensation	Diminished sensation behind medial malleolus may indicate L4 pathology
	Diminished sensation dorsum of foot and first/second web space may indicate L5 pathology
	Diminished sensation lateral aspect of foot and/or posterior calf may indicate S1 pathology
Straight-leg raise (SLR): Positive if reproduction of shooting pain down affected leg (posterior calf) when affected leg is passively raised between 30–70 degrees **Contralateral straight leg raise (cSLR):** Positive if reproduction of shooting pain down affected leg (posterior calf) when unaffected leg is passively raised between 30–70 degrees	If positive, may indicate herniated disk L5–S1 SLR more sensitive (sen/spec 0.80/0.40) cSLR more specific (sen/spec 0.25/0.90)
Anal sphincter tone and perianal sensation	Diminished tone or sensation may indicate cauda equina syndrome

Other Exam Findings and Clinical Implications

- Inflammation and/or joint tenderness may indicate inflammatory arthritis
- Abnormal log roll or windshield wiper test may indicate hip pathology
- Diminished peripheral pulses may indicate peripheral artery disease
- Abdominal tenderness, organomegaly, or mass may indicate referred source of back pain
- Cervical motion tenderness is indicative of PID
- Abnormal findings such as heart murmur, abnormal lung sounds may indicate other sources of infection (e.g., endocarditis, pneumonia)
- Prostate tenderness may indicate prostatitis
- Other abnormal palpation findings may indicate etiology of metastatic cancer (e.g., thyroid, lymph nodes, breast)

Diagnostics

Most diagnosis are made clinically based on history and exam findings alone. If tests are needed, you should order the least invasive and most cost-effective tests that will help you confirm the diagnosis or rule out the do-not-miss diagnosis. For certain conditions, such as lumbar strain, tests are not needed, and the patient can be treated with appropriate pain medications, physical therapy, and lifestyle modifications. In some scenarios you do need more expensive tests, such as MRI, to rule out cord compression or cauda equina syndrome.

Testing	Helpful in Diagnosing the Following Pathology
X-ray lumbar spine	Arthritis or degenerative joint disease Ankylosing spondylitis Fracture Curvature of spine
MRI spine (preferred) or CT spine	All the above *and* Spinal infections, including osteomyelitis, discitis Spinal stenosis Herniated disk Metastatic cancer Cauda equina syndrome
Bone scan (not commonly used, but may be helpful in the listed conditions)	Osteomyelitis Occult fractures Cancer with metastases to bone
Complete blood count (CBC) Erythrocyte sedimentation rate (ESR) C-reactive protein (CRP)	Infection Inflammation
Urinalysis	Kidney stones Urinary tract infection/pyelonephritis
Ultrasound or CT abdomen	Retroperitoneal, intra-abdominal, or pelvic pathology
Electromyogram and nerve conduction studies (EMG/NCS)	Helps identify nerve damage by measuring electrical activity in the nerves and muscles

Management of Low Back Pain

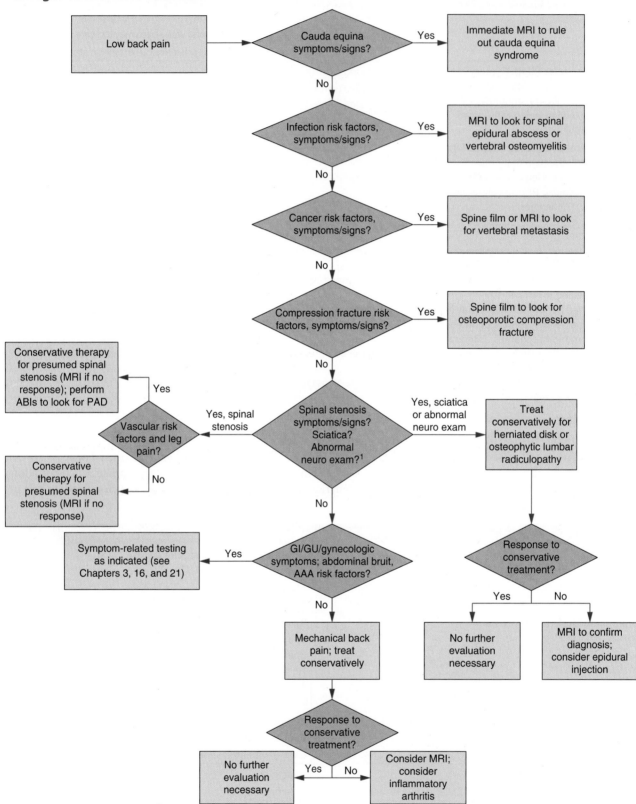

AAA, abdominal aortic aneurysm; ABIs, ankle-brachial index; GI, gastrointestinal; GU, genitourinary; MRI, magnetic resonance imaging; PAD, peripheral arterial disease.

[1]Abnormal neurologic exam means abnormalities consistent with lumbar radiculopathy. Finding any other abnormalities requires consideration of other neurologic causes.

Reproduced with permission from Scott D.C. Stern, Adam S. Cifu, Diane Altkorn. Symptom to Diagnosis: An Evidence-Based Guide, 4e; New York: McGraw-Hill, 2020.

CASE 7 | Herniated Disk

A 60-year-old woman presents with a 2-day history of acute low back pain after she tried to move a sofa at home. The pain is localized to the right lower back with radiation down the posterior aspect of the right leg. She does not have any weakness or bladder/bowel incontinence. Her exam is notable for tenderness over right paraspinal muscles and shooting pain to her right calf when the right leg is raised to 45 degrees (positive SLR). Contralateral straight leg raising is negative. There is no focal spinal tenderness. The right Achilles reflex is absent, and she has diminished sensation in the lateral aspect of her right foot.

Conditions with Similar Presentations	**Cauda equina syndrome:** Symptoms include saddle anesthesia and/or bilateral lower extremity weakness or loss of bowel or bladder control/ **Mechanical low back pain (or lumbar strain):** Paraspinal pain but not shooting pain or positive SLR. **Vertebral fracture** and **spinal infection:** Would present with focal spinal tenderness.
Initial Diagnostic Tests	Clinical diagnosis
Next Steps in Management	Conservative treatment with NSAIDs and early mobilization
Discussion	Disk herniation is a common cause of lumbosacral radiculopathy and low back pain. When a disk herniates beyond its anatomic position, it may compress nearby structures such as nerve roots exiting neural foramina, resulting in symptoms such as pain, weakness, and paresthesias. Intervertebral disks typically herniate posteriorly because the posterior ligament is thinner than the anterior ligament. Symptoms depend upon which disk herniates. 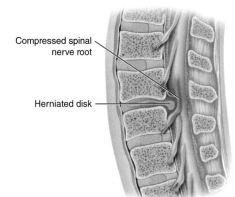Disk herniation. (Reproduced with permission from Edward (Ted) Parks: Practical Office Orthopedics, New York: McGraw Hill, 2018.) **History:** In addition to pain, there may be paresthesias and/or weakness limited to a singular dermatome. Symptoms commonly have a specific onset following a trauma event, bending, or lifting. **Physical Exam:** The SLR is sensitive to disc herniation. cSLR is less specific but is more sensitive. • Physical exam of sensation (pain, temperature, and light touch), strength, and reflexes may help localize the level of the spinal lesion • L3–L4 can lead to weakness of knee extension and a decreased patellar reflex • L4–L5 can cause weakness with ankle dorsiflexion and difficulty with heel walking **Diagnostics:** Diagnosis of a herniated L5–S1 disk with nerve-root impingement (L5–S1 radiculopathy or *sciatica*) is made clinically. MRI can help confirm the diagnosis. **Management:** • Encourage light activity, and palliative measures such as NSAIDs and ice. • If no improvement with conservative treatment or if worsening neurological deficits or symptoms, consider MRI, referring to a spine specialist, and/or physical therapy.
Additional Considerations	**Complications:** Prolonged or permanent disability may result from disk herniation but is uncommon. Red flag symptoms warrant urgent evaluation and include: • saddle anesthesia • progressive nerve damage • progressive pain or weakness • loss of bowel or bladder function **Surgical Considerations:** Severe or progressive low back pain associated with progressing motor weakness is an indication for surgical intervention.

Compressed spinal nerve root

Herniated disk

Back Pain Mini-Cases

Cases	Key Findings
Lumbar Spinal Stenosis (LSS)	**Hx:** Neurogenic claudication is the hallmark of LSS (lower back pain exacerbated by standing and walking, and relieved by sitting, lying down, or flexing the hip). • Other symptoms include discomfort, numbness, tingling, and weakness in the legs • Symptoms in most cases are bilateral but asymmetric Degenerative arthritis is one of the most common causes, followed by RA or ankylosing spondylitis. Risk factors include increasing age (increased likelihood of degenerative arthritis), obesity, and family history. **PE:** The neurologic examination is normal in the majority of patients. • In some patients with LSS, more prolonged or severe nerve root involvement may lead to fixed and/or progressive neurologic deficits • Other signs include positive Romberg, diminished deep tendon reflexes, and wide-based gait • The SLR is positive only in a minority of patients **Diagnostics:** • MRI is the preferred modality • CT is preferred for bony anatomy • Nerve conduction studies can be considered when alternative etiologies are considered • Myelography is invasive but can be considered in patient whom MRI is contraindicated **Management:** Conservative measures including NSAIDs and physical therapy are usually sufficient. • Surgery is considered for progressive disease refractory to conservative treatment • If spondylolisthesis is absent, laminectomy without fusion, percutaneous decompression, or vertebral spacer can be performed • Laminectomy with fusion is considered if concomitant spondylolisthesis is present **Discussion:** Incidental findings of radiographic spinal stenosis without symptoms are relatively common. Conus medularis and cauda equina are rare complications but require immediate surgical intervention.

Compression Fracture from Osteoporosis	**Hx:** Inquire about history of trauma and osteoporosis.
	
	Osteoporosis causes compromised bone strength that increases the risk of fragility fractures even after minimal trauma. Low back pain is the hallmark symptom. Comorbidities that predispose to osteoporosis include:
	• Menopause (increase bone resorption secondary to decreased estrogen levels)
	• Medications
	  • Warfarin (prevents carboxylation of osteocalcin–> cannot incorporate calcium into bone)
	  • Glucocorticoids (increase bone turnover)
	  • Loop diuretics (renal calcium loss)
	  • Antiepileptic drugs, e.g., phenobarbital, phenytoin, carbamazepine (induce P450->increased vitamin D catabolism->increase PTH and bone resorption)
	  • Proton pump inhibitors (decreased gut absorption of calcium)
	  • Thiazolidinediones (decreased osteoblast formation)
	• Poor nutrition, ethanol, caffeine
	• Malabsorption syndromes, vitamin D deficiency
	• Hyperthyroidism
	
	PE:
	• Point tenderness of the dorsal vertebral processes
	• Posture may change to compensate for vertebral deformities resulting from height loss (kyphosis)
	
	Diagnostics:
	• Thoracolumbar films may show diffuse vertebral lucency, decreased cortical thickness (suggestive of osteopenia/osteoporosis), loss of anterior vertebral height, wedge-shaped deformity consistent with vertebral compression fracture
	• Dual-energy x-ray absorptiometry (DEXA) scanning measures bone mineral density, and it is used for diagnosis of osteopenia (T score –1 to –2.5) or osteoporosis (T score < –2.5).

Back Pain Mini-Cases *(continued)*

Compression Fracture from Osteoporosis	**Management:**
	• Pain control and physical therapy for mobility and strength rehabilitation.
	• Osteoporosis is treated with:
	  • Behavioral modifications (exercise, smoking cessation, moderation of ethanol and caffeine)
	  • Medications (calcium, vitamin D, bisphosphonates, teriparatide, selective estrogen receptor modulators [SERMs], denosumab
	
	Discussion: The cause of thoracolumbar compression fractures is most commonly osteoporosis. Osteoporosis is characterized by trabecular and cortical bone loss. As the osteoclastic activity exceeds osteoblastic activity, a generalized decrease in bone density occurs. Deformities resulting from height loss (kyphosis), can result in secondary pain in hips, sacroiliac (SI) joints, and spinal joints.

Cauda Equina Syndrome	**Hx:** Symptom onset can be gradual or sudden, with variable degrees of neurologic dysfunction depending on the involved nerve roots. Pain is usually the first symptom of root compression with radiation into one or both legs. Most of the patients have sensory and/or motor (usually weakness) findings at diagnosis. Bowel and/or bladder dysfunction are later findings. **PE:** • Muscle weakness • Sensory loss in a dermatomal distribution of the affected nerve roots (loss of all sensory modalities) • Anal sphincter paralysis **Diagnostics:** Emergent MRI is indicated **Discussion:** Cauda equina syndrome is a polyradiculopathy resulting from injury to two or more of the 18 nerve roots constituting the cauda equina that are caudal to the conus. Herniation of the intervertebral disc is the most common cause of cauda equina syndrome. Other causes include ankylosing spondylitis, lumbar puncture, trauma, malignant tumor, and infection. Any patient with symptoms of saddle anesthesia, loss of bowel or bladder control, and/or bilateral lower extremity weakness or should undergo immediate imaging and surgical consultation for decompression and intervention to improve outcome.
Mechanical Low Back Pain (Lumbar Strain)	**Hx:** Can sometimes be precipitated by heavy lifting or another source of musculoskeletal stress. Will report non-radiating lower back pain and which can be accompanied by pain and stiffness in buttocks or hips. **PE:** The lower back may be tender to the touch, or spasms in the paraspinal muscles may be palpable. **Diagnostics:** Clinical diagnosis **Management:** • NSAIDs, acetaminophen, muscle relaxants, heat, and early mobility. • Bed rest provides no additional benefit and may prolong pain and recovery times. **Discussion:** Lower back pain is one of the most common causes for office visits in the United States and is commonly due to mechanical causes such as musculoskeletal strain. If there are no red flags, diagnosis can be made clinically and does not require further imaging or testing. Identifying anatomical abnormalities on imaging does not improve clinical outcomes especially in patients with <12 weeks of pain.
Ankylosing Spondylitis (AS)	**Hx:** Gradual-onset back pain that is worse at night and with rest. Morning stiffness (lasting >30 minutes). Stiffness and pain improve through the day, with physical activity and with NSAIDs. It affects men three times more than women, and is seen between ages 15–40 years. Risk factors include family history of AS, Crohn's, or other spondyloarthropathies. **PE:** Decreased range of motion in the back (limited lumbar flexion). Tenderness over SI joints, and possible pain upon external rotation of the hip joints. Stooped posture indicates advanced AS. Other findings can be remembered using the mnemonic **ANKSpOND:** • **A**ortic insufficiency • **N**eurologic (atlantoaxial dislocation, cauda equina syndrome) • **K**idney injury (secondary amyloid) • **Sp**inal fracture, stenosis • **O**cular: anterior uveitis • **N**ephropathy (IgA) • **D**actylitis 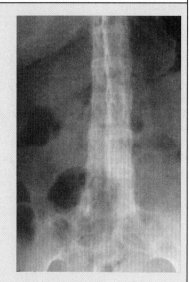 Reproduced with permission from Michael Y.M. Chen, Thomas L. Pope, David J. Ott, Basic Radiology, 2e. New York: McGraw Hill 2011.

Back Pain Mini-Cases *(continued)*

Ankylosing Spondylitis (AS)	**Diagnostics:** • Recognition of the pattern of clinical, laboratory, and imaging findings. • Radiography shows progressive changes characteristic of AS (squaring of the vertebral bodies, syndesmophytes, ankylosis of the facet joints). • ESR and CRP elevated • HLA-B27 (+) in 90% of white individuals with AS, yet it is NOT a diagnostic or prognostic tool. **Management:** Goal is to control symptoms, improve function and prevent structural damage with physical therapy and NSAIDs. If symptoms continue, add TNF or interleukin-17 inhibitors. Glucocorticoids are not effective. **Discussion:** Spondyloarthropathy is a chronic, multisystem inflammatory disorder involving the spine and SI joints. This term covers patients with both radiographic and non-radiographic axial spondylarthritis. It is strongly associated with the HLA-B27 gene. Fusion of the spine in severe AS can lead to restricted chest expansion.

BONE AND CARTILAGE DISORDERS

- The two most tested disorders are osteoarthritis (OA) and Paget's disease.
- OA is the most common type of arthritis caused by progressive damage to articular cartilage
- It is important to differentiate OA from RA as they differ in epidemiology, joint distribution, radiographic findings, and treatment.
- Synovial fluid analysis is very helpful to differentiate various causes of arthritis.

Synovial Fluid Analysis

Characteristic	Normal	Noninflammatory	Inflammatory	Septic	Hemorrhagic
WBC count	<200/mm³	<2000/mm³	2000–50,000/mm³	>50,000/mm³	Variable
PMN leukocyte percentage	<25	<25	>50	>75	50–75
Clarity	Transparent	Transparent	Transparent to opaque	Opaque	Bloody
Color	Clear to yellow	Clear to yellow	Yellow or white	Yellow or white	Red
Clinical associations (examples)		Osteoarthritis Trauma Osteonecrosis	RA SLE Crystalline	Septic arthritis	Trauma TB Coagulopathy Neoplasia PVNS

PMN, polymorphonuclear; PVNS, pigmented villonodular synovitis; RA, rheumatoid arthritis; SLE, systemic lupus erythematosus; TB, tuberculosis; WBC, white blood cell

Reproduced with permission from JB.Imboden, DB. Hellmann, JA. Stone, Current Diagnosis and Treatment in Rheumatology, 4e; NY: McGraw Hill, 2020.

Interpretation of Synovial Fluid

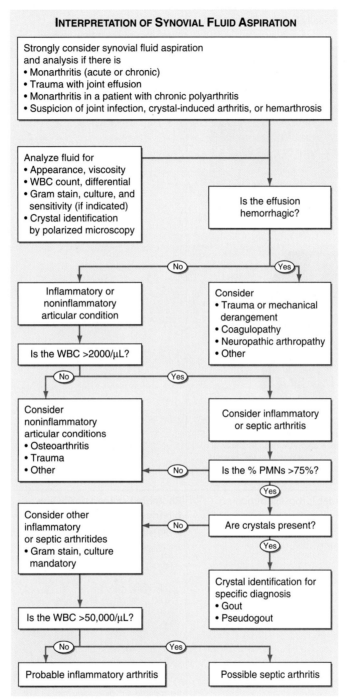

INTERPRETATION OF SYNOVIAL FLUID ASPIRATION

Strongly consider synovial fluid aspiration
and analysis if there is
• Monarthritis (acute or chronic)
• Trauma with joint effusion
• Monarthritis in a patient with chronic polyarthritis
• Suspicion of joint infection, crystal-induced arthritis, or hemarthrosis

Analyze fluid for
• Appearance, viscosity
• WBC count, differential
• Gram stain, culture, and
  sensitivity (if indicated)
• Crystal identification
  by polarized microscopy

Is the effusion hemorrhagic?

No → Inflammatory or noninflammatory articular condition

Yes → Consider
• Trauma or mechanical derangement
• Coagulopathy
• Neuropathic arthropathy
• Other

Is the WBC >2000/µL?

No → Consider noninflammatory articular conditions
• Osteoarthritis
• Trauma
• Other

Yes → Consider inflammatory or septic arthritis

Is the % PMNs >75%?

No → Consider noninflammatory articular conditions
• Osteoarthritis
• Trauma
• Other

Yes → Are crystals present?

No → Consider other inflammatory or septic arthritides
• Gram stain, culture mandatory

Yes → Crystal identification for specific diagnosis
• Gout
• Pseudogout

Is the WBC >50,000/µL?

No → Probable inflammatory arthritis

Yes → Possible septic arthritis

GOUT AND PSEUDOGOUT

Gout and calcium pyrophosphate deposition disease (CPPD, or pseudogout) are arthropathies associated with deposition of insoluble compounds creating crystals inside of joint spaces. Both diseases have a similar pathophysiology, and can be differentiated by joint distribution, radiological features, and synovial fluid analysis.

Diagnosis	History and Exam	Synovial Fluid	X-Ray
Gout	Smaller joints—usually first toe. Tophi often present 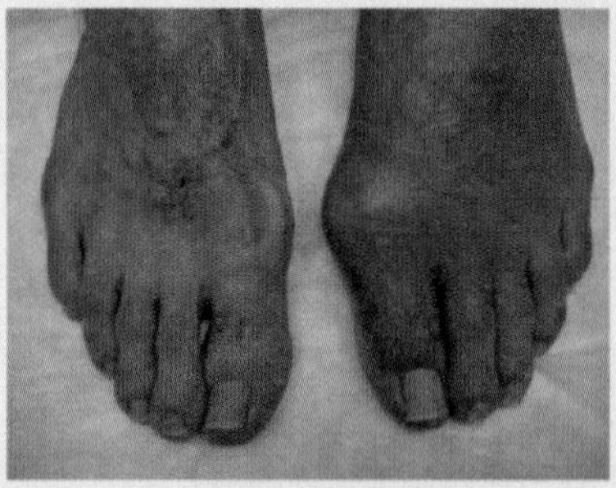 From Manish Suneja, joseph F. Szot, Richard F. LeBlond, Donald D. Brown: DeGowin's Diagnostic Examination, 11e; McGraw Hill 2020. 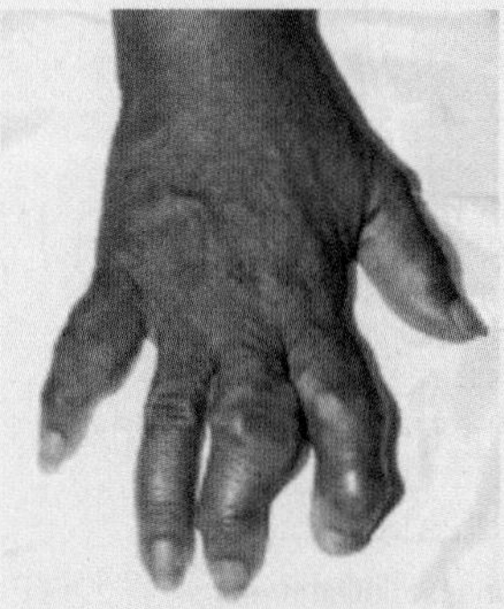 Chronic tophi (From Kevin J. Knoop, Lawrence B. Stack, Alan B. Storrow, R. Jason Thurman, The Atlas of Emergency Medicine, 5e. New York:2021 McGraw Hill. FIGURE 26.2. ISBN 9781260134940. Photo contributor: Kevin J. Knoop, MD, MS.)	Needle-shaped negatively birefringent crystals—yellow under polarized light microscopy	Erosive arthropathy, large tophi (stars) and erosions with overhanging edges (arrows) 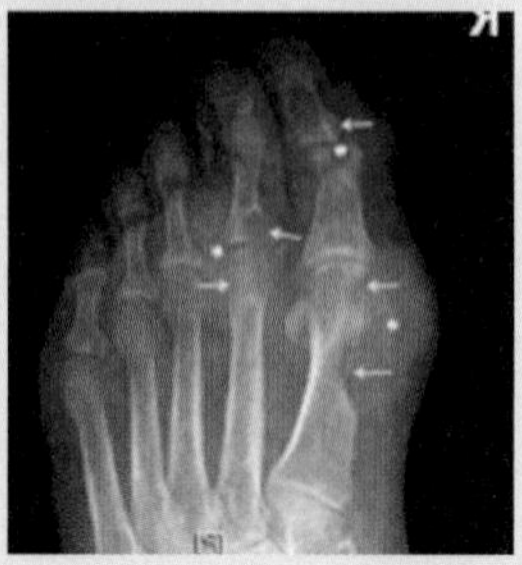 Reproduced with permission from Sylvia C. McKean, John J. Ross, Daniel D. Dressler, Danielle B. Scheurer, Principles and Practice of Hospital Medicine, 2e; McGraw-Hill 2017.
Pseudogout	Larger joints—knee is most common	Rhomboid-shaped positively birefringent crystals—blue under polarized light microscopy 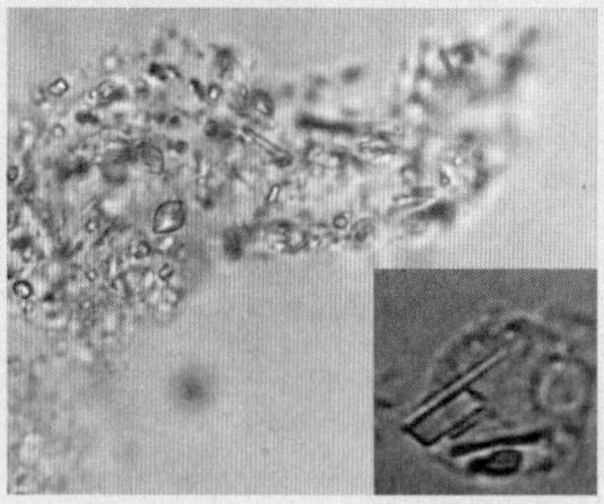 Reproduced with permission from J. Larry Jameson, Anthony S. Fauci, Dennis L. Kasper, Stephen L. Hauser, Dan L. Longo, Joseph Loscalzo, Harrison's Principles of Internal Medicine, 20e; McGraw-Hill 2018.	Linear deposition of CPPD in the meniscus (arrows) 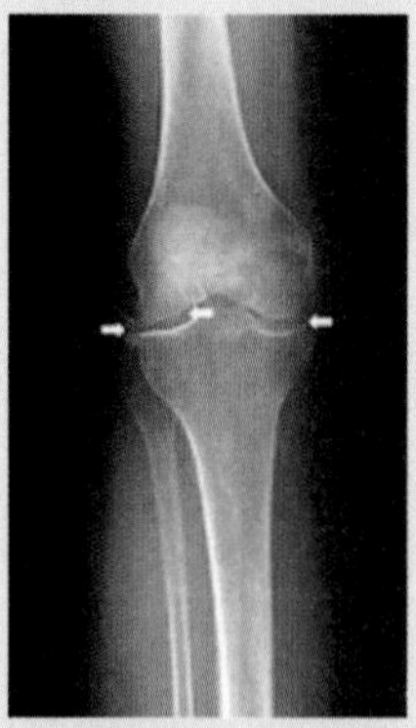 Reproduced with permission from Sylvia C. McKean, John J. Ross, Daniel D. Dressler, Danielle B. Scheurer, Principles and Practice of Hospital Medicine, 2e; McGraw-Hill 2017.

CASE 8 | Gout

A 55-year-old man is started on chemotherapy for Burkitt lymphoma and develops severe right big toe pain and swelling. On exam, his left first MTP joint is erythematous, swollen, warm, and very tender to touch (podagra).

Conditions with Similar Presentations	**Septic arthritis:** Arthrocentesis findings include markedly elevated WBC with predominant neutrophils and positive Gram stain and cultures. **Pseudogout:** Joint aspiration analysis will show rhomboid, positive birefringent crystals.
Initial Diagnostic Tests	Joint aspiration and examination for crystals
Next Steps in Management	High-dose NSAIDs (indomethacin), colchicine, or glucocorticoids (intraarticular or systemic)

Discussion	Gout is caused by deposition of monosodium urate crystals in tissues. Hyperuricemia can occur due to the under secretion of uric acid (most cases), worsened by renal failure or certain medications (thiazides, loop diuretics) or due to overproduction (Lesch-Nyhan syndrome, tumor lysis syndrome, hemolytic anemia).
	
	History: Seen among adult men and postmenopausal women and presents with recurrent attacks of monoarthritis (less frequently, oligoarticular arthritis), and symptoms peak within a day.
	
	Potential triggers: Purine-rich meals (shellfish, red meats), alcohol, high fructose corn syrup–containing drinks, certain medications, or serious medical illnesses.
	
	Risk factors include metabolic syndrome, renal failure, and a family history of gout.
	
	Physical Exam: Joints erythematous, warm, extremely tender to palpation, and swollen.
	• First metatarsophalangeal (MTP) joint most affected, but any joint can be involved.
	• Chronic gout leads to formation of tophi (urate crystal deposition in soft tissues). Can be seen in the joints, external ear, olecranon bursa, and Achilles tendon.
	
	Diagnostics: Joint aspiration will show needle-shaped monosodium urate crystals that are **negatively** birefringent under polarized light.
	• Synovial fluid white count elevated to 2,000–60,000 leukocytes/mm^3
	• Radiography shows soft tissue swelling during an acute gout attack; tophi and erosions with sclerotic margins seen in advanced disease
	• Serum uric acid is not useful in the diagnosis because elevation occurs without gout, and during gout it may be normal
	
	Management:
	• Acute treatment includes high-dose NSAIDs (indomethacin), colchicine, or glucocorticoids, systemic or intraarticular.
	• Lifestyle modifications: limiting alcohol consumption and intake of purines (shellfish, red meat), weight loss
	• For frequent attacks, colchicine may be given prophylactically
	• Long-term urate-lowering therapy indicated for the following patients
	  • One or more subcutaneous tophi
	  • Radiographic damage attributable to gout
	  • Frequent gout flares (>2/year)
	  • First flare and chronic kidney disease stage >3, serum uric acid >9 mg/dL, or kidney stones
	• Options to lower uric acid include xanthine oxidase inhibitors (allopurinol or febuxostat) or probenecid

Additional Considerations	**Complications:** Over time, gout can cause bone erosions and cartilage loss leading to joint destruction. **Conditions associated with hyperuricemia:** • Nephrolithiasis: Uric acid stones can form and are radiolucent on x-ray. Low urinary pH predisposes to their formation • Urate nephropathy

Arthritis Mini-Cases

Calcium Pyrophosphate Deposition Disease (CPPD)	**Hx:** Painful monoarticular inflammatory arthritis (less commonly oligoarthropathy, usually self-limiting. Knee joint is most commonly affected but may occur in joints affected by OA and trauma. Attacks can be acute or subacute and age of onset usually >65 years old. Chronic CPPD presents with stiffness, and patients may also have associated systemic disorders such as hemochromatosis and hyperparathyroidism. **PE:** Tenderness, swelling and warmth of the joint; limited range of motion in chronic CPPD. **Diagnostics:** Synovial fluid is diagnostic: **positively** birefringent rhomboid crystals. • X-ray may show linear calcification of the cartilage • Hook-like osteophytes in the second and third metacarpophalangeal (MCP) joints can be seen in patients with hemochromatosis-associated CPPD disease **Management:** • If multiple joints involved, NSAIDs or colchicine (for frequent attacks, colchicine can be given prophylactically). • Arthrocentesis and intra-articular steroids (after septic arthritis ruled out) **Discussion:** Also known as pseudogout, as acute episodes can mimic gout. More likely than gout to affect larger joints such as knee, shoulder, hip, and wrist. Chronic CPPD can mimic RA (morning stiffness and limited range of motion).
Septic Arthritis	**Hx:** Painful, acute monoarticular arthritis (can be oligo or polyarticular in disseminated gonococcal or Lyme disease but is less common). Most affected joint is the knee. **PE:** Joints are painful, swollen, erythematous, and warm. **Diagnostics:** Arthrocentesis is the gold standard (check synovial fluid for culture, Gram stain, and cell counts). **Management:** Arthrocentesis is both diagnostic and therapeutic. Management consists of both joint drainage and antibiotic treatment. Antibiotics should be started empirically and should cover the most likely pathogens. **Discussion:** Septic arthritis is most caused by bacteria (less commonly fungi and viruses) and is often destructive to the joint. Predisposing factors include pre-existing joint disease (like RA), age, injection drug use, recent surgery or intraarticular joint injection, trauma, adjacent infection such as skin or soft tissue infection, and immunosuppression. Most septic joints develop because of hematogenous seeding.
Osteoarthritis (OA)	**Hx:** Pain often dull and aggravated with use. Located in DIP and PIP joints, the first carpometacarpal (CMC) of the hand, the spine, and weight-bearing joints of the lower extremity. Morning stiffness <30 minutes and stiffness after prolonged immobility (gelling phenomenon). Risk factors: Older age, obesity, previous joint trauma, and family history. **PE:** Crepitus, decreased range of motion, bony enlargement, Heberden (DIP) and Bouchard (PIP) nodes. **Diagnostics:** Clinical diagnosis. • Inflammatory markers normal and synovial fluid is noninflammatory (WBC <2000 cells/mm³) • Radiographs show joint space narrowing, osteophytes, subchondral cysts, and sclerosis 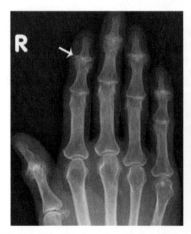 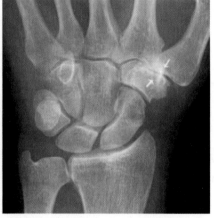 Osteoarthritis. PA view of the right hand in a 73-year-old female shows osteophyte formation and joint narrowing predominantly at the distal interphalangeal joints with "gull-wing" appearance (arrow). Osteoarthritis. PA view of the left hand in a 65-year-old male shows osteophyte formation, joint space narrowing and subchondral sclerosis (arrows) at the first carpometacarpal joint, a favored site of primary osteoarthritis. (Reproduced with permission from Jamshid Tehranzadeh. Basic Musculoskeletal Imaging, 2e; McGraw Hill LLC 2021.)

Arthritis Mini-Cases *(continued)*

Osteoarthritis (OA)	**Management:** • Lifestyle modification (exercise, weight loss) • Physical/occupational therapy • Acetaminophen, topical NSAIDs, duloxetine, and intraarticular steroids for symptomatic relief • Arthroplasty or surgical joint replacement is an option for patients with advanced knee and hip osteoarthritis who cannot tolerate the pain and/or lifestyle limitations of the joint disease **Discussion:** Most common form of arthritis. Slowly progressive degradation of cartilage due to trauma.

CASE 9 | Paget's Disease of Bone

A 65-year-old man presents with right hip pain for the past 6 months. Initially it was intermittently achy but has progressively worsened, is present at rest and with activity, and is worse at night. He also notes headache, hearing loss, and thinks his head has become larger because his hat size has increased. Exam reveals decreased range of motion of the right hip and warmth on the lateral aspect of the proximal thigh. Reduced hearing is noted bilaterally to finger rub.

Conditions with Similar Presentations	**Metastatic disease:** Presents with either lytic or sclerotic lesions (depending on tumor type), more likely to present with new lesions over time **Primary osteosarcoma:** Presents with localized bone pain and overlying soft tissue swelling without the diffuse bone remodeling seen with Paget's disease **Osteomalacia:** Characterized by bone pain without radiographic lytic and sclerotic lesions seen in Paget's disease of bone **OA:** Degenerative disease characterized by joint pain with loss of articular cartilage but would not have elevated alkaline phosphatase levels. **Greater trochanteric pain syndrome (bursitis):** Would have point tenderness over the greater trochanter.
Initial Diagnostic Tests	Check X-ray of the affected area and alkaline phosphatase level
Next Steps in Management	Bisphosphonates
Discussion	Paget's disease is a disorder of bone metabolism marked by accelerated bone turnover resulting in thickened/enlarged bone but with weakened bone strength. Patients are at higher risk of primary bone tumors, specifically osteosarcoma. It is more common in men over the age of 55. **History:** • Often asymptomatic, and an incidental finding • Symptoms depend on site and extent of disease involvement but include pain, warmth, and fracture at sites involved • Commonly involved bones include the skull, spine, pelvis, and long bones of the lower extremity • May have headaches, and narrowing of cranial nerve canals can lead to deafness by impingement on the internal acoustic meatus **Physical Exam:** Bony deformities such as bowing of legs, skull enlargement, and spinal kyphosis. **Diagnostics:** • X-ray of the affected area—mixed lytic/sclerotic lesions with candle flame sign (area of lucency with a V-shaped area of bone destruction extending out of it) • Alkaline phosphatase elevated unless only one site involved • Radionuclide bone scan more sensitive in early disease, can show focal areas of increased uptake due to new bone formation **Management:** • Bisphosphonates (slows bone remodeling and prevents complications such as fracture and OA). IV bisphosphonate if involving weight-bearing sites and the skull. • Denosumab or calcitonin if bisphosphonates are not effective or tolerated.
Additional Considerations	**Complications:** • Fracture and OA are the most common complications • Increased risk of primary bone neoplasms, most commonly osteosarcoma • Hypercalciuria may lead to kidney stones and renal injury

CONNECTIVE TISSUE DISEASES

Connective tissue diseases are a common cause of joint pain and are often autoimmune in nature.

- Can affect the bones, joints, muscles, skin, blood vessels, tendons, ligaments, and other connective tissues.
- Pattern recognition helps to differentiate these disorders, as each will present with a different constellation of symptoms and exam findings.

Key Feature(s) or Associated Symptom(s)	Diagnosis
White, blue, then red color changes in digits precipitated by cold or stress Reproduced with permission from J. Larry Jameson, Anthony S. Fauci, Dennis L. Kasper, Stephen L. Hauser, Dan L. Longo, Joseph Loscalzo, Harrison's Principles of Internal Medicine, 20e; McGraw Hill LLC 2018.	**Raynaud syndrome**
Woman over 50 with progressively worsening bilateral shoulder/hip pain and stiffness and elevated ESR	**Polymyalgia rheumatica** (PMR)
Woman over 50 with PMR, temporal headache with visual loss, jaw claudication, scalp tenderness, tender temporal artery, and elevated ESR	**Giant cell arteritis**
Heliotrope and malar rash (involving nasolabial folds) Heliotrope eruption of dermatomyositis. (From Michael A. Grippi, Jack A. Elias, Jay A. Fishman, Robert M. Kotloff, Allan I Pack, Robert M. Senior, Mark D. Siegel: Fishman's Pulmonary Diseases and Disorders, 5e; by McGraw Hill 2015.) A. Macular erythema plaques (Gottron sign) and erythematous papules (Gottron papules) on extensor surface of fingers and B. elbow. C. Macular erythema plaques over anterior neck and chest (V-sign) and D. the posterior neck, shoulder and upper back (Shawl sign). E. Nail bed changes with dilated capillaries. (Reproduced with permission from J. Larry Jameson, Anthony S. Fauci, Dennis L. Kasper, Stephen L. Hauser, Dan L. Longo, Joseph Loscalzo, Harrison's Principles of Internal Medicine, 20e; McGraw Hill LLC 2018.)	**Dermatomyositis**
Proximal muscle weakness, worsened with repetitive muscle use. Difficulty keeping eyes open, and double vision	**Myasthenia gravis**
History of small cell lung cancer with proximal muscle weakness, diminished or absent reflexes and autonomic symptoms (orthostatic hypotension, dry mouth, erectile dysfunction). Weakness improves with repetitive muscle use	**Lambert-Eaton syndrome**

Key Feature(s) or Associated Symptom(s)		Diagnosis
Sicca (dry eyes and mouth), red fissured tongue with atrophy of papillae	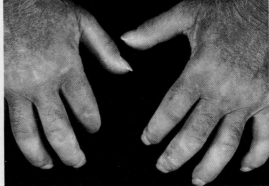	**Sjogren syndrome**
Reproduced with permission from Sewon Kang, Masayuki Amagai, Anna L. Bruckner, Alexander H. Enk, David J. Margolis, Amy J. McMichael, Jeffrey S. Orringer, Fitzpatrick's Dermatology, 9e; McGraw-Hill 2019.		
Calcinosis cutis, **R**aynaud phenomenon, **E**sophageal dysmotility, **S**clerodactyly, and **T**elangiectasias Acral sclerosis and digital ulcers shown Reproduced with permission from J. Larry Jameson, Anthony S. Fauci, Dennis L. Kasper, Stephen L. Hauser, Dan L. Longo, Joseph Loscalzo, Harrison's Principles of Internal Medicine, 20e; McGraw Hill LLC 2018.	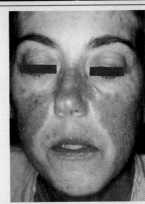	**Scleroderma** (systemic sclerosis, CREST syndrome)
Female of child-bearing age with malar rash (sparing the nasolabial fold), oral ulcers, arthritis, multiple affected organs, cytopenias, and +ANA Lupus erythematosus. A. Systemic lupus erythematosus, with prominent, scaly malar erythema. Involvement of other sun-exposed sites is also common. (Reproduced with permission from J. Larry Jameson, Anthony S. Fauci, Dennis L. Kasper, Stephen L. Hauser, Dan L. Longo, Joseph Loscalzo, Harrison's Principles of Internal Medicine, 20e; McGraw Hill LLC 2018.)		**Systemic lupus erythematosus** (SLE)
Dyspnea/cough and systemic symptoms, uveitis, erythema nodosum, and hilar adenopathy Lupus pernio (chronic inflammatory lesions around nose and eyes) Reproduced with permission from J. Larry Jameson, Anthony S. Fauci, Dennis L. Kasper, Stephen L. Hauser, Dan L. Longo, Joseph Loscalzo, Harrison's Principles of Internal Medicine, 20e; McGraw Hill LLC 2018.	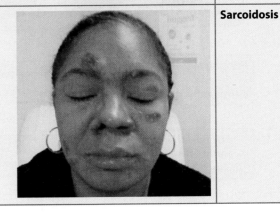	**Sarcoidosis**

Approach to Laboratory Diagnosis of Connective Tissue Disorders

The clinical features of the disease, the morphologic pattern of the ANA test, and the serum titer of the positive ANA test are established.

If the ANA is positive, the pattern of staining suggests the differential diagnosis. The results of specific antinuclear antibody tests often establish the diagnosis.
A negative ANA test can occur in rheumatoid arthritis, inflammatory muscle diseases, and when there are connective tissue manifestations in patients with selected chronic infectious diseases.

The following is an algorithm for the serologic evaluation of autoimmune connective tissue diseases.

If diagnosis is unknown and the ANA is positive, the following test panel is useful:
(a) anti-ds DNA
(b) anti-SS-A (Ro)
(c) anti-SS-B (La)
(d) anti-Sm
(e) anti-U1 RNP
(f) anti-Jo-1
(g) anti-Scl-70

For SLE →
(a) If the ANA is negative, test for anti-SS-A (Ro)
(b) If the ANA is positive, tests for anti-ds DNA, anti-SS-A (Ro), anti-SS-B (La), anti-Sm and, anti-U1 RNP are informative. Anti-ds DNA titers are useful to monitor disease activity.

For Sjogren syndrome →
(a) A positive ANA is supported by positive test results for anti-SS-A (Ro) and anti SS-B (La).

For polymyositis and dermatomyositis →
(a) A positive ANA is supported by a positive anti-Jo-1 test result.

For mixed connective tissue disease →
(a) A positive ANA is supported by a positive result for anti-U1RNP.

For Scleroderma →
(a) If the ANA pattern is the speckled or centromeric, anti-Scl-70 (anti-topoisomerase 1) provides additional diagnostic confirmation.

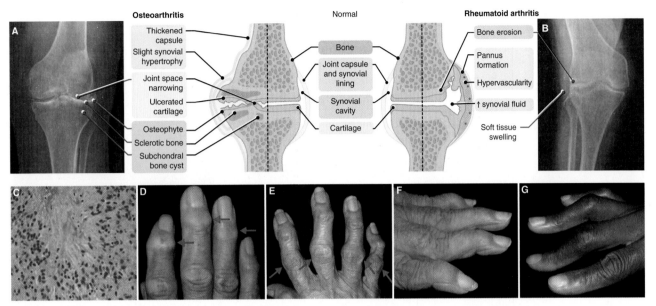

Differences between osteoarthritis and rheumatoid arthritis. (Reproduced with permission from Le, Tao; Bhushan, Vikas; and Sochat, Matthew. First Aid for the USMLE Step 1 2021. New York: McGraw-Hill 2021.)

CASE 10 | Rheumatoid Arthritis (RA)

A 35-year-old bus driver presents with worsening joint pain in bilateral hands, wrists, ankles, and knees for over 4 months. She has morning joint stiffness that lasts approximately 90 minutes. The pain makes it difficult for her to drive but gets better throughout the day. On exam there is swelling, and tenderness of the MCP and PIP joints of the hands as well as the MTP and PIP of the feet.

Conditions with Similar Presentations	**OA:** Has DIP and PIP involvement, while RA spares the DIPs. Pain is in weight-bearing joints after use and improves with rest. X-ray shows osteophytes, joint space narrowing, and subchondral sclerosis.
	Psoriatic arthritis: Can involve DIPs, in addition to skin and nail abnormalities.
	Gout and pseudogout: Typically, monoarticular and acute onset
Initial Diagnostic Tests	Check rheumatoid factor (RF), anti-citrullinated protein antibody (ACPA) and bilateral hand x-rays
Next Steps in Management	• NSAIDs and disease-modifying antirheumatic drugs (DMARDs) with methotrexate as initial choice. • Glucocorticoids for flares, but do not decrease disease progression
Discussion	RA is an autoimmune chronic, systemic inflammatory arthritis with synovial inflammation and proliferation. This leads to synovial hypertrophy and pannus formation. Pannus formation injures bone, cartilage, and tendon, leading to joint destruction, damage, and deformities. There is some association with smoking and major histocompatibility complex (MHC) region coding for certain HLA-DR genes. **History:** • **Symmetric** polyarticular involvement (>3 joints) for ≥ 6 weeks • Morning stiffness (>60 minutes) that improves with activity • Systemic symptoms: fatigue, weight loss, and fevers **Physical Exam:** • Swollen and warm joints • Constitutional symptoms • Joint deformities: swan neck, ulnar deviation, and Boutonniere deformities • Rheumatoid nodules (nontender, firm, subcutaneous)

CASE 10 | Rheumatoid Arthritis (RA) *(continued)*

Discussion	**Diagnostics:**
	• RF and ACPAs positive (10–20% of patients seronegative). ACPA is more specific than RF. • Bilateral hand x-rays may show periarticular osteopenia, marginal erosions, and joint space narrowing. • Normocytic, normochromic anemia, elevated erythrocyte sedimentation rate and C-reactive protein • Synovial fluid inflammatory (WBC 2,000–50,000) **Management:** • NSAIDs and DMARDs (e.g., methotrexate, sulfasalazine, hydroxychloroquine) • Addition of TNF-alpha inhibitors and other biologic agents used for severe cases • Steroids used for short-term relief for acute flares and until onset of action of DMARDs. They do not slow disease progression.

Hand x-ray shows symmetric erosions and joint space narrowing involving the MCP (arrow), carpal (arrowhead), and radioulnar (curved arrow) joints. Ulnar deviation at the MCP joint is also noted. (Reproduced with permission from Le, Tao and Bhushan, Vikas. First Aid for the USMLE Step 2 CK, Tenth Edition. New York: McGraw-Hill Education, 2018. FIGURE2.9-7B. Pg 266. ISBN: 9781260440300., Reproduced with permission from Wolff K, et al. Fitzpatrick's Dermatology in General Medicine, 7th ed. New York,NY: McGraw-Hill; 2008.)

Additional Considerations	**Complications:** **Atlantoaxial Subluxation:** Occurs due to inflammation of ligaments of the atlantoaxial and intervertebral joints and can compress spinal cord and become life-threatening. Obtain cervical spine radiographs prior to procedures that require intubation (necessitating neck hyperextension) **Extra-Articular Manifestations:** Constitutional symptoms, lymphadenopathy, pericarditis, atherosclerosis, pleuritis, lung nodules, interstitial lung disease, amyloidosis, Sjogren syndrome, entrapment neuropathies, osteoporosis, episcleritis and scleritis. • **Caplan syndrome:** Pulmonary fibrosis or pneumoconiosis in RA patients who have inhaled dust (coal miners) or silica, • **Felty syndrome:** RA patients with splenomegaly and neutropenia. Other cytopenias may also be present.

Medications for Rheumatoid Arthritis

Diarrhea, nausea, and abdominal cramping are frequent side effects with many of these medications and are often a significant barrier to adherence. Most of these medications are used as maintenance therapies, as their long-term side effect profiles are preferable compared to steroids except for cyclophosphamide.

Medication	Mechanism	Mild Side Effects	Severe Side Effects	Other Comments
Methotrexate	Dihydrofolate reductase inhibitor; blocks purine synthesis	Nausea, diarrhea, stomatitis, AST/ALT elevation	Myelosuppression, hepatotoxicity, pulmonary fibrosis, renal toxicity at high doses; teratogenic	Monitor CBC, AST/ALT, creatinine Folate reduces side effects
Leflunomide	Pyrimidine inhibition	Nausea, diarrhea, AST/ALT elevation; neuropathy, rash; hypertension	Myelosuppression, hepatotoxicity; teratogenic	Monitor CBC, AST/ALT, creatinine Cholestyramine can reduce side effects
Azathioprine	Purine synthesis inhibitor	Nausea, vomiting, diarrhea, myalgias	Myelosuppression, hepatotoxicity, relative contraindication in pregnancy	Allopurinol and febuxostat require dose adjustments with azathioprine

Medication	Mechanism	Mild Side Effects	Severe Side Effects	Other Comments
Hydroxychloroquine	Anti-inflammatory; modulation of innate immunity	Nausea, vision changes from corneal deposits, rash	Retinopathy; mild QTc prolongation, safe in pregnancy	Monitor with routine eye exams
Mycophenolate mofetil	Inosine monophosphate inhibition (purine synthesis)	Nausea, diarrhea, headache, hypertension	Myelosuppression, lymphoma; teratogenic	Monitor CBC for cytopenia
Sulfasalazine	Unclear, likely via NF-κB	Rash, headache, nausea (less than others), mild ALT/AST elevation	Agranulocytosis, rare hepatotoxicity	Routine CBC and AST/ALT monitoring
Cyclophosphamide	Alkylation of DNA	Nausea, vomiting, abdominal pain, stomatitis, alopecia	Cytopenia, lymphoma, bladder cancer, hemorrhagic cystitis, SIADH, and infertility; rare hepatotoxicity and pulmonary fibrosis; teratogenic	Rarely indicated for autoimmune disease; screen for tuberculosis, hepatitis B and C; routine ALT/AST, albumin, creatinine, CBC

Biologics

The biologic agents in the table below have other indications outside of RA. All patients should be screened for tuberculosis, hepatitis B, and hepatitis C before starting a biologic agent. Rituximab is the biologic most safe to use in patients with tuberculosis.

Class	Medications	Significant Side Effects
Anti-TNF	Etanercept, infliximab,* adalimumab, golimumab*	Infection, including tuberculosis (TB) and hepatitis B reactivation; neutropenia, (rare) heart failure
T-cell co-stimulation (CTLA-4) blocking	Abatacept*	Potential lymphoma; infection including potential reactivation of hepatitis B and TB
IL-1 receptor antagonist	Anakinra	Infection with theoretical risk of TB and hepatitis B reactivation; rare liver toxicity
Anti-IL-6	Tocilizumab, sarilumab	Infection including reactivation of TB and hepatitis B; rare liver toxicity; rare demyelination
JAK inhibitors	Tofactinib, baricitinib, upadacitinib	Infection including reactivation of TB and hepatitis B
Anti-CD20 (B-cell)	Rituximab*	(Safe in TB patients); infection including reactivation of TB, hepatitis B, and BK virus (which can cause progressive multifocal leukoencephalopathy); hypogammaglobulinemia

*IV infusion carries the potential for severe infusion reaction.

CASE 11 | Systemic Lupus Erythematosus (SLE)

A 25-year-old woman presents with headaches, fatigue, and pain in her bilateral hands and knees for a few months. She has noticed her fingers turn blue when she goes out in the cold. On exam, her vital signs are normal, there is an erythematous rash on her cheeks and nose with sparing of the nasolabial fold, along with mild swelling and tenderness of the knees, MCP and PIP joints of the hands bilaterally.

Conditions with Similar Presentations	**Dermatomyositis:** Characterized by proximal muscle weakness and a facial rash that can include and extend beyond the nasolabial folds. May also have rashes in other areas (around eyes, neck, chest, hands).
	Autoimmune hepatitis: Young women mostly affected and can present with polyarthritis, rash, constitutional symptoms, and a positive antinuclear antibody (ANA) (mimicking SLE). Liver manifestations may include acute hepatitis, cirrhosis, and liver failure. Anti-smooth muscle antibodies are positive in two-thirds of patients.
	RA: Symmetrical arthritis that is more likely to be erosive when compared to SLE. Extra-articular manifestations include rheumatoid nodules, serositis, and constitutional symptoms. RF and ANA may be positive in RA patients, but anti-CCP antibodies are more specific.

CASE 11 | Systemic Lupus Erythematosus (SLE) *(continued)*

Initial Diagnostic Tests	• Clinical diagnosis, confirm with ANA, anti-dsDNA (specific and correlates with disease activity), anti-Smith antibodies (specific) • CBC to look for cytopenias • CMP to assess liver and kidney involvement
Next Steps in Management	• Hydroxychloroquine or chloroquine are initial treatments • If there is organ involvement, steroids and other immunosuppressives (e.g., methotrexate azathioprine, mycophenolate) are added.
Discussion	SLE is a chronic multisystem autoimmune disease with damage occurring mostly due to type III hypersensitivity reaction. Autoantibodies are produced and they deposit within the tissues of different organs and fix complement leading to systemic inflammation. Women of child-bearing age and those with genetic predisposition (HLA-DR2/DR3) are more likely to develop SLE. **History: "RASH OR PAIN"** mnemonic: • **R**ash (malar or discoid) • **A**rthritis (non-erosive, peripheral) • **S**erositis (pleuritis and pericarditis) • **H**emolytic disorders (immune cytopenias: hemolytic anemia, leukopenia, lymphopenia, thrombocytopenia) • **O**ral/nasopharyngeal ulcers • **R**enal disorder (lupus nephritis) • **P**hotosensitivity • **A**NA • **I**mmunologic disorder (anti-DNA, anti-smith, or anti phospholipid) • **N**eurologic disorder (seizure or psychosis) • Other symptoms include fever, weight loss, fatigue, hair loss, and history of miscarriages **Physical Exam:** • Skin findings (malar rash sparing nasolabial folds, discoid rash, painless oral or nasopharyngeal ulcers) • Polyarticular arthritis, often symmetric, swan neck deformities • Decreased breath sounds or fine crackles (pleuritis, interstitial lung disease [ILD]) • Lower extremity edema and hypertension (nephritis) **Diagnostics:** At least four of 17 criteria from Systemic Lupus International Collaborating Clinics (SLICC): • Acute cutaneous lupus (malar rash) • Chronic cutaneous lupus (discoid rash with raised erythematous patches with scale) • Nonscarring alopecia • Oral or nasal ulcers • Joint disease • Serositis (pericardial or pleural effusions, pericardial rub, or pericarditis on ECG) • Renal involvement • Neurological involvement (seizures or psychosis) • Hemolytic anemia • Lymphopenia or leukopenia • Thrombocytopenia • ANA (sensitive, not specific) • Anti-dsDNA antibodies • Anti-Sm antibodies (specific, not sensitive) • Antiphospholipid antibodies • Low complement • Direct Coombs test positive Additional Findings: • Complement levels (C3, C4): often decreased • ESR: elevated • CRP: elevated • CBC: may show leukopenia, thrombocytopenia, or anemia (AIHA or anemia of chronic disease) • RPR and VDRL (for syphilis detection) may be falsely positive in patients with antiphospholipid antibodies

CASE 11 | Systemic Lupus Erythematosus (SLE) *(continued)*

Discussion	**Management:**
	• Lifestyle modifications and preventive measures (e.g., smoking cessation, avoidance of UV light, immunizations)
	• Hydroxychloroquine or chloroquine inhibit activation of Toll-like receptors, which decreases immune responsivity.
	• Steroids for acute exacerbations
	• Immunosuppressants for severe disease (azathioprine, mycophenolate, methotrexate)
	• B-cell-directed antibodies (rituximab, belimumab)
	• Specific treatments used for certain complications such as lupus nephritis (cyclophosphamide, mycophenolate mofetil)
	• Topical steroids for skin manifestations
	• NSAIDs for symptom relief
Additional Considerations	**Complications:** Cardiovascular disease (accelerated CAD), kidney disease, and infections are common causes of death in SLE.
	• **Libman-Sacks endocarditis:** Non-bacterial thrombotic endocarditis producing verrucous thrombi on the mitral or aortic valve on the undersurface of the valve.
	• **Lupus nephritis:** May present with nephrotic or nephritic findings (proteinuria or hematuria, respectively).
	• **Neuropsychiatric involvement:** Seizures, strokes, and psychosis.
	• **Antiphospholipid antibody (APLA) syndrome:** Associated with SLE but can occur independently. Should be considered in patients with arterial thrombosis, unprovoked venous thrombosis, thrombosis at unusual sites (e.g., renal vein thrombosis), recurrent fetal loss.
	• Lupus anticoagulant (LA), anticardiolipin antibodies (aCL abs), anti-β2 Glycoprotein I (anti-β2GPI) antibodies should be checked
	• INR and PT normal
	• aPTT may be elevated, due to presence of lupus anticoagulant
	• Treatment with lifelong anticoagulation indicated
	• **Neonatal lupus:** This is a rare acquired autoimmune congenital disorder. Affected infants of mothers who are positive for anti-SSA/Ro and/or anti-SSB/La antibodies often develop a characteristic red rash or skin eruption. They can also develop transaminitis or cytopenias at birth. The most significant potential complication is congenital heart block. Hydroxychloroquine should be given to pregnant women who have positive SSA/SSB, as it helps prevent neonatal lupus.

Connective Tissue Disease Mini-Cases

Drug-Induced Lupus Erythematosus (DILE)	**Hx:** Symptoms include arthralgias, myalgias, rash, constitutional symptoms. History of exposure to drugs associated with DILE (e.g., methyldopa, sulfa drugs, hydralazine, isoniazid, procainamide, phenytoin, etanercept, minocycline).
	PE: Similar to SLE
	• Skin lesions (malar rash)
	• Arthritis
	• Less commonly, serositis
	Diagnostics: Positive ANA; **anti-histone** antibodies can be present (not specific to DILE and can be positive in SLE).
	Management: Discontinue offending drug.
	Discussion: Occurs few weeks to more than a year after exposure to causative drug. Affects men and women equally. Development of drug-induced autoantibodies more common than the development of DILE. Manifestations can range from no clinical symptoms to various presentations of DILE (often dependent on offending agent).
	• Overall prognosis good, and majority of symptoms resolve after stopping the medication
	• NSAIDs help with symptomatic relief
	• Steroids and immunosuppression considered in severe cases

Connective Tissue Disease Mini-Cases *(continued)*

Sjogren Syndrome	**Hx: Sicca syndrome** (dry eyes and dry mouth). Dry eyes can manifest as itchiness, redness, or foreign body sensation in the eyes. Other symptoms include dyspareunia and extra glandular features: arthralgia, fatigue, difficulty swallowing, and Raynaud phenomenon. May have concurrent rheumatological condition.
	
	PE: Findings may include dry oral mucosa, absence of salivary pooling under the tongue, dental caries, parotid gland enlargement.
	
	Diagnostics:
	• Anti-SSA and/or anti-SSB antibodies may be positive.
	• Decreased tear and saliva production assessed by objective markers
	  • Schirmer test in either eye of <5 mm/5 minutes or abnormal ocular surface staining
	  • Dry mouth (sialometry)
	• Biopsy of minor salivary gland showing a chronic lymphocytic infiltrate is the gold standard but is not necessary for diagnosis
	
	Management:
	• Nonpharmacological measures: hydration, reducing caffeine intake, sugar-free gum, lozenges, artificial tears, and smoking cessation counseling
	• Pilocarpine or cevimeline (avoid in narrow-angle glaucoma, asthma and in patients on beta blockers)
	
	Discussion: Autoimmune disease resulting in lymphocytic infiltration of the salivary and lacrimal glands. Can also involve other glands and no glandular organs such as the lungs. It can be primary (idiopathic) or secondary to other rheumatic diseases such as RA, SLE, or systemic sclerosis.
	• Increased risk of lymphoma
	• Increased risk of neonatal lupus or congenital heart block if mother positive for anti-SSA and/or anti-SSB

Scleroderma (Systemic Sclerosis)	**Hx:** Symptoms include skin thickening proximal to the MCP joints, joint pain, fatigue, acid reflux, Raynaud phenomenon (white-≥blue–>red color changes in the digits precipitated by cold or stress), cough, dyspnea (ILD, pulmonary hypertension). **PE:** Findings may include skin thickening of the fingers (sclerodactyly), skin fibrosis proximal to MCP joints, digital ulceration, gangrene, calcinosis cutis, telangiectasias, microstomia (decreased ability to open mouth), crackles, and edema (if cardiac/pulmonary involvement). If a patient is actively experiencing vasospasm, there may be notable color change of the digits during the physical exam (digits may be white [ischemia], blue [hypoxia], or red [reperfusion]). **Diagnostics:** • ANA may be positive • **Anti-scl-70:** Associated with diffuse systemic sclerosis • **Anti-centromere antibody:** Associated with limited systemic sclerosis, formerly known as CREST syndrome (**C**alcinosis cutis, **R**aynaud phenomenon, **E**sophageal dysmotility, **S**clerodactyly, and **T**elangiectasias) **Management:** Tailored to the patient and the specific organ system involved • Proton pump inhibitors for gastroesophageal reflux disease • Calcium channel blockers for Raynaud phenomenon • Immunosuppressants for interstitial lung disease and cardiac disease **Discussion:** Autoimmune disease characterized by collagen deposition with fibrosis that affects the skin and other organs (lungs, kidneys, heart, and GI tract). Subtypes include limited and diffuse sclerosis, and both can cause organ involvement and life-threatening disease. **Diffuse sclerosis:** Skin thickening that extends proximal to the elbows or knees or with truncal involvement. Early onset of pulmonary disease and worse prognosis. **Limited sclerosis** (formerly known as CREST: Skin thickening limited to the neck, face, or distal to the elbows and knees. Less likely pulmonary involvement and better prognosis.

Connective Tissue Disease Mini-Cases *(continued)*

Dermatomyositis	**Hx:** Symptoms include bilateral, proximal muscle pain, weakness (shoulder and pelvic girdle muscles most involved), rash and dysphagia (if pharyngeal and upper esophageal muscles involved).
	PE: Dermatologic manifestations (see above table):
	• Heliotrope rash: erythematous/violaceous rash that affects the eyelids, malar region, forehead, and nasolabial folds
	• V-sign rash: confluent erythematous rash over the anterior chest and neck
	• Shawl-sign rash: erythematous rash over the shoulders and proximal arms
	• Gottron papules: erythematous to purple lesions over the dorsal surface of metacarpals and interphalangeal joints
	• Periungual telangiectasias
	• Calcinosis cutis
	• Malar rash involving nasolabial folds (spared in SLE)
	• Proximal muscle weakness and pain on palpation
	Diagnostics:
	• Creatinine kinase (CK), aldolase, lactate dehydrogenase (LDH), aspartate (AST) and alanine (ALT) aminotransferase, and myoglobin (myoglobinuria can be present in active disease)
	• EMG or MRI of the affected extremity to determine which group of muscles are affected and are appropriate for biopsy.
	• Muscle biopsy: shows perimysial/perivascular inflammation with or without perifascicular atrophy. Inflammatory infiltrate primarily shows CD4+ T cells.
	• Myositis-specific autoantibodies (MSA) help identify clinical subsets and aid in predicting extra muscular presentation, prognosis, and response to therapy
	• Anti-melanoma differentiation–associated gene 5 (MDA-5) is associated with ulceration and rapidly progressive interstitial lung disease
	• **Anti-Jo-1(histidyl tRNA synthetase)** is associated with myositis, rash, seronegative arthritis, Raynaud's, and fever (25%).
	• Anti-transcriptional intermediary factor 1gamma (anti-TIF-1gamma) -associated with increased risk of cancer
	Management: High-dose steroids followed by steroid-sparing agents (methotrexate, azathioprine, or mycophenolate mofetil).
	Discussion: Idiopathic inflammatory myopathy is associated with adenocarcinomas or hematologic malignancies (e.g., breast, lung, pancreas, stomach, colon, ovary, hematopoietic cancer, Hodgkin lymphoma).

CASE 12 | Polymyositis (PM)

A 52-year-old woman with no significant past medical history presents for progressive weakness and fatigue for the last 8 months. She initially had difficulty lifting heavy items onto high shelves and is now having difficulty raising her arms to comb her hair. Her temperature is 36.8, pulse is 78/min, respirations are 16/min, blood pressure is 132/76 mmHg, and SpO$_2$ is 97% on room air. On exam, she has difficulty getting up from her chair. Her grip strength is 5/5 bilaterally, but hip flexion and shoulder abduction are 3/5 bilaterally. Sensation is normal. No rashes or skin lesions are noticed. Reflexes are 2+ bilaterally. Her lab work reveals a creatine kinase (CK) of 1945 (nml <195).

Conditions with Similar Presentations	**Dermatomyositis (DM):** Proximal muscle weakness with skin involvement (e.g., heliotrope rash, Gottron papules, V and shawl sign).
	Inclusion body myositis: Proximal then distal muscle weakness. Much slower onset and often asymmetric. Men affected more than women as opposed to DM and PM. Only minor CK elevations and electromyogram (EMG) shows both myopathic and neuropathic features.
	Myasthenia gravis: Autoimmune neuromuscular disease that causes skeletal muscle weakness. Weakness worse with activity and improves after rest. Usually starts with blurred vision and ptosis. Antibodies against the acetylcholine receptors are positive in 85%, muscle-specific tyrosine kinase (MuSK) antibody positive in 5%.
	Polymyalgia rheumatica: Proximal limb stiffness and pain without weakness and is a precursor to giant cell arteritis (GCA). CK and EMG are normal. ESR and CRP are elevated.
	Hypothyroidism: May have generalized weakness, fatigue, dry skin but muscle enzymes are not elevated.
	Muscular dystrophies: Present at a younger age
	Statin-induced myopathy: Symptoms may be like inflammatory myopathies but would have history of statin use.

CASE 12 | Polymyositis (PM) *(continued)*

Initial Diagnostic Tests	Check CK levels
Next Steps in Management	High doses of steroids initially, then DMARDs
Discussion	PM is an idiopathic inflammatory myopathy characterized by proximal muscle weakness, elevated muscle enzymes, abnormal electromyogram and muscle biopsy. PM is an immune-mediated myopathy. Females are more likely to be affected than males. **History:** Symmetrical proximal muscle weakness: (e.g., difficulty climbing stairs, getting up from a seated position, and/or carrying heavy objects). Dysphagia may suggest esophageal involvement. Cough or shortness of breath may occur due to pulmonary involvement. **Physical Exam:** Evidence of proximal muscle weakness and tenderness. **Diagnostics:** • Muscle enzyme elevation, specifically CK • Other abnormal tests include aldolase, lactate dehydrogenase (LDH), aspartate (AST) and alanine (ALT) aminotransferase, and myoglobin (myoglobinuria can be present in active disease) • EMG is abnormal in PM • MRI shows areas of inflamed muscles which can help identify muscle biopsy location • Muscle biopsy shows perimysial/perivascular inflammation with or without perifascicular atrophy and endomysial inflammation with predominant CD8+ T cells Additional tests: • ESR and CRP are elevated but non-specific • TSH normal anti-Ro/SSA, anti-La/SSB, anti-Sm, and anti-ribonucleoprotein (RNP) antibodies can be positive **Management:** • High-dose steroids initially followed by a steroid taper • Long-term control with steroid-sparing agents (e.g., methotrexate, azathioprine) • In refractory or severe cases IVIG
Additional Considerations	**Screening Considerations:** Associated malignancy may be seen in 10–20% of cases and therefore patients should be appropriately screened/evaluated. Chest radiographs and pulmonary function tests (PFTs) should be performed in all patients to screen for interstitial lung disease.

Polymyositis vs Dermatomyositis

Polymyositis	Dermatomyositis	
Symmetric, progressive proximal muscle weakness and/or pain	Proximal muscle weakness, ⊕ Rash Heliotrope rash: A violaceous periorbital rash (see image A)	A
Difficulty getting up from a seat or climbing stairs		
Difficulty breathing or swallowing (advanced disease)	"Shawl sign": A rash involving the shoulders, upper chest, and back Gottron papules: Papular rash with scales on the dorsa of the hands, over bony prominences (see image B)	 Gottron papule Capillary nail fold changes B

Reproduced with permission from Le, Tao, Bhushan Vikas, First Aid for the USMLE Step 2 CK, 10th ed, New York: McGraw-Hill, 2018. (Images reproduced with permission from Dhoble A, Puttarajappa C, Neiberg A. Dermatomyositis and supraventricular tachycardia. Int Arch Med. 2008;1:25.)

CASE 13 | Polymyalgia Rheumatica (PMR)

A 59-year-old woman is evaluated for progressively worsening shoulder and hip pain and stiffness bilaterally for several months. Stiffness is worse in the morning and lasts greater than 30 minutes. She has difficulty rising from a chair and getting objects from her top kitchen shelves. She denies weakness, but has intermittent fevers, malaise, and has lost about 10 pounds. On exam, vital signs are normal and no rashes or thyromegaly are noted. There is reduced range of motion in the shoulders and hips due to pain. Upper and lower extremity strength and sensation are intact.

Conditions with Similar Presentations	**RA:** Symmetric, inflammatory, peripheral polyarthritis with positive RF and anti-cyclic citrullinated peptide (ACPA). **Polymyositis and dermatomyositis:** Proximal muscle weakness and pain but increased CK, and muscle biopsy is confirmatory.
Initial Diagnostic Tests	• Clinical diagnosis and check ESR • Consider: TSH, CK, ACPA to rule out other causes
Next Steps in Management	Oral corticosteroids
Discussion	PMR is an inflammatory condition characterized by pain and stiffness in the shoulder and hip girdle. It is often seen in women of advanced age, almost exclusively >50, and is common in people of Northern European descent. **History:** Symmetrical proximal joint pain worsens after rest, and morning stiffness is a hallmark of disease. Strength is preserved but other systemic symptoms such as low-grade fever, fatigue, and weight loss may be present and onset of symptoms may be abrupt. **Physical Exam:** • Decreased range of motion of the shoulders, cervical spine, and hips (inability to actively abduct the shoulders past 90 degrees) • Muscle atrophy/weakness may be present due to reduced activity • Distal findings (e.g., clinical synovitis of the wrists and small joints of the hands) may be seen ~50% of patients **Diagnostics:** Clinical diagnosis with elevated ESR/CRP TSH, CPK, RF, and APCA are normal **Management:** • Treat with low-dose oral steroids • Urgent temporal biopsy and higher-dose steroids are indicated if GCA is suspected due to presence of new headache, temporal artery tenderness/pulselessness, jaw claudication, scalp tenderness
Additional Considerations	**Screening:** All patients with PMR should be screened for GCA if signs/symptoms mentioned above are present, as PMR can occur in ~50% of patients with GCA. **Complications:** If GCA is present, vasculitis can progress to stroke or blindness.

SPONDYLOARTHROPATHIES

This is a group of autoimmune, inflammatory disorders involving joints and entheses (sites where ligaments and tendons attach to bones) characterized by being "seronegative," i.e., blood tests such as RF and others are negative. Commonly affect bones in the spine and nearby joints and may present with extra-articular findings such as enthesitis (inflamed insertion sites of tendons, e.g., Achilles) and uveitis. Because they are inflammatory conditions, they present with morning stiffness, which improves with exercise. Examples are ankylosing spondylitis, reactive arthritis, psoriatic arthritis, and joint problems linked to inflammatory bowel disease (IBD) (enteropathy arthritis). There is a strong association with HLA-B27 (look for family history in a question stem).

Key Findings	Diagnosis
Arthritis without rheumatoid factor therefore often called "seronegative." Strong association with HLA-B27 (MHC class 1 stereotype); subtypes below share inflammatory back pain (associated with morning stiffness, improves with exercise), peripheral arthritis, enthesitis, dactylitis (sausage fingers), and uveitis	**Seronegative spondylarthritis**

(Continued)

Key Findings	Diagnosis
Skin psoriasis, nail lesions, asymmetric and patchy involvement, dactylitis and "pencil-in-cup" deformity of DIP, seen in fewer than half 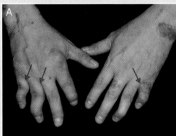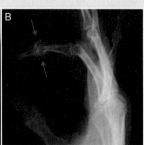 A. Psoriatic arthritis: asymmetric and patchy involvement. B. Dactylitis and "pencil-in-cup deformity" of DIP on x-ray. (Reproduced with permission from Le, Tao and Bhushan, Vikas. First Aid for the USMLE Step 1 2020, 30th rd. New York: McGraw-Hill 2020.)	**Psoriatic arthritis**
Symmetric involvement of spine and sacroiliac joints causing ankylosis (joint fusion) Associated findings: Uveitis, aortic regurgitation; costovertebral and costosternal ankylosis may cause restrictive lung disease, usually in men <50 X-ray: Bamboo spine (vertebral fusion) C. Ankylosing spondylitis: bamboo spine (vertebral fusion). (Reproduced with permission from Le, Tao and Bhushan, Vikas. First Aid for the USMLE Step 1 2020, 30th ed. New York: McGraw-Hill 2020.)	**Ankylosing spondylitis**
Crohn's disease and ulcerative colitis associated with spondylarthritis	**Inflammatory bowel disease**
Classic triad of conjunctivitis, urethritis, and arthritis "Can't see, pee, or bend the knee" Occurs 1–4 weeks after an infection (e.g., *Shigella*, *Campylobacter*, *Escherichia coli*, salmonella, chlamydia, and *Yersinia*).	**Reactive arthritis**

CASE 14 | Psoriatic Arthritis

A 50-year-old man is evaluated for worsening joint pain in his right index finger, right wrist, and right foot over the past 4 months. He has had chronic lower back pain for the past 3 years. He also notes morning stiffness >1 hour. On exam, he has swelling and tenderness of the DIP joint on the right hand with two sausage-shaped digits, and thick red skin patches with silvery scales over the extensor surfaces of the knees and elbows.

Conditions with Similar Presentations	**OA:** Can also present with DIP pain, but no psoriatic skin changes. **RA:** Inflammatory arthritis that spares the DIP, is symmetric, and does not exhibit psoriatic skin changes. **Gout and pseudogout:** Monoarticular and acute onset. **Reactive arthritis:** Can present with asymmetric oligoarthritis, enthesitis; however, occurs several weeks after an infection and may present with urethritis or diarrhea.
Initial diagnostics Tests	Clinical diagnosis
Next Steps in Management	NSAIDs, DMARDs and other nonpharmacological treatments (see below)

CASE 14 | Psoriatic Arthritis *(continued)*

Discussion	Psoriatic arthropathy is an inflammatory spondylarthritis that occurs equally in men and women, usually between the ages of 35–50 years. Peripheral joint disease in 95% of cases is in the form of synovitis, tenosynovitis (dactylitis—sausage digits), and enthesitis.
	Some patients have spinal involvement. Psoriasis predates arthritis in 75% of cases. There is a strong association between all subtypes of spondylarthritis, and genetic expression of HLA-B27 is seen in 10–50%.
	History: • Tenderness and swelling of involved joints, tendons, and ligaments • Psoriasis— family history of psoriasis is present in 40% of patients **Physical Exam:** • Typically asymmetric, multiple joint involvement (DIP, PIP, MCP, MTP, knees, hips, and ankles) and enthesopathy • Sausage digits (dactylitis) caused by tenosynovitis and resorption of distal phalangeal tufts • Axial involvement with back or SI tenderness on palpation • Psoriasis (red patches with silvery scaling on extensor surfaces such as knees and elbows) • Extraarticular manifestations: nail changes (nail pitting, onycholysis, brittle nails, oil drop sign), eye disease (uveitis), and dilatation of base of aortic arch causing aortic insufficiency murmur 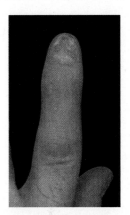 Psoriatic arthritis Dactylitis of index finger. Note sausage-like thickening over interphalangeal joints. There is psoriasis of the nail. (Reproduced with permission from Wolff K, Johnson R, Saavedra AP, Roh EK. Fitzpatrick's Color Atlas and Synopsis of Clinical Dermatology, 8e; McGraw Hill LLC 2017.) **Diagnostics:** Clinical diagnosis • Radiographs: show asymmetric distribution, DIP involvement and distal phalangeal resorption, erosions, and "pencil-in-cup" deformity. May also show spondylosis and SI involvement. • Association with HLA-B27 but not useful as a diagnostic test. • RF and ACPA are negative. **Management:** • Non-pharmacological treatment essential (exercise, physical and occupational therapy, weight loss, use of orthotics, and education on disease management). • NSAIDs: for mild to moderate disease • DMARDs (methotrexate): mainstay of treatment for moderate to severe disease • Biologic DMARDs: if patients do not respond for 3 months to conventional DMARDs or have erosive disease and/or functional limitations
Additional Considerations	Consider concurrent human immunodeficiency virus (HIV) infection when patients present with acute severe psoriasis.

VASCULITIDES

Vasculitis is a systemic process that affects multiple organs. It results from inflammation of the blood vessels and can either occur as a primary disease or can be secondary to an underlying condition. Mimickers of vasculitis include cancers, infections (endocarditis, hepatitis, sepsis), coagulopathies (DIC, TTP, antiphospholipid antibody syndrome), and cholesterol emboli.

History

• Suspect vasculitis in patients who present with symptoms affecting multiple organs (e.g., sinusitis, dyspnea/cough, hematuria) and systemic symptoms (e.g., fever, malaise, weight loss).

• Inquire about HIV, hepatitis, endocarditis, drug abuse (cocaine), previous thrombotic events.

Physical Exam

Examine involved organs and look for rashes, ulcers, asymmetrical or diminished pulses, and/or bruits.

Initial Diagnostic Tests

ESR, CRP, CBC, CMP (renal and liver function), and urinalysis (UA)

Large-vessel vasculitides	Giant cell arteritis (GCA) (temporal arteritis)
	Takayasu arteritis
Medium-vessel vasculitides	Polyarteritis nodosa (PAN)
	Kawasaki disease
Small vessel vasculitides	**ANCA associations:**
	cANCA (anti-proteinase 3, PRO): Granulomatous with polyangitis (GPA)
	pANCA (anti-myeloperoxidase [MPO])
	• Eosinophilic granulomatous with polyangitis (EGPA)
	• Microscopic polyangitis (MPA)
	• Pauci-immune glomerulonephritis
	Immune complex–mediated:
	• IgA vasculitis
	• Henoch Schoenlein purpura (HSP)
	• Cryoglobulinemia
	• Anti-glomerular basement membrane disease (anti-GBM)
Variable-vessel vasculitis	Behçet disease

Vasculitis	Epidemiology and Associations	Main Disease Manifestations	Complications	Diagnostic Tests
Large vessel vasculitis: Affects aorta and its major branches				
GCA • Maxillary artery • Ophthalmic artery	Adults >50 Women > men Polymyalgia rheumatica	New-onset headache, vision loss, jaw claudication; tender temporal and/or occipital arteries	Ophthalmic artery involvement can cause blindness Aortic aneurysm	Temporal artery biopsy (giant cells)
Takayasu • Subclavian artery • Coronary artery • Pulmonary artery • Renal artery • Mesenteric artery	Age <40 Women > men Aorta and its main branches involved	Chest pain Arm claudication Unequal arm pulses and blood pressures Subclavian and/or aortic bruit	Aortic regurgitation Aortic aneurysm Stroke Renal artery stenosis Ischemic colitis	CT or MRI w/ contrast, or arteriogram
Medium vessel vasculitis: Involves main visceral arteries and their branches				
Polyarteritis nodosa (PAN)	Adults >50 Hepatitis B, C and HIV	Many organs involved, especially kidney, skin, and nerves Lungs are spared Livedo reticularis Testicular pain "Rosary bead" microaneurysms on renal angiogram	ESRD Stroke	Neutrophilic infiltration of vessels on biopsy CT or MRI w/ contrast, or arteriogram
Kawasaki disease	Children	Fever >5 days, conjunctivitis, cervical adenopathy, rash	Coronary artery aneurysm	
Small vessel vasculitis: Small intraparenchymal arteries, arterioles, capillaries				
Eosinophilic granulomatous with polyangitis (EGPA)	Age around 40–50 years History of asthma	Asthma Neuropathy Nephritic syndrome Dyspnea, hemoptysis Eosinophilia Rash	ESRD Interstitial lung disease (ILD) Arrhythmia, myocarditis	Clinical findings MPO-ANCA + Biopsy confirms

Vasculitis	Epidemiology and Associations	Main Disease Manifestations	Complications	Diagnostic Tests
Microscopic polyangitis (MPA)	Adults >50 Men/women equally affected	Hemoptysis Hematuria Peripheral neuropathy Nephritic syndrome Rash Sinusitis Dyspnea	ESRD Myocarditis Diffuse alveolar hemorrhage ILD Corneal ulceration Pulmonary-renal syndrome	Clinical findings MPO-ANCA + Biopsy confirms
Granulomatous with polyangitis (GPA)	Men/women equally affected Adults >50	Sinusitis, otitis Oral and ENT ulcers Hearing loss, Tracheal stenosis Hematuria Dyspnea and hemoptysis Nephritic syndrome Rashes	ESRD Myocarditis Subglottic stenosis ILD Corneal ulceration	Clinical findings PR3-ANCA + Biopsy confirms by showing granulomas
Cryoglobulin vasculitis	History of HIV, hepatitis C, and/or connective tissue disease	Purpura, ulcers, Raynaud's, arthralgias, glomerulonephritis peripheral neuropathy	Coronary artery involvement ESRD Malignancy (type II)	Cryoglobulins C4 decreased Biopsy

Management Cutaneous Small Vessel Vasculitis

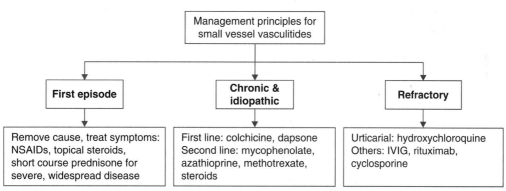

CASE 15 | Giant Cell Arteritis (Temporal Arteritis)

A 69-year-old woman with PMR presents with worsening headaches for the past week. Headaches are new and localized to the left temporal area. She also has jaw pain with chewing gum and reports intermittent blurry vision in her left eye. Her vital signs are normal except for low-grade temperature of 38.1°C. On exam, her left forehead is tender along the temporal artery, and her temporal artery pulse is faint. Her vision is intact but on fundoscopy she has an increased cup-to-disk ratio with blurring of the optic disc margin in her left eye. Her labs show an ESR of 91 (normal <30) and CRP of 39 (normal <10).

Conditions with Similar Presentations	**Migraine headaches, tension headaches, temporomandibular joint (TMJ) syndrome:** Would not present with elevated ESR, tender temporal artery, visual changes, and jaw claudication. **Trigeminal neuralgia:** Allodynia and involvement of other branches of trigeminal nerve distinguishes this from GCA. It can frequently mimic jaw claudication and/or headaches, depending on which division of the trigeminal nerve is involved.
Initial Diagnostic Tests	• Check ESR and CRP • Confirm with temporal artery biopsy
Next Steps in Management	• High-dose oral steroids • Steroids are given intravenously if visual changes are present

CASE 15 | Giant Cell Arteritis (Temporal Arteritis) *(continued)*

Discussion	Giant cell arteritis (GCA), previously known as temporal arteritis, is the most common primary vasculitis, characterized by chronic inflammation of large- and medium-sized arteries (branches of the carotid arteries) and caused by an inflammatory cascade due to an unknown trigger. Granulomatous infiltrates that can form giant cells results from the recruitment of T cells and macrophages by dendritic cells in the vessel wall. Associated risk of blindness in 15% of the cases, which diminishes to 1% if corticosteroid therapy is initiated promptly. Commonly seen in persons >60, and women are more affected than men (2:1).
	History:
	• New onset of headache—usually temporal
	• Jaw claudication—mandibular pain or fatigue triggered by mastication and relieved by stopping
	• Abrupt painless vision loss (transient or permanent)
	• Constitutional symptoms (fever, weight loss, fatigue)
	• 40% of GCA patients have concurrent PMR and report pain and stiffness in proximal limbs
	Physical Exam:
	• Decreased temporal artery pulsation with tenderness
	• Scalp tenderness
	• 10-mm Hg difference in systolic BP between arms due to possible involvement of the aorta and its primary branches
	• Bruit over carotid and subclavian vessels
	• Swollen pale optic disc with blurred margins in patients with arteritic anterior ischemic optic neuropathy
	Diagnostics:
	The American College of Rheumatology defines GCA as having three of the five criteria below:
	1. Onset >50
	2. ESR >50
	3. New headache
	4. Temporal artery tenderness or decreased blood flow
	5. Biopsy with mononuclear or giant cell infiltration
	Management:
	• High-dose oral steroids for 2–4 weeks until symptoms begin to resolve, at which time the steroids can be tapered.
	• Initially IV if vision involvement.
	• Biopsy remains abnormal for several days after steroids are started.
Additional Considerations	**Complications:**
	• Ophthalmic arteritis—can lead to blindness
	• Aortic aneurysm(thoracic aorta more commonly involved) or aortic dissection(rare but fatal). Check CT angiography if clinical suspicion or suggestive x-ray findings.
	• PMR can precede and be concurrent with GCA. Screen all PMR patients for history of headaches, jaw claudication, or vision changes.
	Surgical Considerations: For biopsy, 15- to 20-mm sample of the involved temporal artery is required. If negative, it should be repeated on the other side.

CASE 16 | Polyarteritis Nodosa (PAN)

A 57-year-old woman with chronic hepatitis B presents with right leg numbness, rash, and leg cramps for several months. Her "muscle cramps" are worse every time she walks more than two blocks. On exam, her vital signs are temperature 38.2, pulse 70/min, blood pressure 168/97 mmHg, respirations 14/min. There is a net-like rash over her legs (livedo reticularis) and a tender erythematous nodule on the anterior aspect of the right thigh. Sensation is reduced in the distal right extremity.

Conditions with Similar Presentations	**Granulomatosis with polyangiitis (GPA):** A necrotizing vasculitis with frequent renal and pulmonary involvement.
	Eosinophilic granulomatosis with polyangiitis (EGPA): Similar to GPA, but with peripheral eosinophilia and in tissues on biopsy.
Initial Diagnostic Tests	• Check CBC, creatinine, urinalysis, ESR, CRP
	• Also check imaging based on symptoms
	• Confirm with biopsy

CASE 16 | Polyarteritis Nodosa (PAN) *(continued)*

Next Steps in Management	• High-dose steroids are used initially • If severe/life-threatening organ involvement, treat with cyclophosphamide
Discussion	PAN involves medium-sized arteries and causes segmental areas of blood vessel inflammation, which can lead to aneurysms and micro aneurysms. Vascular inflammation caused by T cell–mediated immune response leads to occlusion of arteries and ischemia/hemorrhage in organs. Inflammation is transmural and causes regions of aneurysmal dilation—"rosary bead" appearance on renal angiography. It spares the lungs, although a wide range of other organs can be affected. The symptoms are due to compromised blood flow and ischemia. **History:** Onset is 50–60 years, and most cases are idiopathic. Risk factors include hepatitis B, C, and HIV. Symptoms may include: • Fever, weight loss, and myalgias • Hematuria, neuropathy, skin lesions • Abdominal pain with eating from mesenteric ischemia • Claudication from ischemia to muscle tissue • Testicular pain or tenderness **Physical Exam:** • New onset hypertension due to altered renal blood flow causing upregulation of the renin-angiotensin-aldosterone axis • Diminished pulses • Skin lesions (livedo reticularis, purpura, painful subcutaneous nodules) • Decreased sensation, or weakness due to neuropathy **Diagnostics:** • Check CBC, ESR, CRP, creatinine (elevated) • Urinalysis shows blood and protein in the urine, but below the threshold for either nephritic or nephrotic syndrome • Screen for hepatitis B, hepatitis C, and HIV • Imaging such as chest x-rays, CT, or MRI, based on symptoms, to determine which blood vessels and organs are affected • Arteriography or cross-sectional (MRI or CT) imaging with contrast "rosary bead" appearance of blood vessels due to small alternating areas of aneurysmal and non-aneurysmal vascular lumen • Biopsy shows fibrinoid necrosis of artery walls with neutrophil infiltration The American College of Rheumatology criteria: Patient has a diagnosis of vasculitis *and* at least three of the following (sensitivity 82%, specificity 87%): • unexplained weight loss ≥4 kg • livedo reticularis • testicular pain • weak or painful muscles • mono or polyneuropathy • new elevation in diastolic blood pressure ≥90 • new kidney dysfunction (BUN >45, creatinine >1.5) • hepatitis B • arteriographic evidence of small aneurysms • biopsy demonstrating neutrophil infiltration of blood vessels **Management:** • Mild disease: NSAIDS for cutaneous involvement, steroids for other areas • End-organ damage: cyclophosphamide. • On remission: steroids tapered, and either azathioprine or methotrexate are used for maintenance
Additional Considerations	**Complications:** Coronary artery disease, ESRD, or stroke

CASE 17 | Granulomatous Polyangiitis (GPA)

A 62-year-old man with no significant past medical history presents with cough, fatigue, and weight loss for the past 2 months. He reports progressive dyspnea, 11 pounds weight loss, and rhinorrhea with occasional blood, and earlier today noted blood in his urine, which prompted him to seek medical care. Vital signs are normal. On exam a few purpuric lesions are noted on his legs; he has nasal crusting and an ulcer in his left nare. On pulmonary auscultation, diffuse crackles are heard.

Conditions with Similar Presentations	**Eosinophilic granulomatosis with polyangiitis (EGPA):** Antineutrophil cytoplasmic antibodies (ANCA) vasculitis presents with hematuria and lung involvement. The main distinguishing factor of EGPA is eosinophilia and eosinophilic infiltration of organs on biopsy
	PAN: Another vasculitis that can present with hematuria. Although both GPA and PAN can affect multiple organ systems, PAN will *not* have lung involvement. PAN is ANCA negative.
	Goodpasture disease: Like GPA, Goodpasture's can present with hematuria and occasionally hemoptysis. However, neither vasculitis nor granulomas will be present. Anti-basement membrane antibody is present.
	Microscopic polyangiitis: Associated with p-ANCA and does not have nasopharyngeal involvement. Unlike GPA, granulomas are not present on biopsy.
Initial Diagnostic Tests	• Check CBC, creatinine, urinalysis, ESR, CRP, ANCA, PR3, myeloperoxidase (MPO) • Imaging based on symptoms • Confirm with lung or kidney biopsy
Next Steps in Management	• Initial: Rituximab, cyclophosphamide, glucocorticoids • Maintenance: Rituximab, methotrexate, azathioprine, mycophenolate
Discussion	GPA, formerly known as Wegener granulomatosis, is a pauci-immune small-vessel vasculitis associated with ANCA. A triggering event leads to production of proinflammatory cytokines which activate neutrophils. ANCA bind to the target antigens exposed on the surface of neutrophils, such as proteinase 3 (PR3) and MPO. Excessive activation of neutrophils leads to granuloma formation which infiltrates organs and vessels, leading to disease manifestations. Affected organs include upper respiratory tract (nose, sinuses, ears), lungs, kidneys, and skin. **History:** Seen in patients >50 years and may present suddenly or slowly over the course of months. • Nonspecific constitutional symptoms (fevers, weight loss) • Sinus pain, rhinitis, epistaxis • Cough which can sometimes be bloody (lung nodules, infiltrates, diffuse alveolar hemorrhage) • Blood in the urine • Hearing loss • Focal neurologic deficits **Physical Exam:** • Sinus tenderness, ulcers in the oropharynx and nares • Cartilage damage and collapse (septal perforation, tracheal stenosis, saddle nose deformity) • Scleritis, conjunctivitis • Stridor, crackles, or wheezing on lung exam • Focal neurologic deficits (sensory neuropathy, cranial nerve defects) • Skin lesions (tender cutaneous nodules, palpable purpura, urticarial and ulcerative lesions) **Diagnostics:** • Initial workup must include creatinine, complete blood count, ANCA (PR3 and MPO), although not part of criteria but can direct to ANCA-associated vasculitis, urinalysis (hematuria and/or proteinuria), ESR, CRP, dsDNA (to rule out SLE), anti-basement membrane (to rule out Goodpasture's) • Imaging such as chest x-rays, CT, or MRI based on symptoms to determine which blood vessels and organs are affected. If respiratory symptoms present, chest CT to look for pulmonary involvement with cavities, nodules, or infiltrates • Biopsy will show blood vessels with necrotizing granulomas without eosinophils infiltrating organs or blood vessel walls which distinguishes it from EGPA • Kidney biopsy will show pauci-immune glomerulonephritis—usually crescentic

CASE 17 | Granulomatous Polyangiitis (GPA) *(continued)*

Discussion	Diagnostic criteria (any four present sensitivity 88%, specificity 92%) (mnemonic "**LUNG**"):
	
	Lung involvement
	    Chest radiograph shows nodules, fixed infiltrates, or cavities
	Urinary sediment abnormalities
	    Microhematuria (>5 red blood cells per high-power field) or red cell casts in urine sediment
	Nasal (or oral) inflammation
	    Oral ulcers or purulent or bloody nasal discharge
	Granulomatous inflammation on biopsy
	    Histology shows granulomatous inflammation in the wall of an artery or in the perivascular or extravascular area (artery or arteriole)
	
	Management:
	• Induction of remission: high-dose steroids and an immunosuppressant
	• Severe organ-threatening ANCA-associated vasculitis (e.g., active glomerulonephritis, pulmonary hemorrhage): rituximab followed by cyclophosphamide
	• Maintenance therapy: methotrexate, rituximab, mycophenolate, and azathioprine

Additional Considerations	**Complications:** ESRD, bronchial or subglottic stenosis, diffuse alveolar hemorrhage.

Vasculitis Mini-Cases

Cases	Key Findings
Eosinophilic Granulomatosis with Polyangiitis (EGPA)	**Hx:** Rare necrotizing vasculitis of the small and medium-sized blood vessels which involves skin, kidney, lungs, nervous system, and nasopharynx. Onset is usually between 40 and 50 years of age. Patients may have history of asthma. Patients can present with fevers, weight loss, fatigue, congestion, rhinorrhea, dyspnea, cough, hemoptysis, arthralgias, myalgias, and GI bleeds. **PE:** New skin lesions such as rashes, purpura, and nodules. Sinusitis and nasal polyps. Focal neurologic deficits—areas of diminished sensation, cranial nerve deficits, or weakness. **Diagnostics:** CBC (peripheral eosinophilia (>10% of WBC), creatinine, urinalysis, ANCA. Biopsy shows extravascular eosinophilic tissue infiltration. Diagnostic criteria (mnemonic "**BLANES**"): Any four sensitivity 85%, specificity 99.7%: • **B**iopsy: extravascular eosinophils (lung or sinus) • **L**ung: infiltrates on chest x-ray • **A**sthma: by history or wheezing on exam • **N**europathy: mononeuritis multiplex or polyneuropathy • **E**osinophilia: >10% • **S**inusitis **Management:** • Treat acute flares with high-dose steroids. • Cyclophosphamide or rituximab are used in severe and life-threatening disease. • For maintenance therapy, steroids should be tapered, and a steroid-sparing agent must be used such as rituximab, methotrexate, azathioprine, or leflunomide. **Discussion:** Multiorgan system disease. It can present with constitutional symptoms, arthralgia, skin involvement, pulmonary involvement, cardiomyopathy, kidney disease, and gastrointestinal involvement. Activated TH2 lymphocytes that produce cytokines are thought to be the key pathogenic factors. The resultant eosinophilic flux causes a necrotizing vasculitis; biopsy of any affected tissue (organ-specific symptoms) shows an eosinophilic infiltrate. Patients also may have allergic rhinitis, nasal polyposis, otitis media, and other upper respiratory manifestations. Lower respiratory manifestations may include pulmonary opacities, pleural effusions, and pulmonary nodules.

Vasculitis Mini-Cases *(continued)*

Cryoglobulinemia	**Hx/PE:** This systemic inflammatory syndrome demonstrates symptoms proportionate to the concentration of deposited immune complexes. Patients may be asymptomatic or symptoms and signs may include: Joint pain, paresthesias, fatigue, rash or other skin lesions, sensory and/or motor deficits from peripheral neuropathy.

> **Hx/PE:** This systemic inflammatory syndrome demonstrates symptoms proportionate to the concentration of deposited immune complexes. Patients may be asymptomatic or symptoms and signs may include: Joint pain, paresthesias, fatigue, rash or other skin lesions, sensory and/or motor deficits from peripheral neuropathy.
> - Type I is associated with livedo reticularis and Raynaud phenomenon.
> - Type II and III are associated with purpura, macules, and ulcers.
>
> **Diagnostics:** Cryoglobulin detection in blood and testing for associated hematologic diseases (Type I) or infection and autoimmune diseases (Type II and Type III).
>
> **Management:** Treat the underlying condition(s) contributing to the cryoglobulinemia (hepatitis, autoimmune disease, malignancy).
>
> **Discussion:**
>
> Cryoglobulins are immunoglobulins (Igs) that precipitate in vitro at temperatures <37°C and dissolve on rewarming. Overproduction of cryoglobulins can bind to other Igs and form complexes that incite vascular inflammation (vasculitis) and organ injury.
>
> Cryoglobulinemia is divided into three types:
> - Type I: The cryoglobulins are monoclonal Igs (IgG or IgM, less commonly IgA). The increased production is due to monoclonal gammopathies seen in Waldenström macroglobulinemia, multiple myeloma, monoclonal gammopathy of undetermined significance (MGUS), or chronic lymphocytic leukemia (CLL).
> - Type II: The cryoglobulins are composed of a mixture of a monoclonal IgM, IgG, or IgA and polyclonal Ig. This is most commonly due to chronic immune stimulation from infectious diseases (hepatitis C most common, but also hepatitis B, HIV) or autoimmune diseases (most commonly SLE or Sjogren syndrome). About 10% of cases have no discernible causation, and this is called essential cryoglobulinemia.
> - Type III: The cryoglobulins are composed of a mixture of polyclonal IgG and polyclonal IgM. Most commonly due to autoimmune diseases (same as Type II) and less commonly infection, particularly hepatitis C.

Type	Composition	Associations
I	Monoclonal Ig	Hematologic monoclones
II	Monoclonal Ig and polyclonal Ig	Infection, autoimmune diseases
III	Polyclonal IgG and polyclonal IgM	Autoimmune diseases, infection

> Treatment and prognosis are dependent on the underlying condition as well as associated lymphoproliferative disorders.

SKELETAL TUMORS

- Primary bone cancers are rare, and range from benign tumors to aggressive and fatal malignancies.
- Unlike most other solid tumors, bone cancers disproportionately affect children and young adults.
- Initial imaging is with x-ray, which may be followed by more advanced imaging.
- Non-malignant bone lesions have a sharp demarcation between the abnormal tissue and the normal bone, whereas malignant lesions will often not.
- Definitive diagnosis is made by bone biopsy
  - An exception is osteochondroma, a benign tumor with characteristic features on x-ray.

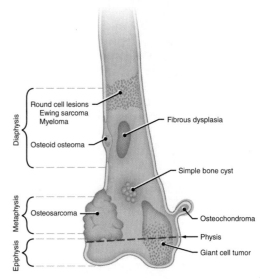

Reproduced with permission from Le, Tao and Bhushan, Vikas. First Aid for the USMLE Step 1 2020, 30th rd. New York: McGraw-Hill, 2020.

Primary bone tumors

Metastatic disease is more common than 1° bone tumors. Benign bone tumors that start with o are more common in boys.

Tumor Type	Epidemiology	Location	Characteristics
Benign tumors			
Osteochondroma	Most common benign bone tumor Males < 25 years old	Metaphysis of long bones	Lateral bony projection of growth plate (continuous with marrow space) covered by cartilaginous cap Rarely transforms to chondrosarcoma
Osteoma	Middle age	Surface of facial bones	Associated with Gardner syndrome
Osteoid osteoma	Adults < 25 years old Males > females	Cortex of long bones	Presents as bone pain (worse at night) that is relieved by NSAIDs Bony mass (< 2 cm) with radiolucent osteoid core
Osteoblastoma	Males > females	Vertebrae	Similar histology to osteoid osteoma Larger size (> 2 cm), pain unresponsive to NSAIDs
Chondroma		Medulla of small bones of hand and feet	Benign tumor of cartilage
Giant cell tumor	20–40 years old	Epiphysis of long bones (often in knee region)	Locally aggressive benign tumor Neoplastic mononuclear cells that express RANKL and reactive multinucleated giant (osteoclast-like) cells. "Osteoclastoma" "Soap bubble" appearance on x-ray
Malignant tumors			
Osteosarcoma (osteogenic sarcoma)	Accounts for 20% of 1° bone cancers. Peak incidence of 1° tumor in males < 20 years. Less common in elderly; usually 2° to predisposing factors, such as Paget disease of bone, bone infarcts, radiation, familial retinoblastoma, Li-Fraumeni syndrome.	Metaphysis of long bones (often in knee region).	Pleomorphic osteoid-producing cells (malignant osteoblasts). Presents as painful enlarging mass or pathologic fractures. Codman triangle (D) (from elevation of periosteum) or sunburst pattern (E) on x-ray (think of an osteocod [bone fish] swimming in the sun). Aggressive. 1° usually responsive to treatment (surgery, chemotherapy), poor prognosis for 2°.
Chondrosarcoma		Medulla of pelvis, proximal femur and humerus.	Tumor of malignant chondrocytes.
Ewing sarcoma	Most common in White patients Generally males < 15 years old	Diaphysis of long bones (especially femur), pelvic flat bones.	Anaplastic small blue cells of neuroectodermal origin (resemble lymphocytes). Differentiate from conditions with similar morphology (eg, lymphoma, chronic osteomyelitis) by testing for t(11;22) (fusion protein EWS-FLI1). "Onion skin" periosteal reaction in bone. Aggressive with early metastases, but responsive to chemotherapy. 11 + 22 = 33 (Patrick Ewing's jersey number).

Bone Lesion Mini-Cases

Cases	Key Findings
Osteochondroma (Benign)	**Hx:** Most commonly occur in younger men. Benign bone tumors (e.g., osteoid osteoma, osteochondroma) are not associated with systemic signs of illness. Lesion may be discovered incidentally on plain radiographs. **PE:** A palpable lump may be identified on physical exam. **Diagnostics:** Plain radiographs demonstrate bony outgrowth of the growth plate characterized by a cartilage-cap. The lesion is contiguous with the marrow space. **Management:** • Observation and reassurance of the low risk of malignant transformation. Lesions grow throughout childhood, then remain static in adulthood after the growth plates close. • New symptoms or tumor growth after adulthood may signal a need for additional workup. **Discussion:** Osteochondroma is the most common benign bone tumor and is classified as a cartilage-producing tumor located at the growth plate and projecting away from the epiphysis. Isolated lesions occur due to mutation of a tumor suppressor gene (*EXT1* or *EXT2*). Multiple lesions occur due to an autosomal dominant condition called hereditary multiple osteochondromas.
Osteoid Osteoma (Benign)	**Hx:** Onset 10–30 years old. Pain worse at night and relieved by NSAIDs. **PE:** Point tenderness with localized swelling. Can present with a limp **Diagnostics:** • X-ray shows radiolucent area of bone cortex with sclerotic margin. • CT scan is used to distinguish from osteoblastoma. Osteoid osteomas will have radiolucent nidus surrounded by dense sclerosis. **Management:** NSAIDs. If symptoms not tolerable, consider surgery. **Discussion:** Osteoid osteomas are nonmalignant bone lesions under 2 cm in size. The central area of an osteoid osteoma produces large amounts of prostaglandins (hence NSAIDs resolve pain quickly). Usually occurs in the metaphysis of a long bone, especially in the lower extremities, but can occur anywhere.
Osteoblastoma (Benign)	**Hx:** Onset 10–30 years old, more common in males. Progressive dull pain, worse at night. Can cause symptoms of nerve compression, depending on the size and location. Minimal relief with NSAIDs. **PE:** Often palpable bone lesion, swelling and tenderness over the lesion—usually involves the posterior spine. **Diagnostics:** X-rays show a lytic lesion >2 cm with a rim of reactive sclerosis, and tends to be expansive but rarely extends into soft tissues. **Management:** Surgical excision is the treatment of choice, with the intention to fully remove tumor to prevent recurrence. **Discussion:** Osteoblastomas are nonmalignant bone lesions >2 cm in size. Most common location is the spinal column, followed by long bones.
Giant Cell Tumor (Benign yet locally Aggressive)	**Hx:** Presenting symptoms include pain and swelling without history of trauma. Slight predominance in women. **PE:** Exam may demonstrate limited range of motion at the affected joint. There may be tenderness to palpation. **Diagnostics:** • Plain radiographs of the primary site demonstrate expansile, eccentrically placed lytic area ("soap bubble" appearance) more commonly at the epiphysis • CT or MRI in symptomatic patients. • Biopsy is required for diagnosis; tumor demonstrates high RANK-L expression. **Management:** • Resection with the intent of complete excision to prevent recurrence, with or without reconstruction is recommended in patients who qualify as surgical candidates. • In patients not considered good surgical candidates, denosumab may be used as neoadjuvant therapy. **Discussion:** These tumors are benign but aggressive. Most cases are solitary. Thinning of cortical bone secondary to the enlarging mass may result in fracture. Tumor size, location, and relationship to nearby structures determine whether the lesion is resectable. A very small number of patients present with pulmonary lesions that are called "implants," not metastases, because the tissue is not malignant.

Bone Lesion Mini-Cases *(continued)*

Brown Tumors	**Hx:** Occurs in the setting of excess osteoclast activity, such as hyperparathyroidism. May also have hypercalcemia with associated symptoms of altered mental status, weakness, bone pain, anorexia, nausea and vomiting, abdominal pain, and constipation. Brown tumor is a type of osteitis fibrosa cystica. Lesions may be painful. Most commonly affects the mandible and the maxilla. **PE:** Exam may demonstrate systemic findings of hypercalcemia. **Diagnostics:** • Plain radiographs of the primary site demonstrate bone cysts. • Biopsy demonstrates a mix of poorly mineralized woven bone and fibrous tissue and are brown due to hemosiderin deposition. **Management:** Treatment of underlying hyperparathyroidism reduces osteoclastic activity, thus improving bony lesions. **Discussion:** Osteitis fibrosa cystica is increasingly rare; however, bone quality not rising to the level of this condition with associated brown tumors is common in hyperparathyroidism. Patients with asymptomatic hyperparathyroidism may demonstrate decreased bone mineral density, as measured with DEXA. Cortical bone is more commonly affected than trabecular bone; such differentiation can be made using advanced imaging techniques (HRpQCT).
Osteosarcoma (Malignant)	**Hx:** Bimodal age distribution—primary osteosarcoma occurs in ages 10–20 years; secondary osteosarcoma occurs >65 years. Pain and swelling are the most common symptoms. Most commonly presents as knee pain due to involvement of femur or tibia. **PE:** Swelling and localized tenderness **Diagnostics:** • X-ray shows medullary and cortical bone destruction. May also show Codman triangle, where the tumor elevates the periosteum above it • Biopsy is diagnostic **Management:** Surgical resection followed by chemotherapy **Discussion:** Osteosarcomas are malignant bone lesions. They represent the second most common primary bone tumor after multiple myeloma. In the pediatric population, osteosarcomas are sometimes ignored as "growing pains," which may delay the diagnosis.

REGIONAL MUSCULOSKELETAL DISORDERS

CASE 18 | Fibromyalgia

A 42-year-old woman with irritable bowel syndrome (IBS) presents with pain all over her body for the past several months. She feels stiff and fatigued all day and feels tired even after a full night of sleep. On exam, she has no synovitis or joint deformities. She has full range of motion of extremities and spine. She is tender along the lower half of her cervical spine, bilateral shoulders, immediately superior to her popliteal fossa bilaterally, and her hips at the greater trochanters bilaterally.

Conditions with Similar Presentations	**Complex regional pain syndrome:** Presents with localized symptoms in an extremity after an injury (fracture, trauma, surgery). There is pain, loss of range of motion, and sensory increase or decrease. **RA:** Would have symmetric, distal evidence of joint inflammation. As opposed to fibromyalgia, there would be increased ESR/CRP, and majority of patients would have RF and ACPA in blood. **Ankylosing spondylitis:** Inflammatory condition affecting SI joints and spine, predominantly in men, and demonstrates decreased flexion of the spine. **PMR:** An inflammatory disorder causing muscle pain and stiffness in the shoulders and hips. These symptoms start quickly and are worse in the morning.
Initial Diagnostic Tests	• Clinical diagnosis • Consider: ESR, RF, ACPA to rule out other causes
Treatment	• Sleep hygiene, exercise • Consider NSAIDs, tricyclic anti-depressants (TCAs), serotonin norepinephrine reuptake inhibitors, and/or gabapentin

CASE 18 | Fibromyalgia *(continued)*

Discussion	Fibromyalgia is a noninflammatory, nonautoimmune central afferent processing, often classified under the term *central sensitization*. It is a chronic diffuse pain disorder. Tenderness is most pronounced at the insertion points of muscle tendons. Unlike other musculoskeletal pain, fibromyalgia is a disease of central pain processing, rather than an inflammatory or peripheral nerve pathology. The disease begins in adulthood and is more common in women.
	History: Diffuse pain for at least 3 months; common comorbidities include IBS, migraines, restless leg syndrome, anxiety, and depression. Symptoms include abdominal cramps, headaches, paresthesias, psychiatric symptoms, fatigue, sleep disturbances, cognitive symptoms
	PE: Tenderness to palpation especially (but not exclusively) in the following tender point locations: • Upper mid-trapezius muscle • Lateral epicondyle • Second costochondral junction • Greater trochanter
	Diagnostics: • Clinical diagnosis: Diffuse pain for at least 3 months with no other disorder that would explain it. • ESR and CRP are normal (can aid in ruling out inflammatory conditions such as polymyalgia rheumatica) • ANA and RF can be positive in healthy individuals and therefore should not be checked unless there is a clinical suspicion for SLE or RA
	Management: • Patient education, exercise, sleep hygiene, and cognitive behavioral therapy are the cornerstones of treatment • Pharmaceutical/adjunctive treatments can include NSAIDs, tricyclic antidepressants (TCA), serotonin norepinephrine reuptake inhibitors, and gabapentin
Additional Considerations	**Screening:** Screen for suicide risk prior to prescribing SNRIs or TCAs.

11

Dermatology

Lead Author: Maria M. Tsoukas, MD, PhD
Contributors: Jonwei Hwang, MD; Yonatan Hirsch, MD; Samantha Hunt, MD

PRINCIPLES OF DERMATOLOGICAL DIAGNOSIS

Most of the information in this chapter is based on the authors expertise and was confirmed using the following sources: American Academy of Dermatology Basic Dermatology Curriculum, DynaMed, Fitzpatrick's Dermatology, 9th edition, Lookingbill and Marks Principles of Dermatology 6th edition and UpToDate.

A Two-Step Approach to Describing a Skin Lesion

Step 1: Characterize the **morphology** of the skin lesion using appropriate terminology.

- Primary skin lesions: Initial reactions that arise de novo due to the internal or external environment.
- Secondary skin lesions: Arise over time as the disease progresses (can be related to scratching, picking, rubbing).
- Growth: Discrete lesion from proliferation of the skin's components.
- Rash: A visible inflammatory process.

Primary Skin Lesions

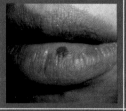	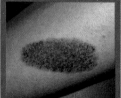	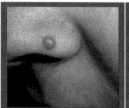	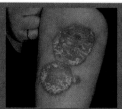	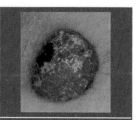
Macule	**Patch**	**Papule**	**Plaque**	**Nodule**
Flat area of discoloration ≤1 cm in maximum diameter	**Flat** area of discoloration >1 cm in maximum diameter	**Elevated** skin lesion ≤1 cm in maximum diameter	**Elevated** solid area >1 cm in maximum diameter "plateau-like"	Elevated, **hard** lesion >1 cm in max. diameter and depth "Tumor" is used to describe elevated hard lesions >2 cm
Reproduced with permission from Le, Tao and Bhushan, Vikas. First Aid for the USMLE Step 2 CK, Tenth Edition. New York: McGraw-Hill Education, 2018. TABLE2.2-1. (Figure A) Pg 56. ISBN: 9781260440300. Reproduced with permission from Dr. Richard Usatine.	Reproduced with permission from Le, Tao and Bhushan, Vikas. First Aid for the USMLE Step 2 CK, Tenth Edition. New York: McGraw-Hill Education, 2018. TABLE2.2-1. (Figure B) Pg 56. ISBN: 9781260440300. Reproduced with permission from Dr. Richard Usatine.	Reproduced with permission from Le, Tao and Bhushan, Vikas. First Aid for the USMLE Step 2 CK, Tenth Edition. New York: McGraw-Hill Education, 2018. TABLE2.2-1. (Figure C) Pg 56. ISBN: 9781260440300. Reproduced with permission from Dr. Richard Usatine.	Reproduced with permission from Le, Tao and Bhushan, Vikas. First Aid for the USMLE Step 2 CK, Tenth Edition. New York: McGraw-Hill Education, 2018. TABLE2.2-1. (Figure D) Pg 56. ISBN: 9781260440300. Reproduced with permission from Dr. Richard Usatine.	Reproduced with permission from Carol Soutor, Maria K. Hordinsky, Clinical Dermatology, 1st ed; by McGraw-Hill 2013.

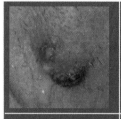	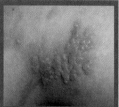	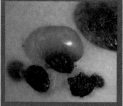	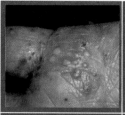	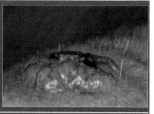
Cyst	**Vesicle**	**Bullae**	**Pustule**	**Telangiectasia**
Nodules filled with expressible material; often under the skin	Elevated, fluid-filled lesion ≤1 cm	Elevated, fluid-filled lesion >1 cm	Elevated, pus-filled lesion Abscess if pustule >1 cm	Enlarged and visible superficial blood vessels; can be seen on a skin lesion or may appear on normal or atrophic skin
Reproduced with permission from Carol Soutor, Maria K. Hordinsky, Clinical Dermatology, 1st ed; by McGraw-Hill 2013.	Reproduced with permission from Le, Tao and Bhushan, Vikas. First Aid for the USMLE Step 2 CK, Tenth Edition. New York: McGraw-Hill Education, 2018. TABLE2.2-1. (Figure E) Pg 56. ISBN: 9781260440300. Reproduced with permission from Dr. Richard Usatine.	Reproduced with permission from Le, Tao and Bhushan, Vikas. First Aid for the USMLE Step 2 CK, Tenth Edition. New York: McGraw-Hill Education, 2018. TABLE2.2-1. (Figure F) Pg 56. ISBN: 9781260440300. Reproduced with permission from Dr. Richard Usatine.	Reproduced with permission from Le, Tao and Bhushan, Vikas. First Aid for the USMLE Step 2 CK, Tenth Edition. New York: McGraw-Hill Education, 2018. TABLE2.2-1. (Figure G) Pg 56. ISBN: 9781260440300. Reproduced with permission from Dr. Richard Usatine.	Reproduced with permission from Carol Soutor, Maria K. Hordinsky, Clinical Dermatology, 1st ed; by McGraw-Hill 2013.

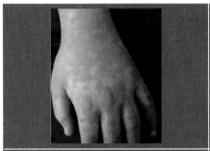

Wheal

Papule or plaque of dermal edema, often with central pallor and irregular borders

Reproduced with permission from Carol Soutor, Maria K. Hordinsky, Clinical Dermatology, 1st ed; by McGraw-Hill 2013

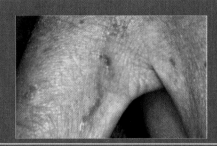

Burrow

Serpiginous tunnel or streak caused by a burrowing mite

Reproduced with permission from Carol Soutor, Maria K. Hordinsky, Clinical Dermatology, 1st ed; by McGraw-Hill 2013.

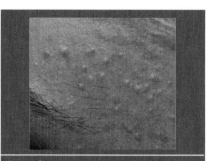

Comedone

Noninflammatory lesion of acne resulting from keratin impaction on outlet of pilosebaceous canal

Reproduced with permission from Carol Soutor, Maria K. Hordinsky, Clinical Dermatology, 1st ed; by McGraw-Hill 2013.

Secondary Skin Lesions

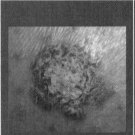

Scale

Visibly thickened stratum corneum; usually whitish

Reproduced with permission from Le, Tao and Bhushan, Vikas. First Aid for the USMLE Step 2 CK, Tenth Edition. New York: McGraw-Hill Education, 2018. TABLE2.2-1. (Figure I) Pg 56. ISBN: 9781260440300. Reproduced with permission from Dr. Richard Usatine.

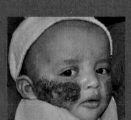

Crust

Liquid debris (serum/blood or pus) that has dried on the skin

Reproduced with permission from Le, Tao and Bhushan, Vikas. First Aid for the USMLE Step 2 CK, Tenth Edition. New York: McGraw-Hill Education, 2018. TABLE2.2-1. (Figure J) Pg 56. ISBN: 9781260440300. Reproduced with permission from Dr. Richard Usatine.

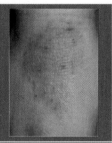

Lichenification

Visible/palpable epidermal thickening with accentuated skin markings

Reproduced with permission from Carol Soutor, Maria K. Hordinsky, Clinical Dermatology, 1st ed; by McGraw-Hill 2013.

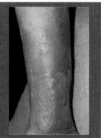

Induration

Dermal thickening resulting in skin that is thicker and firmer than normal

Reproduced with permission from Carol Soutor, Maria K. Hordinsky, Clinical Dermatology, 1st ed; by McGraw-Hill 2013.

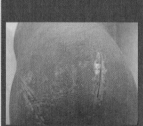

Fissure

Thin, linear tear in epidermis

Reproduced with permission from Carol Soutor, Maria K. Hordinsky, Clinical Dermatology, 1st ed; by McGraw-Hill 2013.

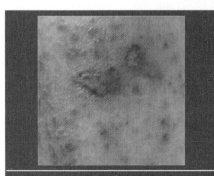

Erosion

Limited loss of epidermis and superficial dermis

Reproduced with permission from Carol Soutor, Maria K. Hordinsky, Clinical Dermatology, 1st ed; by McGraw-Hill 2013.

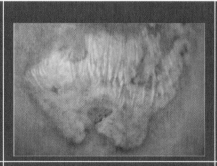

Atrophy

Loss of skin tissue, surface may appear thin and wrinkled

Reproduced with permission from Carol Soutor, Maria K. Hordinsky, Clinical Dermatology, 1st ed; by McGraw-Hill 2013.

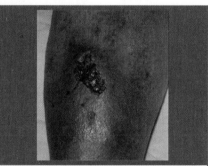

Ulcer

Loss of skin tissue including deeper dermis and may extend to subcutaneous fat

Reproduced with permission from Carol Soutor, Maria K. Hordinsky, Clinical Dermatology, 1st ed; by McGraw-Hill 2013.

Step 2: Describe the distribution and configuration to narrow the differential diagnosis.

- **Distribution** of skin lesions on the body: Describe the initial site, any site of spread, and if involvement is truncal, on extremities, symmetric, or involving flexor or extensor surfaces. For example, a pruritic erythematous patch involving the antecubital fossa is likely atopic dermatitis. The same pruritic erythematous rash on an ear or neck could be allergic contact dermatitis to nickel.
- **Configuration of lesions (if there are multiple):**
    - A line of papules/vesicles is often due to bed bugs.
    - Grouped vesicles in a one-sided dermatomal distribution should raise suspicion for herpes zoster.

Distribution of Dermatologic Lesions

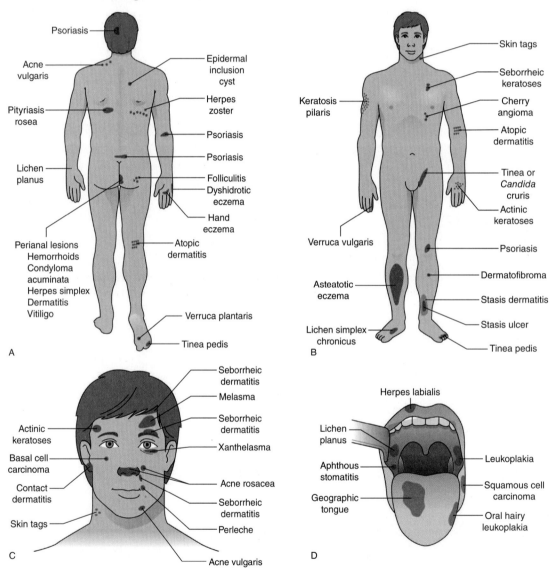

Reproduced with permission from Jameson J, Fauci AS, Kasper DL, Hauser SL, Longo DL, Loscalzo J. eds. Harrison's Manual of Medicine, 20e. McGraw Hill; 2020.

Differential Diagnoses for Common Skin Conditions

A Differential Diagnosis of Common Skin Growths and Raised Lesions Based on Etiology

Malignant and Premalignant	Nonmalignant and Nonvascular	Vascular
Malignant • Basal cell carcinoma • Squamous cell carcinoma • Melanoma • Kaposi sarcoma • Angiosarcoma • Keratoacanthoma **Premalignant** • Actinic keratosis • Sunburns	• Acne • Rosacea • Seborrheic keratosis • Pseudofolliculitis barbae • Herpes simplex and zoster • Molluscum contagiosum • Verrucae/warts • Dermatofibroma • Erythema nodosum • Hairy leukoplakia • Epidermoid cysts • Ganglion cysts • Lipomas • Xanthomas • Melanocytic nevi • Ephelis/ephelides (freckle[s])	• Kaposi sarcoma • Bacillary angiomatosis • Cherry angioma • Strawberry hemangioma • Cystic hygroma • Glomus tumor • Pyogenic granuloma • Angiosarcoma (vascular and malignant)

APPROACH TO RAISED SKIN LESIONS

When evaluating a patient who presents with concern for a raised skin lesion, clinicians should use clues from the patient's history and physical exam to identify lesions that are likely benign and provide reassurance, while also maintaining vigilance for possibly malignant lesions that would require treatment.

- **Characteristics of benign lesions:** Often stable over long periods of time, generally asymptomatic, symmetric, well-circumscribed, homogeneous, and mobile.
- **Characteristics of lesions suspicious for malignancy:** Often rapidly growing, associated with pain, ulceration, bleeding, fixed, non-healing lesions, and color changes. Lesions meeting these characteristics warrant biopsy.

SKIN PIGMENT CHANGES

Variations in skin color largely reflect differences between individuals in the amount of the protein melanin found within their epidermis.

- **Melanocytes:** Dendritic cells which produce pigment, are found within the basal layer of the epidermis and secrete melanin, which is brought to the skin surface via the growth and proliferation of keratinocytes.
- While the number of melanocytes is similar across different races, the amount of melanin produced by melanocytes is greater in darker-skinned individuals.
- Disorders of hypo- or hyperpigmentation, while frequently benign, are often a significant source of distress to patients for cosmetic and/or psychological reasons.
- For patients with skin of color, the effects of such disorders are often more pronounced.
- Treatment will vary depending on the specific diagnosis, but all patients should be counseled on the ways that exposure to ultraviolet (UV) light may affect the course of their disease.

Common Skin Malignancies

The three most common skin cancers are basal cell carcinoma (BCC), squamous cell carcinoma (SCC), and melanoma.

- All three of these cancers are associated with excess sun exposure, lighter skin pigmentation, and genetics.
- While both BCC and SCC are malignant lesions, most BCCs rarely metastasize. However, they are both locally invasive and can lead to disfigurement. SCCs have higher risk than BCC to metastasize. SCC may rapidly grow and metastasize in immunocompromised patients and can be lethal. Melanoma, if not treated at very early stages, can metastasize and is considered the deadliest skin cancer.
- Clinicians can use the ABCDE's of a suspicious mole to determine whether a biopsy may be needed.

ABCDE's of a Suspicious Mole as a General Guideline

A—Asymmetry B—Borders irregular C—Colors changing, or multiple colors present D—Diameter >6 mm E—Evolution of mole/change in mole as per patient	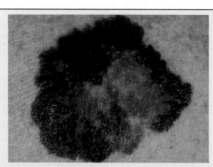 Superficial spreading melanoma, the most common type of melanoma, is characterized by color variegation (black, blue, brown, pink, and white) and irregular borders. (Reproduced with permission from J. Larry Jameson, Anthony S. Fauci, Dennis L. Kasper, Stephen L. Hauser, Dan L. Longo, Joseph Loscalzo, Harrison's Principles of Internal Medicine, 20e; by McGraw Hill LLC 2018.)

Differential Diagnosis of Common Skin Lesions and Rashes Based on Presenting Features

With Fever	No Fever	Blisters or Bullae
• Drug reaction • Cellulitis • Impetigo • Erysipelas • Abscess • Necrotizing fasciitis • Measles • Mumps • Rubella • Rubeola • Secondary syphilis • Rocky Mountain spotted fever • Meningococcal infection • Ecthyma gangrenosum • Disseminated endemic fungi • Toxic shock syndrome • Hemorrhagic fevers	• Atopic dermatitis (eczema) • Allergic contact dermatitis • Seborrheic dermatitis • Psoriasis • Pityriasis rosea • Lichen planus • Dermatitis herpetiformis • Tinea corporis/capitis • Scabies • Urticaria • Scleroderma • Malar rash (SLE)	• Bullous pemphigoid • Pemphigus vulgaris • Dermatitis herpetiformis • Stevens-Johnson syndrome • Erythema multiforme • Drug Rash with Eosinophilia and Systemic Symptoms (DRESS) • Staph • Scalded skin syndrome • Herpes simplex • Varicella zoster

CASE 1 | Acne Vulgaris

A 15-year-old boy presents to clinic with concern for raised skin lesions all over his face for the past few years. These started with puberty and have progressed. Exam is notable for open and closed comedones and erythematous papules and pustules scattered on the central face, forehead, upper back, and chest.

Conditions with Similar Presentations	**Rosacea:** Typically occurs on the face of middle-aged adults with lighter skin pigmentation and is associated with flushing, aggravated by alcohol or other stimuli. Lesions are erythematous papules/pustules like acne, but the presence of telangiectasias without comedones is characteristic. Connective tissue overgrowth, especially of the nose (**rhinophyma**), can occur.
	Malar rash: Spares the nasolabial folds in a butterfly pattern. Seen in patients with systemic lupus erythematosus (SLE) or erysipelas and is characterized by erythematous patches on both cheeks and the bridge of the nose.
	Pseudofolliculitis barbae: Typically occurs in areas that are shaved, related to curving of the hair follicles beneath the skin causing a foreign-body reaction and inflammation
Initial Diagnostic Tests	Clinical diagnosis
Next Steps in Management	• Level of therapy chosen depending on the severity of presenting symptoms and the response to prior therapies. • Options include topical retinoids, topical benzoyl peroxide, topical antibiotics, oral antibiotics, and oral isotretinoin.

CASE 1 | Acne Vulgaris (continued)

Discussion	Acne vulgaris is very common among adolescents, and prevalence generally decreases with increasing age. Main pathogenic factors are as follows: 1. Follicular hyperkeratinization 2. Increased sebum production, stimulated by androgens 3. Infection with *Cutibacterium acnes* 4. Inflammatory response to *C. acnes* **History:** Inquire about risk factors, use of medications that cause acne, and response to any prior therapies. Risk factors include skin trauma, milk consumption, stress, and other causes of hyperandrogenism. Endocrine diseases and steroid use, oral progestin–only contraceptives, phenytoin, and phenobarbital can also increase risk of acne. **Physical Exam:** Usually affects the face, neck, upper back, and chest (areas with large sebaceous glands). There are different subtypes of acne vulgaris: • **Comedonal:** Composed of comedones, closed (whiteheads) and/or open (blackheads). • **Inflammatory** (papulopustular): Composed of erythematous papules and pustules. • **Nodulocystic:** Composed of larger nodules and cysts, often with inflammation. May also be associated with scarring and post-inflammatory hyperpigmentation. **Diagnostics:** Clinical diagnosis **Management:** • All types of acne: • Topical retinoids: Vitamin A derivatives that reduce skin keratinization. Appropriate as initial therapy for all types of acne. Main side effects are xerosis (dry skin) and photosensitivity. • Topical salicylic acid: Keratinolytic agent that can be used in patients who cannot tolerate topical retinoids as a first-line agent. • Mild inflammatory acne • Topical benzoyl peroxide: Comedolytic and antibacterial properties. • Comedonal acne • Topical retinoids. • Moderate inflammatory or nodulocystic acne • Topical antibiotics (clindamycin, dapsone, or erythromycin). • Severe inflammatory or nodulocystic acne • Oral antibiotics (tetracycline, minocycline, doxycycline). • Severe nodulocystic acne, acne conglobata, acne that has not responded to the above therapies: • Oral isotretinoin: highly teratogenic. • Requires patients of childbearing potential to be on two forms of contraception as well as monthly pregnancy checks. Other options for treatment in females include combined oral contraceptives and spironolactone, which have antiandrogenic properties.

CASE 2 | Hidradenitis Suppurativa

A 32-year-old woman with severe obesity and tobacco use presents to the clinic with a 4-month history of painful red bumps with foul-smelling discharge in both armpits and near her groin. She has had these symptoms on and off over the past 7 years but has never been evaluated. On exam, the patient has multiple inflamed and painful papules and nodules in bilateral axilla and inguinal folds. There are also draining sinus tracts and there is significant scarring in the affected areas.

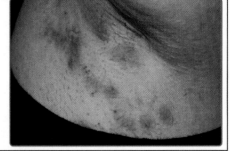

Hidradenitis suppurativa in axilla. (Reproduced with permission from Sewon Kang, Masayuki Amagai, Anna L. Bruckner, Alexander H. Enk, David J. Margolis, Amy J. McMichael, Jeffrey S. Orringer, Fitzpatrick's Dermatology, 9e; by McGraw-Hill 2019.)

Conditions with Similar Presentations	**Skin Infections (e.g., abscesses, cellulitis):** May have more systemic symptoms, such as fever and less likely to be in symmetric configuration. Usually from Gram-positive aerobic cocci (strep and staph) which do not produce an odor. **Cutaneous Crohn's disease:** Draining sinus tracts may be similar, but Crohn's will also be associated with GI symptoms and usually located near anus.

CASE 2 | Hidradenitis Suppurativa *(continued)*

Initial Diagnostic Tests	Clinical diagnosis
Next Steps in Management	Topical antibiotics, lifestyle modifications, and symptomatic treatment (see below for refractory cases)
Discussion	Hidradenitis suppurativa (HS) is a chronic disease characterized by recurrent flares of painful papules, nodules, and abscesses, usually located in the axilla, inguinal folds, and/or anogenital area. These lesions are often accompanied by draining sinus tracts which can secrete foul-smelling pus. These sinus tracts often lead to scarring. HS is more common in females and has a worldwide prevalence of 1–4%. **History:** Inquire about risk factors, family history, frequency of flares, and current pain level. Risk factors include a personal family history (present in 35–40% of patients), obesity, and smoking (60–90% of cases are in smokers). **Physical Exam:** • Lesions can vary in morphology (papules, nodules, abscesses, and/or pustules) and are often tender. • Lesions located in the axillary, inguinal, anogenital, and inframammary areas • Secondary changes include draining sinus tracts and scarring • Unusual to have systemic symptoms such as fever or lymphadenopathy **Diagnosis:** Clinical diagnosis. Staging of lesions through the Hurley system. • Stage 1: Single or multiple abscess formation(s) without sinus tracts or scar formation • Stage 2: Recurrent, widely separated single or multiple abscess(es) with limited sinus tracts and scar formation • Stage 3: Diffuse or near-diffuse involvement with multiple abscesses and interconnected sinus tracts across an entire area **Management:** • Manage symptoms with analgesics and dressings • Initiate treatment with topical antibiotics (clindamycin, doxycycline) • If no response, advance to oral antibiotics (doxycycline, clindamycin and rifampin, or dapsone) • If refractory, consider biologic agent adalimumab (TNF alpha inhibitor) • Can use short oral corticosteroid course to treat acute flares • Procedural treatments such as intralesional corticosteroids or surgical excision for extensive lesions • In addition, discuss lifestyle modifications (e.g., weight loss, smoking cessation, wear loose-fitting clothing)

CASE 3 | Herpes Simplex Virus (HSV) Infection

A 21-year-old man with a history of renal transplant on immunosuppression presents with painful bumps along the sides of his lips with burning and tingling sensation in the area. He has been feeling poorly, with fevers and malaise. On exam, temperature is 99.8°F. There are multiple vesicular lesions on an erythematous base on the lip and face. The anterior cervical and submandibular lymph nodes are enlarged and tender.

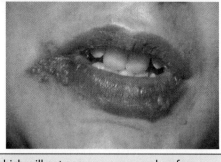

Herpes simplex virus causing herpes labialis. (Reproduced with permission from Carol Soutor, Maria K. Hordinsky, Clinical Dermatology, 1st ed; by McGraw-Hill 2013.)

Conditions with Similar Presentations	**Impetigo:** Is a bacterial infection due to staph or strep species, which will not occur on a mucosal surface. **Varicella zoster:** Can also present with painful/pruritic vesicles, but lesions should be at different stages of healing. • Primary infection (chicken pox) presents with generalized rash • Reactivation (zoster or shingles) presents in a unilateral dermatomal pattern **Verrucae (warts):** Cauliflower-like lesions caused by HPV and are generally not painful **Molluscum contagiosum:** Caused by a poxvirus that induces the epidermis to proliferate and is characterized by multiple 2- to 5-mm flesh-colored papules with central umbilication (dimple in the center) in clusters. Common in children, can be self-inoculated or sexually transmitted in adults.
Initial Diagnostic Tests	• Clinical diagnosis • Can confirm with PCR testing of vesicular fluid

CASE 3 | Herpes Simplex Virus (HSV) Infection *(continued)*

Next Steps in Management	• Treat with antivirals such as acyclovir, famciclovir, and valacyclovir
Discussion	HSV affects >50% of the adult global population. Oral-labial lesions classically occur due to HSV-1, and genital lesions due to HSV-2. However, it is possible to spread HSV-1 to the genital area through oral sex. After primary infection with HSV, the virus survives in latent state in dorsal root ganglia (trigeminal or sacral ganglia) and reactivates during times of stress or in immunocompromised states. During recurrence, the virus travels down the nerve fibers that supply the skin and will replicate, producing the lesion. Recurrent episodes tend to be more mild than initial infection. Autoinoculation can occur from these active lesions. **History:** Risk factors include sexually active adolescents, athletes in contact sports, health care workers, and close contact with another individual with an active HSV infection. • Primary infection: systemic symptoms such as fevers, malaise, painful oral lesions (gingivostomatitis), lymphadenopathy and tingling, numbness, burning, and pain in the affected area • Recurrent HSV can be precipitated by stress, immunodeficiency, trauma, or fever **Physical Exam:** • Primary infection: fever, gingivostomatitis, lymphadenopathy, and pain and/or paresthesias in the affected area • Recurrent infection: lesions are usually localized and progress from vesicles to crusts in a little over a week **Diagnostics:** • If a clinical diagnosis cannot be made, obtain viral culture or PCR • Unroof vesicles before swabbing • Tzank smear has less sensitivity and specificity and shows multinucleated giant cells with or without intranuclear inclusions **Management:** • No permanent cure • Acyclovir, valacyclovir, or famciclovir can reduce synthesis of viral DNA and help reduce severity and viral shedding • Primary infections: antivirals should be given within 72 hours of symptom onset for a 7- to 10-day course • Recurrent infections: antivirals should be given within 48 hours of symptom onset for a 5-day course • Chronic suppression: for patients with severe recurrent disease, especially if they trigger erythema multiforme, eczema herpeticum, or aseptic meningitis
Additional Considerations	**Complications and Related Findings:** • **Herpetic whitlow** is a lesion on the finger • **Erythema multiforme:** target-like lesions with central epidermal necrosis, may also be associated with HSV infection • Patients with atopic dermatitis (eczema) are at risk of developing a superimposed HSV infection, **eczema herpeticum** • HSV infection of the cornea may cause **keratitis**, a leading cause of blindness • Neurologic complications include **temporal lobe encephalitis** (more associated with HSV1) or **aseptic meningitis** (more associated with HSV2) • HSV can cause **esophagitis**, which is characterized by punched-out ulcers, distinguishing it from cytomegalovirus (CMV) esophagitis, which classically presents with linear ulcers **Pregnancy Considerations:** Prophylaxis should be given to pregnant women with a history of genital herpes (without active lesions) to allow for possibility of vaginal delivery. Patients with active lesions will require Caesarean section to avoid passing the virus to the fetus upon delivery.

CASE 4 | Seborrheic Keratosis

A 68-year-old man presents for routine health care and asks if the long-standing skin lesions on his face (shown in figure) are cancerous. The lesions are not itchy or painful. They are well demarcated, circumscribed, hyperpigmented lesions which appear to be "stuck on" and have a waxy texture.

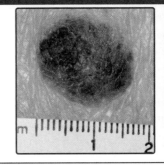 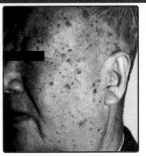

Seborrheic keratosis. (Reproduced with permission from Sewon Kang, Masayuki Amagai, Anna L. Bruckner, Alexander H. Enk, David J. Margolis, Amy J. McMichael, Jeffrey S. Orringer, Fitzpatrick's Dermatology, 9e; by McGraw-Hill 2019.)

CASE 4 | Seborrheic Keratosis *(continued)*

Conditions with Similar Presentations	**Verruca vulgaris:** Small papules that may have variety of colors with small amount of scale (white yellow); can also be present for long periods of time. **Dermal nevi:** Well-circumscribed and may be hyperpigmented; do not often have the described "stuck-on" appearance. **Melanoma:** Have irregular borders and evolve (growing, changing in color) over time. **SCC:** Evolve over time but may grow fast and may have areas of ulceration and potential overlying crusting or scale; may be associated with pain. **BCC:** Smooth nodule or shiny papule ("pearly papule"); may be associated with raised borders or ulcer.
Initial Diagnostic Tests	Clinical diagnosis
Next steps in Management	No treatment needed
Discussion	Seborrheic keratosis affects roughly 90% of adults over the age of 60, and is more common in males. The pathophysiology is not fully understood, but it is a common, benign, pigmented neoplasm that is caused by squamous epithelial proliferation with keratin-filled cysts. **History and Physical Exam:** Usually seen in patients above age 50 and do not itch or cause pain. Characteristic features: Waxy stuck-on appearance; well demarcated, warty texture; color ranges from light brown to black **Diagnostics:** Clinical diagnosis made by visual inspection **Management:** No need for treatment If irritating or present cosmetic concerns, consider removal with cryotherapy, curettage, or conservative shave removal or excision.
Additional Considerations	**Leser-Trélat sign:** Numerous itchy seborrheic keratoses suddenly appear in an asymmetric pattern following skin cleavage planes. It is associated with underlying cancer, most frequently gastric adenocarcinoma.

CASE 5 | Kaposi Sarcoma (KS)

A 34-year-old man with HIV presents for evaluation of multiple purplish lesions that are not itchy or painful. Due to loss of insurance, he has not been able to obtain his anti-retroviral therapy over the past year. On exam, he has a few scattered purplish macules on his palate and multiple red-violaceous macules and papules on his back and legs with patches and plaques.

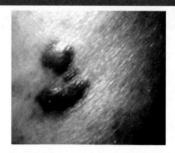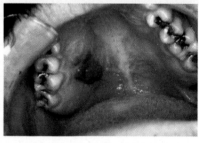

Kaposi sarcoma. (Reproduced with permission from Scott D.C. Stern, Adam S. Cifu, Diane Altkorn, Symptom to Diagnosis: An Evidence-Based Guide, 4e; by McGraw-Hill 2020.)

Conditions with Similar Presentations	**Bacillary angiomatosis:** Caused by *Bartonella* infections; typically occurs in advanced HIV disease. • Papules and nodules look like angiomas: bright red, violaceous, or skin-colored, and can grow up to 3 cm • Biopsy and/or culture with Warthin-Starry silver stain is positive • Histologically, bacillary angiomatosis has a **neutrophilic** infiltrate (indicating bacterial etiology) **Cherry hemangiomas (angiomas):** Benign; occur in the elderly; may increase with age. **Strawberry (infantile) hemangiomas:** Benign; seen in infants, but regress over time.
Initial Diagnostic Tests	Clinical diagnosis confirmed with biopsy
Next Steps in Management	• For patients with AIDS, initiate highly active antiretroviral therapy (HAART) • Local treatment can be considered for solitary lesions • Systemic approaches for multiple lesions

CASE 5 | Kaposi Sarcoma (KS) *(continued)*

Discussion	KS is a human herpesvirus 8 (HHV-8)–associated vascular malignancy and typically involves the skin, GI, or respiratory tracts.
	HHV-8 spreads via sexual contact or can be transmitted through saliva or arthropod bites. Lower CD4 counts are associated more extensive and aggressive KS.
	History:
	Risk factors: Immunosuppression (e.g., AIDS, corticosteroids)
	For patients with HIV, KS is an AIDS-defining illness and is more commonly seen in men who have sex with men. However, any immunosuppressed patients can develop KS.
	Physical Exam: Purplish, reddish, or dark brown/black macules and papules which progress to patches/plaques and/or tumors.
	Diagnostics: Biopsy of lesion is especially important to distinguish KS from bacillary angiomatosis. Biopsy shows lymphocytic infiltrates (Indicating viral etiology).
	Management:
	• In patients with AIDS, start HAART, which has been shown to decrease both the incidence and severity of the disease
	• Important to explore non-adherence
	• Local treatment can be considered for solitary lesions (surgery, radiation, cryotherapy, intralesional, or topical treatment)
	• Systemic approaches (radiation, chemotherapy, medications) may be considered for severe cases/multiple lesions

CASE 6 | Hairy Leukoplakia

A 50-year-old man with a 30-pack-year history of tobacco use presents for evaluation of white painless patches on his tongue and generalized malaise for the past few weeks. He has had unprotected sex with men, and his last HIV test was negative 10 years ago. Oropharyngeal exam reveals bilateral white patches on the lateral tongue, which cannot be scraped off.

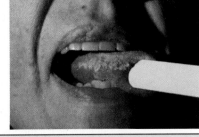

Oral hairy leukoplakia. (From Kevin J. Knoop, Lawrence B. Stack, Alan B. Storrow, R. Jason Thurman, The Atlas of Emergency Medicine, 5e. Copyright 2021 by McGraw Hill. FIGURE 20.4. ISBN 9781260134940. Photo contributor: Kevin J. Knoop, MD, MS.)

Conditions with Similar Presentations	**Oropharyngeal candidiasis** (oral thrush): White patches/plaques on the tongue that can be scraped off and reveal a red base. Seen in immunocompromised patients or those using inhaled steroids.
	Oral leukoplakia: White patches/plaques that cannot be scraped off and are often unilateral. Risk factors include HPV infection, chewing or smoking tobacco, or alcohol use. It is a premalignant lesion that can develop into SCC over time, in contrast to hairy leukoplakia which does not lead to malignancy
Initial Diagnostic Tests	• This is generally a clinical diagnosis in the absence of risk factors • Check: HIV test • Biopsy indicated for diagnosis in this patient given patient's tobacco history
Next Steps in Management	Treat underlying condition
Discussion	Hairy leukoplakia is due to **Epstein-Barr** virus (EBV) infection and typically occurs in immunocompromised patients. Among HIV-positive patients, it is associated with smoking and low CD4 counts.
	History:
	• Immunocompromised state: HIV or solid-organ transplant
	• May be one of the first presenting signs of HIV
	Physical Exam:
	• Non-painful white patches, with fuzzy hair-like projections
	• Often on the lateral aspect of the tongue, bilateral distribution
	• Cannot be scraped off

CASE 6 | Hairy Leukoplakia *(continued)*

Discussion	**Diagnostics:** Clinical diagnosis
	• Rule out HIV
	• Biopsy may be considered in cases suspicious for oral leukoplakia or SCC
	Management:
	• The lesions themselves do not require direct treatment
	• Lesions will improve with resolution of underlying immunodeficiency

CASE 7 | Squamous Cell Carcinoma (SCC) of the Skin

A 72-year-old man who works as a farmer presents for evaluation of a rapidly growing, firm bump on his lower lip. Exam reveals an erythematous ulcerated nodule that is 1.8 cm in diameter.

Squamous cell carcinoma adjacent to the lower lip. (Reproduced with permission from Sewon Kang, Masayuki Amagai, Anna L. Bruckner, Alexander H. Enk, David J. Margolis, Amy J. McMichael, Jeffrey S. Orringer, Fitzpatrick's Dermatology, 9e; by McGraw-Hill 2019.)

Conditions with Similar Presentations	**Actinic keratosis:** Precancerous lesion(s) (usually a papule/plaque of rough, dry, non-healing skin) which can potentially develop into SCC. **Basal cell carcinoma (BCC):** Key distinguishing features on gross examination include a pink, pearly papule with telangiectasias. BCCs more frequently affect the upper lip, medial cheeks, nose, forehead while SCCs affect the lower lip
Initial Diagnostic Tests	Clinical diagnosis confirmed with biopsy
Next Steps in Management	Surgical excision
Discussion	Most SCCs arise in elderly white males and are the second most common type of skin cancer. They are malignant tumors derived from keratinocytes, which may invade past the epidermis into the dermal layers. Most SCCs are associated with DNA mutations caused by excessive exposure to UV radiation. The p53 tumor suppression gene is often implicated, and human papillomaviruses (HPV) are believed to play a role in the development of SCC in immunocompromised patients. SCC can also occur from other chronic cutaneous inflammation, such as a draining sinus from underlying osteomyelitis or Crohn's disease. **History:** Inquire about cumulative sun exposure, prior sunburn, and risk factors for SCC, such as chronic immunosuppression. • History of previous skin cancers or precancerous lesions (actinic keratoses), smoking, lighter skin, and chronic sun exposure • Other risk factors include arsenic exposure, immunodeficiency, h/o solid organ transplant, repeated skin trauma, or rare inherited disorders such as xeroderma pigmentosum (a condition characterized by inability to repair UV-damaged DNA). **Physical Exam:** • In light-skinned individuals, SCC will usually arise in areas of sun-exposed skin • Genital lesions or SCCs in immunocompromised patients are often associated with concurrent HPV presence • Lesions can slowly grow as persistent patch or plaque, usually pink/red, which can bleed or ulcerate

CASE 7 | Squamous Cell Carcinoma (SCC) of the Skin *(continued)*

Discussion	**Diagnostics:** • Always confirm with biopsy—either shave, punch, or excisional • Biopsy will often show keratin pearls (keratinization as well as atypical and mitotic features) • Regional lymph node examination with ultrasound or biopsy if there is extensive tumor spread and concern for metastatic disease. **Management:** • Surgical excision should include a margin of healthy tissue to ensure complete removal of the cancer. • **Mohs surgery** can be utilized, which involves staged circumferential tumor extirpation with horizontal histological frozen sections, removing thin slices of skin, and examining under a microscope to minimize the amount of healthy tissue removed while precisely excising the cancer completely
Additional Considerations	**Keratoacanthoma:** Is a rapidly growing variant of SCC that may spontaneously regress. Standard of care is treatment as for other types of SCCs. **Bowen disease:** Refers to SCC in situ, with no evidence of invasive disease. **Erythroplasia of Queyart:** Refers to Bowen disease involving the penis. **Marjolin ulcer:** Is a SCC developing from sites of chronic wounds or heavy scarring. These are typically very aggressive and have poor prognosis.

Squamous cell carcinoma adjacent to the lower lip. (Reproduced with permission from Sewon Kang, Masayuki Amagai, Anna L. Bruckner, Alexander H. Enk, David J. Margolis, Amy J. McMichael, Jeffrey S. Orringer, Fitzpatrick's Dermatology, 9e; by McGraw-Hill 2019.)

CASE 8 | Basal Cell Carcinoma (BCC)

A 63-year-old man presents for evaluation of a bump on his face. He has a long history of sun exposure as a postal worker and has had multiple severe sunburns as a child. Exam reveals a pink, pearly ulcerated nodule 0.3 cm in size with rolled borders and telangiectasias.

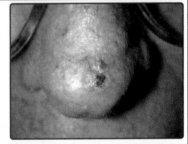

Basal cell carcinoma on nose. (Reproduced with permission from Sewon Kang, Masayuki Amagai, Anna L. Bruckner, Alexander H. Enk, David J. Margolis, Amy J. McMichael, Jeffrey S. Orringer, Fitzpatrick's Dermatology, 9e; by McGraw-Hill 2019.)

Conditions with Similar Presentations	**Dermal nevi:** Well-circumscribed and may be hyperpigmented; do not typically have rolled borders. **SCC:** Evolves over time; may have areas of ulceration and overlying crusting or scale. **Nummular eczema:** Circular plaques, associated with overlying scale and pruritis.
Initial Diagnostic Tests	Clinical diagnosis confirmed with biopsy
Next Steps in Management	Surgical excision and/or topical therapy (imiquimod or 5-fluorouracil).
Discussion	BCC is the most common cancer of the skin and is mostly seen in elderly males. It arises from the basal layer of the epidermis and, while rarely metastatic, can lead to local invasion of the skin and surrounding structures. It occurs due to acquired mutations to the PTCH tumor suppressor gene, often because of UV radiation–induced DNA damage. There are five histological types; the two most common are nodular and superficial. • Nodular types: Pink- or flesh-colored nodules; often have telangiectasias; may have ulceration and a "rolled" border (higher on the sides than in the middle); often found on the face and head • Superficial type: May have a scale; tend to be flatter; often on the trunk **History:** Risk factors include lighter skin pigmentation, sun damage, previous cutaneous injury, arsenic exposure, and genetic predisposition. Compared to SCC, BCC is more correlated with sun exposure at a younger age and intense, intermittent UV exposure.

CASE 8 | Basal Cell Carcinoma (BCC) *(continued)*

| Discussion | **Physical Exam:**
• Most BCC will present on the face and less frequently on the trunk
• Lesions are pink, pearly, papules or nodules with overlying telangiectasias
• Sometimes, the periphery of the lesion will have a rolled border (the outer rim of the lesion is raised)

Diagnostics:
• Should always be confirmed with biopsy
• Biopsy will demonstrate the classic pattern of basaloid cell nests with palisading nuclei, "retraction artifact," between the tumor and dermis and sometimes increased mucin in the surrounding dermal stroma

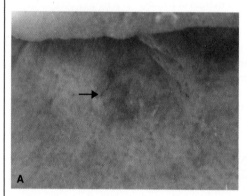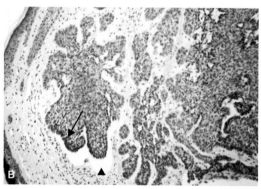
Basal cell carcinoma. A. Pink, shiny papule with telangiectasias (*arrow*) consistent with basal cell carcinoma. B. Blue (basophilic) cells with peripheral palisading (*arrow*) and clefting (*arrowhead*). (Reproduced with permission from Howard M. Reisner, Pathology: A Modern Case Study, 2e; by McGraw-Hill 2020.)

Management:
Mohs micrographic surgery (staged circumferential surgery with concurrent specimen horizontal processing in histology) is the standard of care. If surgical excision applied, 5 mm margin is considered. Other treatment modalities include radiation, electrodesiccation and curettage, or topical therapy (imiquimod or 5-fluorouracil) |
| Additional Considerations | **Preventive:** Advice to patients should include tips on how to limit excessive sun exposure, including preference for shady areas during hours of intense sunlight, the use of sunscreen (SPF 30 or above), and avoidance of tanning beds. |

CASE 9 | Malignant Melanoma

A 55-year-old woman comes in for evaluation of a "mole" on the sole of her foot. She has had it for some time, but it seems to have become bigger. On exam, there is a dark patch on the sole of her foot with irregular borders and various colors that measures 3 cm in diameter.

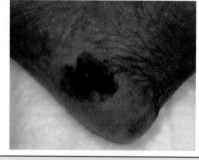

Melanoma. (Reproduced with permission from A. Paul Kelly, Susan C. Taylor, Henry W. Lim, Ana Maria Anido Serrano, Taylor and Kelly's Dermatology for Skin of Color, 2e; by McGraw-Hill 2016.)

| Conditions with Similar Presentations | **Melanocytic nevi (common mole):** Are benign, usually less than 6 mm, uniformly pigmented, and well defined with rounded borders. They can be flat macules (junctional nevi) or papular (intradermal nevi).

Ephelis (freckle): Is an inherited (or acquired), benign, poorly defined, 3- to 10-mm hyperpigmented macule, often arising in patients with lighter skin. They commonly become lighter during the winter months.

Lentigo: Is a benign hyperpigmented lesion, usually less than 5 mm, associated with sun exposure. There are multiple subtypes and, unlike ephelis, these lesions will not fade during the winter months. |

CASE 9 | Malignant Melanoma (continued)

Initial Diagnostic Tests	• Clinical diagnosis, using ABCDE's as well as dermoscopy • Confirm diagnosis with biopsy
Next Steps in Management	Wide local excision.
Discussion	Melanoma is the deadliest form of skin cancer and is the fifth most common type of cancer among both men and women. They occur due to uncontrolled proliferation of melanocytic stem cells from acquired gene mutations (often due to sun damage). Melanomas with a vertical growth phase have the potential to invade through the basement membrane into the dermis, where they can metastasize through the lymphatic system to other organs, particularly the brain and lungs. Most melanomas arise from normal-appearing skin, though roughly 25% arise from precursor lesions such as benign melanocytic nevi, atypical/dysplastic nevi, or atypical solar lentigo. There are four common subtypes: • **Superficial spreading:** Most common and generally, most curable • **Nodular:** Second most common; usually thicker than other subtypes, increasing the risk of malignant invasion and/or metastasis • **Lentigo maligna:** Arises from chronically sun-damaged skin in the elderly and slowly enlarges over years • **Acral lentiginous:** Rare form in general but more common form in patients with darker skin tones. Commonly seen in non-sun-exposed areas such as the palms, soles, and nailbeds **History:** Incidence of melanoma increases significantly with age. Risk factors include personal or family history of skin cancer, numerous benign or atypical nevi, red/blond hair, and lighter skin tones that are susceptible to sunburns. Patients often have a history of easy burning or excessive sun exposure, possibly including the use of tanning beds. **Physical Exam:** Total body skin examination is crucial for identifying lesions suspicious for melanoma • In males, the most common site is the back • In females, the most common site is on the legs • Clinicians should use the ABCDE checklist to identify features that are suspicious for melanoma • Additionally, clinicians should consider the "ugly duckling sign," which describes the observation that one pigmented lesion looks significantly different from the other lesions that a patient may have **Diagnostics:** • Dermoscopy can also be utilized to further evaluate suspicious lesions • Biopsy: Preferred method is an excisional/complete biopsy with 1- to 3-mm margin. • Histopathology will show atypical melanocytes and architectural disorder. • The pathology report should make note of the thickness of the tumor, called the **Breslow depth.** Depth of invasion is most important prognostic factor. **Management:** • Wide local excision. • Mohs micrographic surgery with special stains is used for melanoma in situ (MIS). Margins should be large (5 mm if melanoma in situ, larger margins for head and neck MIS, minimum of 10 mm for invasive melanoma) to ensure complete excision, and pathology reports should demonstrate that the sample has negative margins. Close clinical follow up is required. • Patients who have evidence of regional lymph node enlargement should have those lymph nodes surgically removed. • The presence of a BRAF mutation allows for treatment with targeted BRAF-inhibitors such as dabrafenib, trametinib, and vemurafenib. • Invasion >4 mm has a poor prognosis and palliative chemotherapy and radiation are additional treatments
Additional Considerations	**Screening:** Screening is not indicated for the public but patients of all ages should be counseled to avoid excessive sun exposure. For high-risk patients (personal/family history of melanoma, many dysplastic/atypical nevi, very sun sensitive) an annual total body skin examination (TBSE) should be done by a health care provider and patients should be educated on how to perform self screening and counselled regarding sun protective behavior. **Complications:** Metastatic melanoma most commonly spreads to lymph nodes, liver, lungs, bone, and brain.

SKIN PIGMENT CHANGES

CASE 10 | Vitiligo

A 30-year-old man with diabetes presents with diffuse, white patches on multiple parts of his body for several months. Exam shows discrete white macules/patches on the skin exhibiting depigmentation. There are no associated signs of inflammation.

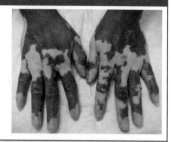

Vitiligo. (Reproduced with permission from Carol Soutor, Maria K. Hordinsky, Clinical Dermatology, 1st ed; by McGraw-Hill 2013.)

Conditions with Similar Presentations	**Tinea (pityriasis) versicolor:** Is caused by fungi (Malassezia globosa is most common species) in hot, sweaty conditions. Patches vary in color, typically occur on back/chest, and can be hyperpigmented/pink/yellow but are classically hypopigmented with associated scale. Will not show complete depigmentation on Wood's lamp as seen in vitiligo.
	Albinism: Is a genetic disorder of decreased production of melanin due to decreased tyrosinase activity or defective tyrosine transport. Patients are at increased risk for skin cancer.
Initial Diagnostic Tests	• Clinical diagnosis • Consider evaluating for additional autoimmune disorders
Next Steps in Management	Glucocorticoids and/or UV light therapy.
Discussion	Vitiligo is an autoimmune disease resulting in well-defined areas of depigmentation. It is characterized by destruction of melanocytes, resulting in focal areas of depigmentation. It is believed to affect around 1% of the world's population, and patients frequently suffer from social stigmatization and low self-esteem. **History:** The peak incidence is in patients in their 20's–30's and is often associated with other autoimmune diseases, such as type I diabetes, Graves' disease, and Hashimoto thyroiditis. **Physical Exam:** • Depigmented, well-defined macules and patches without any signs of inflammation • Lesions can appear anywhere but are most frequently seen on the face, genitals, and hands **Diagnostics:** Clinical diagnosis • Wood's lamp testing may assist with diagnosis, showing well-defined areas of bright blue–white fluorescence • Biopsy is rarely needed, but pathology would show absence of melanocytes with lymphocytic infiltration • Evaluate for additional autoimmune disorders **Management:** There is no cure for vitiligo, and current treatment options yield varying degrees of success • Topical treatments include corticosteroids and calcineurin inhibitors • Phototherapy with UV radiation can help provide a minimal degree of repigmentation, beginning in the hair follicles • Vitiligo can be a significant cause of psychosocial distress, and physicians should ensure that these issues are addressed with patients

Skin Pigment Change Mini-Cases

Cases	Key Findings
Acanthosis Nigricans	**Hx:** History of diabetes, obesity, or insulin resistance **PE:** Hyperpigmented thickening of the skin, usually in axilla, groin, back of the neck **Diagnostics:** Clinical diagnosis **Management:** Treat underlying insulin resistance (e.g., metformin) **Discussion:** Acanthosis nigricans is common in patients with obesity (due to insulin resistance without frank diabetes) and in patients with diabetes. Excess insulin induces rapid proliferation of skin cells with increased melanin production, leading to the darkened appearance. Acanthosis nigricans in a patient without diabetes or obesity can be associated with an underlying adenocarcinoma, usually of the GI or GU tract.

Acanthosis nigricans in neck. (Reproduced with permission from Carol Soutor, Maria K. Hordinsky, Clinical Dermatology, 1st ed; by McGraw-Hill 2013.)

Skin Pigment Change Mini-Cases *(continued)*

Melasma	**Hx:** Pregnant patient or using oral contraceptives **PE:** Bilateral light to dark brown macules and patches, typically on face **Diagnostics:** Clinical diagnosis **Management:** Sun protection, discontinuation of any potential offending agents (e.g., oral contraceptives) **Discussion:** Melasma, also known as chloasma or mask of pregnancy, is an acquired hyperpigmentation on sun-exposed areas seen primarily in women. It has an increased incidence in pregnancy and use of the following medications: oral contraceptive pill (OCP), topical hydroquinone, tretinoin, or steroids. 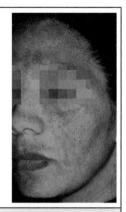 Melasma. (Reproduced with permission from Carol Soutor, Maria K. Hordinsky, Clinical Dermatology, 1st ed; by McGraw-Hill 2013.)
Candida Intertrigo	**Hx:** Overweight/obese, diabetes, history of excessive sweating **PE:** Erythematous and itchy/painful plaques, occasionally with fissuring and peeling; usually located on flexural surfaces and folds in the skin **Diagnostics:** Clinical diagnosis but can be confirmed with microscopy and culture of skin scrapings **Management:** Topical clotrimazole/terbinafine, or oral antifungals if severe **Discussion:** Intertrigo occurs in skin folds, usually a moist environment such as underneath breasts or between the leg creases. It is most frequently seen in obese patients, often with diabetes mellitus or immunodeficiency. 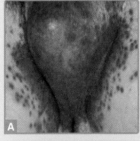 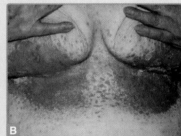 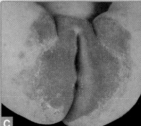 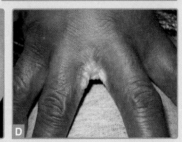 Various presentations of intertrigo. (Reproduced with permission from Sewon Kang, Masayuki Amagai, Anna L. Bruckner, Alexander H. Enk, David J. Margolis, Amy J. McMichael, Jeffrey S. Orringer, Fitzpatrick's Dermatology, 9e; by McGraw-Hill 2019.)
Post-inflammatory Hyperpigmentation	**Hx:** More common on darker skin types, but can occur in anyone **PE:** Hyperpigmented patches at the site of the initial inflamed area **Diagnostics:** Clinical diagnosis **Management:** Sun protection, topical hydroquinone, azelaic acid, vitamin C creams **Discussion:** Post-inflammatory hyperpigmentation is skin darkening in the areas of a prior inflammation/rash/lesion (such as a pimple) and can occur anywhere on the body. Can be more severe in sun-exposed areas. 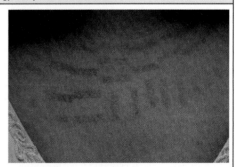 Post-inflammatory hyperpigmentation. (Reproduced with permission from A. Paul Kelly, Susan C. Taylor, Henry W. Lim, Ana Maria Anido Serrano, Taylor and Kelly's Dermatology for Skin of Color, 2e; by McGraw-Hill 2016.)

RASHES (SKIN ERUPTIONS)

A simplified approach to common presentations of rashes is shown below, highlighting classical presentations of the diseases listed. Several other variations of the entities described exist but are rarely tested. Classic presentations are usually tested and will likely stay true to the distribution.

History

Inquire about exposures to new medications, travel history, infections, immunizations, timing (rash onset in relation to fever) and presence of fever, and additional symptoms.

Physical Exam

Type of rash (macular/papular vs. purpuric, localized vs. generalized involvement of palms/soles/mucosal surfaces); evaluate for presence of lymphadenopathy and conjunctivitis; perform an oral exam.

Location and pattern:

- Scalp: psoriasis, seborrheic dermatitis
- Extensor surfaces: psoriasis, dermatitis herpetiformis
- Flexor surfaces: atopic dermatitis, lichen planus
- Herpes zoster will be unilateral dermatomal but can appear anywhere on the body; the first division of the trigeminal nerve is the most common single dermatome. Thoracic dermatomes as an aggregate are more common than cranial, lumbar, or sacral.

The picture/description may not always have vesicles; erosions may be present instead. If unsure, look at the borders.

- Atopic dermatitis is poorly demarcated
- Psoriasis is well demarcated
- Tinea is serpiginous

- Eczematous rashes have a distinct appearance, and the differential is usually atopic dermatitis, urticaria, or contact dermatitis.
- For febrile pediatric rashes the differential is broad: measles, rubella, Kawasaki disease, scarlet fever, erythema infectiosum, roseola, or Rocky Mountain spotted fever.

Approach to Rashes

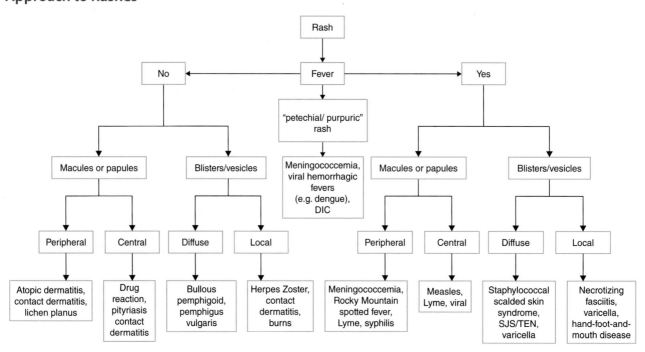

Rash without Fever

CASE 11 | Pityriasis Rosea

A 6-year-old boy is brought in by his mother for evaluation of a rash on his trunk. His mother recalls that her child had a fever, sore throat, and malaise a few weeks ago and a rose-colored oval lesion on his back about 2 weeks ago. This morning he developed multiple smaller lesions on his back. On exam, there is a 3-cm well-demarcated salmon-colored lesion on his lower back as well as multiple small erythematous plaques with fine collarette scales in a "Christmas tree" distribution on his trunk. No lesions were noted on his palms or soles.

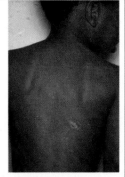

Pityriasis rosea. (Reproduced with permission from A. Paul Kelly, Susan C. Taylor, Henry W. Lim, Ana Maria Anido Serrano, Taylor and Kelly's Dermatology for Skin of Color, 2e; by McGraw-Hill 2016.)

Conditions with Similar Presentations	**Tinea corporis:** Single or multiple lesions; KOH prep would demonstrate fungal hyphae. **Tinea versicolor:** Lesions share a similar distribution to pityriasis rosea, may be hyper- or hypopigmented, but would not have overlying scale. **Secondary syphilis:** Hyperpigmented macules on the palms and soles. **Guttate psoriasis:** Can be confused with pityriasis rosea; however, the scale in psoriasis is thicker and more silvery and the course is longer.
Initial Diagnostic Tests	Clinical diagnosis
Next Steps in Management	• No treatment is necessary, as pityriasis self-resolves within 6 weeks. • Antihistamines can help control itching.
Discussion	Pityriasis rosea is an acute, self-limited, inflammatory skin eruption that is often preceded by a viral syndrome. The rash is due to a type IV hypersensitivity reaction. HSV 6 and 7 have been implicated but the disease does not occur endemically. It is commonly seen in older children and young adults. **History:** Pityriasis rosea can occur at all ages and is most common in teenagers and young adults. It classically begins with a solitary "herald patch." Mild-to-moderate itching is often present, and the patient usually feels well. **Physical Exam:** • Well-demarcated spherical lesion with central clearing closely resembles tinea corporis and ranges from 2–5 cm. • Days to weeks later, multiple pink-colored smaller lesions with peripheral collar-like scales (collarette) emerge on the trunk, neck, and limbs. • Lesions follow the skin cleavage lines (Langer lines) in a pattern that resembles a Christmas tree. **Diagnostics:** Clinical diagnosis Skin biopsy, if done, is nonspecific **Management:** None unless symptomatic Occasionally, antihistamines for pruritus and moisturizing creams for the dryness. UVB and erythromycin may accelerate resolution but are not needed.
Additional Considerations	**Complications:** The disease recurs in approximately 2% of patients. Post-inflammatory hyper/hypopigmentation may occur. **Pregnancy considerations:** If pityriasis rosea occurs in a pregnant woman, she will need close follow-up, as there is a risk of miscarriage.

CASE 12 | Lichen Planus

A 45-year-old man with a history of hepatitis C presents with pruritic bumps on his wrist for several weeks. He denies any new medications or skin products. On exam, vitals are normal, and he has lacy (reticular) whitish lines on the buccal mucosa of his mouth. On the flexor surface of his wrists, forearms, and legs, there are grouped pink-purplish, polygonal, flat-topped (planar), pruritic papules and plaques.

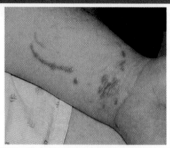

Lichen planus on hand. (Reproduced with permission from Carol Soutor, Maria K. Hordinsky, Clinical Dermatology, 1st ed; by McGraw-Hill 2013.)

Conditions with Similar Presentations	**Lichenoid drug reaction or contact dermatitis:** Should be considered in patients taking new medications or using a new product. **Discoid lupus:** Can be commonly confused when more scale is present; in some cases, the two diseases may overlap. **Secondary syphilis:** Should be ruled out when the palms and soles are involved. **Candidiasis and leukoplakia:** Should be considered when the mucous membranes are involved. Scraping the lesion is helpful; if leukoplakia is suspected, a biopsy must be done to rule out malignancy.
Initial Diagnostic Tests	Clinical diagnosis; biopsy may be performed
Next Steps in Management	• Discontinue any medication that may be a potential cause • Antihistamines and topical steroids
Discussion	Lichen planus is an idiopathic, recurrent, T-cell-mediated, chronic inflammatory condition affecting the scalp, nails, oral mucosa, genitalia, and skin. It commonly occurs in children and adults. See Obstetrics and Gynecology Chapter for genital presentation. **History:** Inquire about risk factors including hepatitis C, medications (e.g., NSAIDs, ACE-I, thiazides), and stress. Patients are often bothered by severe itching, and mucous membrane involvement can cause painful erosions. **Physical Exam:** • Typical lesions are found on flexor surfaces (including the wrists, shins, lower back, genitals). • 6 P's: planar (flat-topped), pruritic, purple, polygonal, papules, and plaques. • Oral mucosal lesions are lacy-reticular whitish lines (**Wickham striae**). • Mucous membrane involvement is common and may be the sole manifestation of disease. Although buccal mucosa is commonly involved, other areas include the tongue, lips, and gums. **Diagnostics:** Clinical diagnosis • Biopsy can confirm. The biopsy shows a dense, "band-like," sawtooth infiltrate of lymphocytes at the dermal-epidermal junction. • Hyperkeratosis, is often seen with thickened granular layer, and degeneration of the basal cell layer. **Management:** • Discontinue any medication that may be a potential cause (e.g., ACE-I, diuretics, NSAIDS). • Mild/localized cases can be treated with antihistamines and topical steroids. • High-potency topical steroids for cutaneous, oral, or genital lesions and systemic steroids for severe widespread disease. • Other options include topical tacrolimus, light therapy, narrowband UV B light (NBUVB), retinoids, or cyclosporine.
Additional Considerations	**Complications:** Although 2/3 of patients spontaneously resolve within 1 year, in some patients the course may be longer. Mucous membrane involvement indicates a more prolonged course. Recurrences are uncommon (<20% of patients). Although serious complications are uncommon, they usually result from mucous membrane involvement and include candidiasis and SCC.

CASE 13 | Psoriasis

A 29-year-old man presents for evaluation of a rash on his lower back and the extensor surfaces of his elbows that has been present for the past few months. The rash is pruritic, and he notes that his skin sometimes bleeds when he scratches the rash. Exam is positive for well-demarcated, erythematous plaques with an overlying silver scale on his lower back and the extensor surfaces of his elbows bilaterally.

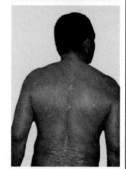

Lesions of psoriasis on back. (Reproduced with permission from A. Paul Kelly, Susan C. Taylor, Henry W. Lim, Ana Maria Anido Serrano, Taylor and Kelly's Dermatology for Skin of Color, 2e; by McGraw-Hill 2016.)

Conditions with Similar Presentations	**Atopic dermatitis:** Typically presents on the flexor surfaces of the body; when chronic, may lead to lichenified plaques that appear like psoriasis; psoriasis involves the extensor surfaces and is less pruritic. **Nummular eczema:** Characterized by well-demarcated, coin-shaped plaques; more pruritic than psoriasis. **Lichen simplex chronicus:** Localized thickening of the skin due to chronic scratching or rubbing; may occur in patients with psoriasis due to scratching.
Initial Diagnostic Tests	Clinical diagnosis
Next steps in Management	Localized psoriasis may be treated with a variety of topical agents including: • Topical steroids • Topical vitamin D analogs • Tazarotene, tar, and calcineurin inhibitors

Discussion	Psoriasis is a chronic inflammatory condition characterized by thick plaques of skin with an overlying silvery scale, and often involves joints. Genetic and environmental factors are thought to play a role.
	
	 The skin thickening and scale seen in psoriatic lesions are results of skin hyperproliferation with complete epidermal turnover in ~4 days instead of the normal 28 days. This increased proliferation is caused by cytokine release from immune cells, and therefore immunomodulators may play a role in the treatment of psoriasis. It often presents before age 40.
	
	 History: Ask about common triggers like drugs, infections, skin trauma, obesity, stress, and other environmental factors.
	 • Patients typically present with raised, erythematous plaques with an overlying scale.
	 • Psoriasis typically waxes and wanes throughout the patient's lifetime, and treatments are used to decrease disease activity.
	
	 Physical Exam:
	 • Psoriatic skin lesions are classically described as well-demarcated, erythematous plaques with an overlying silver scale on extensor surfaces of the skin.
	 • Another form, guttate psoriasis, presents as drop-like plaques with an overlying scale. It classically presents acutely 2–3 weeks after a Group A Streptococcus infection.
	 • The **Koebner phenomenon** is a phenomenon where psoriatic plaques appear in areas of trauma.
	 • **Auspitz sign** is described as pinpoint bleeding from plaques when the overlying scale is removed.
	
	 Diagnostics: Clinical diagnosis; a biopsy may be done in some instances to rule out other conditions
	
	 Management:
	 • Localized disease (<5% body surface area)
	    • Topical steroid with or without a topical vitamin D analog
	    • Tazarotene (a retinoid), tar, and topic calcineurin inhibitors may also be used
	 • Moderate or severe disease
	    • Systemic treatments may be used; options include UV phototherapy, methotrexate, cyclosporine, or biologic agents
	    • Oral steroids should not be used to treat psoriasis, as their discontinuation may lead to flaring
	 See table below for treatment options and side effects.

CASE 13 | Psoriasis *(continued)*

Additional Considerations	**Complications and Associated Findings:**
	Psoriatic arthritis: Is seen in up to 30% of patients with psoriasis. It is important to ask about joint pain in patients with psoriasis.
	Erythroderma: Is widespread inflammation of the skin affecting 90% of the body surface area. It may result from severe psoriasis. Patients present with widespread red, scaly skin and possible fever, chills, and/or malaise and may require hospitalization.

Therapeutic Management of Psoriasis

Type	Medication Name	Adverse Effects	Notes
Topical therapies	Topical steroids	Skin atrophy, telangiectasia, striae, acne, purpura	Various vehicles may be used depending on patient preference and required potency. Examples of vehicles include ointments, creams, gels, foams, and solutions.
	Vitamin D analog (calcipotriene)	Skin redness or irritation, photosensitivity	Used in conjugation with topical steroids.
	Topical retinoid (tazarotene)	Skin redness or irritation, photosensitivity	
	Calcineurin inhibitors	Skin irritation, burning, or itching	Used for areas where steroids may be damaging, such as the face and intertriginous areas of the body.
Systemic therapies	Phototherapy	Skin redness, sunburn-like reaction, stinging, or burning	Treatments are given 2–3 times per week and require patients to come to clinic.
	Methotrexate	Nausea, vomiting, mucositis, fatigue, hepatotoxicity, increased risk for infection	Blood tests are needed to monitor liver function and patients should be monitored for infections. Should not be given to pregnant or breastfeeding women.
	Cyclosporine	Nephrotoxicity, hypertension, hyperlipidemia, hirsutism, neurotoxicity, gingival hyperplasia	Requires monitoring of blood pressure and kidney function.
	Immunomodulators (TNF-α inhibitors, IL 12/23 inhibitors, IL-17 inhibitors)	Skin reactions at injection site, flu-like symptoms, increased risk for infections	Immunomodulators are given as injections or infusions. They require monitoring for infections.

Rash Without Fever Mini-Cases

Cases	Key Findings
Impetigo	**Hx:** Eruptions start as a single lesion and develop into multiple lesions. Other family members may be affected. **PE:** Honey-colored crust is most common, intact pustules are usually not found. Lesions occur around the nose and mouth. **Diagnostics:** Clinical diagnosis. If needed, Gram stain reveals gram-positive cocci. **Management:** Topical antibiotics (mupirocin), systemic antibiotics (dicloxacillin, cephalexin). General hygiene, antibacterial soaps, and changing washcloths/towels are also recommended. **Discussion:** *S. aureus* or *S. pyogenes* are the two most common pathogens. Bacteriologic cure is achieved in 7–10 days in most patients and complications are rare. Impetigo on face. (Reproduced with permission from Scott D.C. Stern, Adam S. Cifu, Diane Altkorn, Symptom to Diagnosis: An Evidence-Based Guide, 4e; by McGraw-Hill 2020.)

Rash Without Fever Mini-Cases *(continued)*

Erythema Migrans	**Hx:** Recent travel to areas endemic for tick-borne illness, may or may not present with fevers and myalgias, followed by development of erythematous rash. **PE:** A central erythematous patch of skin surrounded by clear skin and rings of erythema in a "bull's-eye" appearance. Lesions are usually several cm in diameter. **Diagnostics:** Erythema migrans is diagnosed clinically based on history of possible tick exposure and a classic "bull's-eye" rash in a patient with or without flu-like symptoms. **Management:** • Erythema migrans will self-resolve in about 3–4 weeks. • Patients with erythema migrans and a history of possible tick bite should be treated with appropriate antibiotics to prevent progression of disease. • Serology for Lyme disease is not useful because the skin lesion is diagnostic and serology may be negative at this stage of infection. **Discussion:** Lyme disease is caused by the spirochete *Borrelia burgdorferi*. Erythema migrans is a common dermatologic finding representative of early Lyme disease. It may appear 3 to 30 days after the tick bite (7–14 days on average) at the site of the bite and may expand gradually. See further information about Lyme disease staging and treatment in the Infectious Disease Chapter.	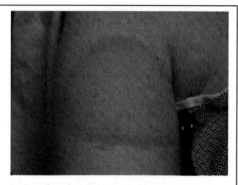 Lesion of erythema migrans with accentuation of erythema at the leading edge. (Reproduced with permission from McKean SC, Ross JJ, Dressler DD, Scheurer DB. Principles and Practice of Hospital Medicine, 2e; McGraw Hill LLC 2017.)
Erythema Nodosum	**Hx:** Females presenting with nodular bumps on lower extremities and may have associated joint pains **PE:** Scattered, warm, erythematous, tender subcutaneous nodules on pretibial surfaces, classically bilateral involvement **Diagnostics:** Clinical diagnosis. Should prompt a work up to determine etiology. **Management:** • Self-limited and commonly resolves with treatment of the underlying cause • Pain may be controlled with NSAIDs **Discussion:** Erythema nodosum is a delayed hypersensitivity reaction leading to inflammation of the subcutaneous fat (panniculitis). It is due to a variety of systemic diseases, medications, or infections. Up to half of cases are idiopathic. Common causes include streptococcal infections, inflammatory conditions such as sarcoidosis, tuberculosis, or inflammatory bowel disease, oral contraceptives, pregnancy, and malignancy	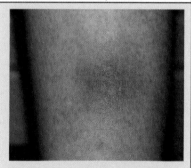 Erythema nodosum. (Reproduced with permission from Carol Soutor, Maria K. Hordinsky, Clinical Dermatology, 1st ed; McGraw-Hill 2013.)

Rash with Fever

CASE 14 | Cellulitis

A 66-year-old man presents with worsening erythema, pain, and swelling of his right leg for the past 3 days. A few days prior he fell after twisting his ankle and sustained a laceration over the right leg. His exam was significant for temperature of 100°F and a warm, tender, swollen, and erythematous right leg with poorly demarcated borders.

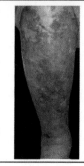

Cellulitis of leg. (Reproduced with permission from Carol Soutor, Maria K. Hordinsky, Clinical Dermatology, 1st ed; by McGraw-Hill 2013.)

CASE 14 | Cellulitis *(continued)*

Conditions with Similar Presentations	**Erysipelas:** Usually confined to superficial layers of skin with more bright red color and distinct demarcation. Lymphangitic streaking may be seen. It usually progresses rapidly over hours instead of days. **Necrotizing fasciitis:** Characterized by pain out of proportion to exam, signs of necrosis, rapid progression (3 cm/hr), and systemic signs. It is the deepest infection, passing down through the subcutaneous fat to the fascia overlying muscles (see Surgery Chapter). **Contact dermatitis:** Rash more eczematous, pruritic (rather than tender), and occurs due to an antigenic exposure (though an exposure history may not be always elicited). **Abscesses:** Collections of pus within deeper layers of skin tissue, most often due to *S. aureus* infection. Abscesses arise from the dermis or subcutaneous tissue. Risk factors for developing an abscess include a break in the skin barrier, peripheral vascular disease, and diabetes.	Erysipelas. (Reproduced with permission from Lowell A. Goldsmith, Stephen I. Katz, Barbara A. Gilchrest, Amy S. Paller, David J. Leffell, Klaus Wolff, Fitzpatrick's Dermatology in General Medicine, 8e; by The McGraw-Hill 2012.)
Initial Diagnostic Tests	Clinical diagnosis	
Next Steps in Management	• Antibiotics targeting *Streptococcus* if non-purulent • If purulent, target *Staphylococcus* species with consideration for community-acquired MRSA	
Discussion	Cellulitis is a deep infection of the skin that involves the deeper dermis and subcutaneous fat. Common pathogens include *S. pyogenes* and *S. aureus*. The source is commonly external but may also be hematogenous. Immunocompetent hosts usually have external sources. Tissue edema predisposes to bacterial proliferation and proteolytic enzymes released by bacteria contribute to the spread of inflammation. **History:** Ask about risk factors including DM, peripheral vascular disease, IV drug use, venous insufficiency, lymphatic disruption, and breaks in the skin from trauma, bites, history of MRSA infections, or tinea pedis. Patients usually feel ill and febrile, and the fever may precede appearance of skin involvement. **Physical Exam:** Red, warm, indurated, and tender area of the skin in a febrile patient. Blisters are rare. **Diagnostics:** Clinical diagnosis • Biopsy is often done in immunocompromised patients who have not responded to antibiotics • Special stains for fungal organisms may also be considered in non-responders **Management:** Antibiotics that target streptococci if purulence is absent, including cephalexin and dicloxacillin • If purulence is present or MRSA is suspected, consider doxycycline, trimethoprim/sulfamethoxazole (TMP-SMX) • IV antibiotics in severe cases include nafcillin (MSSA) or vancomycin (MRSA)	
Additional Considerations	**Complications:** If fever persists beyond 48 hours after treatment initiation, consider a change in antimicrobial therapy. Mortality rate is close to zero in immunocompetent hosts. Residual lymphedema may occur from damage to local lymphatics during an acute episode and may predispose the patient to recurrent cellulitis.	

BLISTERS

Assessment should include the type of blistering, onset, distribution, additional symptoms, comorbidities, patient stability, coexisting infectious factors, biopsy, and serologic testing.

• Remember that different stages of the same disease may be present at the same time

• Flaccid blisters may be eroded

• Mucous membranes may be involved in erythema multiforme, SJS/TEN, pemphigus vulgaris

A general guideline for approaching the diagnosis of a blistering rash is as follows:

Approach to Blisters

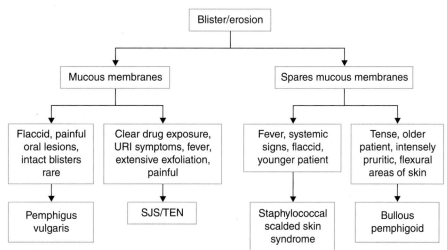

CASE 15 | Pemphigus Vulgaris

A 52-year-old man with heart failure presents for evaluation of a blistering rash. He has painful erosions in his mouth. On exam, he is afebrile and appears uncomfortable. Across his body, there are diffuse blisters and erosions with crusts that ooze and bleed easily. When the skin surrounding the lesion is pulled laterally, there is separation of the epidermis or creation of an erosion (**positive Nikolsky sign**).

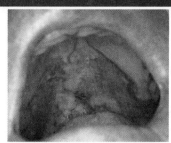

Pemphigus vulgaris involving the oral cavity. (Reproduced with permission from Carol Soutor, Maria K. Hordinsky, Clinical Dermatology, 1st ed; by McGraw-Hill 2013.)

Conditions with Similar Presentations	**Bullous pemphigoid:** Pruritic blisters that spares mucous membranes; negative Nikolsky sign (no separation of epidermis or creation of an erosion when skin surrounding lesion is pulled laterally). **Erythema multiforme:** Multiple types of lesions (macules, papules, target lesions) and can be associated with drugs (sulfa, B-lactams, phenytoin), infections (HSV, *Mycoplasma pneumonia*), autoimmune disease, or cancer. **Dermatitis herpetiformis:** Smaller blisters (papules or vesicles), intensely itchy, in groups (usually on elbows), and is seen in patients with celiac disease.
Initial Diagnostic Tests	• Skin biopsy with direct immunofluorescence • Blood test for indirect immunofluorescence or ELISA
Next Steps in Management	Oral prednisone (60 mg/day).
Discussion	Pemphigus vulgaris is an autoimmune type II hypersensitivity reaction caused by IgG antibodies against desmoglein 1 and desmoglein 3. These antigens are intraepidermal, so inflammation is close to the surface, which is why the blisters rupture easily and are flaccid. **History:** Most seen in adults between the ages of 50 to 60 years, with increased frequency in people of Askhkenazi Jewish ancestry. **Physical Exam:** Blisters are flaccid (positive Nikolsky sign), and oral mucosa may be only involvement. Background skin may be inflamed or noninflamed. Erosions vary in size and are painful, with irregular borders. **Diagnostics:** • Biopsy with immunofluorescence is diagnostic and shows intraepidermal bulla with loss of cell-cell adhesion of keratinocyte • Immunofluorescence staining shows a sawtooth pattern of IgG and complement C3 in the epidermis **Management:** Start systemic corticosteroids and consider the role for an additional immunosuppressive agent, such as rituximab, azathioprine, methotrexate, mycophenolate mofetil.
Additional Considerations	**Complications:** Infection and death if not treated. Morbidity is significant due to complications of therapy.

CASE 16 | Stevens-Johnson Syndrome (SJS)

A 35-year-old woman presents with a progressively worsening, painful, blistering rash over her trunk which is now starting to spread to other areas. She was started on TMP-SMX for a urinary tract infection 4 days ago. Review of systems was positive for fatigue, burning eyes, and sore throat. Her vitals are notable for a temperature of 99°F, pulse of 118/min. Skin exam shows erythematous macules, papules, and some targetoid lesions on the face, trunk, and back that are sloughing. When the skin surrounding the lesion is pulled laterally, there is separation of the epidermis and creation of an erosion (positive Nikolsky sign). There are hemorrhagic crusting lesions on the lips. Bullae and erosions are noted on the oral and genital mucosa. The lesions are tender to palpation. Bilateral conjunctivitis is noted. Greater than 10% of the body surface area is affected.

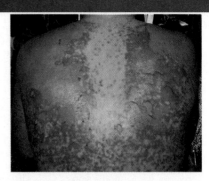

Stevens-Johnson syndrome. (Reproduced with permission from Carol Soutor, Maria K. Hordinsky Clinical Dermatology, 1st ed; by McGraw-Hill 2013.)

Conditions with Similar Presentations	**Staphylococcal scalded skin syndrome (SSSS):** Characterized by fever and an erythematous rash with sloughing of the upper layers of the epidermis and positive Nikolsky sign. Biopsy shows destruction of keratinocyte attachments in the stratum granulosum.
	Drug rash with eosinophilia and systemic symptoms (DRESS syndrome): A hypersensitivity syndrome that is drug-induced and presents with systemic symptoms and, at times, eosinophilia. Patients may present with a morbilliform rash, high fever, lymphadenopathy, eosinophilia, LFT abnormalities, and inflammation of one or more internal organs. Typically presents 2–8 weeks after starting the offending medication (e.g., carbamazepine, phenobarbital, phenytoin, allopurinol, olanzapine, or sulfa drugs).
	Erythema multiforme: Presents with macules, papules, vesicles, and target lesions (rings with dusky red center) in a symmetric pattern on the distal extremities. Most seen with infections (e.g., mycoplasma, HSV), although other causes include drugs (e.g., sulfa drugs, beta-lactams, phenytoin), cancer, or autoimmune disease, and Nikolsky sign is negative.
Initial Diagnostic Tests	Clinical diagnosis
Next Steps in Management	Discontinue drug, admit to the hospital, and initiate aggressive supportive care, potentially in a burn unit.

Discussion	SJS, also known as erythema multiforme major, is a severe, life-threatening, blistering mucocutaneous syndrome. It is thought to be secondary to an immunologic reaction. Cytotoxic T cells and natural killer cells are thought to be the major players in inducing keratinocyte apoptosis. It is more common in males.
	
	History:
	• Risk factors can include HIV, genetics, or underlying immunologic disease or malignancies. Male to female ratio of 1:2. In over one-third of cases, no cause can be identified.
	• It is usually associated with an adverse drug reaction (e.g., allopurinol, NSAIDs, antiepileptics, sulfa drugs, penicillin), exposure to which can occur 7–28 days before the onset of rash.
	• *M. pneumoniae* infection is also a known trigger.
	
	Physical Exam:
	• Patients with SJS are extremely sick, often with systemic signs of shock (fever, hypotension, tachycardia).
	• There is involvement of at least two mucous membranes with erythema usually involving >10% of the body surface area.
	  • **Toxic epidermal necrolysis (TEN)** is a more extensive form of SJS where >30% of the body surface area is affected
	  • If 10–30% of body surface is involved, it is considered an overlap syndrome between SJS and toxic shock syndrome
	• Hemorrhagic crusting of the lips is pathognomonic.
	• There may be atypical target lesions and large epidermal sheets of blistering.
	
	Diagnostics: Clinical diagnosis
	• Biopsy can be done to confirm the diagnosis or rule out other causes, and it would show full epidermal thickness skin separation and epidermal necrosis. However, biopsy should not delay management.
	  • A biopsy cannot differentiate SJS/TEN vs. erythema multiforme vs. fixed drug eruption
	• Peripheral blood eosinophilia is sometimes present and may heighten suspicion.

CASE 16 | Stevens-Johnson Syndrome (SJS) *(continued)*

Discussion	**Management:** • Supportive care: Fluids, nutrition, pain management, and wound care • Adjunctive therapies: Systemic corticosteroids, IVIG, or cyclosporine
Additional Considerations	**Complications:** Mortality is 25% among SJS/TEN patients. Common causes of in-hospital death include sepsis, ARDS, and multiple organ failure. Conjunctivitis may be complicated by secondary bacterial infection and lead to corneal scarring.

Blisters/Vesicles Mini-Cases

Cases	Key Findings
Bullous Pemphigoid	**Hx:** Blistering, pruritic rash usually presents in patients >60 years old; spares mucous membranes. May be precipitated by a new drug (e.g., NSAIDs, furosemide, penicillin). **PE:** Large, tense blisters and bullae; negative Nikolsky sign. **Diagnostics:** Skin biopsy shows separation of epidermis and dermis at the epidermal basement membrane. **Management:** Remove offending agent and start corticosteroids. **Discussion:** Autoimmune, bullous disorder involving IgG antibodies against BP antigen 180 and 230 (components of hemidesmosomes responsible for dermal-epidermal cohesion). Because this is at the base of the epidermis, the entire epidermis is above it and the blisters do not rupture easily (they are tense, not flaccid).
Erythema Multiforme	**Hx:** Recurrent episodes of lesions that appear over 3–5 days and resolve within 1–2 weeks. Asymptomatic or mild prodromal infectious symptoms. **PE:** Round, sharply demarcated, erythematous papules surrounded by blanched areas. Typical targetoid lesions are often seen. May involve mucosa. **Diagnostics:** Clinical diagnosis **Management:** Workup for common triggers (HSV, PCR of throat swabs, *M. pneumoniae*, medication review). Treat underlying cause. Manage symptoms with topical corticosteroids or oral antihistamines. **Discussion:** Self-limiting disease, with up to 50% of cases idiopathic in etiology. Recurrence is seen in 20–25% of patients, and morbidity is higher in patients with mucosal erosions.	 Erythema multiforme. (Reproduced with permission from Carol Soutor, Maria K. Hordinsky, Clinical Dermatology, 1st ed; by McGraw-Hill 2013.)
Dermatitis Herpetiformis	**Hx:** Very itchy blisters on extensor surfaces with spontaneous improvement and cyclic exacerbations. May not have GI symptoms. **PE:** Grouped "herpetiform" vesicles symmetrically distributed on extensor surfaces (elbow, knees, scalp, back, buttocks, tip of nose). May only see erosions and excoriations. **Diagnostics:** Biopsy for H&E and direct immunofluorescence (DIF) followed by anti-tTG IgA and IgG, total IgA, and anti-endomysial IgA, IgG. Immunofluorescence is at the epidermal basement membrane. **Management:** Screen for associated disease (thyroid, glucose). Gluten-free diet. Dapsone for itch. **Discussion:** Dapsone is only for skin manifestations as it does not treat GI manifestations. Gluten-free diet is the essential treatment.	 Dermatitis herpetiformis. (Reproduced with permission from Carol Soutor, Maria K. Hordinsky, Clinical Dermatology, 1st ed; by McGraw-Hill 2013.)

Blisters/Vesicles Mini-Cases *(continued)*

Drug Rash with Eosinophilia and Systemic Symptoms (DRESS)	**Hx:** Fever and cutaneous eruption 2–6 weeks after drug initiation. **PE:** Edema of face is a frequent finding. Morbilliform ("measles-like" macules that may coalesce) eruption that becomes edematous. **Diagnostics:** RegiSCAR or J-SCAR scoring system. Components of scoring system include CBC with differential for eosinophilia, ALT/AST >100, internal organ involvement, fever, and lymphadenopathy. **Management:** Thyroid studies. ECG and echocardiogram to evaluate potential cardiac dysfunction. Oral or IV prednisone with taper. May add topical clobetasol. **Discussion:** Mortality is 2–10%. Patients may develop interstitial nephritis, myocarditis, thyroiditis, interstitial pneumonitis, or myositis. Cutaneous and visceral involvement may persist for weeks to months after drug withdrawal. 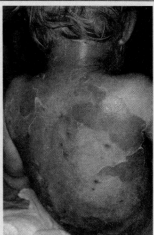 Drug rash with eosinophilia and systemic symptoms (DRESS). (Reproduced with permission from Carol Soutor, Maria K. Hordinsky, Clinical Dermatology, 1st ed; by McGraw-Hill 2013.)
Staphylococcal Scalded Skin Syndrome	**Hx:** Fever, preceding upper respiratory infection (URI); sudden onset of skin tenderness, and development of bullae. **PE:** Large bullae that are easily ruptured and become flaccid (positive Nikolsky). Desquamation of large areas of skin in sheets and ribbons. Face, neck, trunk, axillae, and groin involvement. Mucous membranes are spared. **Diagnostics:** Clinical diagnosis **Management:** Antibiotics for *S. aureus* including MRSA. **Discussion:** Most commonly in children (<6 years old) or adults with chronic kidney disease due to inability to excrete toxin. Good prognosis, spontaneous healing within several days. Staphylococcal scalded skin syndrome (SSSS). (Reproduced with permission from Carol Soutor, Maria K. Hordinsky, Clinical Dermatology, 1st ed; by McGraw-Hill 2013.)

HYPERSENSITIVITY

Hypersensitivity reactions are a result of an exaggerated and/or uncontrolled response by the immune system in response to an antigen. The resultant inflammatory response can lead to significant cellular damage and bodily harm. There are four types of hypersensitivity reactions.

Type	Pathophysiology	Dermatologic Examples
Type I **Allergic/Immediate Hypersensitivity Reaction**	The distinguishing feature is that this is an IgE antibody–mediated reaction. External antigens (e.g., peanut protein, egg protein, Hymenoptera venom) will bind to IgE on mast cells and basophils, causing cross-linking and subsequent release of pro-inflammatory and vasodilatory mediators such as histamine. This reaction occurs in minutes to hours, hence the name immediate.	• Urticaria • Atopic dermatitis • Angioedema
Type II **Cytotoxic/Antibody Dependent**	Rather than IgE, these reactions result from IgG or IgM antibodies binding to self-antigens which are falsely recognized as being foreign. The binding of these antibodies triggers the complement system to attack the host cell. Additionally, the bound antibodies will attract natural killer cells which will release enzymes into the host cell, causing apoptosis.	• Bullous pemphigoid • Pemphigus vulgaris • Idiopathic thrombocytopenic purpura

Type	Pathophysiology	Dermatologic Examples
Type III **Immune-Complex Mediated**	IgG antibodies will bind to circulating antigens, creating a circulating immune complex. These immune complexes can then deposit in various tissues throughout the body and activate the complement cascade, causing a localized inflammatory response wherever that may be.	• Systemic lupus erythematosus • Arthus reaction • Small-vessel vasculitis • Henoch-Schonlein purpura
Type IV **Cell-Mediated or Delayed**	Unique in that it does not involve antibodies. Antigen-presenting cells will present antigens to CD4 helper T-cells, which will release inflammatory mediators. These mediators will activate macrophages and CD8 T-cells which will destroy host cells and further potentiate inflammation. Reaction will occur 48–72 hours after exposure, hence the name delayed.	• Allergic contact dermatitis • Tuberculosis skin test • Delayed drug reactions

CASE 17 | Atopic Dermatitis (Eczema)

A 7-year-old girl is brought in by her parents for evaluation of an intermittent rash in the creases of her elbows and knees. It occasionally involves the wrists and thigh and legs. This rash is associated with intense itching followed by scaly patches and has been present intermittently since the patient was 6 months old. There is no history of use of any new products or exposures. Her mother has a history of hay fever. On exam, the patient has thickened skin with hyperpigmented, scaly patches at the flexor surface of her elbows and knees.

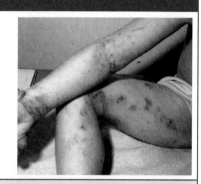

Atopic dermatitis. (Reproduced with permission from Carol Soutor, Maria K. Hordinsky, Clinical Dermatology, 1st ed; by McGraw-Hill 2013.)

Conditions with Similar Presentations	**Allergic contact dermatitis:** Is a type IV hypersensitivity reaction to a particular allergen that results in a localized skin reaction at the site of exposure. Common allergens include metals (nickel), fragrances, poison ivy, and topical antibiotics (e.g., neomycin). Differs from eczema in the acute onset and characteristic distribution in areas in contact with the allergen. 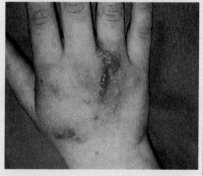 **Psoriasis:** Is a chronic skin condition characterized by erythematous "silvery-scaled" plaques on extensor surfaces and may be associated with arthritis, which tends to involve the DIP joints. Differs from eczema in that it is usually distributed along extensor surfaces (rather than flexor) and differing age of onset. Allergic contact dermatitis. (Reproduced with permission from Carol Soutor, Maria K. Hordinsky, Clinical Dermatology, 1st ed; by McGraw-Hill 2013.) **Tinea corporis:** (commonly from *Trichophyton rubrum*): Can present with pruritic, scaling, red patches. Can be distinguished from eczema by presence of hyphae on KOH microscopy.
Initial Diagnostic Tests	Clinical diagnosis
Next Steps in Management	• Topical corticosteroids during flares • Encourage moisturization with skin emollients
Discussion	Atopic dermatitis, or eczema, is an intensely pruritic, chronic, relapsing, inflammatory skin condition caused by disrupted innate and adaptive immune response, epidermal barrier dysfunction, and altered cutaneous microbiome. This causes epidermal barrier breakdown, dry skin and trans epidermal water loss, penetration of irritants, microbes, and antigens which results in an inflammatory response, predominantly Th2. **History:** Risk factors: History of atopic disease (asthma, allergic rhinitis). It is more common in children and is uncommon in adults without a history of childhood eczema. Pruritus is the predominant symptom.

CASE 17 | Atopic Dermatitis (Eczema) *(continued)*

Discussion	**Physical Exam:** • Dry skin (xerosis) and intense pruritus, leading to scratching and excoriation or eventual thickened skin patches (lichenification, hallmark of chronic disease) • Infants will have vesicles, oozing, crusting, and juicy papules, while adults will have lichenified plaques and scaling • In infants the areas involved are scalp, cheeks, chin, and extensor surfaces of extremities • In adults and older children, it most often involves the flexor surfaces such as the antecubital and popliteal fossae, as well as the face and neck **Diagnostics:** Clinical diagnosis; increased IgE levels support the diagnosis **Management:** • Use of bland moisturizers soon after bathing • Avoidance of irritants (wool clothing, harsh soaps, uncomfortable climate) • Topical steroids for flares and as maintenance if patients have recurrent flares • Steroid-sparing agents include topical macrolides, immunomodulators (tacrolimus, pimecrolimus) • Second-line options include phototherapy (NBUVB) or immunosuppressive medications (azathioprine, cyclosporine, mycophenolate mofetil), biologics (dupilumab)
Additional Considerations	• Most children (90%) outgrow their disease by adolescence • Adults may have localized forms such as in the hand or foot • Atopic dermatitis is frequently complicated by skin infections

Topical Steroids	Potency
Fluocinonide acetonide 0.01% Desonide 0.05% Hydrocortisone 1%	Low
Triamcinolone acetonide 0.1%	Medium
Fluocinonide 0.05%	High
Clobetasol propionate 0.05%	Super High

CASE 18 | Urticaria

A 32-year-old woman presents for evaluation of an "itchy rash" all over her body. She describes that red lesions started to appear on her skin a few days ago, and individual lesions last for a few hours and then resolve. She recently started taking penicillin for a dental infection. She has had no shortness of breath or chest pain. Exam reveals diffuse erythematous papules and wheals scattered across the patient's chest, back, and arms. Vital signs are normal.

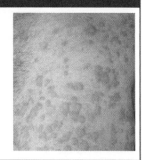

Urticaria. (Reproduced with permission from J. Larry Jameson, Anthony S. Fauci, Dennis L. Kasper, Stephen L. Hauser, Dan L. Longo, Joseph Loscalzo, Harrison's Principles of Internal Medicine, 20e; by McGraw-Hill 2018.)

Conditions with Similar Presentations	**Anaphylaxis:** Is a serious allergic reaction that must be ruled out. Common symptoms of anaphylaxis include respiratory distress, hoarse voice or throat tightness, nausea or vomiting, chest pain, and/or gastrointestinal symptoms and hypotension. Patients may have hives as well, but the respiratory distress and hypotension are the major concerns. **Allergic contact dermatitis:** Should be ruled out in patients using new products. Differs from urticaria in its slower, delayed onset. **Atopic dermatitis:** May also cause pruritic skin lesions. In atopic dermatitis, lichenification and xerosis may be present on physical examination. Differs from urticaria in its chronicity. **Drug eruptions:** Should be considered in patients taking new medications or those who recently have had a change in the dose of their medications. Lesions will persist, while urticaria usually resolves within 24 hours.

CASE 18 | Urticaria *(continued)*

Initial Diagnostic Tests	• Clinical diagnosis • Urticaria may not be present at the time of the exam • A detailed history must be taken to identify possible triggers
Next Steps in Management	Oral antihistamines are first line for the treatment of acute or chronic urticaria.
Discussion	Urticaria is caused by the release of histamine from mast cells that leads to swelling of the upper dermis. Histamine acts on the blood vessels in the skin, leading to arteriolar dilation, venous constriction, and increased capillary permeability. These mechanisms result in the characteristic wheals, which are areas of central edema surrounded by erythema and are associated with itching. The wheals vary in size and time of appearance, and often resolve within 24 hours without scarring. It is often idiopathic but can be triggered by infection and physical factors. **History:** • Urticaria may be classified as acute (<6 weeks) or chronic (>6 weeks). • Ask about infection (rotavirus, rhinovirus, *M. pneumoniae*, and group A streptococcal pharyngitis). • Other triggers for acute urticaria include infections, certain foods, medications, and IV administration of blood products or contrast. • Physical factors, such as temperature changes or skin pressure, infections, medications, or autoimmunity, may cause chronic urticaria. • Many cases of both acute and chronic urticaria are idiopathic. **Physical Exam:** • Patients usually present with blanching, palpable, erythematous wheals anywhere on their bodies. • Wheals usually self-resolve within 24 hours. • Examine to ensure that there is no mucous membrane involvement to suggest anaphylaxis. **Diagnostics:** • Clinical diagnosis • Consider allergy testing of severe cases of chronic urticaria and those that are unresponsive to treatment **Management:** • Daily oral second-generation H1 antihistamines are preferred for the treatment of urticaria, as they cause less drowsiness. • Steroids and omalizumab, a humanized monoclonal anti-IgE antibody, may be effective for chronic urticaria that is unresponsive to high doses of antihistamines.
Additional Considerations	**Angioedema:** May occur with or without urticaria and is caused by the same mechanism as urticaria and presents as swelling of the face or body. The swelling is a result of vascular changes occurring deep in the dermis. It commonly affects the lips and periorbital areas. Angioedema without urticaria should prompt evaluation of acquired C1 inhibitor deficiency, or drug-induced or hereditary angioedema. **Dermatographism:** Is a form of urticaria in which well-demarcated wheals appear on the skin in areas where the skin has been scratched or rubbed.

INFECTIOUS DISEASES OF SKIN

Skin infections are common, with potential sources including bacterial, viral, fungal, and parasitic etiologies. While each of these organisms can exert vastly different effects, there are some common risk factors that can make patients more susceptible to skin infection.

• Skin trauma and open wounds can easily serve as a nidus for infection.

• Chronic skin diseases such as eczema and psoriasis can similarly make one susceptible to superimposed infection.

• Immunosuppression can limit one's ability to fight off opportunistic infections as well.

It should be noted that the skin is not a sterile organ and is home to numerous harmless microorganisms. In fact, excessive skin hygiene may make one more susceptible to skin infection by destroying that protective microbiome and damaging the protective skin barrier.

Viral Diseases

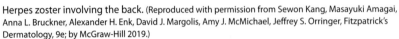

CASE 19 | Herpes Zoster

A 65-year-old man presents for evaluation of a rash on his torso that has been present for the past 4 days. He states that a few days before the rash appeared, he experienced burning and pain in the same area. Exam is notable for erythematous grouped vesicles and pustules scattered in a dermatomal distribution on the patient's torso. The lesions are unilateral and do not cross the midline.

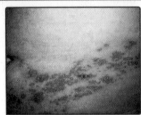

Herpes zoster involving the back. (Reproduced with permission from Sewon Kang, Masayuki Amagai, Anna L. Bruckner, Alexander H. Enk, David J. Margolis, Amy J. McMichael, Jeffrey S. Orringer, Fitzpatrick's Dermatology, 9e; by McGraw-Hill 2019.)

Conditions with Similar Presentations	**HSV:** Grouped vesicles appearing near the groin or around the mouth may signify a reactivation of HSV rather than herpes zoster. **Allergic contact dermatitis:** Consider in a patient using a new product; skin lesions well-defined and appear in the area that made contact with the allergen. **Insect bites:** May appear as linear, erythematous papules anywhere on the body. **Drug eruptions:** Consider in patients who have recently started new medications or had dosage changes.
Initial Diagnostic Tests	Clinical diagnosis based on the classic prodrome of burning and pain followed by the characteristic rash in a unilateral dermatomal distribution
Next Steps in Management	• Rest and pain relief with analgesics • Antivirals such as acyclovir, famciclovir, or valacyclovir may be given within 72 hours of the eruption to reduce the duration and severity of the rash

Discussion	Herpes zoster, also known as shingles, is a vesicular skin eruption arising in a single dermatome, often unilateral and painful due to the **reactivation of the varicella zoster virus** (VZV). The virus remains dormant in the dorsal root ganglia of the patient for life. Upon reactivation, the virus travels in a dermatomal fashion through the sensory nerve and causes an eruption on the skin. Anyone who has been previously infected with VZV (chicken pox) is at risk for developing herpes zoster, and this is usually seen with advancing age.
	 History:
	 • Ask about previous infection with VZV and immunosuppression.
	 • Pain and paresthesias of the skin are usually the first signs of herpes zoster. Patients may experience itching, burning, tingling, or pain that can be severe. These symptoms are usually present 1–3 days before the classic herpes zoster rash appears.
	 • There is also tenderness or hyperesthesia of the skin during the prodromal phase. Patients may also experience fever, headache, and lymphadenopathy at this time.
	 Physical Exam:
	 • The rash of herpes zoster classically appears in a unilateral dermatomal distribution, often including thoracic, lumbar, cervical, and trigeminal dermatomes.
	 • It first begins as unilateral, erythematous macules and papules presenting along the involved sensory nerve.
	 • Within 24–48 hours, vesicles begin to form.
	 • On the third day, vesicles evolve into pustules that then crust over, and the crusted lesions may be present for up to an additional 10 days.
	 Diagnostics:
	 • Clinical diagnosis
	 • Testing is reserved for atypical cases and is usually a PCR of swab from affected area
	 Management:
	 • Pain control
	   • Cool compress to the affected area and take analgesics as needed
	   • Calamine lotion or oral antihistamines may help with itching if present

CASE 19 | Herpes Zoster *(continued)*

Discussion	• Viral control indications
	  • Treatment of all patients, if given within 72 hours can reduce duration of illness and infectivity
	  • All immunocompromised individuals should be treated to prevent dissemination to internal organs (liver, lung, brain)
	  • Patients with disseminated cutaneous zoster should be treated
	  • Disseminated disease is defined as >3 dermatomes or >30 lesions outside of the original dermatome(s)
	• Available antivirals used are acyclovir, famciclovir, and valacyclovir

Additional Considerations	**Complications:** **Postherpetic neuralgia (PHN):** Defined as persistent pain in the area for more than 1 month after the onset of herpes zoster. Patients may present with persistent pain, itching, burning, numbness, or tenderness of the skin. PHN is often self-limited but may be treated with anti-epileptic medications, such as gabapentin, tricyclic anti-depressants, or local anesthetics. The incidence of postherpetic neuralgia is decreased if patients are given antiviral medications as soon as clinical symptoms appear and within 72 hours of the rash. It is not decreased by administering other medications. **Ophthalmic zoster:** Occurs when VSV reactivates along the ophthalmic division of the trigeminal nerve. This rash presents along half of the forehead including the eyelids. Early recognition and management is needed if the tip or side of the nose is involved, as the patient is also at risk for eye involvement, which may lead to corneal ulcerations, infections, and possible vision loss. **Ramsay Hunt syndrome:** Occurs when the VSV reactivates in the geniculate ganglion of cranial nerve VII. It is characterized by unilateral facial weakness and the classic herpes zoster rash within the ear canal, the mouth, or on the same side of the face as the facial palsy.

Other Common Causes of Vesicular or Pustular Lesions

Diagnosis	Description
Dermatophyte	Central clearing of annular lesions with elevated serpiginous, erythematous borders. Removal of vesicle or scale for KOH exam reveals hyphae.
HSV	Clear, grouped vesicles on an erythematous base and recurrence in the same location. Erosions with scalloped borders are also common.
VZV	Multiple stages of healing and diffuse itchy vesicles on an erythematous base.
Atopic Dermatitis	Oozing from inflamed skin leading to crust. History of atopic disease, distribution of rash to characteristic areas such as antecubital fossa.

Viral Infection Mini-Case

Case	Key Findings
Molluscum Contagiosum	**Hx:** Commonly seen among school-aged children, spread via physical contact and through fomites. Can also be seen in adults (less common) and immunocompromised patients. **PE:** Multiple, scattered, skin-colored papules with central umbilication are usually noted across the trunk. If sexually transmitted, may be seen in genital areas and inner thighs. **Diagnostics:** Clinical diagnosis **Management:** The infection is usually self-limited and resolves within 6–12 months • Patients should use measures to decrease transmission and autoinoculation, such as cleaning clothing and towels • If treatment is desired, cantharidin, curettage, or cryotherapy may be used to remove the skin lesions **Discussion:** • Molluscum contagiosum is a benign viral infection of the cutis and subcutaneous layers of skin caused by a **poxvirus** • Patients should avoid sharing clothing, bedding, or towels to prevent transmission to others or autoinoculation	 Molluscum contagiosum. Labial lesions are flesh-colored, dome-shaped papules with central umbilication. (Reproduced with permission from , Hoffman BL, Schorge JO, Halvorson LM, Hamid CA, Corton MM, Schaffer JI. Williams Gynecology, 4e; McGraw Hill LLC 2020.)

Fungal Infections

CASE 20 | Dermatophytes

A healthy 19-year-old man presents with an itchy and scaly rash that has been present on his left lower leg for 2 weeks. He states that he recently began his wrestling season at college and noticed the rash shortly after. Exam is positive for an erythematous, well-demarcated plaque with scaling at the edges on the patient's lower left leg.

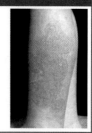

Dermatophyte infection. (Reproduced with permission from Wolff K, Johnson R, Saavedra AP, Roh EK. Fitzpatrick's Color Atlas and Synopsis of Clinical Dermatology, 8e; 2017. by McGraw-Hill)

Conditions with Similar Presentations	**Nummular eczema:** Characterized by well-demarcated, coin-shaped plaques. It commonly presents with multiple skin lesions, while tinea corporis normally has one or few lesions. **Psoriasis:** May present with scaly plaques on extensor surfaces of the body; not itchy. **Allergic contact dermatitis:** Consider in patients who recently started using new products.
Initial Diagnostic Tests	• Clinical diagnosis • KOH examination of skin scrapings can be performed to identify fungal hyphae and spores
Next Steps in Management	• Localized tinea corporis may be treated with topical antifungals such as topical imidazoles or terbinafine • The area should be kept dry

Discussion	Tinea corporis is a superficial fungal cutaneous infection that may appear anywhere on the body except for the scalp, groin, nails, face, hands, and feet. It is one of the many superficial fungal infections caused by dermatophyte fungi. Tinea corporis is caused by dermatophytes of the *Trichophyton* or *Microsporum* genus. These fungi thrive in the warm, moist environment of the skin, infecting the outer layer of the epidermis. Dermatophyte infections are spread through direct skin-to-skin contact or the sharing of fomites, such as towels or clothing, resulting in increased transmission in families.
	
	Other superficial fungal infections include:
	• **Tinea pedis** of the feet
	• **Tinea capitis** of the scalp
	• **Tinea cruris** of the groin area
	• **Tinea manuum** affects the hand and is characterized by red, scaling plaques on the hands
	
	History:
	• Direct skin-to-skin contact and sharing fomites
	• Exposure to infected animals
	• Occupational exposures like wrestling, gyms
	• Immunocompromised conditions
	• Patients with dermatophyte infections typically have a history of exposure to another affected individual through direct contact or fomites. Tinea corporis is commonly seen in athletes who participate in sports with skin-to-skin contact or in patients with house pets.
	• Tinea pedis may be spread through public showers or in gyms.
	
	Physical Exam:
	• Well-demarcated, erythematous plaque with a raised, scaling edge
	• There may be a central area of clearing as the rash grows outward
	• Tinea pedis has multiple types of presentations
	  • The interdigital form presents with red, scaly skin lesions between the toes
	  • There is also a moccasin form, presenting with scaling along the lateral feet
	  • Vesicular form presents with vesicles or bullae on the feet
	
	Diagnostics: Clinical diagnosis
	• If unclear, a skin scraping may be performed with a scalpel to remove some of the scale from the edge of the infection. The sample is then looked at under the microscope with KOH to identify fungal hyphae and spores.
	
	Management:
	• First-line therapies include topical imidazoles, such as clotrimazole, or terbinafine.
	• In addition to medications, patients must keep the area clean and dry. They should take precautions to decrease spreading and autoinoculation, including cleaning clothing and sheets and avoiding direct contact with other individuals or other parts of their own body.
	• Oral therapies (e.g., terbinafine or itraconazole) may be given if patients do not respond to topical treatment.
	• There are two superficial fungal infections in which oral therapies are always used. **Onychomycosis** of the nails and **tinea capitis** are treated with oral agents such as terbinafine or itraconazole.

CASE 20 | Dermatophytes *(continued)*

Additional Considerations	**Onychomycosis:** Is a superficial fungal infection of the nails. The nail appears thickened and discolored with subungual debris. The infection is also diagnosed by KOH examination and is usually chronic. Oral antifungals are used for treatment, but treatment failure is common.

Tinea corporis

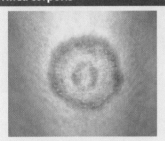

Reproduced with permission from Carol Soutor, Maria K. Hordinsky, Clinical Dermatology, 1st ed; by McGraw-Hill 2013.

Tinea pedis

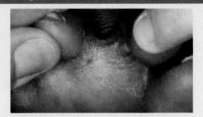

Reproduced with permission from Klaus Wolff, Richard Allen Johnson, Arturo P. Saavedra, Ellen K. Roh, Fitzpatrick's Color Atlas and Synopsis of Clinical Dermatology, 8e; by McGraw-Hill 2017.

Tinea cruris

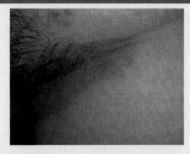

From Maxine A. Papadakis, Stephen J. McPhee, Michael W. Rabow, Current Medical Diagnosis & Treatment 2021; by McGraw Hill 2021. ISBN 9781260469868. EFIGURE 6Ö-9., Used, with permission, from Richard P. Usatine, MD in Usatine RP, Smith MA, Mayeaux EJ Jr, Chumley H, Tysinger J. The Color Atlas of Family Medicine. McGraw-Hill, 2009.

Tinea capitis

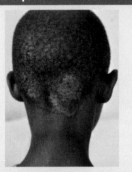

Reproduced with permission from Richard P. Usatine, Mindy A. Smith, E.J. Mayeaux, Jr., Heidi S. Chumley, The Color Atlas and Synopsis of Family Medicine, 3e. Copyright 2019 by McGraw-Hill Education. FIGURE 143-6. ISBN 9781259862045. Reproduced with permission from Richard P. Usatine, MD.

Tinea manuum

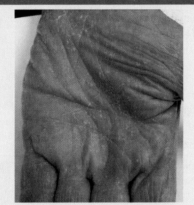

Reproduced with permission from Carol Soutor, Maria K. Hordinsky, Clinical Dermatology, 1st ed; by McGraw-Hill 2013.

Onychomycosis

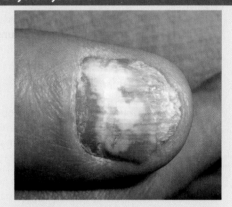

Reproduced with permission from Richard P. Usatine, Mindy A. Smith, E.J. Mayeaux, Jr., Heidi S. Chumley, The Color Atlas and Synopsis of Family Medicine, 3e. Copyright 2019 by McGraw-Hill Education. FIGURE 201-7. ISBN 9781259862045. Reproduced with permission from Richard P. Usatine, MD.

Superficial fungal infections of the skin.

Antifungals

Agent	Indication	Adverse Effects
Nystatin	Mostly used for treatment of Candidiasis. Swish and swallow for oral thrush.	Use limited to oral swish and swallow because of severe side effect profile. Diarrhea, nausea, vomiting, and abdominal pain.
Clotrimazole	Topical use for tinea pedis, corporis.	Hepatotoxicity, nausea, vomiting, diarrhea, and abdominal pain.
Terbinafine	Topical use for tinea pedis, cruris and corporis. Oral use for onychomycosis and tinea capitis.	Hepatotoxicity, headache, diarrhea, dyspepsia.
Griseofulvin	Oral agent used mainly for treatment of tinea capitis.	Rash, urticaria, CYP-450 inducer.
Itraconazole	Oral drug that treats aspergillosis, blastomycosis, and histoplasmosis as well as dermatophytes.	Hepatotoxicity, nausea, vomiting, diarrhea, abdominal pain, hypertension, peripheral edema, and hypokalemia.

Also see Infectious Disease Chapter

Parasitic Infection Mini-Cases

Cases	Key Findings
Scabies	**Hx:** More common in patients who live in congregated populations due to transmission by physical contact and fomites. Often present with a pruritic rash and can occur in patients of all ages. **PE:** May present with pink to red papules near the axillae, breasts, umbilicus, genital area, wrists, and webbed spaces of their fingers. There may be burrows seen between these papules. **Diagnostics:** Scabies can be diagnosed by performing a skin scraping to identify the presence of mites and eggs. **Management:** • Topical agents such as 5% permethrin cream or 5% precipitated sulfur are first-line agents. They are applied from the neck down and kept on overnight. This treatment is repeated 1 week later to ensure all mites are killed. • May use oral ivermectin if topical therapy cannot be used • The patient should wash all clothing and bedding to avoid spreading or reinfection **Discussion:** Scabies infections are caused by *Sarcoptes scabiei* Scabies. (Reproduced with permission from A. Paul Kelly, Susan C. Taylor, Henry W. Lim, Ana Maria Anido Serrano, Taylor and Kelly's Dermatology for Skin of Color, 2e; by McGraw-Hill 2016.)
Bed Bugs	**Hx:** May occur in patients of all ages, presenting generally with an itchy rash after use of either infected bedding, clothing, or furniture. **PE:** Scattered papules on areas of skin that have been exposed to the fomite, often in a **linear array**. May have overlying excoriations. **Diagnostics:** Clinical diagnosis **Management:** • Will resolve in 1–2 weeks • Symptomatic management: Topical steroids and antihistamines • Clean bedding, clothing, or furniture **Discussion:** Commonly caused by *Cimex lectularius* Bed bugs. (Reproduced with permission from Carol Soutor, Maria K. Hordinsky, Clinical Dermatology, 1st ed; by McGraw-Hill 2013.)
Head Lice	**Hx:** More common in children and in patients of all ages in congregated populations. Physical contact and the sharing of fomites, such as brushes, hats, or bedding lead to its spread. Most patients complain of scalp itching, frequently on the retroauricular or occipital scalp. **PE:** Nits (eggs) are commonly seen at the proximal end of the hair shaft near the hairline at the nape of the neck or behind the ear. Live lice may not be visible at the time of the exam, as they tend to avoid light. Hatched nits may be easier to identify, as they are further from the scalp and appear whiter in color. **Diagnostics:** • The diagnosis of an active head lice infection may be confirmed by the presence of viable nits or live lice on the scalp or by combing the head with a fine-toothed comb **Management:** • Topical therapies applied to the scalp are the basis for the treatment of head lice • Most therapies kill hatched lice but not unhatched lice; therefore, retreatment after 7–9 days to kill the newly hatched lice is important • First-line options include permethrin 1% lotion and pyrethrin + piperonyl butoxide which is applied, left for 10 minutes and then rinsed • Those living in the same household as the effected individual should be examined and treated and all clothing, bedding, brushes, and combs should be washed in hot water. • Infected children can return to school after their first round of treatment. **Discussion:** *Pediculus humanus* var. *capitis* is the variety of louse responsible for head lice infections. Head lice. (Reproduced with permission from Richard P. Usatine, Mindy A. Smith, E.J. Mayeaux, Jr., Heidi S. Chumley, The Color Atlas and Synopsis of Family Medicine, 3e. Copyright 2019 by McGraw-Hill Education. FIGURE 148-6. ISBN 9781259862045. Reproduced with permission from Richard P. Usatine, MD.)

EYELID LESIONS

Approach to Common Eyelid Lesions

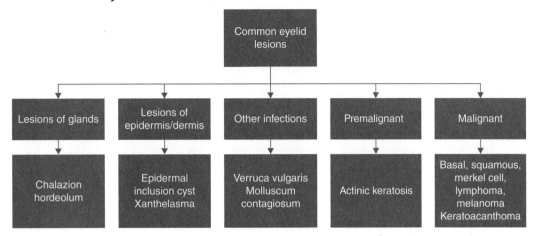

Common eyelid lesions				
Lesions of glands	Lesions of epidermis/dermis	Other infections	Premalignant	Malignant
Chalazion hordeolum	Epidermal inclusion cyst Xanthelasma	Verruca vulgaris Molluscum contagiosum	Actinic keratosis	Basal, squamous, merkel cell, lymphoma, melanoma Keratoacanthoma

Eyelid Lesion Mini-Cases

Cases	Key Findings
Hordeolum	**Hx:** Painful, red "bump" occurring at eyelash line of the eyelid **PE:** Tender, erythematous nodule that presents near the eyelid margin. **Diagnostics:** Clinical diagnosis **Management:** Self-limited • Using a warm compress daily and massaging the area may help to drain the stye • If the stye is persistent, antibiotics may be prescribed and/or incision and drainage may be pursued **Discussion:** • A hordeolum, also known as a stye, is a painful, red lesion that may be internal or external to the patient's eyelid. • They are caused by a bacterial infection (almost always *S. aureus*) of a hair follicle or an oil-producing gland. • When compared to a chalazion, a hordeolum is more painful, red, and tender. They also occur closer to the eyelash line of the eyelid.
Chalazion	**Hx:** Eyelid bump that is not painful. **PE:** Firm, non-erythematous, non-tender nodule located farther back on eyelid, away from the root of the eyelashes. **Diagnostics:** Clinical diagnosis **Management:** Self-limited • Using a warm compress daily may help the clogged oil gland open and drain • Steroid injections may be given if the chalazion is very swollen or painful **Discussion:** • A chalazion is a swollen lesion that appears on the eyelid. • It is caused by a blockage of an oil gland on the eyelid. • Patients initially present with a bump on their eyelid that is not painful. It may occasionally become tender and red as it grows. • Compared to a hordeolum, a chalazion is usually not painful and is more commonly located farther back on the eyelid away from the roots of the eyelashes. Chalazion of upper eyelid. (From Maxine A. Papadakis, Stephen J. McPhee, Michael W. Rabow, Current Medical Diagnosis & Treatment 2021. Copyright 2021 by McGraw Hill. EFIGURE 7Ö. ISBN 9781260469868., From M. Reza Vagefi. Reproduced, with permission, from Riordan-Eva P, Augsburger JJ. Vaughan & Asbury's General Ophthalmology, 19th ed. McGraw-Hill, 2018.)

Eyelid Lesion Mini-Cases *(continued)*

Xanthelasma	**Hx:** Patients with dyslipidemia presenting with painless yellow lesions on eyelids
	PE: Various well-circumscribed yellow macules and papules scattered across bilateral eyelids
	Diagnostics: Clinical diagnosis • Check lipid profile • Consider fasting blood glucose levels, liver, thyroid, and renal function to investigate for an associated condition
	Management: Treat dyslipidemia if present; otherwise, no specific treatment needed unless for cosmetic reasons
	Discussion: • Xanthomas are skin lesions caused by the accumulation of lipids within the macrophages of the skin. • Xanthomas are associated with primary and secondary causes of dyslipidemias. • Xanthelasmas are the most common forms and affect the eyelids. • They typically appear as soft, yellow macules or papules that may enlarge over time. • It is important to work up patients with xanthelasmas for causes of dyslipidemia, though they may appear in patients with normal lipid levels.

DERMATOLOGIC MANIFESTATIONS OF VITAMIN AND MINERAL DEFICIENCIES

CASE 21 | Scurvy

A 57-year-old man presents with bleeding gums for the past 4 hours. He has also felt fatigued over the past few months and has noted a rash on his lower extremities. He is currently undomiciled and has a history of alcohol use disorder. On examination, there is pinpoint bleeding from swollen gingival mucosa. Over the lower extremities, there are petechiae, perifollicular hemorrhages, and corkscrew hairs.

Conditions with Similar Presentations	**Leukocytoclastic vasculitis:** Small-vessel vasculitis that affects postcapillary venules in the dermis. Punctate petechial macules may be seen, but look for palpable purpura that may coalesce over time. **Disseminated intravascular coagulation:** May also present with pinpoint bleeding and petechiae in less acute forms, but patients are usually severely ill; a coagulation workup will help differentiate the diagnosis. **Platelet dysfunction (idiopathic thrombocytopenic purpura, [ITP]):** Is an acquired autoimmune disease, and patients with platelet counts between 10,000–20,000 may have petechia, purpura, or ecchymoses on skin and mucosa. **Vitamin K deficiency:** May present as easy bruising, bleeding, and splinter hemorrhages. Usually in adults it is caused by malabsorption syndromes. PT/INR is elevated.
Initial Diagnostic Tests	• Clinical diagnosis • Vitamin C levels can be confirmatory
Next Steps in Management	Vitamin C replacement
Discussion	Scurvy is a disease that manifests because of a deficiency of **vitamin C**, or **ascorbic acid**, found in vegetables and citrus fruit. This disease historically afflicted sailors who went long periods of time without fresh fruits or vegetables. They made efforts to incorporate citrus juice in their diets, creating the nickname of "limey" to refer to sailors at the time. Vitamin C is essential for the hydroxylation reaction in the synthesis of collagen. Collagen is an important structural protein and integral to the wound-healing process. Without properly functioning collagen, capillaries become fragile, resulting in bleeding. Symptoms of scurvy can appear 1–3 months after inadequate intake. **History:** Inquire about adequate nutrition (housing instability, alcohol use) or malabsorption (Crohn's disease, previous intestinal resection) **Physical Exam:** • Dermatologic manifestations include petechiae, perifollicular hemorrhage, ecchymosis, and corkscrew hairs • Gingival bleeding and edema • Delayed wound healing • Fatigue, myalgias, bone pain **Diagnostics:** Clinical diagnosis with low serum vitamin C level **Management:** • Vitamin C supplementation • Can expect full recovery within 3 months of replacement • Address underlying socioeconomic factors that may be contributing to deficiency

Other Dermatologic Manifestations of Vitamin Deficiencies

Vitamin Deficiency	Dermatologic Manifestations
Vitamin A	Phrynoderma (follicular hyperkeratosis)
	Hair follicle destruction
Vitamin B2	Mucous membrane edema
	Angular stomatitis
	Cheilitis
	Glossitis
	Seborrheic dermatitis
	Angular stomatitis. (Reproduced with permission from J. Larry Jameson, Anthony S. Fauci, Dennis L. Kasper, Stephen L. Hauser, Dan L. Longo, Joseph Loscalzo, Harrison's Principles of Internal Medicine, 20e; by McGraw-Hill 2018.)
Vitamin B3	Pellagra (dermatitis on sun-exposed areas)
	Glossitis
	Cheilitis
	Angular stomatitis
	Pellagra. (Reproduced with permission from Klaus Wolff, Richard Allen Johnson, Arturo P. Saavedra, Ellen K. Roh, Fitzpatrick's Color Atlas and Synopsis of Clinical Dermatology, 8e; by McGraw-Hill 2017.)
Vitamin B6	Stomatitis
	Glossitis
	Cheilitis
	Nasolabial seborrheic dermatitis
	Nasolabial seborrheic dermatitis. (Reproduced with permission from J. Larry Jameson, Anthony S. Fauci, Dennis L. Kasper, Stephen L. Hauser, Dan L. Longo, Joseph Loscalzo, Harrison's Principles of Internal Medicine, 20e. Copyright 2018 by McGraw-Hill Education. FIGURE A4-6. ISBN 9781259644030. Courtesy of Robert A. Swerlick, MD; with permission.)
Vitamin C	Scurvy
	• Petechiae
	• Ecchymoses
	• Perifollicular hyperkeratosis
	• Gingivitis with bleeding gums
	• Dry skin
	• Corkscrew hairs
	• Poor wound healing
	Parafollicular purpura characteristic of scurvy. (Reproduced with permission from Kaushansky K, Prchal JT, Burns LJ, Lichtman MA, Levi M, Linch DC. Williams Hematology, 10e; McGraw Hill LLC 2021.) Clinical features of vitamin C deficiency (scurvy): corkscrew hairs. (Reproduced with permission from McKean SC, Ross JJ, Dressler DD, Scheurer DB. Principles and Practice of Hospital Medicine, 2e; McGraw Hill LLC 2017.)

(Continued)

Vitamin Deficiency	Dermatologic Manifestations	
Zinc	Acrodermatitis enteropathica • Acral and periorificial rash • Diarrhea • Alopecia 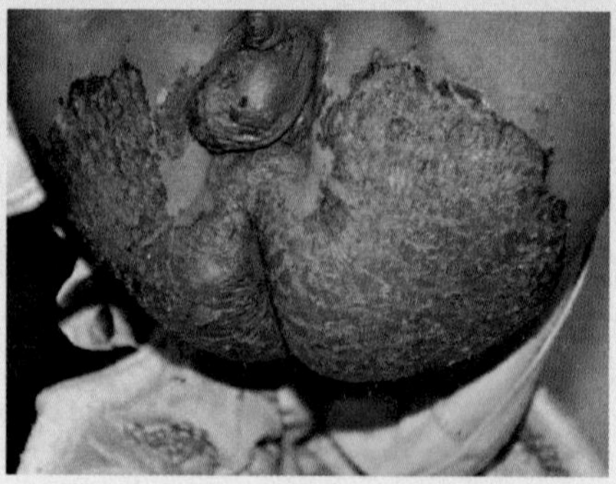 Acrodermatitis enteropathica. (Reproduced from Richard P. Usatine, Mindy A. Smith, E.J. Mayeaux, Jr., Heidi S. Chumley, The Color Atlas and Synopsis of Family Medicine, 3e. Copyright 2019 by McGraw-Hill Education. FIGURE 117-6. ISBN 9781259862045. Reproduced with permission from Richard P. Usatine, MD.)	

12

Nephrology

Lead Authors: Julia Brown, MD; Stephanie Toth-Manikowski, MD, MHS
Contributors: Natalie Meeder, MD; John Hickernell, MD; Ajit Augustin, MD

ACUTE KIDNEY INJURY (AKI)

AKI can be categorized by anatomic location: pre-renal, intra-renal, or post-renal. as shown in the following table.

Causes of AKI

Classification of AKI	Etiology	Examples

Pre-renal	Total body volume depletion	• Hemorrhage
		• Diuresis
		   • Medications
		   • Osmotic (diabetes)
		• Vomiting, diarrhea, sweating
		• Low intake

	Total body volume overload with poor renal blood flow	• Nephrotic syndrome • Hepatorenal syndrome • Cardiorenal syndrome
	Hemodynamic change: Afferent arteriole vasoconstriction	• NSAIDs • Hypercalcemia • Contrast dye
Intra-renal	Glomerular diseases	• Minimal change disease • Focal segmental glomerular sclerosis (FSGS) • Membranous nephropathy • Membranoproliferative glomerulonephritis (MPGN) • Diabetic nephropathy • Amyloid nephropathy • Infection-related glomerulonephritis • IgA nephropathy • Anti-GBM antibody glomerulonephritis • ANCA vasculitis
	Tubulo-interstitial diseases	• Acute interstitial nephritis (AIN) • Acute tubular necrosis (ATN)
Post-renal	Urinary tract obstruction	• Benign prostatic hyperplasia • Kidney stones • Prostate cancer • Ovarian, uterine, cervical cancer

History can help identify the specific etiology:

• IV contrast, NSAIDs, antibiotics, proton pump inhibitors (PPIs), and chemotherapy are associated with specific types of injury.

• Known vasculitides (lupus, ANCA-associated) may lead to intra-renal injury.

• Long-standing diabetes is a very common cause of intra-renal injury and can lead to nephrotic/nephritic syndromes (see below).

Useful labs and tests include:

• Basic metabolic profile (BMP): BUN, creatinine, and serum electrolytes (sodium, potassium)
  • Assesses the degree of renal injury (creatinine)
  • Assists in determining the classification (BUN: creatinine ratio)
  • Assesses potentially serious electrolyte abnormalities
• Urinalysis (UA)
  • Proteinuria and hematuria suggest glomerulonephritis
  • WBCs indicate AIN (especially if eosinophils)
  • Presence of nitrite, blood, leukocyte esterase, and bacteria may indicate urinary tract infection (UTI)
• Urinary sediment is helpful in distinguishing between glomerular and tubulointerstitial lesions causing AKI

Casts in Urinary Sediment	Significance
RBC	Glomerulonephritis
WBC	Acute interstitial nephritis (AIN), infection
Muddy brown, granular	Acute tubular necrosis (ATN)
Hyaline	Prerenal or benign

- Urine sodium, urine creatinine, urine urea are used to calculate fractional excretion of sodium (FeNa) and fractional excretion of urea (FeUrea) (use FeUrea for patients on diuretics, which increase urine sodium).
  - In patients with **oliguria** (defined as <400 mL urine per day, or <0.5 mL/kg/hour), the FeNa can help differentiate between a prerenal state and intrinsic renal damage
  - A FeNa <1% or FeUrea <35% indicates a prerenal state

Laboratory Test	Prerenal AKI	Intrinsic AKI/ATN
Urine Na	<20	>40
FeNa	<1	>2
FeUrea	<35	>35
Urinary casts	Hyaline casts or absence of urinary casts	Granular or "muddy brown casts"

- Renal ultrasound helps identify a post-renal cause by showing evidence of obstruction with hydroureter and/or hydronephrosis, and may demonstrate the etiology of the obstruction (e.g., stone, cancer).

Diagnoses/Conditions and Key Findings

Diagnoses or Conditions	Key Findings
Pre-renal with volume depletion	• Poor renal perfusion due to severe volume depletion or hypotension • Dry mucous membranes, orthostatic hypotension, decreased urine output, decreased skin turgor, absent axillary sweat

Pre-renal with volume overload	• Poor renal perfusion due to poor cardiac output or third spacing
	• Heart failure
	• Hypoalbuminemia
	  • Nephrotic syndrome
	  • Cirrhosis
	  • Protein-losing enteropathy

AIN	• Rash, fever, eosinophils in the urine or blood after drug exposure (e.g., antibiotics, NSAIDs)
Vasculitis, anti-GBM antibody GN	• Upper respiratory tract involvement (sinusitis) • Lower respiratory tract involvement (hemoptysis)
Thrombotic microangiopathy (TMA), hemolytic uremic syndrome (HUS), thrombotic thrombocytopenic purpura (TTP)	• Severe hypertension, livedo reticularis, abdominal pain, mental status changes, fever, thrombocytopenia
Preeclampsia, ATN, cortical necrosis, HELLP syndrome, TMA	• Pregnancy-related emergencies
Glomerulonephritis (GN)	• Proteinuria, hematuria +/– RBC casts, dysmorphic RBCs
Glomerulonephritis secondary to SLE, MPGN, endocarditis, post-streptococcal, hepatitis C, cryoglobulinemia	• Low complements, hematuria, RBC casts, dysmorphic RBCs, proteinuria
Glomerulonephritis secondary to vasculitis, anti-GBM, IgA nephropathy, TMA	• Normal complements. Hematuria, RBC casts, dysmorphic RBCs, proteinuria
Genitourinary (GU) obstruction	• Decreased urine output or sudden onset anuria, suprapubic pain, hematuria, urinary frequency, inability to empty bladder

Approach to a Patient with AKI

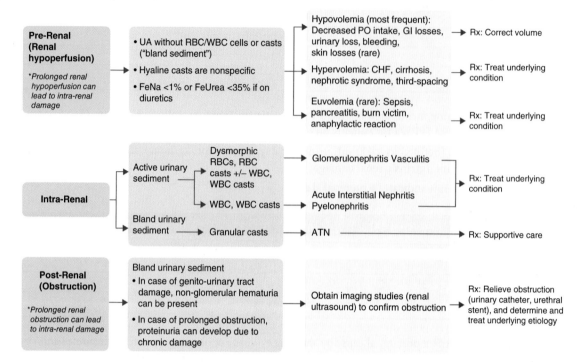

A 58-year-old man with no significant past medical history comes to clinic for evaluation of weakness and lethargy. He was at a picnic a few days ago and developed watery diarrhea and has decreased appetite, weakness and decreased urine output for the past 2 days. He is not on any medications and denies any pain, dysuria, frequency, or hematuria. On exam, he appears tired. Temperature is 37.2°C, respiratory rate 14, and SpO2 98% on room air. Reclining blood pressure is 110/60 mmHg, pulse is 92/min and upon standing, he reports feeling lightheaded and his blood pressure drops to 88/54 and heart rate increases to 116 (orthostatic hypotension). He has dry mucous membranes and decreased skin turgor.

Conditions with Similar Presentations	**Sepsis:** Can also present with oliguria and orthostatic hypotension but would have manifestations of infection including fever, tachycardia, and tachypnea.
	Urinary tract infections: Can also present with weakness and lethargy but would have urinary symptoms including dysuria, frequency and urgency.
	Hepatorenal syndrome (HRS): Can also cause pre-renal AKI but is seen in the setting of chronic liver disease (see mini-case).
	Cardiorenal syndrome: Can also cause pre-renal AKI but is seen in patients with severe heart failure due to renal hypoperfusion from decreased cardiac output. Will have symptoms of heart failure/volume overload: dyspnea on exertion (DOE), paroxysmal nocturnal dyspnea (PND), edema.
Initial Diagnostic Testing	Check: BUN, creatinine, urinalysis, and urine sodium and urine creatinine to compute FeNa.
Next Steps in Management	Fluid resuscitation with oral or IV fluids.
Discussion	Pre-renal AKI is caused by hypoperfusion to the kidneys.
	History: Inquire about poor oral intake, excessive fluid loss (diarrhea, diuretic use, massive hemorrhage, sweating), or other causes of poor perfusion to the kidneys (heart failure, shock, hypoalbuminemia).
	Physical Exam: Signs of volume depletion: decreased skin turgor, dry mucous membranes, orthostatic hypotension, tachycardia.

CASE 1 | Pre-Renal AKI *(continued)*

Discussion	**Diagnostics:** • Increased creatinine compared to patient's baseline. • BUN/Cr > 20:1, FeNa <1%. • May see hyaline casts in the urine but these are nonspecific. • Urinalysis should not have RBCs or WBCs, which could indicate another inflammatory process (e.g., **AIN,** acute **GN**, pyelonephritis) and be an intra-renal cause of AKI. • If serum creatinine worsens despite improved volume status, pre-renal AKI may have progressed to ATN or there may be another cause of the AKI. **Management:** • PO or IV fluids. • Hold diuretics and ACE inhibitors (and ARBs) until volume status and serum creatinine improve.
Additional Considerations	**Complications:** Prolonged and/or severe pre-renal states can lead to acute tubular necrosis (ATN).

CASE 2 | Hepatorenal Syndrome (HRS)

A 62-year-old man with cirrhosis from ethanol use disorder is admitted with a cough and fever for 2 days. He is eating and drinking fluids, and has no change in urine output or frequency, and no hematuria, or dysuria. He has no vomiting or diarrhea. On physical exam he is alert and oriented. Temperature is 38.1, blood pressure 98/66, pulse rate 98, respiratory rate 18. Orthostatics are negative. He has palmar erythema. He has a new left lower lobe infiltrate on CXR and his serum creatinine on admission is 2.9 with a baseline of 1.1. Urinalysis shows no cells, protein, nitrites, or bacteria. Urine Na is 7 and FeNa is 0.5%. Renal ultrasound is normal. He is treated with azithromycin and ceftriaxone for community-acquired pneumonia. His serum creatinine is 3.5 the next day.

Conditions with Similar Presentations	**Pre-renal AKI from other etiologies:** Causes a rise in serum creatinine and a low urine sodium and FeNa but history/exam and clinical data would point to another cause (e.g., vomiting, diarrhea, hemorrhage, heart failure exacerbation). **Intra-renal AKI:** Causes a rise in serum creatinine but would not have a low urine Na or FeNa. **Post-renal AKI:** Causes a rise in serum creatinine, would not have a low urine sodium or FeNa, and renal ultrasound would show obstruction.
Initial Diagnostic Testing	• Clinical diagnosis • Confirm with: Low urine Na and FeNa
Next Steps in Management	IV midodrine, octreotide, albumin ("HRS cocktail")
Discussion	HRS is characterized by an AKI in someone with known cirrhosis, often after a precipitating event such as an infection. Portal hypertension from cirrhosis leads to splanchnic vasodilation from vasodilators like nitrous oxide, leading to decreased systemic vascular resistance and shunting of blood away from the renal arteries. In response to decreased perfusion, activation of the RAAS system and sympathetic nervous system lead to renal vasoconstriction and hypoperfusion of the kidneys. **History:** Patients with cirrhosis and signs and symptoms of a precipitating event including infection (e.g., spontaneous bacterial peritonitis (SBP), pneumonia, UTI), GI bleed **Physical Exam:** No specific findings of HRS, but may have stigmata of cirrhosis (e.g., peripheral edema, ascites, spider angiomas, palmar erythema, gynecomastia) **Diagnostics:** Clincal diagnosis • Diagnosis of exclusion; rule out other causes of AKI including pre-renal, ATN, GN • Rising serum creatinine • Low urine Na and FeNa

CASE 2 | Hepatorenal Syndrome (HRS) *(continued)*

Discussion	**Management:** • IV albumin to increase serum oncotic pressure to increase intravascular volume and renal blood flow • Start medications that cause splanchnic arterial vasoconstriction to shunt blood to the renal arteries (midodrine and octreotide)
Additional Considerations	**Complications:** Failure to respond to initial treatment is a bad prognostic sign. Patients may require hemodialysis and should be evaluated for liver transplantation.

CASE 3 | Post-Renal Obstructive AKI

An 81-year-old man with hypertension and benign prostatic hyperplasia (BPH) is seen in the emergency department (ED) for lower abdominal pain. He has had no nausea or vomiting and notes he has not been able to urinate for over 10 hours. His medications include amlodipine. On examination, vital signs are normal. He has a palpable, tender mass in the suprapubic region. Digital rectal examination (DRE) reveals an enlarged, nontender, smooth prostate. Creatinine is 1.8 with a baseline of 0.8 mg/dL.

Conditions with Similar Presentations	**Prostate cancer:** Can also present with an enlarged prostate. However, usually it grows in the peripheral zone and thus is less likely to obstruct than BPH, which grows in the transition zone that surrounds the urethra. Prostate cancer is more likely to be nodular (vs. smooth) on rectal exam.
Initial Diagnostic Testing	• Confirm diagnosis: Bladder ultrasound or urethral catheter placement • Consider: Renal ultrasound, urinalysis
Next Steps in Management	Urethral catheter placement
Discussion	Suprapubic mass and tenderness in an elderly man with no urine output is suggestive of bladder outlet obstruction from an enlarged prostate causing bladder distension. **History:** • Inability to void to urine • May have symptoms of BPH (chronic): Urinary frequency, urinary hesitancy, nocturia, weak urinary stream, dribbling, and feeling of incomplete emptying. • Less common: May also have history of prior malignancy, retroperitoneal fibrosis **Physical Exam:** • Suprapubic fullness, enlarged prostate on DRE. **Diagnostics:** • Elevated serum creatinine due to AKI. If obstruction has been prolonged, ATN may occur. • Renal ultrasound may show bilateral hydronephrosis. • Urine Na and FeNa both low unless ATN occurs. **Management:** • Immediate decompression of the bladder with a urethral catheter. • Treat BPH
Additional Considerations	**Complications:** Long-standing obstruction may result in ATN and patients may develop post-obstructive diuresis after urethral catheter placement. Fluid and electrolyte replacement will be needed if severe.

CASE 4 | Acute Tubular Necrosis (ATN)

A 32-year-old woman presents with right lower abdominal pain, vomiting, and fever for 3 days. Her only medications include NSAIDs for pain. On examination, she is afebrile, blood pressure is 90/54 mmHg, pulse is 120/min. Her bowel sounds are decreased, and her abdomen is soft, slightly distended, and tender to palpation in the right lower quadrant. Abdominal CT scan with contrast reveals an ovarian abscess, and patient is started on empiric IV antibiotics and taken for surgical intervention. Post-operatively, her urine output decreases to 5 mL/hr and post-void residual urine volume is 3 mL. Labs show BUN 28, serum creatinine 1.52 (baseline 0.82 mg/dL), and UA shows multiple granular and muddy brown casts with 2 RBCs and 4 WBCs. Renal ultrasound is normal. Her FeNa is 2.8%.

CASE 4 | Acute Tubular Necrosis (ATN) *(continued)*

Conditions with Similar Presentations	**Pre-renal AKI:** Also causes an elevated Cr but FeNa would be <1% and is reversible if perfusion to the kidneys is restored early. If the pre-renal state persists, ATN may develop. **Acute glomerulonephritis:** Is inflammation/damage to the glomeruli; urine will demonstrate hematuria and/or proteinuria. May have red blood cell casts. **AIN:** Causes include NSAIDs and antibiotics but takes several days to manifest and UA may show pyuria or eosinophils. **Post-renal AKI:** Also causes elevated Cr but occurs when there is obstruction. Renal ultrasound will show hydronephrosis and an elevated (>200 mL) post-void residual urine volume. FeNa is initially <1% unless ATN ensues.
Initial Diagnostic Tests	• Serum creatinine, urinalysis, urine electrolytes (Na, Cr). • Consider urethral catheter placement and renal ultrasound.
Next Steps in Management	• Treat underlying cause *(In this patient: Intrinsic AKI due to decreased renal perfusion precipitated by the patient's sepsis and made worse by CT contrast administration and NSAIDs (both reduce blood flow to the kidneys)).* • IV fluids
Discussion	Severe or prolonged pre-renal AKI from hypotension results in ATN. ATN is divided into three phases: 1. Initiation phase = initial renal insult 2. Maintenance phase = oliguria or anuria 3. Recovery phase = restoration of tubular cells and significant increase in urine output ("post-ATN diuresis") Pre-renal disease or nephrotoxic injury result in renal ischemia and death of the renal tubular cells. Renal cell death causes sloughing of the tubular and epithelial cells that can be visualized as "muddy brown granular casts" on urinalysis. Urine microscopy, showing muddy brown casts of acute tubular necrosis (ATN). (Reproduced with permission from First Aid Step 1 2022. New York, NY: McGraw-Hill; 2022. pg 627. (Figure A).) **History:** • Risk factors: Volume depletion, hypotension during surgery, shock, use of nephrotoxic agents, cardiorenal or hepatorenal syndrome. • Timing variable, but occurs within 1–3 days after ischemic event or toxic exposure. **Physical Exam:** Hypotension, dry mucous membranes, low urine output. **Diagnostics:** • Elevated BUN, serum Cr • Urine electrolytes and urea to calculate the FeNa and FeUrea to distinguish between pre-renal and intrinsic causes. • Urinalysis and renal/bladder ultrasound to rule out other causes • Urine microscopy with muddy brown casts **Management:** • Treat underlying causes (e.g., infection). • Supportive care including fluid resuscitation, discontinuing nephrotoxic medications (see inpatient considerations) and adjusting medications per eGFR. • If patient remains oliguric/anuric and develops signs of volume overload or electrolyte abnormalities refractory to medical management, hemodialysis should be considered.
Additional Considerations	**Inpatient Considerations:** Medications that inhibit autoregulation of the kidneys (e.g., NSAIDs, diuretics, and ACEIs/ARBs) often worsen the degree of AKI and can precipitate ATN. Therefore, these medications should be held in hospitalized patients until patients are fully volume resuscitated and renal function improves.

Acute Interstitial Nephritis Mini-Case	
Case	**Key Findings**
Acute interstitial nephritis (AIN)	**Hx/PE:** • History of common culprit medication use including NSAIDs, PPIs, antibiotics (e.g., penicillins, cephalosporins, rifampin, fluoroquinolones, and sulfonamides). • Commonly asymptomatic, but can have nonspecific symptoms or signs/symptoms of allergic reaction (fever, rash, nausea, vomiting, or malaise). **Diagnostics:** As most present without clear signs of AIN in the urine or CBC, the diagnosis is often made by a strong clinical suspicion • Elevated serum creatinine • UA with pyuria (WBCs); may also have WBC casts and eosinophils • CBC may show eosinophilia • Renal biopsy makes the definitive diagnosis in select cases **Management:** • Discontinue offending agent • Consider steroids if severe **Discussion:** • AIN is most commonly associated with beta-lactam antibiotics or NSAID use. • Production of antibodies to the offending medication leads to damage of the kidney interstitium. • Timing of AIN depends on drug and usually occurs within 1–2 weeks of antibiotic initiation vs. months to years following NSAID or PPI administration. If drug is readministered, onset is quicker. • The majority (>70%) of AIN in adults is associated with drugs; however, various infections and systemic diseases such as systemic lupus erythematosus (SLE), Sjögren syndrome, and sarcoidosis can cause acute interstitial inflammation of the kidneys. • In patients with normal renal function and relatively short exposure, full recovery of renal function is expected on discontinuation of the medication. In rare circumstances if there is no improvement, steroids can be tried.

CHRONIC KIDNEY DISEASE (CKD)

CKD is decreased kidney function ongoing for > 3 months. Staging is by glomerular filtration rate (GFR) and albuminuria >30 mg/g. The two most common causes of CKD are diabetes and hypertension. It is important to identify CKD early to prevent progression to end-stage renal disease (ESRD).

Stages of Kidney Disease

Stages	GFR (mL/min/1.73m²)	Function
Stage 1	>90	Normal
Stage 2	60–89	Mildly decreased
Stage 3A	45–59	Mildly–moderately decreased
Stage 3B	30–44	Moderately–severely decreased
Stage 4	15–29	Severely decreased
Stage 5	<15	Kidney failure

Complications of Progressive CKD

- Secondary hyperparathyroidism (see figure below)
- Anemia due to decreased erythropoietin production
- Acidosis due to failure to excrete acids (sulfates, phosphates, urates)
- Electrolyte abnormalities (hyperphosphatemia, hypocalcemia, hypermagnesemia)
- Hypervolemia

Secondary Hyperparathyroidism

As CKD progresses, the kidneys fail to excrete phosphate (which complexes with calcium), fail to reabsorb calcium (Ca), and fail to convert 25-hydroxyvitamin D to 1,25-hydroxyvitamin D (its active form). All of these lead to hypocalcemia which stimulates secretion of parathyroid hormone (PTH) (see figure below). This can be managed with phosphate binders and vitamin D analogs like calcitriol.

Hyperparathyroidism in CKD

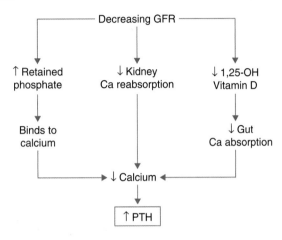

Electrolyte Abnormalities that May Require Urgent Dialysis

	Hyperkalemia	Hypercalcemia
History	Muscle weakness, palpitations, arrhythmia, sudden cardiac death	Nausea, vomiting, abdominal pain, weakness, confusion, lethargy, neurologic changes
Physical exam	Arrhythmias, decreased or absent deep tendon reflexes (extreme)	Altered mental status, signs of dehydration
Diagnostics	↑Serum potassium EKG: peaked T waves, widening of QRS, short QT, prolonged PR	↑Serum ionized calcium EKG: short QT
When to consider hemodialysis	Hyperkalemia refractory to medical management	Severe, symptomatic hypercalcemia (≥14 mg/dL) refractory to medical management (e.g., neurologic symptoms or renal failure caused by severe hypercalcemia)

Renal Replacement Therapy

Renal replacement therapy (RRT) may include hemodialysis, peritoneal dialysis, or kidney transplantation. RRT should be considered in patients with low GFR (typically <10 mL/min/1.73m^2), decreasing urine output, and in "AEIOU" conditions that are refractory to medical management:

Acidosis

Electrolyte imbalance (hyperkalemia, hypercalcemia)

Intoxication (SLIME: salicylates, lithium, isopropyl alcohol, methanol, ethylene glycol)

Overload (Symptomatic fluid overload)

Uremia (pericarditis, encephalopathy)

CASE 5 | Chronic Kidney Disease (CKD)

A 50-year-old man comes to the clinic for a wellness visit. He hasn't seen a doctor in 10 years. He was diagnosed with diabetes and hypertension at his last visit but hasn't been taking medication as he feels fine. He smokes half a pack a day for 30 years. Blood pressure is 167/97, and the rest of the physical exam is normal. Routine labs show a creatinine of 2.1 and BUN of 37. HbA1c is 9.0.

Conditions with Similar Presentations	**AKI:** Can also present with elevated creatinine and BUN but is usually reversible. If an elevated Cr persists for 3 or more months, it is then considered "chronic," or CKD.
Initial Diagnostic Tests	• Additional tests in persons with CKD include BMP (serum K), serum Ca, CBC to look for anemia, urinalysis, urine protein/creatinine ratio. • Consider: Renal ultrasound.
Next Steps in Management	• ACE inhibitor/ARB for HTN and proteinuria. • SGLT2 for diabetes and proteinuria. • Treat risk factors.
Discussion	CKD is kidney damage that lasts for at least 3 months, regardless of etiology. In the United States, the most common causes of CKD are diabetes and hypertension. CKD can progress to ESRD, requiring dialysis or renal transplant. The pathophysiology depends on the cause of CKD. Damage will produce fibrosis/scarring in the kidneys and nonfunctional tissue. This can be seen on biopsy and in advanced CKD, and on imaging kidneys may appear shrunken/atrophic. Some damage to the kidney (such as diabetic) can result in the kidneys adapting by increasing the GFR in the remaining nondamaged/functional nephrons. This is called adaptive hyperfiltration. This adaptation results in normal or near-normal kidney function for a period of time, but eventually leads to glomerular damage and eventually kidney failure. **History:** Patients are usually asymptomatic Risk factors include: HTN, DM, cardiovascular disease, tobacco use, obesity, family history of kidney disease **Physical Exam:** May have hypertension or edema if fluid overloaded or caused by nephrotic syndrome **Diagnostics:** CKD is defined by kidney damage or decreased kidney function for at least 3 months, usually diagnosed w/ urinary albumin to creatinine ratio >30 mg/g or an estimated GFR <60 Also check: • BMP for electrolyte abnormalities and GFR for staging (as above) • CBC for anemia • Urinalysis for hematuria/pyuria • Urine protein/creatinine ratio or urine albumin/creatinine ratio to check for proteinuria and albuminuria • PTH and vitamin D to look for secondary hyperparathyroidism • Renal ultrasound to check for structural abnormalities **Management:** Involves preventing progression, treating complications, and preparing for future hemodialysis or renal transplant. • Avoid nephrotoxic meds (such as NSAIDs) • Control hypertension: ACE inhibitors/ARBs also slow progression of renal damage (and proteinuria) • Managing diabetes slows proteinuria/albuminuria • SGLT2 inhibitors benefit both diabetic and nondiabetic patients in reducing proteinuria/albuminuria • Control risk factors: Encourage smoking cessation, discourage NSAID use, optimize blood pressure, diabetes, and weight control • Optimize conditions that reduce blood flow to the kidneys (liver failure, heart failure) • Plan for possible future hemodialysis
Additional Considerations	**Complications:** The risk of death from cardiovascular disease is significantly greater in patients with CKD than in the general population. Proper treatment of their CKD and comorbidities, especially hypertension, remains crucial in decreasing patient mortality

CASE 6 | Uremia

A 68-year-old woman with uncontrolled hypertension and stage 5 CKD presents for a follow-up appointment after missing her last few monthly appointments. She reports nausea, anorexia, and worsening shortness of breath and fatigue for the past 2 weeks. She also reports pruritis and weight loss. Her husband notes that the patient at times is lethargic and confused. On exam, she has conjunctival pallor, dry skin, a pericardial friction rub, bilateral basilar crackles, 2+ bilateral lower extremity edema, and asterixis. Labs show sodium 132 mEq/L, potassium 6.0 mEq/L, bicarbonate 12 mEq/L, BUN 152 mEq/L, Cr 15 mg/dL, phosphate 7.8 mg/dL.

Conditions with Similar Presentations	**AKI:** Can also cause uremia if severe and prolonged **Hemolytic uremic syndrome (HUS)/thrombotic thrombocytopenic purpura (TTP):** Presents with uremia and AKI but can also include fever, anemia, and neurological symptoms. Will see thrombocytopenia and microangiopathic hemolytic anemia with schistocytes on peripheral smear.
Initial Diagnostic Tests	Clinical diagnosis with uremic signs/symptoms in the setting of markedly elevated BUN
Next Steps in Management	Urgent hemodialysis
Discussion	Uremia is a sign of severe CKD. It occurs when the kidney does not effectively eliminate waste products. It is difficult to predict when uremia will cause symptoms, but it most commonly occurs when the BUN is >90 mg/dL or higher. Uremia typically develops in the setting of CKD but can be seen in severe AKI. The BUN and creatinine are markers of other toxins/waste products that are not measured in the blood but can cause systemic manifestations of uremia including abnormal platelet function (bleeding risk), pericardial inflammation (pericarditis), altered mental status, asterixis, and seizures (uremic encephalopathy). **History:** • Risk factors include HTN, DM, cardiovascular disease, tobacco use, obesity, family history of kidney disease. • Symptoms: GI (nausea, anorexia, dysgeusia [an altered, usually metallic taste in mouth]), weight loss, neurologic (lethargy, fatigue, confusion, seizures) **Physical Exam:** May have altered mental status, signs of volume overload, hyperreflexia, asterixis, pericardial friction rub **Diagnostics:** Clinical diagnosis with any of the following signs/symptoms (nausea, anorexia, dysgeusia, pericarditis, asterixis, encephalopathy, platelet dysfunction) in the setting of markedly elevated BUN (usually >90 mg/dL). • Check BMP (↑Cr and ↑↑BUN) (may have other electrolyte abnormalities including ↑potassium, ↓bicarb) • CBC • Renal ultrasound **Management:** • Urgent hemodialysis if symptomatic uremia (pericardial friction rub, uremic encephalopathy [confusion, asterixis, seizure]), and severe electrolyte abnormalities, e.g., severe hyperkalemia refractory to medication management
Additional Considerations	**Complications:** Uremia usually requires multiple dialysis sessions to determine if symptoms resolve with RRT. If uremic toxins are cleared too quickly, dangerous osmotic shifts can occur in the brain and cause dialysis disequilibrium syndrome.

Indications for Urgent Dialysis Mini-Cases

Cases	Key Findings
Acidosis	**Hx:** Confusion, fatigue, and causes of acidosis (e.g., sepsis, DKA, methanol/ethylene glycol ingestion). **PE:** Depends on underling etiology but may include hyperventilation, rapid and shallow breathing, slurred speech, blurry vision, fruity breath (DKA). **Diagnostics:** • BMP for bicarbonate, anion gap • Arterial blood gas (ABG) for degree of acidosis (pH) **Management:** • Sodium bicarbonate can be used to correct acidemia and attempt to prevent the need for dialysis • Urgent dialysis if pH <7.1 that is refractory to bicarbonate supplementation

Indications for Urgent Dialysis Mini-Cases (*continued*)

Acidosis	**Discussion:** • Severe metabolic acidosis that is refractory to medical management is an urgent indication for dialysis • Patients compensate for metabolic acidosis by hyperventilating to exhale CO_2 to increase the pH • However, the patient can tire out or may not be able to exhale enough CO_2 to maintain an adequate pH. BIPAP can help with ventilation, but intubation may be required
Intoxication/ Ingestion	**Hx:** History or suspicion of substance use **PE:** Confusion, slurred speech, blurry vision, ataxia **Diagnostics:** History and serum levels of suspected toxins: SLIME: salicylates, lithium, isopropyl alcohol, methanol, ethylene glycol **Management:** Urgent dialysis is indicated for severe intoxication of select substances. Some indications for urgent dialysis are as follows: • Aspirin (salicylate) intoxication with altered mental status, pulmonary edema causing respiratory distress, cerebral edema, acute renal dysfunction, or severe acidemia • Serum lithium level >5 mEq/L • Known methanol/ethylene glycol ingestion with high anion gap metabolic acidosis regardless of drug level or evidence of end-organ damage (visual changes, renal failure). Fomepizole is also indicated for treatment. **Discussion:** Dialyzable toxins include methanol, ethylene glycol, lithium, salicylates, theophylline, barbiturates.
Volume Overload	**Hx:** Shortness of breath, orthopnea, PND. **PE:** Signs of volume overload refractory to diuresis including elevated JVP, pulmonary crackles, anasarca, abdominal fluid wave (ascites), peripheral edema. **Diagnostics:** Clinical diagnosis • Elevated BNP, CXR demonstrating pulmonary edema and/or pleural effusion, an increasing oxygen requirement. **Management:** • Dialysis when symptomatic volume overload is refractory to diuresis. **Discussion:** Life-threatening signs of volume overload include pulmonary edema and hypertensive emergency (blood pressure >180/120 + end-organ damage) that does not respond to high-dose antihypertensive medications and/or diuresis.

CASE 7 | Autosomal Dominant Polycystic Kidney Disease (ADPKD)

A 42-year-old woman presents to urgent care with left-sided flank pain for 1 week. She also reports intermittent blood-tinged urine. She has no dysuria but has a history of recurrent UTIs. Her family history is notable for ESRD in her father and a brother who died of a ruptured brain aneurysm at age 34. On exam, she is afebrile, blood pressure is 140/90 mmHg, pulse is 94/min, and abdominal exam is notable for enlarged and palpable kidneys and bilateral flank tenderness.

Conditions with Similar Presentations	**Nephrolithiasis:** May also present with flank pain and tenderness and hematuria but is not associated with palpable kidneys on exam or a family history of brain aneurysms or ESRD. **Benign cysts:** Can be difficult to differentiate from mild ADPKD but typically are not numerous (number increases with age) and do not have a significant family history. **Localized renal cystic disease:** Is usually unilateral. **Von Hippel-Lindeau (VHL)** and **tuberous sclerosis:** Can also have kidney cysts but present with other symptoms (see Chapter 15).
Initial Diagnostic Tests	• CT abdomen/pelvis • Creatinine, urinalysis
Next Steps in Management	• Increased fluid intake • ACE-I

CASE 7 | Autosomal Dominant Polycystic Kidney Disease (ADPKD) *(continued)*

Discussion	Polycystic kidney disease (PKD) is an inherited disorder characterized by cystic expansion of the kidneys, producing progressive kidney enlargement and renal insufficiency. There is also an increased personal and family risk of cerebral berry aneurysms and cysts in other organs (liver, spleen, and pancreas). The disease can be inherited in an autosomal dominant or recessive form. Cystic expansion of the kidneys, especially the collecting ducts, leads to progressive kidney enlargement and renal insufficiency. Autosomal dominant PKD (ADPKD) is most often due to a mutation in *PKD1* on chromosome 16, but can also be caused by a mutation in *PKD2* on chromosome 4. ADPKD is found in 1/1000 live births, with only half being diagnosed during the patient's life. Slow but progressive enlargement leads to renal failure (requiring dialysis) usually by the fifth or sixth decade of life. **History:** • Risk factors: Family history of renal failure, PKD, brain aneurysms • Symptoms: Bilateral flank pain, recurrent nephrolithiasis and/or UTIs **Physical Exam:** Palpable kidneys, bilateral flank tenderness **Diagnostics:** • CT abdomen/pelvis shows enlarged kidneys with numerous cysts replacing normal parenchyma • Elevated creatinine and urinalysis with proteinuria is suggestive of CKD **Management:** • Increase fluid intake (>3 L/day) and follow low-sodium diet. • ACE inhibitors or ARBs slow rate of cyst growth and should be used to target blood pressure <110/75. • ADH antagonists (tolvaptan) also delay cyst growth, slow progression of kidney disease, and should be considered in high-risk patients • Dialysis and renal transplantation for ESRD
Additional Considerations	**Screening:** Renal US is recommended for patients with a family history of ADPKD **Complications:** Hypertension (from increased renin production) and/or extra-renal manifestations, such as liver cysts, berry aneurysms leading to subarachnoid hemorrhage, mitral valve prolapse, and diverticulosis. **Pediatric Considerations:** Cysts can be detected in childhood. Associated with hepatic fibrosis and signs associated with oligohydramnios.

ALBUMINURIA/PROTEINURIA AND NEPHROTIC SYNDROME

An abnormal amount of protein or albumin in the urine indicates the presence of kidney disease even if serum creatinine and GFR are normal. Normally, protein excretion in the urine is <150 mg/day. The albumin fraction is about 20% of the total urinary protein and should be <30 mg/day. The other proteins normally excreted in the urine include tubular Tamm-Horsfall protein and various globulins also found in the blood (e.g., immunoglobulins).

Normal urine protein	<150 mg/day
Albuminuria ("microalbuminuria")*	>30 mg /day
Overt proteinuria**	>150 mg/day
Nephrotic range proteinuria	>3000–3500 mg/day

*Albuminuria or abnormal albumin in the urine (over 30 mg/day or over 30 mg/g) might be detected as the earliest manifestation of the glomerular filtration barrier abnormality, while total urinary protein still remains normal (below 150 mg/day). In fact, the measurements of albuminuria are used routinely for screening diabetic patients for developing diabetic nephropathy and for kidney donors for early detection of kidney disease.

**In pregnancy, urinary protein excretion can increase to up to 300 mg/day.

Proteinuria can be classified as:

• **Glomerular proteinuria:** Damage to the glomerular filtration barrier results in albuminuria, with albumin constituting >50–75% of total protein in urine. Diabetic nephropathy is an example.

• **Tubular proteinuria:** Tubular damage and inflammation. Predominant protein excreted in urine will be Tamm-Horsfall protein produced by the tubular cells. Acute tubular necrosis (ATN) is an example.

- **Overflow proteinuria:** Occurs with significant increase in concentration of filtered serum protein. The most frequent cause is monoclonal light chain immunoglobulin, such as Bence-Jones protein in multiple myeloma.
- **Transient proteinuria:** Does not signify renal pathology. It can occur in congestive heart failure, heavy exercise, and fever.
- **Benign orthostatic proteinuria:** Rare condition of abnormal protein excretion when the patient is in an upright position.

Proteinuria can be measured as follows:

Urine dipstick	Detects urine albumin in semiquantitative fashion (does not detect other proteins)
Spot urine albumin-to-creatinine or protein-to-creatinine ratios	Rough measure of 24-hour total protein excretion Measured in grams or milligrams per gram of creatinine Quick, easy to estimate, and accurate
24-hour urine collection for protein and/or albumin	Most accurate but difficult to obtain Measured in grams or mg/day Simultaneous creatinine collection should be performed to estimate accuracy of the urine collection (kg × 20 mg for men, kg × 15 mg for women)

Nephrotic Syndrome

The hallmark of nephrotic syndrome is nephrotic range proteinuria (excretion of >3.5 g/day). In clinical vignettes, this is often expressed as at least 3+ protein on urine dipstick. Protein loss leads to all of the events that characterize nephrotic syndrome:

- Loss of albumin in the urine leads to hypoalbuminemia (serum albumin <3 g/dL) when the liver can no longer compensate by increasing albumin synthesis sufficiently.
- Hypoalbuminemia leads to decreased oncotic pressure, which results in edema.
- The liver increases production of other molecules to increase oncotic pressure.
  - Increased cholesterol and triglyceride synthesis leads to hyperlipidemia.
  - Increased clotting factors (with the exception of IV and VIII) lead to a hypercoagulable state which is contributed to by loss of anti-thrombin III in the urine (increased risk of renal vein thrombosis).
- Loss of other proteins in the urine leads to:
  - Increased risk of infection (loss of complement and immunoglobulin).
  - Protein malnutrition.

Nephrotic syndrome can be due to two categories of disease processes:

1. Primary (idiopathic) glomerular disease: Diseases intrinsic to the kidney, including minimal change disease (MCD) (most common cause in children), membranous nephropathy (most common cause in adults), and focal segmental glomerulosclerosis (FSGS).
2. Secondary nephrotic syndrome: Associated with diseases outside of the kidney or medications.
   a. Systemic conditions: Endocrine (diabetes mellitus), autoimmune (SLE), infectious (hepatitis B, hepatitis C, HIV, syphilis, poststreptococcal glomerulonephritis), oncological (solid tumors), hematological malignancies (leukemia, lymphoma), amyloid, myeloma, obstructive nephropathy, sickle cell disease, chronic renal allograft rejection, obesity, or obstructive sleep apnea.
   b. Medications:
      - NSAIDs in association with AIN
      - Pamidronate and IVIG can cause collapsing FSGS
      - Interferon, lithium, penicillamine, and sirolimus
      - Vascular endothelial growth factor (VEGF) inhibitors
      - Tobacco use is associated with nephrotic-range proteinuria and nodular glomerulosclerosis
      - Drugs of abuse (e.g., heroin and cocaine) have been associated with significant proteinuria

Below are some of the key features of the different nephrotic syndromes or their associated conditions. Definitive diagnosis of most nephrotic syndromes can only be made with renal biopsy.

Key Feature(s) or Associated Symptom(s)	Diagnoses
Distended bladder, increased post-void residual	FSGS secondary to obstructive uropathy
Class III obesity	FSGS secondary to OSA and/or obesity
Sickle cell disease	FSGS secondary to sickle cell disease
Renal vein thrombosis	Membranous nephropathy
Weight loss, B symptoms (night sweats), malignancy	Membranous nephropathy secondary to lymphoma
Diabetic with diabetic retinopathy and/or neuropathy, poor glycemic control	Diabetic nephropathy
Malar rash, joint pains	Membranous nephropathy secondary to SLE
Macroglossia, bruising, neuropathy	Amyloidosis

CASE 8 | Focal Segmental Glomerulosclerosis (FSGS)

A 25-year-old man with HIV/AIDs, not taking medications, presents with a 12-pound weight gain and bilateral leg swelling over several months. He does not use any over-the-counter medications. He has no history of smoking, alcohol, or other drug use. Vital signs: temperature 37.2°C, pulse 74/min, blood pressure 160/90 mmHg, respiration 18/min, and SaO2 99% on room air. Exam is significant for 2+ lower extremity edema. His urine dipstick is positive for blood and has 3+ protein. His creatinine is elevated from his baseline.

Conditions with Similar Presentations	**Minimal Change Disease (MCD):** Also causes nephrotic-range proteinuria, but is more common in children and less likely to have hypertension, renal insufficiency, or microscopic hematuria. **Membranous and secondary nephrotic syndromes:** Can also present with nephrotic-range proteinuria, but have different histologic lesions and patient histories. See the mini-cases below for more details.
Initial Diagnostic Tests	Check urine protein (urine protein/creatinine ratio, urinalysis) and renal biopsy
Next Steps in Management	ACE-I/ARB, blood pressure and lipid control, low-salt diet
Discussion	Focal Segmental Glomerulosclerosis (FSGS) is a common cause of primary nephrotic syndrome in adults. It may be primary (idiopathic) or secondary to other conditions (e.g., HIV/AIDs, APOL1 gene, obesity, sickle cell disease, chronic obstructive uropathy, illicit drugs, or other medications [e.g., pamidronate, IVIG]). Pathologic lesions of FSGS under light microscopy show focal (some, but not all glomeruli) and segmental (part of, but not the entire glomerulus) sclerosis, and hyalinosis (scarring). **History:** • Often asymptomatic before experiencing leg swelling and weight gain. • Risk factors include obesity, HIV, and APOL1 gene. **Physical Exam:** Hypertension and peripheral edema **Diagnostics:** • Nephrotic-range proteinuria (>3.5 g/day) • Diagnose with renal biopsy showing FSGS. Electron microscopy shows effacement of foot processes similar to MCD **Management:** • As with other nephrotic syndromes, ACE-I/ARB, blood pressure control, lipid control, and diuretics if volume overload is present • Depending on severity, glucocorticoids or calcineurin inhibitors
Additional Considerations	**Complications:** FSGS often leads to ESRD

Nephrotic Syndrome Mini-Cases

Cases	Key Findings
Minimal change disease (MCD)	**Hx:** Frothy urine and leg swelling **PE:** Lower extremity edema, facial swelling with periorbital edema **Diagnostics:** • Renal biopsy shows no findings on light microscopy (thus the name) but electron microscopy shows effacement of foot processes **Management:** Glucocorticoids **Discussion:** • MCD is the major cause of nephrotic syndrome in children (90% of cases of nephrotic syndrome) but is less common in adults (10–25% of cases of nephrotic syndrome) • MCD is often idiopathic, but may be triggered by infection, hypersensitivity reactions, or lymphomas
Diabetic nephropathy	**Hx:** Long-standing history of diabetes, usually with diabetic retinopathy and/or neuropathy. **PE:** Lower extremity edema, facial swelling. **Diagnostics:** • Elevated urine albumin to creatinine ratio (>30 mg/g) with history of diabetes. • Often creatinine increased, indicative of CKD. • Consider ruling out other causes of albuminuria with labs/biopsy. **Management:** • ACE-I or ARB (blood pressure) and SGLT2 inhibitor (diabetes) both can decrease proteinuria and slow disease progression • Optimize glucose control • Diuretics if volume overload **Discussion:** • Hyperglycemia results in nonenzymatic glycation of kidney proteins, resulting in mesangial expansion, thickening of the glomerular basement membrane (GBM), and increased permeability of the glomerulus leading to nephrotic range proteinuria. • Initially presents with albuminuria, and if not aggressively treated, will progress to CKD frequently accompanied by proteinuria in the nephrotic range. • Classical nephrotic syndrome is not always present; proteinuria can range from significantly less to significantly >3.5 g/day. • Kidney biopsy (not necessary for diagnosis) shows mesangial expansion, GBM thickening, and—in more advanced cases—eosinophilic nodular glomerulosclerosis (Kimmelstiel-Wilson nodules).

Membranous nephropathy (MN)	**Hx:** Can present with edema, but typically asymptomatic unless presenting with complaints from sequelae such as renal vein thrombosis (i.e., back pain)
	PE: Normal but may reveal weight gain or edema (e.g., periorbital, bilateral lower extremities)
	Diagnostics:
	• Urine protein >3.5 g/day
	• Renal biopsy:
	  • Electron microscopy: "spike and dome" appearance (subepithelial immune deposits in GBM)
	  • Light microscopy: GBM thickening, little/no cellular infiltration/proliferation
	  • Immunofluorescence staining: diffuse granular GBM staining with IgG and C3
	• Primary MN: Positive anti-phospholipase A2 receptor (aPLA$_2$R) antibody titer in serum, or antigen staining on histology may be positive in many, but not all, cases of primary MN. Negative in secondary MN.
	Management:
	• ACE inhibitor or ARB, low-sodium diet, dyslipidemia treatment, anticoagulation depending on risk of bleed and albumin level <2–2.5 g/dL (thrombosis risk increases as albumin decreases), diuretics for significant edema.
	• Primary MN: If high risk for progression, may treat with rituximab or cyclophosphamide + glucocorticoids or calcineurin inhibitor + rituximab.
	• Secondary MN: Treat the cause, which can include malignancy, infections, SLE, and medications such as NSAIDS and penicillamine.

Nephrotic Syndrome Mini-Cases (*continued*)

Membranous nephropathy (MN)	**Discussion:**
	• MN is usually primary (idiopathic) but can be secondary to another cause.
	  • Primary MN: If left untreated, about 30% will go into complete remission, 30% will go into partial remission, and 30% will develop ESRD.
	  • Secondary MN: Identify and address underlying cause
	• Proteinuria can often be severe, and these patients are at high risk of thrombosis and progression to ESRD.

Amyloidosis	**Hx:** Nephrotic syndrome, renal insufficiency **PE:** Macroglossia, bruising, neuropathy **Diagnostics:** • Renal biopsy with amyloid deposits on Congo red staining with apple-green birefringence under polarized light • Electron microscopy shows extracellular fibrils 9–11 nm in diameter randomly arranged **Management:** • Depends on the cause; refer to oncology for management • In later stages with ESRD, the patient will need hemodialysis or kidney transplantation **Discussion:** • Amyloidosis is a collection of diseases caused by the deposition of beta-sheet fibrils in tissues. The beta-sheet fibrils are formed from abnormal proteins, either from a monoclonal protein (primary amyloid, amyloid light [AL] amyloid) or proteins produced by chronic inflammation (secondary amyloid), genetic mutations (hereditary amyloid producing transthyretin), or hemodialysis-related. These extracellular deposits lead to cellular damage and apoptosis. • Can manifest in kidneys as nephrotic syndrome and can affect other organs (heart failure, arrhythmias, hepatosplenomegaly, macroglossia, and pancytopenia)

HEMATURIA AND NEPHRITIC SYNDROME

- Microscopic hematuria: Presence of ≥3 RBCs/high-power field (hpf) on urinalysis.
- Hematuria can be classified as non-glomerular/extraglomerular (RBCs are smooth and biconcave, as they appear in plasma) or glomerular (dysmorphic RBCs or RBC casts on urine microscopy).
- RBCs from the glomerulus traverse the tubules, where they are exposed to variations in osmolality causing them to be dysmorphic or may be trapped in protein forming RBC casts, resulting in an "active" urinary sediment.
- The finding of glomerular hematuria suggests one of the numerous nephritic syndromes, which may also present with proteinuria (usually <3.5 g/day), hypertension, and/or renal failure.

Possible Causes of Non-Glomerular Hematuria

Etiology	Examples
Malignancy	• Renal cell carcinoma • Urothelial cancer • Prostate cancer • Wilms tumor
Infection	• Pyelonephritis • Cystitis • Urethritis • Prostatitis
Coagulation disorders	• Hemophilia • Thrombotic thrombocytopenic purpura
Obstruction	• Acute urinary retention • Benign prostatic hyperplasia
Trauma	• Urethral stricture • Recent urologic procedure
Medications	• Cyclophosphamide
Other	• Renal papillary necrosis • Hemolytic uremic syndrome

Key Features of Hematuria and Their Associated Diagnoses

Key Findings	Diagnoses
Back or flank pain radiating to groin, costovertebral angle tenderness	Nephrolithiasis, pyelonephritis, papillary necrosis (sickle cell crisis)
Suprapubic tenderness	UTI, urinary retention
Dysuria, irritative voiding symptoms (frequency, urgency, nocturia)	UTI, bladder stone
Pinpoint urethral meatus, dysuria, irritative voiding symptoms, split urinary stream	Urethral stricture
Lower abdominal pain, tobacco history, irritative voiding symptoms	Bladder cancer
Lower urinary tract symptoms (slow stream, frequency, nocturia, incomplete emptying)	Benign prostatic hyperplasia
Gross hematuria, acute anuria	Obstructive uropathy
Nodular and firm prostate on digital rectal exam	Prostate cancer
Hematuria occurring concurrently with respiratory infection (synpharyngitic hematuria)	IgA nephropathy
Skin rashes, joint pains	SLE, vasculitis, Henoch-Schonlein purpura (HSP)
Hemoptysis, epistaxis	Anti-GBM, ANCA-associated vasculitis
Bloody diarrhea	*Escherichia coli* Hemolytic uremic syndrome (HUS)
Fever, mental status changes, low platelets	Thrombotic thrombocytopenic purpura (TTP)
Post-pharyngitis	Post-streptococcal glomerulonephritis (PSGN)

Evaluation of Suspected Nephritic Syndrome

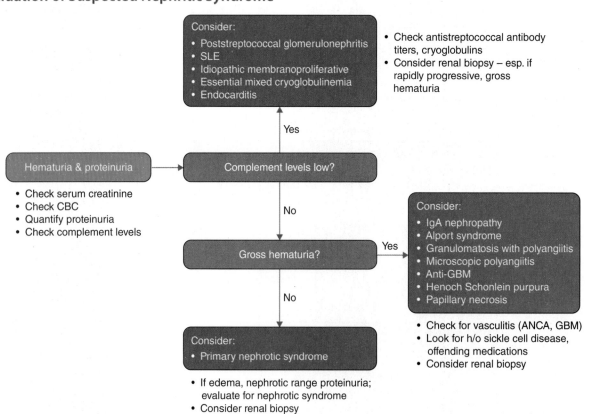

CASE 9 | Renal Papillary Necrosis

A 47-year-old man with sickle cell trait, HTN, and chronic back pain for which he is taking NSAIDS, presents for evaluation of bloody urine. Two days ago, he noted passing "clumps of blood" in his urine. He has no acute flank pain, dysuria, or increased frequency/urgency. He takes ibuprofen three times daily for the past 6 years for his chronic back pain. Labs show sodium 137 mEq/L, potassium 4.5 mEq/L, bicarbonate 24 mEq/L, BUN 36 mEq/L, Cr 1.6 mg/dL. UA shows grossly bloody urine with >50 RBCs/hpf, 15 WBCs/hpf, + +protein, no casts, negative nitrite, negative leukocyte esterase, normal serum complement levels.

Conditions with Similar Presentations	**Glomerulonephritis:** Also presents with proteinuria +/− elevated creatinine, and hematuria, but will have RBC casts and/or dysmorphic RBCs in the urine. **Chronic interstitial nephritis:** Can also occur with NSAID use but typically presents with pyuria (may see eosinophils) rather than hematuria. **Nephrolithiasis:** Can also present with microscopic or gross hematuria, but will have acute-onset severe, sharp, unilateral flank pain. **Pyelonephritis:** Can also present with microscopic or gross hematuria but will typically have dysuria, CVA tenderness, and fever.
Initial Diagnostic Tests	• Clinical diagnosis • UA to confirm presence of RBCs • Consider serum creatinine, urine culture, renal US or CT scan
Next Steps in Management	Discontinue offending agent (ibuprofen).
Discussion	Renal papillary necrosis is caused by ischemic damage to the renal papilla and inner portions of renal medulla from a variety of causes. Pathologically, it is characterized by coagulative necrosis of medullary pyramids and papillae caused by any condition that affects medullary perfusion. A number of conditions can lead to medullary ischemia. Most important of these are diabetes mellitus (nonenzymatic glycosylation of renal vasculature), sickle cell disease (sickled RBCs obstructing small renal vessels), chronic analgesic use such as NSAIDs (decreased prostaglandin synthesis resulting in vasoconstriction of afferent arteriole and renal hypoperfusion), renal transplant rejection, pyelonephritis, and urinary tract obstruction. **History:** • Hematuria; back pain in more severe cases • Risk factors are causes of renal ischemia including sickle cell disease/trait, pyelonephritis, chronic NSAID use, and diabetes mellitus **Physical Exam:** May have CVA tenderness **Diagnostics:** Diagnosis of exclusion • UA with hematuria, mild pyuria, and mild proteinuria. • Elevated creatinine may occur. • Imaging (ultrasound or CT without contrast) may show papillary necrosis. Renal ultrasound is an appropriate first step in evaluation of any hematuria. CT scan is required for definitive diagnosis of papillary necrosis and is helpful in ruling out renal stones or renal vein thrombosis. • Consider urine culture to rule out infection **Management:** Treat or avoid the underlying cause
Additional Considerations	**Complications:** Progression to CKD may occur if the underlying problem is not fixed

Nephritic Syndrome Mini-Cases

Cases	Key Findings
IgA nephropathy	**Hx:** • Typically male in 20s or 30s, but can present at any age • Episodic gross hematuria occurring after or concurrently with a respiratory or GI tract infection, a.k.a. "synpharyngitic hematuria" **PE:** May reveal hypertension, edema

Nephritic Syndrome Mini Cases (*continued*)

IgA nephropathy	**Diagnostics:**
	• UA with hematuria ± proteinuria
	• Elevated creatinine
	• Normal complement levels (C3, C4)
	• Definitive diagnosis is with renal biopsy:
	  • Light microscopy: mesangial proliferation, matrix expansion
	  • Electron microscopy: dense mesangial deposits
	  • Immunofluorescence: IgA deposits in mesangium
	
	Management:
	• ACE inhibitor (or ARB) with goal proteinuria <1 g/day
	• SGLT2 inhibitors
	• Glucocorticoids are indicated if proteinuria <1 g/d is not achieved after 6 months of ACEI (or ARB) therapy
	
	Discussion:
	• IgA nephropathy has identical renal findings to the renal complications of IgA vasculitis (Henoch-Schönlein purpura), which typically occurs in males <15 years old
	• Risk factors for progression to ESRD: HTN, worsening renal function, proteinuria >1 g/d
	• Key factors in distinguishing IgA nephropathy from other nephritic syndromes: Synpharyngitic hematuria, normal complement levels, and renal biopsy findings

Anti-GBM glomerulonephritis	**Hx:**
	• Typically presents with microscopic hematuria and pulmonary symptoms (classically hemoptysis but may be dyspnea or cough)
	• May have systemic signs (fever, weight loss, arthralgias)
	
	PE: May reveal hypertension, edema
	
	Diagnostics:
	• UA: hematuria, proteinuria
	• Positive anti-GBM antibody
	• Definitive diagnosis with renal biopsy
	  • Light microscopy: crescent moon shape (rapidly progressive glomerulonephritis)
	  • Immunofluorescence: linear deposits of IgG
	
	Management:
	• Immunosuppressive therapy: Glucocorticoids + cyclophosphamide
	• Plasmapheresis and/or dialysis may be necessary for patients with severe AKI
	
	Discussion:
	• The presentation of hematuria with concomitant hemoptysis (pulmonary-renal syndrome) is a clue to recognizing anti-GBM glomerulonephritis
	• Positive anti-GBM Ab blood test and linear deposits on immunofluorescence confirm the diagnosis and distinguish it from other causes of RPGN (granulomatosis with polyangiitis, microscopic polyangiitis, PSGN, DPGN)

Alport syndrome (hereditary nephropathy)	**Hx:** • Classic presentation is boy <10 years old with gross hematuria after recent upper respiratory infection • May have hearing loss and lens dislocation ("can't see, can't pee, can't hear a bee") • May have family history of renal failure or hearing loss (usually X-linked) • If undiagnosed in childhood will present with proteinuria, hypertension, and progressive renal dysfunction as adults **PE:** Exam may reveal hypertension, bilateral sensorineural hearing loss, and bilateral white retinal granulations (fleck retinopathy).

Nephritic Syndrome Mini Cases (*continued*)

Alport syndrome (hereditary nephropathy)	**Diagnostics:** • UA revealing hematuria, proteinuria • Elevated creatinine • Normal complement levels (C3 and C4) • Definitive diagnosis with renal biopsy: • Electron microscopy reveals "basket weave" or "lamellar" GBM due to longitudinal splitting **Management:** • Supportive care with ACE inhibitor or ARB to slow disease progression • Consider dialysis or kidney transplant in patients who develop ESRD **Discussion:** • Hypertension, elevated creatinine, and gross hematuria may be absent in early childhood but will develop with time • Key clues to recognizing Alport syndrome include patient's age and sex, family history, and sequential nature of URI followed by hematuria

Lupus nephritis	**Hx:**
	• Typical patient is a female with previously diagnosed SLE or clinical features suggestive of SLE (fever, fatigue, weight loss, arthralgias, rash, pericarditis, pleuritis) presenting with proteinuria, microscopic hematuria, and/or elevated serum creatinine
	
	PE: May reveal hypertension, edema
	
	Diagnostics:
	• UA with hematuria, proteinuria
	• Elevated creatinine
	• Low complement levels (C3 and C4)
	• Double-stranded DNA (dsDNA) antibodies and/or anti-Smith antibodies (both more specific for SLE than ANA and a marker of disease/glomerulonephritis activity)
	• Definitive diagnosis: Renal biopsy, which reveals evidence of focal or diffuse immune-complex glomerulonephritis (classified into LN class I–VI based on disease severity on histopathology):
	  • Light microscopy: wire loop deposits of capillaries
	  • Immunofluorescence: "full house" appearance, meaning IgG, IgM, IgA, C3, and C1q deposits
	  • Electron microscopy: deposits are seen in mesangial, subendothelial, and subepithelial locations
	
	Management:
	• Immunosuppressive therapy: Glucocorticoids + mycophenolate mofetil or cyclophosphamide
	• Dialysis or kidney transplant in patients who develop ESRD
	
	Discussion:
	• Key clues include AKI in a patient with existing SLE and new onset proteinuria and/or hematuria
	• Renal biopsy is required for diagnosis and is notable for its "full house" appearance on immunofixation.

NEPHROLITHIASIS

The hallmark symptoms of nephrolithiasis (kidney stones) are acute flank pain and hematuria. It is important to understand the different conditions associated with flank pain and how they may present.

Etiologies of Flank Pain

Key Findings	Diagnoses
Acute onset, unilateral, colicky pain radiating to groin, unable to get comfortable or relieve pain, hematuria	Nephrolithiasis
Fever, chills, dysuria, costovertebral angle tenderness (CVAT)	Pyelonephritis; infected nephrolithiasis
Missed menses	Ectopic pregnancy
Associated with shortness of breath or cough	Consider pulmonary causes
Associated with specific movements, reproducible tenderness	Consider musculoskeletal causes
Changes in bowel habits	Consider GI cause
Burning, shooting, and tingling unilateral pain, rash	Shingles (varicella Zoster virus)

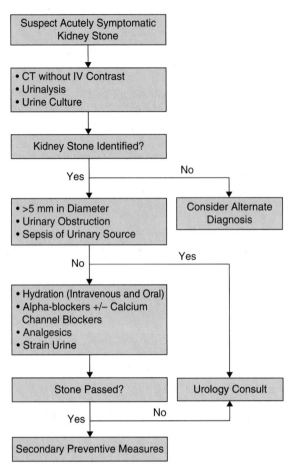

Approach to flank pain suspicious for kidney stone. (Reproduced, with permission, from McKean SC, Ross JJ, Dressler DD, Scheurer DB. Principles and Practice of Hospital Medicine. 2nd ed. New York, NY: McGraw Hill; 2017.)

Characteristics of Different Kidney Stone Types

Stone Type	Causes	Radiopaque	pH	Crystal	Treatment
Calcium oxalate	Hypercalciuria Hypocitraturia Ethylene glycol Vitamin C excess Malabsorption	Y	Not pH dependent	Envelope	Thiazides; citrate; low-sodium, normal calcium diet
Calcium phosphate	Hypercalciuria Elevated urine pH	Y	>6.5		Low-sodium diet, thiazides
Struvite magnesium, ammonium, phosphate ("triple phosphate")	Urease (+) bacteria such as *Proteus, Staph saprophyticus,* or *Klebsiella* produce ammonia, increasing urine pH	Y Staghorn caliculi	>6.5	Wedge	Antibiotics to treat infection, lithotripsy or surgery for stone
Uric acid	Dry climates Acidic urine pH Gout Tumor lysis syndrome	No	<5.5	"Coffin lids"	Alkalinize urine, allopurinol
Cystine	Cystinuria (hereditary, autosomal recessive)	Y (faint)	<5.5	Hexagon	Alkalinize urine (potassium citrate or acetazolamide) and chelators (penicillamines)

CASE 10	Nephrolithiasis
A 34-year-old woman presents with sudden onset of sharp, severe right flank pain with radiation to the groin. She has associated nausea and vomiting, but has no dysuria, hematuria, or fevers/chills. She has never had this pain before and has tried acetaminophen with no improvement. Her father has a history of recurrent kidney stones. On exam, she is in moderate distress, changing body position frequently. Temperature is 37.5°C, pulse 108/min, with mild costovertebral angle tenderness on the right. Her abdomen is non-distended with mild tenderness to palpation in the right mid-lower quadrant. She has no spinal tenderness, straight leg raise test is negative, and her genitourinary exam is unremarkable.	
Conditions with Similar Presentations	**Appendicitis:** May also present with abdominal pain and nausea/vomiting but pain is not in flank and begins periumbilical and migrates to RLQ. Physical exam may have rebound tenderness **Pyelonephritis:** May also present with flank pain and CVA tenderness but will have infectious symptoms of fever and dysuria **Bladder cancer:** Presents as painless gross hematuria with smoking as a major risk factor **Ectopic pregnancy and other pelvic pathology:** Should be considered in females with flank and pelvic pain/tenderness. **Ovarian torsion** should be suspected in females with sudden-onset severe, unilateral lower abdominal pain.
Initial Diagnostic Tests	• Check urinalysis, non-contrast CT abdomen/pelvis. • Also check urine pregnancy test.
Next Steps in Management	IV hydration, pain control.
Discussion	Kidney stones are formed in the urine when stone-forming constituents (calcium, oxalate, uric acid or cystine) reach a concentration above their solubility. **History:** • "Renal colic" = severe flank pain radiating to groin • May include gross hematuria, nausea/vomiting • Risk factors: Hypercalciuria, Crohn's, UTI, gout, and hereditary cystinuria (see table) **Physical Exam:** • CVA or flank tenderness, unable to sit still due to intense pain **Diagnostics:** • UA may show microscopic hematuria (RBCs). Presence of WBCs, leukocyte esterase, and bacteria would raise likelihood of struvite stones • Non-contrast CT abdomen/pelvis will show stone location and size **Management:** • IV fluids • Pain medications: NSAIDs, opioids • Up to 4 weeks of "medical expulsive therapies": 　• Alpha-blockers (tamsulosin, terazosin) to relax ureteral smooth muscle to promote stone passage 　• Calcium channel blockers to relax ureteral smooth muscle to promote stone passage • Antiemetics (metoclopramide, ondansetron) **Complications:** Nephrolithiasis with pyelonephritis and hydronephrosis may warrant antibiotics and urologic intervention to relieve obstruction. **Surgical Considerations:** Stones initially >10 mm, or >5 mm that do not pass after 4 weeks of medical therapy, warrant urologic intervention. **Inpatient Considerations:** Patients with uncontrollable pain, fever, or can't take oral fluids may need to be hospitalized. **Considerations during pregnancy:** Preferred imaging is renal and pelvic ultrasound rather than the non-contrast CT abdomen/pelvis.

ELECTROLYTE DISTURBANCES

Electrolyte disturbances can cause significant physiological disturbances and symptoms across many body systems. Changes to electrolyte levels are commonly caused by loss of body fluids, acute or chronic illness, medications, and kidney disease. The kidney plays a major role in the excretion and/or reabsorption of almost every electrolyte.

Electrolyte Abnormality	Key Findings
Hyponatremia	Confusion, lethargy, seizures
Hypokalemia	Can be seen with use of diuretic medications. Also, with hyperglycemic states (DKA, HHS); though may present with initial hyperkalemia Can cause ileus, bladder dysfunction, hypoventilation ECG: U wave (very specific), prolonged PR, depressed ST
Hyperkalemia	Metabolic acidosis ECG: Peaked T waves, QRS widening, sine wave
Hypercalcemia	"Moans, stones, groans," abdominal pain, constipation, decreased appetite, nausea, vomiting, peptic ulcer disease, bone pain
Hyperphosphatemia	Conjunctival icterus, skin pruritus, calciphylaxis
Hyper- and hypokalemia Hypophosphatemia	Paralysis, weakness, paresthesia, arrhythmias
Hyperkalemia Hyper- and hypophosphatemia	Rhabdomyolysis, muscle pain
Hypocalcemia Hypomagnesemia	Tetany
Hypocalcemia Hypomagnesemia Hypokalemia	ECG: Torsade de pointes

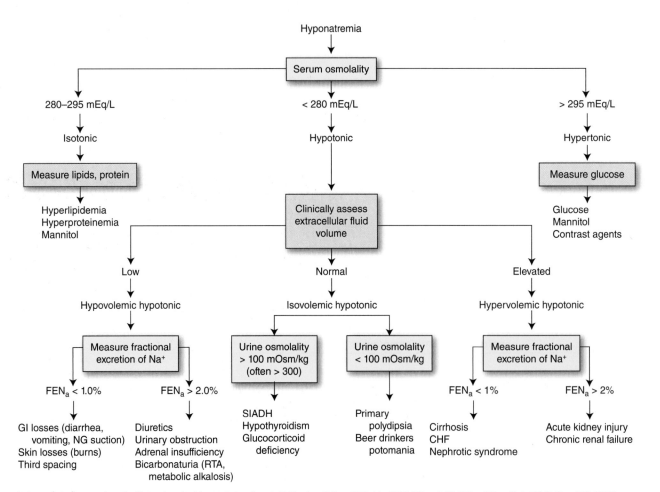

Approach to hyponatremia. (Reproduced, with permission, from Le T, Bhushan V. First Aid for the USMLE Step 2 CK. 10th ed. New York, NY: McGraw Hill; 2019.)

CASE 11 | Hypovolemic Hyponatremia

A 25-year-old man with no past medical history presents to the ED with 5 days of nausea, vomiting, and diarrhea. He is not able to keep anything down and feels lightheaded. On exam, he appears uncomfortable and his orthostatic vitals are as follows: supine blood pressure 110/70 mmHg and pulse is 104/min; standing blood pressure is: 86/58 mmHg and pulse is 118/min. His labs are notable for serum osmolality 262, serum Na 129 mEq/L, BUN 36, creatinine 1.6, FeNa <1%, urine Na <10.

Conditions with Similar Presentations	**Euvolemic hyponatremia:** Also presents as hypotonic hyponatremia, but patients will not have findings of volume depletion (causes include SIADH and hypothyroidism).
	Hypertonic hyponatremia: Also presents as hyponatremia, but with elevated serum osmolality (>295) and is due to the presence of osmotic substances (glucose, mannitol) that increase plasma osmolality and plasma water leading to dilution of Na concentration.
	Hypervolemic Hyponatremia: Also presents as hypotonic hyponatremia, but patients will have evidence of increased body water (edema, ascites) due to decreased oncotic pressure due to hypoalbuminemia (cirrhosis or nephrosis) or increased hydrostatic pressure (heart failure).
Initial Diagnostic Tests	• Assess volume status • Check serum osmolality, serum sodium, and serum creatinine • Check urine osmolality, urine sodium, and urine creatinine
Next Steps in Management	Volume resuscitation with normal saline.
Discussion	Patients with hyponatremia (Na <135 mEq/L) have too much free water in relation to sodium. • Mild hyponatremia: 120–130 mEq/L • Moderate hyponatremia: 110–120 mEq/L • Severe hyponatremia: <110 mEq/L Hypovolemic hyponatremia can be further classified by urine sodium level. • Low urine sodium (FeNa <1.0%) is consistent with loss of total body Na in vomiting, diarrhea, and third spacing. • High urine sodium (FeNa >2.0%) is associated with diuretic use or adrenal/mineralocorticoid insufficiency. **History:** May have a history of gastrointestinal illness, diuretic use, poor PO intake, shifting of fluid into interstitium (third-spacing) (i.e., burns or ascites). **Physical Exam:** May have evidence of dehydration and diminished circulating volume (e.g., hypotension, tachycardia, dry mucous membranes, decreased capillary refill, orthostatic vitals) **Diagnostics:** • Serum Na <135 mEq/L • Low plasma osmolality (<280 mEq/L) to confirm hypotonic hyponatremia; if plasma osmolality is higher, rule out confounding factors such as hyperglycemia, hyperlipidemia, hyperproteinemia. • Assess volume status and classify as hypovolemic, euvolemic, or hypervolemic. • Use urine osmolality or FeNa to help narrow etiologies (see algorithm above). For hypovolemic hyponatremia, FeNa <1.0% indicates extrarenal salt loss (due to GI losses in this patient) and FeNa >2.0% indicates renal salt loss (diuretics, adrenal insufficiency). **Management:** • Rate of Na+ correction should not exceed 6–8 mEq/L in the first 24 hours. • For hypovolemic hyponatremia administer isotonic fluids for intravascular fluid resuscitation. • If significant neurologic symptoms (confusion, obtundation, seizure, coma) from hyponatremia, give 3% hypertonic saline to rapidly increase the serum sodium by 4–6 mEq, which will decrease brain swelling and improve symptoms.
Additional Considerations	**Complications:** **Central pontine myelinolysis:** Overcorrection of hyponatremia can cause demyelination of the pons which can cause "locked-in syndrome" (alert but quadriplegic, mute, but retain blinking and vertical eye movements).

CASE 12 | Nephrogenic Diabetes Insipidus (DI)

A 50-year-old man with bipolar disorder and hyperlipidemia was admitted for an elective cholecystectomy. His only medications are lithium for >10 years and atorvastatin for 5 years. He was made NPO (nothing by mouth) but the surgery got delayed for several hours due to another emergent case. He now has increased thirst but frequent urination. On exam, he is afebrile, has dry mucous membranes, pulse 105/min, and blood pressure 95/52 mmHg.

His urine output in a 24-hour period is 3.5 L and his labs are Na 157 mEq/L, serum osmolality 327 mOsm/kg, urine osmolality 122 mOsm/kg, and urine specific gravity: 1.007. Serum glucose is normal.

Conditions with Similar Presentations	**Central DI:** Also presents with hypernatremia, polydipsia, and polyuria with serum osmolality > urine osmolality. Suspect in patients with head trauma, brain tumor, or post neurosurgery. Unlike nephrogenic DI, a desmopressin challenge will result in increased urine osmolarity and decreased urine output.
	Osmotic diuresis: Can also present with polydipsia, and polyuria, but usually also with hyperglycemia from diabetes mellitus. Classified as a urine osmolality >600 mOsm/kg.
	Primary polydipsia: Presents with polydipsia in patients with psychiatric illness, but will cause euvolemic hyponatremia (not hypernatremia).
Initial Diagnostic Tests	• Check plasma and urine osmolality • Desmopressin challenge to differentiate nephrogenic and central DI after free water repleted. • Consider: Brain MRI
Next Steps in Management	• Low salt and low protein diet to decrease urine output. • Diuretic therapy with thiazide or amiloride.

Discussion	Nephrogenic DI occurs due to resistance to ADH at the renal collecting duct resulting in reduction of urine concentrating capacity. ADH secretion is increased in response to hypernatremia but the kidney does not respond by increasing water reabsorption. Causes include intrinsic renal disease (bilateral obstruction, sickle cell nephropathy, amyloidosis), medications, and genetic causes.
	• Genetic mutations are the most common cause of nephrogenic DI in children
	• Chronic lithium use and hypercalcemia are the most common causes in adults
	• Lithium prevents ADH from inserting aquaporin channels on the luminal side of the collecting tubule, which results in an aquaresis and low urine osmolality. Renal concentrating ability should improve with discontinuation of lithium, but chronic use can result in irreversible damage
	History:
	• Polyuria, polydipsia, and nocturia. Urine will appear colorless due to dilution
	• Risk factors include family history, lithium use, hypercalcemia, CKD
	Physical Exam: Evidence of dehydration and diminished circulating volume including orthostasis, hypotension, tachycardia, and dry mucous membranes may be present
	Diagnostics:
	• **Urine:** Low osmolality with low specific gravity.
	• **Serum:** Increased osmolality (280–310 mOsm/kg); mild hypernatremia may occur.
	• **Water restriction test:**
	  • Differentiates primary polydipsia and diabetes insipidus
	  • If urine osmolality increases above 280 mOsm/kg with water restriction, primary polydipsia is likely
	• **Desmopressin challenge:**
	  • Differentiates nephrogenic and central DI
	  • Nephrogenic DI: can be confirmed with negative response to water restriction and desmopressin challenge.
	  • Central DI: negative response to water restriction and positive (increase) response to urine osmolality to desmopressin administration
	Management:
	Acute treatment:
	• Stop any causative medications (e.g., lithium).
	• Correct any causative electrolyte abnormalities (hypercalcemia, hypokalemia).
	• If orthostatic or hypotensive, fluid resuscitation with hypotonic fluid with 5% dextrose or one-quarter isotonic saline (D5W, ¼ NS). Solutions with higher osmolality run the risk of worsening hypernatremia.
	Chronic treatment:
	• Low-protein diet, sodium restriction, and thiazide diuretics to decrease polyuria (by upregulating aquaporin channels and ENaC channels in the collecting tubules, effectively counteracting the effects of lithium).
	• If insufficient improvement in polyuria or patients continuing lithium therapy, consider adding amiloride for further reduction in urine output. Amiloride can prevent progression of lithium-induced DI and may have a role in improving existing resistance.
	• Sodium restriction results in increased sodium reabsorption at the proximal tubules and less sodium reabsorption at the distal tubules, facilitating water retention.

CASE 12 | Nephrogenic Diabetes Insipidus (DI) *(continued)*

Additional Considerations	**Inpatient Considerations:** Patients with nephrogenic DI should be allowed to drink freely. If patients are NPO, urine output should be matched with 5% dextrose or one-quarter isotonic saline.
	Complications: Lithium-induced DI: Lithium has a narrow therapeutic index so changes in renal function or certain medications can alter the plasma lithium level and cause toxicity. Plasma lithium levels should be monitored frequently and adjusted as needed to maintain a therapeutic level.

Sodium and Water Imbalance Mini-Cases

Cases	Key Findings
Hypernatremia	**Hx:** • Fluid loss through bowel, urine, or skin and without access or ability to ingest water to replace the losses • Presents with increased thirst and, if severe enough, neurologic symptoms: altered mental status, weakness, focal neurologic deficits, confusion, seizures • Patients who are critically ill and/or altered develop hypernatremia if they are not given free water **PE:** Nonspecific; focal neurologic deficits may be seen on exam **Diagnostics:** • Sodium >145 mEq/L • Check urine osmolality (high in extrarenal loss and lower in DI) • If DI is suspected, water deprivation followed by desmopressin administration can help distinguish central vs. nephrogenic causes of DI (see renal case on nephrogenic DI for further details) **Management:** • Correction of hypernatremia, particularly chronic hypernatremia, must be gradual (10 mEq or less in 24 hours) • Rapid correction may result in fluid shifts causing cerebral edema • Treatment is determined by volume status, and the free water deficit must be calculated to determine fluid replacement *Hypovolemic hypernatremia:* Correct hypernatremia once patient is hemodynamically stable by determining the free water deficit: $$\text{Free Water Deficit} = \text{Total Body Water} \times \left(\left[\frac{serum\ Na}{140} \right] - 1 \right)$$ Total Body Water ~ 60% of lean body weight. Replace water deficit with D5W, 0.45% saline, or enteral water. *Euvolemic/hypervolemic hypernatremia:* Treat with water/D5W +/− diuretics to restore sodium-water balance. See nephrogenic DI case for further details. **Discussion:** Hypernatremia is due to excess loss of water or excess retention of sodium. • Excess loss of water is either extrarenal (bowel, skin) or renal (DI, diuretics). • Excess retention of sodium is due to ingestion or administration of high-sodium IV fluids or high mineralocorticoid states (hyperaldosteronism, hypercortisolism).

Central DI	**Hx:** Polydipsia, polyuria.
	PE: Unremarkable.
	Diagnostics:
	• Hypernatremia.
	• Serum osmolality > urine osmolality.
	• Because it is a result of impaired ADH secretion:
	  • Water restriction test: negative, continued low urine osmolality
	  • Desmopressin challenge: ↑urine osmolality and ↓urine output
	• Brain imaging to assess disease of the hypothalamus and/or pituitary should be performed
	Management: Desmopressin
	Discussion: Central DI is either idiopathic or from head trauma, neurosurgery, stroke, or brain tumor.

CASE 13 | Hyperkalemia

A 62-year-old woman with hypertension, diabetes mellitus, and advanced CKD presents for a follow-up blood pressure check after her lisinopril was increased from 10 mg to 40 mg daily. She has no concerns and her other medications include amlodipine 10 mg daily and insulin. On exam, her blood pressure is 122/76 mmHg, pulse is 80/min, and she has 1+ pedal edema. Labs show potassium 6.7 mEq/L (previously 4.8 mEq/L), eGFR 32 mL/min/1.71 m² (at baseline), bicarbonate 24 mEq/L, and glucose 133 mg/dL. Serum osmolality is 277 mOsm/kg and an ECG shows peaked T waves.

Conditions with Similar Presentations	**Rhabdomyolysis:** Can also cause hyperkalemia but usually presents with muscle pain and/or weakness and dark urine (from myoglobinuria). **Hypoaldosteronism:** Also causes hyperkalemia but presents with hyponatremia and hypotension if associated adrenal insufficiency. **Diabetic ketoacidosis (DKA):** Can cause hyperkalemia but would expect symptoms (abdominal pain/nausea, polyuria, polydipsia), elevated glucose, increased serum osmolality, and low serum bicarbonate due to acidosis.
Initial Diagnostic Tests	Check potassium level, BMP, and ECG for peaked T waves, short QT, long PR, QRS widening.
Next Steps in Management	• IV calcium gluconate • Shift potassium into cells: Insulin/glucose, albuterol, bicarbonate • Remove excess potassium from the body (e.g., loop diuretic, potassium binders or dialysis)

Discussion	Hyperkalemia is defined as K+ >5.0 mEq/L. Severe hyperkalemia is defined as K+ >6.5 mEq/L or ECG changes (peaked T waves, short QT, long PR, QRS widening) and can cause fatal arrhythmias and cardiac arrest. The etiology of hyperkalemia is from any of the following processes:
	1. Decreased potassium excretion
	  a. Renal disease with GFR <15 mL/min
	  b. Hypoaldosteronism (primary or due to type IV renal tubular acidosis or due to medications (spironolactone, triamterene, eplerenone) or inhibition of angiotensin II production or binding (ACEi or ARB).
	2. Potassium shift from intracellular to extracellular
	  a. Cell lysis (trauma, rhabdomyolysis, cytotoxic chemotherapy, hypothermia)
	  b. Metabolic acidosis
	  c. Insulin deficiency
	  d. Hyperosmolality
	  e. Beta-2 antagonism
	  f. Genetic defect (hyperkalemic periodic paralysis)
	3. Increased potassium load
	  a. IV administration (K solutions, lysed RBC transfusion, high-dose potassium penicillin)
	  b. Usually only seen with associated renal failure or in infants
	
	History:
	• May be asymptomatic or present with nausea, vomiting, or palpitations
	• Muscle weakness or paralysis at high levels (>7.0 mEq/L)
	• Risk factors: Medications that inhibit RAAS, metabolic acidosis, renal failure, and low aldosterone states
	• Ask about common medications that contribute to hyperkalemia: ACEi, ARBs, potassium-sparing diuretics, digoxin, beta blockers
	
	Physical Exam: Absent or diminished deep tendon reflexes, arrhythmias, and paresthesias
	
	Diagnostics:
	• ↑ Serum K+ level
	• Serum bicarbonate; serum creatinine and GFR to assess renal function
	• ECG changes may include peaked T waves, low amplitude p waves, prolonged PR interval, and widening QRS interval
	
	Management: Treatment depends on the degree of hyperkalemia, presence of cardiac changes, and underlying etiology. ECG changes can occur at any level of elevated potassium and are more often seen with acute change of K+ >6.0 mE/L
	• If ECG changes:
	  • Give IV calcium gluconate immediately
	    • Only a temporizing measure to stabilize the cardiac cell membranes
	  • Shift potassium intracellularly using insulin (w/ glucose), beta agonists (albuterol), and sodium bicarbonate

CASE 13 | Hyperkalemia (continued)

Discussion	• To definitively treat hyperkalemia, need to eliminate potassium from the body
	  • GI tract: cation exchangers (sodium zirconium cyclosilicate, patiromer, or sodium polystyrene sulfonate [Kayexalate])
	  • Kidneys: loop diuretics such as furosemide
	• Refractory hyperkalemia (not responsive to medical management) requires hemodialysis.
	Helpful mnemonic for steps in management: **C BIG K**
	Calcium chloride or gluconate, **B**icarbonate, **β**2-agonists, **I**nsulin + **G**lucose, **K**ayexalate.

Additional Considerations	**Spurious Hyperkalemia:** Due to cell lysis during or after venipuncture. If suspected, obtain a repeat K+ level because hyperkalemia can be due to spurious causes including a hemolyzed specimen or tight/prolonged tourniquet use. **Special Considerations:** DKA often presents with hyperkalemia but total-body hypokalemia. Decreased insulin and acidemia results in potassium shifting extracellularly and potassium is lost in urine due to osmotic diuresis. As a result, patients have elevated serum K+ levels but decreased total body K+ stores. Management of DKA includes K+ repletion once K+ returns to normal throughout initial treatment, as K+ is shifted intracellularly when insulin is administered.

ACID-BASE DISORDERS

Acid-base disorders are divided into four categories: **metabolic acidosis, metabolic alkalosis, respiratory acidosis, and respiratory alkalosis.**

Key components of diagnosis include clinical history, arterial or venous blood gas for pH and PCO_2, BMP for serum HCO_3^- and calculation of anion gap ($Na^+ - [Cl^- + HCO_3^-]$), and identification of any compensatory mechanisms.

- The primary cause of acidosis or alkalosis is determined by looking at the serum HCO_3^- and blood gas PCO_2 in relation to pH.
- Metabolic processes are driven by changes in serum HCO_3^-, while respiratory processes are driven by changes in PCO_2.
- When a metabolic acidosis is identified, the anion gap must be calculated to help identify the cause of acidosis.
- Multiple acid-base derangements may be present if there is more than one primary disorder
- When working properly, the renal or respiratory system can help compensate for the underlying primary disorder.

The following figure outlines a helpful diagnostic approach to acid-base disorders as well as common etiologies.

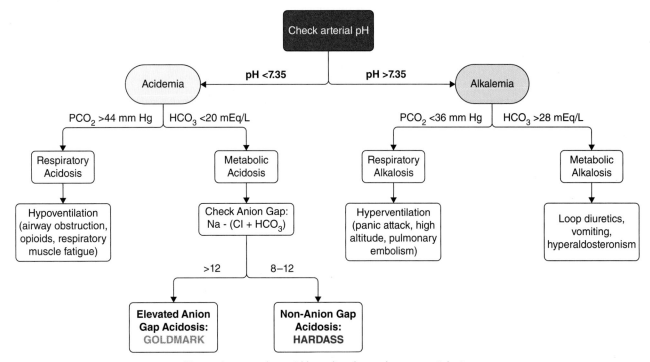

Diagnostic approach to acid-base disorders and common etiologies.

Helpful mnemonics:

- **GOLD MARK (elevated anion gap acidosis)**
  - Glycols (ethylene and propylene), Oxoproline, L-lactate, D-lactate, Methanol, Aspirin, Renal failure (uremia), Ketoacidosis
- **HARDASS (non-anion gap acidosis)**
  - Hyperalimentation, Addison disease, Renal tubular acidosis, Diarrhea, Acetazolamide, Spironolactone, Saline infusion

Compensation in Acid-Base Disorders

When the body undergoes a primary acid-base disturbance, it will try to normalize the body's pH via compensatory mechanisms. Compensation occurs in the respiratory system via alterations in respiratory rate and in the renal system via regulation of acid excretion in the urine. Respiratory compensation occurs immediately, whereas renal compensation requires a few days to take effect. Compensation can produce a near-normal pH, but if the pH is completely normal, there are two primary processes.

1. Respiratory compensation: Hyperventilation decreases PCO_2 in response to metabolic acidosis *or* hypoventilation increases PCO_2 in response to metabolic alkalosis.
2. Metabolic compensation: Increased H^+ excretion in the urine in response to respiratory acidosis *or* H^+ retention in response to respiratory alkalosis.

Renal Tubular Acidosis (RTA)

RTA causes a normal anion gap metabolic acidosis (NAGMA) and can be divided into three subtypes: distal (type 1), proximal (type 2), and hyperkalemic (type 4).

- **Type 1 (Distal) RTA** is the result of impaired acid excretion in the distal tubule and can occur in the setting of certain medications (amphotericin B, lithium), hypercalciuria, or autoimmune diseases.
- **Type 2 (Proximal) RTA** is the result of impaired bicarbonate reabsorption in the proximal tubule and can occur as a primary disorder or secondary to medications or diseases (e.g., carbonic anhydrase inhibitor, multiple myeloma, Fanconi syndrome).
- **Type 4 (Hyperkalemic) RTA** occurs as the result of aldosterone resistance or deficiency in the distal tubule. This lack of aldosterone causes impairment of hydrogen and potassium excretion, resulting in acidosis and hyperkalemia. There is an impaired but not absent ability to eliminate acid in the urine, so urine pH is typically <5.5. This can occur in diabetic kidney disease, sickle cell disease, NSAIDs, and drugs that block/inhibit the effects of aldosterone (e.g., ACEI/ARBs, mineralocorticoid receptor antagonists, amiloride).

The subtypes of RTA are identified by examining serum K^+, urinary pH, and clinical history. The following table outlines the three subtypes of RTA.

	Cause	Serum Potassium	Urine pH	Management	Associated Conditions
Type 1 Distal	Impaired H+ secretion	↓	>5.5	Bicarbonate supplementation	Autoimmune conditions, amphotericin B, ifosfamide, hypercalciuria
Type 2 Proximal	Impaired HCO₃⁻ reabsorption	↓	Variable	Treat underlying cause, electrolyte repletion as needed	Fanconi syndrome, rickets, osteomalacia, multiple myeloma
Type 4	Aldosterone deficiency or resistance	↑	Variable Usually <5.5	Mineralocorticoid and bicarbonate replacement, diuretics as indicated	Hypoaldosteronism, CKD, diabetes, sickle cell, NSAIDs, ACEIs/ARBS, urinary tract obstruction, heparin

History/Physical Exam

RTA presentation can be variable given the above-associated conditions and causes. It is important to note medications (amphotericin, antiepileptics, lithium, carbonic anhydrase inhibitors), current and past medical history, risk factors (e.g., autoimmune disease, amyloidosis, diabetes, sickle cell disease, or multiple myeloma) and exam findings.

Diagnostics

Steps to determining presence of an RTA:

1. Low bicarbonate indicating present of a metabolic acidosis.

2. Confirm non-anion gap metabolic acidosis (NAGMA): Calculate anion gap (AG): $Na - (Cl + HCO_3)$, normal between 8–12.

3. If no AG, then calculate urinary anion gap (UAG) to determine if acidosis is due to renal or gastrointestinal cause. UAG= Urine Na + Urine K – Urine Cl. A positive UAG (>10) suggests a renal cause.

   - Gastrointestinal cause (diarrhea): UAG is ne-GUT-ive

   - Renal cause: UAG is positive

4. Check urinary pH to help distinguish between the different types of RTA

   - Distal RTA urine pH persistently >5.5

   - Proximal RTA urine pH is initially high but the distal tubule can compensate by increasing H+ secretion and urine pH then drops to <5.5

Management

- If caused by medication, discontinue the offending agent.

- For all RTAs, correction of acidosis with alkali agents (sodium bicarbonate) can be beneficial and decrease long-term complications.

CASE 14	Anion Gap Metabolic Acidosis: Lactic Acidosis

A 63-year-old man with chronic myeloid leukemia (CML) currently on chemotherapy is admitted to the intensive care unit (ICU) for management of fever and hypotension due to community-acquired pneumonia. Temperature is 101.6°F. Blood cultures are collected, and he is started on empiric antibiotics. His blood pressure drops to 80/50, and he is started on two vasopressors.

Labs are significant for a sodium of 142, potassium 3.3, chloride of 96, bicarbonate of 16. Anion gap is 30. Creatinine is 1.89, which is increased from the patient's baseline of 0.95. Lactate is 5.7. An ABG shows a pH of 7.26, pCO_2 of 34, and pO_2 of 92.

Conditions with Similar Presentations	**Diabetic ketoacidosis:** Also presents as an anion gap metabolic acidosis but is due to elevated serum beta-hydroxybutyrate and usually presents with polyuria and polydipsia.
	Uremia: Also presents as an anion gap metabolic acidosis but with significantly elevated creatine much greater than this patient.
	Other causes of anion gap acidosis: Are due to ingestion of substances that can often be determined or suspected by history, including methanol, propylene glycol, iron, INH, ethanol, ethylene glycol, and salicylates.
Initial Diagnostic Tests	To confirm anion gap metabolic acidosis from lactic acidosis check: • Basic metabolic panel and calculate anion gap • Serum lactate level and ABG
Next Steps in Management	• Fluid resuscitation and blood pressure support • Treat the underlying cause of the lactic acidosis
Discussion	Lactate is a marker of the adequacy of tissue perfusion and oxygenation. Normal plasma lactate concentration is 0.5–1.5 mmol/L. Elevation of plasma lactate (lactic acidosis) occurs when blood supply to tissues is impaired, such as in conditions leading to shock (hypovolemia, myocardial infarction, sepsis). Lactic acidosis is the most common cause of an elevated anion gap metabolic acidosis in hospitalized patients. Sepsis causes widespread systemic vasodilation which leads to tissue hypoperfusion. When there is not enough oxygen present, tissues are forced to use anaerobic metabolism instead of aerobic metabolism with resultant conversion of pyruvate to lactate.

CASE 14 | Anion Gap Metabolic Acidosis from Lactic Acidosis (continued)

Discussion	**History:** Symptoms suggestive of causes for hypovolemia (fluid losses, hemorrhage), sepsis (site-specific signs of infection), or myocardial infarction (chest pain).
	Physical Exam: Hypotension, reduced urine output, altered mental status.
	Diagnostics:
• BMP to calculate anion gap (normal 8–12 mEq/L). AG = Sodium – (Chloride + Bicarbonate)
• ↑Serum lactate level
• ABG to assess degree of acidosis
	Management:
• Treat underlying cause (i.e., infection, hypovolemia, MI).
• Fluid resuscitation will increase organ perfusion and oxygenation, while antimicrobials must be given to septic patients to treat the source of infection.
• Lactate is not effectively cleared with dialysis, but hemodialysis may be indicated to correct a severe acidosis.

CASE 15 | Non-Anion Gap Metabolic Acidosis (NAGMA): Proximal Type 2 RTA (Fanconi Syndrome)

A 29-year-old man with a history of seizures presents for routine follow-up. His seizures have been well controlled with valproic acid for the past 5 years. He has no other concerns. On physical examination, temperature is 37.4, blood pressure 120/74 mmHg, pulse 74/min, and respirations 14/min. BMI is 24 and the rest of the examination is normal. Labs include sodium 134 mEq/L, chloride 105 mEq/L, bicarbonate 21 mEq/L, potassium 2.7 mEq/L, creatinine 1.2 mg/dL, glucose 98 mg/dL, and phosphate 1.8 mg/dL. Venous blood gas shows pH 7.32, PCO_2 42. UA demonstrates urine pH 5.1, +1 protein, +2 glucose, no RBCs/WBCs, and no casts.

Conditions with Similar Presentations	**Renal tubular acidosis type 1 (distal RTA):** Is characterized by impaired hydrogen ion secretion in the distal tubule. It causes a NAGMA with low serum potassium, but with an elevated urine pH (>5.5).
	Renal tubular acidosis type 4 (hyperkalemic RTA): Is characterized by aldosterone deficiency or resistance. Results in hyperkalemia with lower (<5.5) urine pH.
Initial Diagnostic Tests	Check BMP, urinalysis (look at urine pH), urine sodium/potassium/chloride.
Next Steps in Management	• Replete sodium bicarbonate (and phosphorus as needed).
• Start another antiepileptic and taper off valproic acid.
Discussion	RTA type 2 (proximal RTA) can be genetic or due to an adverse side effect of medications. Type 2 RTA is due to an abnormality in bicarbonate reabsorption in the proximal convoluted tubule (PCT). This impaired reabsorption results in increased bicarbonate excretion in the urine and a non-anion gap metabolic acidosis. RTA type 2 may be an isolated defect in bicarbonate reabsorption or associated with Fanconi syndrome, which is characterized by impaired reabsorption of bicarbonate along with phosphate, glucose, uric acid, and amino acids.
	History: Risk factors for proximal (type 2) RTA include multiple myeloma (due to light chain deposits in PCT), carbonic anhydrase use, and medications that are directly toxic to the PCT (valproic acid, ifosfamide, aminoglycosides)
	Physical Exam: Normal exam.
	Diagnostics: Fanconi syndrome is a clinical diagnosis with following findings:
1. BMP (low bicarbonate and no anion gap consistent with NAGMA, potassium (↓), glucose [normal])
2. Serum phosphorus (↓)
3. Urinalysis (pH <5.5, glucosuria)
4. Urine electrolytes and UAG >10, confirming renal cause of NAGMA
	Management:
• Discontinue offending medication. In this case, start another antiepileptic and taper off valproic acid.
• Replace sodium bicarbonate to a goal of normal (22–24 mEq/L).
• Correct electrolytes as indicated, in this case potassium and phosphorus.

Hyperchloremic NAGMA Mini-Cases

Cases	Key Findings
Diarrhea	**Hx:** Gastroenteritis, *Clostridium difficile* infection, laxative overuse **PE:** Crampy abdominal pain, signs of hypovolemia (dry mucous membranes, decreased skin turgor) **Diagnostics:** • BMP with low bicarbonate and elevated chloride • Calculation of UAG may help identify the etiology (renal vs gastrointestinal loss): • UAG = (Urine Na^+ + Urine K^+) – Urine Cl^- • Negative urine anion gap (UAG <0) is consistent with gastrointestinal bicarbonate loss (think "neGUTive") **Management:** • Supportive care, as diarrhea is usually self-limited (fluid resuscitation) • *C. difficile* infection requires antibiotic treatment with oral vancomycin or fidaxomicin. **Discussion:** Diarrhea is one of the most common causes of NAGMA. Bicarbonate is excreted in stool, so large-volume diarrhea results in excessive loss of bicarbonate and a compensatory increase in chloride anions.
Saline infusion	**Hx:** Large-volume fluid replacement with normal saline (for hypovolemia) **PE:** Nonspecific **Diagnostics:** BMP will show low bicarbonate and elevated chloride in a patient receiving normal saline **Management:** • Use lactated ringers instead of normal saline • Stop fluid resuscitation if no longer clinically indicated **Discussion:** Saline infusion is an iatrogenic cause of NAGMA. High chloride anions in the body result in bicarbonate moving intracellularly to maintain ionic neutrality.

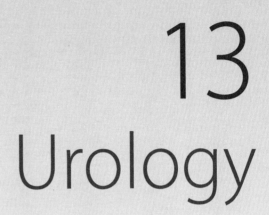

13
Urology

Lead Author: Samuel Ohlander, MD
Contributors: Matthew del Pino, MD; Jonathan Alcantar, MD

UROLOGIC TRAUMA/FLANK PAIN

Urologic injuries usually occur in the setting of multisystem trauma and should be considered in any patient who incurs chest, abdominal, or pelvic trauma. As with all other trauma patients, the initial focus should be on hemodynamic stabilization and managing any life-threatening injuries. History taking and physical examination should identify the mechanism of injury and anatomical sites involved. Accurate diagnosis of a urologic injury usually requires appropriate radiologic imaging, although the hemodynamically unstable trauma patient often is taken directly to the operating room without such studies. In such instances, the suspected urologic injury may be identified during surgical exploration through direct visualization of the affected organ.

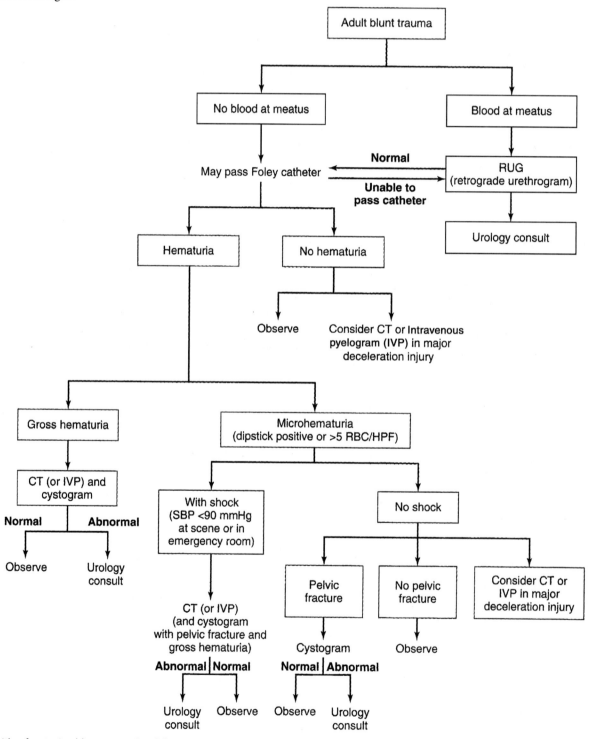

Algorithm for staging blunt trauma in adults. (Reproduced, with permission, from McAninch JW, Lue TF, eds. Smith & Tanagho's General Urology, 19th ed. New York, NY: McGraw Hill; 2020.)

CASE 1 | Bladder Rupture

A 29-year-old man is brought to the ED after a head-on motor vehicle collision in which he was the restrained passenger and airbags were deployed. On transport he was tachycardic, normotensive, complained of abdominal pain, and voided bloody urine. On exam, he has tenderness and crepitus over the pubic bone, and his abdomen is diffusely tender. There are no obvious rib fractures, flank ecchymosis, or blood at the meatus.

Conditions with Similar Presentations	**Renal injury:** Most common urologic injury, often seen after motor vehicle accidents. While gross hematuria would be expected, question stems will usually describe posterior rib fractures or flank ecchymosis (see later). In addition, evidence of pelvic fracture makes bladder injury more likely. **Ureteral injury:** Rare form of genitourinary trauma due to location, mostly seen with penetrating injuries (i.e., gunshot wounds) or iatrogenic causes (i.e., a complication of pelvic or retroperitoneal surgery). CT of abdomen and pelvis with IV contrast and delayed images (urogram) would show contrast extravasation as well as possible ipsilateral hydronephrosis and delayed contrast excretion from the ipsilateral kidney. **Posterior urethral injury:** Posterior urethral injury should be considered in trauma patients with pelvic fractures. The classic presentation will involve blood at the urethral meatus and inability to void. Other findings may include perineal bruising and a high-riding prostate on rectal exam. A retrograde urethrogram will show contrast extravasation from the urethra.
Initial Diagnostic Tests	First identify and treat any life-threatening injuries. See Surgery Chapter. Check: • Retrograde urethrogram to rule out urethral injury, prior to catheterization. • Retrograde cystogram will confirm the diagnosis and distinguish between intraperitoneal and extraperitoneal bladder injury. Consider: Urinalysis (UA), complete metabolic profile, CBC.
Next Steps in Management	• Surgical repair when stable (extraperitoneal bladder ruptures may be managed conservatively)
Discussion	The bladder has the second highest rate of injury among urologic organs, most often due to blunt abdominal trauma. While an empty bladder is protected in the bony pelvis, a full bladder extends into the abdomen, increasing its chance of injury. Bladder injuries are either intraperitoneal (increased intravesical pressure leads to rupture of its weakest point at the superior bladder dome), extraperitoneal (anterolateral bladder wall is most susceptible; almost always associated with pelvic fracture), or a combination of the two. Twenty-nine percent of patients presenting with gross hematuria and pelvic fracture are found to have a bladder injury. One-quarter of bladder injury cases are associated with urethral trauma. **History/Physical Exam:** • Abdominal/pelvic pain and gross hematuria. • May or may not be able to void, depending on the amount of urine diverted out of the bladder through the site of injury. • Guarding and referred shoulder pain can be signs of chemical peritonitis from leaked urine. • Often non-specific but may include abdominal distension, suprapubic tenderness, and altered mental status. • Evidence of pelvic fracture should increase suspicion of bladder and urethral injury. **Diagnostics:** • Retrograde urethrogram done first if a urethral injury is suspected (to make sure contrast does not extravasate through urethra). • Retrograde cystogram (plain film or CT) is the most accurate test for bladder rupture (to make sure contrast does not extravasate from bladder). • CT of the abdomen and pelvis with IV contrast is often done for trauma patients, but this study would not be adequate to exclude bladder injury. • UA (positive for hematuria). • Serum creatinine and BUN may be elevated due to urine absorption after intraperitoneal rupture. **Management:** • Bladder repairs are non-emergent and should be managed expectantly until life-threatening injuries are addressed. • Intraperitoneal bladder ruptures require surgical repair. • Extraperitoneal bladder ruptures may be managed conservatively with urethral catheter drainage and prophylactic antibiotics with gram-negative coverage. • Follow-up cystography should be done to confirm complete bladder healing prior to catheter removal.
Additional Considerations	**Complications:** The most common complication is persistent urinary leakage requiring extended catheter drainage. Other complications include bacterial peritonitis and sepsis, fistula formation if rectum or vagina are involved, and incontinence or neurogenic bladder from pelvic nerve injury.

Flank Pain Mini-Cases

Cases	Key Findings
Renal Trauma	**Hx:** • Flank/back pain and hematuria after blunt trauma involving rapid deceleration (i.e., motor vehicle accident) or significant blow to the flank • Penetrating injuries to the abdomen, flank, or lower chest are other potential causes **PE:** • May note posterior rib fractures (tenderness or crepitus) and flank ecchymosis **Diagnostics:** • CT abdomen/pelvis with IV contrast is gold standard for evaluating renal injuries **Management:** • Hemodynamically stable patients managed conservatively (hemodynamic monitoring, bed rest, ICU admission, and blood transfusions if necessary) with follow-up imaging. • Indications for surgical intervention include hemorrhagic shock due to renal injury, expanding retroperitoneal hematoma, and avulsion of the renal pelvis or ureter. **Discussion:** • Kidneys are the most commonly injured urologic organ and the third most common visceral organ injured in abdominal trauma, only behind the liver and spleen. • Management of renal trauma has shifted away from early operative intervention and now often favors a non-surgical approach early on, even for most intermediate to high-grade renal injuries secondary to blunt trauma. • Complications may include blood loss (can be delayed or associated with AV fistula), urine leak/urinoma, perinephric abscess, renovascular hypertension, and renal insufficiency.
Renal Infarction	**Hx/PE:** • Underlying risk factors for thromboembolism formation (i.e., atrial fibrillation, endocarditis, hypercoagulability), aortorenal vascular pathology (i.e., fibromuscular dysplasia), or a history of renal artery trauma • Can present with abdominal/flank pain, hematuria, hypertension (due to activation of RAAS system), nausea/vomiting, and fever **Diagnostics:** • Leukocytosis, elevated LDH, elevated serum creatinine • UA with hematuria • CT angiogram with wedge-shaped perfusion defect of the affected kidney **Management:** Options include anticoagulation, percutaneous endovascular therapy, and open surgery **Discussion:** • Renal infarction is a rare condition that can occur with blockage or reduction in renal arterial flow • Important clues are the presence of risk factors and imaging findings
Renal Vein Thrombosis (RVT)	**Hx:** • Neonate or an adult with risk factors of hypercoagulability (i.e., congenital, nephrotic syndrome, malignancy, oral contraceptive use) or recent renal transplant. • Gross hematuria, flank pain, nausea/vomiting, and fever. • Renal transplant recipients usually develop sudden anuria and severe abdominal pain over the graft region. **PE:** • Pain overlying the affected kidney and may have leg edema or varicocele with an extensive thrombus. • Neonates will have a palpable flank mass and appear dehydrated or in shock. **Diagnostics:** • Ultrasound (US) is first-line study for diagnosis (enlarged and hyperechogenic kidney without hydronephrosis). • CT and MR angiography studies can be nephrotoxic and are reserved for cases with inconclusive US results.

Flank Pain Mini-Cases (*continued*)

Renal Vein Thrombosis (RVT)	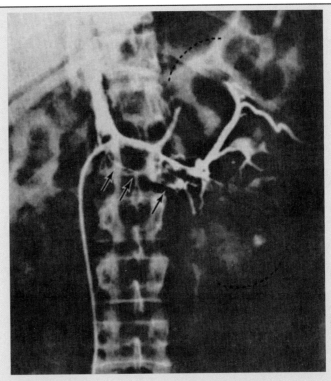 Thrombosis of renal vein. Selective left renal venogram showing almost complete occlusion of vein. Veins to lower pole failed to fill. Note the large size of kidney. (Reproduced, with permission, from McAninch JW, Lue TF, eds. Smith & Tanagho's General Urology, 19th ed. New York, NY: McGraw Hill; 2020.) **Management:** • Oral anticoagulation (heparin; adults bridged to warfarin). • Thrombolysis/thrombectomy considered if acute renal failure. **Discussion:** • RVT is the formation of a blood clot in a major renal vein or one of its tributaries, with the left renal vein affected twice as often as the right. • Since presenting symptoms overlap with other renal pathologies and blood tests will be non-specific, imaging studies are needed to make a definitive diagnosis. • Complications of RVT include hypertension, chronic kidney disease (CKD), pulmonary embolism, and early allograft loss (for renal transplant patients).
Pyelonephritis	See Infectious Disease Chapter.
Renal Stones	See Nephrology Chapter.

HEMATURIA

A patient may present with gross or microscopic hematuria from a variety of different causes. Upper tract sources, such as urolithiasis, glomerulopathies, renal cell carcinoma (RCC), and urothelial carcinoma of the ureters or renal pelvis, and interstitial nephritis, and lower tract causes such as BPH, urethral stricture, and urothelial carcinoma must all be considered during evaluation. Patients who present with gross hematuria require imaging of the upper tract as well as cystoscopy to rule out urothelial carcinoma of the bladder. Microscopic hematuria workup includes risk stratification and is summarized in the following algorithm.

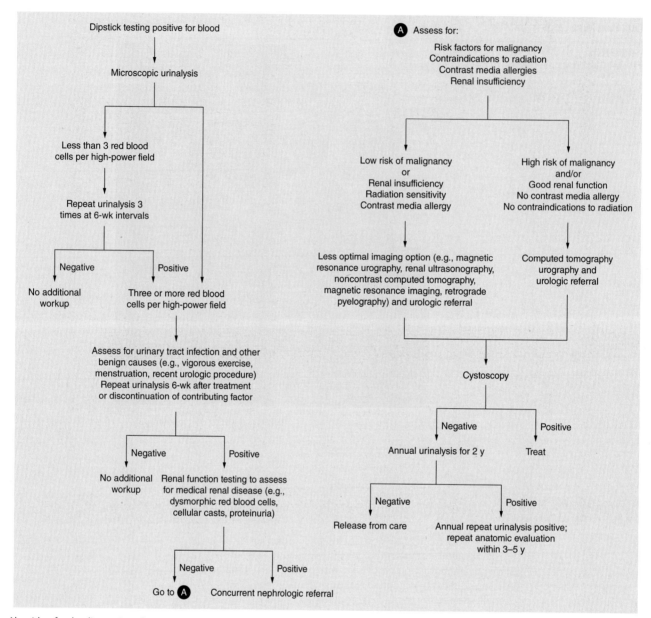

Algorithm for the diagnosis and management of incidentally discovered microscopic hematuria. (Reproduced, with permission, from David JA. Current Practice Guidelines in Primary Care, 2021-2022. New York: McGraw Hill; 2022.)

RENAL MASSES AND URINARY TRACT CANCERS

Renal masses are either benign or malignant, and they are often discovered incidentally in asymptomatic patients. They primarily present in older adults, with the exception of Wilms tumor, which presents in children. Renal masses are classified as solid or cystic (fluid-filled) on imaging, with 80% of solid masses being malignant. The Bosniak classification is used to assign risk of malignancy for cystic masses based on CT findings. Complex features associated with malignancy include contrast enhancement, heterogeneous internal texture, irregular borders, and thick septations. In addition to imaging studies, the evaluation of patients with suspected renal malignancy should include assignment of baseline CKD stage, as renal function may impact management. While active surveillance is a treatment option for many renal masses based on tumor features, primary interventions include surgical resection and ablation. Even in the setting of metastatic disease, radical nephrectomy with adjuvant therapies including VEGF inhibitors, mTOR pathway inhibitors, and immune checkpoint inhibitors have shown to confer a survival benefit.

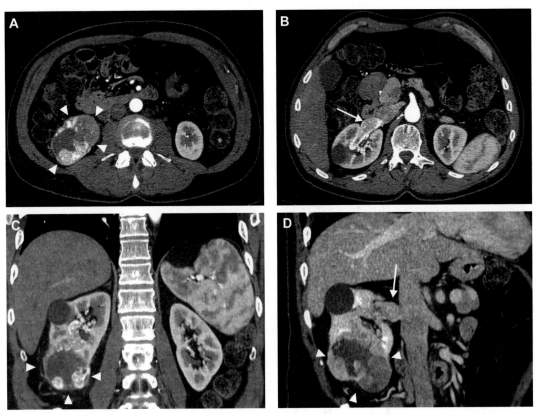

Post-contrast CT scan of the abdomen in axial (A, B) and coronal (C, D) planes of a patient with RCC demonstrated as a hypervascular lesion of the lower pole of the right kidney (*arrowheads*) with extension of the tumor into the renal vein (*arrow*). (Reproduced, with permission, from Elsayes KM, A. Oldham SAA, eds. Introduction to Diagnostic Radiology, New York: McGraw Hill; 2014.)

CASE 2	Renal Cell Carcinoma (RCC)

A 65-year-old man with a 20-pack-year smoking history presents with 3 weeks of right flank pain and recent onset of gross hematuria. He denies dysuria but he has noticed some sweats and has lost 20 pounds over the last month. He also feels more fatigued than usual. On exam, he is febrile, hypertensive, and there is fullness in his right flank and an irregular soft right scrotal mass (varicocele).

Conditions with Similar Presentations	**Simple renal cyst:** Benign growth characterized by a smooth thin wall, homogeneous fluid content with no solid components, and lack of radiocontrast enhancement (avascular) on imaging.
	Oncocytoma: Most common benign solid renal tumor arising from the collecting ducts. These tumors are difficult to distinguish from RCC without pathology.
	Angiomyolipoma: Second most common benign solid renal tumor that appears with patches of dense fat on imaging. Associated with tuberous sclerosis.
	Urothelial carcinoma: Although more often localized to the bladder, this carcinoma may arise in the renal pelvis and present as a central renal mass on imaging.
	Perinephric abscess: Usually a complication of urinary tract infections (UTIs), although it may be due to bacteremia, especially if it is due to *Staphylococcus aureus*. Fever and flank pain would be expected, but not a palpable flank mass or weight loss.
Initial Diagnostic Tests	• Confirm Diagnosis: Abdominal CT (or alternatively MRI) with and without contrast. • Consider: CBC, BMP, transaminases(AST/ALT), UA, chest radiographs for staging.
Next Steps in Management	Urology referral. Active surveillance vs. surgical resection vs. ablation.

CASE 2 | Renal Cell Carcinoma (RCC) *(continued)*

Discussion	RCC originates in the renal cortex and constitutes the majority of primary renal neoplasms. It may be associated with paraneoplastic syndromes such as ectopic EPO, ACTH, PTHrP, and renin excretion. Clear cell carcinoma is the most common histological type of renal malignancy. It is one of the few carcinomas that tends to favor hematogenous spread. Incidence of metastatic disease at presentation is 30% and most common sites of spread are to the lungs, liver, bone, and brain. RCC may extend locally into the renal vein (and may cause thrombosis) or inferior vena cava and present with varicocele due to increased venous pressure within the pampiniform plexus. **History:** • Predominantly occurs in the sixth to eighth decades of life. More common in men. Risk factors include smoking, hypertension, obesity, and end-stage renal disease (ESRD). Hereditary causes of RCC, such as von Hippel-Lindau, are all autosomal dominant, have an earlier age of onset (third to fifth decade), and often present with bilateral and multifocal carcinomas. • Most often asymptomatic. • Classic triad of flank pain, hematuria, and palpable mass is rarely encountered and is an indication of advanced disease. • Patient may have constitutional symptoms of fever, chills, and weight loss. **Physical Exam:** • Exam is often unremarkable, but findings may include a palpable abdominal mass or a unilateral varicocele ("bag of worms") that does not reduce with lying down. • Signs of paraneoplastic syndromes may include hypertension, cachexia, Cushingoid appearance, and fever. **Diagnostics:** • Diagnosis usually suggested by ultrasound and confirmed with multiphase abdominal CT or MRI. • Gross or microscopic hematuria (≥3 RBCs) on UA. • CBC may show anemia from chronic hematuria or secondary polycythemia from excess EPO production. • Other lab findings may include hypercalcemia due to production of PTHrP, transaminitis if there are liver metastases, or elevated alkaline phosphatase if there is liver or bone involvement. • Chest radiographs are recommended for initial detection of metastatic disease, followed up with advanced imaging studies as indicated, including chest CT, nuclear medicine bone scan, and brain MRI. • Core biopsies are not recommended for resectable kidney lesions due to concern for seeding. **Management:** • Small renal masses (<4 cm): Active surveillance (repeat imaging in 3–6 months) followed by partial nephrectomy (removing only the suspicious lesion) if the rate of growth is rapid. • Larger masses (>7 cm) require surgical management, including radical nephrectomy (removal of the entire kidney) or partial nephrectomy. • Thermal ablation is an option for small renal masses (biopsy required to confirm diagnosis) and/or poor surgical candidates. • Targeted adjuvant therapy such as mTOR inhibitors or anti-angiogenesis agents are utilized for metastatic RCC.
Additional Considerations	**Screening:** There are currently no established screening modalities for early detection of RCC. **Complications:** Venous thrombosis involving the renal vein or inferior vena cava occurs in 10% of cases.

CASE 3 | Bladder Cancer

A 65-year-old woman with a 30-pack/year history of smoking presents for evaluation of intermittent blood in her urine for the past 4 months. She has a history of chronic UTIs but denies dysuria or fevers. She has urgency but no pain and denies incontinence or vaginal discharge. On exam, she has no costovertebral angle tenderness or abdominal tenderness and the pelvic exam is normal.

Conditions with Similar Presentations	**UTI:** Usually associated with dysuria in addition to urgency. **RCC:** May also cause painless hematuria but may have flank pain as well. Not associated with urgency. Further studies needed to determine etiology. **Nephrolithiasis:** Causes hematuria but has acute presentation with pain that radiates from the flank to the pelvis. **Hemorrhagic cystitis:** Hematuria usually in the setting of history of transplant (BK virus infection), other symptoms consistent with adenovirus infection, or exposure to chemotherapeutics (cyclophosphamide, iphosphamide toxicity). **Renal papillary necrosis:** Hematuria with flank pain and associated with NSAID use, sickle cell, diabetes mellitus, and/or acute pyelonephritis.

CASE 3 | Bladder Cancer *(continued)*

Initial Diagnostic Tests	• UA with microscopy. • Must evaluate the lower tract (cystoscopy) and the upper tract (imaging). • Cystoscopy with biopsy to confirm diagnosis.
Next Steps in Management	• Transurethral resection of the bladder tumor (TURBT). • If muscular layer invasion, radical cystectomy +/− systemic chemotherapy is indicated.
Discussion	Bladder cancer is the fifth most common malignancy in the United States and the most common genitourinary malignancy, with the most common subtype being urothelial (transitional cell) carcinoma. Urothelial carcinoma rarely involves the renal pelvis, ureter, and/or urethra. Squamous cell carcinoma of the bladder is less common overall but more common in unindustrialized countries with exposure to the parasitic trematode *Schistosoma haematobium* endemic in the Middle East and East Africa. Adenocarcinoma of the bladder rarely occurs and is typically secondary to a urachal remnant and involves the dome of the bladder. **History:** Risk factors include smoking, occupational exposure to aromatic amines (e.g., aniline dyes), aromatic hydrocarbons (e.g., coal tar), formaldehyde, or medications such as phenacetin and cyclophosphamide. Symptoms/Presentations: • Painless hematuria (most common), irritative voiding symptoms (e.g., urinary frequency, urgency, dysuria). • Obstructive symptoms and hydronephrosis are rare but may occur due bladder neck or ureteral obstruction, respectively. **Physical Exam:** Palpable suprapubic mass may be present in advanced cases. **Diagnostics:** • UA and urine culture to confirm presence of RBCs and exclude infectious causes of hematuria. • Flexible cystoscopy with biopsy is gold standard to make the diagnosis and evaluate the lower tract. • CT scan, MRI, or combination of ultrasound with retrograde pyelography is done as an initial diagnostic test to evaluate the upper tract as a potential source of pathology. **Management:** • TURBT can both assist in staging and treatment. • Low to intermediate risk (non-muscular invasive) bladder cancer: intravesical chemotherapy (BCG, mitomycin, and gemcitabine). • Muscle-invasive bladder cancer without positive lymph nodes or distant metastasis: Radical cystectomy with construction of a urinary diversion (neobladder or ileal conduit).
Additional Considerations	**Screening:** There are currently no established screening modalities for early detection of bladder cancer. **Complications:** Bladder cancer may lead to distension and hypertrophy of the bladder, hydronephrosis, impaired renal function, or UTIs. **Surveillance:** Regular surveillance with cystoscopy after diagnosis. Five-year survival of bladder cancer is 90–95% for noninvasive disease and <15% in metastatic disease.

CASE 4 | Prostate Cancer

A 68-year-old man with a history of benign prostatic hyperplasia (BPH) presents with increased difficulty with urination, back pain, and weight loss. He denies dysuria or fevers. The back pain started 1 month ago and wakes him up at night. He denies bowel incontinence, saddle anesthesia, or difficulty walking. His brother has a history of prostate cancer. On exam, he is tender to palpation throughout his spine and bilateral pelvis, but has intact flexion and extension of the spine and normal gait. Genital exam reveals a normal penis without evidence of meatal stenosis. His digital rectal exam (DRE) reveals an asymmetric nodular prostate with different textures.

Conditions with Similar Presentations	**BPH:** May also present with urinary frequency but the prostate is smooth, uniformly enlarged, and nontender. **Prostatitis:** Painful, boggy, tender prostate on DRE.
Initial Diagnostic Tests	• Check DRE and prostate-specific antigen (PSA) levels. • Biopsy will confirm diagnosis. • Consider: UA, urine culture, alkaline phosphatase if bone pain.
Next Steps in Management	Transrectal ultrasound and prostate biopsy.

CASE 4 | Prostate Cancer (continued)

Discussion	The majority of prostate cancers are adenocarcinomas and arise in the peripheral zone (posterior lobe) of the prostate, whereas BPH occurs in the transition zone.

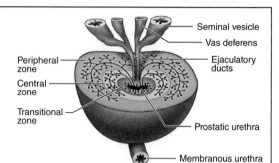

Prostate cancer. (Reproduced, with permission, from Mescher AL. Junqueira's Basic Histology: Text & Atlas, 16th ed. New York: McGraw Hill; 2021.)

The majority of prostate cancers are adenocarcinomas and arise in the peripheral zone (posterior lobe) of the prostate, whereas BPH occurs in the transition zone.

Prostate cancer is the second leading cause of cancer deaths in men in the United States, and typically is seen in older men (>50 years old).

Men with a family history of prostate cancer and African-Americans have a higher risk of developing the disease.

History:
- Early prostate cancer often asymptomatic.
- Advanced prostate cancer may present with weight loss, fatigue, loss of appetite, hematuria, incontinence, urinary retention and hydronephrosis, and signs of metastatic disease such as bone pain, neurological deficits (due to spinal compression), and lymphedema.

Physical Exam:
- DRE may reveal an asymmetric prostate with nodules and different textures, though a normal exam does not preclude the diagnosis.

Diagnostics:
- UA and urine culture to exclude infectious causes of urinary symptoms (i.e., frequency, hesitancy, hematuria).
- **PSA** >4 ng/mL suggests an abnormality and further steps to rule out malignancy are indicated. Notably, PSA can be elevated in other settings such as prostatitis, BPH, and trauma.
- **Ultrasound-guided prostate biopsy** confirms diagnosis.
- Gleason score summarizes the two most dysplastic samples (1–5), with a maximum score of 10.
- Alkaline phosphatase may be elevated if there are bone metastasis.
- Staging with CT/MRI pelvis, spinal x-ray, and possible bone scintigraphy. Prostatic adenocarcinoma may metastasize (osteoblastic), most commonly to pelvic lymph nodes or to the vertebrae of the lumbosacral spine.

Management:
- If localized to the prostate: Radical prostatectomy or radiation.
- Antiandrogen therapy (GnRH agonists [leuprolide], and GnRH antagonists [degarelix]) may be combined with radiation and is not curative.
- Active surveillance and watchful waiting (PSA tracking) may be used in men with low-risk prostate cancer.
- Radiotherapy reserved for patients with a lower life expectancy due to complications.

Additional Considerations	**Screening:** Males aged 55–69 years, shared decision-making regarding PSA screening after a discussion of risks and benefits, and proceeding based upon the patient's wishes.
	Surveillance: Active surveillance typically includes DRE and PSA measurements every 6–12 months and regular repeat biopsies.
	Complications: Of treatment may include erectile dysfunction (ED), urinary incontinence, and infertility secondary to radical prostatectomy. Radiotherapy may lead to proctitis, enteritis, cystitis, or urethritis.

Scrotal Swelling or Mass

A scrotal swelling or mass can present at any age and may or may not be accompanied by pain. Testicular cancer is the most common malignancy in men between the ages of 20–35 years and should be considered in the differential for any scrotal mass in this age group. All scrotal masses should be transilluminated to determine if the mass is cystic (light shines through) or solid (light blocked by the mass). An ultrasound can also help determine if a mass is solid or cystic. Any solid mass requires immediate evaluation for cancer, including tumor markers LDH, AFP, and β-hCG. For masses suspicious for testicular cancer, an orchiectomy should be performed instead of a biopsy (which may cause lymphatic tumor seeding).

It is important to expedite the evaluation of scrotal pain and to rule in or out emergent cases such as testicular torsion from less emergent cases such as epididymo-orchitis or testicular varicocele.

Key Clinical Associations

	Testicular Torsion	Epididymo-Orchitis	Varicocele
Onset	Acute	Gradual	Gradual/chronic
Pain	Severe	Severe	Dull ache
Physical Exam	⊖ Cremasteric reflex	⊕ Cremasteric reflex	Dilated veins of pampiniform plexus (increases with Valsalva), "bag of worms"
	Long axis of testicle is lying horizontally, high riding testicular position in scrotum	Normal testicular position	Veins decompress in recombinant position
Management	Emergent surgery	Antibiotics/anti-inflammatories	Symptomatic management vs. surgical varicocelectomy

While surgical exploration should not be delayed if testicular torsion is suspected, a testicular Doppler ultrasound can help accurately differentiate various pathologies.

Key Ultrasound Findings	Diagnosis
Lack of blood flow	Testicular torsion
Hypervascular, enlarged epididymis	Epididymitis
Anechoic extra-testicular lesion	Spermatocele/epididymal cyst
Retrograde spermatic vein flow with Valsalva	Varicocele
Hypoechoic intratesticular lesion with blood flow	Testicular mass
Inguinal mass, + peristalsis, luminal debris	Inguinal hernia

CASE 5 | Testicular Cancer

A 32-year-old man presents for evaluation of right testicular mass. He is unsure of the duration, but noticed it while in the shower few weeks ago. He denies any pain, urinary symptoms, or trauma. His only past history includes surgical correction of hypospadias as a child. On physical exam, there is a non-tender, non-mobile, solid, firm, homogeneous mass on the anterior aspect of his right testis that does not transilluminate. The left testis is nontender and palpably normal. There is no inguinal lymphadenopathy.

Conditions with Similar Presentations	**Hydrocele:** Transilluminates, soft swelling mass. **Varicocele:** Palpable strands, with "bag of worms" on physical exam. **Inguinal hernia:** Protruding mass, often reducible, auscultation of bowel sounds may also be appreciated on physical exam. **Testicular hematoma:** History of trauma will be present.
Initial Diagnostic Tests	• Scrotal ultrasound with Doppler. • Tumor markers (AFP, hCG, LDH).
Next Steps in Management	• Radical inguinal orchiectomy and possible sperm cryopreservation prior to surgery. • Staging CT abdomen and pelvis to assess for lymph node involvement/metastasis.

CASE 5 | Testicular Cancer *(continued)*

Discussion	Primary testicular cancer is the most common malignancy in males aged 20–35 years and often presents as a firm, unilateral, non-mobile mass that cannot be isolated away from the testicle. Testicular tumors are broadly divided into germ cell tumors (~95%), which develop from sperm-producing germ cells, or sex cord stromal tumors, which develop from derivatives of the embryonic sex cord. Serum tumor markers in testicular tumors can help narrow the differential.

- Most germ cell tumors are malignant, while most sex cord stromal tumors are benign in men.
- Most common testicular tumor and most common germ cell tumor subtype is the **seminoma**. Pathology would show large cells in lobules with a watery cytoplasm and a "fried egg" appearance. Pure seminomas, have normal serum AFP and β-hCG but some also have non-seminomatous elements which may produce β-hCG.
- Other types of testicular **germ cell tumors** include teratomas, embryonal carcinomas, yolk sac tumors, and choriocarcinomas and are often categorized as non-seminomatous germ cell tumors (NSGCT).
- Yolk sac tumors have very high AFP levels, while choriocarcinomas have very high β-hCG levels.
- Non-germ cell tumors, or **sex cord stromal tumors**, include Sertoli cell tumors, Leydig cell tumors, and testicular metastatic lymphoma.
- Following radical inguinal orchiectomy, histology can help identify the specific tumor subtype, and this will help guide subsequent management.
- Testicular tumors have an excellent prognosis and are often curable in metastatic stages.

Hormone levels in germ cell tumors					
	Seminoma	**Yolk Sac Tumor**	**Choriocarcinoma**	**Teratoma**	**Embryonal Carcinoma**
PALP	↑	–	–	–	–
AFP	–	↑ ↑	–	–	–/↑ (when mixed)
β-hCG	–/↑	–/↑	↑ ↑	–	↑

History:

Risk factors: Cryptorchidism (the failure of descent in one or both testes), hypospadias (congenital malformation where urethral opening is not at the tip of the penis), Klinefelter syndrome, trisomy 21, subfertility, contralateral testicular cancer, and family history of testicular cancer.

Symptoms:
- Painless nodule or swelling of a testicle.
- Lower abdominal or scrotal discomfort may be present.
- Metastatic disease may present with respiratory symptoms or bone pain.
- Non-seminomas may present with gynecomastia from hCG or estrogen production, or signs of androgen excess either of which can be present in Sertoli-Leydig tumors.
- Because of structural similarity to TSH, β-hCG can cause paraneoplastic hyperthyroidism and is usually seen in choriocarcinoma.

Physical Exam:
- Negative transillumination test, palpable firm adherent nodule of the testicle.

Diagnostics:
- Scrotal ultrasound with Doppler.
- Serum tumor markers including AFP, hCG, and LDH.
- Trans-scrotal biopsy should not be conducted, as there is a risk of tumor seeding.

Management:
- Orchiectomy via inguinal approach.
- Imaging (e.g., CT scans or MRI) for staging.
- Post-operative staging will guide additional treatment.
- Radiation and/or cisplatin-based chemotherapy is considered for higher stage seminomas.
- Retroperitoneal lymph node dissection and/or multi-agent cisplatin-based chemotherapy are considered for higher stage NSGCT.
- Select patients may be candidates for testis-sparing surgery and is considered for those wishing to preserve gonadal function.

Additional Considerations	**Surveillance:** Monitor serum tumor markers for recurrence

Scrotal Abnormality Mini-Cases

Cases	Key Findings
Varicocele	**Hx:** • Chronic, non-radiating scrotal pain ("dull and heavy") and swelling exacerbated with prolonged standing or increased strenuous activity, improved with lying down • May present with fertility concerns **PE:** • "Bag of worms" on palpation and will not transilluminate • Examining the patient supine and then while standing will demonstrate engorgement with standing or Valsalva **Diagnostics:** • Clinical diagnosis and imaging are not needed • If unsure of diagnosis, scrotal Doppler ultrasound **Management:** • Supportive measures (scrotal support, NSAIDs) and observation if no associated infertility, testicular atrophy, or pain • Surgical ligation or embolization may be indicated if pain or swelling are present or persistent **Discussion:** A varicocele is a dilation of the pampiniform venous plexus and the internal spermatic veins due to increased venous pressure. It is the most common cause of scrotal swelling in the adult male and is usually on the left side due to increased resistance to flow from the right-angle insertion of the left gonadal vein into the left renal vein. This is opposed to the right gonadal vein, which flows directly into the inferior vena cava. Right-sided varicoceles are rare and should raise suspicion for mass in the retroperitoneal space compressing the spermatic vein
Fournier Gangrene	**Hx:** Risk factors: Poorly controlled diabetes, immunocompromised state, alcoholism, IV drug use. Symptoms/presentation: Acute onset of groin pain and a "boil" that is enlarging. **PE:** • Fever, tachycardia, hypotension. • Diffuse swelling and erythema of the scrotum, groin, and/or perineum. May have blisters/bullae. • Classic findings include pain out of proportion to exam (early) and palpable crepitus (late). May see black necrotic tissue and signs of sepsis in advanced infections. **Diagnostics:** • Definitive diagnosis can be made by surgical exploration of the involved area. Obtaining labs and imaging studies should not delay surgery if Fournier gangrene is suspected. • On imaging, air along fascial planes or deeper tissue often present. **Management:** • IV fluid resuscitation, broad-spectrum IV antibiotics, and emergency surgical debridement of devitalized tissue. **Discussion:** • Fournier gangrene is a life-threatening necrotizing soft tissue infection that involves the genitalia and perineum. • It is usually caused by mucosal barrier breakdown in the urethra or colon, which allows for a polymicrobial infection from a mixture of aerobic and anaerobic organisms from fecal flora including *E. coli, Klebsiella,* enterococci, and *Clostridium.* • If left untreated, it can spread rapidly along fascial planes over the course of hours. Mortality rate from resultant sepsis is 20–40%. A patient with Fournier's gangrene of the scrotum. Note the sharp demarcation of gangrenous changes (black portion) and the marked edema of the scrotum and the penis. (Reproduced with permission from Tintinalli JE, Ma O, Yealy DM, Meckler GD, Stapczynski J, Cline DM, Thomas SH. Tintinalli's Emergency Medicine: A Comprehensive Study Guide, 9e. 2020 by McGraw-Hill Education.)

PEDIATRIC URINARY TRACT INFECTION (UTI)

In the pediatric population, UTIs are one of the most common reasons for medical visits. All infants <2 years old with a febrile UTI should have a renal and bladder ultrasound (RBUS) to rule out structural anomalies of the urinary tract. If the RBUS shows abnormalities, such as hydronephrosis or increased cortical echogenicity suggesting scarring, or if a child has a history of two febrile UTIs regardless of RBUS findings, the patient should receive a voiding cystourethrogram (VCUG). VCUG results, along with differentiating symptomatology, help guide diagnosis and treatment decisions. Vesicoureteral reflux (VUR) is graded on a scale from I–V (see figure). In the setting of high-grade reflux, renal scintigraphy with dimercaptosuccinic acid (DMSA) can be used to assess renal cortical function and monitor for renal scarring. The goals of treatment are to prevent the complications of recurrent UTIs and renal injury while minimizing over-treatment. Pediatric UTIs are strongly associated with bladder and bowel dysfunction, and ensuring appropriate elimination habits plays a critical role in prevention and management.

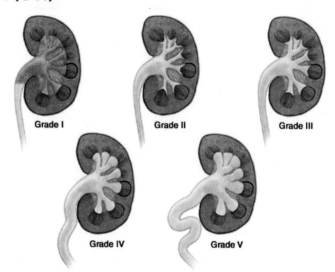

Illustration showing grades of vesicoureteral reflux (VUR). Grade I involves backup of urine into the ureter. Grade II involves backup of urine into the ureter, renal pelvis, and calyces. Grade III begins to involve dilation of the renal pelvis and blunting of the calyces. Grade IV involves more pronounced dilation of the renal pelvis and blunting of calyces. Finally, Grade V involves a tortuous appearance of the ureters. (Reproduced with permission from Elsayes KM, Oldham SA: Introduction to Diagnostic Radiology. New York: McGraw Hill; 2015.)

CASE 6	Posterior Urethral Valve (PUV)
\multicolumn{2}{l}{A 7-day-old newborn boy is brought to the ED for poor urine output and recent fever. Since birth, he has only been having one wet diaper per day. His parents mention that he seems irritable, is breastfeeding less than normal, and vomited once this evening. They deny cough or rhinorrhea. He was born at 39 weeks and spent 2 days in the ICU for respiratory difficulty. Prenatal ultrasounds were notable for decreased amniotic fluid volume. On exam, his temperature is 40°C and he appears lethargic. His chest cavity appears small, abdomen is distended, and a walnut-sized bladder can be palpated.}
Conditions with Similar Presentations	**Primary VUR:** Often present with UTI, but would expect to see unilateral hydroureteronephrosis (if high-grade) and no bladder distension on RBUS. **Ureteropelvic junction obstruction (UPJO):** Although most often asymptomatic in infancy, may present with UTI. Would see isolated hydronephrosis without hydroureter on RBUS (see below).
Conditions with Similar Presentations	**Duplex collecting system:** The most common renal tract anomaly. It may be complicated by VUR, ureteral obstruction, and UTIs in the first year of life. Would see a renal pelvis with isolated superior and inferior poles on RBUS and "drooping lily" appearance on VCUG. **Neurogenic bladder:** Caused by spinal cord–based disorders such as myelomeningocele and traumatic spinal cord injury. Although children may present with UTI and bladder distention from urinary retention, would see sacral bony defects in myelomeningocele and additional neurologic deficits with spinal cord injuries. **Dysfunctional voiding:** Develops in older children with habitual contraction of the urethral sphincter during voiding and is managed with behavioral modifications. While VUR and increased UTIs are often seen in these children, distinguishing features will be a history of urinary frequency, urgency, and incontinence.
Initial Diagnostic Tests	• Check: CBC, BMP, UA, and urine culture with catheterized specimen, blood cultures, and RBUS. • Confirm diagnosis with VCUG after infection is treated.
Next Steps in Management	• Immediate bladder decompression and initiation of antibiotics should be done prior to pursuing confirmation of PUV diagnosis. • Definitive treatment involves endoscopic valve ablation.

CASE 6 | Posterior Urethral Valve (PUV) *(continued)*

Discussion	
	PUV is an obstructing membranous fold within the lumen of the prostatic urethra that impedes urine flow. It is one of the few potentially life-threatening congenital anomalies of the urinary tract during the neonatal period.

PUV is an obstructing membranous fold within the lumen of the prostatic urethra that impedes urine flow. It is one of the few potentially life-threatening congenital anomalies of the urinary tract during the neonatal period.

Increased bladder outlet resistance results in chronically elevated bladder pressures (leads to bladder dysfunction and VUR) and urinary stasis (increases risk for recurrent infections), all of which can contribute to progressive renal failure. PUV only occurs in boys. Between 20–50% of PUV patients will progress to ESRD despite appropriate treatment.

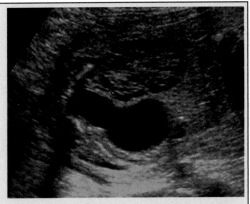

Image of a 19-week fetus with severe bladder outlet obstruction. The bladder is dilated and thick-walled, with dilatation of the proximal urethra resembling a "keyhole." Adjacent to the bladder is an enlarged kidney with evidence of cystic dysplasia, conferring a poor prognosis. (Reproduced, with permission, from F. Gary Cunningham, Kenneth J. Leveno, Steven L. Bloom, Jodi S. Dashe, Barbara L. Hoffman, Brian M. Casey, Catherine Y. Spong, et al, eds. Williams Obstetrics, 25th ed. New York: McGraw Hill; 2018.)

History:
- Newborn boy with delayed/minimal urine output, abdominal mass, poor feeding, lethargy, or urosepsis. Less affected boys can present later with recurrent UTIs, urinary incontinence, or failure to thrive.

Physical Exam:
- Distended abdomen and bladder.
- If renal dysfunction developed in utero, may have a small chest cavity and be in respiratory distress from pulmonary hypoplasia.
- Fever and flank pain are signs of pyelonephritis.

Diagnostics:
- 40–60% of cases are detected by routine prenatal ultrasound showing bilateral hydronephrosis with distended bladder, dilated posterior urethra ("keyhole sign"), and/or oligohydramnios.
- Postnatally, first perform a renal/bladder ultrasound (see bilateral hydronephrosis and distended bladder) followed by a VCUG (may show a thickened, trabeculated bladder, VUR, and a dilated posterior urethra) to confirm the diagnosis.
- Although cystoscopy is the most accurate way to diagnose PUV, radiographic studies usually suffice.

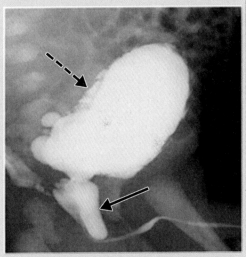

Voiding cystourethrogram shows marked dilatation of the posterior urethra (*black arrow*) with transition to narrow caliber of the bulbous and penile urethra distal to the valve tissue, which is not seen. There is also irregular bladder wall thickening (*dotted arrow*). (Reproduced, with permission, from Elsayes KM, A. Oldham SAA, eds. Introduction to Diagnostic Radiology, New York: McGraw Hill; 2014.)

- BMP and CBC assesses for dehydration, kidney failure (elevated BUN and creatinine), and inflammatory response (leukocytosis). Of note, a serum creatinine nadir of ≥1 mg/dL in the first year of life is a strong predictor of progression to ESRD.
- The presence of ≥10,000 CFU/mL of a single organism in a urine specimen obtained through catheterization or suprapubic aspiration is positive for UTI in neonates and children with urinary tract abnormalities.
- DMSA or mercaptoacetyltriglycine (MAG-3) scans are recommended after 4 weeks of age to assess kidney function.

CASE 6 | Posterior Urethral Valve (PUV) *(continued)*

Discussion	**Management:** • Initiate any necessary resuscitative measures (IV fluid replacement, mechanical ventilation). • Urgent bladder decompression with urethral or suprapubic catheterization. • Start appropriate antibiotics for pediatric febrile UTIs including first-generation cephalosporins and trimethoprim-sulfamethoxazole (avoid in infants <2 months). • Definitive treatment with endoscopic valve ablation to remove the obstruction should be done early after child has been stabilized. • Urinary diversion through vesicostomy or bilateral ureterostomies can be used as a temporizing measure in certain instances, such as premature infants with urethras that are too small to accommodate resectoscope.
Additional Considerations	**Complications:** In severe cases of PUV, where renal function becomes significantly impaired in utero, decreased urine production can result in profound oligohydramnios, leading to Potter sequence (pulmonary hypoplasia, flat facies, limb deformities). Surgical complications may include urethral injury/stricture, post-obstructive diuresis.

Pediatric UTI Mini-Cases

Cases	Key Findings
Ureteropelvic Junction Obstruction (UPJO)	**Hx:** • Most cases are asymptomatic. • Can present with hematuria, UTI, nausea, and renal colic, particularly in settings of increased urine production (hydration while playing sports, caffeine intake, binge drinking) that overwhelms the ability of the UPJ to drain and causes distension of the renal capsule. **PE:** • Often unremarkable, but may note abdominal/flank mass **Diagnostics:** • RBUS (see isolated hydronephrosis without hydroureter) and MAG-3 diuretic renography (see impaired drainage of the affected kidney) to confirm the diagnosis and assess the severity of obstruction. • VCUG is also recommended to assess for reflux. **Management:** • Asymptomatic: Managed conservatively with serial imaging +/- antibiotic prophylaxis, and obstruction often self-resolves. • Surgical reconstruction of renal pelvis with a pyeloplasty indicated for worsening renal function and/or hydronephrosis, recurrent UTIs, nephrolithiasis, and pain. **Discussion:** UPJO is obstruction of urine outflow from the renal pelvis into the proximal ureter, resulting in urine build-up and hydronephrosis. It is usually due to stenosis of the UPJ (more common in infants) or extrinsic compression by a lower pole renal vessel that crosses the pelvis (more common in older children), although poor peristalsis of the UPJ is another cause.
Duplex Collecting System	**Hx:** • Most often asymptomatic and discovered incidentally. • May present with UTI or even chronic pyelonephritis in the first year of life, and dribbling incontinence in girls (if ectopic ureter inserts into the vaginal vault). **PE:** • Often unremarkable, but may detect palpable mass in cases of severe hydronephrosis or protruding ureterocele. **Diagnostics:** • Often incidentally found on prenatal or postnatal ultrasound. • Diagnosis is confirmed with IV urography using computed tomography (CTU) or magnetic resonance (MRU).

Pediatric UTI Mini-Cases (*continued*)

Duplex Collecting System	**Management:** • A duplex collecting system does not require treatment per se, but associated complications may necessitate intervention. • Surgical management may include ureterocele incision to relieve ureteral obstruction, ureteral reimplantation if there is VUR, and removal of a nonfunctioning upper pole by heminephrectomy. If the upper pole moiety of a duplex kidney is noted to still have renal function, a ureteropyeloanastomosis can be considered (connects the upper pole ureter to the renal pelvis that drains the lower pole). **Discussion:** • A duplex collecting system is characterized by incomplete fusion of the upper and lower poles of a single kidney, resulting in two separate collecting systems that drain into a single ureter (partial duplication) or two separate ureters (complete duplication). • There is a 1–5% incidence in children investigated for urinary tract symptoms, making it the most common collecting system anomaly. • Complications include VUR, obstruction, or ureterocele (cystic dilatations of the terminal ureter, usually draining the upper pole).
Vesicoureteral Reflux (VUR)	**Hx:** • Most often asymptomatic, may present with recurrent UTIs. • Risk factors include having a first-degree relative with VUR. • Consider diagnosis if routine prenatal ultrasound shows hydronephrosis. **PE:** • Often unremarkable; however, may have flank/abdominal pain associated with voiding. **Diagnostics:** • RBUS may detect hydronephrosis along with dilation of the ureter. • VCUG is the diagnostic test of choice for VUR and retrograde reflux of contrast into the ureters during micturition confirms the diagnosis. **Management:** • Conservative management, which includes active surveillance with or without daily antibiotic prophylaxis, is generally indicated at presentation for children 1–5 years of age. • Recognizing and managing bladder and bowel dysfunction (e.g., constipation) is important in preventing breakthrough infections. In the setting of high-grade primary VUR that persists after toilet training and management of bladder/bowel dysfunction, surgical correction with ureteral reimplantation or injection of bulking agents near the UVJ may be indicated, particularly for children with abnormal kidney function or frequent breakthrough UTIs. • Secondary causes of VUR must be addressed prior to anti-reflux surgery to ensure optimal outcomes. **Discussion:** Of infants and young children with a febrile UTI, 30–40% are diagnosed with VUR. VUR is the retrograde flow of urine from the bladder to the upper urinary tract. • Primary VUR: Due to an incompetent valve at the ureterovesical junction (UVJ). • Secondary VUR: Due to high bladder pressures (secondary to bladder outlet obstruction, neurogenic bladder, or dysfunctional voiding) or other congenital anomalies of the urinary system associated with UVJ deficiency (such as ureterocele, ectopic ureter, and horseshoe kidney). • Up to 80% of low-grade VUR cases (reflux reaches the renal pelvis but does not cause significant dilatation of the ureter or collecting system) will spontaneously resolve, compared to only 12% of high-grade cases (reflux causes dilatation of the ureter and/or collecting system). • Screening with RBUS indicated if first-degree relative has VUR or there is presence of hydronephrosis on prenatal ultrasound.

URINARY RETENTION/LOWER URINARY TRACT SYMPTOMS (LUTS)

Urinary retention is the inability to voluntarily empty the bladder that leads to elevated postvoid residual (PVR) or, in more extreme cases, complete retention. The differential diagnosis for urinary retention is broad and spans multiple organ systems (see following chart). In essence, it is either caused by anatomical obstruction (more common in men), or impairment of bladder contractility and/or bladder outlet relaxation due to neurogenic or pharmacologic causes (equally common across both sexes). Acute urinary retention presents with a sudden inability to pass urine with associated suprapubic pain and bladder overdistension. In contrast, chronic urinary retention is usually painless and is associated with recurrent UTIs or bladder stones due to urinary stasis. If not alleviated, urinary retention can cause bladder rupture (in the acute setting) or overflow incontinence (in the chronic setting) from bladder overfilling leading to increased intravesical pressure that overcomes the outlet resistance. Both acute and chronic urinary retention can result in post-obstructive renal injury.

Differential Diagnosis for Patients Presenting with Urinary Retention

Neurogenic	Obstructive	Pharmacologic
• Spinal cord injury • Multiple sclerosis • Stroke • Diabetes mellitus • Cauda equina syndrome • Spinal anesthesia • Parkinson disease • Spina bifida	• Urethral stricture • Benign prostatic hyperplasia • Prostatitis • Urinary tract infection • Prostate cancer • Pelvic organ prolapse • Pelvic mass • Bladder diverticulum • Constipation • Hematuria (clot retention) • Bladder stone • Bladder cancer	• Anticholinergics • Antihistamines • Antidepressants (i.e., TCAs) • Antipsychotics • Anesthetics • Alpha-adrenergic agonists • Opioids • Benzodiazepines

Medications used to treat BPH/LUTS

Medications	Mechanism	Side Effects/ Contraindications	Additional Considerations
Alpha-adrenergic-antagonists (i.e., terazosin, tamsulosin)	Smooth muscle relaxation in the prostate and bladder neck	Orthostatic hypotension, headache, dizziness, retrograde ejaculation	Used as first-line therapy for symptomatic BPH (Terazosin is a nonselective α-1 antagonist and is also used in the treatment of hypertension)
5-alpha-reductase inhibitors (i.e., finasteride, dutasteride)	Reduced conversion of testosterone to DHT leading to decreased prostate size	Erectile dysfunction, decreased libido	Takes 3–6 months to achieve desired effect Causes a reduction in PSA
Antimuscarinics (i.e., oxybutynin tolterodine)	Inhibition of detrusor contractions	Urinary retention, dry mouth, constipation, blurry vision, confusion (avoid use in the elderly)	Used to treat associated bladder overactivity
Beta-3 agonists (i.e., mirabegron)	Relaxes detrusor muscle, increasing bladder storage and decreasing sensation for micturition	Urinary retention, hypertension	Used to treat associated bladder overactivity

CASE 7 | Benign Prostatic Hyperplasia (BPH)

A 68-year-old man without significant past medical history presents with abdominal pain and inability to urinate. He has only been able to urinate small drops the entire day and denies any similar episodes in the past. He does not take any medications. Review of systems is positive for nocturia three times nightly and a several-month history of weak stream, frequency, hesitancy, and postvoid dribbling. He is in moderate distress and his vital signs are T 98.8, BP 138/84, HR 94, and RR 14. On exam, his bladder is markedly distended, palpable, and tender; he does not have any costovertebral angle tenderness and his urethral meatus is normal and patent. On DRE, the prostate is smooth, uniformly enlarged, nontender, and non-nodular.

Conditions with Similar Presentations	**Urethral stricture:** Usual presentation in younger males in setting of injury, instrumentation, or radiation treatment. Prostate exam would be normal (see below). **Acute prostatitis:** Would also have infectious symptoms such as dysuria, fever, and recurrent UTIs. DRE would reveal a tender, swollen prostate (see below).

CASE 7 | Benign Prostatic Hyperplasia (BPH) *(continued)*

Conditions with Similar Presentations	**Prostate cancer:** DRE may reveal presence of nodules, areas that are harder than the rest of the gland, or different textures. **Neurogenic bladder:** Any nervous system disturbance that causes detrusor overactivity or underactivity, or detrusor sphincter dyssynergia (simultaneous activation of detrusor muscle and urethral sphincter). On physical exam, would expect other sensation/reflex abnormalities in the S2–S4 distribution.
Initial Diagnostic Tests	Clinical diagnosis. Consider: UA, bladder ultrasound, basic metabolic panel.
Next Steps in Management	• Acute bladder decompression with urethral or suprapubic catheterization • α_1-antagonists (e.g., terazosin, tamsulosin) and/or 5α-reductase inhibitors (e.g., finasteride).
Discussion	BPH is a non-neoplastic condition caused by hyperplasia of epithelial and smooth muscle cells within the transitional zone of the prostate gland, stimulated by circulating androgens. The transitional zone surrounds the urethra as it passes through the prostate, so hyperplasia in this area can cause difficulties with urination. BPH is the most common cause of urinary retention in men. Age is the biggest risk factor. Nearly 50% of men have BPH by 60 years of age, and prevalence continues to increase by ~10% per decade. **History:** • Obstructive symptoms: Weak/intermittent urinary stream, incomplete emptying, hesitancy, straining to void, postvoid dribbling. • Irritative symptoms: Urinary frequency, urgency, nocturia, urge incontinence. **Physical Exam:** • DRE: Prostate smooth, uniformly enlarged, nontender, and non-nodular. • Acute urinary retention: Suprapubic tenderness and bladder distension. **Diagnostics:** • UA and urine culture, to exclude infectious causes as reasons for retention. • Imaging not routinely necessary, but renal and bladder ultrasound in the setting of acute urinary retention can help to assess the bladder volume and upper urinary tracts for hydronephrosis. Evaluation of PVR volume will allow for an assessment of the patient's ability to empty their bladder. A PVR over 200 mL indicates inadequate bladder emptying. • BMP should be considered to assess renal function if there is evidence of hydronephrosis on renal US or if bladder is distended >1 L. **Management:** • Asymptomatic patients managed conservatively. • If complete obstruction or PVR >200 mL, decompress with urinary catheterization. • Symptomatic patients initially managed with pharmacotherapy. 　• α_1-antagonists (e.g., terazosin, tamsulosin) cause prostate and bladder neck smooth muscle relaxation. No effect on progression of BPH. Adverse effects include hypotension and ejaculative dysfunction. 　• 5α-reductase inhibitors (e.g., finasteride, dutasteride) block conversion of testosterone to DHT, a potent stimulator of prostate proliferation. These agents decrease prostate volume over several months. Adverse effects are decreased libido, ED, and gynecomastia. 　• Phosphodiesterase-5 inhibitor (tadalafil) decreases smooth muscle tone in the prostate. Adverse effects include dizziness, back pain, headache, and nasal congestion. • Patients whose symptoms are not improved by pharmacotherapy are candidates for bladder outlet obstruction surgery such as transurethral resection of the prostate (TURP).
Additional Considerations	**Complications:** BPH may lead to distension and hypertrophy of the bladder, hydronephrosis, impaired renal function, or increased risk of UTIs. BPH does not predispose to prostate cancer. Risks of surgery include dilutional hyponatremia (TUR syndrome), urethral stricture, incontinence, impotence, and retrograde ejaculation.

Urinary retention/LUTS Mini-Cases

Cases	Key Findings
Urethral Stricture	**Hx:** • Incomplete emptying, weak stream, split stream, dysuria, and frequency. • May have a history of straddle injury or urethral instrumentation (transurethral procedures, foley catheter placement), urethritis, lichen sclerosis, or radiation therapy. **PE:** • Suprapubic tenderness in acute obstruction. **Diagnostics:** • Bladder US shows elevated PVR volume. • Diagnosis is made by retrograde urethrography (RUG), VCUG, or cystourethroscopy. **Management:** • Urethroplasty or urethral dilation. **Discussion:** Urethral strictures are a fibrotic narrowing of the urethra typically occurring in the bulbous region. Although often idiopathic, they may occur secondary to a urethral insult. Urethral strictures present similarly to BPH but often are presented as younger males on examinations.
Acute Prostatitis	**Hx:** • Pain may be suprapubic, perineal, testicular, penile, or involving the lower back, with difficulty urinating, dysuria, and painful ejaculation. • Systemic infectious symptoms (fever, malaise) and lower urinary tract symptoms (i.e., dysuria, frequency, weak stream). • Risk factors: Genitourinary intervention (prostate biopsy, urethral instrumentation), voiding dysfunction/obstruction, indwelling catheters, and sexual contact with persons with gonorrhea and/or *Chlamydia*. **PE:** • DRE reveals an exquisitely tender, enlarged, and boggy prostate. **Diagnostics:** • Clinical diagnosis (systemic symptoms, exquisitely tender prostate). • Supporting labs include UA and urine cultures. PSA is not necessary and will be falsely elevated during active inflammation of the prostate. Prostatic massage is contraindicated due to risk of bacteremia. **Management:** UA and urine culture should guide selected antibiotic treatment. • Older men: Gram-negative organisms (*E. coli*.), trimethoprim-sulfamethoxazole or fluoroquinolone for 4–6 weeks. • Men <35 years: Acute prostatitis less common and usually secondary to an STI (*C. trachomatis* or *N. gonorrhea*), ceftriaxone IM once + doxycycline for 14 days. • If acute urinary retention is present along with persistent fever, urgent catheterization is indicated. **Discussion:** Acute prostatitis is caused by bacterial infection of the prostate. The key to differentiate prostatitis from a UTI or cystitis is the presence of systemic symptoms (usually not present with a UTI or cystitis) and a tender, edematous prostate on DRE.
Chronic Bacterial Prostatitis	**Hx:** • Recurrent UTIs that temporarily resolve with antibiotic treatment. • Symptoms persist >3 months, are typically less severe compared to acute prostatitis, but may also include pain with ejaculation and hematospermia. **PE:** • DRE may be normal or with tender enlarged prostate. **Diagnostics:** • UA and urine culture of two urine collections, obtained before and after a prostatic massage. Presence of significantly more organisms in the post-massage specimen localizes the infection to the prostate. **Management:** Fluoroquinolone for 6 weeks. **Discussion:** Chronic prostatitis is usually a gram-negative infection of the prostate. May be secondary extension of genitourinary tract infections or direct seeding after prostate biopsy.

Urinary retention/LUTS Mini-Cases (*continued*)

Chronic Nonbacterial Prostatitis/ Chronic Pelvic Pain Syndrome	**Hx:** • Several month history of urinary frequency, hesitancy with pelvic pain and painful ejaculation. • May also include diffuse perineal, penile, and/or scrotal pain, hematospermia, and ED. **PE:** • DRE often normal or with possible tender enlarged prostate. **Diagnostics:** • Diagnosis of exclusion facilitated by a negative urine culture. **Management:** • Alpha blockers, 5-alpha reductase inhibitors, NSAIDs, antimuscarinics, Sitz baths, and possibly antibiotics if secondary to prior infections. **Discussion:** Nonbacterial chronic prostatitis can be related to prior infections, neurologic in origin, autoimmune, or secondary to chemical irritation from urinary reflux. Treatment is focused on supportive measures.

URINARY INCONTINENCE

Incontinence results from derangements to the micturition cycle that impair the ability of the bladder to sufficiently empty or hold urine. An intact micturition cycle consists of:

• A filling phase: bladder is relaxed while the sphincter is contracted (low-pressure bladder filling).

• An emptying phase: bladder contracts while the sphincter relaxes (emptying of the bladder).

• The average adult bladder capacity is 500 mL, and normal voiding frequency is every 3–4 hours during wakeful hours. Waking overnight once to void is considered normal.

Urinary Incontinence Types

Diagnosis	Etiology	Treatment
Stress incontinence	Dysfunctional urinary storage due to weakness of the urethral sphincter and/or support of urethral tissues (or, e.g., following prostatectomy or vaginal delivery)	• Weight loss (if obese) • Kegel exercises • Pelvic floor physical therapy • Urethral bulking agents • Urethral sling; artificial urinary sphincter
Urgency incontinence	Dysfunctional urinary storage due to detrusor muscle hyperactivity (e.g., bladder spasm, neurogenic bladder in multiple sclerosis)	• Behavior modification (timed voiding, diet modification) • Bladder retraining • Pelvic floor physical therapy • Antimuscarinics (i.e., oxybutynin tolterodine) • Beta-3 agonists (i.e., mirabegron) • Onabotulinum toxin-A (Botox) bladder injections • Sacral neuromodulation
Mixed incontinence	Shared stress and urge components, usually with a predominant symptom profile of one or the other	• Behavior modification • Bladder retraining; pelvic floor physical therapy • Combination of treatments noted above for stress and urgency incontinence
Overflow incontinence	Incomplete emptying often due to bladder outlet obstruction (e.g., BPH, vaginal prolapse, constipation) or urine leaking from a distended, hypoactive bladder (e.g., neurogenic bladder due to peripheral nerve or spinal cord injury [i.e., cauda equina syndrome])	• Treat underlying cause of retention • Intermittent catheterization
Nocturnal enuresis	Urinary incontinence while asleep; may be due to bladder spasm, overflow, or significant evening fluid intake	• Behavior modification (fluid restriction, scheduled voiding) • Moisture alarms • Desmopressin

Patient history may point to simple or complex etiology (e.g., postoperative sphincter injury vs. diabetic neuropathy). A voiding diary may provide insight to patient drinking and voiding behavior.

Diagnostic studies are generally limited and include:

- UA and urine culture are helpful to assess for UTI or hematuria.
- Postvoid ultrasound of the bladder to assess for significant volume of residual urine (indicates inability to voluntarily empty the bladder consistent with overflow incontinence).
- Interventional diagnostic studies include cystoscopy to evaluate for physical causes of bladder irritation (e.g., tumor) or urethral obstruction (e.g., stricture).
- Urodynamic studies provide a functional assessment of the bladder and sphincter during the micturition cycle. Typically done for complicated cases, notably (mixed components or involving neurogenic etiology).

Key Associated History Findings and Incontinence Differential Diagnosis

Incontinence with Key Associated History Findings	Diagnosis
Chronic constipation	Overflow incontinence due to neurogenic dysfunction or outlet obstruction
Incontinence with increased abdominal pressure (e.g., laugh, cough, sneeze)	Stress urinary incontinence, overflow incontinence
Urinary frequency and/or urgency	Overactive bladder, urgency incontinence, overflow incontinence
Small volume voids and/or weak urinary stream	Possible overflow incontinence due to outlet obstruction
History of prostatectomy or endoscopic urethral procedure	Stress incontinence due to sphincteric injury with insufficiency
History of diabetes or spinal cord injury or other neuropathy	Stress, urge, or mixed incontinence due to neurogenic bladder

Key Associated Exam Findings and Incontinence Differential Diagnosis

Incontinence with Key Associated Exam Findings	Diagnosis
Palpable bladder, abdominal fullness (constipation)	Overflow incontinence due to neurogenic dysfunction or outlet obstruction
Bladder or vaginal prolapse, urethral stenosis, hypertonic pelvic floor muscle tone	Overflow incontinence due to outlet obstruction
Hypotonic pelvic floor muscle tone	Possible stress incontinence or overflow incontinence due to neurogenic bladder

CASE 8 | Overactive Bladder (OAB)

A 32-year-old woman presents with urge to urinate every 20–40 minutes, and urinates 10–12 times per day. She denies dysuria or incontinence with cough. She wakes up three to four times per night to urinate. She drinks tea throughout the day and has no history of frequent UTIs or tobacco use. Her vital signs and general exam are normal. Her external genital exam and pelvic floor tone on bimanual exam are also normal.

Conditions with Similar Presentations	**UTI:** In addition to urgency and frequency, would also have dysuria.
	Diabetes mellitus: When not controlled, hyperglycemia may cause an osmotic diuresis with frequency, but would not cause urgency.
	Diabetes insipidus: Produces frequent urination but would not cause urgency.
	Bladder cancer or stones: May have urgency and frequency from uroepithelial inflammation but this should cause dysuria and often hematuria.
	Prolapse: Usually presents with stress incontinence (due to weakness in the vaginal muscles surrounding the urethra). As prolapse worsens, the uterus can compress the urethra and cause overflow incontinence.
	Neurogenic bladder: Dysfunction of the urinary bladder due to disease or injury of the central nervous system or peripheral nerves involved in the control of urination. Conditions associated with neurogenic bladder include spinal cord injury, multiple sclerosis, or stroke.

CASE 8 | Overactive Bladder (OAB) (continued)

Initial Diagnostic Tests	Clinical Diagnosis: Voiding diary helpful in making diagnosis. Consider: UA, urine culture, postvoid bladder ultrasound to rule out other causes.
Next Steps in Management	• Behavior modifications (e.g., cutting down on caffeinated products, regular scheduled voiding). • Anticholinergics are first-line medications.

Discussion	OAB reflects a complex of lower urinary tract symptoms, primarily involving urinary urgency, with or without associated urge incontinence. Urinary retention is uncommon, with normal postvoid bladder ultrasound volumes.
	
	History: Urinary urgency and frequency without dysuria.
	
	Physical Exam: Normal.
	
	Diagnostics: Clinical diagnosis.
	• Voiding diary (may demonstrate significant daily fluid intake, urinary frequency, and urgency).
	• Check: UA and urine culture and postvoid bladder ultrasound (no retention for OAB) to rule out other causes
	• Urodynamic studies (may demonstrate detrusor instability) usually performed for complex cases after medication therapy has failed or where diagnosis is in doubt.
	
	Management:
	• Cut down on caffeinated products, spicy food, and other bladder irritants—especially before bedtime.
	• Regular scheduled voiding.
	• Pharmacotherapy may be initiated if behavioral modification fails.
	  • Antimuscarinic (oxybutynin, tolterodine). Adverse effects are dry eyes, dry mouth, constipation, confusion. Avoid using in geriatric population because of potential for confusion.
	  • Beta-3 agonist (mirabegron). Adverse effects include hypertension, headache.
	• Before initiating pharmacotherapy, obtain a PVR to rule out underlying urinary retention, as treatment of OAB may cause complete urinary retention in at-risk patients.
	• If pharmacotherapy fails, more invasive options include intravesical botulinum toxin injections or sacral neuromodulator implantation.

Urinary Incontinence Mini-Cases

Cases	Key Findings
Neurogenic Bladder	**Hx:** • Flaccid bladder—urinary retention, incontinence (overflow), weak stream, dribbling, recurrent UTI, loss of sensation that bladder is full. • Spastic bladder—urinary frequency, small volume voids, incontinence (urgency incontinence). **PE:** • Often normal. May present with sequelae of underlying disorder (e.g., paraplegia from spinal cord injury). • If in retention, may have palpable bladder. **Diagnostics:** • Bladder ultrasound may demonstrate elevated PVR or bladder stones from urinary stasis. • Serum creatinine to assess renal function. • UA and culture to rule out infection. • Urodynamics allow for evaluation of urinary storage and evacuation. Video urodynamics offer the ability to assess for ureteral reflux and assess the contour of the bladder wall. Urodynamics may demonstrate a large capacity, hypotonic bladder (i.e., diabetes) or a small, poorly compliant, spastic bladder (i.e., suprasacral spinal cord injury). **Management:** • Bladder decompression with indwelling foley catheter or clean intermittent catheterization. • If there is poor bladder compliance, antimuscarinics may be used for bladder relaxation and decrease of intravesicle pressures. • A primary goal of bladder decompression and maintenance of low pressures is avoidance of ureteral reflux and renal deterioration. • If unable to tolerate antimuscarinics, or if they are ineffective, more invasive measures such as intravesical botulinum toxin injections or bladder augmentation may be considered.

Urinary Incontinence Mini-Cases (*continued*)

Neurogenic Bladder	**Discussion:** Neurogenic bladder is a dysfunction of the urinary bladder due to disease or injury of the central nervous system or peripheral nerves involved in the control of urination. Conditions associated with neurogenic bladder include spinal cord injury, multiple sclerosis, or stroke. The lesion location is associated with patient symptoms. For example, suprasacral lesions may lead to bladder spasticity and irritative symptoms similar to OAB, while peripheral lesions lead to bladder atonia and urinary retention with elevated postvoid bladder volumes. Patients are at high risk for UTIs and bladder stones, so a regimen of regular, complete bladder emptying is essential. Low-pressure storage is essential for protection of the kidneys as well as urinary continence. High-pressure bladders with upper tract reflux may lead to pyelonephritis, renal scarring, and deterioration of renal function.
Stress Incontinence	**Hx:** • Urinary leakage with coughing, laughing, exercise, or other activities that increase intra-abdominal pressure. • May be associated with history of vaginal deliveries in females or prostatectomy in males. **PE:** • Loss of urine with coughing or Valsalva. May be done in lithotomy (female) or standing (male or female). **Diagnostics:** • Urethral mobility may be assessed with Q-tip test (female). A Q-tip is placed in the urethral meatus and patient is asked to Valsalva. More than 30 degrees change from horizontal classifies urethral hypermobility. • Postvoid bladder ultrasound to rule out significant PVR urine and overflow incontinence. **Management:** • Initially non-pharmacologic with weight loss (if obese), limiting alcoholic and carbonated beverages. • Kegel exercises and pelvic floor physical therapy may assist with pelvic floor strengthening; biofeedback. • Depending upon the underlying pathology, pessaries or urethral bulking agents may be considered but often represent a bridge between conservative options and more invasive surgical options. • Surgery for definitive treatment and if prolapse is present. • Synthetic and autologous slings • Artificial urinary sphincters (treatment of choice for large volume stress incontinence following prostatectomy) **Discussion:** Stress incontinence is a dysfunction of bladder storage due to weakness in the intrinsic urethral sphincter, its support, or denervation. Urine is lost during conditions that increase intraabdominal pressure such as coughing, sneezing, or laughing.

PENILE PATHOLOGIES

Erectile dysfunction (ED) is the inability to achieve or maintain an erection sufficient for satisfactory performance. It affects up to 50% of men over the age of 40 with associated perturbations in quality of life. The physiology of normal erections is complex and, as such, ED tends to be multifactorial in etiology. It can be broadly categorized as either organic or psychogenic, with pure psychogenic causes being rather rare.

ED Differential Diagnosis

Vascular	Intrinsic	Psychiatric	Miscellaneous
• Non-coronary atherosclerosis • Cardiovascular disease and risk factors (e.g., HTN, DM, smoking) • Penile fracture	• Neurological conditions (Parkinson disease, MS, GBS, diabetic neuropathy) • Anatomical conditions (Peyronie disease, hypospadias)	• Performance anxiety • Depression	• Endocrine disorders • Drug interactions (antihypertensives, antidepressants) • Hypogonadism • Alcohol use disorder

CASE 9	Erectile Dysfunction (ED)

A 54-year-old man with a 20-pack year history of smoking presents with difficulty attaining and maintaining an erection sufficient for penetration over the past 8 months. He denies any nocturnal erections and states that he is still sexually attracted to his partner. He has no history of previous surgeries or pelvic trauma. He is not on any medications and drinks two to three beers a night. On physical exam, both testes are easily palpable in the scrotum and they are of normal size and consistency. He is circumcised and his penile shaft is without palpable penile scarring.

CASE 9 | Erectile Dysfunction (ED) *(continued)*

Conditions with Similar Presentations	**Psychogenic ED:** Presents as situational ED (e.g., worse with intercourse than with masturbation) with nocturnal erections still occurring.
	Hypogonadism: May have symptoms and signs of low testosterone such as decreased muscle mass, decreased libido, loss of body hair, or gynecomastia.
	Penile fracture: Presents with pain, "pop," acute loss of erection, bruising, swelling; eggplant deformity.
	Penile hematoma: Pain, "pop," no immediate loss of erection, bruising, swelling.
	Medication side effects: Such as beta blockers or antidepressants may cause ED.
	Peyronie disease: An abnormal penile curvature or scarring on exam.
Initial Diagnostic Tests	Clinical diagnosis.
	Consider: Serum testosterone, TSH, HbA1c, and lipid profile.
Next Steps in Management	Trial of oral phosphodiesterase type 5 (PDE5) inhibitors (sildenafil, vardenafil, tadalafil).
Discussion	ED is the inability to sustain or achieve an erection for at least 6 months. It is the most common sexual disorder and treatment is often guided by the underlying etiology. The autonomic erection center provides parasympathetic (S2–S4) and sympathetic (T12–L2) input to the pelvic plexus, including the cavernous nerves, which regulate penile blood flow. The cavernous nerves deliver high local concentrations of nitric oxide (NO), which initiates a biochemical cascade resulting in smooth muscle relaxation. With smooth muscle relaxation comes increased blood flow to the penis. One of the key regulators to this biochemical cascade is phosphodiesterase enzymes (PDEs), specifically PDE-5. PDEs inactivate cGMP, resulting in smooth muscle contraction leading to detumescence.
	History: Look for risk factors (see above table).
	Physical Exam: Often normal exam, look for signs of hypogonadism (small testes).
	Diagnostics:
	• Clinical diagnosis by detailed history and physical.
	• Testing to rule out other possible causes: Serum testosterone, TSH, A1c, and lipid profile are used to determine endocrine abnormalities or cardiovascular risk factors that may be contributing to the presentation.
	• Nocturnal tumescence monitoring (philography) can aid in ruling in or out psychogenic causes of ED.
	• Duplex US or arteriography with injection of vasodilatory agents can aid in detection of arterial insufficiency or venous leaks, as well as allow for the quantification of any potential penile curvature.
	Management:
	• PDE-5 inhibitors (sildenafil, vardenafil, tadalafil) are first-line treatment (contraindicated in patients taking nitrates, as this may cause severe hypotension).
	• Psychotherapy may be beneficial in patients with psychogenic ED.
	• Testosterone supplementation alongside PDE-5 treatment for patients with hypogonadism.
	• Intracavernous injection or intraurethral suppositories of alprostadil (prostaglandin-E1 agonist) are a second-line treatment option.
	• Mechanical methods (vacuum pump) are a second-line treatment option.
	• Surgical treatment with penile prosthesis is typically last-line therapy for ED.

Penile Abnormality Mini-Cases

Cases	Key Findings
Ischemic Priapism (IP)	**Hx:** • Painful erection lasting >4 hours, persisting after or presenting without sexual stimulation. • Most common risk factors include drugs (i.e., intracavernous injection, PDE5 inhibitors, psychotropics, beta-blockers, cocaine) and blood dyscrasias (i.e., sickle cell disease, leukemia). **PE:** • Rigid and tender corpora cavernosa with soft glans is pathognomonic. **Diagnostics:** • Cavernosal blood aspirate will be dark, with pO_2 <30, pCO_2 >60, and pH <7.25. • Penile Doppler US shows minimal blow flow in the cavernous artery.

Penile Abnormality Mini-Cases (*continued*)

Ischemic Priapism (IP)	**Management:** • High-risk patients should be placed on telemetry and treatment should be initiated emergently. • Initial interventions include corporal aspiration/irrigation and intracavernosal sympathomimetic agent (phenylephrine) injections, with creation of a surgical shunt reserved for refractory cases. **Discussion:** • Medical emergency that accounts for 95% of priapism cases. It is due to persistent cavernous venous occlusion (low outflow) that starts to decrease arterial inflow, eventually leading to penile compartment syndrome. • The feared complications of corporal fibrosis and permanent ED become increasingly likely if IP lasts longer than 24–36 hours. • >50% of cases are idiopathic. Regardless of the cause, the most important step in assessment is distinguishing ischemic from non-ischemic priapism,* as their management differs markedly.
	*__Non-ischemic priapism (NIP)__ is a rare, non-emergent form of priapism usually associated with recent perineal or penile trauma that results in formation of a fistula between the cavernosal artery and corpus cavernosum. Patients present with a partially erect, non-tender penis. The high inflow, high outflow state that is characteristic of NIP can be identified by a normal cavernosal blood gas (pO_2 90, pCO_2 <40, pH 7.4) and high peak systolic velocity in the cavernosal artery seen on penile Doppler. It is initially treated conservatively (perineal compression, active surveillance), as 62% of cases spontaneously resolve. Selective arterial embolization is reserved for refractory cases.
Penile Carcinoma	**Hx:** • Enlarging painless ulceration or mass of the penis with or without inguinal lymphadenopathy. • Negative screenings for syphilis (RPR). Risk factors for this disease include, phimosis,* human papillomavirus, HIV, and tobacco use. • Circumcision is a protective factor. **PE:** • Painless mass or ulceration of the penis typically near or involving the glans, inguinal lymphadenopathy, possible phimosis obstructing the lesion. **Diagnostics:** • Excisional biopsy. • Staging is accomplished with fine-needle aspiration, which may require a follow-up sentinel node biopsy or inguinal lymph node dissection as well as CT pelvis and MRI/US.
Penile Carcinoma	**Management:** • Small tumor: Local excision, laser ablation, and/or radiation. • Large invasive tumors: Partial or total penectomy, inguinal lymph node dissection, and adjuvant chemotherapy. **Discussion:** • Primary squamous cell carcinoma of the penis is rare but most commonly presents in elderly men. • The prognosis is determined by lymph node involvement, and the 5-year survival rate ~85% in locally confined tumors.
	*__Phimosis__ is tight foreskin unable to be fully retracted from the glans penis. It is an independent risk factor for penile carcinoma and it can be, post-infectious, congenital, or iatrogenic due to scarring from circumcision or trauma. It can be treated conservatively with topical corticosteroids and stretching exercise, but may require surgery. It may become complicated by paraphimosis, a urological emergency characterized by inability to reduce the foreskin and signs of penile ischemia (i.e., blue skin, firm glans).

14

Obstetrics and Gynecology

Lead Authors: Catherine Wheatley, MD; Leslie Ballard MD
Contributors: Jacquelyne Anyaso, MD; Jasmine Solola, MD;
Olivia Murray, MD; Alexandria N. Young, MD, PhD

INTRODUCTION

Female reproductive health care includes physiologic health support and maintenance (e.g., annual gynecologic care, prenatal care, contraceptive support), along with a broad range of pathology in both the gynecologic and obstetric patients. As is the case in much of medicine, a focus on foundational elements like maternal-fetal physiology, the physiologic menstrual cycle, and pelvic anatomy lends clarity to build understanding of the various concerns in female reproductive healthcare. Most of the content in this chapter is based on the authors expertise and information from American College of Obstetricians and Gynecologists Practice Bulletins and Committee Opinions, DynaMed, Williams Obstetrics, 25e, 2018 and Williams Gynecology, 4e, 2020.

OBSTETRICS

Obstetrics is a branch of medicine that specializes in the health and well-being of the pregnant individual and fetus. Through this chapter we will present the practical aspects of obstetrics in a manner that is useful for the medical student at the bedside while preparing for the USMLE Step 2 exam.

PREGNANCY

Definitions

Pregnancy: The period in which the fetus develops in utero, typically 280 days, which is about 40 weeks from the last menstrual period (LMP) or 38 weeks from conception for the patient with a 28-day menstrual cycle. This is divided into three trimesters:

- First trimester: 0 to 13+6 weeks
- Second trimester: 14+0 to 27+6 weeks
- Third trimester: beyond 27+6 weeks

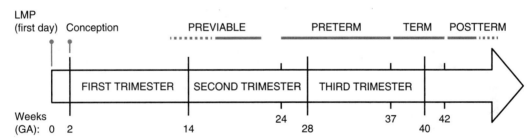

Pregnancy timing and dating. (Modified from Cunningham F, Leveno KJ, Bloom SL, Dashe JS, Hoffman BL, Casey BM, Spong CY. Chapter 7. Embryogenesis and Fetal Development. Williams Obstetrics, 25th ed. 2018.)

- Gestational age (GA) is the period of time from the first day of the last menstrual period expressed in weeks.
- The conceptus is called an embryo until 10 weeks, thereafter termed fetus until delivery.
- A neonate delivered during the time periods illustrated above is either preterm, term, or postterm.
- A neonate delivered before 23–24 weeks is considered pre-viable, as they generally cannot survive extrauterine life with the current medical interventions available.

Gravida: Number of times a patient has ever been pregnant, including current pregnancy.

Para: Refers to the outcomes of each pregnancy.

　　Term (37+ weeks' gestational age)

　　Preterm (20–36+6 weeks' gestational age)

　　Abortion or early pregnancy losses (prior to 20 weeks' gestational age)

　　Living children (any age).

For example, a patient who has been pregnant five times, with two term deliveries, one preterm delivery, a first-trimester miscarriage, an induced abortion at 15 weeks, and three living children would be described as G5P2123.

Nulliparous: Has not previously been pregnant

Primiparous: First pregnancy

Multiparous: Has had at least 1 prior pregnancy

Physiologic Changes in Pregnancy

Weight gain	25–35 pounds weight gain is expected in a patient with a singleton pregnancy and prepregnancy BMI between 18.5–25
Renal	Increased renal flow and GFR by ~50%
Cardiovascular	Increase in heart rate (~10 bpm), stroke volume and cardiac output (~40%), decreased systemic vascular resistance, with gradual decrease in blood pressure in second trimester
Hematology	Increase in blood volume by 15%, slight decrease hematocrit, hypercoagulable state (increased clotting factors, decreased proteins C and S)
Pulmonary	Increase in tidal volume and respiratory minute volume (results in a respiratory alkalosis that facilitates transfer of CO_2 from fetus), respiratory rate and vital capacity unchanged but gradual decrease in expiratory reserve
Gastrointestinal	Increase in gastric emptying and transit time and decrease in all sphincter tone, decreased gallbladder contractility

Symptoms of Pregnancy

- Amenorrhea in a healthy patient of reproductive age with cyclic menstrual bleeding is one of the earliest symptoms suggestive of pregnancy.
- Nausea, breast tenderness, and fatigue occur early in pregnancy
- Perception of fetal movements usually starts at 18- to 20-weeks' gestation.
- As the uterine size increases, round ligament and back pain are common, often through the second and third trimesters.
- Some mild lower extremity edema (symmetric, resolved with elevation), can also be normal in the later third trimester.

Signs of Pregnancy

Breast	• Breast engorgement • Areolar hyperpigmentation • Prominence of veins around the areola
Skin (does not happen to all patients)	• Darkening of forehead, bridge of nose, cheekbones (chloasma) • Darkening of lower midline from umbilicus to pubis (linea nigra) • Striae (silver) • Spider angiomata • Palmar erythema
Vagina	• Bluish discoloration of the vagina due to congestion of pelvis (Chadwick sign) • Increased physiologic discharge
Cervix	• Cervical softening and dilation of the external os
Uterus	• Widening and softening of the body of the uterus—seen at 6–8 weeks (Hegar sign) • At 10–12 weeks the uterus is at the pubic symphysis • At 16 weeks it is at the midpoint between the pubic symphysis and umbilicus • At 20 weeks the uterus is palpated at the umbilicus, and the fundal height in centimeters will be approximately the same as the number of weeks of pregnancy from here forward • After 37 weeks, as the fetal head descends into the pelvis, the fundal height may decrease
Fetal heart tones via Doppler	Typically heard ~10–12 weeks, normal rate of 110–160 beats/minute
Musculoskeletal	• Lordosis • Gait changes later in pregnancy • Diastasis recti

Initial Diagnostic Tests

Early pregnancy tests measure the level of hCG subunit, which is detected in maternal serum as early as 20–22 days after the last menstrual period. These levels return to normal 21–24 days after delivery. Urine studies will detect hCG as low as 20–25 mIU/mL, so urine hCG is the initial test for pregnancy.

Ultrasound is used to confirm intrauterine pregnancy and to rule out ectopic pregnancy and other pathology. The gestational sac is visible ~5 weeks on transvaginal ultrasound (TVUS).

Dating:

- Commercially available pregnancy tests are sensitive enough to detect human chorionic gonadotropin (hCG) around the time of the missed menstrual cycle (~4–5 weeks).
- Ultrasound may detect pregnancy beginning with the gestational sac containing a yolk sac around 5 weeks and the fetal pole with cardiac motion around 6 weeks.

Estimation of Due Date (estimated date of confinement [EDC] or estimated date of delivery [EDD]):

- Menstrual dating: add 280 days from certain LMP or 266 from date of certain ovulation.
- Ultrasound: There should not be a difference in due date by USG from due date by LMP of more than 1 week in first trimester, 2 weeks in second trimester, or 3 weeks in third trimester.
  - Crown-rump length (CRL) in first trimester is most accurate (6–12 weeks)
  - Other biometrics are used after 13 weeks (biparietal diameter [BPD], abdominal circumference [AC], femur length [FL])
- Assistive reproductive technology: calculated based on date of embryo transfer.

Prenatal Counseling

Routine prenatal care counseling includes discussion on:

- Healthy weight gain based on prepregnancy body mass index
- Healthy diet and safe exercise, including discussion on foods/drinks/medications to avoid (see below tables)
- Obstetric "warning signs:"
  - Early pregnancy: severe cramping and pain, vaginal bleeding, and severe vomiting with inability to tolerate any intake
  - After 20 weeks: focused on contractions, leakage of fluid, vaginal bleeding, absence or significant decrease in fetal movements, persistent headache, right upper quadrant (RUQ)/epigastric pain, visual disturbances, and severe/progressive edema
- Peripartum mood disorders (along with screening during pregnancy and postpartum)
- Vaccination recommendations (influenza, COVID, pertussis)
- Travel recommendations (considerations about Zika virus, tips for safe car and flight travel)
- Genetic screening options
- Postnatal considerations including plans for neonatal feeding (breast vs. formula) and contraceptive plans

Substance Use Disorders in Pregnancy

Substance	Fetal Associations	Management
Alcohol	Fetal alcohol syndrome—pre- and postnatal growth restriction, mid-face hypoplasia, microcephalus, microphthalmia, renal and cardiac defects, intellectual disability • Consuming >6 drinks per day increases risk • Has been described after ingestion of >2 oz daily	Avoid use • Counseling programs have been shown to be beneficial • Barbiturate management of withdrawal symptoms (benzodiazepines are avoided due to teratogenicity) • Nutrition counseling and supplementation due to risk of nutritional deficiency
Caffeine	• Known teratogen in animal models • Human data is lacking	• Avoid excessive caffeinated intake (e.g., coffee, tea, soda)

Substance Use Disorders in Pregnancy

Substance	Fetal Associations	Management
Cocaine	Crosses the placenta and has vasoconstrictive and hypertensive effects that may result in: • Spontaneous abortion • Preterm birth • Abruptio placentae • Fetal growth restriction • Bowel atresia • Heart, limb, face abnormalities • CNS complications • Developmental delay	• Avoid use • Distinguish cocaine use from preeclampsia in patients presenting with hypertension
Cannabis	• Crosses the placenta and found in breast milk • Low birth weight • Preterm birth, stillbirth • Impaired neurocognitive development	Avoid use
Methamphetamines	• Low birth weight • Neurodevelopmental delay • Intrauterine fetal demise	Avoid use Methamphetamine may cause maternal: • Hypertension • Cardiomyopathy • Cardiac arrhythmias • Paranoia and psychosis
Tobacco/ cigarette smoking	• Spontaneous abortion • Preterm delivery • Abruptio placentae • Low birth weight • Sudden infant death syndrome • Respiratory illness of childhood	Avoid use Smoking cessation programs and resources should be provided to patients in the preconception period
Opioids	• Not known to be teratogenic • Opioid withdrawal is associated with miscarriage, preterm delivery, and fetal death • Neonatal abstinence syndrome • Opioid withdrawal may be more dangerous than exposure	• Pregnant patients should be enrolled in a maintenance program, usually with methadone or buprenorphine • Neonatology should be prepared to manage neonatal abstinence syndrome if it occurs after delivery

Prenatal Exposures/Teratogens

Drug(s)	Fetal Abnormality
ACE inhibitors	Renal tubular dysplasia, renal failure, oligohydramnios
Androgens	Male fetus: Advanced genital development Female fetus: Virilization
Carbamazepine	Neural tube defects, microcephaly, IUGR, fingernail hypoplasia
Diethylstilbesterol	Adenocarcinoma of the cervix or vagina, abnormal uterus, cervix, or testes
Lithium	Ebstein anomaly and congenital cardiac defects
Phenytoin	Dysmorphic craniofacial features, cardiac defects, intellectual disability, growth retardation, fingernail hypoplasia
Tetracycline	Yellowish-brown discoloration of deciduous teeth and hypoplasia of enamel
Thalidomide	Limb deficiencies, microtia, GI and cardiac abnormalities
Vitamin A analogues	Microtia, thymic agenesis, cleft lip, cleft palate, craniofacial dysmorphism, cardiovascular defects, intellectual disability
Valproic acid	Spina bifida and other neural tube defects

Routine Exam in Pregnancy

Routine obstetric physical exam varies depending on the stage of pregnancy and patient's concerns.

- All visits should include an assessment of maternal vital signs and weight.
- After 12 weeks' gestation, the fetal heart tones can be detected by portable Doppler monitor. These are obtained at every visit beyond that point.
- After 20 weeks' gestation:
  - Fundal height can be measured
  - Speculum exam may be performed if the patient is due for cervical cancer screening or has concerns about discharge/leakage of amniotic fluid
  - Cervical exam may be performed if the patient is experiencing contractions or pressure
  - Additional maneuvers will be performed related to patient-specific concerns

Routine Tests in Pregnancy

First visit	CBC
	HIV
	RPR
	Hep B/C
	Type and screen
	Urine culture
	Gonorrhea, chlamydia and trichomonas
	Rubella
	Varicella
	Pap (if due for screening)
	Dating ultrasound
10 weeks	Noninvasive prenatal genetic screening (based on patient preference)
	Nuchal translucency ultrasound
15 weeks	Alpha-fetoprotein (AFP)
18–20 weeks	Anatomy ultrasound
24–28 weeks	Glucose challenge test (1 hour)
28 weeks	HIV
	RPR
	CBC
36 weeks	GBS (group B strep test)

CASE 1 | Normal Pregnancy

A 23-year-old presents with 3 weeks of nausea, vomiting, bilateral breast tenderness, and is concerned that her period is late. Her last menstrual period (LMP) was 9 weeks ago. She has vaginal sex with a male partner and uses condoms inconsistently. On exam, abdomen is flat and non-tender with normal bowel sounds. Bimanual exam reveals a non-tender, enlarged uterus (~10 weeks' size).

Conditions with Similar Presentations	**Other causes of amenorrhea:** Can be distinguished from pregnancy by absence of nausea, vomiting, breast tenderness, and negative hCG. See "Chief Concerns Specific to Pregnancy" table at the end of the case for more pregnancy-related differentials.
Initial Diagnostic Tests	Urine hCG (urine pregnancy test [UPT])

CASE 1 | Normal Pregnancy *(continued)*

Next Steps in Management	• Pregnancy options—counseling • Prenatal vitamins • Obtain first-visit routine labs
Discussion	Conception is likely to occur in 30% of couples in the first month of unprotected sexual intercourse, and rates of conception increase to 75% and 90% after 6 months and 1 year, respectively. Knowledge of maternal-fetal physiology can assist understanding of pathologic conditions that can arise in pregnancy. **History:** Consider diagnosis in reproductive-age females who have vaginal sex with male partners. Initial symptoms include amenorrhea, fatigue, breast tenderness, nausea, and constipation. Later symptoms include dyspnea, lower extremity edema, urinary frequency, musculoskeletal aches and pains. **Physical Exam:** See Introduction for more details. • Fundal height (FH) changes: Start to measure at week 20 • Fetal heart tones (FHTs): Heard by Doppler starting at 12 weeks **Diagnostics:** • Urine hCG detected 8 days after conception • Obtain first-visit routine labs—see "Routine Tests in Pregnancy" table above **Management:** Prenatal visits should occur: Every 4 weeks from diagnosis to 28 weeks Every 2 weeks from 28-36 weeks Every week after 36 weeks • See "Routine Exam in Pregnancy" section above for details. • Counseling: See "Prenatal Counseling" section above. • Sexual activity has no adverse outcomes during pregnancy. If postcoital spotting, cramping, or bleeding occurs, sexual activity should be avoided until further evaluation. Nutrition: • Caloric requirement: additional 340 and 450 kcal/day in the second and third trimesters if not overweight or obese at baseline. • Protein: 1 g/kg/day. • Calcium: 1000–1300 mg/day • Elemental iron: 30mg/day during the second and third trimester • Folic acid: 0.4 mg per day 1 month before conception and 3 months after delivery. Immunization: • Killed virus, recombinant vaccines, and toxoids are safe during pregnancy • Influenza vaccine and COVID vaccine should be given • Tetanus toxoid and acellular pertussis (TDaP) given in the third trimester of each pregnancy
Additional Considerations	**Screening:** All reproductive-age females should be assessed and receive counseling regarding sexual activity and potential pregnancy plans. If applicable, counsel on prevention options and safe-sex practices. **Complications:** See below table for pregnancy-related concerns; complications will be covered in subsequent cases. *Patients instructed to seek advice if the following occur:* Decreased fetal movement, contractions, vaginal bleeding, rupture of membranes, progressive swelling of hands and/or face, persistent headache, visual disturbances, persistent RUQ or epigastric pain.

Pregnancy-Related Concerns and Key Points

Concern	Key Points
Nausea and vomiting	Classically in first trimester and can occur at any time throughout the day (though colloquially known as "morning sickness") May occur due to progestin relaxation effect on GI smooth muscle, decreased gut motility, and/or loss of lower esophageal sphincter (LES) tone with gastroesophageal reflux Treatment goals: Maintain adequate hydration and nutrition, correct electrolyte abnormalities, and antiemetics as needed *Intermittent Mild Symptoms:* • Avoid triggering foods/drinks and ingest smaller, more frequent meals • Temporarily hold prenatal vitamin and only take folate • Trial ginger, pyridoxine, doxylamine, and/or acid reflux treatments *Persistent Mild Symptoms:* • All of the above plus promethazine or prochlorperazine *Moderate to Severe Symptoms:* • All of the above plus ondansetron and/or metoclopramide • IV fluid and electrolyte replacement if evidence of dehydration or electrolyte imbalance *Refractory Symptoms:* • Trial of IV methylprednisolone • Consider parenteral nutrition until symptoms improve **Hyperemesis gravidarum:** • Severe persistent vomiting causing greater than 5% body weight loss and electrolyte disturbance • Occurs due to excessive hCG (multifetal gestation, molar pregnancy)
GERD	May occur due to relaxation of LES and decreased transit time from progesterone effect Treatment: • Smaller more frequent meals, avoidance of triggering foods, and avoiding lying down after eating • Antacids, H_2 blockers, or proton pump inhibitors if severe
Constipation	May occur from decreased bowel motility due to progestin relaxation effect Treatment: • Oral hydration, stool softeners, bulking agents/fiber • Laxatives if needed (generally avoided in the third trimester due to the risk of preterm labor [PTL])
Hemorrhoids	May occur due to increased venous stasis due to inferior vena cava compression and/or increased abdominal pressure from constipation Treatment: • Hydration, stool softeners, increased dietary fiber intake • Topical anesthetics and/or topical steroids
Biliary colic/ gallstones	May occur due to increased estrogen (increased cholesterol secretion), increased progesterone (relaxation of biliary motility), and/or bile salt secretion, which causes further cholesterol concentration Treatment: • Supportive treatment, pain control, and avoidance of dietary triggers • Severe or complicated courses may require cholecystectomy (optimally performed in second trimester) Rule out other causes of RUQ/epigastric pain (e.g., preeclampsia, Hemolysis, Elevated Liver enzymes, Low Platelets (HELLP) syndrome, and acute fatty liver of pregnancy)
Round ligament pain	Occurs in the mid-late second trimester due to pulling/stretching from growing uterus with fetal or maternal movements.] Treatment: Heat, acetaminophen, and/or pregnancy support belt
Low back pain	May occur due to mass effect from the growing uterus, temporary increased lumbar lordosis, and/or stretching of ligaments from effect of relaxin in third trimester Treatment: • Exercise/stretching, massage, heat • Acetaminophen; muscle relaxants • Physical therapy for severe symptoms

Pregnancy-Related Concerns and Key Points (*Continued*)

Concern	Key Points
Urinary frequency	May occur due to increased intravascular volume, increased renal flow and GFR, and/or compression of the bladder by the growing uterus Treatment: Reassurance that increased frequency is normal and to continue hydration Rule out UTI, *pyelonephritis* (more common in pregnancy due to urinary stasis)
Dyspnea of pregnancy	May occur due to respiratory center stimulation (from increased fetal CO_2) leading to chronic hyperventilation Treatment: Reassurance and treat the underlying cause Rule out other causes of dyspnea (e.g., asthma exacerbation, pulmonary embolism [pregnancy is a hypercoagulable state]), peripartum cardiomyopathy)
Peripheral edema	May occur due to compression of inferior vena cava by the growing uterus and/or increased plasma volume. Treatment: • Elevation of lower extremities, lying on side when sleeping • Compression stockings Assess for *preeclampsia* or *VTE* if other associated symptoms
Varicose veins	May occur due to venous stasis, increased intravascular volume and/or venous smooth muscle relaxation Treatment: • Elevation, compression stockings • Surgical treatment if severe and no improvement/resolution postpartum
Carpal tunnel syndrome	May occur due to decreased tunnel caliber and compression of the median nerve from interstitial edema Treatment: • Wrist splinting • Corticosteroid injection or surgical release if severe
Dermatologic changes	Spider angiomata and palmar erythema—due to increased estrogen Hyperpigmentation of the face [*melasma/chloasma*], areolae, abdominal midline [*linea nigra*], umbilicus, and perineum, are caused by increased melanocyte-stimulating hormone and steroid hormones Treatment: • Reassurance • Topical treatment and/or postpartum dermatology referral if discoloration persists and is bothersome

Abnormalities Specific to Pregnancy

Symptom or Sign	Differential Diagnosis
Abdominal pain	Preterm labor, labor, ectopic pregnancy, miscarriage (missed, incomplete, spontaneous), threatened miscarriage, placental abruption, uterine rupture, preeclampsia, eclampsia, acute fatty liver of pregnancy
Depressed mood	Postpartum blues, peripartum depression
Hypertension	Gestational hypertension, molar pregnancy, preeclampsia, eclampsia, HELLP syndrome
Nausea and/or vomiting	Normal pregnancy, hyperemesis gravidarum
Postpartum hemorrhage	Infection, uterine atony, uterine rupture or trauma, retained placenta, morbidly adherent placenta, Disseminated intravascular coagulation (DIC)
Uterine size less than dates	Incorrect dating, oligohydramnios, fetal growth restriction
Uterine size greater than dates	Incorrect dating, polyhydramnios, fetal macrosomia, molar pregnancy, multiple fetal gestation
Vaginal bleeding	Preterm labor, labor, implantation bleeding, ectopic pregnancy, molar pregnancy, miscarriage (missed, incomplete, spontaneous), threatened miscarriage, premature rupture of membranes, placental abruption, placenta previa, vasa previa

LABOR & FETAL MONITORING

Labor is defined as regular uterine contractions resulting in effacement and dilation of the cervix, ending with delivery of the neonate and expulsion of the placenta. Biochemical connective tissue changes in the cervix and biomechanical changes in the myometrium precede the onset of labor. The three "P's" of labor are as follows:

- **Power:** The force generated by uterine contractions
  - When measured internally, contractions can be quantified by Montevideo units (a rough measure of area under the curve of the contraction on the monitor)
  - The presence of 3–5 contractions in 10 minutes is considered an adequate contraction pattern and often adds up to at least 200 Montevideo units (minimum measure for adequacy)
- **Passenger:** The successful passage of the fetus (passenger) through the pelvic canal depends on:
  - Fetal size
  - Fetal lie and presentation
  - Position of the fetal head in the pelvis
- **Pelvis:** Adequacy of the maternal bony pelvis and soft tissue also play a role in successful vaginal birth

Stages of Labor

Normal labor is a continuous process and is divided into distinct stages as given below:

- **Stage 1:** From onset of labor until 10 centimeters (cm) of cervical dilation
  - *Latent phase*: Onset of labor up to 6cm of cervical dilation
    - Duration unpredictable (usually <20 h in primiparous, and <14 h multiparous patients), usually longer than active phase
  - *Active phase*: 6–10 cm of cervical dilation
    - Faster and more predictable pattern of progression
    - Inadequate contractions or protraction may be augmented with oxytocin and/or amniotomy
- **Stage 2:** From the time of achieving 10 cm until delivery of the neonate
  - <3 h in a primiparous and <2 h in multiparous patients (may be an additional hour in each group if received an epidural)
- **Stage 3:** From delivery of the neonate until delivery of the placenta, <30 minutes for all patients

  Signs of placental separation from the uterus include:
  - Elongation of the umbilical cord
  - A gush of blood
  - A feeling of fundal rebound as the placenta releases

Stages of Labor

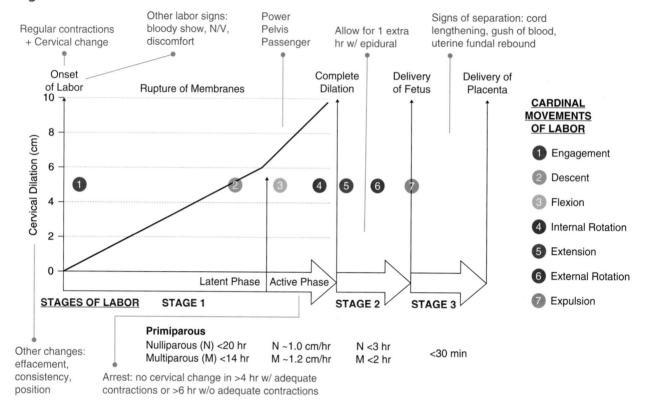

Regular contractions + Cervical change

Other labor signs: bloody show, N/V, discomfort

Power
Pelvis
Passenger

Allow for 1 extra hr w/ epidural

Signs of separation: cord lengthening, gush of blood, uterine fundal rebound

Onset of Labor

Rupture of Membranes

Complete Dilation

Delivery of Fetus

Delivery of Placenta

CARDINAL MOVEMENTS OF LABOR

1 Engagement
2 Descent
3 Flexion
4 Internal Rotation
5 Extension
6 External Rotation
7 Expulsion

Cervical Dilation (cm)

Latent Phase | Active Phase

STAGES OF LABOR   STAGE 1   STAGE 2   STAGE 3

Other changes: effacement, consistency, position

Primiparous
Nulliparous (N) <20 hr   N ~1.0 cm/hr   N <3 hr
Multiparous (M) <14 hr   M ~1.2 cm/hr   M <2 hr   <30 min

Arrest: no cervical change in >4 hr w/ adequate contractions or >6 hr w/o adequate contractions

Other Definitions in the Setting of Labor

Ferning: The formation of a fern-like pattern (arborization) of crystallization when amniotic fluid from the posterior fornix of the vagina is air-dried on microscope slide. When this is seen in vaginal fluid in pregnant patients it confirms spontaneous rupture of membranes.

Pooling: The term used to describe when amniotic fluid collects in the posterior fornix of the vagina.

Station: This term indicates the location of the most leading part of the fetus in the pelvis. The ischial spines (palpable at 4 and 8 o'clock on the side of the vaginal canal) are the reference points for fetal station. When the presenting fetal part reaches this point, this position is designated as station "0." Negative numbers are assigned when the presenting part is above this point, positive numbers when past (closer to the introitus). +3 corresponds to visible scalp at the introitus, suggestive of impending delivery.

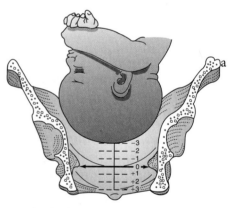

Reproduced with permission from AH De Cherney, Lnathan et al., CURRENT Diagnosis & Treatment: Obstetrics & Gynecology. 12th ed, New York: McGraw Hill, 2019 and Reproduced with permission from Benson RC. Handbook of Obstetrics & Gynecology. 8th ed; Los Altos, CA: McGraw Hill 1983.

Induction of Labor

Common Indications for Induction	Methods for Induction
• Late-term or postterm gestational age; can also offer electively at 39+0* • Preeclampsia, chronic and gestational hypertension • Diabetes (pregestational and gestational) • Category II fetal tracing, abnormal antenatal testing, and/or fetal growth restriction	"Ripening" the cervix with • Prostaglandins [gel (PGE₂), dinoprostone insert (PGE₂), or misoprostol (PGE₁M)] • Mechanical balloon dilation of the cervix
	After ripening, contractions are induced with IV oxytocin (Pitocin)
	Artificial rupture of membranes (ROM) or amniotomy can also assist the induction process

*The desire to no longer be pregnant without other comorbidities is NOT an indication for elective induction prior to 39+0 weeks, as early term (37+0 to 38+6) neonates have higher rates of neonatal morbidity.

Pain Management Options in Labor

Option	Comment	Phase of Labor
Systemic	Narcotics: • Fentanyl • IM morphine sulfate • Nalbuphine	• May be used in early labor • Not in active phase (to avoid neonatal respiratory depression)
Pudendal nerve (PN) block	• PN can be infiltrated with anesthetic bilaterally where it passes posterior to the ischial spine • Provides perineal analgesia	• During second stage or for perineal repair
Epidural anesthesia	The catheter is placed in the epidural space via the L3–L4 interspace There is a risk of postdural puncture headache (PDPH), which can occur after an unintentional dural puncture PDPH is thought to be secondary to decreased CSF pressure due to loss of CSF in epidural space	• Can use any time in labor • May provide continuous infusion of anesthetic throughout labor and delivery • Must block T10–L1 for first stage of labor and extend to S2–S4 during late first stage and second stage of labor
Spinal anesthesia	A one-time anesthetic bolus is administered directly into the spinal canal	• Cesarean delivery
Inhaled nitrous oxide	Patient-controlled inhaled pain option	• Can be used throughout labor
Non-pharmacologic	• Meditation • Focused breathing • Doula/support person • Aromatherapy	• Can be used in all stages

Delivery of Neonate

Most deliveries are approached via vaginal route unless there are contraindications.

Contraindications to Vaginal Delivery

- Maternal or fetal instability
- Placental abnormalities (previa, placenta accreta spectrum)
- Cephalopelvic disproportion—a potential cause of arrest disorders (dilation and descent)
- Prior uterine surgery in active uterine segment (prior classical cesarean and/or transmural myomectomy)
- Fetal malpresentation
- Prolonged and/or arrested labor
- Risk of vertical transmission for specific infections (e.g., active HSV II)

Cesarean Route of Birth

- Results in delivery of the fetus from an abdominal approach; performed when vaginal delivery is contraindicated or there is fetal intolerance to labor
- Most are performed via a low-transverse incision on the uterus
- Complications include infection, hemorrhage, and, if over three or more cesareans, subsequent need for cesarean birth in all future pregnancies with attendant risk of significant adhesive disease and abdominal visceral injury

Trial of Labor After Cesarean (TOLAC)

TOLAC is a safe option for many patients after a prior cesarean birth. The most worrisome complication of attempt at vaginal birth after prior cesarean is uterine rupture. People who are at increased risk for uterine rupture include:

- Those who have had multiple cesarean sections
- Prior uterine incision in the active segment of the myometrium
- Short interval (<18 months) since last cesarean

- Those being induced
- Those with prior uterine infection at the time of cesarean

FETAL MONITORING

The basis of both antepartum and intrapartum fetal monitoring is the premise that events affecting the fetus will cause measurable adaptive responses. Ambulatory-based antepartum fetal surveillance is utilized preemptively in settings where the fetus is being monitored for chronic maternal and/or fetal pathologies. During labor, intrapartum fetal monitoring is used to guide interventions, including potential for cesarean birth if fetal intolerance to labor.

Antepartum Fetal Surveillance (Outside of Labor)

This is commonly done starting at 32–34 weeks when the risk for fetal demise is elevated due to a fetal and/or maternal condition.

Test	Comment
Fetal movement count	• Recommended for all patients • Patient instructed to track number of fetal movements over 1 hour (average ~10 movements over 2 hours) and report any decrease
Nonstress test (NST)	• External fetal heart rate (FHR) and contraction monitoring • Considered reactive if two accelerations in 20 minutes • Nonreactive NSTs require further assessment, usually with BPP
Biophysical profile (BPP)	• Scoring done based on NST plus four ultrasound findings (fetal tone, breathing, movement, amniotic fluid volume) • Categories are scored 2 (normal) or 0 (abnormal) and added up • BPP of 8–10 is normal and 0–4 worrisome for asphyxia; 6 is equivocal and requires further assessment
Amniotic fluid volume or index (AFI)	• Measure of fluid volume by ultrasound • Can assess for oligohydramnios (AFI <5 cm) or polyhydramnios (AFI >25 cm)
Contraction stress test (CST)/ Oxytocin challenge test (OCT)	• Performed at or after 34+0 weeks • When delivery is indicated, contractions are provoked by nipple stimulation or IV oxytocin, and the fetus' ability to tolerate contractions is assessed with a fetal heart monitor
Doppler velocimetry	• Doppler assessment of umbilical artery (in setting of fetal growth restriction) and/or fetal middle cerebral artery (in setting of fetal anemia/alloimmunization) • Decreased, absent, or diastolic reversal of umbilical artery flow is worrisome for fetal compromise/acidosis
Percutaneous umbilical blood sampling (PUBS)	• Used when an accurate fetal hematocrit (fetal anemia) needs to be obtained • Can also be used for fetal transfusion, karyotyping, and assessment of other blood cell types (i.e., platelets in fetal thrombocytopenia)

Fetal heart rate (FHR) monitoring or cardiotocography (CTG):

- Can be conducted externally (Doppler ultrasound) or internally (fetal scalp electrode) and can be monitored continuously or intermittently in patients with no significant obstetric risk factors.
- Each small square in the CTG chart is equal to 10 seconds and large square is one minute.
- Always requires a measure of contractions to interpret fully.

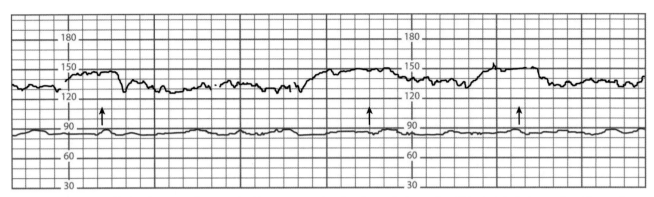

Reactive nonstress test. Notice there are at least two fetal heart rate accelerations (arrows) of more than 15 beats/min for longer than 15 seconds. The black line reflects fetal heart rate, whereas the purple line reflects the mother's. (Reproduced with permission from Cunningham F, Leveno KJ, et al., Williams Obstetrics, 26e, New York: McGraw-Hill Education; 2022.)

- Tocometry: Measures the frequency and duration of uterine contractions.
- Intrauterine pressure catheters measure the frequency, duration, and intensity of contractions but are invasive and can be done only after the rupture of membranes, so most patients undergo external monitoring.

Assess contractions for the following:

- **Duration:** Length of time the contractions last
- **Intensity:** Strength of contractions—can only be calculated when an internal pressure catheter is being used. The intensity is calculated by subtracting the base pressure of the contraction from the peak pressure of the contraction and adding the sum of each contraction in a 10-minute period.

Based on monitoring and interpretation of the findings, a category is assigned conveying the risk of fetal hypoxia:

- **Category I:** Normal tracing and low risk of fetal hypoxic acidemia
- **Category II:** Indeterminate tracing, needs close monitoring to assess trends
- **Category III:** Abnormal tracing and increased risk of fetal hypoxic acidemia, indicating immediate delivery if unable to quickly resolve

FHR interpretation includes several key components and must be assessed in reference to contraction pattern.

Rate:

- Normal FHR: 110–160 beats per minute (bpm) (assessed over a 10-minute window)
- Fetal bradycardia is <110 bpm. Etiologies include severe hypoxia, congenital heart malformations/blocks.
- Fetal tachycardia is >160 bpm. Etiologies include hypoxia, infection, tachyarrhythmia (usually >200), fetal anemia, maternal fever/infection, hyperthyroidism, medications/drugs (e.g., beta-agonists, atropine, cocaine), abruption.

Variability: Beat-to-beat difference (variation) of FHR fluctuates over time and does not include accelerations and decelerations.

FHR Tracings and Key Points

Finding	Description	Tracing	Significance/Etiology
Absent	Appears as a flat line	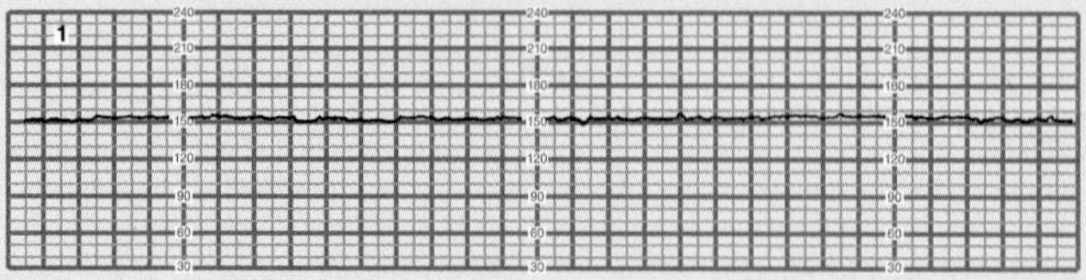	When occurring with recurrent late or variable decelerations, indicates severe fetal distress and is a category III tracing
Minimal	Beat-to-beat changes only 1–5 bpm off the baseline	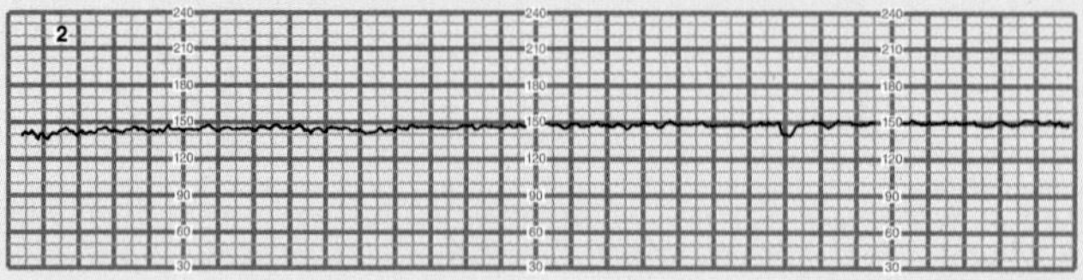	Sign of hypoxia but can occur in setting of fetal sleep cycles or from medications (e.g., magnesium, opioids)
Moderate	Beat-to-beat changes range from 6–25 bpm off the baseline	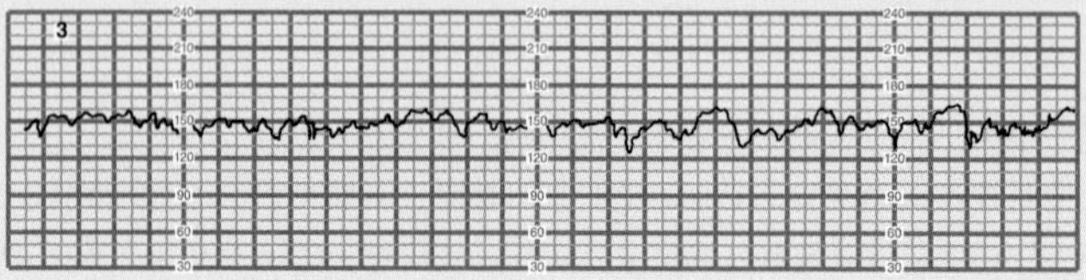	Suggestive of normal fetal acid-base status
Marked	Beat-to-beat changes >25 bpm off the baseline	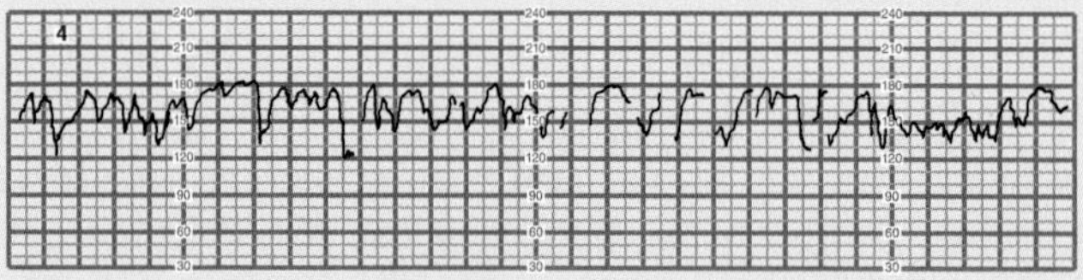	Very rare, may indicate hypoxia
Sinusoidal	Saw-toothed/ sine-wave tracing pattern	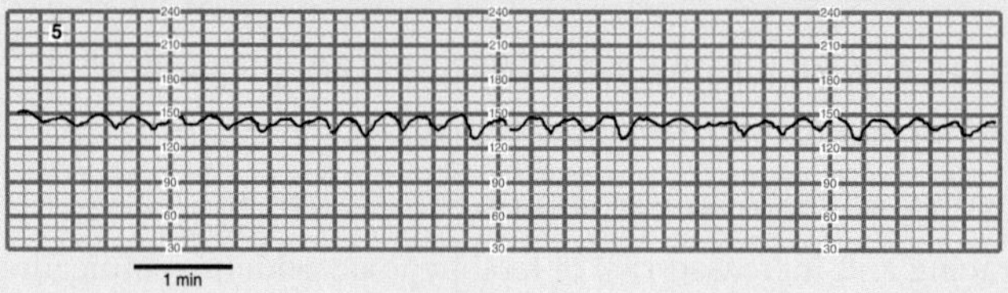	Signifies serious fetal anemia (e.g., Rh alloimmunization, parvovirus B19 infection, massive feto-maternal hemorrhage, thalassemia) and is a category III pattern

Reproduced with permission from Intrapartum Assessment In: Cunningham F, Leveno KJ, et al., Williams Obstetrics, 25e; New York: McGraw Hill, 2018.

Accelerations:

- An increase in FHR >15 bpm over the baseline for at least 15 seconds in length, after 32+0 weeks (prior to this gestational age, expect only 10 bpm over 10 seconds).
- Reassuring sign, indicating appropriate fetal response to environment.
- If lasting >2 minutes, termed "prolonged" and if >10 minutes is considered a change in baseline.

Decelerations:

- Decelerations (decels) are based on when they occur in relation to contractions.
- They can be defined as recurrent if present with >50% of contractions.
- There are four types of decelerations, as shown in the table below.

Deceleration Types	Description	Graph
Early	• A gradual decrease in FHR and return to baseline • Nadir of the deceleration *mirrors* the peak of the contraction • Onset >30 seconds and may last up to 2 minutes • Due to vagal response with compression of the fetal head	
Variable	• An abrupt/quick decrease in FHR ≥15 bpm below baseline lasting ≥15 seconds –2 minutes • The timing of the deceleration is independent of contraction (can occur randomly in the tracing or before, during, or after a contraction) • Due to compression or prolapse of the umbilical cord or oligohydramnios	
Late	• A gradual decrease in FHR and return to baseline • The nadir of the deceleration occurs *after* the peak of the contraction • Onset >30 seconds and may last up to 2 minutes • Appearance is very similar to that of an early decel, highlighting the importance of contraction monitoring to interpret the findings • Due to uteroplacental insufficiency (e.g., abruption, preeclampsia), vessel rupture (vasa previa), maternal factors (e.g., hypotension, hypoxemia/acidemia, vasculopathy, acute respiratory changes [e.g., pneumonia, asthma exacerbation])	
Prolonged	• A deceleration that lasts over 2 minutes is prolonged. • One that is >10 minutes is a change from baseline and may require immediate attention if consistent with terminal fetal bradycardia • Multifactorial contributors, but may be seen with acute compromise, like placental abruption, cord prolapse, hypotension, uterine rupture, fetal heart block, or rapid fetal descent	Prolonged deceleration example due to uterine hypertonicity (fetal heart monitor = top panel, intrauterine pressure catheter = bottom panel).

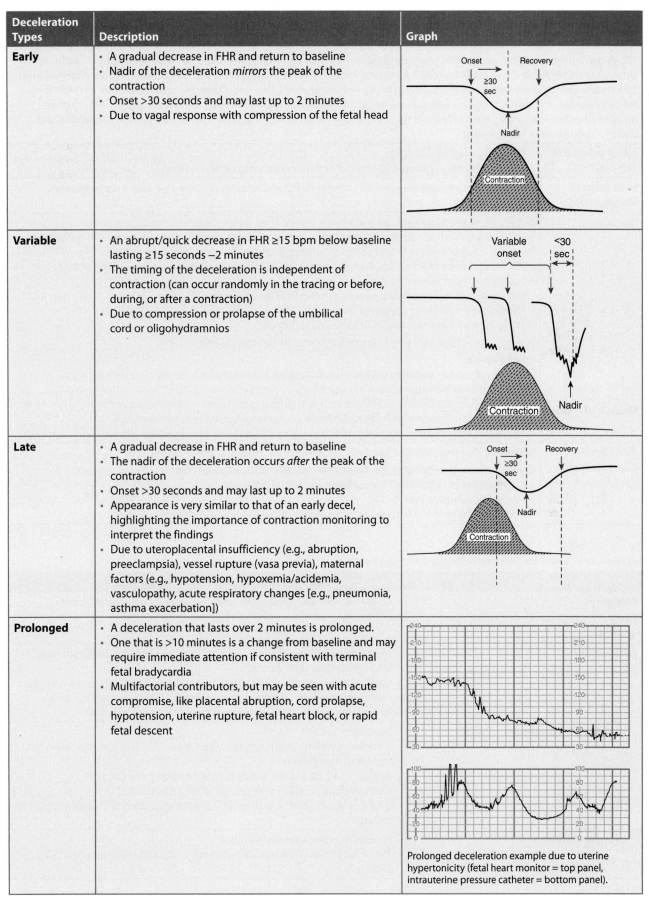

Reproduced with permission from Cunningham F, Leveno KJ, et al., Williams Obstetrics, 25e; New York: McGraw Hill, 2018.

CASE 2 | Fetal Surveillance during Labor

A 20-year-old G1P0 at 37+3 weeks is admitted in labor. Rupture of membranes is confirmed with ferning and positive pooling. The estimated fetal weight is about 3400 grams by palpation and fetus is cephalic. A continuous fetal heart monitor and external tocometer are placed. The FHR is 145 bpm with moderate variability. Three accelerations and no decelerations are observed after 15 minutes. Contractions are occurring regularly at 4- to 5-minute intervals. Two hours later, the contractions are not recording well and several variable decelerations with minimal variability are now noted. An attempt is made to reposition the patient; however, the decelerations do not resolve, and the contractions remain difficult to trace. The cervical exam is unchanged and there is no evidence of cord prolapse.

Initial Diagnostic Tests	• Continuous fetal monitoring • Tocodynamometry/tocometry (internal or external pending clinical factors)
Next Steps in Management	• Placement of intrauterine pressure catheter (IUPC) and infusion of saline to improve the heart rate (amnioinfusion)
Discussion	Monitoring of the fetal heartbeat and uterine contractions during labor is common practice to determine fetal tolerance of labor. The fetal heart patterns help providers determine if an intervention in the birthing process is needed to prevent fetal compromise. Factors that affect fetal heartbeat include maternal or fetal pathology or issues affecting the extraembryonic tissues that connect the two (i.e., placenta or umbilical cord). Stressors can cause: • Oxygenation deficit leading to fetal hypoxemia (low blood oxygen) • Hypoxia due to reduced oxygen to tissues • Acidosis (from hypercapnia and/or increased lactic acid) See the above chart for review of contributors to different tracing abnormalities. **Management:** • In cases of sudden anoxia to the fetus (i.e., abruption, cord occlusion), delivery is necessary within <10 minutes to avoid permanent hypoxic injury. • In cases where there is not an immediate threat to fetal or maternal morbidity and/or mortality (i.e., arrest of descent), intrapartum cesarean section may be warranted, but not as emergently. • The management of delivery based on the category of fetal heart rate monitoring is given in below table.
Additional Considerations	**Screening:** See table "Antepartum Fetal Surveillance (Outside of Labor). " above. **Complications**: Unscheduled/emergent cesarean delivery is associated with: • Increased risk of postpartum hemorrhage and postop infection • Anesthetic complications • Accidental injury to the fetus or maternal organs of the pelvis and abdomen.

Management Based on Fetal Heart Rate Monitoring Findings

FHR Monitoring Category	Management
Category I (normal tracing; low risk of fetal hypoxic acidemia)	• Continue monitoring and expectant management of labor/induction
Category II (indeterminate tracing; not category I or III)	• Moderate variability or spontaneous accelerations lowers suspicion of fetal acidosis but does not rule it out • Tracings that convert back to category I do not require further intervention • May need to reduce or discontinue uterotonic drugs (i.e., oxytocin for augmentation/induction) to improve uteroplacental blood flow
• **Variable decelerations**	• Reposition patient • If pre-labor patient, assess amniotic fluid index (AFI) and consider ruling out rupture of membranes • In labor, examine patient to rule out cord prolapse and consider amnioinfusion (instillation of normal saline around fetus) • If cord prolapse present, elevate fetal head and proceed to emergent cesarean delivery
• **Late decelerations**	• Reposition patient, assess hydration • Assess for causes of uteroplacental insufficiency and treat identified cause directly

Management Based on Fetal Heart Rate Monitoring Findings

FHR Monitoring Category	Management
• **Prolonged or recurrent decelerations**	• Verify that the heart rate is fetal and not maternal by having continuous maternal HR monitoring and repositioning the external monitor or placing a fetal scalp electrode • Reposition patient • If maternal hypotension is the cause, initiate IV hydration and ephedrine; assess for anesthetic causes • For tetanic (sustained) uterine contraction or tachysystole, treat with terbutaline • Prepare for cesarean delivery if unresolved
• **Fetal tachycardia**	• Assess for maternal/fetal infection • Review maternal exposures (beta-agonists, atropine, cocaine)
• **Minimal variability (w/o decelerations)**	• Assess fetal status (fetus may be in sleep cycle) • Perform fetal scalp stimulation to provoke an acceleration (if found, probability of concurrent fetal acidosis is <10%) • Review maternal exposures (opioids, magnesium sulfate, CNS depressants)
Category III Tracing (abnormal tracing [absent variability with recurrent late or variable decelerations, bradycardia, or sinusoidal tracing]—increased risk of fetal hypoxic acidemia; indication for immediate delivery)	• Extrauterine resuscitation measures as above may be attempted • Immediate delivery is indicated if unresolved rapidly, usually by emergent cesarean delivery unless vaginal birth (especially if could be assisted by vacuum or forceps) is imminent
• **Sinusoidal (fetal anemia)**	• Prophylactic anti-D immune globulin (Rhogam) to prevent RhD alloimmunization when Rh (−) patient has reduced the instance of fetal anemia • If fetal anemia is recognized early enough in pregnancy, consider intrauterine fetal transfusion • In the setting of a sinusoid tracing, resuscitation and/or delivery should not be delayed • The pediatric team should be notified to prepare for their own resuscitative measures given potential for profound anemia in the neonate

FETAL ABNORMALITIES AND COMPLICATIONS

Genetic Considerations

- Genetic screening and diagnostic testing should be offered in all pregnancies.
- Genetic assessments include both maternal carrier screening and aneuploidy screening.

Carrier Screening

Only needs to occur once in a person's lifetime

- All patients are recommended for cystic fibrosis (CF) and spinal muscular atrophy (SMA) screening.
- Additional genetic carrier condition screening is based on individual risk.
- Optimally, this is done preconception but can be obtained any time in pregnancy.

Maternal Serum Markers

- Can be utilized in screening for fetal aneuploidies and body wall defects (e.g., gastroschisis or neural tube defects [NTD]).
- Screening can also be completed via cell-free fetal DNA (cffDNA).

Causes of Abnormal Levels of Maternal Serum Alpha-Fetoprotein (MSAFP)

Elevated msAFP	Low msAFP
Underestimation of gestational age	Overestimation of gestational age
Multiple gestations	Aneuploidies (Down syndrome, trisomy 18, trisomy 13)
Abdominal/body wall defects	Molar pregnancy
Decreased maternal weight	Increased maternal weight
Oligohydramnios	Fetal death
Cystic hygroma (Turner syndrome)	
Sacrococcygeal teratoma	
Neural tube defects	

Aneuploidy Screening

- Assesses for trisomies 13, 18, 21, and sometimes monosomy X based on assay used.
- The risk of aneuploidy increases with advancing maternal age.
- Abnormal genetic screening should prompt discussion of further diagnostic testing with chorionic villus sampling (CVS) or amniocentesis for diagnosis, though patients can select diagnostic testing directly if they prefer.

Serum Marker Levels in Aneuploidies

Serum Marker	Description	Trimester	Trisomy 21	Trisomy 18	Trisomy 13
β-hCG (human chorionic gonadotropin, β subunit)	Produced by placenta, signals corpus luteum to produce progesterone	first	↑	↓	↓
		second	↑	↓	Normal
PAPP-A (pregnancy-associated plasma protein A)	Produced by fetus and placenta, limits maternal immune system recognition of fetus, and angiogenesis	first	↓	↓	↓
AFP (alpha-fetoprotein)	Produced by fetus: ↑ in neural tube defects (NTD), ↓ in chromosomal aneuploidies	second	↓	↓	Normal
Estriol	Produced by the placenta, large increase occurs during pregnancy	second	↓	↓	Normal
Inhibin A	Produced by placenta, corpus luteum, and fetus; negative feedback on FSH	second	↑	↓ or Normal	Normal

Neural Tube Defects

- Closed NTDs: spinal column abnormality due to malformation of bone, fat, or membranes
- Open NTDs: defect in vertebrae and/or skull resulting in exposure of spinal cord or brain

Open neural tube defects (NTD) are the most common side effect of folate deficiency, and include the following:

Name	Description	Features
Spina Bifida Occulta	The caudal neuropore fails to close but there is no herniation of neural tissue or meninges	• Most benign and common form of NTD • There is often associated a hair tuft or dimpling of skin at the level of the bony defect • Most often at lower vertebral levels
Meningocele	Failure of the caudal neuropore to close with herniation of meninges	• More severe manifestation
Meningomyelocele	Herniation of meninges and neural tissue	
Anencephaly	Failure of the cranial (or rostral) neuropore to close	• Results in no forebrain with an open calvarium

CASE 3 | Neural Tube Defects (NTD)

A 24-year-old G2P0010 at 19+6 with a history of housing instability and food insecurity presents for a routine prenatal visit. Fetal ultrasound reveals a meningocele.

Conditions with Similar Presentations	See table above on conditions with low and high maternal serum alpha-fetoprotein. These conditions can be distinguished from neural tube defects by ultrasonography.
Initial Diagnostic Tests	Check fetal ultrasonography and/or serum, amniotic fluid AFP
Next Steps in Management	Referral to genetics and maternal-fetal medicine
Discussion	NTDs occur in 1 in 300 to 1 in 1000 pregnancies worldwide and are one of the most common congenital abnormalities of the central nervous system (CNS). They occur due to failed closure of the neural tube, which begins to form 3–4 weeks after fertilization. Depending on whether the NTD is caused by failure of fusion of the cranial or caudal neuropore, the deficits observed in the fetus or neonate will occur in the cranium or spinal column, respectively. Because this occurs early in gestation, patients of reproductive age should ideally initiate folate prior to conception, with continuation during pregnancy. **History:** Risk Factors: Family history of or prior pregnancy affected by spina bifida or anencephaly, inadequate maternal intake of folate, diabetes, exposure to valproic acid or carbamazepine **Diagnostics:** Second-trimester fetal two-dimensional ultrasonography (US) findings suggestive of NTD include: • Lemon- or acorn-shaped skull • Small biparietal diameter and head circumference • Parallel cerebral peduncles • Caudal displacement of metencephalon • Intracranial translucency • Reduced fronto-maxillary facial angle • Abnormal brainstem diameter/brainstem to brainstem occipital • Non-visualization of cisterna magna • Posterior displacement of the aqueduct of Sylvius • Abnormal "four-line" sign Additional tests: • ↑ Maternal serum AFP (msAFP), ↑ amniotic fluid AFP, ↑ acetylcholinesterase • If obtained, amniocentesis would not show any chromosomal abnormalities. **Management:** Offer pregnancy options including: • Maternal-fetal medicine consult • Amniocentesis • Induced abortion if desired • Fetal surgery (depending on the defect) • Neonatal surgical intervention (for insertion of a ventriculoperitoneal shunt for ventriculomegaly/hydrocephalus)
Additional Considerations	**Preventive:** USPSTF recommends all people that can become pregnant to take 0.4–0.8 mg of folate daily (Grade A).

Fetal Abnormality Mini-Case	
Case	**Key Findings**
Trisomy 21 (Down Syndrome)	**Hx:** Risk factors include advanced maternal age
	PE: Neonate: with flat occiput, upslanting palpebral fissures and epicanthal folds, flat nasal bridge, large tongue, hypotonia, short fingers, single palmar crease
	Diagnostics:
	Antepartum tests:
	• Serum QUAD screen: $\downarrow$ AFP, $\downarrow$ estriol, $\uparrow$ β-hCG, $\uparrow$ inhibin
	• Fetal ultrasound may show: major cardiac abnormalities (e.g., tetralogy of Fallot, AV canal defects, septal defects), thickened nuchal fold, echogenic bowel, renal pelvis dilation, shortened long bones, or cardiac echogenic foci may be present.
	• Confirm diagnosis with amniocentesis or CVS: trisomy of chromosome 21 on karyotyping
	Management:
	Antepartum:
	• Offer genetic counseling, diagnostic testing, and discuss option of induced abortion if the patient does not want to continue pregnancy.
	• Perform fetal ultrasound and surveillance throughout pregnancy.
	• Plan for a prenatal neonatal consult.
	See Pediatrics chapter for additional discussion.
	Discussion: Down syndrome (trisomy 21) is an autosomal trisomy involving the presence of three copies of chromosome 21. The condition is the most common viable chromosomal disorder and cause of non-inherited genetic intellectual disability, most often due to maternal meiotic nondisjunction. In addition to trisomy 21, the other two potentially viable autosomal trisomies include trisomy 13 (Patau syndrome) and 18 (Edwards syndrome). Risk of aneuploidy increases with advancing maternal age, but all pregnant patients should be offered aneuploidy screening regardless of risk

ANTEPARTUM COMPLICATIONS OF PREGNANCY

Some early pregnancy complications include ectopic implantation of the pregnancy, miscarriage, and molar pregnancy. Late pregnancy risks include fetal growth abnormalities, multifetal gestations, vaginal bleeding, venous thromboembolism, fetal infections, and malpresentation. Abdominal pain and vaginal bleeding in pregnancy will be discussed toward the end of the obstetrics section.

Uterine Size Unequal to Dates

When the fundus measures greater or lesser than expected, this may suggest pathology. However, inaccurate dating should always be ruled out first.

- Initial evaluation includes assessing if stated gestational age is accurate and ruling out multifetal gestation, via ultrasound (most optimally in first trimester).
- Fundal height (FH) can help track fetal growth in singleton pregnancies after 20 weeks' gestation.

Multifetal Gestations

- Ovulations that produce two ova will result in dizygotic twins if both are fertilized.
- Monozygotic twins occur when a single fertilized ovum splits. Depending on the timing of the split, various possibilities exist regarding whether the fetuses will have separate or shared extraembryonic tissues (see below figure). Specifically, the fetuses may share a fused placenta, amnion (innermost membrane enclosing the embryo/fetus), and/or chorion (outermost membrane). When division occurs very late, it is incomplete and results in conjoined twinning.

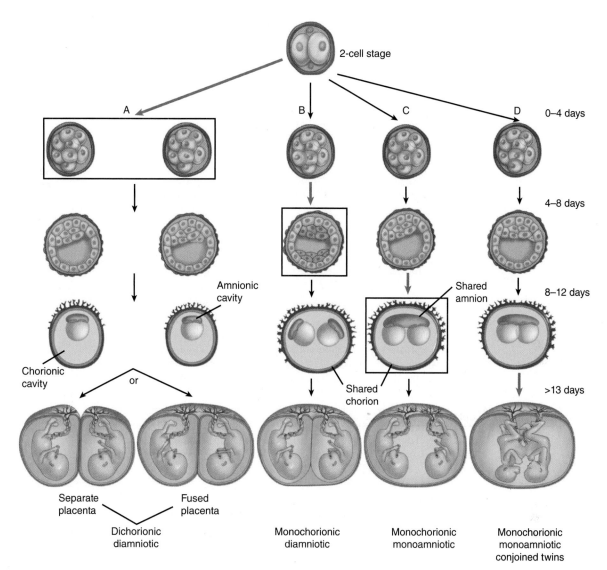

2-cell stage

A   B   C   D   0–4 days

4–8 days

Amnionic
cavity

Chorionic
cavity

or

Shared
amnion

Shared
chorion

8–12 days

>13 days

Separate
placenta

Fused
placenta

Dichorionic
diamniotic

Monochorionic
diamniotic

Monochorionic
monoamniotic

Monochorionic
monoamniotic
conjoined twins

Reproduced with permission from Multifetal Pregnancy In: Cunningham F, Leveno KJ, et al., Williams Obstetrics, 25e; New York: McGraw Hill, 2018.

CASE 4 | Fetal Growth Restriction (FGR)

A 36-year-old G2P1001 at 34+2 weeks with dichorionic-diamniotic twin gestation presents for routine prenatal care and scheduled fetal growth surveillance ultrasound. On the prior assessment, twin A was in the 30th percentile for estimated fetal weight (EFW) and twin B was in the 26th percentile. The pregnancy has been unremarkable to date.

Repeat ultrasound shows that twin A is stable at the 30th percentile for EFW; however, twin B is now at the 8th percentile for EFW. Given the new growth restriction, Doppler velocimetry and a biophysical profile (BPP) were completed showing normal umbilical artery Dopplers for both twins and BPP of 10/10 and 8/10 for each twin, respectively.

Conditions with Similar Presentations	• Constitutionally small fetus, inaccurate dating of pregnancy, and oligohydramnios can present with uterine size less than expected dates. • The term small for gestational age (SGA) refers to a neonate after delivery measuring below the expected curve for gestational age at birth and should not be used antenatally.
Initial Diagnostic Tests	Monitor with serial antenatal fetal surveillance, growth ultrasound, and weekly Doppler velocimetry

CASE 4 | Fetal Growth Restriction (FGR) *(continued)*

Next Steps in Management	Delivery planning based on developing findings
Discussion	FGR is a prenatal diagnosis and is classically defined as EFW below the 10th percentile for gestational age, though a newer definition also includes specifically decelerated growth of the abdominal circumference below the 10th percentile.
	• Prior to 20 weeks, growth is hyperplastic, or driven by cellular division and the increasing number of cells. An insult occurring in this phase will likely impact cell division globally and cause symmetrically decreased growth.
	• After 20 weeks, growth is hypertrophic, or driven mainly by increasing cell size without ongoing rapid addition of cells. Insults impacting this phase, especially those that are chronic, will result in nutrients and oxygen being preferentially shunted to the most vital organs, namely the brain. Growth restriction in the hypertrophic phase may cause asymmetric restriction.
	History: Risks include conditions that affect fetal, maternal, and/or placental condition: pregestational diabetes, renal disease, chronic and pregnancy-related hypertensive disorders, autoimmune conditions, chronic substance use/tobacco use, multifetal gestations, TORCH infections/teratogen exposure.
	Physical Exam: Fundal height may be smaller than expected for the gestational age.
	Diagnostics:
	• Doppler velocimetry, serial growth, and antenatal fetal surveillance
	• If FGR is diagnosed early (at or before 20 weeks), patient should also be screened for TORCHes infections, aneuploidy, and other causes of global growth restriction
	• For those patients and fetuses that are especially at risk, continuous inpatient monitoring may be warranted
	Management: Decision-making is based on risk of continuation of pregnancy.
	• Preterm delivery is indicated for patients with abnormal umbilical Doppler velocity, especially reversed end diastolic flow, as it is associated with high risk of intrauterine fetal demise
	• Fetuses with normal Doppler velocimetry should be monitored closely with serial assessments as per above
	• Corticosteroids can be administered to accelerate fetal lung maturity in anticipation of early labor (prior to or at 34 weeks)
	See below for specific treatment notes regarding selected conditions.
	• *Substance use disorders:* Discuss and aid in cessation-based treatments prior to pregnancy when possible
	• *Vascular disorders* (placental insufficiency, preeclampsia, collagen vascular disorders): Low-dose daily aspirin
	• *Clotting disorders* (history of prior placental thrombosis, thrombophilias, anti-phospholipid antibody syndrome): Heparin with or without corticosteroids
	• Multifetal gestation and intrauterine fetal demise: Discussed in mini-case below
Additional Considerations	**Screening:**
	• Monitor fetal growth with FH at regular intervals starting 24 weeks of gestation.
	• If FH differs by >2 centimeters from expected, confirm with estimated fetal weight calculation by ultrasound and verify the accuracy of the pregnancy's dating.
	• This measurement can be challenging with multifetal gestations and central adiposity in patients with elevated BMI, so screening can also be conducted with serial growth ultrasound every 4 weeks.
	Complications:
	Fetuses with FGR have increased risk of:
	• Fetal demise or neonatal death
	• Neonatal morbidity—respiratory distress syndrome, retinopathy of prematurity, sepsis
	• Adverse neurodevelopmental outcomes—cognitive impairment, cerebral palsy
	• Later development of elevated BMI, metabolic dysfunction, insulin sensitivity, type 2 diabetes mellitus, cardiovascular and renal disease are thought to be attributed to alterations in fetal metabolic homeostasis, endocrine function, and cardiac remodeling in utero

Pregnancy Complication Mini-Cases

Cases	Key Findings
Oligohydramnios	**Hx:** Exposure to ACEI, ARBs, and NSAIDs, presence of pregestational hypertension or diabetes, rupture of membranes, decreased fetal movements. **PE:** Small for date fetus, leakage of amniotic fluid. **Diagnostics:** • Ultrasound reveals a low amniotic fluid index (AFI) <5 cm. • Rule out rupture of membranes (ROM) • Assess for FGR, markers of aneuploidy, and placental insufficiency **Management:** Treat the underlying cause; delivery if term gestation. **Discussion:** Oligohydramnios means low amniotic fluid and frequently presents in the late third trimester and can be associated with ROM or placental insufficiency. When seen earlier, it may be due to fetal anomalies such as renal agenesis or posterior urethral valves. Preterm diagnosis of oligohydramnios requires close surveillance and, if severe, can necessitate iatrogenic preterm birth. At term, the treatment is delivery. Longstanding severe oligohydramnios can lead to the **Potter sequence**, a specific fetal phenotype including clubbed feet, pulmonary hypoplasia, and compressed facial features.
Fetal Hydrops	**Hx:** Recent infection with parvovirus (can see with TORCH infections, parvovirus most common), presence of some ABO antibody groups (Kell is most severe), or prior pregnancy with Rh (+) fetus in patient with either unknown or Rh (−) status. **PE:** Fundal height > gestational age **Diagnostics:** • Ultrasound to detect polyhydramnios • Middle cerebral artery Doppler of fetus • Fetal heart tracing to detect for anemia or asphyxia **Management:** Mild cases may be observed, while severe cases can be treated with intrauterine umbilical transfusion. **Discussion:** Hydrops fetalis is defined as the excessive accumulation of fluid in two or more fetal compartments. The most common nonimmune, infectious cause is parvovirus, while the most common immune cause is Rh isoimmunization. Fetal anemia or asphyxia with ultimate fetal demise are the most feared complications of hydrops fetalis, which can manifest as a sinusoidal heart rate pattern on fetal heart tracing.
Multifetal Gestation	**Hx:** Family or personal history of dizygotic twins, infertility treatment, advanced maternal age. Symptoms related to elevated beta-hCG levels in multifetal gestations (e.g., severe nausea and vomiting, reflux) **PE:** Increased uterine growth, weight gain, and blood volume expansion **Diagnostics:** • US is used for the detection of multifetal gestation, the number of chorions (chorionicity) and the number of amnions (amnionicity). Multifetal gestation can be classified by the number of fertilized ova (zygosity), chorionicity, and amnionicity. **Management:** • Expectant management. • Timing and method of delivery is determined based on chorionicity, amnionicity, number of fetuses, and presence of complications.

Pregnancy Complications Mini-Cases *(continued)*

Multifetal Gestation	**Discussion:** Multifetal gestations are associated with increased complications. • Maternal: Hyperemesis, anemia, gestational diabetes, hypertension, preterm labor/PPROM, cesarean delivery, hemorrhage, and postpartum depression. • Fetal complications: Early pregnancy losses are due to: congenital anomalies and spontaneous miscarriage. Late complications are due to: preterm complications, cord entanglement, and **twin-twin transfusion syndrome** (TTTS): • TTTS occurs when blood from a donor twin is transfused to a recipient twin due to aberrant flow in deep arteriovenous anastomoses in the placenta. Oxygenated blood is then preferentially shunted to one twin, which will experience volume overload (polyhydramnios, hypervolemia, heart failure, polycythemia, possibly thrombosis) and the other twin will develop conditions attributable to hypovolemia, including oligohydramnios, growth restriction and contractures, pulmonary hypoplasia, premature rupture of the membranes, and heart failure. Treatment options include amnioreduction, laser ablation of vascular anastomoses, selective feticide, and septostomy.
Intrauterine Fetal Demise (IUFD)	**Hx:** Loss of pregnancy symptoms, absent fetal movement **PE:** May find size < expected dates **Diagnostics:** IUFD is confirmed with US revealing absent fetal cardiac motion **Management:** The treatment is based on gestational age at discovery and can include dilation and curettage/evacuation or induction of labor with prostaglandins or high-dose oxytocin. **Discussion:** Intrauterine fetal demise is associated with several medical and obstetric conditions, including placental abruption, infection, rheumatologic or hypertensive disease, and postterm pregnancy. Retained IUFD for longer than 3–4 weeks may result in the release of thromboplastic substances and hypofibrinogenemia, leading to DIC. Efforts are usually made to identify an etiology for the IUFD through maternal and fetal testing, including autopsy, but many cases will remain without an identified cause.
Preterm Prelabor Rupture of Membranes (PPROM)	**Hx:** Leakage of fluid before 37 completed weeks of pregnancy **PE:** Uterine contractions are usually absent, amniotic fluid pooling in vagina and positive Valsalva sign (fluid leaking from the cervical os during Valsalva maneuver) are seen on sterile speculum exam **Diagnostics:** • If pooling of amniotic fluid is not seen, low amniotic fluid index on ultrasound and/or a positive fern test on microscopic exam is presumptive of PPROM • May use nitrizine paper to test pH, will be generally >7.5–8 **Management:** • In patients <34 weeks' gestation, antibiotics (azithromycin × 1 day and ampicillin for 5 days), corticosteroids, and fetal surveillance are indicated. • In the absence of spontaneous labor, complications that would prompt induction or augmentation of labor include intraamniotic infection or placental abruption. • Induction of labor is indicated once at 34 weeks (or at diagnosis when after this gestational age). **Discussion:** PPROM refers to the rupture of the amniotic membrane before the onset of labor, and occurs <37 weeks of gestation. The most significant consequence of PPROM is intrauterine infection, a risk that increases with the duration of membrane rupture. Routine antibiotic treatment in patients with PPROM reduces neonatal and maternal complications. Around 50% of patients with PPROM will enter labor within 2–7 days after PPROM.

Pregnancy Complications Mini-Cases *(continued)*

Cervical Insufficiency	**Hx:** History of prior cervical surgery, prior mechanical cervical dilation, prior preterm birth, recurrent second-trimester pregnancy loss; presenting without contractions, having pelvic pressure, cramping, or vaginal spotting in current pregnancy **PE:** Cervical dilation before 24 weeks' gestation in the absence of contractions; prolapsed fetal membranes **Diagnostics:** TVUS cervical length <25 mm prior to 24 weeks' gestation in singleton gestation **Management:** Vaginal progesterone supplement or cerclage placement (if severe cervical shortening, <10 mm) **Discussion:** Cervical insufficiency should be considered in those who experience painless cervical dilation. Any cervical intervention, such as excisional procedures, can weaken the cervical stroma and impair its ability to retain a pregnancy. The goal of treatment is to prevent further cervical dilation. In the setting of patients with a history of cervical insufficiency, history-indicated cerclage can be offered at the start of the second trimester to reduce the risk for repeat pregnancy loss.

Abdominal Pain in Pregnancy

An important aspect of evaluation of any clinical symptom in a pregnant patient is to consider both obstetric and non-obstetric etiologies.

First Trimester (0–13 + 6 weeks)	Second Trimester (14–27 + 6 weeks)	Third Trimester (28 weeks and beyond)
Ectopic pregnancy	Miscarriage	Preterm labor or labor
Miscarriage	Preterm labor	Intraamniotic infection
	Placental abruption	Placental abruption
	Uterine rupture	Uterine rupture
	Preeclampsia/eclampsia	Preeclampsia/eclampsia
	Acute fatty liver of pregnancy	Acute fatty liver of pregnancy

Obstetric Etiologies of Abdominal Pain

Diagnosis	Symptoms and Signs	Labs/Imaging
Ectopic pregnancy	Abdominal pain and vaginal bleeding following a missed period in the first trimester	$\uparrow$ serum HCG Ultrasound: absent intrauterine pregnancy, may have mass in adnexa with free fluid in pelvis
HELLP	Abdominal pain, nausea, jaundice, and $\uparrow$ blood pressure	Hemolysis, $\uparrow$ liver enzymes, and $\downarrow$ platelets
Acute fatty liver of pregnancy	Acute right upper quadrant pain, nausea, vomiting seen in the second and third trimester	Labs show $\uparrow$ liver enzymes and $\uparrow$ bilirubin, $\uparrow$ creatinine, hypoglycemia, coagulopathy Ultrasound shows fatty changes in the liver
Uterine rupture	Abdominal pain in the second and third trimester with vaginal bleeding, often with history of prior uterine surgery, loss of fetal station, and possibly palpation of fetal parts in the abdomen	Imaging (ultrasound or CT) shows dehiscence and hematoma
Placental abruption	Acute abdominal pain in the second and third trimester, vaginal bleeding, elevated uterine tone on palpation and tocometry	Clinical diagnosis Confirm with visual inspection of placenta after delivery

CASE 5 | Preterm Labor (PTL)

A 32-year-old G2P0101 at 31+0 weeks' gestation presents with lower abdominal pain and persistent pelvic pressure. The pain was waxing and waning, but now severe intermittent cramps are occurring every 15–20 minutes for the past 3 hours. There is no preceding trauma, but patient reports a small amount of vaginal spotting. Her prior pregnancy was complicated by preterm birth at 33 weeks. On physical exam, abdomen is gravid with palpable contractions, cervix is dilated to 3 cm, and is 50% effaced.

Conditions with Similar Presentations	**Braxton-Hicks contractions:** Do not result in cervical change. These contractions typically occur at an irregular pattern and can resolve with rest and hydration. **Acute cholecystitis:** Will be associated with RUQ pain, nausea/vomiting. **Gastroenteritis:** Will have vomiting and/or diarrhea. May have illness in close contacts. **Nephrolithiasis:** Pain is unilateral, colicky. May radiate to the groin, and may have hematuria.
Initial Diagnostic Tests	Clinical diagnosis (see below for details)
Next Steps in Management	• Tocolytic treatment: Tocolytics inhibit uterine contractions and prolong pregnancy, which allows time for administration of antenatal steroids. • See chart below for discussion on options.
Discussion	Regular uterine contractions that occur between 20 and 36-6/7 weeks of gestation leading to cervical change is termed PTL. In PTL, decidual activation (which consists of paracrine signaling from the fetus through amniotic fluid and across membranes to underlying maternal decidua and myometrium) triggers contractions prematurely due to genetic and environmental factors. PTL is seen in 12% of all births in the United States; it occurs in 50% of twin births and 90% of all higher-order multiple births **History:** Risk Factors: Prior preterm birth, multifetal gestation, tobacco and/or other substance use, bacterial vaginosis, and sexually transmitted infections (STIs). Symptoms: Regular uterine contractions, menstrual-like cramping, low back pain, pelvic pressure, vaginal discharge and/or mucus, or light spotting. **Physical Exam:** Cervix dilation, contractions on tocometry **Diagnostics:** Clinical diagnosis • Start fetal heart monitoring and obtain a transabdominal ultrasound for fetal and placental position. Additional tests to consider: • TVUS for cervical length. Increased risk of preterm birth is associated with a short cervix before 34 weeks of gestation (<30 mm) • Fetal fibronectin (fFN): Extracellular matrix protein present at the junction of the amniotic sac and the uterine lining. Disruption of this interface due to uterine contractions releases fFN into cervicovaginal secretions. • Urinalysis and culture, vaginal samples in symptomatic patients to assess for bacterial vaginosis and STIs, and rectovaginal culture in unscreened patients to assess for group B *Streptococcus*. **Management:** • Tocolytics are administered up to 34 weeks to inhibit uterine contractions and prolong the pregnancy to allow for interventions that can reduce morbidity of the premature neonate; contraindicated if abnormal NST/fetal tracing, severe preeclampsia or eclampsia, maternal hemorrhage, PPROM, and intraamniotic infection. • Antenatal steroids: A single course of IM betamethasone or dexamethasone is given for PTL to improve fetal lung maturity and surfactant production. • Magnesium sulfate administration is indicated if <32 weeks' gestation and concern for delivery within the next 12 hours for fetal neuroprotection, as it reduces the occurrence of neurological disorders such as cerebral palsy. • Antibiotics for group B *Streptococcus* prophylaxis are recommended in PTL for patients who are confirmed GBS positive or GBS unknown.

6

CASE 5 | Preterm Labor (PTL) (continued)

Additional Considerations	**Screening:** If previous history of PTL in a prior pregnancy, patient can be placed on progesterone injections as early as 16 weeks to be continued through 36 weeks and should also have a TVUS to assess cervical length from 16 to 24 weeks. **Complications:** Fetal: Premature birth increases the risk for neonatal hypoglycemia and feeding difficulties, necrotizing enterocolitis, lung immaturity and attendant respiratory complications and intraventricular hemorrhage. Maternal: If cesarean birth is indicated, severe prematurity (24–28 weeks) is a risk factor for a vertical uterine incision, which increases perioperative morbidity and creates a need for future cesarean births due to the increased risk of uterine rupture. **Surgical Considerations:** Indications for cesarean delivery in PTL are no different than any other pregnancy and can include malpresentation, tracing abnormalities, and arrest disorders.

Medications for PTL

Medications	Mechanism	Adverse Reactions/Contraindications
Nifedipine (instant-release)	Binds to L-type calcium channels located on the vascular smooth muscle and causes smooth muscle relaxation	**Maternal:** Dizziness, flushing, hypotension **Fetal:** No known adverse effects **Contraindication:** Hypotension
Indomethacin	Inhibition of COX-1 and COX-2, which leads to decreased formation of prostaglandins	**Maternal:** Esophageal reflux, nausea, gastritis. **Fetal:** In utero constriction of ductus arteriosus, necrotizing enterocolitis in preterm neonates, oligohydramnios **Contraindications:** Gestational age >32 weeks, platelet dysfunction or bleeding disorder, hepatic dysfunction, renal dysfunction, peptic ulcer disease
Terbutaline	Beta-2 agonist that causes smooth muscle relaxation leading to relaxation of uterine contractions	**Maternal:** Tachycardia, hypotension, palpitations, tremor, pulmonary edema, shortness of breath, hypokalemia, hyperglycemia **Fetal:** Tachycardia **Contraindications:** Tachycardia-sensitive maternal cardiac disease and poorly controlled diabetes
Magnesium sulfate	Decreases uterine muscle intracellular calcium, which leads to decreased uterine contractility	**Maternal:** Flushing, diaphoresis, respiratory depression, nausea, loss of deep tendon reflexes **Fetal:** Neonatal depression **Contraindications:** Myasthenia gravis

Abdominal Pain Mini-Cases

Cases	Key Findings
Ectopic Pregnancy	**Hx:** Right or left lower quadrant pain/tenderness, vaginal bleeding, adnexal tenderness within context of missed menstruation Paradoxical adnexal tenderness and bleeding from vagina. **Diagnostics:** Serum hCG positive, and TVUS showing no intrauterine pregnancy **Management:** If the patient is stable, medical (methotrexate) or surgical therapies can be explored. • Surgical management indicated: when there are symptoms of ruptured ectopic pregnancy, intraperitoneal bleed, or hemodynamic instability • Medical management with intramuscular methotrexate is appropriate for stable patients with an unruptured ectopic pregnancy **Discussion:** Ectopic pregnancy is the leading cause of maternal death in the first trimester, and results from implantation of the fertilized ovum in a location other than the endometrial lining of the uterus. Most ectopic pregnancies are implanted in the ampulla of the fallopian tube.

Abdominal Pain Mini-Cases *(continued)*

Uterine Rupture	**Hx:** Sudden, severe abdominal pain late in pregnancy which is persistent between contractions and not relieved by previously adequate analgesia; sudden change in uterine contraction pattern **PE:** Maternal: Tachycardia, hypotension, change in abdominal contour, uterine tenderness, new abdominal distension Fetus: Inability to detect fetal heart rate at old transducer site, loss of fetal station **Diagnostics:** • Clinical diagnosis by tracing and exam • Fetal heart tracing: Recurrent late decelerations or fetal bradycardia **Management:** Treat shock and emergent cesarean delivery **Discussion:** Uterine rupture results from disruption of the myometrium during labor. It is most common in those who have had prior cesarean birth or other transmural uterine surgery (myomectomy). Labor contractions cause the stretching of the scarred and weakened myometrium, which increases the chances of rupture. Other causes include uterine anomalies, history of abnormally invasive placenta in prior pregnancy, and fetal malpresentation. Complications include postpartum hemorrhage, peripartum hysterectomy, and fetal compromise/hypoxia, including potential for fetal demise.
Acute Fatty Liver of Pregnancy	**Hx:** >20 weeks' gestation with progressive intense pruritis, nausea, vomiting, RUQ abdominal pain and lethargy. **PE:** Jaundice, tenderness to palpation in RUQ of the abdomen, absence of skin rash **Diagnostics:** ↓ Blood glucose, ↑ serum creatinine, abnormal liver tests (↑ transaminases, ↑ bilirubin, abnormal coags) **Management:** Delivery **Discussion:** Acute fatty liver of pregnancy is a rare condition that involves microvesicular steatosis of the liver. It presents as RUQ pain, acute renal failure, hypoglycemia, coagulopathy, and fulminant liver failure with altered mental status. It should be suspected in the presence of hyperbilirubinemia, acute renal failure, and hypoglycemia.

VAGINAL BLEEDING IN PREGNANCY

Bleeding in pregnancy can have several etiologies, both obstetric and non-obstetric.

• The first step in evaluating a pregnant patient with bleeding is to assess vital signs and to hemodynamically stabilize the maternal patient in setting of acute hemorrhage.

• Non-obstetric causes of bleeding in pregnancy include severe cervicitis, cervical polyps/dysplasia/cancer, vaginal laceration/trauma, abdominal or pelvic trauma, bleeding disorder, mistaken bleeding from rectum (e.g., hemorrhoids, fissure) or bladder.

• Determining gestational age for the pregnancy is useful, as obstetric etiologies of bleeding may differ based on trimester.

Obstetric Causes of Vaginal Bleeding

First Trimester	Second Trimester	Third Trimester	Postpartum
Ectopic pregnancy	Miscarriage (<20 weeks)	Preterm labor	Tone (uterine atony)
Threatened miscarriage	Preterm labor (>20 weeks)	Placental abruption	Trauma (lacerations, uterine rupture)
Incomplete miscarriage	Placental abruption	Premature rupture of membranes	Tissue (retained placenta)
Complete miscarriage	Premature rupture of membranes	Placenta previa	Thrombin (disseminated intravascular coagulopathy)
Molar pregnancy	Placenta previa	Vasa previa	Endometritis (delayed postpartum hemorrhage)
Implantation bleeding	Vasa previa		

Miscarriages are categorized based on timing, dilation of cervix, and if there has been any passage of tissue. Most will present with crampy lower abdominal pain and vaginal bleeding. For each of these, the **initial diagnostic testing** is **transvaginal ultrasound** and **β-hCG**. Classification of the type of miscarriage is important as it will guide management for the patient.

Types of Miscarriages and Key Features

Type	History	Exam	Management	Key Notes
Threatened miscarriage	Crampy lower abd pain Vaginal spotting	Closed cervix Intrauterine pregnancy	Expectant management Repeat tests (ultrasound, β-hCG) if ongoing pain	Vaginal bleeding occurs in patients <20 weeks gestation. In most cases, bleeding will stop, and a viable pregnancy will continue.
Inevitable miscarriage	Crampy lower abd pain Vaginal bleeding	Dilated cervix	Dilation/curettage, vaginal misoprostol, or expectant management	Cervix has dilated without other passage of tissue, making pregnancy loss inevitable
Incomplete miscarriage	Crampy lower abd pain Vaginal bleeding Passage of tissue	Dilated cervix	Dilation/curettage, vaginal misoprostol, or expectant management	Some products of conception have passed but not all. Goal is to help eliminate retained tissue to prevent bleeding & infection
Complete miscarriage	Crampy lower abd pain and vaginal bleeding, peaked and then subsided Passage of tissue	Pending timing of exam to event, cervix may be closed or dilated	If setting of pregnancy of unknown location (never had confirmed intrauterine gestation) or concern for molar pregnancy, follow β-hCG to undetectable level	All products of conception have passed without medical intervention Most pregnancy losses are due to genetic errors but can arise from poorly controlled maternal comorbid conditions β-hCG levels should be followed closely to ensure complete expulsion of pregnancy tissue and because of the risk of developing choriocarcinoma Rh alloimmunization is indicated after abortion if patient is Rh (−)
Missed miscarriage	No classic symptoms, though may describe sudden loss of "normal pregnancy symptoms" like nausea, breast tenderness	Closed cervix	Dilation/curettage or vaginal misoprostol; may consider expectant management unless concern for long duration of pregnancy loss at time of diagnosis.	Pregnancy <20 weeks gestation with embryonic or fetal demise without any maternal symptoms, such as cramping or bleeding.

Antepartum Vaginal Bleeding Mini-Cases	
Cases	**Key Findings**
Hydatidiform Mole	**Hx:** Significant nausea, emesis, and vaginal bleeding **PE:** Uterus is larger than expected for dates, hypertension, absent fetal heart tones **Diagnostics:** Pelvic ultrasound shows uterine cysts ("honeycombed," "snowstorm," or "cluster of grapes") and no fetal parts. Quantitative hCG is very elevated. TSH is low, free T4 is high. No FHTs detected. **Management:** • Dilation and curettage • Serial monitoring of hCG to confirm resolution of the molar pregnancy • Monitor for progression to gestational trophoblastic neoplasia **Discussion:** Gestational trophoblastic diseases such as choriocarcinoma, hydatidiform moles, and gestational trophoblastic neoplasias are other causes of an elevated hCG. A hyperthyroid state may occur, possibly due to the structural similarity between β-hCG and TSH. Hydatidiform molar pregnancy is caused by the abnormal proliferation of trophoblastic epithelium with the absence of a viable fetus.

Antepartum Vaginal Bleeding Mini-Cases (continued)

Hydatidiform Mole	Complete hydatidiform mole: • Typically caused from a single sperm and an enucleated ovum. • The paternal DNA from the sperm is subsequently duplicated, so the karyotype of a complete mole is 46XX but can see 46XY if two sperm enter enucleated ovum. Partial hydatidiform moles: • Typically form from two sperm and a nucleated ovum, giving rise to a characteristic triploid karyotype of 69XXX, 69XXY, or 69XYY. • Partial moles will have elevated hCG and they often show presence of fetal parts on imaging.

Placental Abruption	**Hx:** Risk Factors: Prior abruption, uncontrolled/acute hypertension, multiparity, advanced maternal age, use of cocaine or tobacco, intraamniotic infection, and trauma.
	Symptoms: Sudden-onset severe lower abdominal pain and vaginal bleeding in third trimester, decreased fetal movement.
	PE: Fundus is firm and tender, brisk vaginal bleeding is present, and fetal heart tracing is abnormal. Severe abruption may cause hypotension.
	Diagnostics: Fetal monitoring, CBC, PT/PTT, fibrinogen level (to assess for DIC)
	Management: Delivery
	• If hemodynamically stable with a normal fetal heart rate, trial of labor with goal for vaginal delivery is appropriate.
	• If a patient is hemodynamically unstable or has fetal tracing abnormalities:
	  • Resuscitation with fluids, packed red blood cells, fresh frozen plasma, and platelets if needed
	  • Once the maternal patient is stable, emergent cesarean delivery
	Discussion: Placental abruption is the premature separation of a normally implanted placenta. Abruption may be complete or partial; bleeding may be concealed or apparent.
	Complications: Hemorrhagic shock, DIC, uterine atony, fetal hypoxia, and maternal and/or fetal death.

Placenta Previa	**Hx:** Sudden, painless vaginal bleeding in the third trimester of pregnancy (≥20 weeks' gestation), postcoital bleeding. Risk Factors: Include prior cesarean birth, multiple gestations, prior placenta previa, and prior uterine curettage. **PE:** If mild bleeding, usually patient is hemodynamically stable, and normal fetal heart tones will be seen on tracing. If bleeding is severe, maternal hypotension, tachycardia, and abnormal fetal tracing may be present. **Diagnostics:** Confirm diagnosis with TVUS **Management:** Expectant management can be pursued if bleeding is not excessive and is first episode; cesarean birth should be scheduled for 36–37 weeks' gestation unless there are ongoing episodes of bleeding. **Discussion:** Placenta previa occurs when the placenta implants over the cervical internal os. Any form of vaginal manipulation can induce bleeding, such as intercourse or a cervical exam. Patients with multiple prior cesarean births and the presence of placenta previa are at high risk for abnormally invasive placenta (accreta-spectrum disorders).
Vasa Previa	**Hx:** Painless vaginal hemorrhage in third trimester of pregnancy **PE:** TVUS **Diagnostics:** Category III fetal heart tracing **Management:** If diagnosed prenatally, close monitoring with Doppler ultrasound and non-stress testing until 34 weeks' gestation and then scheduled cesarean section. If vessels are already ruptured, emergent c-section should be performed **Discussion:** Vasa previa is when the fetal vessels rupture as the cervix begins to dilate because of the abnormal location of the vessels over or near the birth canal. The main cause of vasa previa is velamentous insertion, which is when the umbilical cord inserts directly into the membranes and the vessels connect to the placenta unprotected.
Bloody Show	**Hx:** Cramping, pelvic pressure, contractions, and vaginal bleeding in late pregnancy **PE:** Presence of blood and mucus on pelvic exam, cervix may be dilated. Hemodynamically stable mother and fetus. **Diagnostics:** Clinical diagnosis **Management:** Expectant management **Discussion:** Bloody show is a normal event that occurs at the start of labor. It occurs because the cervix softens and begins to dilate.

Intrapartum Complications

Complications during labor can be due to:

- Uterine contractions that are not adequately strong or coordinated to cause effacement and dilation of the cervix
- Abnormalities in the fetal presentation, anatomy, or position which can slow progress
- Abnormalities of the pelvis and the lower reproductive tract that obstruct fetal descent or expulsion from the maternal patient

CASE 6	Arrest of Labor
A 30-year-old G1P0 at 39+2 weeks presents with regular, painful contractions occurring every 5 minutes. She denies leakage of fluid and reports fetal movement. On initial exam, the fetus is found to be cephalic, and the patient is 6 cm dilated with 90% effacement and a −2 fetal station (6/90/−2). FHTs are category I, and her contractions occur regularly every 4 minutes. The patient is admitted in active labor, and rupture of membranes occurs spontaneously as she is admitted. After 2 hours, the cervix is unchanged, so a uterine pressure catheter is placed. The contractions measure 210 Montevideo units, occurring every 2–3 minutes. Four hours later, her cervix is unchanged despite the same power of contractions.	
Conditions with Similar Presentations	**Pre-labor contractions:** Prodromal or "false" labor occurs when irregular (sometimes noted as Braxton-Hicks) contractions occur without cervical change. **PTL:** Labor is considered preterm if contractions with cervical change begin prior to 37+0 weeks. See Case 5 (PTL) above for further discussion on this topic.
Initial Diagnostic Tests	Clinical diagnosis
Next Steps in Management	Cesarean delivery
Discussion	In the active phase of the first stage of labor, arrest of labor is diagnosed after ≥4 hours without cervical change WITH adequate contractions or ≥6 hours without cervical change WITHOUT adequate contractions. **History:** Advanced maternal age, elevated BMI, and/or diabetes **Physical Exam:** Unchanged cervical dilation despite adequate contractions **Diagnostics:** Clinical diagnosis with continued serial cervical examination and fetal heart/contraction monitoring **Management:** Cesarean delivery is indicated for arrest of labor

Intrapartum Complications Mini-Case	
Case	**Key Findings**
Shoulder Dystocia	**Hx:** Prolonged or precipitous labor, macrosomia, diabetes, elevated maternal BMI **PE:** "Turtle sign"—retraction of the fetal head against the maternal perineum after head delivered, inability to deliver shoulder with normal gentle downward traction **Diagnostics:** Clinical diagnosis—noted only at delivery of the fetal head with inability to complete rest of delivery **Management:** Instruct patient to stop pushing and perform the following maneuvers, which are effective in the majority of cases: • McRoberts maneuver: hyperflexion and abduction at the maternal hips • Suprapubic pressure (NOT fundal pressure) • Delivery of posterior arm • Axillary traction

Intrapartum Complications Mini-Case *(continued)*

Shoulder Dystocia	**Discussion:** Most shoulder dystocias occur without an identified risk factor. See below table on common complications of this condition.
	Complications of Shoulder Dystocia

Fetal	
Brachial plexus injuries	**Erb palsy:** Affects the C5–C6 roots, resulting in abnormality of internal rotation, adduction, and extension of the arm ("waiter's tip")
	Klumpke palsy: Affects the C8–T1 roots, resulting in abnormality of extension at the metacarpophalangeal (MCP) joints and flexion at the distal interphalangeal (DIP) and PIP joints ("claw hand")
Clavicular fracture	Findings include tenderness and crepitus at the site of fracture, and decreased movement of the arm that is affected with an asymmetric Moro reflex
Fetal asphyxia	May occur due to compression of the umbilical cord or fetal neck vessels leading to cerebral venous obstruction, excessive vagal stimulation, and bradycardia
Maternal	Hemorrhage, higher-order perineal laceration (third and fourth degree)

POSTPARTUM COMPLICATIONS

Late-Term and Post-Term Gestation

Late term is defined as ≥41 weeks of gestation; post term is ≥42 weeks of gestation.

- Maternal risk associated with late- and post-term pregnancy include postpartum hemorrhage, increased risk for cesarean birth, and infection.
- Fetal risks include fetal dysmaturity syndrome, macrosomia, stillbirth, meconium aspiration syndrome, and oligohydramnios.
- Labor induction is recommended at 41+0. However, if patient chooses expectant management, then twice-weekly antenatal fetal surveillance is recommended.

Postpartum Vaginal Bleeding Mini-Cases

Case	Key Findings
Placenta Accreta	**Hx:** Severe, persistent hemorrhage following delivery with abnormally adherent placenta despite attempts to manually extract **Risk Factors:** Include prior uterine surgery, prior cesarean birth, placenta previa, multiple gestations, Asherman syndrome **PE:** Adherent placenta; in presence of severe hemorrhage, maternal hemodynamic instability/DIC can be seen **Diagnostics:** Obtain TVUS MRI is considered before delivery in the stable patient to better characterize degree of invasion **Management:** Hysterectomy **Discussion:** Placenta accreta is the least invasive form of abnormally invasive placental disorders. It is the invasion of the placenta into the myometrium, beyond the decidua basalis layer of the endometrium. **Placenta increta** is the invasion of the placenta into greater than 50% of the myometrium, and **placenta percreta** is the invasion of the placenta through the myometrium into uterine serosa, which can then invade nearby viscera, such as the bladder and bowel. All three present similarly, though percreta may have associated hematuria or hematochezia if visceral involvement.
Postpartum Hemorrhage	**Hx:** Cramping, pelvic pressure, contractions, and vaginal bleeding within 24 hours of delivery **PE:** Hemodynamic instability with tachycardia and hypotension, presence of blood on pelvic exam **Diagnostics:** Clinical diagnosis Obtain CBC, PT, PTT, type and screen

Postpartum Vaginal Bleeding Mini-Cases *(continued)*

Postpartum Hemorrhage	**Management:** • Fluid resuscitation, shock management, transfusion, and arrest of the source of hemorrhage, all occurring concurrently. • When retained placental tissue is suspected, evacuation with exploration is recommended. • If uterine compression or tamponade, and other conservative measures have failed to control bleeding, surgical methods can be lifesaving and include artery ligation, and in refractory cases hysterectomy. **Discussion:** Postpartum hemorrhage is the leading cause of maternal mortality worldwide. Primary postpartum hemorrhage is defined as blood loss of ≥1000 mL or sufficient blood loss causing signs and symptoms of hypovolemia occurring within 24 hours of delivery. Etiology: Four T's: • **T**one uterine atony—80% of all cases of postpartum hemorrhage • **T**rauma—maternal lacerations • **T**issue—retained placenta • **T**hrombin—coagulation defects
Uterine Atony	**Hx:** Risk factors: Include prolonged labor, macrosomia, grand-multiparity (≥5 births), or uterine infection. **PE:** Tachycardia, hypotension from profuse bleeding, and the uterus is boggy **Diagnostics:** Clinical diagnosis. CBC, PT/PTT, and bimanual exam to assess for retained placenta. **Management:** Uterine massage, uterotonics such as oxytocin, prostaglandin F2 alpha, misoprostol, or methylergonovine maleate. **Discussion:** The most common cause of postpartum hemorrhage is uterine atony. The myometrium has not contracted to cut off the uterine spiral arteries that supplied the placental bed.

Medications for Management of Postpartum Hemorrhage

Medication	Mechanism	Adverse Reactions/Contraindications
Oxytocin	Binds to uterine receptors and releases intracellular calcium causing uterine muscle contraction	Tachyarrhythmias
Methylergonovine	Stimulates increased tone, rate, and amplitude of contractions	Contraindicated in hypertensive patients
Misoprostol	Prostaglandin E1 agonist that induces uterine contraction	Can cause diarrhea, abdominal pain, and headache
Caboprost	Prostaglandin F_2-alpha agonist that induces uterine contraction	Contraindicated in patients with asthma or patients with active cardiac, renal, or hepatic disease
Tranexamic acid	Displaces plasminogen from fibrin, thus decreasing fibrinolysis	Can cause thromboembolic events, abdominal pain, altered color vision, headache, and anaphylaxis

CASE 7 | Postpartum Depression

A 28-year-old G1P1001 presents for her 6-week postpartum visit. She had a full-term spontaneous vaginal delivery complicated by postpartum hemorrhage of 750 mL. The patient is breastfeeding. She reports that since her baby has been born, she has been restless and unable to sleep through the night. She reports decreased appetite and while speaking, she becomes tearful saying, "I used to love going out to lunch with my friends and catching up, but now I'm making excuses to cancel on them. I just feel so tired throughout the day. I feel like a terrible mother!" Her exam is normal.

Conditions with Similar Presentations	Lack of sleep, hypothyroidism, and anemia can also cause fatigue, low energy. **Postpartum blues:** A temporary condition, characterized by mood lability and mild depressive symptoms, that resolves within 2 weeks of delivery. **Postpartum psychosis:** Hallucinations or delusions, accompanied by symptoms of a depressive or manic episode. The patient needs to be separated from their child(ren) and started on antipsychotic medication.

CASE 7 | Postpartum Depression *(continued)*

Conditions with Similar Presentations	**Sheehan syndrome (postpartum pituitary infarct) resulting in hypothyroidism:** • The pituitary is enlarged during pregnancy which makes it more susceptible to ischemia and infarction. • Excessive hemorrhage and hypovolemia during delivery can result in infarction. • Can be differentiated by the presence of amenorrhea (decreased luteinizing hormone, LH), inability to breastfeed (decreased prolactin), symptoms of hypothyroidism (decreased TSH) and MRI findings. • Treatment is replacement of hormones.
Initial Diagnostic Tests	Clinical diagnosis based on DSM-5 criteria (See Chapter 16, Psychiatry) Consider checking: CBC, TSH
Next Steps in Management	• Assess risk for suicidal/homicidal ideation • Psycho/behavioral therapy and/or selective serotonin reuptake inhibitors (SSRIs)
Discussion	Postpartum depression refers to minor depressive symptoms, mood disorders, or unipolar major depressive disorder which occurs in the postpartum period (the first 12 months after delivery). The rapid decline in estrogen and progesterone in the postpartum period is thought to play a role. This is seen in 6.5–20% of all postpartum patients. **History:** Risk Factors: for postpartum depression include prior depression or family history of perinatal depression and anxiety, a traumatic birth experience or preterm birth, low levels of social support, adolescence. Symptoms: DSM criteria for depression and suicide risk. Ask about infant sleep pattern and personal and family history of depression. **Physical Exam:** May have a flat or constricted affect. **Diagnostics:** Criteria for postpartum depression are the same as for major depressive disorder: five or more symptoms during the same 2-week period that are a change from previous functioning. Symptoms may include depressed mood, loss of interest/pleasure, insomnia or hypersomnia, weight loss or gain, psychomotor agitation or retardation, feeling worthless or having excessive/inappropriate guilt, fatigue, decreased concentration, thoughts of death/suicide. • Depressed mood and/or loss of interest/pleasure must be present. • The symptoms must result in clinically significant distress or impairment in occupational, social or other important areas of functioning. • The episode should not be attributable to another medical condition or physiological effects of a substance. • The provider should also rule out any psychotic disorder or history of manic or hypomanic episodes. **Management:** • Psycho/behavioral therapy is the first line for mild to moderate postpartum depression. • Antidepressants are considered for patients who meet criteria for major postpartum depression, with SSRI being the first-line medication. • Although most medications are found in breast milk, they are present at very low levels and do not produce clinically relevant effects in the neonate. • For patients who breastfeed monitoring serum levels in the neonate is not recommended. • Psychiatric referral is recommended for those who do not respond to 6 weeks of therapy.
Additional Considerations	**Screening:** All patients should be screened at least once during the perinatal period for depression and anxiety symptoms using a standardized, validated tool, such as the Patient Health Questionnaire 9 or Edinburgh Postnatal Depression Scale. A full assessment of emotional well-being and mood should be done during the first postpartum visit for all patients. **Inpatient Considerations:** A suicide risk assessment should be performed on all patients with depression, and patients who are suicidal must be stabilized and treated in a hospital.

CARDIOPULMONARY EMERGENCIES IN PREGNANCY

Cardiopulmonary collapse in pregnancy can be caused by various insults and should always be treated emergently. Some of the common causes of cardiac collapse during pregnancy are given below.

Diagnosis	Symptoms and Signs	Lab findings/Imaging
Amniotic fluid embolism (AFE)	Sudden catastrophic cardiovascular collapse during labor up to 30 minutes after delivery of the placenta	Disseminated intravascular coagulopathy (DIC)
Pulmonary thromboembolism (PE)	Sudden obstructive shock	Hypoxemia CT scan or VQ scan confirm diagnosis
Air embolism	Sudden obstructive shock with provoking factor (i.e., instrumentation, central line insertion) Can be associated with a "mill-wheel" murmur	Air can be visualized with bedside echocardiography
Anesthetic accident (high spinal anesthesia, local anesthetic toxicity)	Distributive shock	
Myocardial infarction (MI) or peripartum cardiomyopathy	Cardiogenic shock Crushing substernal pain	ECG-ST wave changes Echocardiography with regional wall motion abnormality pericardial effusion, valve rupture
Septic shock	Hypotension, fever; infectious source	Leukocytosis with left shift DIC may be present
Acute respiratory distress syndrome (ARDS)	Difficulty breathing Precipitating factors may be present.	Hypoxemia Chest x-ray shows findings of ARDS

Causes of Disseminated Intravascular Coagulopathy (DIC)

- **Pregnancy complications:** Amniotic fluid embolism, placental abruption, HELLP syndrome, severe preeclampsia/eclampsia, septic abortion, postpartum hemorrhage
- **Acute hemolytic transfusion reaction (ABO incompatibility)**
- **Sepsis**
- **Liver disease/failure**
- **Vascular malformations:** Peritoneovenous shunt, abdominal aortic aneurysm, giant hemangioma
- **Cancer:** Procoagulant state (Trousseau syndrome), acute leukemia
- **Trauma:** Severe head injury, crush injury, complicated surgery, burns
- **Exposure/substance:** Heat stroke, amphetamines, snake venom

CASE 8 | Amniotic Fluid Embolism (AFE)

A 27-year-old G4P2103 at 35+2 weeks undergoes induction of labor for preeclampsia with severe features. The patient suddenly becomes agitated with the following vitals: T 37.0°C, P 50, BP 85/60, R 20, and there is a sudden drop in SPO_2 to 72%. Oxygen and IV fluids are initiated, but maternal pulse becomes undetectable, and the fetal heart rate is bradycardic. While the team is performing resuscitative measures, the patient begins to bleed spontaneously from the IV sites.

Conditions with Similar Presentations	**Pulmonary embolism:** Presents with dyspnea, hypoxia but not DIC **Septic shock:** Presents with fevers and signs of infection at primary site. **Peripartum cardiomyopathy:** Presents with signs and symptoms of heart failure confirmed by echocardiogram.
Initial Diagnostic Tests	• Clinical diagnosis. High pulmonary artery pressures on TEE support diagnosis • Also check: CBC, ABG, BMP, BNP, coagulation profile to exclude other diagnosis and establish a baseline
Next Steps in Management	• Cardiopulmonary resuscitation • Emergent cesarean delivery • DIC management including replacement of products (massive transfusion protocol)

CASE 8 | **Amniotic Fluid Embolism (AFE)** *(continued)*

Discussion	AFE, usually presents as sudden cardiopulmonary collapse (hypoxia and hypotension, noncardiogenic pulmonary edema) with or without DIC. AFE is thought to be a massive anaphylactoid response to fetal debris in the maternal circulation. Vasoactive and procoagulant substances elevate pulmonary pressures, causing ventilation/perfusion mismatch, pulmonary edema, hypoxemic respiratory failure, and increased right ventricular pressure, leading to heart failure. Maternal inflammatory mediators are activated, setting off the coagulation cascade and causing DIC. AFE is exceedingly rare, with some estimates as infrequent as 1 in 80,000 births. The majority (70%) occur during labor, 11% occur within 30 minutes of delivery of the placenta, and 19% occur during cesarean births. Onset is abrupt, catastrophic, and rapidly progressive in 90% of cases.
	History: Symptoms include agitation, chills, nausea/vomiting, dyspnea, bleeding from IV sites. One-third of patients may have a prodrome, including agitation and sense of impending doom.
	Physical Exam:
	Rapidly destabilized vitals: sudden hypotension, bradycardia, and drop in oxygen saturation. Sudden bleeding from IV sites is indicative of DIC.
	Diagnostics: Clinical diagnosis aided by the exclusion of other diagnoses
	• Coagulation changes occur within 30 minutes of cardiopulmonary compromise)
	• D-dimer: ↑ (but nonspecific, often elevated in pregnancy)
	• CBC: thrombocytopenia and possible anemia secondary to hemorrhage and/or ↑WBC (nonspecific, as may be elevated in labor)
	• Fibrinogen: ↓ (usually <200 mg/L)
	• ECG: May show sinus tachycardia or arrhythmia
	• Arterial blood gas (ABG): Profound hypoxemia, possibly hypercapnia
	CXR: Initially may be normal, followed by bilateral pulmonary infiltrates.
	• Echocardiography: Increased pulmonary pressures followed by left ventricular failure, possible right ventricular enlargement
	The Society for Maternal-Fetal Medicine and AFE Foundation developed diagnostic criteria for AFE: All four below must be present:
	1. Sudden cardiorespiratory arrest OR hypotension (systolic BP <90 mmHg) with evidence of respiratory compromise
	2. DIC
	• Platelet count: >100,000/mL = 0, <100,000/mL = 1, <50,000/mL = 2
	• Increased PTT or INR: <25% = 0, 25–50% = 1, >50% = 2
	• Fibrinogen level: >200 mg/L = 1, <200 mg/L = 1
	3. Onset within 30 minutes of placental delivery
	4. Absence of fever (T ≤38C)
	Management:
	Emergent management of unstable patients:
	• Perform CPR and initiate multidisciplinary resuscitative efforts (e.g., crystalloid IV fluids if hemorrhage is not present or until blood products arrive, supplemental oxygen or intubation, vasopressors)
	• Control hemorrhage and reverse coagulopathy: Administer tranexamic acid, crossmatch and screen blood products, and activate massive transfusion protocol
	• CBC, BUN/Cr/Ca/Mg/phosphate, ABG, PT/PTT, troponin, BNP, ECG, and imaging (bedside echocardiography, ultrasound, CXR)
	• Emergent cesarean delivery is indicated, which ideally should occur within 4 minutes of cardiovascular collapse to prevent neurologic deficits in the neonate.
	Care of stable patients:
	• Care is mainly supportive
	• Close follow-up testing with labs and CXR to monitor for worsening or complications as indicated
	• Delivery
Additional Considerations	**Complications:** AFE has a poor maternal prognosis. Cause of death is most commonly cardiac arrest/cardiogenic shock (85%) and/or hypoxemia (50%), resulting in death usually within the first hour. The fetal mortality rate is 20–60%, and 50% of surviving neonates have neurologic deficits.

HYPERTENSION IN PREGNANCY

Hypertensive disease in pregnancy spans a spectrum of severities and symptoms. Diagnosis can be determined by the timing of onset of elevated blood pressures and other associated symptoms/findings. Antihypertensives used in pregnancy are labetalol, nifedipine, and methyldopa (less common); in acute hypertensive treatment, may also use hydralazine.

Definitions

Chronic Hypertension

Diagnosis of hypertension prior to pregnancy, elevated blood pressure present before 20 weeks' gestation, or persistent 12 weeks after delivery.

Gestational Hypertension

Elevated blood pressure (Systolic BP ≥ 140 and/or diastolic BP ≥ 90) *after* 20 weeks' gestation in a patient with previously normal blood pressures *without* proteinuria or other signs/symptoms of end-organ damage.

Preeclampsia

- Elevated blood pressure *after* 20 weeks' gestation in a patient with previously normal blood pressures *with* proteinuria (≥300 mg/dL of protein in 24 hours) and/or signs/symptoms of end-organ damage (<20 weeks suggests molar pregnancy)
- Classified as severe if any of the following criteria are met: Severe-range blood pressure (systolic ≥160 or diastolic ≥110), creatinine >1.1mg/dl or twice baseline, AST/ALT twice the upper limit of normal or twice baseline if underlying hepatic disease, platelets <100,000, persistent headache unresolved with acetaminophen, visual disturbances, persistent RUQ or epigastric pain not responding to medication and pulmonary edema.

HELLP Syndrome

- Subset of preeclampsia
- **H**emolysis, **E**levated **L**iver enzymes, **L**ow **P**latelet count

Eclampsia

- Preeclampsia plus maternal seizures

CASE 9	Preeclampsia	
	A 35-year-old G1P0 presents at 38+1 weeks' gestation with persistent headache not relieved by analgesics, and visual disturbances. Her blood pressure is 170/95 mmHg and she has bilateral 3+ LE edema to the knee.	
Conditions with Similar Presentations	**Chronic (pregestational) hypertension:** Onset prior to pregnancy	
	Gestational hypertension: Absence of proteinuria or end-organ damage.	
	HELLP: Abnormal CBC with smear (↓ platelets, schistocytes) and abnormal liver tests (↑ transaminases, ↑ bilirubin).	
Initial Diagnostic Tests	• Confirm with urine protein • Check CBC, serum electrolytes and creatinine, serial blood pressure	
Next Steps in Management	• Magnesium sulfate • Antihypertensive medications • Prompt delivery	
Discussion	Preeclampsia is diagnosed when there is new hypertension after 20 weeks of gestation and new-onset proteinuria. It can be diagnosed in the absence of proteinuria if the patient presents with severe features (see below). It is linked to abnormal remodeling of the placental spiral arteries, causing widespread endothelial dysfunction, vasoconstriction, and spasm leading to ischemia.	
	Preeclampsia is considered severe if it has the following features: • Systolic >160 or diastolic ≥110 • Platelet count <100 K • Liver transaminase levels 2 × upper limit of normal • Doubling of serum creatinine or >1.1mg/dl • Severe RUQ/epigastric pain or headache unrelieved with medication • Pulmonary edema	

CASE 9 | Preeclampsia *(continued)*

Discussion	**History:** Risk Factors: DM, CKD, preexisting HTN, autoimmune disorders, primigravid patients. Patients may be asymptomatic or present with severe persistent RUQ pain, severe persistent headache, visual disturbances **Physical Exam:** Elevated blood pressure, retinal hemorrhages, papilledema, pulmonary edema, pedal edema **Diagnostics:** • Urine protein: elevated (≥300 mg/dL of protein in 24 hours or protein-creatinine ratio 0.3 or greater) • CBC with smear to detect thrombocytopenia, schistocytes, serum electrolytes, creatinine and albumin to assess for hepatic and/or renal dysfunction. **Management:** Delivery is the definitive treatment. • Delivery at 37 weeks or, if severe features, delivery at 34 weeks or any time after diagnosis. • Magnesium sulfate is the prophylactic anticonvulsant of choice. (Monitor for magnesium toxicity—loss of deep tendon reflexes, respiratory depression, cardiac arrhythmias/arrest.) • Severe hypertension must also be controlled with antihypertensive medication (e.g., labetalol, hydralazine) to reduce risk for stroke.
Additional Considerations	**Screening:** BP measurements at each prenatal visit. **Complications:** Pulmonary edema, renal failure, coagulopathy, HELLP syndrome, uteroplacental insufficiency, and placental abruption. Progression to **eclampsia** is one of the most serious complications of preeclampsia and it is diagnosed by the presence of maternal seizures.

High Blood Pressure during Pregnancy Mini-Cases

Cases	Key Findings
HELLP Syndrome	**Hx:** Nausea, vomiting, RUQ/abdominal pain in pregnancy >20 weeks' gestation with elevated blood pressure **PE:** Elevated blood pressure; tenderness to palpation is noted in the RUQ of the abdomen. **Diagnostics:** • CBC (↓ Hb, ↓ platelets) with smear showing schistocytes indicative of microangiopathic hemolytic anemia • ↑ reticulocyte count • Abnormal liver tests (↑ transaminases, ↑ bilirubin) Also consider checking: • PT, INR, aPTT • Urine protein/creatinine ratio (to assess for proteinuria) • Abdominal US **Management:** Administer magnesium sulfate, and delivery. **Discussion:** HELLP syndrome is on the spectrum of hypertensive disorders of pregnancy, and it is an extreme manifestation of severe preeclampsia. The diagnosis of HELLP syndrome requires the presence of the following: 1. *Hemolysis*, related to microangiopathic hemolytic anemia is characterized by the presence of schistocytes on peripheral smear 2. Elevated *Liver* enzymes at least above 2 times the upper limit of normal 3. Low *Platelet* count <100,000/mm³ 4. Elevated total bilirubin due to indirect hyperbilirubinemia related to hemolysis If left untreated, it can progress to DIC and subcapsular hematoma of the liver. Delivery is the only known treatment.
Chronic Hypertension in Pregnancy	**Hx:** Elevated blood pressure in pregnant patient present before 20 weeks of gestation, maybe asymptomatic **PE:** No abnormal physical exam findings **Diagnostics:** Repeat blood pressure. Check urine protein, liver function tests, CBC with platelet count, and serum creatinine. **Management:** Antihypertensives (e.g., labetalol, nifedipine, methyldopa) **Discussion:** Chronic hypertension is blood pressure of 140/90 before pregnancy or before 20 weeks of gestation. It should be managed with non-teratogenic antihypertensives. Left untreated, increases the risk of developing preeclampsia and HELLP.

INFECTIOUS DISEASE CONSIDERATIONS IN PREGNANCY

Pregnant people carry the same risk of exposure to infectious diseases as the general population. Many have unique considerations related to potential for teratogenicity and vertical transmission in labor.

Transmission of Infectious Diseases during Pregnancy and Postpartum Care

Infectious Agent	Transplacental	During Delivery	Breast Milk
HIV	x	x	x
Herpes simplex (HSV)	x	x	x
Varicella Zoster virus (VZV)	x		
Cytomegalovirus (CMV)	x		x
Rubella	x		
Parvovirus 19	x		
Treponema pallidum	x		
Listeria monocytogenes	x		
Toxoplasma gondii	x		
Zika virus	x		
Hepatitis viruses	x	x	
Neisseria gonorrhea		x	
Chlamydia trachomatis		x	
Group B *Streptococcus* (GBS)		x	
Human papillomavirus (HPV)		x	
Covid-19		x	
Human T cell lymphotropic viruses (HTLV)			x

Infectious Diseases Occurring in Pregnancy

TORCHes

Infection	Transmission	Fetal findings
Congenital toxoplasmosis	• Undercooked meat and occasionally cat feces	• Neonatal infections with chorioretinitis, hydrocephalus, and intracranial calcifications
Congenital syphilis	• Sexual • Routine testing first trimester	• Stillbirth, hydrops fetalis • Prematurity • Congenital deafness • Facial abnormalities—notched teeth, saddle nose • Most are asymptomatic at birth
Congenital cytomegalovirus (most common congenital viral infection)	• Contact with children, such as in daycare facilities	• Sensorineural hearing loss, seizures • "Blueberry muffin" rash • Periventricular calcifications
HSV	• Perinatally acquired during vaginal delivery	• Localized mucocutaneous disease—vesicles that may lead to scarring and eye damage • CNS disease • Disseminated disease

TORCHeS: **T**oxoplasmosis, **O**ther, **R**ubella, **C**ytomegalovirus (CMV), **H**erpes simplex virus (HSV), **S**yphilis

Pregnancy and HIV

HIV in Pregnancy	Recommendations
Maternal	• Administer vaccines not yet received (including hepatitis A, hepatitis B) • Start or continue combination antiretroviral therapy • Discuss delivery route and breastfeeding • If viral load (VL) <1000 copies/mL, vaginal birth is a safe option • If VL is >1000 copies/mL, offer cesarean delivery (reduces the transmission rate by 80%) and plan intrapartum zidovudine
Fetus	• Administer prophylactic antiretroviral therapy • With access to safe formula preparations, advise against breastfeeding (transmission risk as high as 20%) • Breastfeeding benefit is outweighed by risk in low-resource settings (e.g., low or no access to clean water, high risk for malnutrition)

CASE 10 | Rubella in Pregnancy

A 33-year-old primigravida at 18+4 weeks' gestation presents with fever and macular rash which started on her face. On exam, vitals are P 98, BP 110/80, T 101°F, R 18. The rash is localized to the face and trunk, is pink, maculopapular, and blanches with pressure but does not coalesce. There is generalized lymphadenopathy.

Conditions with Similar Presentations	**TORCH Infections and other infections** such as Varicella (VZV), Parvovirus, HIV, and HBV differentiated by history, exam, and testing. **Congenital toxoplasmosis:** Most mothers asymptomatic, transmitted via undercooked meat and occasionally cat feces. **Congenital cytomegalovirus:** Most mothers asymptomatic; transmitted via contact with children, such as in daycare facilities.
Initial Diagnostic Tests	• Rubella-specific IgM antibodies • Fetal ultrasound
Next Steps in Management	Symptomatic management
Discussion	Rubella is transmitted via airborne droplets. Eighty percent vertical transmission noted in the first trimester. Since the onset of consistent vaccination against rubella, infection in pregnancy is rare. Titers are routinely checked in early pregnancy to establish a patient's immunity status. **History:** Symptoms include fever, malaise, rash, and arthralgias; 20–50% may be asymptomatic. **Physical Exam:** Macular, blanching rash that begins on face and trunk; lymphadenopathy **Diagnostics:** Diagnosis confirmed with Rubella-specific IgM antibodies **Management:** • Symptomatic management • Check fetal ultrasound
Additional Considerations	**Screening:** Titers are routinely checked in early pregnancy to establish a patient's immunity status; should be checked for immunity with preconception care, so patients can be vaccinated if susceptible. **Complications:** Most infants are asymptomatic but may develop symptoms over time. Fetal infection is associated miscarriage, intrauterine growth restriction, eye defects, sensorineural hearing loss, purpuric "blueberry muffin" rash, patent ductus arteriosus, and cerebral palsy. The classic triad consists of cataracts, deafness, and congenital heart disease.

Infections during Pregnancy Mini-Cases

Cases	Key Findings
Herpes Simplex Virus (HSV)	**Hx:** May have history of HSV or recurrent painful, itchy ulcers, swollen lymph nodes **PE:** May have active vesicular lesions **Diagnostics:** Clinical diagnosis, confirm with swab of unroofed vesicle **Management:** • Daily prophylaxis with acyclovir, valacyclovir starting 36+0 weeks until delivery • Cesarean delivery if active lesions during labor or induction **Discussion:** Cesarean birth is indicated in patients with active genital lesions or prodrome at the time of labor, as these symptoms suggest viral shedding and risk of neonatal herpes infection, which carries significant neonatal morbidity and mortality. Administration of antiviral prophylaxis at 36 weeks helps reduce need for cesarean birth.

Infections during Pregnancy Mini-Cases (continued)

Hepatitis B Virus (HBV)	**Hx:** Risk Factors: Include IVDU, unprotected intercourse. Usually asymptomatic. If symptomatic may have abdominal pain, jaundice, nausea, fatigue. **PE:** Jaundice, RUQ tenderness, hepatomegaly **Diagnostics:** Hepatitis B surface antigen **Management:** Neonates of seropositive patients should receive hepatitis B immune globulin within 12 hours of delivery and should begin the hepatitis B vaccination series before discharge **Discussion:** Pregnant people who are hepatitis B surface antigen–positive transmit the virus transplacentally ~90% of the time. Newborns and young children face higher rates of morbidity and mortality, so prevention is important. Routine serum screen with initial prenatal visit is recommended.
Human Papillomavirus (HPV)	**Hx:** May be asymptomatic or have itchiness and/or genital warts **PE:** May have genital warts **Diagnostics:** Cervical specimen for HPV via PCR testing **Management:** • If high-risk strain present (e.g., HPV 16 and 18), may obtain pap and colposcopy during pregnancy to assess for cervical dysplasia or cancer. • Low-risk HPV (e.g., 6, 11) are associated with genital warts/condyloma acuminata which may be treated to prevent potential obstruction of the vaginal canal using trichloroacetic acid, cryoablation, laser therapy, or surgical removal for large/obstructive warts. **Discussion:** Treatment options do not reduce vertical transmission. If HPV transmission occurs during delivery, papillomas may occur on mucosal, conjunctival, or laryngeal surfaces in early childhood. Podophyllin, interferon, and fluorouracil are contraindicated in pregnancy.
Neisseria gonorrhoeae (GC)	**Hx:** Often asymptomatic. Symptoms include mucopurulent discharge, itchiness, foul odor, pelvic pain, dyspareunia, dysuria if urethral involvement. **PE:** Discharge and inflammation of cervix may be noted on pelvic exam **Diagnostics:** • Routine NAAT testing of vaginal or cervical swab with initial prenatal visit • Consider repeat in third trimester based on risks • In pregnancy, test of cure is recommended at 4 weeks **Management:** • IM ceftriaxone. Add presumptive treatment for *Chlamydia* with azithromycin if NAAT testing for it is not immediately available. • Treatment of sexual partners should be administered where expedited partner therapy (EPT) is an option. **Discussion:** Neonates with intrapartum infection can develop ophthalmia neonatorum 5–10 days postpartum, causing irreversible visual impairment. This is the rationale for universal prophylactic topical erythromycin at birth. GC in pregnancy may also cause preterm PPROM, intraamniotic infection, PTL, and neonatal and/or maternal postpartum sepsis.
Chlamydia trachomatis (CT)	**Hx:** Watery discharge, itchiness, foul odor, pelvic pain, dyspareunia, dysuria if urethral involvement **PE:** Discharge and inflammation of cervix on pelvic exam **Diagnostics:** Vaginal swab to perform NAAT test **Management:** • Oral azithromycin • If neonatal conjunctivitis is suspected, administer azithromycin eye drops in newborn. **Discussion:** Neonates exposed during delivery may develop neonatal conjunctivitis (within 2 weeks; most common cause of neonatal conjunctivitis) or pneumonia (within 3–4 months). CT in pregnancy may also cause PPROM, PTL, low birth weight, and neonatal death.
Group B Streptococcus (GBS)	**Hx:** Usually asymptomatic or generalized flu-like symptoms, lethargy, irritability, difficulty feeding in neonate **PE:** Signs of sepsis in neonate: hypotension, fever, irregular breathing, and cardiac activity **Diagnostics:** Vaginal and rectal swab indicated between 35 and 37 weeks

Infections during Pregnancy Mini-Cases *(continued)*

Group B *Streptococcus* (GBS)	**Management:** • Routine screening via vaginal and rectal swab at 35–37 weeks • If positive, or if unknown status with certain criteria (preterm gestational age in setting of labor, rupture of membranes [ROM] for >18 hours, previous GBS in another pregnancy, GBS bacteriuria any time in pregnancy, or temperature >100.4°F), treat with IV penicillin G or ampicillin • Negative GBS results are valid for 5 weeks **Discussion:** GBS can cause neonatal sepsis, maternal UTI, intraamniotic infection, and endometritis in pregnancy (outside of pregnancy, generally an asymptomatic colonizer).

CASE 11 | Intra-amniotic Inflammation and Infection

A 25-year-old G3P2002 at 39+0 weeks' gestation comes to the hospital in labor. She had spontaneous rupture of membranes 24 hours ago. She reports good fetal movement and regular contractions. On physical exam, patient's temperature is 38.8°C, pulse is 114, respirations are 20/min, blood pressure is 104/69 mmHg and SpO_2 is 98% on room air. There is tenderness to palpation over the uterine fundus. The cervix is 4 cm dilated, 50% effaced, and fetal station −2.

Conditions with Similar Presentations	**Postpartum endometritis:** Infection of the decidua is a common cause of postpartum fever and patients presents *after* delivery with fever, uterine tenderness, and purulent lochia. **Prelabor rupture of membranes (PROM):** Membrane rupture before labor, and patients present with leakage of fluid from the vagina without regular contractions producing cervical change.
Initial Diagnostic Tests	• Clinical diagnosis (see below) • Monitor maternal and fetal vitals
Next Steps in Management	• Antibiotics • Antipyretics • Continue toward delivery with labor augmentation

Discussion	Intraamniotic inflammation and infection ("triple I"), known previously as chorioamnionitis, is an infection with inflammation involving any combination of the fetus, fetal membranes, placenta, amniotic fluid, or decidua. The infection is ascending bacterial invasion originating from the vaginal flora, usually polymicrobial, involving aerobic and anaerobic bacteria.
	History:
	Risk Factors include:
	• Prolonged labor and/or rupture of membranes
	• Multiple digital cervical exams
	• Presence of certain genital tract pathogens like group B streptococcal infection, and sexually transmitted infections
	Physical Exam: Fever, maternal and/or fetal tachycardia, uterine tenderness
	Diagnostics:
	• Clinical diagnosis: Maternal intrapartum fever and one or more of the following: fundal tenderness, purulent cervical drainage, maternal and/or fetal tachycardia, and maternal leukocytosis.
	• Check CBC
	• Consider blood, urine, and vaginal cultures to rule out other causes
	Management:
	Start antibiotics and antipyretics to reduce fever, and supportive care (e.g., IV fluids)
	• Intrapartum antibiotics
	  • Gold standard: Ampicillin and gentamicin
	  • Cefazolin and gentamicin (if mild penicillin allergy)
	  • Clindamycin and gentamicin (if severe penicillin allergy)
	• For patients undergoing cesarean deliveries, an additional dose of antibiotics after delivery is recommended for anaerobic coverage
	• Intraamniotic infection alone is not an indication for cesarean delivery unless worsening of infection or other usual indications for cesarean birth

Additional Considerations	**Complications:** Neonatal complications: Pneumonia, meningitis, sepsis, bronchopulmonary dysplasia, and cerebral palsy Maternal complications: Postpartum uterine atony/hemorrhage and postpartum endometritis

ENDOCRINE DISORDERS IN PREGNANCY

Endocrine Disorders in Pregnancy Mini-Cases	
Cases	**Key Findings**
Pregestational and Gestational Diabetes	**Hx:** Increased thirst, urination, and fatigue Risk factors: History of fetal macrosomia, gestational diabetes in previous pregnancies, elevated BMI, hypertension, PCOS, and/or other conditions associated with the metabolic syndrome **PE:** May have acanthosis nigricans, elevated BMI, possible fundal height/size greater than dates Fetal findings: Macrosomia **Diagnostics:** • Screening test: 1-hour oral glucose challenge test (50 g at 24–28 weeks) if blood sugar (BS) ≥140 mg/dL, needs diagnostic assessment • Diagnostic test: 3-hour oral glucose tolerance test (100 g), presence of ≥2 of any of the following abnormal results confirms the diagnosis of gestational diabetes: first hour, BS ≥180 mg/dL, second hour ≥155 mg/dL, third hour ≥140 mg/dL **Management:** • Nutrition counseling and lifestyle modifications (diet, exercise) • Prenatal counseling regarding fetal macrosomia • Blood glucose goals in pregnancy: Fasting plasma glucose <95 mg/dL and 2 hours postprandial <120 mg/dL • Antihyperglycemic therapy if not managed with diet alone • Insulin: Gold standard of treatment in pregnancy; requirements often increase between 28–32 weeks; does not cross the placenta • Metformin is safe in pregnancy **Discussion:** Gestational diabetes: Two important fetal complications include macrosomia and shoulder dystocia. Pregestational diabetes: Seen in 2% of all pregnancies • Increased risk of abnormal fetal outcomes with either type 1 or type 2 diabetes—especially if poor glucose control at the time of conception Possible abnormal fetal outcomes include cardiac defects (most common of all defects [e.g., ventriculoseptal defect, transposition of the great arteries]), cleft lip/palate, and neural tube defects
Hyperthyroidism	**Hx:** Weight loss, excessive sweating, anxiety, palpitations, heat intolerance, insomnia, and hyperdefecation **PE:** Can be normal or present with diaphoresis, exophthalmos, postural hand tremor, goiter, thyroid nodules **Diagnostics:** • ↓TSH, May have ↑free T4, ↑free T3 • (↑Thyroid-stimulating immunoglobulin level distinguishes Graves' disease from other causes) **Management:** • Give propylthiouracil or methimazole at lowest possible dose (both cross placenta) to achieve TSH between 0.5 and 2.5 • Repeat labs every 6–8 weeks • Fetal survey at 18–20 weeks and fetal ultrasound in third trimester to assess for fetal goiter • Non-stress testing antenatally to look for signs of fetal hyperthyroidism (i.e., tachycardia) **Discussion:** In normal early pregnancy, T3 and T4 levels are elevated and TSH levels are low. One to three percent of pregnant people have transient gestational thyrotoxicosis, and 0.2% have Graves' disease (the most common cause of hyperthyroidism). Complications can include preeclampsia, heart failure, and PTL. Fetal and neonatal hyperthyroidism can occur.

Endocrine Disorders in Pregnancy Mini-Cases *(continued)*

Hypothyroidism	**Hx:** Weight gain, excessive fatigue, cold intolerance, constipation
	PE: Coarse dry skin, bradycardia
	Diagnostics: ↑TSH, ↓T4, ↓T3
	Management:
	• Oral levothyroxine is the recommended treatment
	• Increase baseline levothyroxine dose by 25–30% (due to increased volume of distribution, binding globulins, renal clearance, and metabolic rate)
	• Maintain TSH at low normal level
	• Repeat labs each trimester or 4 weeks after medication changes
	Discussion: Hypothyroidism in pregnancy is defined as TSH levels above the normal limit of pregnancy-specific range. Thyroid autoantibodies are present in 30–60% of patients, and prevalence of hypothyroidism is 2–3% of all pregnancies. Hashimoto thyroiditis is the most common cause in pregnancy. The fetus does not produce thyroid hormone for 12–14 weeks and is dependent on the parent for thyroid hormone.

OTHER COMORBID CONDITIONS IN PREGNANCY

Comorbid Conditions in Pregnancy Mini-Cases

Cases	Key Findings
Seizure Disorders	**Hx/PE:**
	Risk Factors: Personal or family history of seizure disorders, or congenital malformation. In a patient with seizures, number of seizures in the year prior to pregnancy is the best predictor of seizure frequency in pregnancy. Antiepileptic drug (AED) use and adherence should be assessed.
	Diagnostics: AED: Check prepregnancy levels, monitor and maintain therapeutic levels monthly during pregnancy and at the time of labor.
	Management: Shared decision-making is ideally performed at a preconception appointment.
	• Aim to transition to the lowest possible dose of AED monotherapy with the lowest teratogenicity (e.g., lamotrigine, levetiracetam, or oxcarbazepine).
	• Maternal serum alpha-fetoprotein screening test at 16 weeks and detailed anatomy ultrasound if needed
	• Vitamin K supplementation in late pregnancy is recommended if taking an AED, which is an inducer of P450 enzymes that metabolize vitamin K. Recommend supplemental folate to prevent neural tube defects.
	Discussion:
	• Pregnant patients with epilepsy have a greater baseline risk of fetal malformation, which must be weighed again the risk of fetal congenital abnormalities associated with antiepileptic drugs (AEDs).
	• Epilepsy also confers a higher risk of spontaneous abortion, perinatal death, and patients may see an increase in seizure activity during pregnancy.
	• The hormonal (estrogen is epileptogenic) and physiologic (increased intravascular volume and renal function, sleep deprivation) changes of pregnancy may affect AED pharmacokinetics (estrogen increases the function of cytochrome P_{450} enzymes in the liver, has a greater volume of distribution and greater renal clearance), so levels must be monitored closely.
	• Fetal hydantoin syndrome: Spectrum of disorders with facial, hand, and phalangeal abnormalities, microcephaly, ocular defects, intrauterine growth restriction, congenital heart defects, and variable systemic abnormalities involving the nervous, renal, and gastrointestinal systems caused by in utero exposure to phenytoin.
	• Valproate: Associated with neural tube defects.
	• Phenobarbital: Associated with cardiac defects.
	• Topiramate and zonisamide: Associated with low birth weight.
	• Levetiracetam and lamotrigine: Lowest teratogenic risk, and are first line if medication is initiated during pregnancy.

Comorbid Conditions in Pregnancy Mini-Cases *(continued)*

Systemic Lupus Erythematosus (SLE)	**Hx:** Review personal course of SLE with focus on frequency of flares (patients who do not have flares immediately prior to pregnancy have a better course), history of antiphospholipid antibody syndrome, obstetric history (including prior spontaneous abortions), history or symptoms of other autoimmune disease, current medications, and adherence **PE:** May have malar rash (see Chapter 10, Rheumatology and Musculoskeletal disorders) **Diagnostics:** Patients with SLE have higher risk for preeclampsia; therefore, monitoring with the following baseline tests recommended: • 24-hour urine studies for proteinuria • Blood counts, coagulation studies, liver and renal tests If concern for flare: Check for active urine sediment and reduced complement levels of C3 and C4 **Management:** *Maintenance:* • Continue medications such as hydroxychloroquine for arthritis and skin manifestations. • If antiphospholipid antibodies present and/or recurrent pregnancy losses, initiate antepartum prophylaxis with low-dose aspirin and heparin in first trimester. *Lupus flares:* • Low-dose corticosteroids if not adequately controlled with acetaminophen or hydroxychloroquine. • Manage severe flares with high-dose corticosteroids and/or cyclophosphamide. **Discussion:** • SLE confers a high risk of thrombosis, infection, transfusion, cesarean birth, PTL, preeclampsia, fetal loss, and maternal mortality for pregnant patients. • Placental thrombosis causes a higher rate of second trimester loss. • There is also a risk of FGR leading to intrauterine fetal demise (IUFD), so antenatal testing indicated starting at 32+0 weeks. • Prognosis of SLE during pregnancy follows a rule of thirds: one-third improve, one-third worsen, and one-third have unchanged disease. • Signs and symptoms of lupus flares (CNS lupus, hypertension, pulmonary edema, renal disease, hepatitis, thrombocytopenia, hemolytic anemia) are often difficult to distinguish from symptoms of preeclampsia/eclampsia. Lupus flares typically have reduced C3 and C4 complement levels and active urine sediment. **Neonatal lupus:** Antinuclear antibodies (specifically anti-Ro/SSA and anti-La/SSB) can cross the placenta and cause fetal skin lesions, hepatosplenomegaly, cytopenias, and heart block. Management includes serial fetal monitoring and fetal electrocardiogram, and treatments include corticosteroids, plasmapheresis, and IV immunoglobulin. Because these antibodies are also seen in Sjogren syndrome, similar sequelae can occur.

GYNECOLOGY

The realm of gynecologic care includes trauma-informed and comprehensive health maintenance for the patient with female reproductive anatomy, along with management of several unique conditions that can impact the anatomy and physiology of the female reproductive tract. Gynecologic pathology is common and can lead to loss of quality of life if inadequately assessed and treated.

THE MENSTRUAL CYCLE AND DISORDERS OF MENSTRUATION

Normal Female Reproductive Physiology

Normal menstrual cycle

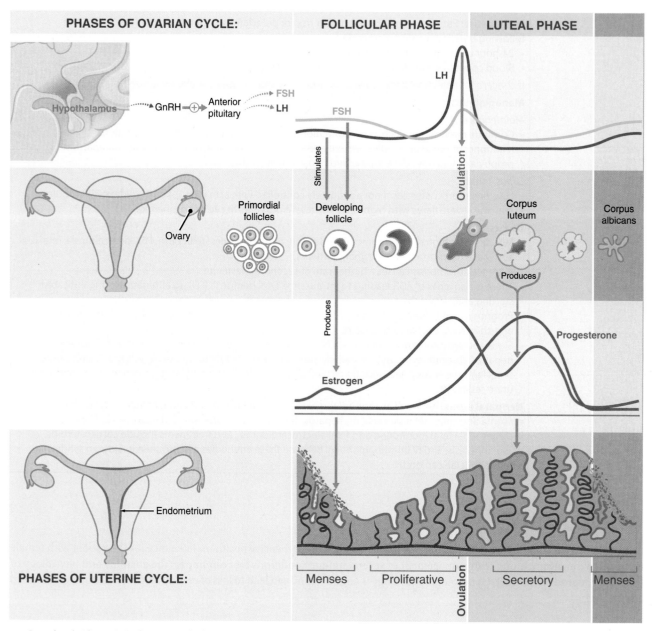

Reproduced with permission from Le Tao, Bhushan Vikas, Sochat Matthew, First Aid for the USMLE Step 1 2021, 31st ed. New York: McGraw-Hill Education, 2021.

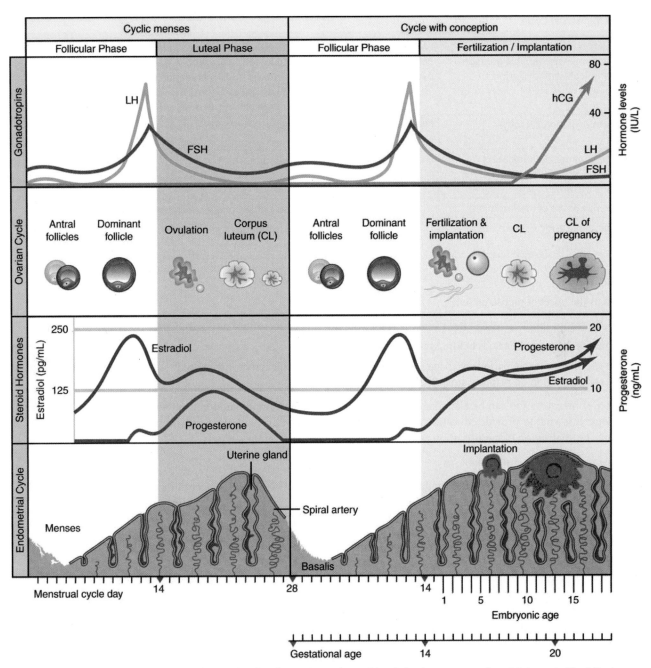

Gonadotropin control of the ovarian and endometrial cycles. The ovarian-endometrial cycle has been structured as a 28-day cycle. The follicular phase (days 1 to 14) is characterized by rising estrogen levels, endometrial thickening, and selection of the dominant "ovulatory" follicle. During the luteal phase (days 14 to 21), the corpus luteum (CL) produces estrogen and progesterone, which prepare the endometrium for implantation. If implantation occurs, the developing blastocyst begins to produce human chorionic gonadotropin (hCG) and rescues the corpus luteum, thus maintaining progesterone production. FSH = follicle-stimulating hormone; LH = luteinizing hormone. (Reproduced with permission from Cunningham F, Leveno KJ, et al., Williams Obstetrics, 25e; New York: McGraw Hill, 2018.)

Normal Menstrual Cycle

Follicular Phase (Days 1–13)	Ovulation (Day 14)	Luteal Phase (Days 15–28)
Starts with menses; variable duration as only completes with ovulation	Release of mature ovum	Without luteinizing hormone (LH) or human chorionic gonadotropin (hCG) stimulation (as seen in pregnancy), the corpus luteum lasts from days 15 to 28, and then involutes; set duration (always 14 days)
Ends with ovulation/LH surge	Development of the corpus luteum	Corpus luteum produces progesterone and some estradiol
Increase gonadotropin-releasing hormone (GnRH), follicle-stimulating hormone (FSH), estrogen	Increase LH	Progesterone > estrogen
Proliferative phase of uterine lining		Secretory phase of uterine lining
Dominant follicle increases in size		If no fertilization or implantation, sloughing of endometrial lining

Menarche

Defined as the onset of menstruation.

- Usually occurs about 2.5 years after thelarche (onset of puberty or breast development), with a mean age of 12 years
- Premature menarche: Periods before age 8
- Delayed menarche: No periods until age 15 if other secondary sexual characteristics are present, or until age 13 if they are not (see the section on primary amenorrhea)

Initiation of menstruation can be alarming for a patient, particularly if unprepared and undereducated about this normal physiology. It is vital to provide education and support early on, including providing reassurance, a safe environment for questions, normalization of menstruation as a process, and menstrual hygiene support.

Normal symptoms of menstruation:

- Characterized by generally mild to moderate bothersome symptoms including but not limited to headache, weight fluctuation or bloating, breast tenderness, fatigue, generalized back and abdominal discomfort,
- Irritability, restlessness or feeling out of control, or depressed/anxious mood
- Symptoms occur in the 1–2 weeks prior to menstruation and resolve at the onset of menstruation

Contraception

There are several prescribed and non-prescribed methods of contraception. Birth control methods act based on how they target key elements of the conception process:

- Methods that provide a physical barrier to or deny proximity for the meeting of the gametes
- Methods that stop or decrease sperm motility before contact
- Methods targeted at prevention of follicle development/oocyte release
- Methods that alter the endometrial environment, making it unfavorable to implantation if a zygote is formed

    Several methods may act in multiple ways to prevent pregnancy.

Contraceptive Options

Method and effectiveness*	Comment
Non-Prescribed/Non-Purchased	
Abstinence 100% effective when strictly followed	If only choice (as is in the setting of abstinence-only education programs), proven to be an ineffective method
Fertility awareness 77–98%	User tracks menstrual cycle to be aware of their most fertile (ovulatory) window and avoids intercourse during these times, or may also use another method during ovulatory window

Contraceptive Options

Method and effectiveness*	Comment
Withdrawal 80%	Pulling out the penis before ejaculation is not as effective as other methods: • May be incomplete or occur too late • Pre-ejaculate fluid may still contain sperm
Lactational amenorrhea temporarily effective if all three conditions are met: • Amenorrhea • Fully breastfeeding • <6 months after delivery	Following birth and during breastfeeding, there is partial or total suppression of ovulation because of hyperprolactinemia on the hypothalamic-pituitary-ovarian (HPO) axis • May be difficult to predict when nadir of this effect reached and when ovulation may resume (particularly during the weaning process)
Barrier Methods	
External/internal condoms 87% External condoms 79% Internal condoms	Worn over the penis or inside the vagina and reduce STI transmission risk • Consider latex allergy/sensitivity
Cervical cap/diaphragm 71–86%	Placed vaginally and obstructs the cervix • Most effective when used with spermicide • Higher risk for failure if improperly fitted
Sponge 73–86%	Placed vaginally and is pretreated with spermicide • Least effective of the barrier options, as it is highly susceptible to fit issues and improper use
Sperm-Disruptive Methods	
Spermicide/vaginal pH attenuator 79%	Non-hormonal; available in multiple forms (i.e., gels, films, foams) • Acts by halting sperm motility prior to passing through the cervix • Not very effective if used alone; improved efficacy if used jointly with other options • Maybe a topical irritant for some patients
Hormonal Methods	
Combined hormonal contraceptives (CHCs): Oral: Daily Transdermal patch: Weekly Vaginal ring: Monthly and annual options available 93%	Mechanism of action: Ovulatory suppression, thickening of cervical mucus to impede sperm progress, endometrial changes that make implantation unfavorable Contraindications: • H/O venous thromboembolism or cardiovascular disease • Tobacco use age>35 years • Migraine with aura • Liver disease (e.g., cirrhosis, hepatitis, hepatic adenomas) • Pregnancy or undiagnosed vaginal bleeding • Breast cancer Caution: • Hypertension (poorly controlled) • Dyslipidemia (hypertriglyceridemia) • Diabetes with complications
Progestin-only pill contraceptives (POPs): Every day 93%	Mechanism of action: Ovulatory suppression, thickening of cervical mucus, endometrial atrophy Comments: • Reliant on strict daily use within a narrow window of time for best effectiveness • Good option if breastfeeding • Can cause breakthrough bleeding
Progestin injectable (medroxyprogesterone): Subcutaneous or intramuscular Administered every 3 months 96%	Mechanism of action: Ovulatory suppression, thickening of cervical mucus, endometrial atrophy Comments: • Can cause low bone density with prolonged use • Can cause unscheduled vaginal bleeding and amenorrhea

Contraceptive Options (*Continued*)

Method and effectiveness*	Comment
Subdermal progestin implant: Long-acting reversible contraception (LARC) (Nexplanon) Administered every 3 years 99.9%	Mechanism of action: Ovulatory suppression, thickening of cervical mucus, endometrial atrophy Comments: • Unscheduled vaginal bleeding—is main reason patients discontinue this method
Progestin intrauterine device (IUD): LARC lasting 3–7 years 99.2–99.9%	Mechanism of action: Ovulatory suppression, thickening of cervical mucus, endometrial atrophy, changes in tubal cilia and sperm motility Comments: • Unscheduled vaginal bleeding or reduction in or complete cessation of menses with the devices
Copper intrauterine device (IUD): Only non-hormonal prescribed method Approved for 10 years of use 99.2–99.9%	Mechanism of action: Local inflammatory response in the uterus that disrupts sperm function and implantation Comments: • Can increase the amount and duration of menses (avoid in patients with baseline non-cyclic or heavy menses) • Avoid in patients with Wilson disease • Can be used for emergency contraception
Permanent Contraception	
Tubal and vas deferens sterilization	• Works by disrupting the pathway between the gametes • Sterilization is highly effective in preventing pregnancy but still not 100% effective • With female procedure, relative increase in the proportion of ectopic pregnancies that may occur if fertilization takes place • Assisted-reproductive techniques and re-anastomoses procedures can allow a patient with previous sterilization to potentially consider future pregnancy

*Based on % of patients who had unintended pregnancy within the first year of typical use.

Source: From Williams Gynecology, 4e. McGraw Hill; 2020, bedsider.org.

https://www.cdc.gov/reproductivehealth/unintendedpregnancy/pdf/family-planning-methods-2014.pdf

Emergency Contraception

Method	Comment
High-dose combination pills, progestin-only pills levonorgestrel (plan B), or ulipristal acetate (progesterone receptor modulator)	• Work primarily by suppression or delay of ovulation • Can act on endometrium to prevent implantation • Can be associated with nausea due to the amount of hormone in a single dose • Should optimally be used within 72 hours of unprotected event
Copper IUD	• Endometrial and sperm dysfunction are the primary mechanisms of action • Can be inserted within 5 days of unprotected sex

These methods must be used within 72 to 120 hours of unprotected intercourse to be most effective.

CASE 12 | Contraception

A 17-year-old G0 presents to clinic after a recent episode of unprotected intercourse. She states she has been sexually active with one male partner for the past few months. They use male condoms every time, but 2 days ago, the condom broke during vaginal intercourse after her partner had ejaculated. The patient has cyclic menses every 29 days, lasting 4 days in duration. Her last menstrual period was 3 weeks ago. She has no known medical history and has no current medication use.

Initial Diagnostic Tests	• Urine pregnancy test • STI screening
Next Steps in Management	• Offer and counsel on emergency contraceptive (EC) options • Discuss alternatives to barrier method for post-EC contraception per patient preference • If pregnancy test is positive, offer pregnancy options counseling

CASE 12 | Contraception *(continued)*

Discussion	The importance of adequate access to and education on contraceptive methods is highlighted by the fact that around 50% of pregnancies in the United States are unintended. Discussions on contraception can be complex and require an understanding of the patient's goals, preferences, and medical history. This is a crucial time to employ shared decision-making and empower patients to make the choice that best fits their individualized needs. **History:** If considering hormonal options, also inquire about contraindications (e.g., personal or family history of venous thromboembolism, vascular disease, migraines with an aura, liver disease, abnormal vaginal bleeding) **Physical Exam:** Obtain baseline blood pressure (hormonal contraceptives can raise blood pressure) **Management:** Contraceptive options: See the table above for details • Discuss proper usage, adverse reactions, and potential risks/complications • Encourage adherence and offer follow-up in few months to assess for any adverse reactions or concerns
Additional Considerations	*Use of contraceptive medications for other indications:* **Prevention of STIs:** External and internal condoms prevent transmission of common STIs **Non-Contraceptive Benefits:** Hormonal contraceptives may reduce symptoms associated with: • Functional ovarian cysts • Premenstrual dysphoric disorder and syndrome • Menstrual migraines • Some can also offer menstrual manipulation and reduction of menstrual episodes **Disease Risk-Reduction:** • Ectopic pregnancy • Osteoporosis • Endometrial and ovarian cancers **Treatment of Disease:** • Abnormal and heavy uterine bleeding • Anovulatory conditions • Dysmenorrhea • Endometriosis • Acne and hirsutism

Menstrual Disorder Mini-Cases

Premenstrual Dysphoric Disorder (PMDD)	**Hx/PE:** Episodes of depressed mood, fatigue, lack of concentration, and somatic symptoms that coincide with menstruation; resolution of symptoms in between menstruation **Diagnostics:** Clinical diagnosis **Management:** SSRIs are first-line treatment **Discussion:** The etiology is not well understood. The symptomatology of PMDD is much more profound than premenstrual syndrome (PMS) and has a DSM 5 diagnostic criteria set that includes presence of five or more of the following in the week before menses, with resolution shortly after start of the period: At least one of the following must be present: • Marked affective lability • Marked irritability, anger, or increased interpersonal conflicts • Marked depressed mood, feeling of hopelessness, or self-deprecating thoughts • Marked anxiety, tension And at least one of the following additional symptoms must be present: • Feeling of being overwhelmed • Decreased interest • Difficulty concentrating • Easy fatigability, low energy • Increase or decrease in sleep • Physical symptoms such as breast tenderness, muscle or joint aches, "bloating" or weight gain *Note:* Criteria must be present for most menstrual cycles in the preceding year.

Menstrual Disorder Mini-Cases *(continued)*

Dysmenorrhea	**Hx:** Mild-moderate cramping at the beginning of menses, improved with NSAIDs, most common in those who recently started menstruating
	PE: Normal vitals on exam, no abdominal masses or tenderness
	Diagnostics: Clinical diagnosis
	Consider pelvic ultrasound to rule out other causes if pain is unimproved after trial of management
	Management:
	• Start NSAIDs 2 days preceding start of menses and continue for first 1–2 days of menses
	• Discuss/offer adjunctive symptom management with non-pharmacologic options such as local heat, exercise, massage, acupuncture, and transcutaneous electrical nerve stimulation (TENS)
	Discussion:
	Primary dysmenorrhea is presence of pain during periods since menarche. The pain is often described as cramping, and in the setting of primary is secondary to local prostaglandin effect on the myometrium leading to shedding of the non-implanted endometrium.
	Secondary dysmenorrhea, or pain during periods that starts after the onset of menses, is more closely associated with structural and/or inflammatory pathologies. Therefore, initial workup including pelvic exam, ultrasound, and possible vaginal cultures is indicated. Common etiologies for secondary dysmenorrhea include uterine fibroids, endometriosis and adenomyosis, endometrial polyps, and endometritis.

Menopause

Clinical diagnosis, defined as cessation of menses for 12 months.

- Age-related reduction of ovarian follicles leads to declining estrogen levels
- Most common menopausal symptoms are vasomotor symptoms (e.g., hot flashes, flushes, night sweats)
- Other symptoms and concerns include vaginal atrophy, dyspareunia, and sleep disturbance
- Postmenopausal patients have an increased risk for osteoporosis and coronary artery disease

Menopause is NOT diagnosed by laboratory criteria. Patients without menopause may have increases in FSH and decline in estrogen before menstrual cessation.

CASE 13 | Menopause

A 49-year-old female presents with episodes of sudden sensation of heat and sweats which come on intermittently and have affected her quality of life. For the last 3 years her menses had been irregular, occurring every 3–6 months, and then completely stopped for the last 13 months. She denies weight loss, fevers, chills, or other focal findings. On exam, vital signs are normal and pelvic examination reveals thin and pale vaginal mucosa with loss of rugae and discomfort on placement of the speculum. The rest of the exam, including thyroid and lymph node exam, is normal.

Conditions with Similar Presentations	**Diaphoresis or night sweats:** Can be due to a variety of causes, including infection or malignancy, but will also have other findings such as weight loss, cough, lymphadenopathy, or other focal findings.
	Secondary amenorrheic states: Can be caused by other conditions, such as pregnancy, oral contraceptive use, thyroid disease, increased prolactin levels (prolactinoma/antipsychotics), and can be differentiated by history, age, and lab testing.
	Primary ovarian insufficiency: Is defined by the cessation of menses before the age of 40 years.
Initial Diagnostic Tests	• Clinical diagnosis • Consider checking pregnancy test, TSH, and/or consider prolactin level (if indicated) to rule out other causes of secondary amenorrhea
Next Steps in Management	Provide reassurance to patient and discuss treatment options for debilitating symptoms

CASE 13 | Menopause *(continued)*

Discussion	Menopause is a physiologic process defined as 12 months of amenorrhea and occurs due to a reduction of ovarian follicles with age, leading to decreased hormonal secretion of estrogen and progesterone.
	• Median age of onset in the United States is ~51 years.
	• Perimenopause symptoms can begin 5–10 years before cessation of menses.
	• Decline in estrogen levels can cause myriad of symptoms, including vasomotor symptoms, mood instability, and symptoms related to vulvovaginal atrophy (genitourinary syndrome of menopause).
	• Most effective treatment for hypoestrogenic symptoms of menopause is hormone replacement therapy (HRT).
	• Benefit of HRT should be balanced with the risks of breast cancer, venous thromboembolism (VTE), stroke, and cardiovascular disease.
	• When treating with systemic estrogen and the patient still has their uterus, a progestin should always be used to avoid endometrial hyperplasia or malignancy. The lowest necessary dose possible should be prescribed and used for the shortest duration of time needed.
	
	History: Absent menses in the perimenopause window. Symptoms include hot flashes, sleep disturbances, vaginal dryness, vaginal irritation/discharge, dyspareunia.
	
	Physical Exam: May have vaginal atrophy and/or pain on exam, vaginal discharge.
	
	Diagnostics:
	• Clinical diagnosis, labs not needed unless diagnosis uncertain.
	• Can consider the following tests to confirm hormone status:
	  • FSH ($\uparrow$), typically >40 mIU/mL
	  • LH ($\uparrow$), estrogen ($\downarrow$), progesterone ($\downarrow$)
	  • Testosterone and prolactin levels will be normal
	  • Tests to rule out other causes of secondary amenorrhea (e.g., hCG, prolactin, TSH)
	
	Management: First step is to provide diagnosis, reassurance and treat bothersome symptoms, if present.
	
	Vasomotor symptoms (hot flashes) can be treated with:
	• Lifestyle modifications (relaxation techniques, fans, air-conditioning, dressing in layers)
	• Medications, including HRT (see table below)
	• Cognitive behavioral therapy
	
	Genitourinary syndrome of menopause can be treated with:
	• Vaginal moisturizers/lubricants or vaginal estrogen products

Additional Considerations:	**Complications:** **Osteoporosis:** Decreased estrogen levels lead to bone resorption and an imbalance of bone formation and resorption resulting in bone loss and postmenopausal osteoporosis. • Screen with DEXA scan starting at age 65, earlier if risk factors • Advise calcium, vitamin D, and weight-bearing exercise • HRT may help reduce the risk to develop the condition • Treat with bisphosphonates (anti-resorptive), parathyroid hormone–receptor agonists, and/or sclerostin inhibitors **Heart disease:** Risk of heart disease increased two- to threefold after menopause. However, both primary and secondary prevention studies have not shown benefit of HRT

Medication	Indications	Discussion
Hormone replacement therapy (HRT)	Best treatment option for vasomotor symptoms	Estrogen replacement is a patient-centered decision; it is generally safest and most effective in the early years of menopause In patients with intact uterus, must also treat with progestin to decrease risk of endometrial cancer. Avoid in patients with significant risk factors or the following conditions: CAD, stroke, venous thromboembolism, or breast cancer

(Continued)

Medication	Indications	Discussion
SSRI/SNRI	Option when HRT is contraindicated Consider if symptoms with concomitant depression	When discontinuing, taper medication to avoid rebound symptoms
Vaginal estrogen	Genitourinary syndrome of menopause or vulvovaginal atrophy	Systemic absorption is minimal but can occur, so use with caution when oral estrogens are contraindicated
Calcium and vitamin D	To prevent osteoporosis	If dietary intake is inadequate, supplemental calcium and vitamin D is recommended to meet daily minimum requirements (calcium: 1200 mg/day; vitamin D: 600 IU/day)

PRIMARY AND SECONDARY AMENORRHEA

Primary Amenorrhea

- Failure to initiate menarche by age 13 with absence of any other pubertal milestones (secondary sex characteristics), including growth spurt, adrenarche, thelarche (initiation of mature breast development) *or*
- No menarche by age 15 in the presence of other normal pubertal milestones

Approach to Evaluation of Primary Amenorrhea

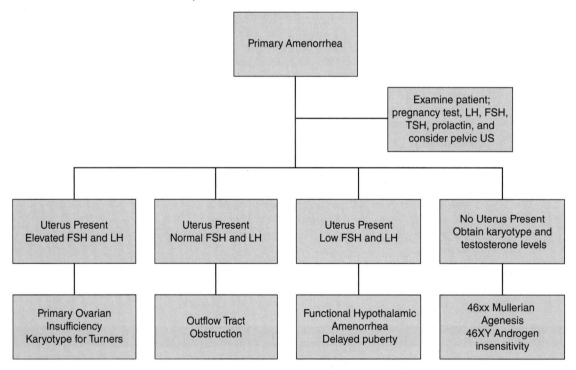

Secondary Amenorrhea

- The cessation of menses in a patient who previously had menstrual bleeding
- If a patient had prior monthly *cyclic* menstrual bleeding, this is defined by cessation of menses for ≥3 months
- If they previously had *non-cyclic* menstrual bleeding, then cessation of menses for ≥6 months is classified as secondary amenorrhea
- Depending on the patient's history and age, discontinuation of menses for ≥12 months may ultimately represent menopause or primary ovarian insufficiency.

Approach to Evaluation of Secondary Amenorrhea

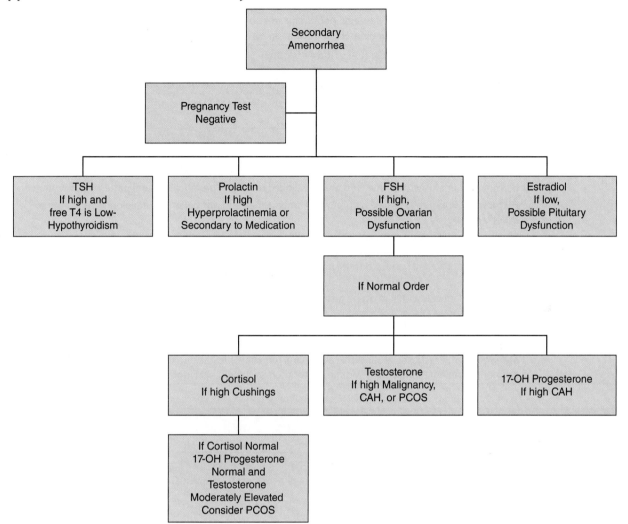

Hypergonadotropic Hypogonadism (Primary Hypogonadism)

- Occurs due to inadequate response of gonads to FSH and LH
- Condition is characterized by ↓ estrogen, ↑ GnRH, and ↑ LH/FSH

Hypogonadotropic Hypogonadism (Secondary Hypogonadism)

- Arises from dysfunction at the level of hypothalamus or pituitary gland
- Characterized by ↓ estrogen, ↓ GnRH, and ↓ to normal LH/FSH
- Etiology may be hypothalamic or pituitary in origin or due to excessive exercise or nutritional problems

Eugonadotropic Hypogonadism

- Characterized by anovulation due to immaturity in the hypothalamus-pituitary-ovarian axis (in adolescents) or problems with estrogen receptors
- ↑ Estrogen/↓ progesterone, ↑ or ↓ GnRH, and normal LH/FSH levels are seen.

CASE 14 | Androgen Insensitivity Syndrome

A 16-year-old who identifies as a girl presents for evaluation of primary amenorrhea. She has Tanner stage 4 breasts and phenotypic female external genitalia with a short vagina. No uterus or adnexa is palpated on bimanual exam.

Conditions with Similar Presentations	Congenital adrenal hyperplasia (CAH), Turner Syndrome, 5-alpha-reductase deficiency, Müllerian agenesis, complete XY gonadal agenesis (Swyer syndrome), Kallmann syndrome can present with amenorrhea. These conditions are differentiated based on labs, presence of female pelvic anatomy, and karyotype testing.
Initial Diagnostic Tests	• Initial tests include pelvic ultrasound, serum testosterone, LH, FSH • Confirm diagnosis with karyotype testing
Next Steps in Management	• Symptomatic management • Psychosocial support and counseling
Discussion	Androgen insensitivity syndrome occurs due to the unresponsiveness of androgen receptors to circulating hormones, namely testosterone, and has an X-linked recessive (genetically male) pattern of inheritance. **History:** Phenotypically female with primary amenorrhea and normal breast development at time of expected puberty. **Physical Exam:** Sparse or absent pubic and axillary hair (secondary to the inability of androgen receptors to respond to circulating hormones), undescended testes which may be palpated in inguinal canal, absent uterus, short or absent vagina, normal breast development. **Diagnostics:** • Confirm diagnosis with karyotype testing (46, XY with female phenotype) • Pelvic US shows absence of a uterus • Serum testosterone and LH (comparable to XY individuals) • FSH is normal **Management:** Psychosocial support/counseling, removal of testes due to increased risk for malignancy, hormone supplementation, and vaginal dilator therapy for vaginal lengthening.

Amenorrhea Mini-Cases

Cases	Key Findings
Müllerian Agenesis	**Hx:** Failure of menses in ≥15 years in presence of normal secondary sex characteristics **PE:** Absent uterus (can rarely have small rudimentary horn or uterus), absent cervix with a short or absent vagina, functional ovaries **Diagnostics:** • Clinical diagnosis, confirm with karyotype testing (46, XX genotype) • Transvaginal and abdominal ultrasound to visualize pelvic structures. **Management:** • Psychosocial support/counseling • Neovagina surgery • Evaluate for renal tract abnormalities, fertility concerns, and possible gestational surrogacy **Discussion:** Müllerian agenesis, also known as **Mayer-Rokitansky- Kuster-Hauser Syndrome**, results from the incomplete development of the embryologic paramesonephric ducts leading to absence of a functional vagina and commonly cervical and uterine agenesis. It is characterized by normal functional ovarian development resulting in normal female secondary sex characteristics so is usually asymptomatic prior to expected menarche. It may be associated with renal or skeletal anomalies.
Complete XY Gonadal Agenesis	**Hx:** Failure of menses in ≥15 years and absence of some secondary sex characteristics **PE:** Phenotypically female patient with female external genitalia, uterus, and fallopian tubes; pelvic exam notable for small uterus and enlarged clitoris **Diagnostics:** Clinical diagnosis; karyotype analysis reveals 46, XY genotype **Management:** • Lifelong estrogen and progesterone replacement therapy • Surgical removal of streak gonad **Discussion:** Nonfunctional gonads in Complete XY Gonadal Agenesis **(Swyer Syndrome)**, fail to produce estrogen resulting in failed menarche and causing failed development of some secondary sexual characteristics, such as breasts.

Amenorrhea Mini-Cases *(continued)*

5-Alpha Reductase Deficiency	**Hx:** Failure of menses in ≥15 years and absence of some secondary sex characteristics, enlarged clitoris, presence of acne on face, back, and arms **PE:** Short vagina, palpable testes, clitoromegaly on pelvic exam **Diagnostics:** • Hormonal analysis: Normal or ↑ testosterone, ↓ dihydrotestosterone (DHT), normal estrogen and FSH, and normal or ↑ LH • Karyotype analysis: 46, XY genotype **Management:** • If the patient endorses female identity, may perform gonadectomy. • Regardless, gender-affirming measures are indicated, with robust psychosocial support. **Discussion:** Defective 5-alpha-reductase leads to decreased conversion of testosterone to dihydrotestosterone (DHT). With ↓ DHT, masculinization of external genitalia will not occur. Patients most often demonstrate ambiguous genitalia until puberty, when virilization leads to growth of the external genitalia, often resulting in a more male phenotypic appearance.
Congenital Adrenal Hyperplasia: 17-α-Hydroxylase Deficiency	**Hx:** Indiscernible genitalia in genotypical male neonate; vomiting, diarrhea, and dehydration **PE:** Hypertension, hypoglycemia, and hyperpigmentation of the skin **Diagnostics:** ↓ 17-hydroxyprogesterone and potassium; ↑ 11-deoxycorticosterone, corticosterone, and sodium; metabolic alkalosis present **Management:** • Glucocorticoid and estrogen replacement therapy, spironolactone • Hydrocortisone is indicated in neonates and children • Fluid resuscitation may be required, depending on the patient's status **Discussion:** Congenital Adrenal Hyperplasia (CAH) is a disorder characterized by the deficiency of one of the enzymes needed to produce adrenal hormones. In genotypically XX patients, Müllerian development remains normal with presence of the uterus, cervix, and vagina. But genotypically XY patients often present with external genitalia of unclear male or female phenotype. The adrenal insufficiency can cause vomiting, diarrhea, and dehydration.
Turner Syndrome	**Hx:** Failure of menses ≥15 years and absence of secondary sex characteristics **PE:** Short stature, webbed neck, high arched palate, widely spaced nipples, absence of breast tissue, bilateral distal ulnar protrusions on wrist **Diagnostics:** • Karyotype is 45, XO. • Check for associated congenital malformations such as horseshoe kidney with renal ultrasound and coarctation of the aorta or bicuspid aortic valve with echocardiogram. • CT abdomen/pelvis shows streak gonads **Management:** Treat with growth hormone (when diagnosed in early childhood) and estrogen replacement. **Discussion:** Turner syndrome (45, XO) is the commonest cause of primary amenorrhea and is caused by chromosomal non-disjunction leading to ovarian agenesis and consequent primary hypogonadism. Plasma levels of gonadotropins (LH, FSH) are markedly elevated. Signs of adrenarche such as pubic hair are present because the hypothalamus and pituitary are unaffected and are activated at puberty.

ABNORMAL UTERINE BLEEDING

The term abnormal uterine bleeding (AUB) is defined as anything the patient feels is abnormal, and it should be assessed accordingly. The amount of blood loss is quantified by determining the number of pads or tampons used or frequency of menstrual cup change in a day at the peak of menses. Typical normal findings are:

- Menstrual cycle is 28 days (+/− 7 days) with little intra-cycle variability
- Menses last from 2–7 days
- Light to moderate passage of blood without clots or flooding

Patterns of AUB

Terms	Definition
Heavy menstrual bleeding (formerly called menorrhagia)	• Menstrual bleeding that lasts >7 days duration *or* • Blood loss >80 mL over the menstrual event or that patient defines as excessive • May be cyclic or non-cyclic
Irregular menses (formerly called metrorrhagia)	• Non-cyclic/unpredictable occurrence of the menstrual cycle • May represent anovulatory bleeding; may also come from medications or comorbid conditions
Intermenstrual bleeding	• Episodes of vaginal/uterine spotting or bleeding that occur outside of the cyclic menstrual period
Frequent or infrequent menses (formerly called poly- or oligomenorrhea)	• Menses occurring <21 days or >35 days apart, respectively
Severe acute bleeding	• Bleeding that requires more than one pad/tampon per hour, or changes in vital signs indicating hypovolemia

Differential for AUB

PALM (Structural)		COEIN (Nonstructural)	
P	Polyp (endometrial)	C	Coagulopathy
A	Adenomyosis	O	Ovulatory dysfunction
L	Leiomyoma (fibroid)	E	Endometrial dysfunction
M	Malignancy/hyperplasia	I	Iatrogenic
		N	Not yet classified

Approach to Abnormal Uterine Bleeding

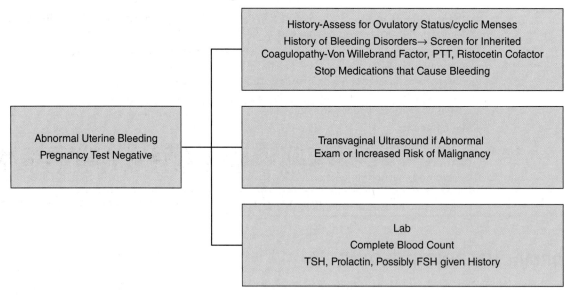

CASE 15 | Leiomyoma (Fibroids)

A 40-year-old presents with heavy menstrual bleeding, pelvic pressure, and fatigue. She reports that her menses have always been heavy. She is not sexually active and her LMP was 3 weeks ago. On exam, vital signs are stable and the abdomen is soft and non-tender, but the uterus is palpable just above the pubic symphysis and is irregular in contour. On bimanual exam, there is an enlarged, irregularly shaped, firm, non-tender uterus; no adnexal masses are noted.

Conditions with Similar Presentations	**Adenomyosis** and **endometrial polyp** can cause heavy bleeding but can be differentiated by exam and/or ultrasound
Initial Diagnostic Tests	• Confirm diagnosis with plain or saline-infused pelvic ultrasound • Also check CBC and iron studies if microcytic anemia present
Next Steps in Management	• Hormonal and/or surgical management • Ferrous sulfate if iron deficiency anemia present
Discussion	Leiomyomata are benign hormone-sensitive submucosal, intramural, or sub-serosal smooth muscle tumors of the myometrium, and on pathology there is a whorled pattern of smooth muscle bundles with borders that are well-demarcated. They are sensitive to estrogen and can increase in size with pregnancy or decrease with menopause. The overgrowth of smooth muscle can also lead to vascular proliferation and, depending on position, increase in the surface area of the endometrium, hence a risk for heavier menses (as seen in submucosal fibroids). **History:** Risk Factors: Nulliparity, early menarche, elevated BMI, reproductive age, alcohol consumption. Symptoms: Asymptomatic or pelvic pain, prolonged menses, and/or heavy menstrual bleeding. "Bulk" symptoms (due to tumor size) include urinary frequency, incontinence, bloating and lower abdominal fullness, pelvic or back pain, or infertility. **Physical Exam:** Enlarged or irregular uterus may be present on bimanual physical exam. **Diagnostics:** • Confirm presence of fibroids with ultrasound • Check CBC to assess for anemia • Consider TSH to rule out other causes of menstrual irregularity **Management:** • If fibroids are found incidentally and patient is asymptomatic, no treatment is needed • Treatment options include medical vs. procedural interventions and should be selected based on patient goals (i.e., control bleeding vs. bulk symptom management, fertility goals) • Medical: contraceptives or tranexamic acid for heavy menstrual bleeding • Procedural: myomectomy, uterine artery embolization, hysterectomy
Additional Considerations	**Complications:** Severe bleeding may lead to iron-deficient anemia and in some cases, leiomyomas may cause infertility. **Leiomyosarcoma** is a malignant smooth muscle tumor of the myometrium. The malignant transformation of leiomyoma is very rare (~0.1%). Leiomyosarcoma usually are aggressive and demonstrate mitotic activity, cellular atypia, areas of necrosis, and invade nearby tissues.

Abnormal Uterine Bleeding Mini-Case

Case	Key Findings
Adenomyosis	**Hx:** Cyclic but heavy and/or prolonged menses, pelvic discomfort/fullness, dyspareunia, severe cramping/pain. Risk Factors: Prior uterine surgery, such as dilation and curettage, and high parity. **PE:** Uniformly enlarged, globular-shaped and boggy uterus **Diagnostics:** • Imaging: pelvic ultrasound, MRI • Definitive diagnosis only with pathology at hysterectomy **Management:** • Analgesia for pain control • Hormonal birth control to lessen heavy bleeding and pain. • In cases of severe and refractory pain and/or heavy bleeding, hysterectomy can be curative. **Discussion:** Adenomyosis is caused by the extension of glandular endometrial tissue into the myometrium. Anemia is a potential complication caused by prolonged and/or heavy menses.

CASE 16 | Polycystic Ovarian Syndrome (PCOS)

A 27-year-old G0 comes in for evaluation of severe acne, infrequent and irregular menses since menarche, and hirsutism. She is sexually active and currently does not want to get pregnant. Her LMP was 8 weeks ago; she uses condoms and denies any history of blood clots. Her BMI is 36 and she has acne over face and back, acanthosis nigricans, androgenic alopecia, and hirsutism.

Conditions with Similar Presentations	**Thyroid dysfunction:** Can present with irregular menstrual cycles, and/or infertility, and be differentiated by abnormal TSH (high or low). **Hyperprolactinemia:** Can present with infrequent or absent menses, infertility, and can be differentiated by prolactin levels and galactorrhea. **Congenital adrenal hyperplasia (CAH):** Usually diagnosed in younger patients, may present with androgen excess and can be differentiated by ↑ serum 17-hydroxyprogesterone (17OHP) before 8 a.m.
Initial Diagnostic Tests	• Check pelvic ultrasound and serum testosterone • Also check urine pregnancy, LH, FSH, TSH, prolactin, DHEA-S, 17-OH progesterone, cortisol level to rule out other causes
Next Steps in Management	Hormonal contraception
Discussion	PCOS is one of the common causes of anovulation and infertility in patients and is characterized by excess testosterone and estrogen levels. The exact etiology is unclear, but likely related to altered LH action, insulin resistance, and predisposition to hyperandrogenism. **History/Physical Exam:** Menstrual irregularities, weight gain, symptoms or signs of insulin resistance—acanthosis nigricans, elevated BMI with central distribution, hirsutism, oily skin and/or acne, androgenic alopecia. **Diagnostics:** • Pelvic US to confirm diagnosis and rule out androgen-secreting ovarian tumor • Testosterone level (↑) One classic schema for diagnosis is the *Rotterdam criteria*, in which patients must meet two out of three of the following: 1. Ovulatory dysfunction (e.g., infrequent or absent menses) 2. Clinical or laboratory hyperandrogenism: Testosterone (↑) 3. TVUS with polycystic-appearing ovaries (ovaries containing multiple small follicles forming a "pearl necklace" sign and/or increased ovarian volume) *Consider checking*: • LH and FSH (LH/FSH ratio typically elevated in PCOS) • DHEA-S (rule out adrenal tumor) • 17-OH progesterone (rule out nonclassical CAH) • Cortisol level (rule out Cushing syndrome) • TSH (rule out thyroid disorders) • Lipids and A1C or glucose tolerance test to assess for dyslipidemia and diabetes **Management:** Management is driven by the patient's goals *If not planning pregnancy*: The primary goal is endometrial protection from prolonged unopposed estrogen. Options include: • Cyclic oral progestin therapy • Hormonal birth control methods (e.g., combined oral contraceptives, levonorgestrel IUD) *If desiring pregnancy*: Weight reduction of even 5–10% can help promote ovulation and therefore more cyclic menses. • Clomiphene citrate first line for ovulation induction *For metabolic abnormalities* (obesity, dyslipidemia): • Lifestyle modifications (e.g., diet, exercise weight-loss first line) • Metformin can be used to treat insulin resistance and can help with ovulatory dysfunction *For hirsutism*: Options include OCPS (first line), antiandrogens (spironolactone, finasteride), metformin
Additional Considerations	**Complications:** Increased risk for diabetes, cardiac disease, infertility, and endometrial cancer (due to unopposed estrogen secretion).

Infertility

Infertility is defined as the inability to conceive after 12 months of regular unprotected penile-vaginal intercourse.

- If >35 years old, this time frame is shortened to 6 months
- Primary: Patient with no prior pregnancy
- Secondary: Patient with at least one prior conception
- For conception to occur, a well-choreographed sequence of events is required, as below. Anomaly in even one of these steps can prevent successful conception.
  - Ovulation must occur and intercourse must be timed appropriately to allow joining of the female and male gamete
  - There needs to be an adequate number of functionally motile, high-quality sperm so that this union can occur in the fallopian tube
  - The tube itself must be patent to allow for this meeting and subsequent fertilization, along with presence of normal cilia to promote movement of the fertilized ovum to the endometrial cavity
  - There must be a prepared and available intrauterine site for the blastocyst to implant

Female reproductive factors involved in infertility include:

- Tubal/cervical/uterine factors
- Ovulatory dysfunction—hypothalamic/pituitary causes, PCOS, primary ovarian insufficiency

Male reproductive factors involved in infertility include:

- Sperm/testicular/post-testicular abnormalities
- Hypothalamic/pituitary causes

Treatment may involve:

- Hormonal or surgical correction *and/or*
- Intrauterine insemination
- In vitro fertilization
- Patients may ultimately benefit from reproductive endocrinology and infertility (REI) specialist

Infertility Evaluation

Female	Male
Menstrual history, basal body temperature, TSH, prolactin, anti-Müllerian hormone, day 3 FSH, day 3 estradiol, day 21 progesterone, pelvic exam, saline-infused ultrasound and/or hysterosalpingogram	Testicular exam, semen analysis, LH, FSH, testosterone, estradiol, TSH, prolactin, karyotype

Infertility Mini-Cases

Cases	Key Findings
Elevated BMI	**Hx:** Persistently irregular menses in context of elevated BMI; inability to conceive **PE:** Hemodynamically stable, elevated BMI; acanthosis nigricans may be present **Diagnostics:** Check TSH, prolactin, serum testosterone, pelvic ultrasound **Management:** • Weight loss is the first-line management for menstrual changes secondary to elevated BMI. • For a patient who meets indications (BMI >40 without comorbidities, BMI >35 with comorbidities), weight loss surgery should be discussed as an option. **Discussion:** Elevated BMI is a common finding in PCOS and patients with endometrial hyperplasia—both causes of AUB and infertility. However, it can independently contribute to aberrations of the normal menstrual cycle and ultimately ability to conceive. People with elevated BMI also have higher risks for pregnancy complication regardless of other comorbid conditions, so achieving a healthy weight is important as a preconception consideration.

Infertility Mini-Cases *(continued)*

Prolactinoma	**Hx:** Change in menses, headaches, visual changes, inability to conceive Female patients: Galactorrhea, amenorrhea, infertility, reduced bone density Male patients: Erectile dysfunction, reduced libido, infertility **PE:** Bitemporal hemianopsia, evidence of estrogen deficiency **Diagnostics:** ↑ Serum prolactin levels, (↓ testosterone or estradiol levels in males or females respectively), brain MRI with pituitary mass **Management:** • Dopamine agonists (↓ size and ↓ secretion of prolactinomas) • Consider surgery if large mass or unresponsive to therapy **Discussion:** Prolactinomas are prolactin-secreting pituitary tumors and are a cause of hypogonadotropic hypogonadism (↑ prolactin levels and ↓ gonadotropin levels).
Kallman Syndrome	**Hx:** Infertility, may have primary amenorrhea, hyposmia, or anosmia **PE:** Decreased sense of smell, normal visual field testing, possible congenital defects such as midline facial anomalies Female patients: May have delayed secondary sexual characteristics **Diagnostics:** • In male patients: Lack of GnRH results in ↓ LH and ↓ FSH, resulting in ↓ testosterone and ↓ sperm counts • In female patients: Lack of GnRH results in ↓ LH, ↓ FSH, and ↓ estradiol • Also consider: Pelvic ultrasound, karyotype testing, and brain MRI to rule out other causes. **Management:** The goal is to replace hormones not produced by the disrupted hormonal axis. • Prepubertal and adult female patients: Treat with exogenous estrogen to ensure initiation of secondary sexual development and to develop and sustain normal bone and muscle mass • Male patients: Treat with human chorionic gonadotropin (hCG), which acts as LH analog to stimulate testes and initiate testosterone production and spermatogenesis. **Discussion:** Kallmann syndrome is a form of hypogonadotropic hypogonadism that presents with delayed or absent puberty in male or female patients and has associated anosmia. Secondary gonadal failure occurs due to impaired GnRH-releasing neuron migration from the hypothalamus to the anterior pituitary. This results in failed stimulation of the pituitary by GnRH and subsequent hypogonadism. It is more common in male patients.
Primary Ovarian Insufficiency	**Hx:** Amenorrhea, hot flashes, dyspareunia, and mood disturbances ≤40 years **PE:** Atrophic changes of the vaginal mucosa **Diagnostics:** • ↑ FSH levels (>30–40 mIU/mL) and at least two ↓ estradiol levels (<50 pg/mL) 1 month apart. • Consider TSH, prolactin levels and karyotype tests to rule out other causes. **Management:** HRT **Discussion:** Primary Ovarian Insufficiency (previously known as Premature Ovarian Failure) is defined by failure of ovarian function before the age of 40 leading to premature menopause and associated symptoms (vaginal dryness, night sweats, "hot flashes," dyspareunia, mood changes), amenorrhea, and infertility/sub-fertility.
Intrauterine Adhesions (Asherman Syndrome)	**Hx:** Inability to conceive for ≥12 months, history of uterine surgery that may have resulted in scarring (i.e., dilation and curettage), absent or significantly decreased menses post-procedure, recurrent pregnancy loss **PE:** Normal pelvic exam **Diagnostics:** • Saline-infused ultrasound (may reveal severe adhesions) • Hysteroscopy to directly visualize adhesions • Consider additional female infertility workup (hysterosalpingogram, laboratory assessment) **Management:** Resection of adhesions **Discussion:** Adhesions and fibrosis of endometrium can occur due to prior dilation and curettage or due to post-inflammatory syndrome following pelvic inflammatory disease or endometritis.

Infertility Mini-Cases *(continued)*

Sertoli Leydig Tumor	**Hx/PE:** Palpable mass on pelvic exam
	Excess testosterone causes rapid virilization, amenorrhea, new facial acne, hair on upper lip and chin (hirsutism), temporal hair loss or thinning, clitoral enlargement, infertility.
	Excess estrogen causes irregular or heavy menstrual bleeding, endometrial polyps, hyperplasia.
	Diagnostics: Ultrasound with ovarian mass; check androgen levels.
	Management: Surgical resection, possible chemotherapy, depending on stage.
	Discussion: This is a rare sex cord–stromal ovarian tumor.

PELVIC PAIN

A female patient presenting with pain requires consideration of multiple pathophysiologic processes ranging from benign to infectious or malignant. It is also imperative to evaluate for and include non-GYN etiologies of pain in the differential, as female patients are at risk for delay in care if excessive focus is placed on GYN-only causes. Despite the need for a wide differential, GYN-specific causes of pelvic pain are common and may be a primary or co-contributing etiology of pain in persons with a female reproductive anatomy.

The chart below suggests an initial differential diagnosis based on the anatomic location of pain.

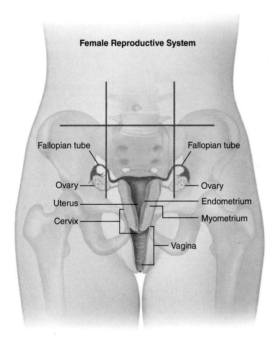

Female Reproductive System

Fallopian tube — Fallopian tube
Ovary — Ovary
Uterus — Endometrium
Cervix — Myometrium
Vagina

R Lumbar	Umbilical	L Lumbar
• UTI • Pyelonephritis	• Pregnancy	• UTI • Pyelonephritis
R Iliac/Lower Quadrant	**Suprapubic**	**L Iliac/Lower Quadrant**
• Ovarian Torsion • Ectopic Pregnancy • Appendicitis	• Menstrual Pain • Endometriosis • Endometritis • Adenomyosis • Leiomyoma • Pelvic Inflammatory Disease • UTI	• Ovarian Torsion • Ectopic Pregnancy • Diverticulitis

Compartments of Pelvic Pain

Gynecologic	Urologic	Gastrointestinal	Musculoskeletal	Neuropsychiatric
Pregnancy (normal and abnormal)	Painful bladder syndrome	Inflammatory bowel disease	Osteoporosis of hip and lower back	History of trauma/abuse
Endometriosis	Infection	Irritable bowel syndrome	Pelvic floor tension myalgia	Neurogenic pain
Fibroids	Nephrolithiasis	Diverticulitis	Abdominal wall hernia	Depression
Ovarian masses (benign or cancerous)		Appendicitis		Nerve entrapment
Ovarian torsion		Gastroenteritis		Fibromyalgia
Ovarian cyst		Constipation		
Vulvodynia				
Infections:				
STIs				
Pelvic inflammatory disease (PID)				
Vaginitis				
Ovarian abscess				

Emergent and Nonemergent Causes of Pelvic Pain in the Nonpregnant Patient

Pelvic Pain	Acute	Chronic	Secondary to Infections
Emergent/serious	Ovarian torsion Ectopic pregnancy	Cancers (ovarian, cervical, endometrial, vulvar)	Pelvic inflammatory disease (PID) Ovarian abscess
Nonemergent	Ruptured ovarian cyst (unless evidence of acute blood loss)	Endometriosis Fibroids Vulvodynia Adenomyosis Intrauterine adhesions Nonmalignant ovarian masses	STIs Vaginitis

Approach to Acute Pelvic Pain

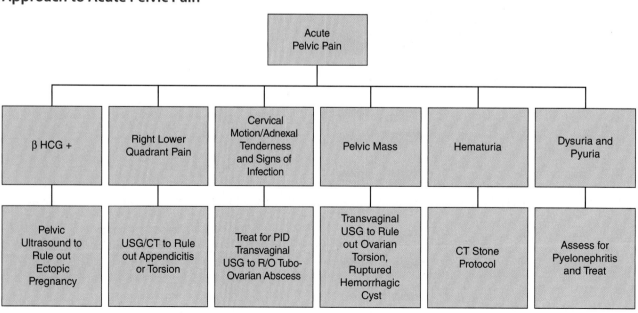

CASE 17 | Ovarian Torsion

A 25-year-old female presents with acute onset of left lower abdominal pain associated with nausea and vomiting. On exam, the patient is in the fetal position; vital signs are normal except for heart rate of 100. Pelvic exam reveals tenderness in the left lower quadrant and left adnexal tenderness without cervical motion tenderness or vaginal discharge. Pregnancy test is negative.

Conditions with Similar Presentations	**Appendicitis:** Typical pain location is RLQ. **Diverticulitis:** Can present with LLQ pain, fever, but is usually seen in older patients. **Ectopic pregnancy:** Would have positive pregnancy test.
Initial Diagnostic Tests	• Confirm with transvaginal Doppler ultrasound • Check urine hCG to rule out pregnancy
Next Steps in Management	Laparoscopic surgery if suspect current torsion
Discussion	Ovarian torsion is a surgical emergency and occurs due to twisting of the ovary on the infundibulopelvic ligament (also known as the suspensory ligament of the ovary). This causes vascular compression of the ovarian vessels, edema, ischemia, and necrosis of the ovary if untreated. **History:** Risk Factors: Biologically female patients of all ages—more common in reproductive age group. Prior torsion, ovulation induction, ovarian cysts, enlarged adnexal mass (e.g., teratoma) Symptoms: Acute onset, severe, unilateral abdominal or pelvic pain, nausea, and vomiting **Physical Exam:** Tenderness in lower abdomen and adnexa on bimanual exam. Ovary may be enlarged and palpable **Diagnostics:** • Clinical diagnosis, confirmed surgically by direct visualization of the rotated ovary. • TVUS: Presence of an adnexal mass; flow is not a reliable indicator of acute torsion and should not strictly guide management. • Check: Urine hCG to rule out pregnancy. **Management:** • Emergent surgery with detorsion of the ovary if still viable • Oophorectomy if ovary is nonviable

CASE 18 | Endometriosis

A 33-year-old G0P0 presents for evaluation of severe pelvic pain. She reports dyspareunia with deep penetration, along with painful periods over the past 10 years. Recently, she has started to have pelvic pain outside of menses. She has been unable to conceive despite unprotected intercourse with her partner for over a year. On exam, she is afebrile and vital signs are normal. On pelvic exam, there is no vaginal discharge; the uterus is not enlarged but is tender to palpation, and there are palpable adnexal masses in addition to uterosacral ligament nodularity.

Conditions with Similar Presentations	**Adenomyosis (extension of glandular endometrial tissue into myometrium):** Can also cause pelvic discomfort and heavy and/or prolonged menses but typically presents with a uniformly enlarged, globular, and "boggy" uterus. **Endometritis (infection or inflammation of the endometrium):** Can also cause pelvic pain and abnormal bleeding but typically occurs in the setting of retained products of conception after delivery, miscarriage, or intrauterine procedure. **Leiomyomata:** The uterus is typically enlarged, and does not always cause pain.
Initial Diagnostic Tests	Pelvic US to rule out other causes followed by laparoscopy
Next Steps in Management	Symptomatic management with nonsteroidal anti-inflammatory agents (NSAIDs), and combined oral contraceptive (COCs)
Discussion	Endometriosis is a condition in which endometrial tissue is found outside of the endometrial cavity often involving the uterus, ovaries, and pelvis. This may result in pain and/or infertility. The etiology is likely multifactorial, and the leading theory is that retrograde menstruation causes implantation of menstrual tissue on pelvic structures. This tissue triggers estrogen-stimulated inflammatory response. Pain and subfertility likely due to chronic inflammation of the lesions.

CASE 18 | Endometriosis *(continued)*

Discussion	**History:** Risk factors: Menarche <10 years, menstrual cycle <28 days, reproductive age group, reproductive tract abnormalities, nulliparity. Symptoms: Chronic pelvic pain, dysmenorrhea, dyspareunia, dyschezia (ineffective defecation), and infertility. Pain is most intense in the days immediately preceding and at the beginning of menses **Physical Exam:** Tenderness on pelvic exam; nodularity over uterosacral ligament and rectovaginal fascia **Diagnostics:** Obtain: Ultrasound as first-line imaging test (though not common to visualize pathology in endometriosis unless endometrioma present) to rule out other pathology • Consider MRI to assess for deeply-infiltrating lesions • Confirm diagnosis with laparoscopy and biopsy of endometriotic lesions **Management:** • First line—symptomatic treatment with NSAIDs, COCs • Extended cycle combined hormone contraception, progesterone agents, GnRH analogues. • Surgical management for unresponsive pain and endometriosis-related infertility

CASE 19 | Chronic Pelvic Pain

A 21-year-old female presents for evaluation of severe pain in her genital region when penetration was attempted during intercourse. She has been unable to use tampons due to vaginal pain. She becomes tearful and explains that 2 years ago she was sexually assaulted by a college friend. On pelvic exam, there are no vulvar skin changes, signs of atrophy, or evidence of abnormal discharge. Placement of a lubricated speculum elicits intense pain, and further exam is deferred for patient comfort.

Conditions with Similar Presentations	**Vulvodynia:** Pain that affects the vulva and often elicited with external touch. Symptoms may be described as burning, stinging, irritation, and rawness which can be localized or general. **Endometriosis:** Patients report deep dyspareunia and have associated dysmenorrhea. Physical exam may reveal nodular thickening of uterosacral ligament and a fixed, nonmobile uterus. **Genitourinary syndrome of menopause:** Most common cause of dyspareunia in menopausal patients and associated symptoms include vaginal dryness, burning, pruritus, discharge, and possible urinary tract symptoms. Vaginal mucosa is atrophic, thin, and with little or no rugae. **Painful Bladder Syndrome (formerly known as interstitial cystitis):** Diagnosis of chronic bladder pain in the absence of other etiologies. The most common presenting feature is an increase in discomfort with filling of bladder and experiencing relief with voiding. This condition is commonly seen with irritable bowel syndrome or fibromyalgia. **Genitopelvic pain/penetration disorder:** Involuntary spasm of vaginal musculature that prevents or causes difficulty in vaginal penetration of any kind. **Female sexual interest/arousal disorder:** A lack of interest in sexual activity, as opposed to an aversion due to anticipated pain.
Initial Diagnostic Tests	• Clinical diagnosis • Consider: Urinalysis and urine culture, STI screening to rule out other conditions
Next Steps in Management	Desensitization therapy
Discussion	Chronic pelvic pain and associated dyspareunia often arises from a combination of causes, both of which should be addressed in the treatment plan. Individuals with sexual pain disorders have genital pain just before, during, or after sexual intercourse or other sexual activities that involve the clitoris, vulva, vagina, and/or perineum. **History:** Risk Factors: Include a history of sexual trauma, lack of sexual knowledge, and history of abuse. **Physical Exam:** Patients have no tenderness on external examination but will be averse to vaginal penetration (including nonsexual such as gynecologic examinations or tampons) due to actual or anticipated pain. **Diagnostics:** • Clinical diagnosis • Physical examination helps to rule out infections or inflammatory dermatitis, which can trigger pain. • Tests are generally not helpful and should be used based on the individual patient's symptoms and physical examination findings. • Consider checking: Urinalysis and urine culture, STI screening, TVUS to rule out other causes

CASE 19 | Chronic Pelvic Pain *(continued)*

Discussion	**Management:** • Desensitization therapy and trauma support are the cornerstone of treatment. • Pelvic floor physical therapy and cognitive behavioral therapy or sex therapy, alone or in combination, helps manage the myofascial and psychosocial causes of pain and dyspareunia. In patients with genito-pelvic pain/penetration disorder: • Desensitization techniques include Kegel exercises and use of dilators. • Goal of dilator therapy is desensitization, and not the physical enlargement of the vaginal opening.

Pelvic Pain Mini-Case

Case	Key Findings
Sexual Trauma/ Assault	**Hx/PE:** History of sexual assault or trauma. May have abrasions or wounds **Diagnostics:** • Pregnancy test • STI testing (e.g., trichomonas, gonorrhea, and chlamydia, HIV, syphilis, hepatitis B) • Urine toxicology to assess for substances used to incapacitate a victim. **Management:** Trauma-informed care or approach, which includes partnering with the patient and shared decision-making regarding: • Oral or uterine emergency contraceptive • Empiric treatment for sexually transmitted infections • HIV post-exposure prophylaxis • Forensic examination • Police report • Vaccination for hepatitis B and HPV are recommended if indicated • Perform assessment of psychological status and referral to trauma-appropriate mental health services if desired **Discussion:** Assault should be suspected in patients whose wounds or abrasions do not exactly match their history. The incidence of assault is higher in pregnant patients. Consent for the medical evaluation and for evidence collection and release must be obtained from the sexual assault victim before initiating a medical forensic examination. Documentation should include details of the assault, relevant medical history, including obstetric and gynecologic conditions and current pregnancy or risk of pregnancy, and a detailed examination of the entire body for injuries. Mandatory reporting of assault of a child or elderly patient is required in all states. Otherwise, it is up to the patient to decide if they would like to report, and the responsibility of the provider to facilitate the process.

Vaginitis and Gynecologic Infections

The timing of menstrual cycle, pregnancy, use of hormones, and infection can cause changes in the normal vaginal ecosystem in the reproductive age. These changes in the ecosystem can cause variations in the amount, color, and consistency of the vaginal discharge. See Infections Disease Chapter for additional STI cases.

Approach to Vaginal Discharge

	Bacterial Vaginosis	Vulvovaginal Candidiasis	Trichomoniasis
Etiology	*Gardnerella, Mobilincus*	*Candida albicans*	*Trichomonas vaginalis*
Presentation	Amine odor	Vulvar redness and itching	Profuse discharge
pH	>4.5	<4.5	>4.5
Wet prep	Clue cells	Pseudohyphae	Trichomonads
KOH prep	Amine odor	Pseudohyphae	Not diagnostic

Evaluation of a Vaginal Concern

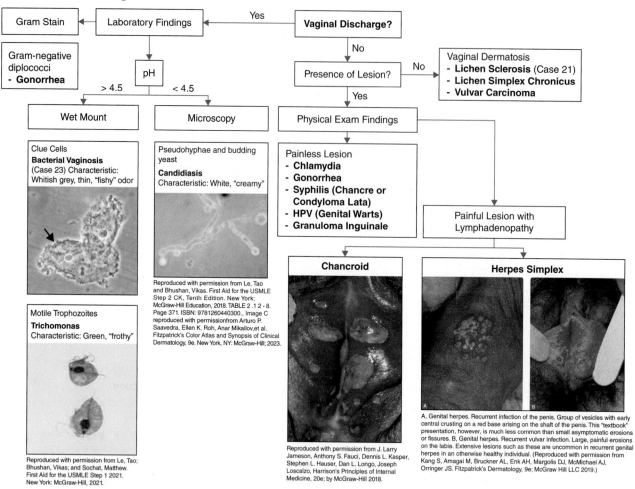

Clue Cells

Bacterial Vaginosis
(Case 23) Characteristic: Whitish grey, thin, "fishy" odor

Motile Trophozoites

Trichomonas
Characteristic: Green, "frothy"

Reproduced with permission from Le, Tao; Bhushan, Vikas; and Sochat, Matthew. First Aid for the USMLE Step 1 2021. New York: McGraw-Hill, 2021.

Pseudohyphae and budding yeast

Candidiasis
Characteristic: White, "creamy"

Reproduced with permission from Le, Tao and Bhushan, Vikas. First Aid for the USMLE Step 2 CK, Tenth Edition. New York: McGraw-Hill Education, 2018. TABLE 2 .1 2 - 8. Page 371. ISBN: 9781260440300., Image C reproduced with permission from Arturo P. Saavedra, Ellen K. Roh, Anar Mikailov,et al. Fitzpatrick's Color Atlas and Synopsis of Clinical Dermatology, 9e. New York, NY: McGraw-Hill; 2023.

Chancroid

Reproduced with permission from J. Larry Jameson, Anthony S. Fauci, Dennis L. Kasper, Stephen L. Hauser, Dan L. Longo, Joseph Loscalzo, Harrison's Principles of Internal Medicine, 20e; by McGraw-Hill 2018.

Herpes Simplex

A, Genital herpes. Recurrent infection of the penis. Group of vesicles with early central crusting on a red base arising on the shaft of the penis. This "textbook" presentation, however, is much less common than small asymptomatic erosions or fissures. B, Genital herpes. Recurrent vulvar infection. Large, painful erosions on the labia. Extensive lesions such as these are uncommon in recurrent genital herpes in an otherwise healthy individual. (Reproduced with permission from Kang S, Amagai M, Bruckner AL, Enk AH, Margolis DJ, McMichael AJ, Orringer JS. Fitzpatrick's Dermatology, 9e; McGraw Hill LLC 2019.)

CASE 20	Genital Herpes

A 21-year-old presents with pain, itching, and burning sensation on the labia. Symptoms started 5 days after her last sexual encounter and were followed by the appearance of small bumps. On exam, there are bilateral clusters of erythematous vesicles on the labia majora that are tender to light palpation, and associated inguinal lymphadenopathy.

Conditions with Similar Presentations	**Chancroid:** Painful genital ulcer with exudate and associated inguinal lymphadenopathy (*Haemophilus ducreyi*). **Granuloma inguinale:** Painless, red papules or ulcer with sparing of regional lymph nodes (*Klebsiella granulomatis*). **Lymphogranuloma venereum:** Painless genital ulcers with painful lymphadenopathy that appear as buboes (*Chlamydial trachomatis* L1–L3). **Condyloma accuminata:** Bumps are non-painful, scaly, verrucous lesions that may vary in size and are itchy. It is sexually transmitted and arises from low-risk HPV 6 and 11.
Initial Diagnostic Tests	• Clinical diagnosis • Confirm with PCR assay of the unroofed vesicle
Next Steps in Management	Acyclovir (or its pro-drugs, valacyclovir or famciclovir)

CASE 20 | Genital Herpes *(continued)*

Discussion	Genital herpes is the most common sexually transmitted infection. HSV is transmitted via sexual activity, saliva, or direct contact, and lesions occur 4–7 days after exposure. The virus enters through mucous membrane and replicates in epithelial cells at the site of entry. It is highly infectious and has a recurrence >70% for symptomatic HSV-1 and 20–50% for symptomatic HSV-2. Both HSV-1 and HSV-2 can cause genital herpes, though historically HSV-2 has been more common in the genital area. HSV-1 also causes gingivostomatitis, keratoconjunctivitis, herpes labialis, and temporal lobe encephalitis. Both types remain latent in sensory ganglia and can reactivate causing recurrent disease. HSV-1 typically reactivates from the trigeminal ganglia and causes cold sores or keratitis. HSV-2 reactivates from the lumbosacral dorsal root ganglia causing genital herpes. **History:** Pain, burning, itching, dysuria, or tingling prior to the outbreak of vesicles. **Physical Exam:** Clusters of papules and vesicles on erythematous base on external genitalia **Diagnostics:** • Clinical diagnosis • Confirm with swab from base of unroofed genital lesion - for PCR assay for HSV–1 and HSV–2 DNA • Consider: HIV test and other STI testing to rule out other co-existing infections. **Management:** • Sitz bath, analgesics • Treat episodes with acyclovir, famciclovir, or valacyclovir for 7 days for the first episode and 2–5 days for recurrent infection • Treatment should be given within 3 days of initial infection or 2 days of recurrent infection, otherwise there is no benefit • Can consider daily antiviral medication for suppression if frequent recurrences or recurrences associated with erythema multiforme, eczema herpeticum, or aseptic meningitis
Additional Considerations	**Prevention:** Counsel patient and sexual partners about sexual transmission—abstinence during prodromal phase and when lesions present. Daily valacyclovir reduces transmission. **Pregnancy Considerations:** In pregnancy, the presence of prodromal symptoms or genital lesions warrants a cesarean birth to prevent vertical transmission.

CASE 21 | Bacterial Vaginosis

A 35-year-old sexually active patient presents for evaluation of a malodorous vaginal discharge. Her last menstrual period was 2 weeks ago. On pelvic exam, there is a whitish-gray thin discharge with fishy odor. There is no vulvar inflammation or cervical motion tenderness.

Conditions with Similar Presentations	**Candida:** Discharge is odorless, thick, white, cottage-cheesy, and pseudohyphae can be seen on wet mount. Often vulvar erythema and itching. The vaginal pH is normal (4–4.5). Treat with azoles (e.g., intravaginal clotrimazole, oral fluconazole). **Trichomoniasis:** Discharge is frothy, malodorous thick, greenish, and motile flagellated trichomonads can be seen on wet mount. Vaginal pH is elevated (>4.5). May have "strawberry cervix." Treat patient and partner with oral metronidazole × 7 days. **Cervicitis:** Typically caused by *Neisseria gonorrheae* or *Chlamydia trachomatis* and associated with cervical discharge, pruritis, and dyspareunia.
Initial Diagnostic Tests	• Check wet mount/microscopy for clue cells • NAAT testing for altered microbiome if available • Consider NAAT to rule out other STI
Next Steps in Management	Intravaginal or oral metronidazole or clindamycin.

CASE 21 | Bacterial Vaginosis *(continued)*

Discussion	Bacterial vaginosis (BV) is caused by an overgrowth of *Gardnerella vaginalis* and other bacteria in the vagina due to the loss of lactic acid-producing lactobacilli. Clue cells (vaginal epithelial cells stippled with *Gardnerella*) are seen on microscopy. Fishy odor can be enhanced with the addition of 10% potassium hydroxide (KOH) to the vaginal discharge ("amine whiff test").
	History:
	Risk factors: Vaginal douching, smoking, new or multiple sexual partners, unprotected intercourse
	Symptoms: Painless, malodorous vaginal discharge
	Physical Exam: Grey vaginal discharge with fishy odor
	Diagnostics: Presence of three of four Amsel criteria:
	1. Homogenous thin white-gray discharge
	2. Vaginal fluid pH >4.5
	3. >20% clue cells on saline microscopy
	4. Positive KOH whiff test result
	Consider screening patients for other co-existing STI.
	• All female patients <25 years old should be screened for asymptomatic chlamydia and gonorrhea
	• All patients should be screened at least once for HIV
	Management:
	• Intravaginal or oral metronidazole or clindamycin
	• If treating with metronidazole, counsel patients not to use alcohol, as it can cause disulfiram reaction
	• Counsel patients to avoid douching
Additional Considerations	**Complications:** Left untreated, can lead to endometritis, pelvic inflammatory disease.
	Pregnancy: BV can cause complications such as PTL or PPROM in pregnant patients.

CASE 22 | Pelvic Inflammatory Disease (PID)

A 28-year-old presents with lower abdominal pain with malodorous thick yellow vaginal discharge. The patient has had multiple male sexual partners and uses condoms intermittently. Vitals P 100, BP 115/78, R 12, T 101°F. On exam, she has tenderness in the lower abdomen, cervical motion, and bilateral adnexal tenderness, along with yellow mucopurulent cervical discharge and a friable cervix.

Conditions with Similar Presentations	**Ovarian torsion:** Presents with acute unilateral pelvic pain and associated nausea and vomiting. May have an adnexal mass; would not have vaginal or endocervical discharge.
	Ectopic pregnancy: Presents with abdominal pain and/or vaginal bleeding with a positive hCG.
	UTI: Presents with dysuria, frequency, +/– suprapubic/flank pain.
Initial Diagnostic Tests	• Clinical diagnosis
	• NAAT for chlamydia/gonorrhea
	• Consider quantitative hCG and TVUS to rule out other causes
Next Steps in Management	Ceftriaxone and doxycycline
Discussion	PID is an infection of the upper genital tract, often polymicrobial, and caused by ascending infection from the vagina and endocervix. It may be due to fecal flora or an STI from *Chlamydia trachomatis* or *Neisseria gonorrhoeae*.
	History:
	Risk Factors: Multiple partners, history of PID or STI, inconsistent condom use, vaginal douching, being within 3 weeks of IUD insertion, and intimate partner violence, rape.
	Symptoms: Lower abdominal or pelvic pain, dyspareunia, back pain, abnormal vaginal discharge, postcoital bleeding, vaginal itching, and odor.
	Physical Exam: Vaginal discharge, uterine, adnexal or cervical motion tenderness.

CASE 22 | Pelvic Inflammatory Disease (PID) *(continued)*

Discussion	**Diagnostics:** • One of the following: Adnexal tenderness, uterine tenderness, cervical motion tenderness • If diagnosis is unclear, ultrasound imaging or abdominal/pelvic CT can be performed. • Test for *Neisseria* and *Chlamydia*; perform a wet mount to evaluate for vaginitis/vaginosis **Management:** • Hospitalize if unable to take oral meds, pelvic abscess on ultrasound, pregnant, failure of prior oral antibiotics. Treat with an IV cephalosporin (ceftriaxone, cefoxitin, cefotetan) and doxycycline. Add metronidazole if ceftriaxone is used to cover anaerobes. Transition to oral outpatient therapy to complete a 14-day course. • Outpatient treatment includes a cephalosporin plus doxycycline, and metronidazole for 14 days. • Treatment with antibiotics should not be postponed while waiting for culture confirmation. • Treat male sexual partners with treatment effective against gonorrhea and chlamydia regardless of patient's test results.
Additional Considerations	**Complications:** Infection/inflammation can cause endometritis, pelvic peritonitis, salpingitis, chronic pelvic pain, infertility, ectopic pregnancy, tubo-ovarian abscess, and/or perihepatitis (Fitz-Hugh-Curtis syndrome). **Fitz-Hugh-Curtis syndrome** causes "violin string" adhesions of peritoneum to liver and presents as pleuritic RUQ pain, referred to the right shoulder, and can be diagnosed with ultrasound. It is treated with ceftriaxone and doxycycline.

CASE 23 | Toxic Shock Syndrome (TSS)

An 18-year-old presents with fever, chills, myalgia, nausea, vomiting, and generalized rash. The patient placed a tampon at the start of menses 3 days ago but did not replace it. Vitals show a temperature of 39.0°C, PR 100, and BP 80/50 mmHg. There is tenderness over the suprapubic area and pelvic exam reveals vaginal hyperemia with malodorous discharge and a retained tampon. A fine erythematous macular rash is present over the chest and extremities. Serum creatinine is 2.1mg/dl and platelet count is 61,000.

Conditions with Similar Presentations	**Fever with rash on palms and soles:** *Rocky Mountain spotted fever (RMSF):* History of possible tick bite; rash is petechial. *Secondary syphilis:* Sexually active, may have had symptoms of primary or secondary syphilis; does not present with shock. **Fever with acute abdominal/pelvic pain:** Pelvic inflammatory disease, appendicitis, diverticulitis, intraabdominal abscess. These would not have a rash.
Initial Diagnostic Tests	• Clinical diagnosis: triad of fever, shock, and rash along with at least three organ systems involved. • Check CBC, CMP, blood, and vaginal cultures • Consider urine culture and serologies to rule out other causes
Next Steps in Management	• Removal of foreign body • Management of septic shock with IV antibiotics, fluids, and supportive care
Discussion	TSS is caused via infection by or colonization of exotoxin-producing strains of staphylococcus resulting in a severe, abrupt-onset systemic illness. TSS is classified as menstrual or non-menstrual. Menstrual-related cases are classically attributed to prolonged retention of a vaginal foreign body, usually a tampon. Approximately one-half of TSS cases are due to non-menstrual causes such as postoperative wound infections and burns. Toxic shock syndrome toxin-1 (TSST-1) and enterotoxins act as superantigens to disrupt immunomodulation and initiates a cascade of toxic events. Blood cultures are often negative in TSS. **History:** History of tampon use or retained foreign body in vagina.

CASE 23 | Toxic Shock Syndrome (TSS) *(continued)*

Discussion	Symptoms: Fever >38.9°C (102°F) and rash, and any of the symptoms of organ involvement (see below).
	Physical Exam: Erythematous, sunburn-like rash, including palms, soles, fingers, and toes. Vaginal exam may show retained foreign object and malodorous discharge and vaginal wall erythema.
	Diagnostics:
	Triad of:
	• Fever ≥102°F (38.9°C)
	• Hypotension
	• Diffuse macular erythematous rash (desquamation, 1–2 weeks after onset of rash)
	And involvement of three or more organ systems:
	• Nausea, vomiting, diarrhea
	• Myalgia and/or elevated CK
	• Liver transaminase and/or bilirubin elevation
	• Thrombocytopenia
	• Altered consciousness
	Management:
	• Source control (removal of retained object when applicable)
	• Sepsis management (see Chapter 20, Emergency Medicine)
	• Empiric vancomycin (until methicillin susceptibilities known from cultures) and clindamycin to inhibit ribosomal production of toxins.

ADNEXAL MASSES

Adnexal masses may be found incidentally or during workup of pelvic concerns, and are usually benign. Many masses in the ovary are cystic and arise in response to normal cyclical changes like the follicular and corpus luteum cysts. They are generally benign and resolve spontaneously but can cause pelvic pain due to torsion or rupture.

Physiologic Masses

• Arise in response to normal cyclic changes in ovarian physiology

• Include follicular and corpus luteum cysts

• Are benign and resolve spontaneously

• Can cause acute pelvic pain if they undergo torsion or rupture with intraperitoneal hemorrhage

Complex Adnexal Masses

These include endometrioma, hemorrhagic cyst, ovarian malignancy, mucinous cystadenomas, metastases from other primary tumors (i.e., Krukenberg tumor), ovarian fibromas, pedunculated sub-serosal uterine fibroids, GI diverticula, ectopic pregnancy, tubo-ovarian abscess, and are differentiated based on imaging and labs.

Approach to Evaluation of Adnexal Mass

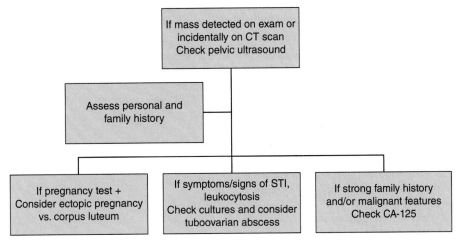

Types of Ovarian Cancer

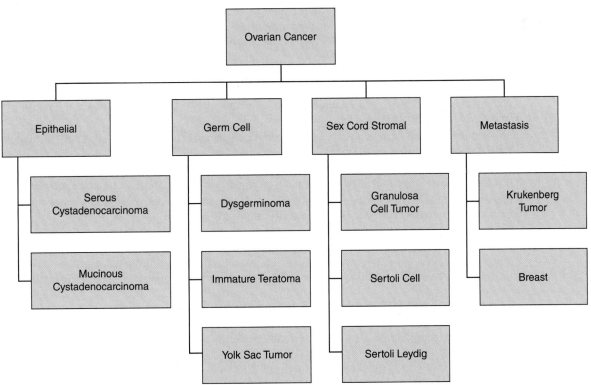

CASE 24	Ovarian Cancer

A 57-year-old G0 presents to clinic with early satiety and progressive abdominal bloating. She has significant ascites and a fixed and nodular adnexal mass.

Conditions with Similar Presentations	**Colon malignancy** with local spread, **leiomyosarcoma** or other malignancies differentiated based on labs, imaging, and pathology
Initial Diagnostic Tests	• Pelvic ultrasound • CA-125 • Abdominal CT scan

CASE 24 | Ovarian Cancer *(continued)*

Next Steps in Management	Pending imaging findings and patient condition, initial debulking surgery vs. neoadjuvant chemotherapy

Discussion	Ovarian malignancies are notorious for later stage at diagnosis given the lack of adequate screening tools, poor symptom specificity, and potential for an asymptomatic window until great disease progression. Ovarian cancer often spreads locally within the peritoneum, resulting in ascites and omental seeding. Surface epithelial (stromal) tumors are the most common form of ovarian cancers (90%).
	
	Ovarian cancers are classified by the site of origin:
	• Epithelial
	   • **Serous cystadenocarcinomas:** Typically aggressive, bilateral, and have **psammoma bodies** on pathological examination
	   • **Mucinous cystadenocarcinomas:** Rare primary ovarian tumors (usually metastatic from the GI tract—resulting in pseudomyxoma peritonei)
	• Germ cell
	   • **Immature teratomas:** Also aggressive, arise from germ cells, have fetal tissue and neuroectoderm on pathology.
	   • **Dysgerminomas:** Occur in adolescents, present with elevation in LDH and hCG, and show **sheets of "fried-egg"** cells on pathological exam.
	• Sex cord-stromal cell
	   • **Granulosa cell tumors:** Usually occur in patients in their 50s; most common tumors originating from the stromal tissue of the ovary, often produce estrogen and/or progesterone and can present with postmenopausal or other abnormal uterine bleeding because of the unopposed estrogen on the endometrium.
	
	History:
	Risk Factors: Early menarche, late menopause, older age, nulliparity or older age at first pregnancy (>35), endometriosis, PCOS, family history, BRCA1 or BRCA2 mutations, HNPCC, and DES exposure in-utero (specifically clear cell ovarian cancer).
	
	Risk-Reductive Factors: Increasing parity, breastfeeding, combined oral contraceptive use, hysterectomy, and tubal ligation.
	
	Symptoms: Are typically non-specific, and they may present as abdominal or pelvic pain, bloating, nausea, fatigue, unintentional weight loss with paradoxical increase in waist circumference, and lack of appetite/early satiety.
	
	Physical Exam: Concerning features for malignancy: a fixed, nodular mass on pelvic exam and nodularity in or loss of the posterior cul-de-sac on rectovaginal exam, and/or ascites.
	
	Diagnostics:
	• Ultrasound/CT scan findings may include papillary projections, thick septations, and other stigmata of malignancy, including ascites, omental thickening/caking, and paraaortic lymphadenopathy.
	• CA-125 may be useful in creating the differential diagnosis and monitoring for response to treatment and recurrence.
	• Consider CA 19-9 and CEA (helpful in ruling out other primary malignancies of the abdomen and pelvis, particularly in more advanced disease when imaging may reveal mass of unknown origin).
	
	Management: Surgical resection/debulking and chemotherapy (generally with at least a platinum-based agent).
	• Early stage: Cytoreductive (debulking) surgery, which includes total abdominal hysterectomy with bilateral salpingo-oophorectomy, possible adjuvant chemotherapy.
	• Advanced ovarian cancer: May initiate neoadjuvant chemotherapy prior to any surgical resection if more advanced disease that cannot be optimally resected or patients with severe comorbidity that precludes safe surgical approach.

Additional Considerations	**Complications:** Ascites, malignant pleural effusion, bowel obstruction.

Adnexal Tumor Mini-Cases

Cases	Key Findings
Teratoma	**Hx:** Asymptomatic or symptoms of hyperthyroidism (palpitations, weight loss, anxiety, polyphagia) **PE:** Fullness in adnexal region, mobile uterus, and non-tender to palpation **Diagnostics:** Confirm with pelvic ultrasound

Adnexal Tumor Mini-Cases *(continued)*

Teratoma	**Management:** • Surveillance via pelvic ultrasound and torsion precautions • Surgery is considered for large masses, symptoms, increase in size of mass, or if there is suspicion of malignancy. **Discussion:** Ovarian mature cystic teratomas (also known as dermoid cyst) are typically benign and represent the most common benign tumor found in the ovary. These arise from abnormal differentiation of totipotent germ cells in the ovary. They may contain single or multiple mature tissues. The most common form is a **struma ovarii**, which can cause severe hyperthyroidism. In rare cases, a teratoma can give rise to paraneoplastic syndromes such as anti-NMDA receptor encephalitis. Possible complications include adnexal torsion, spontaneous rupture, and malignant transformation.
Krukenberg Tumor	**Hx:** Abdominal fullness, increased urinary frequency, may have history of gastric cancer **PE:** Abdominal or adnexal mass palpated on pelvic exam **Diagnostics:** Pelvic ultrasound shows bilateral, solid, well-demarcated adnexal masses with "moth-eaten" appearance and normal appearing anteverted uterus. CEA is elevated. **Management:** Treat the primary cancer and surgical excision of the tumor. **Discussion:** When a cancer metastasizes to the ovary from another primary site (e.g., GI tract), it is referred to as a Krukenberg tumor. The definitive diagnosis of Krukenberg tumor is made with surgical pathology, which typically reveals mucin-filled, signet ring cell adenocarcinoma. When metastasized to the ovary, cystic mass effect may cause urinary symptoms, abdominal distention, early satiety, or pelvic pain.
Granulosa Cell Tumor	**Hx:** Development of secondary sex characteristics ≤8 years old, abdominal fullness **PE:** Distended abdomen with palpable pelvic mass on bimanual exam **Diagnostics:** Pelvic ultrasound **Management:** • Consider unilateral salpingo-oophorectomy (fertility-preserving surgery) for earlier stages • Chemotherapy for more advanced stages. **Discussion:** Granulosa cell tumors (GCTs) are the most common malignant sex-cord stromal tumor. These sex-cord stromal tumors arise from the granulosa cells, which are somatic cells that support the growth and maturation of the developing oocytes within the ovaries. They secrete estrogen and/or progesterone, causing precocious pubertal development. Given the malignant potential, GCTs should be ruled out in *any* young female patient presenting with a pelvic mass.

VULVAR AND VAGINAL CONDITIONS

Vulvar Dermatoses/Lesions

The vulva is also prone to a unique group of conditions classified as the vulvar dermatoses. These three "lichens" are: (1) sclerosis, (2) planus, and (3) simplex chronicus.

Symptoms include classic triad: vulvar pruritis, burning. and dyspareunia.

Diagnosis is made clinically by history and exam, and biopsy may be done to confirm.

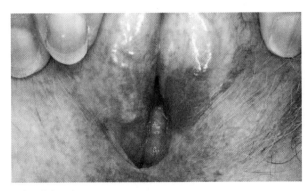

Lichen Sclerosis

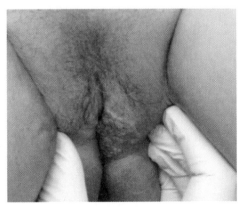

Vulvar Carcinoma

Reproduced with permission from Le, Tao; Bhushan, Vikas; and Sochat, Matthew. First Aid for the USMLE Step 1 2021. New York: McGraw-Hill, 2021.

CASE 25 | Lichen Sclerosus

A 68-year-old presents with 6 months of progressively worsening intermittent vulvar itching, burning, and dyspareunia. On vulvar examination, the labia minora are fused to the labia majora and there are atrophic white patches located around the vaginal introitus. The skin in the area has a thin and crinkled appearance.

Conditions with Similar Presentations	**Lichen planus:** Has an association with hepatitis C infection and certain medications; may occur on vulva or present as "lacy" rash in other areas (e.g., oral mucosa, scalp, nails, wrist). Vulvar variant has violet/red erosive-appearing plaques with reticulated white lines or overlying Wickham striae. Pain is more significant than itching.
	Lichen simplex chronicus: Asymmetric thickening of skin, labia majora, or other areas. Caused by environmental factors such as heat, moisture, irritation, or longstanding dermal infection and characterized by intense vulvar itching that sometimes results in bleeding, change in vulvar skin color resulting in hyperpigmentation and thickened, hyperkeratotic skin and excoriations, scaling, and a lichenified, thick, leathery plaque due to chronic scratching. In addition to mild topical corticosteroids, treatment involves removal of stimuli.
	Vulvar carcinoma: History of HPV infection; leukoplakia, exophytic mass on vulva.
Initial Diagnostic Tests	• Clinical diagnosis • Consider vulvar biopsy if atypical presentation or unresponsive to therapy
Next Steps in Management	Ultrapotent topical steroids (clobetasol)
Discussion	Lichen sclerosis is a chronic inflammatory condition of unknown etiology often affecting postmenopausal patients and associated with autoimmune disorders. It is caused by inflammation and abnormal fibroblast function and leads to fibrosis of the dermis and commonly involves the skin of the genitalia. It is a progressive condition that can lead to scarring and dyspareunia. **History:** Symptoms: worse at night; triad of vulvar pruritis, burning, and dyspareunia. **Physical Exam:** • Labial agglutination, clitoral phimosis • White atrophic plaques ("parchment paper appearance") • Hourglass distribution, sparing the perineal body **Diagnostics:** • Clinical diagnosis • Can confirm with punch biopsy. Histology shows epidermal atrophy. **Management:** Ultrapotent topical steroids.
Additional Considerations	**Complications:** Up to 5% of genital lichen sclerosis will undergo malignant transformation to squamous cell carcinoma. **Surgical Considerations:** Surgery for refractory cases with severe obstructing adhesions.

Vulvar Tumor Mini-Case

Vulvar Carcinoma	**Hx:** New vulvar lesion that itches, burns, or bleeds with manipulation, history of HPV, typically postmenopausal **PE:** May have leukoplakia (thickened mucocutaneous white/gray patches), visible exophytic lesion on vulva, and/or inguinal lymphadenopathy **Diagnostics:** Biopsy to confirm **Management:** Resection with radical vulvectomy +/− radiotherapy and chemotherapy **Discussion:** The major risk factors associated with vulvar cancer are history of HPV, chronic lichen sclerosis, history of smoking, vulvar dystrophy, and presence of cervical intraepithelial neoplasia. It often presents with leukoplakia in postmenopausal patients and has a poor prognosis.

Vaginal Masses

A mass in the vagina can be diagnosed based on a comprehensive history and focused pelvic exam, as vaginal and vulvar cancers are exceedingly rare. Biopsies are done only if the etiology is unclear. These masses can be classified as below:

Classification of Vaginal Lesions by Etiology

Etiology	Vaginal Lesion
Congenital	Vaginal septum, vaginal outlet obstruction
Inflammatory	Post-surgical/radiation changes, fistula formation
Benign	Gartner's duct cyst, Bartholin's gland cyst, urethral diverticulum, leiomyoma
Malignant	Rhabdomyosarcoma, vaginal carcinoma, melanoma

CASE 26 | Pelvic Organ Prolapse

A 60-year-old G5P5005 presents with a 3-month history of increased pelvic pressure. She reports that sometimes she feels like there is a bulge coming out of the vagina when she coughs. She has a long history of stress urinary incontinence managed conservatively with pelvic floor exercises. However, she reports that recently she must insert a finger into the vagina to void completely. On pelvic exam, a smooth, flesh-colored mass emerges to the level of the introitus with Valsalva maneuver.

Conditions with Similar Presentations	**Urethral diverticulum:** May present with localized outpouching of the urethral mucosa, tender anterior vaginal wall mass, and/or postvoid dribbling of urine. **Uterine fibroids:** May present with pelvic pain and urinary or defecatory symptoms, menorrhagia, and uterus may be enlarged on bimanual exam. **Adnexal mass:** Pain or pressure on the affected side.
Initial Diagnostic Tests	Clinical diagnosis
Next Steps in Management	Vaginal pessary
Discussion	The descent of one or more aspects of the vagina and uterus is termed pelvic organ prolapse. The loss of connective tissue and muscular support of the pelvic floor causes displacement of the pelvic organs and prolapse. The anterior vaginal wall, posterior vaginal wall, the uterus, or the apex of the vagina may descend permitting the nearby organs to herniate into the vaginal space. Anterior vaginal wall defect and cystocele is most common. It becomes a problem if it causes pressure, pain, or urinary/defecatory abnormalities. **Cystocele:** An anterior vaginal prolapse which occurs when the supportive tissues around the bladder and vaginal wall stretch and weaken allowing the bladder and vaginal wall to collapse into the vaginal canal. **Rectocele:** A posterior vaginal prolapse which occurs when the thin wall of tissue that separates the vagina from the rectum weakens, allowing the vaginal wall to bulge. **Complete procidentia:** Is the process by which complete prolapse has occurred (involves apex, anterior, and posterior walls); the uterus will be prolapsed completely outside of the vaginal introitus. **History:** Risk Factors: Parity, vaginal delivery, elevated BMI, connective tissue disorders, post-menopausal status, and chronic constipation. Symptoms: • Vaginal or pelvic pressure and/or the sensation of a vaginal bulge or something "falling out" of the vagina • Stress incontinence • Advanced prolapse may lead to obstructed voiding • Defecatory symptoms such as constipation and a feeling of incomplete emptying • Some patients will report having to manually reduce (called splinting) the prolapse to urinate or have a bowel movement

CASE 26 | Pelvic Organ Prolapse *(continued)*

Discussion	**Diagnostics:** Clinical diagnosis based on complete gynecologic, urologic, and defecatory history and physical examination. Consider: • Post void residual—if the prolapse is advanced or the patient has voiding symptoms • Urine analysis—if urinary urgency or other lower urinary tract symptoms • Urodynamic testing—to distinguish between prolapse and voiding dysfunction **Management:** • Treat if prolapse is causing bothersome symptoms • Vaginal pessary—effective nonsurgical treatment • Surgical intervention if significant apical prolapse, anterior prolapse, or both and/or conservative treatment not effective
Additional Considerations	**Complications:** Recurrence of pelvic organ prolapse is common after surgery, with rates of up to 30%.

Vaginal Mass Mini-Cases

Cases	Key Findings
Bartholin Cyst	**Hx:** Asymptomatic, or dyspareunia, vaginal pain **PE:** Presence of unilateral, non-tender fluctuant mass with protrusion near vaginal introitus **Diagnostics:** Clinical diagnosis **Management:** • Incision and drainage if evidence of abscess. • Sitz bath in warm water may improve mild symptoms. **Discussion:** The Bartholin glands (greater vestibular glands) are small glands located just inside the vaginal introitus on each side (approximately 4 and 8 o'clock). Bartholin gland cysts develop due to accumulation of normal secretions in setting of blockage of the Bartholin gland duct. A complication is Bartholin's abscess, which can present with increased pain on the side of the cyst, fever, and dyspareunia. Bartholin Cyst. (Reproduced with permission from Le, Tao; Bhushan, Vikas; and Sochat, Matthew. First Aid for the USMLE Step 1 2021. New York: McGraw-Hill, 2021.)
Vaginal Cancer	**Hx:** Unusual vaginal bleeding, especially postmenopausal bleeding, discharge, presence of vaginal lump or mass **PE:** Presence of vaginal lump or mass, irritation **Diagnostics:** Biopsy and imaging to assess metastases **Management:** Chemoradiation is the mainstay of therapy, with radical surgery playing a lesser role. **Discussion:** • **Squamous cell carcinoma:** Associated with a history of squamous cell cervical cancer. It can spread hematogenously, lymphatically, or via direct invasion. • **Primary vaginal clear cell adenocarcinomas:** Associated with diethylstilbestrol exposure in utero, though these are now exceedingly rare given discontinuation of use of this drug • Most cases of **adenocarcinoma** of the vagina are metastatic
Sarcoma Botryoides	**Hx:** Vaginal bleeding, vaginal discharge, vaginal irritation **PE:** Presence of pelvic mass on exam **Diagnostics:** Clinical and pathology **Management:** Excision and chemotherapy **Discussion:** Sarcoma botryoides is a rare embryonal rhabdomyosarcoma variant seen in infants and children. Mean age of diagnosis is 2–3 years, and on exam, a mass resembling a **cluster of grapes** may be noted protruding from the vaginal apex

GYNECOLOGIC ONCOLOGY AND GYNECOLOGIC PROCEDURES, INDICATIONS AND COMPLICATIONS

There are several unique malignant conditions of the female reproductive tract. Some have been addressed in sections above, with remaining conditions of note discussed below.

Gynecologic Procedures, Indications and Complications

Procedure	Possible Indications
Colposcopy	Abnormal Pap (cytologic abnormalities and/or presence of high-risk HPV—depending on patient age)
Hysteroscopy	Intracavitary lesions (submucosal leiomyomata, endometrial polyps), retained foreign body (IUD), uterine septum
Endometrial biopsy	Postmenopausal bleeding, abnormal uterine bleeding in any patient >45 years or with risk factors for endometrial cancer/chronic anovulation
Hysterectomy	Gynecologic premalignant and malignant conditions, abnormal uterine bleeding and/or pain refractory to medical management, peripartum hemorrhage uncontrolled by other interventions

Complications of Gynecologic Procedures

Possible Nerve Injuries	Key Findings
Iliohypogastric and Ilioinguinal Nerves	Damage to these nerves is most likely in the context of recent abdominal hysterectomy due to incision site and retractor use or entrapment by sutures at lateral sides of transverse fascial incisions. The ilioinguinal nerve is more likely to be damaged than the Iliohypogastric nerve. Patients may report paresthesia and sharp, burning pain from incision to suprapubic area, labia, or thigh. Most symptoms self-resolve, although paresthesias may persist
Femoral Nerve	Femoral nerve damage is most likely in the setting of deep pelvic surgery, when deep or lateral placement of the retractor blades cause compression of the nerve against pelvic wall at the site where it exits the psoas muscle and before exiting the pelvis at the inguinal ligament. Risk factors for the nerve damage include wide incision, thin subcutaneous fat layer, poorly developed rectus muscles, and narrow pelvis. Patients may present with neuropathy with associated sensory and motor impairment, anesthesia along anterior and medial thigh, and weakness in quadriceps and iliopsoas in context of recent abdominal hysterectomy. Treatment is expectant management and physical therapy.
Genitofemoral and Lateral Femoral Cutaneous Nerve	Because these nerves are so superficial, anything that causes compression, such as obesity or pelvic surgery, can lead to damage. Injury to the lateral femoral cutaneous nerve is most commonly termed meralgia paresthetica, and results in pain and paresthesias that radiate down the anterior and posterolateral portion of the thigh. May occur in the setting of pelvic surgery that involves dissection of external iliac lymph nodes, mobilization of iliac vessels, or removal of mass adherent to pelvic sidewall, morbid obesity. Treatment is expectant management, but nerve blocks may be considered.
Obturator Nerve	Surgeries associated with obturator nerve damage include deep excision of endometriosis, paravaginal defect repair, and obturator bypass. Usage of trocar in areas of sacrum, pelvic brim, or obturator canal or pelvic lymph node dissection in obturator fossa increases the risk and patients may present with numbness of inner thigh, weakened adduction of thigh. Treatment is expectant management, postoperative physiotherapy, and possible microsurgical repair
Peroneal Nerve	In a gynecologic setting, the peroneal nerve is most often damaged after prolonged dorsal lithotomy positioning with foot rests. May present with acute foot drop (difficulty dorsiflexing foot), paresthesias, and/or sensory loss over dorsum of foot and lateral shin. Expectant management and ankle foot orthotic.
Pudendal Nerve	Pudendal nerve injuries/entrapment are most associated with procedures that involve the placement of sutures in the arcus tendinous fasciae pelvis during sacrospinous ligament fixation or pelvic reconstructive procedures. The most distinct feature of this damage is pain in the vulvar area that worsens when seated. Surgical decompression is preferred, but pudendal nerve block provides relief

CASE 27 | Squamous Cell Carcinoma of the Cervix

A 44-year-old woman presents with vaginal bleeding with intercourse for the last several months. She has a 15-pack-year history of smoking, has multiple sexual partners, and has had a normal Pap smear after delivery 13 years ago. Exam is notable for a friable ulcerated mass on the posterior lip of the cervix. This is non-tender, and there are no other masses on bimanual exam.

Conditions with Similar Presentations	**Cervical dysplasia or cervical intraepithelial neoplasia (CIN):** Histologic abnormalities that precede invasive cancer; usually not associated with masses but may have visualized surface changes. **STI:** May result in postcoital or contact bleeding due to inflammation of cervix, would not have friable mass.
Initial Diagnostic Tests	• Pap smear with HPV DNA co-testing • Colposcopy • Cervical biopsy
Next Steps in Management	• Depends on stage (see below)
Discussion	Most cervical carcinomas are squamous cell cancers. Pap smears can detect dysplasia before it progresses to invasive cancer. Infection with human papillomavirus (HPV) subtypes 16 or 18 lead to significant risk of developing cervical metaplasia and cancer. **History:** Risk Factors: Multiple sexual partners, immunosuppression, history of STI, in-utero diethylstilbestrol (DES) exposure, cigarette smoking. Symptoms: Asymptomatic or abnormal vaginal or postcoital bleeding; with advanced disease: malodorous brown discharge due to necrosis and possible fistula formation, sciatic pain, leg swelling, and hydroureter due to compression on surrounding structures. **Physical Exam:** Ulceration of cervix on speculum exam **Diagnostics:** • Initial test: Pap smear with HPV DNA Co-testing (CIN with +high risk HPV (16 and/or 18) • Confirm with colposcopy and biopsy (squamous cell carcinoma with koilocytes) • Obtain CT of chest, abdomen, and pelvis for staging • Consider tests to rule out STI **Management:** • Depending on stage, cervical conization or radical hysterectomy may be an appropriate initial step • Radiation therapy for local disease and chemotherapy for systemic disease • Advanced disease is treated with chemoradiation first to avoid macro-invasive surgery like pelvic exenteration when possible
Additional Considerations	**Screening:** USPSTF recommends the following age-based guidelines: 21–29 years: Pap smear every 3 years 30–65 years: Pap smear with HPV co-testing or primary HPV testing every 5 years Cancer screening surveillance frequency for patients with risk factors (e.g., immunocompromised, high risk HPV infection, HIV) or abnormal results depends on calculated risk of developing carcinoma.

CASE 28 | Endometrial Carcinoma

A 67-year-old G0 with history of breast cancer treated with tamoxifen for 5 years presents with vaginal bleeding. Her last menstrual period was over 15 years ago. Pelvic exam reveals an enlarged uterus.

Conditions with Similar Presentations	**Endometrial hyperplasia:** Also presents with postmenopausal bleeding. It is a premalignant condition distinguished on pathology (hyperplastic proliferation of the endometrium). **Atrophic vaginitis, cervical cancer, or other lesions:** May cause vaginal bleeding, and can be distinguished by exam and further testing.
Initial Diagnostic Tests	Any patient with postmenopausal bleeding should be initially evaluated with an ultrasound to assess endometrial thickness

CASE 28 | Endometrial Carcinoma *(continued)*

Next Steps in Management	Endometrial biopsy
Discussion	Endometrial cancer mostly affects post-menopausal patients and is the fourth most common cancer in female patients after breast, lung, and colorectal. Endometrial hyperplasia leads to excess estrogen stimulation causing abnormal endometrial gland proliferation, predisposing patients to increased risk of endometrial cancer, especially if nuclear atypia is present. Often presents first with abnormal or postmenopausal bleeding. Biopsy shows endometrial adenocarcinoma. **History:** Risk Factors: Include unopposed estrogen, elevated BMI, diabetes, nulliparity, hormone replacement therapy (tamoxifen), PCOS, and Lynch syndrome Symptoms: Postmenopausal bleeding **Physical Exam:** Pelvic exam is typically normal **Diagnostics:** Obtain: • Pelvic ultrasound: thickened endometrial stripe >5 mm • Endometrial biopsy: neoplastic proliferation of endometrial tissue, consistent with adenocarcinoma • CT of chest, abdomen, and pelvis to assess for metastatic disease **Management:** • Early-stage disease is treated with total hysterectomy and bilateral salpingo-oophorectomy. • Locally advanced disease should be treated with surgery followed by local radiation therapy. • Systemic disease is typically treated with chemotherapy.

BREAST DISORDERS

Breast disorders arise from several etiologies, most of which are benign. However, breast cancer is the most common invasive malignancy in genetic females worldwide, affecting about one in eight. This section only addresses lactation-associated breast disorders. For all other breast disorders please refer to Chapter 19 (Surgery).

History/Physical Exam

Many benign breast conditions are hormonally mediated (i.e., estrogen and progestin) from the menstrual cycle, pregnancy, exogenous hormone administration (e.g., birth control, hormone replacement), and/or thyroid or /prolactin imbalances. Therefore, in addition to inquiring about location, onset, duration, and nature of symptoms, it is important to elicit if symptoms are related to the menstrual cycle. Patients can present with breast pain, a detectable lump, nodularity, and/or nipple discharge.

The risk of breast cancer increases with age, obesity, XX chromosomes, high estrogen levels, nulliparity (or older age with first pregnancy), alcohol consumption, and family history of breast cancer or certain mutations (e.g., *BRCA*). The risk of breast cancer can be reduced by breastfeeding. Breast cancer can present with a hard "rock-like" mass, nipple discharge, thickening of the skin, skin erythema, or dimpling (peau d'orange). If the cancer has metastasized, patients may present with axillary lymphadenopathy and/or systemic symptoms depending on the organ involved (e.g., back pain with bone involvement, abdominal pain or jaundice with liver involvement, headache or neurological findings with brain involvement).

There are three general components to the breast examination:

• Visual inspection: checking for symmetry, skin changes, nipple retraction
• Palpation: for masses or asymmetric/irregular densities, nipple drainage; should be done while patient is supine with ipsilateral arm above head
• Exam for adenopathy: axilla and supraclavicular regions

A Broad Classification of Breast Disorders is Given Below

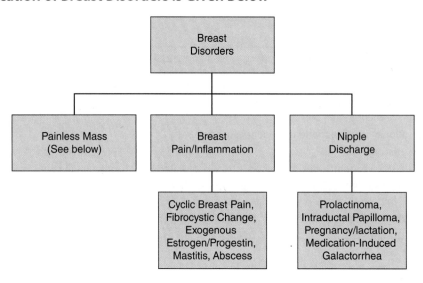

Patients with abnormal findings on initial clinical examination (palpable breast mass, asymmetric thickening or nodularity, skin changes, or nipple discharge) require further evaluation with imaging studies. The appropriate diagnostic imaging study is determined based on the patient's age.

- <30 years with a palpable mass, ultrasonography (US) is the preferred initial test.
- ≥30 years with a palpable mass, diagnostic mammography and possible US should be obtained.

CASE 29	Galactocele

A 28-year-old G2P2002 presents for evaluation of a mass in her left breast that she noted about 1 week ago. She is breastfeeding and had an uncomplicated vaginal delivery 1 month ago. She cannot recall any preceding trauma to the area. On physical exam, breasts are symmetric and there is a 3 × 3 cm fluctuant, non-tender mass in the lateral aspect of the left breast. The area is not warm or erythematous.

Conditions with Similar Presentations	It is important to differentiate the following breast masses from galactoceles, which usually present as a firm, *non-tender* mass usually in the subareolar region. **Acute mastitis:** Presents with breast pain and erythematous, warm, tender breast and possible fever due to bacterial infection (often by *Staphylococcus aureus*) during lactation. Treat with antibiotics (e.g., dicloxacillin, cephalexin, amoxicillin, and clavulanate), warm compresses, and continued breastfeeding or breast pumping to prevent milk stasis. An abscess that develops should be drained.
Conditions with Similar Presentations	**Fibrocystic changes:** Present with pain that may be exacerbated by menstruation and chocolate or caffeine consumption; lumpy, irregular breast texture ("lumpy and bumpy"), and tenderness to palpation from cysts and fibrosis. **Inflammatory breast cancer:** Presents with erythema, swelling, pain of breast and peau d'orange skin due to plugging of the dermal lymphatics. This can mimic acute mastitis, and patients who do not improve with antibiotics should have further evaluation. **Fibroadenoma:** The commonest cause of breast masses in adolescents and young adults. Patients present with a painless, firm, mobile, "rubbery" nodule. It is usually small (1–2 cm), firm, well-circumscribed and mobile. The mass composed of a proliferation of epithelial and stromal elements. On ultrasound, the fibroadenoma appears as a solid mass helping differentiate it from a simple cyst. **Fat necrosis:** A benign condition of the breast that produces a mass and is often accompanied by skin or nipple retraction. This condition can be mistaken for carcinoma. The most common causes are trauma and surgery and tenderness may or may not be present. When untreated, the mass due to fat necrosis disappears.

CASE 29 | Galactocele *(continued)*

Initial Diagnostic Tests	• Clinical diagnosis • Can confirm with needle aspiration • Consider: Breast ultrasound
Next Steps in Management	• Continue breastfeeding • If signs of infection—needle aspiration of contents and antibiotics
Discussion	A galactocele, or milk-retention cyst, is caused by blockage of a milk duct. Acute mastitis can result from an infected galactocele. **History:** Lactating patient presenting with a painless lump in breast. **Physical Exam:** A galactocele is a soft, non-tender, firm, discrete, freely moveable cystic mass. **Diagnostics:** Clinical diagnosis Confirm with ultrasonography: Galactocele may demonstrate a simple milk cyst. **Management:** • Galactoceles are sterile collections that resolve on cessation of lactation. Recurrence is unlikely to occur. • Ultrasound-guided FNA is both diagnostic and therapeutic and is done with gram-positive antibiotic coverage. • Breast massage helps prevent and treat galactoceles.
Additional Considerations	**Complications:** Severe infection/abscess requiring incision and drainage.

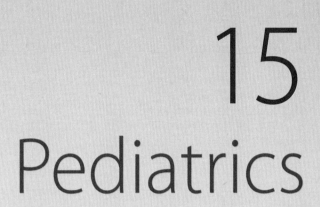

15
Pediatrics

Lead Authors: Claudia C. Boucher-Berry, MD; Daphne L. Vander Roest, MD
Contributors: Julie Conrad, MD; Kathryn Ospino, MD; Margaret M. Van Der Bosch, MD; Maya McKeown, MD; Mahi Singh, MD; Nidhi Suthar, MD; Joseph R. Geraghty, MD, PhD

Pediatric Genetics

18. Classic Galactosemia
19. Phenylketonuria (PKU)
20. Tay-Sachs Disease
21. Glycogen Storage Disease Type I (Von Gierke Disease)
    Glycogen Storage Disease Mini-Cases
       Type V (McArdle Disease)
       Type II (Pompe Disease)
22. Prader-Willi Syndrome
    Chromosomal Genetic Disorders Associated With Intellectual Impairment Mini-Cases
    Angelman Syndrome
    Rett Syndrome
23. Trisomy 21 (Down Syndrome)

Pediatric Immunology

24. X-linked (Bruton) Agammaglobulinemia
25. Severe Combined Immunodeficiency (SCID)
26. DiGeorge Syndrome
    T Cell Deficiency Mini-Case
       Hyper IgE Syndrome
    Phagocytic Defect Mini-Cases
       Chronic Granulomatous Disease
       Leukocyte Adhesion Defect

Pediatric Infectious Disease

27. Streptococcal Pharyngitis/Scarlet Fever
28. Epiglottitis (Secondary to *H. influenzae* type b)
29. Acute Otitis Media
    Cough Mini-Cases
       Bronchiolitis (RSV)
       Laryngotracheitis (Croup)
       Pertussis (Whooping Cough)
30. Kawasaki Disease

Pediatric Pulmonology

31. Foreign Body Aspiration
32. Cystic Fibrosis
    Recurrent Lung Infection Mini-Case
       Primary Ciliary Dyskinesia

Pediatric Nephrology

33. Acute Post-Infectious Glomerulonephritis (Post-Streptococcal Glomerulonephritis [PSGN])
34. IgA Nephropathy (Berger Disease)
35. Hemolytic Uremic Syndrome (HUS)
36. Minimal Change Disease (MCD)
37. Urinary Tract Infection (UTI) in Infant

Pediatric Neurology

38. Chiari II Malformation
39. Cerebral Palsy
40. Spina Bifida/Meningocele
41. Germinal Matrix Hemorrhage-Intraventricular Hemorrhage
42. Tuberous Sclerosis Complex
43. Childhood Absence Epilepsy
44. Febrile Seizures
    Breath-Holding Spells Mini-Case

Pediatric Hematology

45. Iron Deficiency Anemia
46. Hemophilia A (Factor VIII Deficiency)
47. Von Willebrand Disease, Type 1

Pediatric Oncology

48. Acute Lymphoblastic Leukemia (ALL)
49. Retinoblastoma
50. Neuroblastoma
51. Wilms' Tumor (Nephroblastoma)

INTRODUCTION

It is important to note that children are not "small adults." Pediatric medicine is its own field that is unique and very separate from internal medicine. Although the majority of medical students have a limited exposure to pediatrics, there are a significant number of questions on the Step 2 CK examination on pediatrics (20–25% of items). Most questions focus on separating "pathology" from "reassurance" or "normal." We start this chapter with "normal" routine, well-child care, and then introduce cases of pathology to help with this distinction separated out primarily by body systems. Most pediatric content essential for USMLE Step 2 CK preparation is covered in this chapter; however, additional pediatric considerations are also embedded at the end of some cases throughout the remainder of the book.

WELL-CHILD CARE

Well-child care begins in the hospital after the birth of a newborn. Below is the routine screening in all newborns that is completed in the hospital prior to discharge from the newborn nursery.

Recommendations for Newborn Screenings

Screening	Methods	Next Steps if Abnormal
Congenital heart defect	Measure pre- and post-ductal oxygen saturation 24 hours after delivery	Echocardiography
Genetic and metabolic disorders	Obtain blood for newborn screening after 24 hours of age (specific conditions in newborn screen vary by state)	Evaluate and stabilize infant if needed; refer to subspecialists for further evaluation depending on results
Hearing impairment	Auditory brainstem response testing	Referral to audiology
Hyperbilirubinemia	Obtain transcutaneous or serum bilirubin level after 24 hours of age if no risk factors Assess risk using hour-specific nomogram	Repeat bilirubin testing based on previous level and risk factors, phototherapy if indicated

Well-child visits occur frequently early on and then are spaced out regularly. Additional visits are added as needed, especially if newborn screenings are abnormal or there is concern for significant weight loss from birth weight that does not appear to be recovering. Newborns can lose up to 10% of their birth weight but should regain that weight by 2 weeks of life. The following times are standard for well-child visits: 2–3 days, 1 month, 2 months, 4 months, 6 months, 9 months, 12 months, 18 months, 24 months, 30 months, 3 years, and then yearly.

Overall components of all well-child visits include:

- Observation of parent-child interaction
- Vitals (including growth parameters) and physical exam
- Screening
- Developmental surveillance—assessment of age-specific gross motor, fine motor, language, and social/cognitive milestones
- Immunizations
- Anticipatory guidance

Vital signs in pediatrics vary based on the age of the patient, as shown in the below table. Children do not reach the normal range of vital signs expected in adults until around age 12.

Pediatric Vital Signs Based on Age of Patient

Age	Blood Pressure (mmHg, listed as SBP/DBP)	Pulse Rate (beats/min)	Respiratory Rate (breaths/min)
Premature infants (born <37 weeks)	55–75/35–45	110–170	40–70
0–3 months	65–85/45–55	110–160	35–55
3–6 months	70–90/50–65	110–160	30–45
6–12 months	80–100/55–65	90–160	22–38
1–3 years	90–105/55–70	80–150	22–30
3–6 years	95–110/60–75	70–120	20–24
6–12 years	100–120/60–75	60–110	16–22
>12 years	110–135/65–85	60–100	12–20

Weight and height are measured at every well-child visit.

- Infants <10th percentile at birth are considered small for gestational age (SGA) and require preprandial blood glucose monitoring after birth for 24 hours.
- Infants >90th percentile at birth are considered large for gestational age (LGA) and require preprandial blood glucose monitoring after birth for 12 hours.
- The WHO growth chart is used until age 2 years and the CDC growth chart is used for children >2 years old. There are specific growth charts for prematurity as well as some specific medical conditions.
- Overweight is defined as a BMI ≥85th percentile. Obesity is a BMI ≥95th percentile.

Head circumference is monitored at every well-child visit from 0 to 2 years of age.

- Microcephaly is a head circumference <2 SD below the mean (usually <3rd percentile though definitions can differ)
- Macrocephaly is a head circumference >2 SD above the mean (usually >97th percentile though definitions can vary)

Childhood Vaccines

Absolute contraindications for all vaccines:

- Severe allergic reaction is the one absolute contraindication to any vaccine.
- Live vaccines (indicated in table) are contraindicated in pregnancy and in severely immunocompromised patients.

Relative contraindications for all vaccines:

- Current moderate to severe illness. (Mild illness should not stop the administration of vaccines)

Routine Childhood Vaccination Schedule and Indications

Tables such as that below can be helpful to memorize, but typically are tested in a case-based manner (see examples at the end of this section).

Vaccine	Routine Indications	Special Indications/Considerations
Hepatitis B	3 doses: Birth, 1–2 months, and 6–18 months	• First dose should be given within 24 hours after birth if baby is >2 kg or within 2 hours if mother +HBsAg
Rotavirus	2–3 doses: 2 months, 4 months, +/– 6 months (depending on formulation)	• Contraindicated in patients with history of intussusception
Diphtheria, tetanus, acellular pertussis (DTaP) <7 years	5 doses: 2 months, 4 months, 6 months, 15–18 months, 4–6 years	• For all wounds except clean and minor wounds, administer DTaP if more than 5 years since last dose of tetanus-toxoid-containing vaccine and child <7 years old • Contraindicated in patients with encephalopathy without known cause within 7 days of vaccine administration
***Haemophilus influenzae* type B (HiB)**	3–4 doses: 2 months, 4 months, +/– 6 months (depending on formulation), 12–15 months	None
Pneumococcal conjugate (PCV 13)	4 doses: 2 months, 4 months, 6 months, and 12–15 months	None
Inactivated poliovirus	4 doses: 2 months, 4 months, 6–18 months, and 4–6 years	None
Influenza (IIV4 or LAIV4)	Yearly starting at 6 months of age	• LAIV4 is live vaccine, contraindicated with chronic lung disease • Precaution in those with egg allergy (though not absolute contraindication)

Vaccine	Routine Indications	Special Indications/Considerations
Measles, mumps, rubella (MMR)	2 doses: 12–15 months and 4–6 years	• Live vaccine
Varicella	2 doses: 12–15 months and 4–6 years	• Live vaccine
Hepatitis A	2 doses: given between 12–23 months (6 months apart)	• Can be given as early as 6 months of age if traveling to high-risk area
Tetanus, diphtheria, and acellular pertussis (Tdap) ≥7 years	1 dose: 11–12 years	• For clean and minor wounds, administer if more than 10 years since last dose of tetanus-toxoid-containing vaccine; for all other wounds, administer if more than 5 years since last dose of tetanus-toxoid-containing vaccine
Human papillomavirus	2 or 3 dose series depending on age at initial vaccination (recommended 9–14 years of age)	None
Meningococcal ACWY	2 doses: 11–12 years and 16 years	• Given starting at 2 months of age in patients with anatomic or functional asplenia (including sickle cell disease), HIV infection, complement component deficiency, and those traveling to high-risk areas
Meningococcal B	2-doses: 16–23 years Timing based on shared decision-making of risk (living in crowded situation)	• Given starting at 10 years in patients with anatomic or functional asplenia (including sickle cell disease), HIV infection, complement component deficiency, and those traveling to high-risk areas
Pneumococcal polysaccharide (PPSV23)	Not a routine vaccination	• Indicated in chronic heart disease, chronic lung disease (including asthma treated with high-dose, oral corticosteroids), diabetes mellitus, cochlear implant, hemoglobinopathies, anatomic or functional asplenia, immunodeficiency, chronic renal failure, nephrotic syndrome, malignancies, and solid organ transplantation
SARS-CoV-2 (COVID-19)	2-dose series starting at 6 months of age	

Major Developmental Milestones of Infancy and Early Childhood

Age	Motor	Fine Motor	Social	Language
2 months	Chest up in prone position Head bobs	Hands begin to unfist	Social smile	Coos Responds to sound
4 months	Props on forearm when prone Head steady Rolls front to back	Plays with rattle	Smiles spontaneously	Imitates speech sounds Laughs To and fro alternating vocalizations
6 months	Props on forearm when prone Sits without support momentarily	Places hands on bottle	Recognizes familiar vs. unfamiliar people	Babbles Listens, vocalizing when person stops talking
9 months	Crawls Pulls to stand Stands while holding on Immature grasp	Bangs objects together	Separation anxiety Follows someone's point	Says Mama/Dada Enjoys peek-a-boo
12 months	Stands well with wide gait	Pincer grasp Attempts to stack 2 blocks	Points to wants	Speaks 2-3 words Follows 1-step command

Major Developmental Milestones of Infancy and Early Childhood (*Continued*)

Age	Motor	Fine Motor	Social	Language
15 months	Stoops to pick up a toy while standing	Releases pincer grasp Builds 3-4 block tower Scribbles	Shows empathy	Speaks 3-5 words Points to one body part
18 months	Runs well	Able to imitate a vertical line	Pretend play begins	Speaks 10-25 words Can imitate animal sounds
2 years	Kicks Ball Walks down stairs holding onto a rail	Opens door using knob Takes off own clothes	Parallel play	Speaks 50+ words 2- word sentences 50% of speech intelligible to stranger Follows 2-step command
3 years	Goes up stairs alternating feet	Copies a circle	Starts to share Imaginative play	Speaks 200+ words 3-word sentences 75% intelligibility
4 years	Hops on one foot	Copies a square	Deception begins	300-1000 words Tells stories 100% intelligibility

Elements of Well-Child Visits from 0–3 Years

Observation	Parent-child interaction Screening for postpartum depression in mother Family adjustment, adequate resources, childcare
Developmental surveillance	Ages & Stages Questionnaire—given routinely at 9-month, 18-month, 2-year, and 2.5-year visits but available for many other ages
Vitals and exam	Includes growth parameters: weight, length, and head circumference are measured from 0–2 years of age and plotted on growth charts Temperature, respiratory rate, and heart rate are essential vitals Blood pressure measurement begins at 3 years of age for low-risk patients
Screening	**Oral health**—tooth brushing to begin as soon as first tooth is present, all children to see a dentist by 2 years old. Dental caries are the most common chronic disease in children. Oral fluoride for all children >6 months who do not have a consistent fluorinated water source **Lead screening**—usually performed first with capillary (fingerstick) specimen, can follow up with venous lead level if screen is positive **CBC for anemia**—usually iron deficiency. Common in children who are picky eaters or drink too much milk **Tuberculosis risk factors**—children who have traveled to endemic areas, have a parent who is incarcerated or works at a jail or in health care and has not been tested, should all be tested for tuberculosis even if asymptomatic
Immunizations	Most immunizations are administered within the first 3 years of life (see details in separate table)
Anticipatory guidance	Depending on child's developmental phase, especially focused on safety and injury prevention **Car**—children should be placed in a rear-facing car seat in the back row of the car and should remain in rear-facing car seat until they exceed the weight or height limits set by the car seat manufacturer or reach 2 years of age (whichever comes last) **Home**—medications and toxic household products should be out of reach, power outlets covered, furniture mounted to wall, safety gates installed on stairs, smoke detectors installed, and small objects that pose choking hazards avoided **Firearms**—if present in the home, should be stored unloaded in a locked location separate from ammunition **Water**—fences installed around pools, use of life jackets, adult supervision near water at all times, swimming instruction

Early Childhood Well-Child Visits (3–11 Years): School readiness and performance

Vitals and exam	Weight, length, and BMI become primary focus. Temperature, respiratory rate, heart rate, and blood pressure are essential vitals.
Screening	Vision Hearing Lead screening Tuberculosis risk factors Dyslipidemia: American Academy of Pediatrics (AAP) recommends a screening fasting lipid profile once for all children 9–11 years of age.
Immunizations	Boosters for measles, mumps, rubella, varicella, diphtheria, tetanus, pertussis, polio, and yearly influenza vaccination HPV vaccine can be given as young as 9 years old. Meningococcal and Tdap vaccines are given at 11–12 years of age (see table for further details).
Anticipatory guidance	Safety and injury prevention, obesity prevention

Adolescent Well-Child Visits (12–21 Years): Independence and preparation for self-care away from family

History	Risk assessment should occur both with and without guardian in the room to ensure confidentiality. Includes HEADSS assessment (Home, Education/employment, Activities, Drugs, Sexuality, Suicidality)*
Vitals and exam	Weight, length, and BMI. Temperature, respiratory rate, heart rate, and blood pressure
Screening	Vision—universal screening until 15 years of age Hearing—universal annual screening Tuberculosis risk factors Cardiac disease risk factors (see case below for further discussion) Dyslipidemia—the AAP recommends a screening fasting lipid profile once more for all children 17–21 years of age regardless of risk for hyperlipidemia Sexually transmitted diseases—assessment of risk factors (e.g., sex workers, men who have sex with men, participation in high-risk sexual behaviors). Universal HIV screening recommended once at 15–18 years of age regardless of risk factors. Alcohol and drug use—universal screening Depression screening—should be universal, using validated screening tool like Patient Health Questionnaire (PHQ)-9 Pregnancy prevention, contraception discussion recommended for all ages
Immunizations	Boosters for meningococcus HPV vaccine if not yet given
Anticipatory guidance	Risk-taking behaviors, mental health

*Cohen E, Mackenzie RG, Yates GL. J Adolesc Health. 1991 Nov;12(7):539-544.

CASE 1 | Non-Accidental Trauma (NAT)

A 6-year-old previously healthy boy presents for his annual well-child visit with his mother. His mother states that he eats, eliminates, and sleeps well. On exam, he looks well and meets all developmental milestones for his age. Exam shows bruises on his chest and torso and tenderness near his rib cage, which his parent attributes to him falling from his bike. Chest radiograph shows several posterior rib fractures of different stages of healing.

Conditions with Similar Presentations	**Bleeding disorders** (e.g., von Willebrand factor deficiency, hemophilia): Can also present with easy bruising from minor injuries, but would not have fractures.
	Connective tissue disorders: Due to genetic deficiency and/or abnormal collagen production may also present similarly with several bone injuries/fractures. Examples include **osteogenesis imperfecta** (may also have blue sclera, and/or loose joints) and **Ehlers-Danlos** (may also have hypermobility, abnormal scar formation, stretchy skin, loose joints, and/or vascular deformities).
	Rickets: Vitamin D deficiency leading to skeletal deformities, dental problems, fragile bones, bone pain.

CASE 1 | Non-Accidental Trauma (NAT) *(continued)*

Initial Diagnostic Tests	• Confirm diagnosis by obtaining a detailed history and physical exam. • Also check skeletal survey to detect occult fractures and consider other imaging (see below).
Next Steps in Management	• Report any cases of suspected NAT to Child Protection Services • Consult a multidisciplinary team • Treat injuries as indicated
Discussion	NAT is injury purposefully inflicted on a child and affects children of all backgrounds and ages. This includes neglect and physical, emotional, mental, psychological, and sexual abuse. Around 1% of children are victims of NAT. Neglect is the most common type of NAT (75% of reports) with biological parent as perpetrator under 1 year old. **History:** Assessment should consider: • Caregivers (caregiver history of child abuse, young or single parents, substance use, psychiatric condition) • Home environment (divorce or conflict, financial insecurity, intimate partner violence) • Victims themselves (physical or intellectual disability, unwanted child) Often the history may be incomplete, variable, or not consistent with the child's developmental age or physical exam findings. Pay special attention to the story given by the family and whether this fits the injuries seen. For example, a 2-month-old rolling off a bed and getting a scalp hematoma should be questioned, as 2-month-olds cannot yet roll. **Physical Exam:** When performing a physical exam, assess for: • Interactions between patient and family (lack of emotional interaction, arguing, confessions) • Signs that may reveal the method of injury (burns from cigarettes, immersion burns from submersion in hot water, bite marks) • Multiple fractures with different stages of healing, long bone fractures in children who cannot walk, posterior rib fractures, subdural hematomas, bruises (TEN-4: trunk, ear, or neck in children age <4) • Genital injuries or signs of sexually transmitted infections **Diagnostics:** Clinical Diagnosis • Obtain detailed history of trauma from parent • Obtain detailed history of trauma from patient with parent not in the room • Perform a detailed physical exam If there is suspicion for abuse, the child should be referred directly to the emergency department (ED) for further testing: • Complete skeletal survey to detect occult fractures of different healing stages, metaphyseal corner fracture, or abnormal locations (e.g., posterior ribs, skull, or femur in a non-ambulatory infant) • For children <1 year, an ophthalmologic exam to evaluate for retinal hemorrhage Consider: • Head CT and cervical spine MRI to evaluate for brain and spinal injury (e.g., intracranial bleeding such as subdural hematoma) • Spine x-ray to assess for vertebral injury • CT abdomen and pelvis with contrast and liver tests for intraabdominal injury **Management:** • All medical professionals are federally mandated to report any cases of suspected NAT to Child Protective Services, which will conduct a thorough investigation • Consultation with a multidisciplinary team including child abuse specialist, general pediatrician, social worker, nurse, and the family while case is open • Acute management of specific injuries

CASE 2 | Abnormal Adolescent Sports Physical

A 16-year-old previously healthy boy presents to clinic for his annual appointment and needs a pre-participation sports physical form completed. On review of systems, he reports occasional chest pressure and feels like his heart was beating "way too hard" when he pushed himself at football practice. Family history is notable for maternal uncle who unexpectedly drowned in a swimming pool at age 27, despite being a strong swimmer. On exam, vital signs were normal. Cardiovascular exam findings: normal S1, S2, without any murmurs or extra heart sounds. Rest of physical exam was also normal.

| Conditions with Similar Presentations | **Familial hypercholesterolemia:** Seen in families with positive history of premature cardiovascular disease.

Long QT syndromes: Disorder of ventricular myocardial repolarization that can lead to symptomatic ventricular arrhythmias or sudden cardiac death. May have family history of known long QT.

Hypertrophic cardiomyopathy (HCM): Hypertrophy of the left ventricle outflow tract that increases risk of morbidity and sudden cardiac death. |

CASE 2 | Abnormal Adolescent Sports Physical (continued)

Initial Diagnostic Tests	• Check ECG • Consider lipid screening if significant in family history (or universal screening has not been performed at appropriate age)
Next Steps in Management	Refer to cardiology given symptoms and family history concerning for sudden death.
Discussion	A preparticipation physical evaluation is mandatory prior to children and adolescents participating in organized sports. Although rare, sudden cardiac death in young, apparently healthy athletes can occur and any presentation that suggests a cardiac condition should be thoroughly evaluated prior to further sports participation. **History:** • A detailed history should be taken, exploring family history of any cardiac diseases, seizures, or sudden unexplained death (including sudden infant death, unexplained motor vehicle accidents, drownings, or other unexplained deaths at a young age). • Inquire about personal history of syncope, near-syncope, chest pain, palpitations, or excessive dyspnea or fatigue on exertion. • Post-exertional syncope, common and nearly always benign, should be carefully differentiated from syncope during exertion. **Physical Exam:** Vital signs and cardiac exam to assess for murmurs and extra heart sounds. Four-limb blood pressure and orthostatic vitals should be considered (to assess for coarctation of the aorta). **Diagnostics:** • If risk factors or any symptoms are present, obtain an ECG looking for signs of LV hypertrophy, QT abnormalities, and arrhythmias. • An abnormal ECG should be followed up by a transthoracic echocardiogram (TTE). • Consider lipid screening if significant family history (or if universal screening has not been performed at appropriate age) **Management:** • Refer to cardiology given symptoms and family history concerning for sudden death before clearing for sports participation. • Family members should also be alerted of this family history and tested as appropriate. • Further management will depend on the diagnosis. • Patients with HCM are restricted to low-static/low-dynamic sports like golf, as primary prevention is the only management at this time.

Developmental Milestones Mini-Cases

These are examples of cases that will be presented to evaluate your knowledge of developmental milestones.

Cases	Key Findings
Developmental Milestone Delays	**Hx/PE:** 15-month-old boy is brought to clinic for a well-child visit and with parental developmental concerns. He was born full term via normal spontaneous vaginal delivery (NSVD) with no complications. Has been doing well, following routine immunizations but parents note that he is not yet walking and does not recognize his own name. He has repetitive babbling but is not saying any words, and does not point to objects of interest. On physical exam, vitals and growth are normal. He is babbling throughout the appointment. He sits in mom's lap eating cereal, occasionally gets down to crawl or stand for a few seconds before sitting back down. He does not point to objects and when mom asks him to give her some cereal, he does not follow her instructions. **Diagnostics:** • This patient's gross motor skills are not concerning at this point. • His speech is delayed as is his social/emotional development, which raises the concern for autism spectrum disorder. • He should be referred to audiology, ophthalmology, speech and occupational therapy. **Management:** Behavioral and educational interventions are indicated and improve developmental outcomes. Psychopharmacology can be added to target specific symptoms if needed. **Discussion:** Early developmental milestone delays require evaluation for intellectual disabilities, learning disorders, autism spectrum disorder, attention deficit hyperactivity disorder (ADHD), and visual and hearing disorders. Autism spectrum disorder usually presents in the first 2 years of life with deficits in multiple areas including social skills, lagging behind in communication milestones (responding to name, pointing at objects), tantrums, lack of eye contact, and repetitive language (echolalia) or movements (rocking, flapping hands, spinning in circles). Please see Chapter 16 (Psychiatry) for additional information.

Developmental Milestones Mini-Cases *(continued)*

Doing Poorly in School	**Hx/PE:** An 8-year-old girl is brought for evaluation as she is doing poorly in school. She was born full term via NSVD, had no complications, and has no other medical problems. She has been doing poorly in school over the past 2 years and is frequently sent to the principal's office for disruptive behavior and not following instructions. At home, she is unable to sit still at the dinner table and is constantly running around. Mom is very worried, but dad says "she is just a kid." On physical exam, vitals and growth are normal. She answers questions appropriately but is constantly interrupting and asking questions or fidgeting. **Diagnostics:** • An evaluation for ADHD is warranted in this patient. This is a clinical diagnosis that requires an impairment in two different locations (e.g., school and home) and has two core symptoms: hyperactivity/impulsivity and inattention. A validated scoring tool such as the Vanderbilt ADHD Diagnostic Rating Scale should be given to multiple caregivers and returned to the physician. • A specific learning disability should also be considered, which can be diagnosed by neuropsychiatric testing. • A vision and hearing screen should also be performed. **Management:** Stimulant therapy and psychotherapy are the mainstays of treatment of ADHD. The patient should have an individualized educational plan completed by the school to accommodate the learning disability. **Discussion:** Children who perform poorly in school should be evaluated for cognitive and behavioral disorders as soon as possible to minimize their effect on future learning. ADHD is one of the most common behavioral disorders and is diagnosed in approximately 10% of all children up to the age of 17 in the United States (U.S.). It can be diagnosed using standardized testing tools and treated with medications and psychotherapy. Even with treatment, affected children are more likely to have impaired academic performance. In addition, they are more likely to have other life events such as self-injury and motor vehicle accidents as well as substance use disorders, and develop antisocial personality. Please see Chapter 16 (Psychiatry) for additional information.

PEDIATRIC ENDOCRINOLOGY

The endocrine system consists of multiple organs throughout the body connected through hormonal pathways. Disorders of the endocrine system arise from states of excess or deficiency of hormones. The specific symptoms of a particular disorder may be different dependent on the age of the child (e.g., growth hormone excess in a child compared to growth hormone excess in a post-pubertal teen). For more information, including discussion of physiology and detailed descriptions of adult endocrine disorders, please see Chapter 9 (Endocrinology).

Sexual Development

Genitalia, pubic hair, and breast development are assigned Tanner stages.

Tanner Stages

	Stage 1 pre-pubertal	Stage 2 ~8–11.5 y	Stage 3 ~11.5–13 y	Stage 4 ~13–15 y	Stage 5 >15 y
Biologic Sex					
Both	No pubic hair	Pubic hair appearance (pubarche)	Pubic hair coarsening	Pubic hair increases, but spares thighs	Pubic hair crosses over to thigh
Female (menarche: 10–16 years)	Flat chest, raised nipple	Breast buds (thelarche)	Breast enlargement	Raised areola, increased breast enlargement	Adult breast contours, areola flattens
Male		Testicular enlargement	Penis size/length increases	Penis width/glans increase	Penis/testes adult size

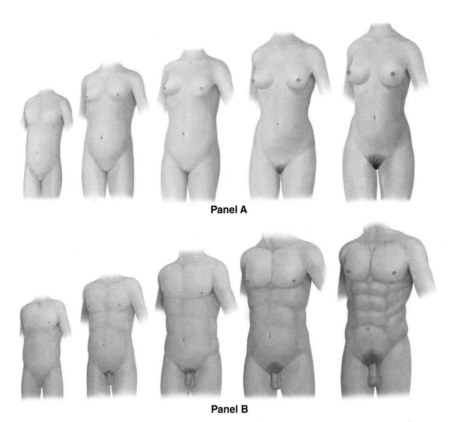

Panel A

Panel B

A. Tanner stages 1 to 5 of pubertal development in females. B. Tanner stages 1 to 5 of pubertal development in males. (Reproduced with permission from Variants of Pubertal Progression In: Sarafoglou K, Hoffmann GF, Roth KS. Pediatric Endocrinology and Inborn Errors of Metabolism, 2e; New York: McGraw Hill, 2017.)

Endocrine Factors Affecting Growth

Short stature in children is defined as height below the third percentile. Short stature can be due to pathological causes (i.e., growth hormone deficiency, hypothyroidism) and nonpathological causes (i.e., familial short stature, constitutional delay of growth and puberty).

Growth failure is usually pathologic and is defined as an abnormal growth velocity for age. Growth failure in children may be multifactorial and requires a comprehensive workup to identify the cause.

Causes of Growth Failure

Cause	Growth Velocity	IGF-1	Bone Age X-Ray	Treatment
Nutritional deficiency: Poor weight gain due to ↓ caloric intake or a condition leading to malabsorption will lead to failure to thrive which will affect the weight initially, then lead to poor growth. Poor weight gain could be due to ↓caloric intake or could be a sign of a systemic condition leading to malabsorption.	↓ or normal	↓ or normal	Delayed or normal for age	Increase caloric intake; treat any underlying disorder
Psychosocial deprivation: Due to parental/caregiver neglect or psychological abuse. Insulin-like growth factor (IGF-1) and growth velocity will be ↓ (due to temporary GH deficiency), Once the child is removed from the environment, normal growth resumes and IGF-1 levels return to normal.	↓	↓	Delayed or normal for age	Remove the child from the current environment and place in a supportive, loving environment and normal growth will resume

Causes of Growth Failure (*Continued*)

Cause	Growth Velocity	IGF-1	Bone Age X-Ray	Treatment
Growth hormone deficiency: Due to ↓growth hormone secretion from the pituitary gland. Can be congenital (due to anatomic defects of the pituitary gland) or secondary to pituitary tumor (i.e., craniopharyngioma). In addition to growth failure (↓growth velocity), children may present with ↓muscle mass and ↑body fat.	↓	↓	Delayed	Growth hormone injections until growth plates have fused, assess for and remove any pituitary tumor
Constitutional delay in growth and puberty: Non-pathologic growth variant that is due to slowed tempo of growth in children. There is usually a family history of "late bloomers."	Normal	Normal	Delayed	Provide reassurance; child will reach adult height potential without intervention
Familial short stature	Normal	Normal	Normal	Provide reassurance

Pituitary Gland

Control of the endocrine system begins in the hypothalamus. Hormones secreted from the hypothalamus either stimulate or inhibit pituitary hormone secretion. The pituitary gland then secretes hormones that stimulate the end organs in the endocrine system.

Pituitary disorders in children are either congenital or secondary to masses that affect pituitary function. Congenital defects of pituitary secretion may result from anatomic malformations resulting in pituitary hypoplasia or aplasia. Please refer to Endocrinology Chapter for additional cases.

CASE 3	Hypopituitarism (Craniopharyngioma)

	A 12-year-old boy presents with concerns about poor growth. According to his mother, he has not grown over the past year and his height has declined in percentiles. They are concerned because he was previously one of the tallest students in the class and now the other children are outgrowing him. He also notes increased fatigue, constipation, cold intolerance, and daily headaches. On exam, his blood pressure is 99/58 mmHg and he has cool and dry skin, central obesity, and prepubertal testicles. Visual acuity is normal, but visual field confrontation testing reveals bitemporal hemianopsia.
Conditions with Similar Presentations	**Prolactinomas:** Characterized by prolactin levels >200. Usually do not compress the pituitary gland or cause hypopituitarism. Patients present with complaints associated with mass effect (headache, blurry vision, hemianopsia) or the effects of elevated prolactin levels (galactorrhea, delayed puberty, amenorrhea). **Primary hypothyroidism:** Can lead to fatigue, cold intolerance, poor growth in children, but TSH would be elevated.
Initial Diagnostic Tests	• Evaluate for hormone deficiency: TSH, free T4, ACTH, cortisol, IGF-1, prolactin. Consider LH/FSH for patients who are at the pubertal age. • Check MRI of the pituitary gland.
Next Steps in Management	• Replace any pituitary hormone deficiencies (i.e., thyroxine, hydrocortisone) • Transsphenoidal pituitary surgery

Discussion	Craniopharyngiomas are rare benign brain tumors that are slow growing but can present with mass effect and hormonal disruption. Craniopharyngiomas have a bimodal age distribution: presentation in children is usually between 5 and 15 years of age. Adults can present between 45 and 60 years of age.
	
	Craniopharyngiomas arise from remnants of Rathke's pouch in the sellar region. The proximity of the tumor to the pituitary gland can cause pituitary hormone deficiencies. The tumor can also compress the optic nerve and cause visual abnormalities.
	
	History:
	• Symptoms due to mass effect: headaches and visual field defects
	• Symptoms associated with pituitary hormone deficiencies:
	  • Polyuria, polydipsia (central diabetes insipidus)
	  • Fatigue, constipation, dry skin (hypothyroidism)
	  • Growth suppression (growth hormone deficiency)
	  • Delayed puberty (gonadotropin deficiency)
	  • Weight loss, loss of appetite (ACTH deficiency)

CASE 3 | Hypopituitarism (Craniopharyngioma) *(continued)*

Discussion	**Physical Exam:**
	• Vital signs may show hypotension and bradycardia; growth velocity will be low for age
	• Visual field testing—bitemporal hemianopsia, papilledema
	• Dry skin
	• Delayed deep tendon reflexes
	
	Diagnostics: Blood tests are used to diagnose pituitary hormone deficiencies. Imaging is used to assess the presence and features of the craniopharyngiomas.
	• MRI of the pituitary gland—multilobulated, multicystic mass
	• Pituitary function
	  • TSH, free T4: in central hypothyroidism the TSH will be low or inappropriately normal in the presence of a low free T4.
	  • Insulin-like growth factor 1(IGF-1): used to assess growth hormone secretion. IGF-1 levels will be low in growth hormone deficiency.
	  • ACTH, cortisol: central ACTH deficiency will present with low or inappropriately normal ACTH level in the presence of low cortisol.
	  • LH, FSH: gonadotropin levels will be low
	  • Prolactin: usually normal
	  • BMP, urine osmolality, serum osmolality: if central diabetes insipidus is present, the serum sodium level will be elevated, with an elevated serum osmolality and a low urine osmolality.
	• Ophthalmologic examination to assess visual fields
	
	Management:
	• Transsphenoidal surgery for tumor resection
	• Hormonal replacement

CASE 4 | Gigantism/Acromegaly

A 15-year-old girl is brought to clinic by her mother for tall stature. According to the mother, the patient started having a growth spurt around 13 years of age and has not stopped growing since. She is now the tallest girl in her class and is being ridiculed by other students. She had her first menses at 14 years of age but has not had a period over the past 6 months. Her mother is buying larger shoes and bigger clothes every 2 months. On physical examination, her BP is 150/95 with a heart rate of 90. She has frontal bossing, a prominent jaw, and large hands and feet.

Conditions with Similar Presentations	**Obesity due to increased caloric intake:** Excessive weight gain will promote increased growth velocity. Insulin resistance leads to elevated insulin levels, which promote growth acceleration. Patients will also have clinical signs of insulin resistance, such as acanthosis nigricans and elevated insulin levels.
Initial Diagnostic Tests	Confirm Diagnosis: • Biochemical: IGF-1 level, GH level, abnormal GH suppression test • Imaging: MRI of the pituitary Consider: • Measure other pituitary hormone levels (TSH, ACTH, LH/FSH, prolactin) • Visual field assessment
Next Steps in Management	Transsphenoidal surgery
Discussion	Acromegaly/gigantism is caused by a growth hormone-producing adenoma. In children when the growth plates are open, the excess growth hormone causes increased linear growth (gigantism). Once the growth plates close, excess growth hormone leads to change in facial features (acromegaly). Growth acceleration in gigantism tends to occur around 13 years of age. **History:** History of excessive growth, change in facial appearance, headaches, visual abnormalities, delayed puberty **Physical Exam:** Frontal bossing, large hands and feet, coarse facial features, large tongue, deep voice, and excessive sweating **Diagnostics:** • Elevated IGF-1 level, elevated GH, and abnormal GH suppression test (failure of GH to suppress to <1 ng/mL 2 hours after glucose load) • MRI shows pituitary adenoma

CASE 4 | Gigantism/Acromegaly *(continued)*

Discussion	**Management:** • Transsphenoidal surgery is the first-line therapy. • Medical therapy if surgery is not possible or curative. Agents used are somatostatin receptor ligands (octreotide, lanreotide) or GH receptor antagonists (pegvisomant).
Additional Considerations	Gigantism can be seen as a manifestation of multiple endocrine neoplasia type 1 (pituitary, pancreas, parathyroid).

Adrenal Glands

Enzyme Defects Causing Congenital Adrenal Hyperplasia

	21-hydroxylase	11β-hydroxylase	17α-hydroxylase
Pathway decreased	MC, GC	GC	GC, SH
Pathway increased	SH	MC, SH	MC
Result	Hypotension Hyponatremia Hyperkalemia AG if XX	Hypertension Hypokalemia AG if XX	Hypertension Hypernatremia Hypokalemia AG if XY
Diagnosis	Elevated 17-hydroxycortisol	Elevated 11-deoxycortisol Decreased cortisol	Elevated 11-deoxycortisol, corticosterone, and deoxycorticosterone
Treatment	GC ± MC	GC	GC + SH
% of CAH cases	70%	5%	1%

Abbreviations: MC, mineralocorticoid; GC, glucocorticoid; SH, sex hormones (mainly androgens); AG, ambiguous genitalia.

CASE 5 | Congenital Adrenal Hyperplasia (21-hydroxylase deficiency)

A newborn infant is delivered by vaginal delivery to a 25-year-old mother at 38 weeks gestational age. The pediatrics team is called to the delivery room due to concerns for ambiguous genitalia. The physical exam shows a midline phallic-like structure which measures 2.5 cm in length. Testicles are not palpated. The genitalia appear hyperpigmented, with fusion of the labioscrotal folds. The infant is alert with a strong cry and no signs of respiratory distress.

Conditions with Similar Presentations	**Placental aromatase deficiency:** Placental aromatase converts androgens to estrogen. When there is a deficiency of the aromatase enzyme, there are increased androgen levels in both the fetus and the mother, resulting in ambiguous genitalia in female infants. **Ovotesticular disorder of sexual differentiation:** Presence of both ovarian and testicular tissue. The presence of testicular tissue can lead to virilization in an XX infant and ambiguous genitalia.
Initial Diagnostic Tests	• Confirm with 17-hydroxyprogesterone level, karyotype, and pelvic ultrasound • Also check BMP
Next Steps in Management	• Glucocorticoid replacement (e.g., hydrocortisone) • Mineralocorticoid replacement (e.g., fludrocortisone)
Discussion	Congenital adrenal hyperplasia (CAH) is a group of autosomal recessive disorders that have defects in adrenal steroidogenesis. The most common form of CAH is 21-hydroxylase deficiency. The 21-hydroxylase enzyme is responsible for converting progesterone and 17-hydroxyprogesterone into 11-deoxycorticosterone (precursor to corticosterone and aldosterone) and 11-deoxycortisol (precursor to cortisol), respectively (see figure). Defect in this enzyme therefore leads to accumulation of progesterone and 17α-hydroxyprogesterone. Since 21-hydroxylase is not involved in the biosynthesis of sex hormones, excess of these precursors is then shunted towards increased synthesis of sex hormones. The lack of aldosterone and cortisol accompanied by increased sex hormones accounts for the clinical manifestation of this disease. Low aldosterone results in hyponatremia and hyperkalemia, and low cortisol results in hypotension and hypoglycemia. Excess androgens can result in ambiguous genitalia with virilization in females, while males may have normal-appearing external genitalia. Classic CAH will present in the neonatal period. In most cases, both parents are heterozygote for the mutation. Most states test for 21-OH deficiency on the newborn screen.

CASE 5 | Congenital Adrenal Hyperplasia (21-hydroxylase deficiency) *(continued)*

Discussion	

History: Newborn XX infant with ambiguous genitalia.

In severe cases, infants will present at 1–3 weeks of age with failure to thrive, poor feeding, lethargy or irritability, dehydration, hypotension, hyponatremia, and hyperkalemia. When the diagnosis is delayed or missed, severe CAH can be fatal.

Physical Exam: Newborn girls will present with ambiguous genitalia: clitoromegaly, fused labia minora, common urogenital sinus, hyperpigmentation of the vaginal area.

Diagnostics:
- ↑↑ 17α-hydroxyprogesterone levels
- Genetic testing
- Pelvic ultrasound: In patients who are 46, XX, ultrasound will show uterus and ovaries

Also check:
- Serum sodium, chloride, bicarbonate, glucose (all may be low)
- Serum potassium (high)
- ↓ Cortisol, ↓ aldosterone
- ACTH stimulation test if above results are equivocal

Management:

For adrenal crisis:
- Fluid resuscitation with NS and then administer D5NS
- Stress dose hydrocortisone

For maintenance therapy:
- Glucocorticoid replacement
- Mineralocorticoid replacement
- Sodium chloride supplementation in infants

Additional Considerations	**Nonclassic CAH** is also caused by a deficiency of 21-hydroxylase deficiency. In the nonclassic form, the enzyme deficiency is mild, so there is enough enzymatic activity to prevent adrenal crisis. However, there is not enough enzymatic activity to prevent shunting to androgen production. These patients present at a later age with signs of androgen excess (acne, irregular menses, excessive growth).

Congenital Adrenal Hyperplasia Mini-Cases

Cases	Key Findings
17α-Hydroxylase Deficiency	**Hx:** Endocrine consult is placed for a 1-day-old infant with micropenis. Prenatal testing showed a karyotype of 46, XY. The baby is clinically stable, but the blood pressures have been at the upper limit of normal. **PE:** On exam, the phallic structure is midline and measures 1.5 cm in length. Testicles are not palpated and the scrotum appears underdeveloped. **Diagnostics:** ACTH stimulation test reveals elevated levels of corticosterone and deoxycorticosterone with the absence of DHEA.

Congenital Adrenal Hyperplasia Mini-Cases *(continued)*

17α-Hydroxylase Deficiency	**Management:** Glucocorticoid (hydrocortisone) **Discussion:** 17α-hydroxylase deficiency prevents the formation of both glucocorticoid and sex hormone precursors, and shifts precursors toward elevation of mineralocorticoids. The compensatory increase in ACTH, due to the failure of cortisol production, stimulates the over-production of 11-deoxycorticosterone and corticosterone, which leads to hypertension and hypokalemia. Affected males present with ambiguous genitalia and intra-abdominal undescended testes, while females may present with primary amenorrhea or delayed puberty and hypertension. The treatment is glucocorticoid (hydrocortisone) and sex hormone replacement.
11β-Hydroxylase Deficiency	**Hx:** A newborn infant presents with ambiguous genitalia. Prenatal karyotype revealed 46, XX chromosomes. Pelvic ultrasound showed uterus and ovaries. **PE:** Ambiguous genitalia in a 46, XX infant. Blood pressure is elevated. **Diagnostics:** ACTH stimulation test will reveal elevated levels of 11-deoxycortisol, deoxycorticosterone, and DHEAS. **Management:** Glucocorticoid replacement **Discussion:** 11β-hydroxylase deficiency involves a defect in 11β-hydroxylase, which prevents the conversion of 11-deoxycortisol to cortisol and 11-deoxycorticosterone to corticosterone; this leads to low cortisol and low aldosterone levels. The resulting increase in ACTH secretion causes the accumulation of 11-deoxycortisol and 11-deoxycorticosterone, increased sex steroid synthesis, and adrenocortical hyperplasia. Infants will have elevated androgen levels, which cause the virilization of the female fetus. Patients may present with hypertension and hypokalemia secondary to increased 11-deoxycorticosterone level. If not diagnosed at birth, this will present with signs of premature adrenarche (body odor and axillary and pubic hair growth).

Thyroid Gland

CASE 6	Congenital Hypothyroidism
	A 2-week-old girl is brought to the pediatrician by her parents who are concerned due to constipation that has been present since birth. The parents have noticed that the child is sluggish and not easily arousable. With stimulation, the infant awakens but has a hoarse-sounding cry and is noted to have macroglossia. Vital signs are normal.
Conditions with Similar Presentations	**Beckwith-Wiedemann syndrome (BWS):** Infants can present with macroglossia. Infants with BWS may also have an omphalocele and hypoglycemia which are not associated with congenital hypothyroidism. **Down syndrome:** Infants with Down syndrome may also present with macroglossia and an umbilical hernia. These infants also have other syndromic features including upward-slanting eyelids, flattened nasal bridge, transverse palmar crease, and hypotonia.
Initial Diagnostic Tests	Check TSH, free T4
Next Steps in Management	Treat with levothyroxine
Discussion	Congenital hypothyroidism is a developmental abnormality in thyroid hormone production resulting in decreased thyroid hormone levels. Most cases are not hereditary and result from thyroid dysgenesis (most common cause in the U.S.). Other causes include inborn errors of thyroid hormone synthesis and iodine deficiency. Most cases are identified by newborn screening (NBS) in the first week of life. Congenital hypothyroidism occurs in 1 in 4000 infants and is seen more predominantly in countries where there is iodine deficiency. **History:** Difficulty feeding, sleeping through feeds, poor weight gain, hoarse cry **Physical Exam:** Wide anterior and posterior fontanelles, feeding difficulties, enlarged tongue, constipation, umbilical hernia, and decreased tone in the extremities **Diagnostics:** ↑ TSH, ↓ free T4 **Management:** • Thyroid hormone replacement with levothyroxine. • Infants with congenital hypothyroidism should be monitored closely for signs of developmental delay. • If congenital hypothyroidism goes undetected there is slowing of physical and mental development.
Additional Considerations	If the free T4 is low and the TSH is low or normal, consider central hypothyroidism. If present, in addition to hormone replacement with levothyroxine, other hormones should be assayed and replaced, and an MRI of the brain performed to evaluate for pituitary abnormalities or masses.

Parathyroid Gland and Bone

Serum calcium levels are regulated by vitamin D, parathyroid hormone (PTH), and calcitonin. Vitamin D deficiency can occur in infants who are primarily breastfed, as breast milk is low in vitamin D, so breastfed babies should routinely be started on oral vitamin D supplementation after birth.

CASE 7	Vitamin D-Deficient Rickets	
	A 16-month-old boy is brought to his pediatrician by his mom due to concerns of difficulty with walking. He is breastfeeding three to four times a day and eating some baby foods. Mom reports that he is not taking any medications. Exam shows bowing of the legs.	
Conditions with Similar Presentations	**Child abuse:** Should be considered if child presents with multiple fractures. **Osteogenesis imperfecta:** Connective tissue disorder that presents with multiple fractures and blue sclera. **Hypophosphatemic rickets:** See other causes of rickets in the following discussion.	
Initial Diagnostic Tests	Check 25-OH vitamin D, calcium, PTH, phosphorus and X-ray of the long bones	
Next Steps in Management	• Calcium supplementation • Vitamin D supplementation	
Discussion	Vitamin D-deficient rickets is a condition due to deficient mineralization of cartilage in the epiphyseal growth plates and is caused by malabsorption, decreased sun exposure, poor diet, or chronic kidney disease. Risk factors for vitamin D deficiency are breastfeeding without vitamin supplementation, lack of sun exposure, or medications that interfere with calcium, pigmented skin, or vitamin D absorption. The average age of presentation is 15 months old. **History:** Seizures (due to hypocalcemia), tetany, delayed motor development, difficulty with ambulation, pain in the legs **Physical Exam:** Short stature, bowing of the legs, enlarged wrists or knees, enlarged costochondral joints (rachitic rosary) **Diagnostics:** • ↓ 25-OH vitamin D • ↑ PTH level • ↓ Phosphorus level • ↓ Calcium level • Long bone x-rays—cupping and fraying of metaphyses—due to under-mineralization of the bones **Management:** • Calcium supplementation • Calcitriol (D3) supplementation or D2 supplementation	 Rickets. There are bilateral lower extremity varus deformities in the 18-month-old with rickets. The metaphyses are irregular and cupped. The growth plates are wide. (Reproduced with permission from Robert G. Wells, Diagnostic Imaging of Infants and Children; by The McGraw-Hill 2013.)

Rickets Mini-Case	
Case	**Key Findings**
Hypophosphatemic Rickets	**Hx:** Most children will present with bowing of the legs as they start weight-bearing, and bone pain. May have pseudofractures (an area of decreased bone mineral density that forms alongside the surface of the bone). **PE:** Short stature with bowing of the extremities, frontal bossing, and tooth decay **Diagnostics:** • ↓ Phosphorus level • Normal 25-OH vitamin D • Normal calcium level • ↑ PTH level • ↑ Alk Phos • ↑ Urinary phosphorus excretion • Long bone x-rays will show rachitic changes: cupping and fraying of the metaphyses

Rickets Mini-Case *(continued)*

Hypophosphatemic Rickets	**Management:** • Oral phosphate and calcitriol to replace low phosphorus levels • In patients with X-linked hypophosphatemic rickets, burosumab might be used (an FGF23 monoclonal antibody which binds to and decreases the activity of FGF23, thus reducing phosphorus excretion). **Discussion:** Hypophosphatemic rickets is a genetic disorder caused by decreased renal tubular reabsorption of phosphorus. There are multiple genetic forms of hypophosphatemic rickets. The genetic defect in the X-linked form is due to increased activity of fibroblast growth factor 23 (FGF23). FGF23 increases phosphorus excretion from the kidneys, which results in low serum phosphorus levels. Due to the abnormal phosphorus levels, there is deficient bone mineralization and thus the rachitic bone abnormalities develop.

CASE 8 | Pseudohypoparathyroidism Type 1A (Albright Hereditary Osteodystrophy)

A 6-year-old girl is brought to clinic for evaluation because her mother is concerned that her daughter is shorter than the rest of the family and has been gaining weight excessively. She noted that her daughter has been on calcium and vitamin D for the past 3 years, which was prescribed by her previous pediatrician. Vital signs are normal, except the girl's hand shows carpal spasms when the cuff is inflated when taking the blood pressure. On physical exam, the patient has short stature, obesity, round facies, shortened 4th/5th digits, and subcutaneous calcifications.

Conditions with Similar Presentations	**Pseudopseudohypoparathyroidism:** Mutation in the paternal allele of the *GNAS1* gene will result in a condition with phenotypic features of pseudohypoparathyroidism (short stature, round face, short 4th/5th digits) but will have normal calcium, phosphorus, and PTH levels. **Progressive osseous heteroplasia:** Also have hypocalcemia but the resistance to PTH is only in the kidney without the phenotype of pseudohypoparathyroidism.
Initial Diagnostic Tests	• Check Parathyroid hormone, calcium, phosphorus level • Consider checking 25-OH Vitamin D
Next Steps in Management	• Calcium supplementation • Calcitriol (D3) supplementation
Discussion	Pseudohypoparathyroidism type 1A is an autosomal dominant condition with maternal inheritance of an inactivating mutation in the *GNAS1* gene, which encodes a Gs protein α-subunit. Defects in this gene result in end-organ resistance to PTH. Maternal inheritance of a defective gene results in resistance to PTH with ensuing hypocalcemia, hyperphosphatemia, and elevated PTH. Pseudohypoparathyroidism is more common in females than males. It is usually identified during childhood due to obesity. **History:** Short stature, obesity, and developmental delay **Physical Exam:** Shortened 4th/5th digits, short stature, obesity, round face, developmental delay, and subcutaneous calcifications. **Diagnostics:** Confirm with: • ↑PTH level • ↑phosphorus level • ↓calcium level **Management:** • Calcium supplementation • Calcitriol (D3) supplementation

Pancreas

CASE 9 | Type 1 Diabetes Mellitus (DM)

An 11-year-old girl is brought in for evaluation of fatigue and frequent urination without dysuria. She says she is always hungry and has been drinking a lot of water and has lost over 5 pounds in the last two weeks. On exam, she appears tired, has dry mucous membranes, is afebrile with normal blood pressure and respirations. Her heart rate is 98 bpm, her orthostatic vitals are normal, and the rest of the exam is normal.

CASE 9 | Type 1 Diabetes Mellitus (DM) *(continued)*

Conditions with Similar Presentations	**Diabetes insipidus:** Due to absence of or resistance to vasopressin (ADH). Patients also present with frequent urination and increased thirst, but the blood sugars will be normal. **Type 2 DM:** Hyperglycemia is due to insulin resistance. There is usually weight gain instead of loss. Pancreatic autoantibodies will be negative. **Nocturnal enuresis:** Common in young patients but would not have any other symptoms or daytime frequent urination
Initial Diagnostic Tests	• Check plasma glucose testing or HbA1C • Consider Urinalysis (UA), BMP
Next Steps in Management	• Start insulin therapy • If the anion gap is elevated, check an ABG and serum ketones to confirm and treat diabetic ketoacidosis (DKA).
Discussion	Type 1 diabetes mellitus (T1DM) is the most common form of diabetes in childhood. It is characterized by autoimmune destruction of pancreatic islet β cells due to a combination of genetic and environmental factors. Patients will have low or absent levels of endogenously produced insulin and be dependent on exogenous insulin to prevent development of DKA and systemic complications of chronic diabetes. Autoantibodies such as anti-glutamic acid decarboxylase, anti-islet cell, and anti-insulin antibodies are present. T1DM is associated with other autoimmune diseases such as thyroiditis, celiac disease, and Addison's disease. Inheritance is polygenic, with an increased risk associated with the HLA-DR4 and HLA-DR3 haplotypes. Girls and boys are almost equally affected, and peaks of presentation occur in two age groups: 5–7 years, and at the time of puberty. **History:** • Classic symptoms: Polyuria, polydipsia, polyphagia, and weight loss. • Children may also experience enuresis, fatigue, difficulty concentrating. • Some patients with T1DM initially present in DKA (above symptoms as well as altered mental status, vomiting, fruity odor to breath) **Physical Exam:** Vital signs may show signs of dehydration: tachycardia, orthostasis, dry mucous membranes on exam. May have **Kussmaul respiration** (pattern of breathing with deep, rapid breaths) to compensate for underlying acidemia by allowing the body to excrete as much acid as possible in the form of CO_2 **Diagnostics** (any one of): • Fasting plasma glucose ≥126 mg/dL • Random plasma glucose ≥200 mg/dL with classic symptoms • Plasma glucose ≥200 mg/dL 2 hours after consumption of 75 g of glucose in water. • Hemoglobin A1C ≥ 6.5% (reflects average blood glucose for the past 3 months) • T1DM and T2DM can usually be differentiated based on clinical presentation (T1DM can present with DKA and T1DM can present with hyperosmolar hyperglycemic state). • In addition, the presence of **autoantibodies to pancreatic β cells** indicates T1DM • C-peptide levels may be measured as a marker for endogenous insulin production; low or undetectable in T1DM, normal or elevated in T2DM **Management:** • Rehydration • Insulin therapy is required due to little or no endogenous production • Frequent injections or via insulin pump
Additional Considerations	**Screening considerations:** American Diabetes Association (ADA) recommends screening all T1DM patients for autoimmune thyroid disease soon after diagnosis, as well as celiac disease if GI symptoms are present **Complications:** see *Endocrine Chapter* for details **Neurocognitive effects:** T1DM in children associated with poorer neurocognitive performance and lower school completion rates **Diabetic Ketoacidosis:** Serious complication of T1DM and is characterized by anion gap acidosis. See *Endocrine Chapter*

NEWBORN CARE

While the majority of newborns are born healthy and well, a high index of suspicion must be maintained for various abnormalities. All mothers and infants remain in the hospital for a minimum of 24 hours to be monitored closely and to allow for education of new parents.

APGAR scores are the "vital signs" of the newborn after delivery, and higher scores indicate a better outcome. Points are given for **A**ppearance, **P**ulse, **G**rimace, **A**ctivity, and **R**espiration 1 and 5 minutes after delivery. If the score is <7 at 5 minutes, immediate further evaluation is needed, as there can be an increased risk of neurologic damage.

The APGAR Score

Points	Appearance	Pulse (beats per minute)	Grimace	Activity/Tone	Respiration
0	Blue	None	Silence	Limp	None
1	Blue extremities (acrocyanosis)	<100 bpm	Whimpering	Moderate	Irregular
2	Pink	>100 bpm	Crying	Active	Regular

Respiratory Distress in the Newborn

It is important to recognize signs of respiratory distress in the newborn. These include tachypnea, cyanosis, nasal flaring, intercostal and subcostal retractions, and grunting. Clues to the etiology can be found in the history of the patient. In addition to the mini-cases below, neonatal sepsis, pneumothorax, meconium-aspiration syndrome, and cyanotic congenital heart disease must also be considered in the differential diagnosis.

Respiratory Distress Mini-Cases	
Cases	**Key Findings**
Transient Tachypnea of the Newborn	**Hx:** Transient signs of respiratory distress most commonly in a <2-hour-old full-term infant. More often in babies born via C-section. Other risk factors include prematurity and maternal diabetes.
	PE: Signs of respiratory distress (tachypnea, cyanosis, nasal flaring, intercostal retractions, and grunting) usually lasting <24 hours of life (though may be up to 72 hours).
	Diagnostics: • Clinical diagnosis • Consider CXR: will show increased lung volume, flat diaphragm (hyperinflation), prominent interstitial vascular markings in a sunburst pattern, and fluid in the interlobar fissures.
	Management: • Supplemental oxygen by hood or nasal cannula to maintain O_2 saturations >90% if there is hypoxia. • Other supportive care such as maintaining normothermia and providing adequate nutrition are also important.
	Discussion: Transient tachypnea of the newborn (TTN) is a benign and self-limited condition caused by delayed resorption and clearance of alveolar fluid after birth.
Respiratory Distress Syndrome (RDS)	**Hx:** Almost always in preterm (<37 weeks gestational age) infants, though other risk facts include infants of diabetic mothers, inaccurate dating of gestational age, and certain genetic conditions. Within first minutes to hours of life, baby will develop signs of respiratory distress that progress and worsen if left untreated, ultimately leading to respiratory failure.

Respiratory Distress Mini-Cases *(continued)*

Respiratory Distress Syndrome (RDS)	**PE:** Signs of respiratory distress, increased work of breathing, cyanosis, breath sounds coarse and decreased on auscultation. **Diagnostics:** • Clinical diagnosis. • CXR will show low lung volume and diffuse reticulogranular ("ground glass") appearance with air bronchograms. **Management:** • Prevention with antenatal corticosteroid therapy in women (usually 23–34 weeks' gestation) prior to delivery decreases severity of symptoms • Assisted non-invasive ventilation (often with nasal CPAP), close monitoring, surfactant therapy, and supportive care (nutrition and thermoregulation in particular) • Intubation, mechanical ventilation, and therapy with exogenous surfactant are used in severe or refractory cases **Discussion:** RDS is due to surfactant deficiency in preterm neonates, leading to high alveolar surface tension. This results in collapse of alveoli, low lung volumes, decreased compliance, a ventilation/perfusion (V/Q) mismatch, and right-to-left intrapulmonary shunting whereby deoxygenated blood is delivered to the left heart. This can evolve into bronchopulmonary dysplasia, which is defined as a need for oxygen supplementation either at 28 days of life or 36-week corrected gestational age.	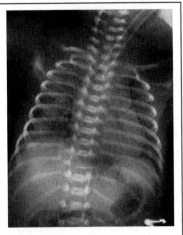 Chest radiograph of an infant with respiratory distress syndrome. An endotracheal tube is present. Despite the application of positive pressure, the lung volume is reduced with the diaphragm at the eighth interspace. The lung parenchyma has a diffuse reticulogranular pattern, and air bronchograms are present. (Reproduced with permission from Kawasaki Disease In: Tenenbein M, Macias CG, et al., Strange and Schafermeyer's Pediatric Emergency Medicine, 5e, New York: McGraw Hill; 2019.)
Persistent Pulmonary Hypertension of the Newborn (PPHN)	**Hx:** Most often in term or post-term infants with prenatal history sometimes showing signs of asphyxia. Often seen in babies born with meconium-stained amniotic fluid. Babies will present with respiratory distress in the first 24 hours of life and are unresponsive to conventional treatments. Usually, low APGARs are present at birth. Other risk factors include infection (pneumonia) or lung hypoplasia (e.g., secondary to congenital diaphragmatic hernia). Increased risk in infants born to mothers who were taking SSRIs during the second half of pregnancy. **PE:** Signs of respiratory distress, cyanosis. May have meconium staining of the skin/nails. Cardiac exam may show prominent precordial impulse, narrowly split and loud S2. **Diagnostics:** • Pulse oximetry demonstrating >10% difference between pre- and post-ductal oxygen saturation and arterial blood gas (ABG) will show low PaO_2. • CXR is normal • Diagnosis is made by echocardiography showing structurally normal cardiac anatomy with signs of pulmonary hypertension. **Management:** • Supportive cardiorespiratory care (almost always requiring intubation, possible inhaled nitrous oxide, or extracorporeal membrane oxygenation [ECMO]). **Discussion:** Caused by abnormal persistence of high pulmonary vascular resistance (PVR) after birth leading to right-to-left shunting through the fetal circulatory system across the ductus arteriosus. Consider this diagnosis in a full-term infant in severe respiratory distress with a normal CXR and structurally normal heart.

Neonatal Extracranial Birth Injuries

Delivery can result in several traumatic injuries to the neonate, most of which are benign and will self-resolve, while others may be life-threatening. Extracranial injuries to the scalp, subcutaneous tissue, and skull present with swelling of soft tissue or bleeding. It is important to differentiate these injuries from the less common but life-threatening intracranial injuries such as subdural hematoma or subarachnoid hemorrhage, both of which would result in abnormal neurologic findings on exam.

Types of Extracranial Birth Injuries

	Caput Succedaneum	Cephalohematoma	Subgaleal Hemorrhage
Location	Subcutaneous edema and swelling above the periosteum that is rarely hemorrhagic	Subperiosteal swelling between periosteum and skull, caused by rupture of subperiosteal vessels	Blood accumulation in the space between the periosteum and aponeurosis
Timing	Present at birth	Develops hours after birth	Develops after delivery, expands over days due to continued bleeding
Physical Exam Findings	Soft, boggy, poorly demarcated, crosses suture lines	More firm, non-fluctuant, well-demarcated, does not cross suture lines (contained within periosteum). May be accompanied by discoloration	Diffuse, soft, fluctuant swelling that is often large and shifts with movement, crosses cranial sutures, and may have associated scalp bruising
Risk Factors	Prolonged engagement of fetal head in vertex delivery, vacuum extraction	Forceps and/or vacuum extraction	Occurs due to vessel shearing due to traction during delivery (often difficult operative delivery)
Treatment	Benign and self-limited, resolving over several days	Resolves spontaneously within a month, although may be complicated by calcification and bony swelling that can persist longer. Increased risk of unconjugated hyperbilirubinemia as RBCs degrade over time	High mortality rates due to potential for massive blood loss. Requires serial monitoring of hemoglobin, transfusions to correct ongoing bleeding and coagulopathy, as well as rare neurosurgical intervention
Diagram			

Drawing of caput succedaneum (A), cephalohematoma with corrections (B), and subgaleal hemorrhage (C). (Reproduced with permission from Birth Injury In: Zaoutis LB, Chiang VW. Comprehensive Pediatric Hospital Medicine, 2e; New York: McGraw Hill, 2017 and Reproduced with permission from Cunningham FG, Leveno KJ, et al. Williams Obstetrics. 23rd ed; New York: McGraw-Hill, 2010.)

Neonatal Hyperbilirubinemia

The ultimate concern with elevated bilirubin levels is the transport across the blood-brain barrier causing central nervous system injury. Acutely, patients can develop reversible symptoms of bilirubin encephalopathy (i.e., drowsiness, decreased activity, decreased feeding). Chronic high levels of bilirubin can affect the basal ganglia/brainstem nuclei and cause permanent choreoathetosis, spasticity, and hearing loss.

Neurotoxicity risk factors: Isoimmune hemolytic disease, G6PD deficiency, asphyxia, significant lethargy, temperature instability, sepsis, acidosis, albumin <3.0 g/dL.

In dealing with hyperbilirubinemia in neonates, first differentiating conjugated from unconjugated hyperbilirubinemia is essential. Conjugated hyperbilirubinemia is defined as a conjugated bilirubin >1 mg/dL if the total bilirubin is <5 mg/dL or more than 20% of the total bilirubin if the total bilirubin is >5 mg/dL.

- **Conjugated hyperbilirubinemia** is never normal, always requires investigation, and cannot be treated with phototherapy. The primary diagnosis to consider is biliary atresia, and this needs to be ruled out first.
- **Unconjugated hyperbilirubinemia** has several causes. Most commonly, it is benign and referred to as "physiologic" and requires no further investigation. The nomogram helps to distinguish physiologic vs. non-physiologic jaundice and can characterize patients into high, intermediate, and low-risk zones. Separate phototherapy and exchange therapy charts are used for management. Risk factor assessment helps determine etiology, which then informs treatment. It is essential to understand the mechanism for bilirubin production, clearance, and excretion.

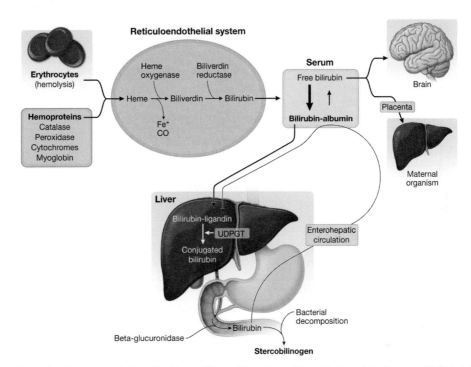

Reticuloendothelial system. (Reproduced with permission from Physiology of Neonatal Unconjugated Hyperbilirubinemia In. Stevenson DK, Maisels M, Watchko JF. Care of the Jaundiced Neonate, New York: McGraw Hill, 2012.)

Hyperbilirubinemia risk factors include: jaundice in first 24 hours, ABO or Rh incompatibility with positive direct Coombs, known hemolytic disease, prematurity, prior sibling requiring phototherapy, cephalohematoma or bruising, and exclusive breastfeeding, especially with poor feeding or weight loss.

The differential diagnosis is determined by the etiology of the hyperbilirubinemia: increased production (hemolysis such as from isoimmune hemolytic disease), decreased clearance (Crigler-Najjar and Gilbert syndromes), or increased enterohepatic circulation (breast milk jaundice, intestinal obstruction, or lactation failure jaundice).

Commonly tested and confused etiologies of unconjugated hyperbilirubinemia are lactation failure (breastfeeding) jaundice vs. breast milk jaundice.

Key Differences between Lactation Failure Jaundice and Breast Milk Jaundice

	Lactation Failure (Breastfeeding) Jaundice	Breast Milk Jaundice
Etiology	Supply/demand issue (e.g., from poor latch of baby or low mother milk supply), leading to reduced intake of fluids/calories. Decreased intake also leads to slower bilirubin elimination and increased enterohepatic circulation.	Unknown. Likely related to high concentration of beta-glucuronidase in breast milk leading to low level of beta-D-glucuronic acid and increased intestinal absorption of unconjugated bilirubin.
Timing of onset	Within first week of life (usually 2–5 days).	Starts to rise at 3–5 days of life, peaks at 2 weeks.
Treatment	Establishment of successful breastfeeding. Phototherapy if needed.	Continue breastfeeding, usually self-limited.

CASE 10 | Classical Vitamin K Deficiency Bleeding in Infancy

A 5-day-old baby boy born to a 26-year-old G2P2 mother is brought to clinic for the initial newborn visit. Mother states that the baby has been eating, eliminating, and sleeping well. Exam notable for minor bleeding around the mouth, nose, and umbilical stump. Medical records indicate that the mother refused vitamin K prophylaxis at birth and takes anticonvulsants due to history of seizures.

Conditions with Similar Presentations	**Familial bleeding disorders:** History often includes frequent familial bleeding or bleeding disorders. Examples include hemophilia, von Willebrand disease. **Non-accidental trauma (NAT):** Injury purposefully inflicted upon a child. Exam notable for possible fear in being examined, evidence of neglect, 4-TEN (bruising on child less than 4 years on **t**runk, **e**ars, **n**eck), evidence of head trauma. **Disseminated intravascular coagulation:** Severely ill, increased fibrin degradation products , skin ecchymoses, occult hemorrhage. Risk factors include prematurity, low birth weight, sepsis, and low Apgar scores.
Initial Diagnostic Tests	• Clinical diagnosis • Check PT and INR • Diagnosis confirmed with normalization of PT and INR after vitamin K given
Next Steps in Management	• Administer IV phylloquinone (vitamin K) as soon as suspected • If severe or CNS bleeding, administering fresh frozen plasma (FFP) or prothrombin complex concentrate (PCC)
Discussion	Vitamin K deficiency bleeding (VKDB) was previously termed hemorrhagic disease of the newborn, and usually occurs at 2–7 days of life due to insufficient vitamin K. Vitamin K is a fat-soluble vitamin, and is a necessary cofactor for the activation of factors II, VII, IX, X, protein C, and protein S. Vitamin K deficiency is rare in adults, but more common in newborns due to insufficient production from gut flora, immaturity of the newborn liver, and minimal transfer of vitamin K in breastmilk. Based on the age at which it occurs, it is divided into early-onset, classic, and late-onset, with classic being the most common. The timing of when VKDB presents informs its etiology.

Types of Vitamin K Deficiency

	Early Onset	Classic	Late
Timing	First 24 hours of life	2–7 days of life	8 days to 6 months of life
Etiology	Maternal medications	Vitamin K not received in the hospital	Neonatal hepatobiliary dysfunction

History/Physical Exam:

Risk Factors: Maternal history of medication use, exclusive breastfeeding (low vitamin K content in breastmilk), malabsorption, no newborn Vitamin K prophylaxis

Symptoms/Signs: Bleeding of skin, mucosa, GI tract, umbilical stump, intracranial/extracranial bleed, lethargy, fussiness, easy bruising, lethargy, hypotonia, abdominal swelling

Diagnostics:
• Clinical diagnosis based on history of vitamin K prophylaxis not being given
• Elevated PT and INR that normalizes within 3 hours of administration of IV phylloquinone
• Also check CBC and aPTT (usually normal but low aIX and aX may lead to elevated aPTT, and CBC may show anemia)

Consider:
• Imaging depending on the location of the bleeding
  • CT/MRI brain if neurological signs present such as hypotonia or lethargy
  • CT abdomen if distended
• Screening for bleeding disorders if family history of frequent bleeding

Management:
• IV phylloquinone (vitamin K)
• Fresh frozen plasma or prothrombin complex concentrate for severe or CNS bleeding
• Encourage breastfeeding
• May discharge with close follow-up if:
  • No major signs of bleeding or neurological signs
  • Normalization of coagulation factors

Additional Considerations	**Screening:** Consider if no prophylactic vitamin K administration, family history of bleeding disorders **Complications:** Severe internal bleeding, neurological complications (seizures, hearing and visual disturbances, developmental delay, motor problems, sleep problems), failure to thrive, death

Non-Infectious Neonatal Rashes

Type	Morphology	Distribution	Treatment	Image
Milia	1- to 2-mm pearly white or yellow papules due to keratin retention	Forehead, cheeks, nose, and chin	Self-limited	Reproduced with permission from Neil S. Prose, Leonard Kristal, Weinberg's Color Atlas of Pediatric Dermatology, 5e; by McGraw-Hill 2017.
Miliaria crystallina	Small, thin-walled vesicles	Face, scalp, intertriginous areas	Self-limited	The lesions in miliaria crystallina are small, clear, thin-roofed vesicles that develop when the sweat duct is obstructed within the stratum corneum. They occur after sunburn or in response to excessive sweating in high environmental heat and humidity. Fever may also be a cause. (Reproduced with permission from Neil S. Prose, Leonard Kristal, Weinberg's Color Atlas of Pediatric Dermatology, 5e; by McGraw-Hill 2017.)
Miliaria rubra	Known as "heat rash"; small erythematous papules and vesicles	On covered portions of the skin	Self-limited	Miliaria rubra (prickly heat) is the most common form of miliaria. It occurs when there is plugging of the eccrine ducts and release of sweat into the adjacent skin. It is characterized by discrete erythematous papules and papulovesicles. The forehead, upper trunk, and intertriginous areas are commonly affected. Unlike miliaria crystallina, miliaria rubra is characterized by spasmodic pricking sensations. A decrease in environmental heat and humidity is the only treatment required. (Reproduced with permission from Neil S. Prose, Leonard Kristal, Weinberg's Color Atlas of Pediatric Dermatology, 5e; by McGraw-Hill 2017.)

Non-Infectious Neonatal Rashes (*Continued*)

Type	Morphology	Distribution	Treatment	Image
Seborrheic dermatitis	Erythema and greasy scales, most likely due to *Malassezia furfur*	"Cradle cap" (mainly affects the scalp), intertriginous areas, diaper area	Self-limited, but if not resolved can use anti-fungal cream	 Seborrheic dermatitis is a scaly, crusting, and erythematous eruption that is most common in infancy (ages 2–12 weeks), where it tends to favor the scalp, diaper area, and intertriginous folds. This figure is an illustration of the process in the scalp, where it is often referred to as "cradle cap." (Reproduced with permission from Neil S. Prose, Leonard Kristal, Weinberg's Color Atlas of Pediatric Dermatology, 5e; by McGraw-Hill 2017.)
Acne neonatorum	Open comedones, inflammatory papules, pustules	Forehead, nose, cheeks	Self-limited, but can use benzoyl peroxide lotion if unresolved	 Neonatal and infantile acne. Mild comedonal acne is fairly common in the newborn. The typical eruption consists of closed comedones. Open comedones, inflammatory papules and pustules, and small cysts may also occur. Neonatal acne is due to the stimulation of sebaceous glands by androgens from both mother and infant. (Reproduced with permission from Neil S. Prose, Leonard Kristal, Weinberg's Color Atlas of Pediatric Dermatology, 5e; by McGraw-Hill 2017.)
Erythema toxicum neonatorum	Erythematous, 2- to 3-mm macules and papules that evolve into pustules Surrounded by erythema "flea-bitten" appearance	Face, trunk, proximal extremities; no palm and sole involvement	Self-limited	 The lesions are erythematous macules, within which papules and pustules may develop. The trunk is the most common site, but all other body surfaces, except for the palms and soles, may be involved. In rare cases, these lesions may occur in plaques. (Reproduced with permission from Neil S. Prose, Leonard Kristal, Weinberg's Color Atlas of Pediatric Dermatology, 5e; by McGraw-Hill 2017.)

CASE 11 | Neonatal Opioid Withdrawal Syndrome

A 5-day-old girl born to a 30-year-old G1P1 mother with opioid use disorder presents for a follow-up newborn checkup and weight check. Baby was born at 39 weeks with no prenatal or labor complications, with a weight of 3500 g and length of 50 cm. Parent states that the baby has more than 10 dirty diapers/day, at least five episodes of emesis/day, inconsolable crying and irritability, and excessive yawning and sneezing. On exam, vital signs are normal. Weight is 3450 g. There is hypotonia of all extremities, minor tremor, excessive sucking, and diaphoresis.

Conditions with Similar Presentations	**Sepsis:** Important to always rule out sepsis due to variable presentations in neonates. Additional symptoms include fever/hypothermia and history of parental fever, premature rupture of membranes, chorioamnionitis. **Hyperthyroidism:** Maternal history of hyperthyroidism usually present. **Hypocalcemia:** More likely if premature, intrauterine growth restriction, asphyxia, or maternal diabetes. **Hypoglycemia:** More likely if premature, large for gestational age, maternal diabetes. **Withdrawal from other substances:** Most common withdrawal seen in neonates is from opioids, but must rule out other substances, including alcohol and cocaine.
Initial Diagnostic Tests	• Clinical diagnosis • Check urine cord, or meconium drug tests
Next Steps in Management	• Use Eat, Sleep, Console (ESC) approach to determine newborn's ability to function • Pharmacological care when infant is not improving

Discussion	Maternal use of opioids should always be asked about and addressed to minimize risk of neonatal opioid withdrawal syndrome (NOWS), previously called neonatal abstinence syndrome. Opioids cross the placenta and bind to CNS μ-receptors. Timing of when NOWS presents depends on the type, amount, and frequency of opioid use. Withdrawal increases various neurotransmitters in the brain, including norepinephrine, dopamine, and serotonin, that contribute to the symptom complex.
	
	History:
	Risk factors: Maternal history of opioid use, lack of prenatal follow-up, low parental socioeconomic status, unstable social environment, and babies born in developing countries.
	Symptoms: Include hyperirritability, diaphoresis, hyperphagia, diarrhea, high-pitched uncontrollable crying, seizures if severe.
	Physical Exam: Vital sign instability, hypotonia, tremor, mottling, perianal skin excoriation secondary to excessive loose stools.
	Diagnostics:
	• Clinical diagnosis in known or suspected maternal opioid use
	• Laboratory confirmation: Urine, cord, or meconium drug test
	• Consider labs (e.g., TSH, glucose and calcium levels) to rule out other diagnosis
	Management:
	• Gold standard: ESC system
	  • Eat:
	    • Day of life 1–2: Less than 1 ounce per feeding
	    • Day of life 3 and greater: 1 or more ounces per feeding
	    • Breastfeeding: "good" defined by mother and medical team
	  • Sleep: Undisturbed for at least 1 hour
	  • Console: Consoled within 10 minutes
	• Pharmacological therapy if no improvement.
	  • Synthetic drug addiction: morphine or methadone
	  • Non-synthetic drug addiction: phenobarbital
	• Involve Child Protective Services in the case and care of the patient
	• Close follow-up with family to ensure stable social environment and neonate is healthy
	• Connect mother with treatment for opioid use disorder
	• No restrictions on breastfeeding
	• Discharge home with family when:
	  • No major signs of withdrawal, feeding well, sleeping well, gaining weight, stable ESC with minimal medication support
	  • Parental education of drug abuse and resources from a social worker provided
	• Close follow-up must be ensured prior to discharge

CASE 11 | Neonatal Opioid Withdrawal Syndrome *(continued)*

Additional Considerations	**Screening:** Screen at birth if maternal history of opioid use. If there is concern for NOWS, child protective services will need to be contacted to assess whether the home is safe for the newborn to return to upon discharge.
	Complications: Severe dehydration, neurological complications (seizures, hearing and visual disturbances, developmental delay, motor problems, sleep problems), failure to thrive, sudden infant death syndrome.

Abnormal Fetal Findings

Abnormal fetal findings discovered in the intrapartum period are varied in presentation and origin. Genetic abnormalities, infections, maternal conditions and morbidities, and teratogenic exposures prior to or during pregnancy can all affect the development of the fetus. Teratogens are substances that have the potential to cause anatomic and/or physiologic abnormalities to an exposed fetus. The risk of congenital anomalies from teratogen exposure is highest from 2 to 8 weeks of gestation, a time of the most intensive fetal organogenesis. In general, the earlier the disturbance in normal embryonic and fetal development occurs, the more severe the abnormalities are. Please refer to Obstetrics and Gynecology Chapter for additional information.

Conditions That May Affect Fetal Development

Infections	*Transplacental infections* **(ToRCHHeS):**	*Streptococcus agalactiae* (Group B strep)
		Escherichia coli
	Toxoplasma gondii	*Listeria monocytogenes*
	Rubella	Tuberculosis
	Cytomegalovirus (CMV)	Parvovirus B19
	Human immunodeficiency virus (HIV)	Varicella zoster virus
	Herpes simplex virus (HSV)	Malaria
	Syphilis	Fungal
Prescription Teratogens	ACE inhibitors	Folate antagonists (trimethoprim, sulfamethoxazole, methotrexate)
	Alkylating agents	Isotretinoin
	Aminoglycosides	Lithium
	Antiepileptic drugs (valproate, carbamazepine, phenytoin, phenobarbital)	Methimazole
	Diethylstilbestrol (DES)	Tetracyclines
		Thalidomide
		Warfarin
Maternal Conditions	Lack of prenatal care	Iodine excess/deficiency
	Diabetes mellitus	Methylmercury ingestion (seen with some types of seafood)
	Alcohol use	
	Cocaine use	Vitamin A excess
	Tobacco use	Vitamin deficiency
Genetic Defects	Trisomy 13 (Patau syndrome)	Monosomy X (Turner syndrome)
	Trisomy 18 (Edward syndrome)	
	Trisomy 21 (Down syndrome)	

PEDIATRIC CARDIOLOGY

The diagnosis of cardiac disorders in children relies on a thorough history and physical examination. The presenting symptoms and signs will differ dependent on the age of the patient.

Age Group	Most Common Etiologies	Presentation of Cardiac Disorders
Infant	Congenital heart disease	Failure to thrive—weight is primarily affected, then height and head circumference Feeding difficulties Easy fatigability Vomiting Lethargy Rapid breathing Increased perspiration
Older children	Acquired or infectious causes	Easy fatigability Shortness of breath Dyspnea on exertion

Fetal to Neonatal Circulation

Understanding cardiac physiology as it changes from fetal to the neonatal period is an important step to help connect the presenting symptoms with the pathology of the infant. Infants with cardiac disease can initially be asymptomatic due to the presence of a patent ductus arteriosus (PDA) and thus some treatment regimens include keeping the PDA open to help delay symptomatology until further treatment can be initiated.

In the fetal circulation (see figure), the ductus arteriosus remains open. The right ventricle is the predominant ventricle that supplies oxygenated blood. The open ductus arteriosus allows blood oxygenated by the placenta to enter the systemic circulation from the right ventricle without going through the lungs. At the time of delivery, when the infant takes their first breath, the resistance in the pulmonary vasculature decreases and blood flows from the right ventricle through the lungs for oxygenation. At this point, the ductus arteriosus starts to constrict and close, which should happen within 1 day after birth. Please refer to Chapter 4 (Cardiology) for additional information.

Circulation in the fetus. Most of the oxygenated blood reaching the heart via the umbilical vein and inferior vena cava is diverted through the foramen ovale and pumped from the aorta to the head, while the deoxygenated blood returned via the superior vena cava is mostly pumped through the pulmonary artery and ductus arteriosus to the feet and the umbilical arteries. (Reproduced with permission from Circulation Through Special Regions In: Barrett KE, Barman SM, Brooks HL, Yuan JJ. Ganong's Review of Medical Physiology, 26e; New York: McGraw Hill, 2019.)

High-Yield Findings in Pediatric Cardiology Diagnoses

Diagnoses	Key Associated Findings
Tricuspid atresia Total anomalous pulmonary venous return Hypoplastic left heart syndrome Coarctation of aorta	• Progressive cyanosis in the first 2 weeks of life (usually due to closure of the PDA)
Transposition of great arteries	• Cyanosis at birth, hypoxia, tachypnea, failure to thrive within the first hours or days • Loud P2 because of anteriorly displaced aorta • Murmur may be absent or a faint systolic murmur may be present • CXR with an oval- or egg-shaped cardiac silhouette with a narrow superior mediastinum
Total anomalous pulmonary venous return	• Cyanosis, hypoxia, tachypnea, failure to thrive in the first week, with prominent neck veins • "Figure-of-eight" or "snowman" on CXR refers to small cardiac silhouette with large pulmonary vascularity
Tetralogy of Fallot	• Dyspnea with feeding, poor growth, and sudden hypercyanotic "tet" spells; cyanosis improves with squatting • Harsh systolic murmur at the left upper sternal border with a single heart sound (S2); prominent right ventricular impulse and systolic thrill may be noted • Boot-shaped heart on CXR
Truncus arteriosus	• Cyanosis • Wide pulse pressure and bounding arterial pulses • Harsh systolic murmur with a palpable thrill along left sternal border, loud and single S2
Atrial septal defect	• Mid-systolic murmur at the left upper sternal border (secondary to increased flow across the pulmonic valve) • Wide and fixed S2 • Palpable right ventricular heave, left sternal border
Ventricular septal defect	• High-pitched, holosystolic murmur, best heard in third, fourth, and fifth left intercostal space • PMI is hyperdynamic • Cyanosis a late finding secondary to Eisenmenger physiology
Eisenmenger syndrome	• History of childhood left-to-right shunt: ventricular septal defect (VSD)/atrial septal defect (ASD), patent ductus arteriosus (PDA) • Exam findings: elevated jugular venous pressure (JVP), hepatomegaly, lower extremity edema, left parasternal heave, pulmonary crackles, cyanosis, clubbing, loud P2 with increased S2 splitting, holosystolic murmur at left sternal border from tricuspid regurgitation
Coarctation of aorta	• Intermittent claudication on exercise in older children • Exam findings: suprasternal notch pulsations, hypertension, reduced lower extremity pulses, brachial-femoral delay (femoral pulse occurs after brachial pulse), lower blood pressure in lower extremities compared to upper extremities, ejection systolic murmur in back or can be continuous

Cyanotic Heart Conditions

An approach to the differential diagnosis of cyanosis is to stratify etiologies by age.

Differential Diagnosis Based on Age

Age	Diagnosis
Infants	Cyanosis that begins in the first hours to days of life is seen with right-to-left shunt congenital heart diseases. These include transposition of great arteries, persistent truncus arteriosus, tetralogy of Fallot, total anomalous pulmonary venous return, Ebstein anomaly, hypoplastic left heart syndrome, and tricuspid atresia. Congenital heart disease can have variable presentations and can become more evident once the PDA begins to close, because the PDA allows for left-to-right circulation and can partially compensate for the defect.

Differential Diagnosis Based on Age

Age	Diagnosis
Toddlers	If Tetralogy of Fallot (ToF) does not present as cyanosis in infancy, it may present later in toddlers. It may be described as a toddler who cannot keep up with his classmates at recess and has to squat when catching their breath. Hypercyanotic "Tet" spells may be noted.
Young adults	Difficult-to-control hypertension in young adults should raise suspicion for coarctation of the aorta. They may also have claudication on exertion, and lower extremity cyanosis secondary to an associated PDA.
Any age	Right ventricular failure symptoms may indicate untreated congenital heart disease that has progressed to Eisenmenger syndrome (chronic left-to-right shunt leading to pulmonary hypertension and cyanosis when shunt reverses). Individuals with surgical corrections of congenital heart disease who have been lost to follow-up may present with symptoms of right- and left-sided heart failure later in life.

CASE 12 | Tetralogy of Fallot

An 8-month-old boy is brought to the clinic for evaluation because he turns blue when he cries or feeds. On exam, he is underweight, and clubbing is noted in upper extremities. A systolic thrill along the left sternal border and a sustained right ventricular impulse along the left sternal border is noted. On auscultation, there is a loud and harsh systolic ejection murmur radiating to the pulmonary and aortic areas, with a single S2. His lungs are clear to auscultation bilaterally.

Conditions with Similar Presentations	**Hypoplastic left heart syndrome:** Congenital anomaly that results in underdeveloped left ventricle. May also present with cyanosis, but the murmur on examination is a continuous murmur. **Ebstein anomaly of the tricuspid valve:** Congenital anomaly that results in downward displacement of the tricuspid valve. May also present with cyanosis and poor feeding. Associated murmur is a pansystolic murmur heard best at the left sternal border. S2 has a wide split due to associated right bundle branch block. **Transposition of the great arteries:** Congenital anomaly in which the pulmonary artery and the aorta are switched. The degree of cyanosis is based on the pathology. Does not have a detectable murmur.
Initial Diagnostic Tests	• Confirm diagnosis with transthoracic echocardiogram (TTE) • Consider: ECG, CXR
Next Steps in Management	Surgical repair
Discussion	ToF is the most common cyanotic congenital cardiac defect and is characterized by a tetrad of pulmonary infundibular stenosis, right ventricular hypertrophy (RVH), an overriding aorta, and a ventricular septal defect (VSD). ToF is usually identified in the neonatal period. The degree of pulmonary infundibular stenosis predicts prognosis and severity of symptoms. Children will often "learn" the behavior of suddenly stopping during activity and squatting. This maneuver increases afterload, which decreases the right-to-left shunt and improves hypoxia. **History:** Although most commonly diagnosed prenatally with fetal echocardiography, infants or young children with undiagnosed ToF will have a history of cyanosis that worsens with exertion like crying or eating and that improves with squatting. **Physical Exam:** On exam, there is a loud and harsh systolic ejection murmur radiating to the pulmonary and aortic areas, a RV heave along the left sternal border, and a single S2. **Diagnostics:** • Echocardiogram shows an overriding aorta, VSD, pulmonary infundibular stenosis, and RVH. • ECG shows right axis deviation and RVH. • CXR shows a "boot"-shaped heart due to RV enlargement. **Management:** Surgical repair, usually performed before 6 months of age. 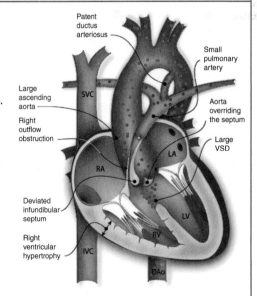 Tetralogy of Fallot. (Reproduced with permission from Suspecting Congenital Heart Disease In: Shahab Noori, Pierre Wong, Practical Neonatal Echocardiography, New York: McGraw Hill, 2018.)

CASE 11 | Tetralogy of Fallot *(continued)*

Additional Considerations	**Screening:** ToF is more common in patients with Down syndrome, DiGeorge syndrome (thymic aplasia, 22q11 deletion), and fetal alcohol syndrome.
	Complications: Following repair, patients have chronic pulmonary regurgitation and eventually require pulmonary valve replacement. Patients are also at greater risk of arrhythmias and sudden cardiac death than the general population.

Cyanotic Congenital Heart Condition Mini-Cases

Cases	Key Findings
Hypoplastic Left Heart Syndrome (HLHS)	**Hx/PE:** Newborn baby appears cyanotic and tachypneic with a loud and single second heart sound due to hypoplastic aortic valve making no contribution. Pulses are very weak or absent. Cyanosis does not improve with supplemental oxygen. There may be an ejection systolic flow murmur across the pulmonary valve and/or a pansystolic murmur of tricuspid regurgitation.
	Diagnostics: Most cases diagnosed prenatally with fetal echocardiography showing hypoplastic left ventricle, abnormal mitral and aortic valves, and small ascending aorta.
	Management: Three-stage palliative surgery (the Norwood procedure during the first week of life, the bidirectional Glenn procedure at 3–6 months, and the Fontan procedure at 2–5 years).
	Discussion: HLHS is characterized by a small, underdeveloped LV, left-sided valves, and ascending aorta that cannot support systemic circulation. This condition is universally fatal without surgery, and even with surgery has high rates of morbidity and mortality.
Truncus Arteriosus (TA)	**Hx/PE:** Newborn with poor feeding, lethargy, grunting, and respiratory distress. Bounding peripheral pulses, harsh systolic ejection murmur along left sternal border, loud and single S2. 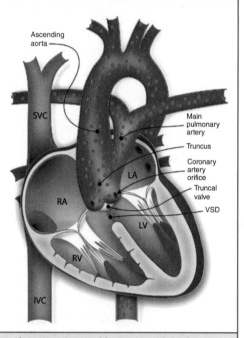
	Diagnostics: • Can be diagnosed with prenatal echocardiography, but diagnosis is challenging and often missed. • Postnatal echocardiography will show a single great vessel overriding the heart, generally larger in diameter than a healthy aorta.
	Management: Surgical repair
	Discussion: In TA, the aorta and pulmonary arteries fail to septate during development, resulting in a single truncal valve and vessel that gives rise to both the aorta and the pulmonary arteries. In patients with TA, 20–25% have comorbid 22q11.2 deletions. Without correction, severe pulmonary hypertension develops. Diagram of truncus arteriosus with MPA arising from ascending trunk close to the truncal valve. (Reproduced with permission from Suspecting Congenital Heart Disease In: Shahab Noori, Pierre Wong, Practical Neonatal Echocardiography, New York: McGraw Hill, 2018.)
Total Anomalous Pulmonary Venous Return (TAPVR)	**Hx/PE:** Newborn with severe respiratory distress, cyanotic, hypotensive, and hypoxic, with tachypnea, grunting, and nasal flaring. May also have hepatomegaly, diminished peripheral pulses, cool extremities, and a prominent and fixed S2. A systolic ejection flow murmur over the pulmonic valve and a diastolic rumble across the tricuspid valve can be heard. 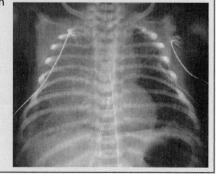 Total anomalous pulmonary venous return. This 6-hour-old infant with obstructed supracardiac total anomalous pulmonary venous return had oxygen saturations of less than 50% despite supportive measures. Radiographic evaluation shows severe pulmonary edema and normal heart size. There is a right pleural effusion; the left effusion has been drained. (Reproduced with permission from Robert G. Wells, Diagnostic Imaging of Infants and Children; by The McGraw-Hill 2013.)

Cyanotic Congenital Heart Condition Mini-Cases *(continued)*

Total Anomalous Pulmonary Venous Return (TAPVR)	**Diagnostics:** • Echocardiography is diagnostic test of choice. • CXR shows pulmonary edema, and in older infants and young children it may show the classic "figure-of-eight" or "snowman." **Management:** Surgical intervention to restore pulmonary return to the left atrium. **Discussion:** In TAPVR, all four pulmonary veins plug into the systemic venous circulation rather than into the left atrium, usually with an associated ASD. Because the right side of the heart is receiving both systemic and pulmonary venous return, there is significant right-sided overload. There are two types: with and without obstruction of pulmonary venous return. TAPVR with obstruction presents earlier with more severe symptoms and causes severe pulmonary hypertension. Neonates with unobstructed return may have only mild cyanosis at birth and present as an infant or toddler with failure to thrive and right heart failure.
Transposition of the Great Arteries (TGA)	**Hx/PE:** Newborn with tachypnea, cyanosis, and hypoxia. Exam is significant for cyanosis that is not worsened by exertion or improved with supplemental oxygen. Murmurs are not a prominent feature. There is a single loud S2 from the anteriorly displaced aorta. **Diagnostics:** • Echocardiography is diagnostic. • Prenatal screening with fetal ultrasound can often identify this abnormality, but occasionally it can be missed. • CXR shows an enlarged, globular, egg-shaped heart (called "egg on a string"). **Management:** Prostaglandin E1 (PGE1) to maintain the patency of the ductus arteriosus until surgical repair can be performed. **Discussion:** TGA is a cyanotic congenital heart malformation in which the aorta arises from the right ventricle and the pulmonary artery from the left ventricle. The result is two parallel circulations, one that sends deoxygenated systemic venous blood through the right atrium and ventricle to the aorta and back to the body, and the other that sends oxygenated pulmonary venous blood through the left atrium, left ventricle, and pulmonary artery back to the lungs. This condition is well tolerated in utero but is incompatible with life after birth without some connection between the circuits such as a PFO, PDA, ASD, or VSD. The ductus arteriosus is maintained patent until surgical correction can be performed. 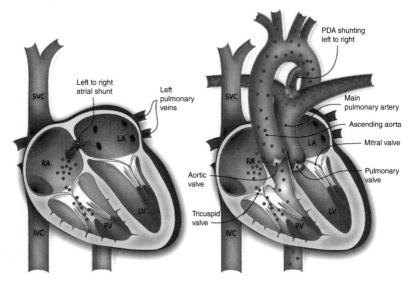 Diagram of D-transposition of the great arteries, atrial septal defect, and patent ductus arteriosus. (Reproduced with permission from Suspecting Congenital Heart Disease In: Shahab Noori, Pierre Wong, Practical Neonatal Echocardiography, New York: McGraw Hill, 2018.)

Cyanotic Congenital Heart Condition Mini-Cases *(continued)*

Tricuspid Valve Atresia	**Hx/PE:** Newborn with cyanosis and breathing fast.
	Physical exam is significant for central cyanosis and a single S2. Associated murmurs depend on whether there is an associated VSD (holosystolic at left lower sternal border) or PDA (continuous murmur).
	Diagnostics:
	• Diagnosis is frequently made prenatally with echocardiography.
	• ECG shows left axis deviation, small or absent R waves in the precordial leads, and evidence of LVH.
	Management:
	• PGE1 to maintain the PDA until a shunt can be placed
	• Three-stage palliative surgical correction is performed, similar to HLHS
	Discussion: TV atresia is characterized by congenital atresia of the TV. Because there is no communication between the RA and RV, the RV and pulmonary outflow tract are hypoplastic. This condition is incompatible with life without associated PFO, ASD, or VSD.

Acyanotic Conditions

Acyanotic congenital heart disease is a group of disorders characterized by normal oxygenation of the blood but abnormal flow throughout the body.

CASE 13 | Ventricular Septal Defect (VSD)

A 15-year-old boy with a history of an unrepaired "hole in his heart" presents with worsening exertional dyspnea for the last several months. On exam, his vital signs are normal. There is JVD, a sternal lift, and a laterally displaced PMI. On auscultation, there is a harsh holosystolic murmur and palpable thrill at lower left sternal border and bibasilar crackles in the lungs.

Conditions with Similar Presentations	**Patent ductus arteriosus:** A congenital anomaly in which the connection between the aorta and the pulmonary artery remains open. Infants may be asymptomatic but will have a continuous murmur at the left sternal border.
	Tetralogy of Fallot: Cyanotic congenital heart disease with loud and harsh systolic ejection murmur radiating to the pulmonary and aortic areas, with a single loud S2.
	Coarctation of aorta: Congenital defect that results in narrowing of the aorta leading to decreased blood flow to the lower extremities. BP is lower in legs than arms, pulse is delayed in legs vs. arms, and pulses are diminished in legs. May present with signs of heart failure.
Initial Diagnostic Tests	• Confirm diagnosis with echocardiography • Consider CXR, ECG
Next Steps in Management	Percutaneous closure device or surgical repair
Discussion	VSDs are the most common congenital cardiac defect. The prevalence of VSDs in the U.S. is 1 in every 240 newborns. Most VSDs are diagnosed after birth, and they most commonly occur in the membranous septum.

VSDs are the most common congenital cardiac defect. The prevalence of VSDs in the U.S. is 1 in every 240 newborns. Most VSDs are diagnosed after birth, and they most commonly occur in the membranous septum.

Small VSDs may close spontaneously in childhood, but some persist asymptomatically into adulthood. Chronic left-to-right shunting can result in pulmonary hypertension and RVH, as in this patient, causing reversal of the shunt to a cyanotic right-to-left shunt. This is called **Eisenmenger syndrome** and results in cyanosis and heart failure.

History/Physical Exam: Most commonly presents as an asymptomatic infant with a harsh holosystolic murmur over the left lower sternal border and a loud S2. The murmur is sometimes not heard in the neonatal period while pulmonary vascular resistance remains high.

Perimembranous and muscular ventricular septal defects. (Reproduced with permission from Suspecting Congenital Heart Disease In: Shahab Noori, Pierre Wong, Practical Neonatal Echocardiography, New York: McGraw Hill, 2018.)

CASE 13 | Ventricular Septal Defect (VSD) (continued)

Discussion	**Diagnostics:** • Echocardiography: shows a VSD with significant intracardiac shunt and RVH • CXR may show cardiomegaly and increased pulmonary vascular markings **Management:** Large or symptomatic lesions require percutaneous closure or surgical repair.
Additional Considerations	**Complications:** There is an increased risk of endocarditis and a long-term risk of heart failure and pulmonary hypertension in patients with unrepaired lesions.

Acyanotic Congenital Heart Disease Mini-Cases

Cases	Key Findings
Atrial Septum Defect (ASD)	**Hx:** Most infants and children are asymptomatic, and the ASD may be diagnosed incidentally or in the workup of a murmur. If the ASD does not close spontaneously in childhood, adults may eventually develop fatigue, exercise intolerance, and sometimes overt heart failure from chronic left-to-right shunting resulting in pulmonary hypertension. **PE:** Exam is significant for a wide, fixed S2. Flow across the ASD is too low in velocity to be heard as a murmur, but you may hear a mid-systolic ejection murmur from increased blood flow across the pulmonic valve. **Diagnostics:** Echocardiography **Management:** Most ASDs close spontaneously in childhood, but surgery or transcatheter closure is indicated for symptomatic patients. **Discussion:** ASD is a communication between the atria of the heart. It can occur in several locations, most commonly in the septum secundum, but also seen in the septum primum and the sinus venosus. • Long-term complications can include Eisenmenger syndrome and "paradoxical emboli" which move from the venous system through the defect to the cerebral circulation, causing strokes (also seen in patent foramen ovale). • ASD is also associated with other congenital heart defects such as tricuspid atresia and total anomalous pulmonary venous return, or seen as part of fetal alcohol syndrome or trisomy 21.
Ebstein Anomaly	**Hx:** Presentation is widely variable, ranging from cyanotic newborns to asymptomatic adults. Symptoms may include poor feeding, increased sleepiness, and fast breathing. There is an association with maternal lithium use during pregnancy. **PE:** Holosystolic murmur best heard over the left lower sternal border, with widely split S1 and S2. There is tachypnea and hepatomegaly. **Diagnostics:** Echocardiogram: dilated right atrium and right ventricle, tricuspid regurgitation, and significant apical displacement of the valve in the RV. **Management:** • Asymptomatic patients should be monitored for development of arrhythmias and symptoms of heart failure. • Surgical repair is indicated for symptomatic individuals. **Discussion:** Ebstein anomaly is a congenital heart abnormality characterized by inferior displacement of the tricuspid valve, artificially "atrializing" the ventricle. It is associated with right-sided heart failure, tricuspid regurgitation, and arrhythmias arising from accessory conduction pathways. It can also be associated with mild to severe intra-atrial shunt, which can cause cyanosis. Diagram of Ebstein anomaly of the tricuspid valve. Markedly enlarged RA including the atrialized portion of RV is displayed. Right-to-left atrial shunting leading to various degrees of cyanosis may be present. (Reproduced with permission from Suspecting Congenital Heart Disease In: Shahab Noori, Pierre Wong, Practical Neonatal Echocardiography, New York: McGraw Hill, 2018.)

PEDIATRIC GASTROENTEROLOGY

The clinical manifestations of pediatric GI disease will help dictate the differential diagnosis depending on the age of the patient.

Timing of Presentation of Pediatric GI Pathologies

Timing	Key Findings	Diagnostic Consideration(s)
Birth to 24 Hours	Drooling; Difficult feeding	Esophageal atresia ± tracheoesophageal fistula
	Abdominal wall defects	Gastroschisis, omphalocele
	Scaphoid abdomen, respiratory distress	Congenital diaphragmatic Hernia
	Bilious emesis	Malrotation with volvulus Duodenal Atresia Intestinal (jejunal/ileal) atresia
	Failure to pass meconium	Meconium ileus Small bowel obstruction Hirschsprung disease Small left colon syndrome
First Few Weeks of Life	Failure to pass stool regularly	Hirschsprung disease
	Non-bloody, non-bilious emesis	Hypertrophic pyloric stenosis
	Persistent jaundice Conjugated hyperbilirubinemia	Biliary atresia
	Abdominal distension, bilious emesis, bloody stools, sepsis	Necrotizing enterocolitis
Late Infancy and Childhood	Hematochezia, painless	Meckel's diverticulum
	Hematochezia, intermittent abdominal pain	Intussusception
	Abdominal mass	Wilms tumor Neuroblastoma
	Difficulty feeding and respiratory problems	Vascular ring

Emesis

Emesis is a common presentation in newborns and children, and causes can include physiologic, infectious, or anatomic etiologies. Emesis may be broadly categorized as bilious or non-bilious and workup depends upon this categorization. Bilious emesis is always pathologic and suggestive of obstruction distal to the ampulla of Vader.

CASE 14	Bilious Emesis in a Newborn (Malrotation with Volvulus)
	A 5-day-old old boy presents with bilious emesis, passage of one bloody stool, and refusal to feed for 10 hours. He appears lethargic, has a distended abdomen, and gross blood is seen on digital rectal exam. His vital signs are currently stable. IV fluids are begun, and a nasogastric (NG) tube is placed to decompress his stomach.
Conditions with Similar Presentations	**Intestinal malrotation with volvulus:** Congenitally abnormal positioning of the bowel loops within the peritoneal cavity. Predisposes infant to midgut volvulus. **Duodenal atresia:** Failure of the duodenum to recanalize. Inability to swallow will lead to polyhydramnios in utero. Associated with Down syndrome. Abdominal x-ray will show "double bubble sign" (distended stomach and proximal duodenum) with absent distal intestinal gas. **Annular pancreas:** Failure of apoptosis in utero. Presentation is similar to duodenal atresia but is not associated with Down syndrome. **Jejunal atresia:** Etiology attributed to vascular disruptions in utero. Associated with maternal cocaine use. Abdominal x-ray may demonstrate "triple bubble sign" and multiple air-fluid levels.

CASE 14 | **Bilious Emesis in a Newborn (Malrotation with Volvulus)** *(continued)*

Conditions with Similar Presentations	**Necrotizing Enterocolitis:** Seen in preterm or ill infants who develop mucosal or full thickness intestinal necrosis. May present with abdominal distention, intolerance to feeding, vomiting, blood in the stools or diarrhea. **Incarcerated hernia:** May develop any time after birth but most often occurs in babies < 1 year old. May present with irritability, vomiting, poor appetite, tenderness of the groin area and abdominal distention. **Meconium ileus:** Caused by obstruction of the terminal ileus by meconium and comprises 33% of neonatal small bowel obstructions but can also be an early manifestation of cystic fibrosis. May present with abdominal distension, bilious vomiting, no passage of meconium in the first 12 to 24 hours of life, and can be associated with malrotation and intestinal atresia. **Imperforate anus (or anal atresia):** Neonates may also have VACTERL (*v*ertebral anomalies, *a*nal atresia, *c*ardiac malformations, *t*racheoesophageal fistula, *e*sophageal atresia, *r*enal anomalies and *r*adial aplasia, and *l*imb *a*nomalies). If absence of the anus is missed on exam and the baby is fed, signs of bowel obstruction will occur. **Hirschsprung's disease:** Congenital aganglionosis of the lower GI tract, most often the colon, results in partial or total bowel obstruction. May present with inability to pass gas or stool, abdominal distention, and vomiting. Rectal suction biopsy will show the absence of ganglion cells.
Initial Diagnostic Tests	• Plain abdominal x-ray (may demonstrate non-specific obstructive findings) • Transabdominal ultrasound • Upper GI series (barium swallow) may reveal abnormal positioning of the bowel upper GI obstruction at the level of distal duodenum
Next Steps in Management	NPO, suction decompression, surgical intervention if needed

Discussion	Any obstruction distal to the ligament of Treitz can present with bilious emesis. Midgut volvulus is the result of malrotation of a segment of the small intestine around the superior mesenteric artery, which can lead to obstruction, ischemia, and infarction. Failure of complete midgut rotation leads to the small bowel on the right side of the abdomen. Fibrous bands (Ladd bands) can develop and cause duodenal obstruction. Midgut volvulus is a surgical emergency.
	
	History: Bilious emesis, abdominal distension, and hematochezia in an infant
	
	Physical Exam:
	• Abdominal distension and tenderness, with decreased bowel sounds
	• Signs of bowel ischemia and perforation (peritonitis, rigid abdomen, hematochezia)
	
	Diagnostics:
	• Abdominal X-ray: not diagnostic but can exclude acute perforation (which would show pneumoperitoneum); will show dilated loops of bowel and air-fluid levels
	• Transabdominal US: not diagnostic but may show third part of the duodenum is not in the normal retromesenteric position or abnormal position of the superior mesenteric vein (should be anterior or to the left of the superior mesenteric artery)
	• Upper GI series is the gold standard test
	  • Ligament of Treitz on the right side of the abdomen
	  • Duodenum with "corkscrew" appearance
	  • "Beaked" duodenal appearance
	
	Management:
	• NPO with IV fluids
	• Decompression via orogastric or NG tube
	• Emergent surgical repair if patient shows signs of clinical instability (skip imaging and go straight for diagnostic laparotomy or laparoscopy)
	
	Midgut volvulus. Left lateral decubitus radiographs of a 2-month-old infant with a 1-day history of vomiting and progressive abdominal distension show an ileus pattern, with generalized dilation of the intestine and multiple air–fluid levels. (Reproduced with permission from Robert G. Wells, Diagnostic Imaging of Infants and Children; by The McGraw-Hill 2013.)

Additional Considerations	**Surgical Considerations:** Goals of surgery are to relieve the volvulus by turning the bowel counterclockwise and opening the narrow mesenteric pedicle to prevent volvulus from recurring (Ladd procedure). An appendectomy is also performed at the time of the procedure to prevent future diagnostic confusion.

CASE 15 | Hypertrophic Pyloric Stenosis

A 4-week-old boy is brought for evaluation of non-bloody, nonbilious, projectile vomiting after each feed for the past 24 hours. The baby previously had normal feeds. He has no fever or diarrhea. After vomiting, the infant appears hungry and wants to feed, only to vomit again. On exam, a small abdominal mass is palpated in the epigastric area.

Conditions with Similar Presentations	**Tracheoesophageal fistula (TEF):** Non-bilious emesis and drooling starting at day 1 of life. Diagnose with coiling of NG tube on x-ray. Most common type is blind-ending esophagus (esophageal atresia) with Distal TEF. Assess for "VACTERL" anomalies (**V**ertebral defects, **A**nal atresia, **C**ardiac defects, **TE**F, **R**enal defect, **L**imb defects). Requires surgical correction via disconnection of the fistula, closure of hole in the trachea, and anastomosis of the two segments of esophagus.

Gastroesophageal reflux (GER): Physiologic in newborns due to weakened lower esophageal sphincter (LES).

Annular pancreas and intestinal atresia: Can present similarly with vomiting, abdominal distention, and feeding intolerance in this age group. Intestinal atresia would present with bilious vomiting, however duodenal atresia typically presents with non-bilious vomiting and is associated with Down's syndrome.

Gastric Volvulus: this condition is commonly due to rotation of the stomach around the axis running from the cardia to the pylorus. Suspicion is raised if the combined chest/abdominal x-ray shows a left hemidiaphragm abnormality. Abdomen is often soft and non-tender in the early presentation.

Elevated Intracranial Pressure: neonatal brain tumors, diagnosed in the first 4 weeks of life, can present with nonbilious vomiting however they may also have a bulging fontanelle, seizures, focal motor deficits, or other neurological findings. |
Initial Diagnostic Tests	Check abdominal ultrasound and BMP
Next Steps in Management	Hydrate, correct electrolyte abnormalities, then surgery
Discussion	Pyloric stenosis occurs due to a hypertrophied muscularis propria of the pylorus, resulting in gastric outlet obstruction. Typical age at presentation is 2–12 weeks old because it takes time for the muscle to hypertrophy. It is more common in premature births, and first-born male infants are disproportionately affected. Erythromycin and azithromycin treatment are associated with a higher risk of hypertrophic pyloric stenosis. 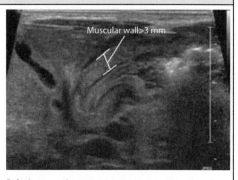 Pyloric stenosis. (Reproduced with permission from C. Keith Stone, Roger L. Humphries, Dorian Drigalla, Maria Stephan, CURRENT Diagnosis & Treatment: Pediatric Emergency Medicine; by McGraw-Hill 2015.) **History:** Persistent, projectile vomiting after feeds **Physical Exam:** Olive-shaped mass and visible peristaltic waves **Diagnostics:** • Abdominal ultrasound will reveal hypertrophied pylorus muscle. • BMP/CMP to evaluate for electrolyte and liver abnormalities. Hypokalemia, hypochloremia, and metabolic alkalosis may occur due to loss of gastric HCl and potassium via emesis. Paradoxical aciduria may occur as the kidneys attempt to retain sodium at the expense of hydrogen ions. **Management:** • Hydrate with IV fluids and correct electrolytes abnormalities • Once rehydrated and electrolytes normalized, treat with surgical pyloromyotomy (laparoscopic or open)

CASE 16 | Hirschsprung Disease

A 24-hour-old boy with trisomy 21 presents with failure to pass meconium, bilious emesis, and abdominal distention.

On physical exam, he has a palpable colon. Digital rectal exam is notable for a tight anal sphincter and explosive passage of stool upon withdrawal of the examining finger.

Conditions with similar presentations	**Imperforate anus:** No anal opening (this is why you should never do the first temperature check rectally!) **Meconium ileus:** Usually associated with cystic fibrosis. Treat and diagnose with water-contrast enema (shows microcolon). Follow up with sweat chloride test, supplement with fat-soluble vitamins (vitamins A, D, E, and K), and pancreatic enzymes.

CASE 16 | Hirschsprung Disease *(continued)*

Initial Diagnostic Tests	• Abdominal x-ray and contrast enema • Confirm with rectal suction biopsy
Next Steps in Management	IV fluids, decompression, and surgical resection
Discussion	Hirschsprung disease is due to a *RET* mutation that causes failure of ganglion migration in the Auerbach and Meissner plexuses. These inhibitory neurons are thus unable to innervate the distal colon, leading to increased tone. The severity of disease is associated with how proximal the de-innervation is. Ninety-nine percent of healthy newborns will pass meconium within the first 24 hours of life, and virtually all healthy newborns will pass meconium within 48 hours of life. Hirschsprung disease is more common in male infants and is associated with Down syndrome. **History:** • Failure to pass meconium in the first 48 hours of life • Symptoms of obstruction due to disinhibited smooth muscle contraction • In less severe cases, can present later in childhood with chronic diarrhea from overflow incontinence **Physical Exam:** • Positive "squirt sign" (explosive passage of stool upon withdrawal of the examining finger) • Palpable colon due to colonic distention proximal to the transition zone **Diagnostics:** • Abdominal x-ray: shows dilation of proximal bowel with absence of air in the rectum • Contrast enema: funnel-shaped transition zone • Rectal suction biopsy (gold standard): absence of ganglion cells in Auerbach and Meissner plexuses and increased tone in the distal colon **Management:** • IV fluids • Decompression and surgical resection of the aganglionic segment of bowel
Additional Considerations	**Surgical Considerations:** The pull-through procedure involves removal of the aganglionic colon and subsequent end-to-end anastomosis of the normal colon to the rectum. Patients with Hirschsprung disease should be assessed for other VACTERL anomalies (see Case 15).

Abdominal Pain

CASE 17 | Intussusception

A 2-year-old boy is brought to the ED for evaluation of acute lower abdominal pain. The mother says the patient started crying inconsolably with legs drawn up to his abdomen 4 hours ago. The pain subsided after 2 hours but recurred an hour later. The mother noted stool with mixed mucous and blood in the toddler's diaper. Of note, the patient recovered from a mild upper respiratory infection 2 weeks ago. On exam, vitals are unremarkable. The patient's abdomen is rigid with diffuse abdominal tenderness. A sausage-shaped abdominal mass is palpated in the RUQ.

Conditions with Similar Presentations	**Constipation:** Due to introduction of solid food, cow's milk, or low-fiber diet (see Constipation mini-case). **Meckel diverticulum:** Is the most common congenital abnormality of the small intestine, which results from incomplete closure of the vitelline (omphalo-mesenteric) duct. Although Meckel diverticulum can be a lead point causing intussusception, the typical presentation is painless hematochezia in a child (see Meckel Diverticulum mini-case).
Initial Diagnostic Tests	Ultrasound of the abdomen
Next Steps in Management	Air enema or reduce telescoping bowel via hydrostatic edema (contrast/saline) with or without ultrasound/fluoroscopic guidance.

CASE 17 | Intussusception *(continued)*

Discussion	Intussusception is the result of telescoping of a part of the intestine into itself and often occurs at the ileocecal junction. When the ileum telescopes into the cecum, pain, obstruction, edema, and compression of blood vessels occur. This leads to bowel ischemia and subsequent rectal bleeding ("currant jelly" stools).	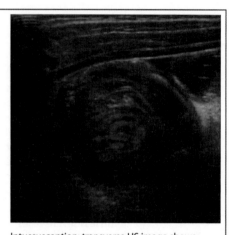
	Most cases occur in infants/toddlers. A lead point can be from Meckel diverticulum (children), Peyer patch hypertrophy, mass/tumor (adults), or idiopathic. Can be associated with Henoch-Schönlein purpura (HSP), rotavirus vaccine, or a recent viral infection.	Intussusception: transverse US image shows target sign (concentric rings of hyperechogenicity and hypoechogenicity). (Reproduced with permission from Warren P. Bishop, Pediatric Practice: Gastroenterology; by The McGraw-Hill 2010.)
	History: The classic triad is crampy/intermittent abdominal pain, vomiting, and currant jelly stools.	
	Physical Exam: Diffuse abdominal tenderness, sausage-shaped abdominal mass, relief of pain by drawing legs up to chest.	
	Diagnostics: Ultrasound is the diagnostic method of choice and can show "target sign," which is a cross-section of the telescoping bowel.	
	Management: • Initial treatment is reduction with enemas • Surgery is indicated if enemas fail, if symptoms are worrisome for perforation or peritonitis, or there is repeated recurrence of intussusception • Surgery would require resection of the telescoped bowel due to ischemia.	

Abdominal Pain Mini-Cases

Case	Key Findings
Constipation	**Hx/PE: Risk factors:** Cow's milk consumption >24 oz a day, low-fiber diet, or recent potty training. Symptoms: Difficulty defecating and producing small, pellet-like stools. May have abdominal tenderness, specifically in LLQ
	Diagnostics: Clinical diagnosis
	Management: • Limit cow's milk to <24 oz a day • Take a break from potty training • Increase fiber and water intake • Consider stool softeners and behavioral changes (sitting on the toilet after each meal). • If persistent and severe, consider disimpaction under anesthesia.
	Discussion: Recent initiation of solid food or cow's milk is a risk factor. School entry is also a risk factor and may contribute to voluntary holding due to fear of pain or embarrassment. Patients with cognitive impairment at higher risk. Patient may have overflow incontinence or encopresis.
Incarcerated Inguinal Hernia	**Hx/PE:** Often present in infancy with symptoms of bilious vomiting May have abdominal distention, inguinal or scrotal mass or fullness
	Diagnostics: • Abdominal X-ray will demonstrate a mechanical bowel obstruction and thickened inguinal-scrotal fold with or without bowel gas in the hemiscrotum
	Management: • Requires emergent reduction and can be attempted manually if patient is stable. • Manual reduction has a high success rate, and surgical repair is done electively afterward.
	Discussion: • Incarceration of inguinal hernias is one of the most common causes of bowel obstruction in infancy. • Inguinal hernias occur due to a patent processus vaginalis and are more frequent in premature than term infants and the ratio in boys to girls is 8:1. • Due to high risk of incarceration, inguinal hernias are surgically repaired even when asymptomatic

Hematochezia

Hematochezia Mini-Cases

Cases	Findings
Necrotizing Enterocolitis	**Hx/PE:** Preterm newborn with feeding intolerance, abdominal distension, and bloody stools. May have lethargy, signs of septic shock, abdominal distension and tenderness. **Diagnostics:** X-ray showing pneumatosis intestinalis (air in the wall of the bowel) and/or pneumoperitoneum. **Management:** • Bowel rest (NPO), gastric decompression • Start on TPN and broad-spectrum IV antibiotics. • Consider surgery if no improvement or worsening condition (free air on imaging, persistent acidosis, peritonitis – all which suggest ischemic or necrotic bowel). • Resection of necrotic bowel is necessary but can result in short-bowel syndrome, defined as <30cm of viable small bowel remaining Necrotizing enterocolitis, with portal venous gas. There is extensive gas within the portal veins (*arrows*) on this abdominal radiograph of a 3-week-old infant. There is distention of the bowel with gas, but only minimal pneumatosis intestinalis. (Reproduced with permission from Robert G. Wells, Diagnostic Imaging of Infants and Children; by The McGraw-Hill 2013.)
Meckel Diverticulum	**Hx/PE:** Painless hematochezia in a child. Physical exam is normal, unless there are complications associated with the diverticulum. Complications may present as abdominal distension or tenderness. Blood may be present on rectal exam. **Diagnostics:** Meckel scan showing uptake of 99m technetium pertechnetate by ectopic gastric mucosa. 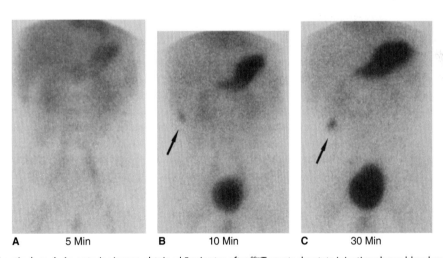 A 5 Min B 10 Min C 30 Min Meckel diverticulum. A. An anterior image obtained 5 minutes after 99mTc-pertechnetate injection shows blood pool activity and normal early accumulation in the stomach wall. B. At 10 minutes, there is a small focus of abnormal uptake in the right upper quadrant (*arrow*). Blood pool activity has faded and there is normal accumulation in the stomach and urinary system. C. The 30-minute image demonstrates progressive uptake in the ectopic gastric mucosa. (Reproduced with permission from Robert G. Wells, Diagnostic Imaging of Infants and Children; by The McGraw-Hill 2013.) **Management:** Surgical resection of the diverticulum **Discussion:** Most common malformation of small bowel, can be a lead point causing intussusception. Rule of twos: • 2% of the population, though only 2% are symptomatic • Location within 2 feet of the ileocecal valve • 2 inches in length • 2 types of heterotopic mucosa: gastric and pancreatic • Presentation before the age of 2.

Congenital GI Defects

	Pathophysiology	Symptoms	Diagnosis	Treatment
Diaphragmatic hernia (Bochdalek)	Opening in diaphragm allows bowel in chest, leading to hypoplastic lung development	Scaphoid abdomen, bowel sounds in chest, respiratory distress; most common on left.	X-ray	Corticosteroids to help develop the lung. Surgical repair of the diaphragm
Gastroschisis	Paraumbilical herniation, usually to right of umbilicus	Bowel protruding outside of abdominal wall, not contained in a membrane	Clinical	Sterile wrap around bowel, surgery via primary closure if possible. Otherwise silicone silo used to cover the defect.
Omphalocele	Failure of midgut to return to abdominal cavity	Bowel protruding out midline, contained in a membrane	Clinical	Sterile wrap around bowel, surgery via primary closure if possible. Otherwise silicone silo used to cover the defect
Exstrophy of bladder	Unknown	Midline defect that is wet with urine, shiny, red	Clinical	Surgical repair
Biliary atresia	Obliteration of extrahepatic biliary system	Jaundice, dark urine, pale stools, hepatomegaly, conjugated hyperbilirubinemia, elevated transaminases	RUQ US showing paucity of ducts, HIDA scan after 7 days of phenobarbital	Hepatoportoenterostomy (Kasai procedure)
Cleft lip/palate	Failure of growth plates to properly fuse	Failure to thrive due to inability to latch, recurrent infections	Clinical	Surgery

PEDIATRIC GENETICS

Genetic conditions in the pediatric population are causes of acute and chronic diseases, and timing of presentation will vary depending on the pathophysiology of the condition. Genetic abnormalities may produce structural disorders, metabolic derangements, or disorders associated with intellectual impairment. Focus on illness scripts and pattern recognition.

Chromosomal abnormalities may arise de novo or may be inherited from one or both parents. Most chromosomal abnormalities will result in spontaneous abortions, thus it's important to obtain a maternal obstetric history. Although a genetic condition may be present at birth, the symptomatology may present over time. In counseling the parents, it is important to provide anticipatory guidance on what other signs and symptoms may present at different times in childhood. It is also important to inform the parents on their risk of producing a child with a similar condition in future pregnancies.

Inborn Errors of Metabolism

Inborn errors of metabolism are a heterogeneous group of disorders that may be inherited or may occur spontaneously. These varied conditions share an inability to break down or store carbohydrates, fatty acids, and proteins. These disorders can present at any age and symptoms are dependent on which organ systems are involved. When an infant or child presents with symptoms suggestive of an inborn error of metabolism, it is important to obtain a thorough family history and organize the presenting symptoms so that the appropriate workup can be performed and the appropriate cause of the symptoms identified.

Infants with inborn errors of metabolism which affect the brain may present with microcephaly, developmental delay, abnormalities of tone, and seizures. Inborn errors of metabolism may also negatively affect nutritional status, leading to recurrent emesis and failure to thrive. These infants may present with hypoglycemia or sequelae of hypoglycemia or lethargy. Laboratory tests and lab abnormalities are specific to the condition that is presenting. Some inborn errors of metabolism will present with elevated ammonia levels or metabolic acidosis.

Inborn Errors of Metabolism Tested on Newborn Screen

CASE 18	Classic Galactosemia
A 1-week-old girl who is breastfed is brought in for evaluation due to poor feeding, vomiting, and lethargy. Physical exam is notable for hepatomegaly, jaundice, and presence of opacification of the lens in each eye.	
Conditions with Similar Presentations	**TORCH infections:** Can present with congenital cataracts. Not associated with hepatomegaly. **Hereditary fructose intolerance:** Hereditary disorder due to the absence of aldolase B enzyme. In the absence of this enzyme, patients are unable to digest fructose. This can also lead to hypoglycemia, but presents later than galactosemia once fruit or fructose is added to the diet.
Initial Diagnostic Tests	Confirm diagnosis with erythrocyte galactose-1-phosphate uridyl transferase (GALT) enzyme activity and molecular genetic testing for the *GALT* gene. • Also check serum glucose, AST/ALT.
Next Steps in Management	• Remove lactose and galactose from the diet. • In infants, switch to soy-based formula.
Discussion	Galactosemia is an inherited disorder of carbohydrate metabolism that prevents the body from converting galactose to glucose and presents a few days after birth. Classic galactosemia is an autosomal recessive disorder due to the absence of the rate-limiting enzyme of galactose metabolism, galactose-1-phosphate uridyltransferase. Patients with galactosemia become hypoglycemic within several hours of exposure to galactose, a breakdown product of the lactose present in both breast milk and most formulas. **History:** Newborn infant develops failure to thrive, jaundice, hepatomegaly, infantile cataracts, and eventually intellectual disability. **Physical Exam:** Hepatomegaly, jaundice, and bilateral cataracts **Diagnostics:** Presence of galactose in the blood and urine. Check: • Erythrocyte GALT enzyme activity • Molecular genetic testing for *GALT* gene Additional tests: low glucose, elevated transaminases **Management:** • Lactose-free formula in the neonatal period • Lifelong elimination of lactose and galactose • Referral to ophthalmology
Additional Considerations	**Screening:** Newborn screening in all 50 states includes testing for classic galactosemia. **Complications:** Classic galactosemia predisposes infants to *E. coli* sepsis because there is impairment of cellular release of superoxide ion by galactose, and this leads to inhibition of leucocyte bactericidal activity.

CASE 19	Phenylketonuria (PKU)
A 2-year-old boy is brought in for evaluation of progressive developmental delays and growth retardation over the last year. He was born at term after an uneventful pregnancy. His parents have noticed a distinct musty body odor. On physical exam, his height and weight are below the fifth percentile for age, and he has light-colored hair and eyes.	
Conditions with Similar Presentations	**Tetrahydrobiopterin deficiency:** Genetic disorder that results in the inability to break down phenylalanine due to the absence of tetrahydrobiopterin, which is a cofactor for phenylalanine hydroxylase. Infants are normal at birth, but the increased phenylalanine leads to intellectual disability, movement disorders, and seizures.
Initial Diagnostic Tests	• Check phenylalanine, tyrosine and tetrahydrobiopterin levels • Perform genetic testing
Next Steps in Management	• Restrict phenylalanine in the diet. • Increase tyrosine and tetrahydrobiopterin cofactor.
Discussion	PKU is the most common inherited defect in amino acid metabolism and is an autosomal recessive disorder involving a mutation in the enzyme phenylalanine hydroxylase (PAH), which converts phenylalanine to tyrosine. PKU can also be caused in rare instances by disorders of tetrahydrobiopterin (BH4) synthesis, which is a PAH cofactor.

CASE 19 | Phenylketonuria (PKU) *(continued)*

Discussion	**History:** • Newborns have no symptoms due to clearance of phenylalanine by the placenta • Delayed development, seizures, a musty body odor due to increased concentrations of phenylacetic acid, and behavioral problems **Physical Exam:** Microcephaly, developmental delay, hypopigmentation (due to deficiency of tyrosine, the starting point of melanin synthesis) **Diagnostics:** Confirm Diagnosis: • ↑ Serum phenylalanine levels • Urine is positive for phenylketones • ↓Serum tyrosine and ↓tetrahydrobiopterin levels • Genetic testing shows a mutation in phenylalanine hydroxylase **Management:** • Restrict phenylalanine and increase tyrosine in the diet. • Tetrahydrobiopterin cofactor supplementation.
Additional Considerations	**Screening:** Newborn screening is widely practiced, allowing initiation of a phenylalanine-restricted diet before the onset of neurological damage. **Complications:** Dietary management generally reverses all signs of PKU except cognitive impairment that developed prior to initiation of treatment.

Lysosomal Storage Diseases (LSDs)

LSDs are inborn errors of metabolism characterized by excess production of substrates due to abnormalities in the body's lysosomes. LSDs may be due to an enzyme defect or dysfunction in a membrane protein. Due to the genetic defect, there is an accumulation of toxic substances in specific organs which leads to the symptomatology. Signs and symptoms may be more severe in children than in adults due to the effects of the accumulated substances on the developing brain.

Early diagnosis can be helpful in preventing the morbidity associated with some LSDs. Many states in the U.S. screen for these diseases at birth. Treatment options differ depending on the diagnosis. While there is currently no cure for LSDs, some can be treated by replacing the missing enzyme or through stem cell transplants.

Lysosomal Storage Disease	Deficient Enzyme	Accumulated Substance	Clinical Findings	Treatment
Tay-Sachs disease	Hexosaminidase A	Ganglioside	Cherry red spot in the macula, seizures, developmental delay, "onion skin" lysosomes	Supportive care
Niemann-Pick disease	Sphingomyelinase	Sphingomyelin	Cherry red spot in the macula, hepatosplenomegaly, progressive neurodegeneration, foam cells	Supportive care
Gaucher disease	β-glucocerebrosidase	Glucocerebroside	Onset by 2 years of age, aseptic necrosis of the femur, lytic bone lesions, Gaucher cells, hepatosplenomegaly	Enzyme replacement
Fabry disease	α-galactosidase A	Ceramide trihexoside	Older age of onset—around 5 years of age, peripheral neuropathy, angiokeratomas	Enzyme replacement
Krabbe disease	Galactocerebrosidase	Glucocerebroside	Severe developmental delay, hypotonia, optic atrophy	Supportive care; early hematopoietic stem cell transplant is associated with longer survival
Metachromatic leukodystrophy	Arylsulfatase A	Cerebroside sulfate	Regression of motor skills, ataxia, hypotonia, seizures, intellectual impairment, or dementia	Supportive care

CASE 20 | Tay-Sachs Disease

A 10-month-old infant is brought in for evaluation of new-onset seizures and gradual loss of skills like sitting and grasping. She has become less interactive and has lost interest in eating. On exam, she is underweight and her funduscopic exam reveals a central area of reddening in the retina bilaterally (see image). She has exaggerated reactions to loud noises and muscle weakness.

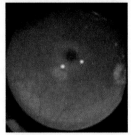

Reproduced with permission from Gregg T. Lueder, Pediatric Practice: Ophthalmology; by The McGraw-Hill 2011.

Conditions with Similar Presentations	**Niemann-Pick disease:** Patients will also have a cherry-red spot on the macula but will have hepatomegaly, which is not seen in Tay-Sachs. **Krabbe disease:** Autosomal recessive neurodegenerative disorder due to a deficiency in galactocerebrosidase enzyme. Presents similar to Tay-Sachs with onset in infancy and progression to death by 2 years of age. Genetic testing helps differentiate between the two.
Initial Diagnostic Tests	• Check levels of hexosaminidase A in serum and genetic testing • Consider MRI of the brain
Next Steps in Management	Supportive care
Discussion	Tay-Sachs is an autosomal recessive lysosomal storage disorder caused by a defect in the enzyme hexosaminidase A, resulting in accumulation of GM2 ganglioside, especially in neurons, where they are toxic and lead to neurodegenerative symptoms. Onset of symptoms occurs during infancy and progresses to death by 3–5 years of age. The late onset and adult forms have slower progression. **History:** Infant with new-onset seizures, exaggerated startle, and gradual loss of strength and developmental skills. There may be a family history of neurodegenerative diseases. **Physical Exam:** On exam, patients have a "cherry-red spot" on the macula (as seen in preceding image). Other features include hypotonia, seizures, blindness, macrocephaly, hyperreflexia. **Diagnostics:** Confirm Diagnosis: • Low serum levels of hexosaminidase A activity • Biopsy of affected tissue shows lysosomes with an "onion skin" morphology • Genetic testing reveals HEXA mutation **Management:** • There is no definitive treatment. • Supportive care: Provide adequate nutrition, physical and speech therapy. • Death is usually secondary to pneumonia and occurs on average between ages 2 and 5.
Additional Considerations	**Screening:** Pre-conception genetic testing should be offered to couples with higher risk, including those with a family history consistent with Tay-Sachs, or for couples where at least one member is of Ashkenazi Jewish, French-Canadian, or Louisiana Cajun descent. It may also be offered to members of the Pennsylvania Dutch community.

Glycogen Storage Disorders (GSD)

GSDs are a group of conditions caused by a defect in enzymes used to break down glycogen. Glycogen is primarily stored in the liver and is broken down into glucose when the body needs an energy source. GSDs primarily affect the liver and/or skeletal muscle.

The inability to break down glycogen leads to glycogen accumulation in the liver and ensuing hepatomegaly. Glycogen accumulation in muscle tissue will lead to easy fatigability during exercise and muscle damage. Additionally, the inability to break glycogen down into glucose will lead to the development of hypoglycemia. Similar to lysosomal storage disorders, no curative treatment exists for GSDs.

Disorder (GSD Type)	Deficient Enzyme	Clinical Findings	Treatment
Von Gierke (Type I)	Glucose-6-phosphatase	Doll-like facies, hypoglycemia, hepatomegaly	Corn starch, allopurinol, G-CSF
Pompe (Type II)	Lysosomal acid maltase	Hypotonia, macroglossia, hepatomegaly, hypertrophic cardiomyopathy	Enzyme replacement therapy
Cori (Type III)	Debranching enzyme	Hepatomegaly, hypoglycemia	High-protein diet; liver transplant
Andersen (Type IV)	Glycogen branching enzyme	Failure to thrive, hypoglycemia, liver failure	Liver transplant
McArdle (Type V)	Muscle phosphorylase deficiency	Fatigability, myoglobinuria during exercise, second-wind phenomenon	Sucrose before exercise

CASE 21 | Glycogen Storage Disease Type I (Von Gierke Disease)

A 4-month-old infant is brought to the ED with irritability, rapid breathing, and cold-like symptoms. Parents report that episodes of fussiness occur when the baby doesn't feed for >4 hours. Exam is notable for hepatomegaly. Labs show hypoglycemia and lactic acidosis.

Conditions with Similar Presentations	**Cori disease:** Also presents with hypoglycemia and hepatomegaly. The main symptom will be muscle weakness.
	Galactosemia: May also present with hepatomegaly and hypoglycemia but infants will usually be jaundiced.
Initial Diagnostic Tests	• Confirm diagnosis with genetic testing • Also check fasting glucose, BMP, lipid panel, lactic acid level, uric acid level and abdominal ultrasound
Next Steps in Management	Frequent oral glucose and limit intake of lactose, galactose, fructose, and sucrose
Discussion	Patients with Von Gierke disease have an autosomal recessive defect in the glucose-6-phosphatase enzyme, preventing glucose-6-phosphate from being converted into glucose during gluconeogenesis. Affected patients present between 3–6 months of age, around the time when they increase the spacing of their feeds (when they start sleeping through the night). **History:** Symptoms of hypoglycemia (irritability, tachypnea, tremors, or seizures), poor growth, and protuberant abdomen. **Physical Exam:** Exam is significant for prominent hepatomegaly. There may also be doll-like facies (fat cheeks), growth failure with thin legs, and hypotonia. **Diagnostics:** • Labs show hypoglycemia, lactic acidemia, hypertriglyceridemia, and hyperuricemia • Genetic testing reveals mutation in the genes that code for synthesis of or transport of glucose 6-phosphatase (glucose-6-phosphatase, or glucose-6-phosphate translocase). • A liver biopsy is rarely necessary. If performed, the liver biopsy will show prominent storage of glycogen and steatosis but minimal fibrosis. **Management:** • Frequent feedings or cornstarch • Avoid fruit juices, high-fructose corn syrup, and sorbital • Limit intake of lactose, galactose, fructose, and sucrose as these also depend on glucose-6-phosphatase for metabolism
Additional Considerations	**Screening:** Genetic testing should be performed in patients with suggestive history, physical exam, and constellation of lab findings described earlier
	Complications: Renal disease, pulmonary hypertension, osteoporosis hepatic adenomas (with rare conversion to hepatocellular carcinoma) are known long-term complications of GSD I and should be screened for.
	Surgical Considerations: Liver transplant may be indicated in patients with poor metabolic control, liver failure, or hepatocellular carcinoma.

Glycogen Storage Disease Mini-Cases

Case	Key Findings
Type V (McArdle Disease)	**Hx:** A 17-year-old boy presents with years of myalgias, cramps, and poor endurance. Symptoms are worse with moderate exercise and improve after a brief period of rest. He also notes red urine after moderate activity. **PE:** Muscle stiffness, pain, and weakness are inducible with exercise, but exam is otherwise unremarkable. **Diagnostics:** • Blood glucose is normal. • Forearm exercise test (patient performs maximal effort handgrips for 1 minute, then blood samples drawn) show inability to produce lactate. **Management:** While no cure is available, diet and exercise strategies like consuming sucrose before low to moderate activity can help control symptoms. **Discussion:** Glycogen storage disease type V (McArdle disease) is an autosomal recessive deficiency of skeletal muscle glycogen phosphorylase (myophosphorylase). Because it only involves skeletal muscle, blood glucose levels are unaffected (unlike in Von Gierke disease). The key features are exercise intolerance and myoglobinuria with exercise. There is a characteristic "second wind" phenomenon, improvement in symptoms about 10 minutes into exercise. This is due to an enhanced sympathoadrenal response and improved delivery of free fatty acids and glucose to working muscles.
Type II (Pompe Disease)	**Hx:** A newborn is noted to have hypotonia and a heart murmur after an uncomplicated birth. **PE:** On physical exam, notable findings include macroglossia, hepatomegaly, and severe hypotonia **Diagnostics:** • Echocardiogram shows severe biventricular cardiac hypertrophy. • Labs show normal glucose and increased serum lactate, CK, AST, and ALT. • Lysosomal enzyme acid-α-1,4-glucosidase activity is low. **Management:** Enzyme replacement therapy with alglucosidase alfa **Discussion:** Pompe disease (GSD Type II) is an autosomal recessive condition involving deficiency in the lysosomal acid α-1,4-glucosidase (acid maltase) enzyme. Early-onset Pompe disease presents in the first year, as a floppy-baby with severe hypotonia and cardiac abnormalities including cardiomegaly and hypertrophic cardiomyopathy. Other symptoms include exercise intolerance, hypotonia, failure to thrive, hepatomegaly, and other systemic findings such as respiratory failure, which can lead to early death. Glucose levels are normal in Pompe disease, helping differentiate it from Von Gierke disease.

Genetic Disorders Involving Chromosomes

CASE 22 | Prader-Willi Syndrome

A 14-year-old boy is brought to clinic for evaluation of hypotonia and intellectual disability. His mother notes that he had feeding difficulties as an infant, but since then has developed an insatiable appetite and behavioral problems. The boy has dysmorphic facial features and is obese with a BMI of 31 kg/m².

Conditions with Similar Presentations	**Autism spectrum disorder (ASD):** Patients with ASD have developmental delay, but lack the polyphagia seen in PWS and would not have dysmorphic facial features. **Fragile X syndrome:** Will also present with obesity and intellectual disability. Patients with Fragile X do not have the facial features associated with PWS or the neonatal history of poor feeding.
Initial Diagnostic Tests	• Confirm Diagnosis: Genetic testing • Consider: TSH, free T4, ACTH, hemoglobin A1c to rule out other causes or identify comorbid conditions
Next Steps in Management	• Strict supervision of food intake • Genetic counseling and growth hormone supplementation

CASE 22 | Prader-Willi Syndrome *(continued)*

Discussion	Prader-Willi Syndrome (PWS) is a genetic disorder that results in obesity, developmental delay, and polyphagia. PWS is a disorder of genomic imprinting. The maternal copy of chromosome segment 15q11-13 is normally methylated so that only the paternal copy is expressed. In PWS, the paternal copy is missing or mutated, and the maternal copy is imprinted as usual, resulting in a lack of expression of the segment 15q11-13. About 25% of cases are caused by uniparental disomy, in which the child receives two maternal copies and both are silenced through genetic imprinting.
	History: Patients present with hypotonia, lethargy, and feeding difficulties at birth, which gradually resolve. Prenatally there is often decreased fetal movement, small for gestational age, polyhydramnios, and breech positioning. At birth there is a weak suck. Hyperphagia develops by 2 years of age which often results in obesity. Other features include intellectual disability and late acquisition of major milestones such as walking and talking.
	Physical Exam: Physical exam reveals characteristic facies and features (almond-shaped eyes, narrow forehead, short stature, small hands and feet), diminished muscle tone, hyporeflexia, and hypogonadism.
	Diagnostics: Genetic testing shows deletion of the paternal chromosome 15q11-13, and DNA methylation studies show methylation on maternal chromosome 15q.
	Management: • Symptomatic treatment and strict supervision of food intake • Genetic counseling • Growth hormone supplementation to address short stature. Growth hormone will also help decrease body fat and increase muscle mass.
Additional Considerations	**Complications:** Significant obesity and related complications often develop, including type 2 diabetes mellitus and sleep apnea. Hypothyroidism and osteoporosis may also develop.

Chromosomal Genetic Disorders Associated with Intellectual Impairment Mini-Cases

Angelman Syndrome	**Hx:** A 2-year-old girl presents for evaluation of new-onset tonic-clonic seizures. Parents report that she is a happy child who frequently laughs and smiles, and that she is fascinated with water. She has a history of developmental delay and microcephaly.
	PE: Exam reveals a child with a smiling demeanor who sits flapping her hands repeatedly. She has an ataxic gait and microcephaly.
	Diagnostics: Genetic testing reveals absence or mutation of maternal alleles on chromosome 15, most commonly *UBE3A*.
	Management: Treatment is supportive, focused on seizure and sleep disorder management. Physical, occupational, and speech therapy are recommended.
	Discussion: Angelman syndrome is a disorder of genomic imprinting resulting from the absence or mutation of maternal alleles on chromosome 15. Normally, the paternally derived copy is methylated and silenced, and the maternally derived copy is expressed. In Angelman syndrome, there is a mutation or deletion in the maternal copy. Clinical features include severe intellectual disability, movement disorders, seizures, developmental delays, learning disabilities, ataxia, and decreased to absent speech. There is a distinct pattern of unprovoked episodes of laughter and smiling.
Rett Syndrome	**Hx:** A previously healthy 2-year-old girl is brought to the clinic for concerns of increasing clumsiness. Additionally, the patient was initially speaking, but she is no longer using words and appears less interested in interacting with her parents. Parents report that the patient used to feed herself and play well with toys, but she no longer seems able to.
	PE: Review of the patient's growth curve shows deceleration of head growth, and exam shows repetitive hand motions.
	Diagnostics: Genetic testing reveals X-linked mutation in *MECP2*.
	Management: Treatment is supportive, including management of seizures and sleep disorders, careful nutritional monitoring, and monitoring of the QTc due to increased frequency of prolonged QT syndrome.
	Discussion: Like Angelman syndrome, Rett syndrome is seen almost exclusively in girls. Key differences include lack of episodes of inappropriate laughter seen in Angelman syndrome. Males with Rett syndrome die in utero or shortly after birth.

CASE 23 | Trisomy 21 (Down Syndrome)

A newborn baby boy born to a 42-year-old mother is noted to have hypotonia and dysmorphic features. He has a flat occiput with bilateral epicanthal folds, a short neck, and short, broad hands with a single horizontal palmar crease. A 3/6 systolic ejection murmur is auscultated at the upper left sternal border.

Conditions with Similar Presentations	**Edwards syndrome (trisomy 18):** After Down syndrome, this is the second most common viable chromosomal abnormality (1 in 5,00 live births). It is an autosomal trisomy characterized by three copies of chromosome 18 due to meiotic nondisjunction, translocation, or mosaicism. Infants with trisomy 18 are born with multiple congenital anomalies. Most notable are low birth weight, prominent occiput, low-set ears, a small jaw (micrognathia), and tightly clenched fingers. Congenital malformations, especially congenital heart disease, are common. First-trimester screening shows decreased alpha-fetoprotein, decreased beta-HCG, decreased estriol, and decreased or normal inhibin A. Clenched fists and rocker bottom feet are often seen on ultrasonography and after birth. Death usually occurs by age 1. **Patau syndrome (trisomy 13):** The rarest viable autosomal trisomy. Infants with trisomy 13 are born with low birth weight and have multiple congenital anomalies, affecting the heart (congenital heart disease), brain (holoprosencephaly), and kidneys (polycystic kidney disease). Most notable are facial anomalies, including hypotelorism (eyes are closer together than normal), cleft lip and palate, microphthalmia (small eyes), and microcephaly. There may be cutis aplasia (areas of absent skin in the scalp), polydactyly. The first-trimester screen shows decreased free beta-HCG and decreased PAPP-A. Death usually occurs by age 1.
Initial Diagnostic Tests	Confirm diagnosis with chromosomal karyotype
Next Steps in Management	Supportive measures
Discussion	Trisomy 21 is an autosomal trisomy characterized by three copies of chromosome 21. Nondisjunction during meiosis leads to three copies of chromosome 21. It is the most common viable chromosomal disorder (1 in 730 live births) and the most common cause of non-inherited genetic intellectual disability. Most cases occur de novo, but risk is increased with advancing maternal age. **History:** Newborns with hypotonia and characteristic facies should raise suspicion for trisomy 21. Congenital heart defects (especially endocardial cushion defects), duodenal atresia, and Hirschsprung disease are all associated with trisomy 21. **Physical Exam:** Characteristic physical features include flat facies, prominent epicanthal eye folds, furrowed tongue, atlantoaxial instability, short fingers and toes, clinodactyly (curved fifth finger), and a wide space between the first and second toes. **Diagnostics:** Diagnosis is often made via prenatal screening but is confirmed with a karyotype. Karyotyping shows 47, XY+21 or 47, XX+21. **Management:** Supportive measures, including early occupational, physical, and speech therapy referrals and screening for common complications including cardiac and GI conditions.
Additional Considerations	**Screening:** All women should be offered aneuploidy screening in early pregnancy. Cell-free DNA from maternal serum is a useful first-trimester screening test. First-trimester ultrasound will show increased nuchal lucency and hypoplastic nasal bone. Second-trimester labs from maternal serum show decreased alpha-fetoprotein, increased beta-HCG, decreased estriol, and increased inhibin A. **Complications:** There is an increased risk of leukemia (AML and ALL). In adulthood they are at risk for early-onset Alzheimer disease because amyloid precursor protein is found on chromosome 21. Patients are also at risk for thyroid disease, vision and hearing difficulties, obstructive sleep apnea, and obesity.

PEDIATRIC IMMUNOLOGY

Children with primary immunodeficiencies will present with recurrent infections. In the neonatal period, immunoglobulins are transferred from mother to child through the placenta. Therefore, some immunodeficiencies will not present until these immunoglobulins are no longer present at 4–6 months of age. The recurrent infections that occur in children with primary immunodeficiencies tend to occur in the respiratory system, GI tract, or the skin.

Type of Immunodeficiencies and Examples	Common Presentations	Causative Organisms
B-cell deficiencies • *X-linked agammaglobulinemia*	Sinopulmonary infections (otitis media, sinusitis, pneumonia)	• *Streptococcus pneumoniae* • *Haemophilus influenzae* • *Staphylococcus aureus*
T-cell deficiencies • *Severe combined immunodeficiency (SCID)* • *DiGeorge syndrome* • *Hyper-IgE syndrome*	Sinopulmonary infections (otitis media, sinusitis, pneumonia) Skin infections	• *Streptococcus pneumoniae* • *Haemophilus influenzae* • *Staphylococcus aureus* • *Candida albicans* • *Pneumocystis jirovecii* • Toxoplasmosis • Viral infections

Phagocytic Disorders
 • *Chronic granulomatosis disease (CGD)*
 • *Leukocyte adhesion deficiency (LAD)*
	Mucous membrane infections, poor wound healing	• Catalase-producing organisms
		   • *S. aureus*
		   • *Aspergillus*
		   • *Serratia*
		   • *Nocardia*

B Cell Defects

CASE 24	X-Linked (Bruton) Agammaglobulinemia (XLA)

An 18-month-old boy is brought to clinic for fever and right ear pain over the past 2 days. Review of his medical records reveals frequent visits for otitis media and several episodes of pneumococcal pneumonia over the last 12 months. In addition, his maternal uncle had many infections as a child, one of which ultimately led to his death. The patient's temperature is 39.2°C, pulse is 138/min, respirations are 26/min, and blood pressure is 100/52 mmHg. Bulging of the right tympanic membrane with obscured landmarks is present. Examination of the oropharynx reveals very small tonsils. No skin lesions are noted.

Conditions with Similar Presentations	Other B cell deficiencies such as transient hypogammaglobulinemia of infancy (THI), hyper IgM syndrome, common variable immunodeficiency (CVID), and cystic fibrosis (CF) may present with recurrent sinopulmonary infections with encapsulated organisms (*Haemophilus influenzae, Streptococcus pneumoniae, Neisseria meningitidis*) in children. **THI:** Similarly characterized by increased susceptibility to infections at around 6 months of age, when transplacental maternal IgG is no longer active. B-cell levels are normal and THI spontaneously resolves around age 2–5 years. **CVID:** Characterized by decreased plasma cells with resultant immunoglobulins of all classes. It presents later in life (15–35 years) and is less severe than XLA, however patients are at increased risk for autoimmune disease, lymphoma, and bronchiectasis. **Hyper-IgM syndrome:** Presents as recurrent infections at a young age due to defective CD40L on T-helper (Th) cells. B cells cannot undergo class switching and thus only continue to produce IgM. This leads to low levels of IgA, IgG, and IgE, and thus poor opsonization and insufficient antibody response to protein and polysaccharide. **CF:** Often diagnosed on the newborn screen. In children >1 year of age, CF can present similarly with failure to thrive (FTT) and recurrent respiratory infections. Meconium ileus at birth may occur.
Initial Diagnostic Tests	Check: • CBC with differential • Quantitative serum immunoglobulin levels (IgG, IgA, and IgM)
Next Steps in Management	• IVIG and prophylactic antibiotics
Discussion	XLA is a B-cell deficiency found in boys characterized by severe hypogammaglobulinemia, and increased susceptibility to infection. Defects in Bruton tyrosine kinase (BTK) gene lead to failure of B-cell development. Immunoglobulins of all classes are decreased, and patients are prone to recurrent bacterial, enteroviral, and giardia infections, especially after 6 months of age when maternal immunoglobulins have decreased. Infection from encapsulated organisms like *S pneumoniae*, *Pseudomonas*, and *Haemophilus* can be life-threatening.

CASE 24 | X-Linked (Bruton) Agammaglobulinemia (XLA) *(continued)*

Discussion	**History:** • Patients present with recurrent and chronic sinopulmonary infections and sequelae, including chronic cough, chronic rhinitis, and postnasal drainage. • Up to 40% of patients have had an affected male family member. **Physical Exam:** • Growth charts should be examined for evidence of FTT/growth delay. • Lymphoid hypoplasia (e.g., small tonsils, absent lymph nodes) due to a lack of germinal centers in their lymph nodes. **Diagnostics:** • Low immunoglobulin levels (all classes) and absence of B cells in peripheral blood. **Management:** • Treat with immune globulin replacement therapy (often IVIG) at regular intervals • Consider prophylactic antibiotics and immediate antibiotics at the first sign of possible infection • Avoid live vaccines
Additional Considerations	**Screening:** XLA is not included on most newborn screens

T-Cell Defects

CASE 25 | Severe Combined Immunodeficiency (SCID)

A 6-month-old boy is brought to clinic with fever and tachypnea over the past 2 days. Review of his medical records reveals frequent visits for recurrent diarrhea, two episodes of otitis media, and oral thrush. In addition, his maternal uncle had many infections as a child and required a hematopoietic stem cell transplant. The patient's temperature is 39.2°C, pulse is 180/min, respirations are 55/min, and blood pressure is 90/54 mmHg. Diffuse crackles are present in all lung fields.

Conditions with Similar Presentations	**HIV:** Family history, such as maternal HIV status or exposure, compliance with anti-retroviral medications in pregnancy, and/or ecological factors like emigration from a country with a high rate of HIV/AIDS, may point toward HIV as the cause of recurrent infections and severe immunodeficiency.
Initial Diagnostic Tests	Check: • CBC with differential to detect lymphopenia. • Flow cytometry to assess numbers of T cells, B cells, and NK cells • Test T-cell receptor excision circle (TREC) activity or review TREC results from newborn screening exam Consider: • CXR, quantitative serum immunoglobulins and adenosine deaminase (ADA) level • HIV nucleic acid test
Next Steps in Management	• Treat any active infection and give IV immune globulin (IVIG) replacement therapy • Begin prophylactic antibiotics and avoid live vaccines and nonirradiated blood products. • Hematopoietic stem cell transplant (HSCT) can be curative.
Discussion	SCID presents in early infancy and is more common in boys. SCID is a combined immunodeficiency characterized by impaired or absent T-cell response to infection with or without impaired B cell and/or natural killer cell responses. SCID can be X-linked due to a defective IL-2R gamma chain or autosomal recessive due to an ADA. Both mutations limit the proliferation of immune cells, most commonly T cells. Additional mutations have been identified to cause SCID, and de novo mutations are common. **History:** Patients present within the first few months of life with failure to thrive, chronic diarrhea, thrush, and recurrent infections from viruses, bacteria, fungi, and protozoa. Family history of immunodeficiency may be present. **Physical Exam:** Poor overall growth, rash, sparse hair, small or absent tonsils, lack of lymph nodes, oral ulcers, coarse facial features, microcephaly, hepatosplenomegaly

CASE 25 | Severe Combined Immunodeficiency (SCID) (continued)

Discussion	**Diagnostics:** Check: • CBC: Absolute lymphocyte counts <2000 cells/mm³ • Flow cytometry: Immunoglobulins and NK cells low or absent, depending on the type of mutation • TREC activity, indicative of thymic T-cell receptor rearrangement, will also be decreased Consider: • ADA activity might be low • CXR may show absence of a thymic shadow • Lack of germinal centers may be present on lymph node biopsy • HIV nucleic acid test. (Antibody tests do not establish the presence of HIV in infants because of transplacental transfer of maternal HIV antibodies.) **Management:** In the absence of treatment, death by infection occurs by age 1–2 years. Acute treatment: • Treat any active infection • Give IV immune globulin (IVIG) replacement therapy at the earliest opportunity, as early as 1 month of age. • Begin prophylactic antibiotics for *Pneumocystis jiroveci* pneumonia (PJP) with trimethoprim-sulfamethoxazole. • Consider fungal prophylaxis with fluconazole • Consider RSV prophylaxis with palivizumab • Consider HSV prophylaxis with acyclovir Long-term management: • HSCT can be curative. Infants transplanted before 3.5 months have a 94% survival rate. • Avoid live vaccines and nonirradiated blood products. • Gene therapies and polyethylene glycol (PEG)-conjugated ADA are newly developing treatment options in ADA+ SCID
Additional Considerations	**Screening:** Several states have adopted the TREC assay as part of routine newborn screening programs. TREC screening will identify the majority of infants with common forms of SCID.

CASE 26 | DiGeorge Syndrome

A newborn girl is observed by a nurse to have a seizure. The infant has been experiencing poor feeding and a "bluish" appearance to the skin, especially when the child becomes agitated. The patient's temperature is 37.3°C, pulse is 160/min, respirations are 42/min, and blood pressure is 90/52 mmHg. She appears sleepy, has mild cyanosis of the lips, and a harsh systolic murmur is heard at the left upper sternal border.

Conditions with Similar Presentations	**Congenital heart diseases:** May present with cyanosis and harsh systolic murmur; however, a concomitant seizure in a neonate indicates additional or alternative pathology. **Neonatal hypoglycemia:** Infants of diabetic mothers (IDM) may present with cardiac defects due to uncontrolled pre-gestational diabetes. At birth, neonates with increased insulin secretion due to excess maternal glucose prenatally are at risk for seizures, coma, and long-term brain damage if hypoglycemia is unrecognized and untreated. **Neonatal meningitis:** Often due to group B streptococcus, neonatal meningitis can present with seizures in addition to temperature instability, irritability, lethargy, poor tone, and/or bulging anterior fontanelle. **Hypoxic-ischemic encephalopathy (HIE):** Neonatal encephalopathy occurring as the result of hypoxia-ischemia or birth asphyxia is the most common cause of neonatal seizures and can also lead to cerebral palsy.
Initial Diagnostic Tests	• Check: glucose, CBC with differential, serum calcium, phosphorus, PTH levels and echocardiography • Diagnosis confirmed with genetic testing for 22q11 deletion • Consider: CXR
Next Steps in Management	• Treat seizure and hypocalcemia with calcium gluconate • Administer oxygen
Discussion	DiGeorge Syndrome (DGS) is the most common microdeletion syndrome and is autosomal dominant, with a known prevalence of about one to two cases per 10,000 live births. DGS results in failure of development of the third and fourth pharyngeal pouches and thus an absent or scant thymus and parathyroid glands. Thymic hypoplasia in DGS results in diminished T cells and increased susceptibility to recurrent viral and fungal infections. Newborns may present (as in this case) with seizures due to hypocalcemia (secondary to absent parathyroids), episodes of cyanosis, and a harsh murmur (due to ToF).

CASE 26 | DiGeorge Syndrome *(continued)*

Discussion	**History:**
	• Tetany and/or seizures within the first few days of life
	• Feeding difficulties due to palatal abnormalities
	• Recurrent infections throughout childhood
	• Developmental delays, especially speech delay, is common
	Physical Exam:
	• Craniofacial abnormalities (small chin, overfolded ear helices, ocular hypertelorism, long face, microcephaly)
	• Palatal or laryngotracheal abnormalities
	• Heart murmurs due to conotruncal heart defects, commonly ToF, truncus arteriosus, or interrupted aortic arches
	Diagnostics:
	Check:
	• Point-of-care glucose to evaluate possible hypoglycemia
	• CBC with differential: low or absent absolute T-lymphocyte quantity
	• Labs: low calcium, low PTH, elevated phosphorus
	• Echocardiography to evaluate conotruncal cardiac anomalies
	• Confirm with genetic evaluation:
	• Comparative genomic hybridization will detect the 22q11.2 deletion
	• Fluorescent in situ hybridization will also detect the deletion
	Consider:
	• CXR to evaluate absence of a thymic shadow
	• Other pertinent workup should include evaluation of craniofacial abnormalities affecting feeding
	Management:
	Acute management:
	• Focused on treating hypocalcemia and its complications (e.g., seizures) with calcium gluconate
	• Identify and treat congenital cardiac defects: Administer oxygen and give prostaglandin therapy to maintain PDA prior to surgical repair for ToF
	• Identify and treat immunodeficiency status and acute infections
	Long-term management:
	• Possible thymic or hematopoietic cell transplantation, depending on severity.
	• Complete immunodeficiency may be managed with IVIG and hematopoietic cell transplantation.
	• Prophylactic antibiotics, such as PCP prophylaxis, are warranted and prompt treatment of infections is needed.
	• Surgical management may be necessary for cardiac and/or craniofacial anomalies.
	• Hypoparathyroidism should be managed with calcitriol (active form of vitamin D) and oral calcium replacement. Infants are also placed on a low-phosphorus formula to help prevent hyperphosphatemia.
	• Patients should be monitored for developmental and behavioral difficulties.

T-Cell Deficiency Mini-Case

Case	Key Findings
Hyper IgE Syndrome	**Hx:** A 3-year-old girl is brought for evaluation and treatment of sinusitis. This is her third case of sinusitis within the last 6 months. Past medical history is relevant for severe eczema diagnosed within the first year of life. She recently underwent incision and drainage of an abscess on her lower back.
	PE: Exam reveals diffuse eczema with some pustules, small abscesses on the lower extremities, and coarse facial features with prominent forehead and broad nose.
	Diagnostics:
	• Clinical diagnosis: Quartet of symptoms—eczema, recurrent sinopulmonary and skin infections, high IgE, and eosinophilia—is highly suggestive of hyper-IgE syndrome.
	• Genetic testing is confirmatory.
	Management:
	• Antibiotic prophylaxis with trimethoprim-sulfamethoxazole to prevent infections
	• Early identification and treatment of any active infections.
	Discussion: Hyper-IgE syndrome consists of the combination of atopic dermatitis, recurrent infections, eosinophilia, and elevated serum IgE. Children with this condition have recurrent infections with *S. aureus*, *H. influenzae*, *Candida*, and *Aspergillus*. There are different genetic variants which may have additional symptoms. Therapy is aimed at early treatment and prevention of infections.

Phagocytic Defect Mini-Cases

Cases	Key Findings
Chronic Granulomatous Disease (CGD)	**Hx:** A 5-month-old infant is brought for evaluation of respiratory distress and fever and is diagnosed with pneumonia. He has a past medical history of failure to thrive. The infant has had recurrent upper and lower respiratory infections requiring hospitalization since birth. **PE:** Exam shows growth failure and poor weight gain, diffuse lymphadenopathy, hepatosplenomegaly, and multiple cutaneous abscesses. **Diagnostics:** • Measurements of neutrophil superoxide are low. • Confirmation of diagnosis with genetic testing of genes encoding one of the six proteins required to make nicotinamide adenine dinucleotide phosphate (NADPH) oxidase genes. **Management:** • Antimicrobial prophylaxis • Immediate management of acute infections with antibiotics • Hematopoietic stem cell transplant can be curative. **Discussion:** CGD is a disorder of neutrophils that results from an ineffective respiratory oxidative burst leading to inadequate killing of microbial pathogens, especially catalase-positive organisms such as *S. aureus*, *Aspergillus*, *Serratia*, and *Nocardia*. The most common genetic form is due to X-linked mutations in the genes encoding the six proteins in the NADPH oxidase complex. Children with the X-linked form present with recurrent infections, abscesses, and growth failure before 5 years of age.
Leukocyte Adhesion Deficiency (LAD)	**Hx:** A 3-week-old infant is brought by parents who are concerned that the umbilical cord stump still has not completely separated and the area appears red and infected. **PE:** Physical exam shows signs of delayed wound healing of the umbilicus but no pus. **Diagnostics:** • CBC will show marked leukocytosis (neutrophils >100,000 cells/mL) during infections. • Flow cytometry to measure phagocyte surface molecules. • Molecular genetic testing. **Management:** • Antibiotic treatment for acute infections. • Hematopoietic stem cell transplant can be curative. **Discussion:** LAD is a group of genetic disorders that lack proteins necessary for effective leukocyte trafficking to sites of infection. There are three distinct syndromes that have varying presentations. Common to all is LAD, an increased susceptibility to recurrent bacterial and fungal infections. They have delayed wound healing and thus infants present with delayed detachment of the umbilical cord stump. The absence of pus at infection sites is a hallmark of LAD.

PEDIATRIC INFECTIOUS DISEASE

The treatment of infectious disease in the pediatric population requires an understanding of the epidemiology and risk factors associated with each infection and the age of the child. Susceptibility of specific populations to each infection is based on the environmental risk factors as well as the developmental stage of the immune system. Please refer to Infectious Diseases Chapter for additional information and cases.

Age	Key Factors
Neonatal infections	• Adequacy of prenatal care • Gestational age of the infant • Maternal risk-taking behavior
Daycare/school-aged children/teenagers	• Immunization history • Living conditions • Exposure to infected adults or children • Travel • Exposure to insects, animals, or exotic pets • Sexual activity

Pediatric Rashes

Viral Exanthems of Childhood

Viral Illness	Etiology	Symptoms	Rash Appearance and Progression	
Chickenpox	Varicella zoster virus	Generalized pruritic vesicular rash and fever. Lesions at various stages of progression.		Top: In rare cases of chicken pox, lesions occur primarily in sun-exposed areas. Figure shows an example of photo-related varicella, with a concentration of lesions on the sun-exposed areas of the mid-upper chest. Bottom: The classic lesion of chickenpox has been described as a "dewdrop on a rose petal." Over days, the vesicles rupture and then crust. The rash begins on the chest and back and spreads to involve the face, scalp, and the extremities. Since crops of macules, papules, vesicles, and crusts are successive and overlapping, lesions at all stages of development are seen. (Reproduced with permission from Prose NS, Kristal L. Weinberg's Color Atlas of Pediatric Dermatology, 5e; McGraw Hill LLC 2017.)
Erythema infectiosum (Fifth disease)	Parvovirus B19	"Slapped cheek" and maculopapular rash. May have pruritus.		The appearance has been given the suggestive description of "slapped cheeks." During the second stage, the facial rash begins to fade, and a maculopapular, urticarial, or morbiliform exanthem develops on the extremities and trunk. (Reproduced with permission from, Kane K, Nambudiri VE, Stratigos AJ. Color Atlas & Synopsis of Pediatric Dermatology, 3e; McGraw Hill LLC 2016.)
Roseola infantum (Sixth Disease)	HHV-6 and HHV-7	High fever, with nonpruritic, blanchable rash on trunk and neck. May have pharyngitis and cervical adenopathy.		Most cases of Roseola occur during the first year of life. The disease is characterized by 3–5 days of high fever accompanied by minimal constitutional symptoms and light pink, blanchable rash. (Reproduced with permission from Neil S. Prose, Leonard Kristal, Weinberg's Color Atlas of Pediatric Dermatology, 5e; by McGraw-Hill 2017.)
Measles	Measles virus	Prodrome of fever, cough, coryza, conjunctivitis. Red maculopapular rash, Koplik spots.		Measles is brief and self-limited for most children, and the treatment is supportive. Rash starts on head and spreads downward. The incidence of complications is higher, however, than in other childhood exanthems. Otitis media is the most common. Serious complications include bronchopneumonia and encephalitis. Subacute sclerosing panencephalitis is a late sequela of measles. (Reproduced with permission from Neil S. Prose, Leonard Kristal, Weinberg's Color Atlas of Pediatric Dermatology, 5e; by McGraw-Hill 2017.)
Rubella	Rubella virus	Fever, red maculopapular rash. Fainter than measles rash and does not coalesce.		Rubella affects both children and young adults. The rash typically begins on the face and neck and spreads to the trunk and extremities over 1 or 2 days. The lesions are small pink macules and maculopapules, which rapidly coalesce and then fade. The rash is evanescent that it may begin to disappear on the face before developing on the trunk and extremities. (Reproduced with permission from Neil S. Prose, Leonard Kristal, Weinberg's Color Atlas of Pediatric Dermatology, 5e; by McGraw-Hill 2017.)

Viral Exanthems of Childhood (*Continued*)

Viral Illness	Etiology	Symptoms	Rash Appearance and Progression	
Hand-foot-mouth disease	Coxsackie virus	Maculopapular or vesicular rash, painful oral lesions, fever.		Vesicular lesions arise on the soft palate, tongue, buccal mucosa, and uvula. The lips are usually spared. Occasionally, these lesions may be painful and cause some difficulty in eating. The cutaneous lesions develop 1 or 2 days after those in the mouth. They consist of asymptomatic round or oval vesiculopustules that evolve into superficial erosions. The edges of the palms and soles are a favored location. (Reproduced with permission from Neil S. Prose, Leonard Kristal, Weinberg's Color Atlas of Pediatric Dermatology, 5e; by McGraw-Hill 2017.)
Molluscum contagiosum	Poxvirus	Flesh-colored, pearly umbilicated papules, may be pruritic.		Molluscum contagiosum is a benign viral infection that appears as crops of discrete, slightly umbilicated, flesh-colored, or shiny papules on the trunk, extremities or head and neck. It is common among children and may be seen in several children within a family. The lesions may become inflamed if traumatized or infected and sometimes become inflamed spontaneously as they resolve. (Reproduced with permission from Neil S. Prose, Leonard Kristal, Weinberg's Color Atlas of Pediatric Dermatology, 5e; by McGraw-Hill 2017.)

Fever and Sore Throat Differential Diagnosis

Diagnosis	Key Feature(s) or Associated Symptom(s)
Adenovirus	High fevers Conjunctivitis School-age child
Coxsackie	Herpangina: Fever, papulovesicular pharyngeal lesions in infants and young children Hand-foot-mouth disease: Low-grade fever, anterior tongue, buccal mucosa, and hand and foot lesions in children
Streptococcus pyogenes (Streptococcal pharyngitis, aka "strep throat")	Tonsillar exudates in a school-age child Scarlatiniform rash if scarlet fever
Infectious mononucleosis (EBV) ("kissing disease")	Exudative pharyngitis, extreme fatigue Posterior cervical lymphadenopathy, hepatosplenomegaly, atypical lymphocytosis Teens to young adults
Corynebacterium diphtheriae, aka diphtheria (obstruction of airway secondary to pseudomembranes)	Grayish-white membranes (pseudomembranes) in oropharynx; lymphadenopathy, myocarditis, arrhythmias Airway obstruction Unvaccinated patient
Epiglottitis (classically due to *Haemophilus influenza* type b)	Drooling, difficulty breathing leading to respiratory distress "Hot potato" voice "Tripod" or "sniffing" posture; "cherry red" epiglottis Unvaccinated patient

Fever and Sore Throat Differential Diagnosis

Diagnosis	Key Feature(s) or Associated Symptom(s)
Gonococcal pharyngitis (*Neisseria gonorrhoeae*)	Men who have sex with men, history of anogenital gonorrhea
	May be exudative
Peritonsillar or retropharyngeal abscess	Neck swelling, trismus
	"Hot potato" voice

CASE 27 | Streptococcal Pharyngitis/Scarlet Fever

An 8-year-old girl is brought to clinic for evaluation of fever and sore throat for 2 days. She has no cough. She has had no recent travel and is up to date on her vaccinations. On exam, her temperature is 39.2°C, pulse is 112/min, respirations are 14/min, and blood pressure is 110/68 mmHg. She has white exudates on her tonsils bilaterally and her posterior oropharynx is erythematous. Her anterior cervical lymph nodes are palpable and tender. She has a red, "sandpaper" diffuse raised rash on her trunk and extremities.

Conditions with Similar Presentations	**Adenovirus:** Fever and sore throat, but patients have a viral prodrome, other sick contacts, and conjunctivitis.
	Diphtheria: Grayish-white exudates in the posterior oropharynx. Rarely seen in vaccinated children. Not associated with a rash.
	Peritonsillar abscess: Deeper infection of the head and neck. Presents with a "hot potato" voice and uvula deviation away from the enlarged tonsil. The pain is more severe on one side of the neck than the other and there can be referred pain to the ipsilateral ear. Not associated with a rash.
Initial Diagnostic Tests	• Check rapid streptococcal antigen test • Send for throat culture, if rapid test negative (as false-negative rate of ~20%)
Next Steps in Management	Treat with penicillin V or amoxicillin
Discussion	Streptococcal pharyngitis is caused by *Streptococcal pyogenes* (group A strep), a gram-positive cocci in chains. Strep pharyngitis is typically in children >3 years old and most commonly in children 6–12 years old. Scarlet fever is a syndrome induced by the pyrogenic exotoxin secreted by some *S. pyogenes*, and presents with a blanching sandpaper-like body rash, circumoral pallor, and a strawberry tongue. Non-infectious sequelae such as rheumatic fever and post-strep glomerulonephritis (PSGN) are caused by host antibody production to the streptococcal M protein, which shows molecular mimicry with various proteins, including those on heart valves.
	History: Pain is rapid in onset and fever is typically greater than 38.3°C. Absence of viral symptoms (cough, coryza, conjunctivitis, diarrhea). The rash of scarlet fever is found on the neck, armpits, and groin.
	Physical Exam: Fever, tonsillar exudates, tender anterior cervical lymphadenopathy, macular sandpaper rash.
	Diagnostics: Rapid streptococcal antigen test has an 80% sensitivity and 95% specificity. Therefore, if rapid antigen test is negative but there is high clinical suspicion for streptococcal pharyngitis, send a throat culture.
	Management: • Antibiotic treatment is warranted for all cases of streptococcal pharyngitis in order to prevent rheumatic fever. • If rapid Ag is negative and awaiting culture (which can take up to 48 hours), therapy can be withheld pending results without increasing the risk of local or immunologic sequelae.
Additional Considerations	**Complications:** Peritonsillar abscess, rheumatic fever, post-streptococcal glomerulonephritis, toxic shock syndrome, reactive arthritis, acute otitis media, bacteremia, pneumonia.

CASE 28 | Epiglottitis (Secondary to *H. influenzae* type b)

A 3-year-old unvaccinated boy is brought for evaluation of sore throat, fever, and drooling for 1 day. His parents report that he has had increased difficulty breathing and sounds hoarse but has not had a cough. On exam, the patient is acutely ill and anxious. His vitals are temperature 38.9°C, pulse 128/min, respirations 30/min, and blood pressure 100/64 mmHg. When examined, he refuses to lay back, appears anxious, and has intercostal retractions and audible inspiratory and expiratory stridor at rest. He speaks as if he has a hot potato in his mouth.

Conditions with Similar Presentations	**Retropharyngeal abscess:** History of pharyngitis with exudates and lack of improvement with antibiotics. Pain becomes unilateral. Trismus may be present.
	Croup: Typically present with "seal bark" cough, inspiratory stridor, and hoarse voice.
	Respiratory syncytial virus (RSV) bronchiolitis: Typically seen in patients <2 years of age and present with wheezing/ dyspnea in winter months

CASE 28 | Epiglottitis (Secondary to *H. influenzae* type b) *(continued)*

Initial Diagnostic Tests	• Clinical diagnosis, secure the airway immediately • Lateral neck x-ray and laryngoscopy —can help confirm the diagnosis
Next Steps in Management	Stabilize airway and start IV antibiotics
Discussion	Epiglottitis is most commonly caused by the gram-negative rod *Haemophilus influenzae* type b (Hib). This is rare in the modern era following the widespread use of Hib vaccination. *H. influenzae* is transmitted by respiratory droplets. Epiglottitis may occur at any age and has no seasonal predilection. Most *Haemophilus* infections in vaccinated patients come from nontypeable strains. Any child with the three D's—dysphagia, drooling, and distress (respiratory)—should be suspected to have epiglottitis and impending airway obstruction, which needs to be treated urgently. Lateral radiograph of the neck shows diffuse swelling of the epiglottis (arrow), representing the thumb sign in a patient with epiglottitis. (Reproduced with permission from Elsayes KM, Oldham SA. *Introduction to Diagnostic Radiology*; McGraw Hill LLC 2015.) **History/ Physical Exam:** • High fever, severe sore throat, and odynophagia with drooling. • Patients have severe respiratory distress (often with stridor) requiring them to sit in a "tripod" position (trunk leaning forward, elbows on knees, neck extended, and chin forward to maximize air intake). • May have hot potato voice. This is because the base of the tongue insets proximate to the epiglottis so the patient talks with as little tongue movement as possible. **Diagnostics:** • High index of clinical suspicion is required. • Confirmation of diagnosis may be required using a fiberoptic laryngoscope, but it must be undertaken after the airway is stabilized. Nasolaryngoscopy reveals a cherry-red, edematous epiglottis • Lateral neck radiograph shows a "thumb sign" due to an enlarged epiglottis with narrowing of the airway. **Management:** • Stabilize the airway with endotracheal/nasotracheal intubation or tracheostomy. • Begin IV third-generation cephalosporin. • Consider using IV corticosteroid to limit pharyngeal edema and airway obstruction.
Additional Considerations	**Complications:** *H. influenzae* can also cause meningitis, otitis media, and pneumonia.

CASE 29 | Acute Otitis Media

A 3-year-old boy is brought to clinic by his mother for 3 days of ear pain following recent URI symptoms. The boy has been tugging at his right ear and has had difficulty sleeping due to the pain. Patient's temperature is 38.8°C (101.9°F), pulse is 100/min, respirations are 20/min, blood pressure is 100/61 mmHg, and SpO₂ 98% on room air. Physical exam is notable for a bulging, erythematous tympanic membrane, and loss of light reflex on otoscopic exam.

Conditions with similar presentations	**Otitis media with effusion:** Otalgia and middle ear effusion *without* acute inflammatory signs (tympanic membrane is not bulging or erythematous). **Otitis externa:** Pain with movement of outer ear, erythematous external ear canal, otorrhea, recent history of swimming.
Initial Diagnostic Tests	Clinical Diagnosis
Next Steps in Management	Observation with close follow-up, or oral amoxicillin treatment
Discussion	Otitis media can be acute or with effusion. Acute otitis media (AOM) is a suppurative infection of the middle ear. Otitis media with effusion (OME) is a chronic inflammatory condition presenting with a collection of fluid in the middle ear without acute signs or symptoms. Otitis media can be caused by bacteria (most commonly *S. pneumoniae,* then *H. influenzae* and *M. catarrhalis*) or viruses (influenza A, parainfluenza, RSV).

CASE 29 | Acute Otitis Media *(continued)*

Discussion	Younger children are more predisposed to middle ear infections because they have narrower and straighter eustachian tubes. AOM often follows an upper respiratory infection (URI), as nasopharyngeal inflammation leads to obstruction of the eustachian tube inflammation orifice.
	History:
	Risk factors include cigarette smoke exposure, day care attendance, and formula feeds.
	Symptoms: ear pain, fever, crying, fussiness in infants, ear tugging in children, decreased hearing.
	Physical Exam: Middle ear effusion and bulging tympanic membrane (TM), loss of light reflex, immobile tympanic membrane on pneumatic insufflation
	Diagnostics: History and appearance of tympanic membrane are diagnostic
	Management:
	• In a child >2 years old and without severe symptoms, treatment is either observation or oral amoxicillin.
	• If infection reoccurs within 1 month, treat with amoxicillin-clavulanic acid to cover beta-lactamase producing strains.
	• Tympanostomy tubes provide middle ear decompression and are indicated in children with three or more episodes of acute otitis media in 6 months or four or more episodes in 12 months.
Additional Considerations	**Complications:** Complications are rare, but may include:
	• Perforation of the TM; conductive hearing loss; development of chronic otitis media potentially requiring placement of tympanostomy tubes.
	• Mastoiditis: fever, mastoid inflammation, anterior displacement of the ear.
	• Brain abscess/meningitis: severe headache, seizures, vomiting, focal neurologic deficits after episode of acute otitis media, and mastoiditis.
	• Cholesteatomas can develop as a result of chronic ear infections. A cholesteatoma is an abnormal cutaneous cyst that can invade the middle ear and damage the bone. This can lead to pain and loss of hearing. Treatment is with surgical removal.
	Surgical Considerations: Mastoiditis and brain abscesses require surgical drainage.

Cough Mini-Cases

Cases	Key Findings
Bronchiolitis (RSV)	**Hx:** A previously healthy 9-month-old infant is brought to the ED in January because of cough, wheezing, and poor feeding for the past 2 days. He had a runny nose and a low-grade fever (100.8°F) 5 days ago.
	PE: Bilateral crackles, wheezing, increased work of breathing, intercostal retractions, tachypnea, nasal flaring, low O_2 saturation.
	Diagnostics:
	• Clinical diagnosis based on history and physical exam alone. (Key findings: Age <2 years, wheezing/dyspnea in winter).
	• Respiratory viral panel can confirm RSV as cause, or other common pathogens such as rhinovirus, enterovirus, and human metapneumovirus.
	• CXR shows hyperinflation with patchy atelectasis but should not be ordered unless clinical course is inconsistent with bronchiolitis.
	Management:
	• Supportive (oxygen, IV fluids, nasal bulb suction) and hospitalization if the patient is in respiratory distress and unable to drink.
	• Bronchodilators, epinephrine, or steroids should only be used if infection has triggered underlying asthma.
	• Palivizumab (a RSV-specific monoclonal antibody) can be used as prophylaxis in preterm infants with congenital heart disease or lung disease, or those who are immunocompromised.
	Discussion: RSV can cause inflammation of the small airways/bronchioles, leading to bronchiolitis. RSV occurs more commonly in winter months and is spread in daycare centers or other sick contacts.

Cough Mini-Cases *(continued)*

Laryngotracheitis (Croup)	**Hx:** A 1-year-old girl is brought to the ED in October because of a loud, "barking" cough and hoarse voice for the last 3 days. She had rhinorrhea and a low-grade fever (100.6°F) 5 days ago. **PE:** Inspiratory stridor **Diagnostics:** • Clinical diagnosis based on history and physical exam. (Key findings: "Seal bark" cough, inspiratory stridor, hoarse voice). • Respiratory viral panel can confirm parainfluenza virus infection (most common viral etiology) but should be ordered routinely • CXR: "steeple sign" from narrowing of upper trachea. **Management:** • If mild, use cool mist and corticosteroids. • If there is stridor at rest or respiratory distress, nebulized racemic epinephrine. **Discussion:** Croup is caused by a viral infection of the larynx and trachea (most commonly parainfluenza). The inspiratory stridor and barking cough are due to inflammation and narrowing of the proximal trachea (subglottis). If a child is suspected to have croup but does not respond to racemic epinephrine, consider bacterial tracheitis.	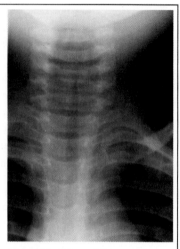 Croup. Classic "steeple" sign seen on an anteroposterior radiograph of the neck showing subglottic tracheal narrowing. (Reproduced with permission from Mark W. Kline, Rudolph's Pediatrics, 23e; by McGraw-Hill 2018.))
Pertussis (Whooping Cough)	**Hx:** A 5-year-old boy who recently immigrated to the U.S. presents to clinic for episodes of severe coughing and post-tussive emesis after 2 weeks of rhinorrhea, low-grade fever, and dry cough. **PE:** Coughing spells (paroxysms) with loud inspiratory whoops **Diagnostics:** • Clinical diagnosis (Key findings: Coughing spells with inspiratory "whoop" preceded by vague viral URI symptoms). • Pertussis throat culture or PCR. **Management:** • Treat with a macrolide. • Everyone with exposure to this patient should receive macrolide post-exposure prophylaxis, regardless of their immunization status. **Discussion:** Whooping cough is caused by the bacteria *Bordetella pertussis*. Catarrhal phase (1–2 weeks): rhinorrhea, low-grade fever, mild cough. Paroxysmal phase (2–6 weeks): whooping cough, classically so severe that the patient vomits. Convalescent (weeks to months): resolution of symptoms gradually. Pertussis vaccination should be given to all children according to the schedule (see Immunizations section). Uncontrolled seizures or encephalopathy within 2 weeks of receiving the vaccine are a true contraindication to the pertussis component of the DTaP vaccine.	

CASE 30 | Kawasaki Disease (KD)

A 3-year-old boy is brought to clinic for evaluation of fevers for 6 days, decreased appetite, malaise, and rash. He is otherwise healthy, vaccinations are up to date, and there have been no sick contacts. On exam, he is very irritable and clings to his mother. Vital signs are temperature of 39°C, pulse of 148/min, blood pressure of 85/55 mmHg, and O$_2$ saturation of 94% on room air. Bilateral conjunctival injection, a strawberry tongue, dry mucous membranes, and cracked red lips are present. He has an extensive erythematous rash with desquamation, involving both palms and soles and his groin. His hands and feet are swollen, and he has nontender anterior cervical lymphadenopathy bilaterally. He is tachycardic, but no murmurs are heard.

Conditions with Similar Presentations	**Stevens-Johnson syndrome (erythema multiforme major):** Hypersensitivity reaction to infections (HSV as cause in 60%), drugs (sulfa and penicillins most common) and after immunizations that presents with flu-like symptoms followed by a multiforme and mucosal involvement.
	Scarlet fever: Due to infection with group A *Streptococcus*. The rash is a diffuse macular sandpaper rash with circumoral pallor. Also causes a strawberry tongue. Group A strep antigen or throat culture positive.

CASE 30 | Kawasaki Disease (KD) *(continued)*

Initial Diagnostic Tests	• Clinical diagnosis when patient meets criteria (see Discussion section). • Consider checking: CBC, viral panel, blood cultures, transaminases, and echocardiogram
Next Steps in Management	• IV immunoglobulin • Aspirin
Discussion	KD is a mucocutaneous lymph node syndrome and involves acute necrotizing vasculitis of the medium- and small-sized vessels and can cause coronary artery disease in children. It is more common among children less than 5 years, male children, and with a higher incidence in Japan. There is a seasonal predominance, with peaks in late winter-spring, suggesting a possible underlying infectious trigger. Mucocutaneous changes and lymphadenopathy are early manifestations and there can be other multiorgan injury (see Additional Considerations). **History:** Fever and a constellation of other symptoms including rash, conjunctival injection, fissuring of lips, and swollen hands and feet. **Physical Exam:** Fever, bilateral conjunctival injection, strawberry tongue, cracked red lips, erythematous rash involving the palms and soles, swollen hands and feet, cervical lymphadenopathy. **Diagnostics:** Clinical diagnosis using the Kawasaki criteria: • Fever for ≥5 days and at least four of the following five manifestations: 　• Bilateral conjunctivitis 　• Lip injection or fissures, or strawberry tongue 　• Red and/or swollen palms or soles 　• Polymorphous rash 　• Cervical lymphadenopathy 　• Other lab findings include anemia, leukocytosis and thrombocytosis, negative viral panel and blood cultures, and elevated AST, ALT, and creatinine. 　• Echocardiogram may initially be normal, and ECG may show sinus tachycardia. **Management:** IV immunoglobulin and aspirin Algorithm for diagnosing Kawasaki disease. (Reproduced with permission from Kawasaki Disease In: Tenenbein M, Macias CG, et al., Strange and Schafermeyer's Pediatric Emergency Medicine, 5e, New York: McGraw Hill; 2019.)
Additional Considerations	**Complications:** Coronary artery vasculitis, which can present as aneurysm, calcification, or stenosis, is the most serious complication. Systemic inflammation of other organs can also occur, such as meningitis, myocarditis (resulting in heart failure), pericardial effusions, and pericarditis and valvular vegetations. **Surgical Considerations:** In children who develop coronary artery disease, coronary stents and coronary bypass surgery may eventually be necessary.

PEDIATRIC PULMONOLOGY

Pediatric pulmonology focuses primarily on asthma managements as well as management of other childhood illnesses of the respiratory tract. There is a lot of overlap with pediatric pulmonology and infectious diseases, so please reference those sections and Chapters in particular.

CASE 31 | Foreign Body Aspiration

An 18-month-old boy is brought to the urgent care facility for evaluation of wheezing and low-grade fever. He has no personal or family history of reactive airway disease. On exam, he is mildly tachypneic with focal right-sided wheezing and intermittent coughing. Symptoms do not improve despite treatment with nebulized albuterol.

Conditions with Similar Presentations	**Asthma:** Would have bilateral expiratory wheezing and should respond to albuterol.
	Pneumonia: Presents with cough and fever and would have focal findings on lung exam.
Initial Diagnostic Tests	CXR
Next Steps in Management	Bronchoscopy for visualization and removal of foreign body
Discussion	Foreign body aspiration (FBA) is most commonly seen in children <3 years of age. Aspiration of the foreign body is unintentional and usually prevented by protective reflexes such as coughing. When foreign bodies are aspirated, they tend to settle in a bronchus and thus cause unilateral findings, but if it is large and lodges more proximally it may cause death from suffocation. Persistent/recurrent infection may occur if the obstruction is partial and the diagnosis is missed. The most commonly aspirated items include small, round foods like nuts and seeds, hardware, and pieces of toys.
	History: Caregivers may seek medical attention after a witnessed choking episode, but children more commonly present sometime after the event has occurred with cough, dyspnea, wheezing, or fever.
	Physical Exam: Patient may have normal vital signs or have tachypnea, tachycardia, and fever. Lung auscultation may initially be normal but eventually reveals signs of obstruction such as wheezing and asymmetric breath sounds.
	Diagnostics: Chest radiograph may show hyperinflation, atelectasis, or infiltrate. Most aspirated objects are radiolucent, and they are most commonly found in the right mainstem bronchus because it is on less of an angle of the trachea than the left mainstem bronchus.
	Management: Traditional choking relief methods such as back slapping and chest thrusts in the head-down position (or abdominal thrusts for older children) may relieve the obstruction. Otherwise, children should be transferred without delay to the nearest facility with pediatric airway and bronchoscopy capacity.
Additional Considerations	**Complications:** Children with an undiagnosed obstruction are at risk of death from suffocation or of recurrent or persistent lung infections.
	Surgical Considerations: Children who fail bronchoscopy may require thoracotomy to relieve the obstruction.

CASE 32 | Cystic Fibrosis

An 8-month-old boy who was born at home presents with a cough productive of dark brown, thick sputum. His past medical history is significant for pneumonia 1 month ago. On exam, the patient is fussy, underweight, febrile and tachycardic, tachypneic and grunting. Oxygen saturation is 89% on room air. He has decreased breath sounds, crackles, and dullness to percussion in the left lower lung field.

Conditions with Similar Presentations	**Primary ciliary dyskinesia (immotile cilia syndrome):** Inherited defect of airway ciliary function. Also presents with cough, recurrent pulmonary infections, hypoxemia, and tachypnea. However, sweat test will be normal.
	Asthma: Chronic inflammatory disorder of the airway. Presents with wheezing and respiratory distress that is responsive to bronchodilators. PFTs show reversible airway obstruction.
Initial Diagnostic Tests	Check CXR and confirm diagnosis with sweat chloride testing followed by genetic testing
Next Steps in Management	• Treat pneumonia with antibiotics • Start chest physiotherapy, inhaled DNAase, inhaled hypertonic saline, and inhaled albuterol • Consider CFTR modulators
Discussion	Cystic fibrosis (CF) is an autosomal recessive disorder involving a defect in the cystic fibrosis transmembrane conductance regulator (*CFTR*) gene on chromosome 7, commonly at codon 508. *CFTR* encodes an ATP-gated chloride channel involved in the secretion of chloride in the lungs and GI tract and the reabsorption of chloride in sweat glands. The abnormal chloride regulation results in thick secretions. In the lungs, thick secretions increase susceptibility to infection. In the GI tract, they can lead to pancreatic insufficiency (steatorrhea, fat-soluble vitamin deficiencies). Abnormal chloride channels in the sweat glands lead to excessive sodium chloride loss in sweat.

CASE 32 | Cystic Fibrosis *(continued)*

Discussion	CF is usually diagnosed in the newborn period. There is a higher prevalence of disease in those with European ancestry.
	History: Most infants are diagnosed via the newborn screen. When the diagnosis is not made at birth, infants, or young children may present with meconium ileus, failure to thrive, or history of recurrent respiratory infections.
	Physical Exam: May show focal lung abnormalities consistent with pneumonia, tachypnea, increased work of breathing, failure to thrive. Digital clubbing may be seen with increasing age.
	Diagnostics:
	Check CXR: Findings consistent with pneumonia
	Confirm Diagnosis of CF:
	• Sweat chloride test is the initial step.
	• If abnormal, confirm diagnosis with genetic testing to detect mutations of the *CFTR* gene (over 200 known). Fecal elastase is low.
	• Nasal transepithelial potential difference is elevated.
	Management: Treatments for patients with CF are aimed at:
	1. Improving airway clearance with dornase alfa and/or hypertonic saline and chest physiotherapy.
	2. Treating obstructive airway disease with inhaled beta-2 agonists.
	3. Decreasing airway inflammation with azithromycin in selected patients.
	4. Urgent treatment of all respiratory infections.
	5. Genetic modulation is indicated; in patients with certain *CFTR* mutations, *CFTR* modulators can be used. These include lumacaftor, which helps correct misfolding of the CFTR protein, ivacaftor, which helps promote opening of chloride channels, and tezacaftor and elexacaftor, which facilitate processing of mature CFTR protein.
Additional Considerations	**Screening:** Newborn screening for cystic fibrosis is required in all 50 states.
	Complications: Pancreatic insufficiency with or without diabetes mellitus, biliary cirrhosis, liver disease, infertility, nasal polyps.
	Surgical Considerations: Patients with advanced lung disease should be considered for lung transplant. Transplant discussions should begin well before the patient's condition is end-stage.

Recurrent Lung Infection Mini-Case

Cases	Key Findings
Primary Ciliary Dyskinesia	**Hx:** Most commonly presents with recurrent sinus infections and/or recurrent infections of the lower respiratory tract. Affected individuals may present with productive cough with thick sputum and thick nasal discharge. They may also report a decreased sense of smell.
	PE: On exam, nasal mucosa is not visible due to thick nasal secretions, and bilateral sinus tenderness is present. If situs inversus is present, the apical impulse is on the right fifth intercostal space and hepatic dullness is percussed on the left side.
	Diagnostics:
	• CT sinuses show mucosal thickening.
	• Biopsy of sinus cavities or airway shows ciliary abnormalities.
	• Semen analysis in male patients will show immotile spermatozoa.
	Management:
	• Airway clearance therapy to help loosen thick mucus.
	• Antibiotics to treat respiratory, sinus, or ear infections.
	Discussion: Primary ciliary dyskinesia (**Immotile Cilia Syndrome**) is caused by autosomal recessive mutations that affect the proteins involved in the dynein arm of cilia leading to various degrees of ciliary movement defects or complete absence of cilia. These lead to frequent middle ear, sinus, and lung infections, and conductive hearing loss. In men there may be infertility due to immotile sperm, and in women there is an increased risk of ectopic pregnancy. Headache, anosmia, and corneal abnormalities can also occur. About 50% of the time, situs inversus is present. When situs inversus, chronic sinusitis, and bronchiectasis occur together, it is known as **Kartagener syndrome**.

PEDIATRIC NEPHROLOGY

Hematuria

Hematuria can be classified as gross hematuria (able to be seen with the naked eye) and microscopic hematuria (visible only on microscopic examination). Gross hematuria in the absence of a negative microscopic examination suggests that the urine is discolored by medication (e.g., orange-red colored urine with rifampin) or the breakdown of hemoglobin or myoglobin (e.g., rhabdomyolysis).

Proteinuria

Healthy children can have a small amount of protein in their urine. The first step in evaluating proteinuria is to determine whether the protein is transient or persistent. Protein can be found in the urine in children after exercise, standing for long periods of time, or during acute febrile illness. These episodes of proteinuria are transient and tend to resolve spontaneously. Persistent protein in the urine should be evaluated further. Nephrotic range proteinuria in children is defined as protein greater than 1 g/m^2 of body surface area per day.

Hematuria	Proteinuria	Edema	Differential Diagnosis
No	Yes	No	• Exercise • Orthostatic • Fever
No	Yes	Yes	• Minimal change • Nephrotic syndrome • Focal segmental glomerulosclerosis
Yes	Yes	No	• IgA Nephropathy • Henoch-Schonlein purpura • Hemolytic-uremic syndrome
Yes	Yes	Yes	• Membranoproliferative glomerulonephritis
Yes	No	No	• Benign hematuria • Sickle cell disease

CASE 33 | Acute Post-Infectious Glomerulonephritis (Post-Streptococcal Glomerulonephritis [PSGN])

A 9-year-old girl is brought to clinic by her parents after reporting brown urine and swelling in her legs. A few weeks ago, she had a sore throat but her symptoms improved within a few days of starting antibiotics. Her temperature is 37°C, pulse is 90/min, respirations are 18/min, blood pressure is 135/84 mmHg, and SpO_2 is 98% on room air. Physical exam is notable for 2+ bilateral lower extremity edema.

Conditions with Similar Presentations	**IgA nephropathy:** May present with gross hematuria several days after an URI, unlike PSGN that occurs weeks later. Age range typically 15-30 years. **Henoch-Schoenlein purpura** (HSP): May present with gross hematuria in children but typically have other findings such as palpable purpura, abdominal pain, arthralgias **Nephrolithiasis:** Nephrolithiasis can cause hematuria; however, it is associated with flank pain and will not have edema. **Urinary tract infection (UTI):** Presents with dysuria, urgency, frequency, and/or abdominal/flank pain. A history of UTIs or risk factors may also be present.
Initial Diagnostic Tests	• Check urinalysis (UA), CMP (serum creatinine, albumin) • Also check C3 and C4 complement levels and anti-streptolysin O (ASO) and/or anti-DNAse titers • Consider: CBC, ESR, CRP
Next Steps in Management	Supportive care: Treat any hypertension and volume overload

CASE 33 | PSGN *(continued)*

Discussion	PSGN is a common cause of nephritic syndrome in school-aged children and typically occurs 2–4 weeks after GAS infection (pharyngitis or impetigo). It occurs due to subepithelial immune complex deposition along the glomerular basement membrane leading to hypercellular inflamed glomeruli with complement deposition. This results in thickening of the GBM, decreased GFR, volume overload, and nephrotic syndrome.

History:
- Patients may be asymptomatic or present with "cola-colored" urine (hematuria) and/or report occasional oliguria.
- If severe hypertension, may have symptoms of encephalopathy or acute pulmonary edema.
- Consider diagnosis in patients 2-4 weeks after GAS infection.

Physical Exam:
- Patients present with symptoms from volume overload such as periorbital, pedal, abdominal or pulmonary edema.
- Skin findings may include impetigo.

Diagnostics:
- UA shows proteinuria, microscopic or gross hematuria, and RBC casts.
- Low serum C3 and C4 due to immune complex formation
- Elevated ASO and anti-DNAse B titers indicate previous group A streptococcal infection and rise 1–2 weeks after infection. They can remain elevated for several months.
- Serum creatinine elevated
- CBC may show leukocytosis with neutrophilia and normocytic normochromic anemia.
- ESR and CRP may be elevated.
- Renal biopsies are not necessary for diagnosis unless there are atypical features.

Management:
- Treatment is supportive and focuses on management of hypertension and volume overload with antihypertensive agents, sodium restriction and as needed loop diuretics.
- Most patients will recover from acute symptoms within 2 weeks; however, hematuria may persist for up to 6 months.
- Renal function and low complement levels improve within 4–8 weeks.
- Repeated episodes of acute PSGN are rare.

Additional Considerations	**Complications:** • Poorly managed or advanced PSGN may develop into rapidly progressive glomerulonephritis, although this is more common in adults. Children rarely progress to renal failure.

CASE 34 | IgA Nephropathy (Berger Disease)

A 17-year-old boy comes to urgent care due to tea-colored urine. Three days ago, he developed low-grade fever, cough, and rhinorrhea that have only mildly improved. His temperature is 36.8°C, pulse is 110/min, respirations are 20/min, blood pressure is 140/90 mmHg, and SpO$_2$ is 99% on room air. He has no acute physical exam findings.

Conditions with Similar Presentations	**Henoch-Schönlein purpura (HSP):** HSP is a spontaneous systemic small vessel vasculitis causing similar IgA deposition in the kidneys and hematuria. However, it also presents with a non-blanching palpable purpuric rash on the thighs and buttocks without thrombocytopenia that is commonly preceded by up to 2 weeks of joint or abdominal pain.
	PSGN: Presents similarly with macroscopic hematuria but arises 2–4 weeks after group A *Streptococcal* infection (pharyngitis or impetigo).
	UTI: Presents with dysuria, urgency, frequency, and/or abdominal/flank pain. A history of UTIs or risk factors may also be present.
	Nephrolithiasis: Nephrolithiasis can cause hematuria; however, it is more often associated with flank pain.
Initial Diagnostic Tests	• Check: UA, CMP (serum creatinine, albumin) • Consider checking: C3 and C4 complement and CBC, ESR, CRP • Consider biopsy (see below)

CASE 34 | IgA nephropathy (continued)

Next Steps in Management	If hypertensive, optimize blood pressure

Discussion	IgA nephropathy is the most common type of primary glomerulonephritis (GN).
	
	Primary IgA nephropathy most commonly affects young adults ages 16–35 and is seen in men more than women. Symptoms often arise during or after minor acute illnesses or stressors. Primary IgA nephropathy is due to the deposition of IgA immune complexes in the mesangial cells of glomeruli. This leads to podocyte and tubulointerstitial injury causing glomerulosclerosis and fibrosis which can result in loss of renal function.
	
	Of note, the vasculitis of HSP has renal manifestations and histology that are pathologically the same as IgA nephropathy. Renal involvement ranges from none to mild GN with microhematuria to severe GN with associated nephrosis and renal insufficiency. However, HSP has joint pain, purpura, and abdominal pain. Secondary IgA nephropathy, more common in adults, occurs as a complication of various other illnesses:
	• GI and liver diseases: hepatitis B and C
	• Infections: HIV, Lyme disease
	• Autoimmune diseases: IBD, celiac disease
	• Respiratory tract diseases: CF, idiopathic pulmonary fibrosis
	• Neoplasia: lymphomas
	
	History:
	• Dark urine, dysuria, edema, or flank pain
	• Concurrent URI, infection may be present
	
	Physical Exam:
	• May reveal hypertension, edema, or flank tenderness
	
	Diagnostics:
	• UA consistent with IgA nephropathy shows small amounts of nephrotic range proteinuria, microscopic or gross hematuria, and RBC casts.
	• Notably, complement levels are normal in contrast to PSGN and other causes of glomerulonephritis.
	• ESR and CRP may be elevated due to inflammation.
	• Confirmatory renal biopsy is not needed unless severe proteinuria, hypertension, or renal insufficiency develop. Biopsy results will show:
	  • Light microscopy: mesangial proliferation, matrix expansion
	  • Electron microscopy: dense mesangial deposits
	  • Immunofluorescence: IgA deposits in mesangium
	
	Management:
	• Treatment not necessary if blood pressure is normal, GFR is within the normal range, and urinary protein-to-creatinine ratio is <0.2.
	• For hypertension use ACE inhibitors or ARBs with goal of <1 g proteinuria per day.
	• Additional management for blood pressure control: Modify salt intake, weight reduction, alcohol, and smoking cessation.
	• Gross hematuria resolves within days, and there are no serious sequelae in 85% of children.
	• If severe renal insufficiency develops, consider corticosteroids and other immunosuppressive drugs after confirmatory biopsy.
	• For patients with secondary IgA nephropathy (more common in adults), treat the underlying cause.

Additional Considerations	**Complications:** IgA nephropathy leads to chronic kidney disease and end-stage renal disease (ESRD) in approximately 40% of patients at 20 years after diagnosis. **Surgical Considerations:** Refer patients who have ESRD for kidney transplant evaluation.

CASE 35 | Hemolytic Uremic Syndrome (HUS)

A 4-year-old girl is brought to the ED after 1 day of fatigue, pallor, and periorbital edema. She recently had 3 days of abdominal pain and bloody diarrhea after eating an undercooked hamburger. Her temperature is 37.5°C, pulse is 110/min, respirations are 20/min, blood pressure is 150/90 mmHg, and SpO$_2$ is 99% on room air. On exam, she is pale with periorbital edema.

Conditions with Similar Presentations	**Thrombotic thrombocytopenic purpura (TTP):** Occurs due to antibody to or genetic deficiency of ADAMTS13, a metalloprotease that cleaves large von Willebrand fragments when they are released from vascular endothelium to prevent them from macroaggregating platelets. It most often occurs in 30- to 40-year-old women and presents with a similar triad of thrombocytopenia, microangiopathic hemolytic anemia, and acute kidney injury (AKI). However, it may also be accompanied by fever and mental status changes.
	Immune thrombocytopenia (ITP, formerly known as idiopathic thrombocytopenic purpura): Is due to the development of anti-Gp IIb/IIIa antibodies which facilitate opsonization by splenic macrophages. It can be idiopathic or secondary to drug administration or underlying disease like lupus, HIV, hepatitis C, or malignancies. In children it most frequently presents between 1 and 7 years old with an abrupt onset of bleeding: petechia, purpura, gingival bleeding, epistaxis, or menorrhagia. ITP would not cause renal failure.
	Disseminated intravascular coagulation (DIC): Is a serious condition characterized by both platelet activation and coagulation factor consumption which can lead to thrombosis, bleeding, emboli, and end-organ dysfunction such as kidney damage. It is never a primary illness and is always secondary to another condition such as sepsis, malignancy, or trauma. It can be distinguished from HUS by coagulation studies.
Initial Diagnostic Tests	• Check: Stool studies (PCR or culture) for Shiga toxin–producing *Escherichia coli* (STEC) or Shiga toxin itself • Also check: BMP, CBC, blood smear, reticulocyte count • Consider checking: lactate dehydrogenase, haptoglobin, direct anti-globulin test (Coombs)
Next Steps in Management	• Supportive care: Early IV fluid resuscitation • Transfuse red blood cells if hemoglobin < 7 g/dL
Discussion	Hemolytic uremic syndrome (HUS), most often caused by STEC infection from the O157:H7 strain (85–90% of cases), is characterized by thrombocytopenia, microangiopathic hemolytic anemia, and AKI. It is the most common cause of AKI in children, and usually affects those <5 years. Other Shiga toxin–producing pathogens like *Shigella dysenteriae* type 1 can also cause HUS. Shiga toxin-producing bacteria infect the large intestine causing colitis, which results in bloody diarrhea. The toxin then enters circulation and causes endothelial damage leading to microvascular occlusion and thrombotic microangiopathy with subsequent hemolysis. Contributing to this is that the endothelial damage causes increased release of large molecular weight vWF which consumes ADAMTS13, resulting in platelet aggregation as seen in TTP. This causes ischemia in rich vascular beds such as the kidney, resulting in a range of clinical outcomes from mild AKI to renal failure. Risk factors for STEC infection include: • Ingestion of contaminated food (e.g., undercooked ground beef, raw produce) or water sources • Close contact with an infected person (e.g., daycare or school settings) • Contact with animals in their environment (e.g., farms) **History:** Patients present with recent gastroenteritis symptoms about 2–5 days after potential exposure to toxin-producing bacteria. History may reveal risk factors listed earlier. Symptoms may include: • Diarrhea: non-bloody initially but becomes bloody after 1–4 days. • Abdominal pain, nausea, vomiting • Oliguria or anuria, edema • Pallor, easy bruising weakness, shortness of breath • Fever is paradoxically absent • Neurological involvement (lethargy, altered mental status, headache) is present in up to 20% of cases **Physical Exam:** May have hypertension, pallor, edema, abdominal tenderness

CASE 35 | Hemolytic Uremic Syndrome (HUS) *(continued)*

Discussion	**Diagnostics:**
	• HUS from STEC will be confirmed by stool studies detecting presence of Shiga toxin by PCR or enzyme immunoassay (EIA).
	• Labs will likely show acute kidney injury:
	  • Elevated creatinine and BUN
	  • Alterations of Na and/or K
	• Labs will be consistent with microangiopathic hemolytic anemia.
	  • Anemia, thrombocytopenia, schistocytes on blood smear, elevated LDH, low haptoglobin, increased reticulocyte level
	  • Coombs will be negative, as destruction is mechanical and not antibody mediated
	• Leukocytosis and elevated inflammatory markers like ESR and CRP.
	
	Management:
	• Early IV fluid reinfusion to reduce the risk of nervous system involvement, oliguric renal failure, and long-term renal and extrarenal sequela.
	• However, if the patient is severely hypervolemic, hypertensive, or anuric, consider:
	  • Fluid restriction and diuretics
	  • Antihypertensives such as amlodipine or labetalol
	• To prevent complications from anemia, transfuse red blood cells if hemoglobin is <7 g/dL.

Additional Considerations	**Complications:** Mortality is about 4%. Most patients will have a full recovery from the disease after supportive treatment, but about 30% of patients may have long-term renal or neurologic impairment.

CASE 36 | Minimal Change Disease (MCD)

A 6-year-old boy is brought to clinic for evaluation of bilateral lower extremity and facial swelling and frothy urine for 1 week. His temperature is 37.1°C, pulse is 108/min, respirations are 20/min, blood pressure is 100/80 mmHg, and SpO$_2$ is 99% on room air. On exam, he has periorbital edema and 3+ bilateral lower extremity pitting edema.

Conditions with Similar Presentations	**Focal segmental glomerulosclerosis (FSGS):** Presents similarly with nephrotic syndrome but may have a clearer cause (e.g., HIV, parvovirus, CMV, EBV infections, medications, heroin, or genetic causes). Both MCD and FSGS can have hypertension and edema but failure to respond to steroids should prompt a renal biopsy to confirm FSGS. **Membranoproliferative glomerulonephritis (MPGN):** Commonly presents with edema but also features of nephritic syndrome like gross hematuria. There may be a history of recent URI, treatment with alpha interferon, or of hepatitis B, hepatitis C, or HIV history which may cause secondary MPGN. Renal biopsy is required for diagnosis.
Initial Diagnostic Tests	• Check: UA, urine protein to creatinine ratio (UPCR), serum creatinine, albumin • Consider: C3 and C4 complement levels
Next Steps in Management	Corticosteroids
Discussion	Minimal change disease (MCD) is the most common cause of nephrotic syndrome in children and is often seen in preadolescent males. Unlike other renal injuries, it does not have hematuria, persistent hypertension, or renal failure. **History/Physical Exam:** Risk factors include: Use of NSAIDs, hematologic malignancy, URI, allergic reactions to bee sting, recent vaccinations Symptoms and signs: • Fatigue, irritability, reduced exercise tolerance, depression • Facial, extremity, abdominal ascites or vulvar or scrotal edema • Normal blood pressures in 60%

CASE 36 | Minimal Change Disease (MCD) *(continued)*

Discussion	**Diagnostics:**
	Initial labs will be consistent with nephrotic syndrome
	• Nephrotic range proteinuria
	• Early morning urine dipstick 3–4+ protein
	• Random protein to creatinine ratio >2 mg/mg
	• Urine albumin excretion >40 mg/m^2/hour
	• Hypoalbuminemia
	• Hyperlipidemia
	Other lab findings may include:
	• Anemia on CBC
	• Elevated BUN, low serum total calcium (due to hypoalbuminemia)
	• Normal serum complement levels
	The diagnosis is confirmed with disappearance of proteinuria after steroid treatment. Treatment failure would prompt concern for a different cause of nephrotic syndrome and necessitate renal biopsy. If done, biopsy of MCD would show:
	• Light microscopy: no findings
	• Electron microscopy: podocyte effacement
	• Immunofluorescence: no findings
	Management:
	Treatment with immunosuppressive therapy. Children with MCD have excellent response to prolonged course of corticosteroids. Over 70% of children with MCD reach adulthood without renal injury or urinary abnormality.
Additional Considerations	**Complications:** Acute renal failure (more likely in older patients or adults), thromboembolic events, and hyperlipidemia secondary to nephrotic syndrome, increased susceptibility to infections.

Urinary Tract Infections

CASE 37 | Urinary Tract Infection (UTI) in Infant

A 4-month-old uncircumcised boy is brought to the ED with one day of fever, irritability, and decreased urinary output. His temperature is 38.5°C, pulse is 122/min, respirations are 42/min, blood pressure is 84/46 mmHg, and SpO$_2$ is 99% on room air. On exam, he is warm and diaphoretic with palpable bladder.

Conditions with Similar Presentations	In infants less than 3 months old presenting with fever, it is important to consider other causes of infection in addition to UTI, such as meningitis, acute otitis media, gastroenteritis, and pneumonia. None of these would have a palpable bladder.
Initial Diagnostic Tests	• Check: Straight catheterized UA, urine culture and renal and bladder ultrasound if concern about obstruction or urinary retention • Consider: CBC, CMP, blood cultures and voiding cystourethrogram
Next Steps in Management	• Empiric antibiotics with plan to narrow once susceptibilities are obtained • Antipyretics • Supportive care: IV fluids if voiding
Discussion	UTIs or infections of the urethra, ureter, bladder, or kidneys are the most common bacterial infections in children under 2 years old. Most UTIs are caused by bacterial infection from retrograde ascending organisms from periurethral colonization. They are most often caused by: *E. coli* (over 80% of first-time UTIs), *Klebsiella, Proteus, Enterococci, Enterobacter, Citrobacter, Serratia, Pseudomonas* or *Chlamydia trachomatis.* **History:** There are many risk factors for UTIs in infants and children:

CASE 37 | Urinary Tract Infection in Infant (continued)

Discussion	Age: • Infants <60 days • 0–6 months: more common in uncircumcised males • >6 months: more common in females Anatomy: • Urinary tract abnormalities or urethral obstructions • Posterior urethral valves (PUVs) are congenital obstructions caused by a malformation of the posterior urethra. • Vesicoureteral reflux, hydronephrosis • Renal dysplasia • Labial adhesions or phimosis • Fistula between bladder/urethra and GI tract or vagina Historical: • History of UTIs • Recent or frequent urinary tract catheterization, instrumentation, or surgery Other: • Immunodeficiency • Diabetes • Neurogenic bladder • Constipation, bladder withholding behaviors • Foreign body (i.e., toilet paper) Symptom presentation will vary depending on age, development, and severity. In infants and toddlers under 3 years old, parents may report: • Fever, hypothermia, or temperature instability • Irritability or lethargy • Tachycardia or tachypnea • Hematuria or malodorous urine • Flank pain or tenderness • Vomiting, poor feeding, or failure to thrive • Decreased urinary output In children over 3 years old, symptoms include: • Notably, fever may be absent • Dysuria, frequency, hesitancy, urgency, or cloudy, malodourous urine • Lethargy • Nausea, vomiting **Physical Exam:** Findings may include: • Hypertension, tachycardia, and tachypnea • Palpable bladder from urinary retention or urethral obstruction • Abdominal distension from constipation • Suprapubic or flank tenderness infection • Sacral dimples, pits, or hair tufts concerning for congenital anomalies associated with neurogenic bladder • Labial adhesions, vulvitis, phimosis, or epididymo-orchitis, which could contribute to urinary retention **Diagnostics:** Obtain a urine sample prior to starting antibiotics for presumed UTI. High-quality clean-catch midline urine samples are preferred but may be difficult to obtain depending on age. Sterile bladder catheterization and suprapubic aspirations are preferred methods of obtaining urinary specimens in children who are not potty trained. Bagged specimens are frequently contaminated by skin or genital flora. To diagnose a UTI, both UA and urine culture findings are needed. • UA: Positive nitrite (if nitrite-producing organism); + leukocyte esterase; ≥10 white blood cells • Urine culture: ≥50,000 CFU/mL of a uropathogen in a catheterized sample or >100,000 CFU/mL in a clean-catch specimen

CASE 37 | Urinary Tract Infection in Infant *(continued)*

Discussion	Imaging studies are recommended in specific populations.
	• Renal and bladder ultrasound to assess for structural anomalies or exclude obstruction of upper and lower urinary tract is recommended in:
	• Infants <24 months with first febrile UTI
	• Children ≥24 months with more than one UTI
	• Voiding cystourethrogram is recommended in patients with a recurrent UTI as well as a first UTI and:
	• Abnormal findings on ultrasound
	• Findings suggestive of high-grade VUR or obstructive uropathy
	• Severe illness, decreased GFR, hypertension, poor growth, or atypical pathogens.
	Management:
	Ill-appearing children should be treated immediately.
	Once urinary specimens are collected, empiric antibiotics should be started.
	Antibiotics should be narrowed based on cultures and susceptibilities.
	Treatment with an antibiotic that the organism is susceptible to should be given for 7–14 days
Additional Considerations	**Complications:** Renal scarring may develop. Bacteremia occurs in ~5% of cases.

PEDIATRIC NEUROLOGY

Pediatric neurology is a broad specialty. The primary focus remains on epilepsy and seizure disorders as well as congenital abnormalities. Understanding a normal neurologic exam by age is important (reference back to developmental milestones) in helping to distinguish pathologic illness vs. normal development. Refer to Neurology and Obstetrics and Gynecology Chapters for further information and cases.

CASE 38 | Chiari II Malformation

A 6-hour-old male infant was born via spontaneous vaginal delivery to a 23-year-old G1P1 mother. The patient's Apgar scores were 8 and 9 at 1 and 5 minutes, respectively. The mother had no prenatal care during the pregnancy and takes no medications. The infant's temperature is 37°C, pulse is 142/min, and respirations are 35/min. His head circumference is on the 85th percentile with a full fontanelle. Weight is at the 30th percentile. On exam, infant is noted to have a large meningomyelocele on his lower back. Pulmonary exam shows stridor and cardiac exam is unremarkable. The abdomen is soft without masses or organomegaly. Bilateral upper extremities are flaccid and the infant barely moves during the exam.

Conditions with Similar Presentations	**Chiari I malformation:** Most common subtype of Chiari malformation, and involves protrusion of the cerebellar tonsils 5–10 mm through the foramen magnum into the spinal canal without herniation of other cerebellar structures. This malformation can be asymptomatic or present in adolescence or adulthood with headaches and/or syringomyelia.
	Chiari III malformation: Rare malformation associated with an encephalocele and has a high mortality rate due to respiratory failure in infancy.
	Spinal tumor: A spinal cord tumor such as an astrocytoma can present with neurologic deficits at or below the level of the tumor, such as unilateral or bilateral weakness or mild spasticity.
Initial Diagnostic Tests	• MRI is the best imaging modality, though antepartum ultrasound can identify early cerebellar abnormalities
Next Steps in Management	• Surgery to decompress the malformation and treat any associated meningocele • Ventriculoperitoneal shunt to treat associated hydrocephalus
Discussion	Chiari malformations are a congenital structural defect of the cerebellar fossa, which lies above the foramen magnum. These malformations result in a downward displacement of the contents of the fossa such as the cerebellum and cerebellar tonsils. Symptoms are dependent on the degree of cerebellar and brainstem herniation. **Chiari I malformation** is often asymptomatic in children and may be identified incidentally by imaging. It may present with pain, headache, or with associated syringomyelia.

CASE 38 | Chiari II Malformation *(continued)*

Discussion	**Chiari II (Arnold-Chiari) malformation** is nearly always associated with a meningomyelocele.
	History: Usually detected at birth. Symptoms reflect the degree of cerebellar and brainstem herniation below the foramen magnum and can include paresthesia, weakness, headache, and ataxia. Infants may have breathing difficulties, difficulty swallowing or feeding, failure to thrive, or arm weakness.
	Physical Exam: Macrocephaly, stridor, meningomyelocele (Chiari type II), neurologic deficits such as flaccid extremities
	Diagnostics: Confirm Diagnosis: • Antenatal ultrasound can reveal abnormalities in the cerebellar shape and possible ventriculomegaly • MRI of the brain is the best imaging modality for Chiari malformation, and would show low-lying cerebellar vermis and tonsils, extending below the foramen magnum and into the vertebral canal • In Chiari I, cervical and thoracic spine MRI may reveal a cystic cavity at C8–T1, indicative of syringomyelia
	Management: • Decompressive surgery is the initial treatment to reduce pressure of the herniation and potentially close the defect. • Some children may require repeat operations as they grow • In the case of hydrocephalus, ventricular shunting may be necessary to improve brainstem function • Additional surgery is required to close the associated myelomeningocele
Additional Considerations	Chiari malformations can be associated with: • **Neurofibromatosis type I:** a neurocutaneous disorder associated with angiofibromas and optic gliomas • **Noonan syndrome:** an autosomal dominant disorder associated with dysmorphic facial features and short stature

Chiari II malformation. A sagittal T2-weighted image of a 15-day-old infant shows a small posterior fossa, marked enlargement of the foramen magnum, and inferior displacement of the medulla and cerebellar vermis into the cervical spinal canal. (Reproduced with permission from Robert G. Wells, Diagnostic Imaging of Infants and Children; by The McGraw-Hill 2013.)

CASE 39 | Cerebral Palsy (CP)

A 15-month-old girl presents to clinic for delay in walking. She was born at 32 weeks, and her prenatal course was notable for intra-amniotic infection. The infant has a history of delayed motor milestones, including difficulty sitting without support at 9 months. On exam, the patient has hypertonia in all extremities, most prominent in the lower extremities with resistance to passive muscle stretch. She has a positive Babinski reflex bilaterally

Conditions with Similar Presentations	**Spinal muscular atrophy (SMA):** This is an autosomal recessive disorder that presents with weakness in proximal muscles and delayed motor milestones. Patients present with hypotonia rather than hypertonia given LMN dysfunction in SMA.
	Fetal alcohol syndrome (FAS): Maternal alcohol use is a risk factor for both CP and FAS, which both involve developmental delay. However, FAS has characteristic facial features including short palpebral fissures, a thin vermillion border, and smooth philtrum.
Initial Diagnostic Tests	Clinical diagnosis
Next Steps in Management	• Physical and occupational therapy. • Screening of vision, hearing, and cognition. • Manage medical and developmental comorbidities as the child matures.
Discussion	CP is the most common movement disorder of childhood. The prevalence of CP is higher in preterm infants and increases with decreasing gestational age. CP is due to prenatal insults to the nervous system resulting in nonprogressive motor dysfunction. Prematurity and complications during delivery that disrupt oxygen supply to the infant, such as placental abnormalities or antepartum hemorrhage, increase the risk for CP. Most commonly, patients have no known risk factors or identified etiology for their CP, so a thorough history and physical is necessary for any infant presenting with delayed motor milestones or spasticity.

CASE 39 | Cerebral Palsy (CP) *(continued)*

Discussion	**History:** • Risk factors include: prenatal insult to the fetus such as maternal tobacco or alcohol use, maternal obesity, intrauterine infections, and perinatal stroke. • May have delay in reaching motor milestones • May have had abnormal behavior early in infancy, including irritability and difficulty sleeping **Physical Exam:** • Increased tone and signs of upper motor neuron dysfunction (hyperreflexia, clonus, Babinski sign) • Spasticity of extremities, difficulty extending limbs, and contractures • Lower extremities are more affected than the upper extremities **Diagnostics:** • Cerebral palsy is a clinical diagnosis • Consider: Brain MRI may reveal periventricular leukomalacia (necrosis of white matter due to infection or ischemia) or germinal matrix bleeding. **Management:** • The neurologic damage due to CP is permanent and nonprogressive, though the presentation of symptoms may change as the CNS develops. • Treatment goals involve maximizing current motor function via a multidisciplinary approach including physical and occupational therapy. • Motor dysfunction should be monitored regularly over time. • In the case of spasticity and hyperreflexia, patients may be treated with anti-spasticity drugs, such as baclofen or diazepam.
Additional Considerations	**Obstetrics Considerations:** Pregnant women who experience preterm labor at <32 weeks gestational age are at higher risk of having a fetus with cerebral palsy. To reduce this risk, magnesium sulfate is given for fetal neuroprotection.

CASE 40 | Spina Bifida/Meningocele

A newborn male born at 38 weeks' gestation is noted to have a large membranous sac over his lumbosacral area. His mother received no prenatal care but is noted to have a history of seizures adequately managed by carbamazepine. On physical exam, the infant has full range of motion of his upper extremities and paralysis of his lower extremities. He also has bilateral club feet.

Conditions with Similar Presentations	**Anencephaly:** A severe open NTD resulting in absent cranium, cerebrum, or abnormalities in the cerebellum and brainstem. Polyhydramnios is noted during prenatal ultrasound. This condition is incompatible with life.
Initial Diagnostic Tests	• Clinical diagnosis • Consider: MRI of the spine and brain to delineate spinal cord malformations
Next Steps in Management	Surgical repair of the defect if needed to preserve neurologic function
Discussion	Spina bifida is a birth defect in which the spinal column is either absent or did not completely form. Subtypes include spina bifida occulta, meningocele, and myelomeningocele. Maternal folate deficiency, particularly in the first trimester of pregnancy during which the neural tube closes, is a risk factor for NTD. Folate deficiency can be due to inadequate intake, metabolic abnormalities, or folate antagonist medications (e.g., methotrexate, carbamazepine). There is a genetic component as well as an association with many chromosomal disorders (e.g., trisomy 13 and 18). NTDs are more common in regions without access to prenatal care and screening programs or lack of access to folate-fortified foods. **History:** Assess maternal folate intake and medication history (particularly use of drugs that interfere with folate metabolism) **Physical Exam:** • **Spina bifida occulta:** Minor defect in fusion of vertebrae, and neural tissue is unexposed. May have sacral dimple above the gluteal cleft, patch of hair, or dark pigmentation. • **Meningocele:** Open neural tube defect (NTD) with protrusion of meninges from spinal column. Presents as a cyst covered with skin or meninges. • **Myelomeningocele:** Open NTD with cyst-like protrusion of meninges and spinal cord. Often associated with Chiari II malformation and obstructive hydrocephalus. Neurologic deficits are noted distal to the lesion, such as bowel or bladder incontinence.

CASE 40 | Spina Bifida/Meningocele *(continued)*

Discussion	**Diagnostics:** • Clinical diagnosis • Consider: MRI of the spine and brain to delineate spinal cord malformations **Management:** • Management during the prenatal period includes discussions surrounding serial imaging, potential termination of pregnancy, and possibility of fetal surgery. • After birth, surgical repair of the defect should be considered in the case of meningomyelocele. • For obstructive hydrocephalus, a ventriculo-peritoneal shunt is required.
Additional Considerations	**Obstetrics Considerations:** Due to the strong association of NTD with folic acid deficiency, all women should begin folic acid 0.4 mg daily supplementation at least 1 month prior to conception. Patients who require continued drugs that interfere with folate metabolism require a higher dosage of 4 mg daily.

CASE 41 | Germinal Matrix Hemorrhage-Intraventricular Hemorrhage (GMH–IVH)

An 8-hour-old boy presents with seizure. The infant was born via vaginal delivery at 30 weeks and is small for gestational age. The infant's upper extremities are flaccid. His breathing is irregular, and cardiac exam reveals tachycardia. On physical examination, the infant is found to have bulging fontanelles and depressed respirations.

Conditions with Similar Presentations	**Hypoglycemia:** May also present with neonatal seizures. There may be a history of maternal diabetes mellitus. It would not have bulging fontanelles. **Periventricular leukomalacia:** Brain injury that leads to damage of white matter tissue around the ventricles. Also more common in premature infants. Presents with weakness but is greater in the lower extremities and often not present at birth. Is not associated with seizures.
Initial Diagnostic Tests	Cranial ultrasound showing intraventricular hemorrhage (hyperechoic lesions) and dilation of ventricles
Next Steps in Management	• Supportive care • Manage seizures with antiepileptic medication
Discussion	GMH-IVH are neurologic injuries that can rarely occur in premature infants. The germinal matrix is an embryological structure in the fetal brain that is located between the caudate nucleus and the thalamus at the level of the foramen of Monro. It is a highly vascular area with thin-walled vessels which rupture easily. Rupture is associated with neural injury and also bleeding into the adjacent intraventricular space. **History:** Risk factors include prematurity, neonatal stress, and very low birth weight. Usually presents within 7 days of birth. Most cases are asymptomatic. **Physical Exam:** Hypotension, bulging anterior fontanelle, respiratory distress **Diagnostics:** Presentation of a germinal matrix hemorrhage can range from asymptomatic to catastrophic (seizures, apnea, stupor, or coma). Therefore, routine cranial ultrasound screening is performed on all preterm infants <30 weeks to screen for brain injury. • Grade 1—bleeding limited to germinal matrix • Grade 2—intraventricular hemorrhage without ventricular dilation • Grade 3—intraventricular hemorrhage with ventricular dilation • Grade 4—bleeding into surrounding cerebral tissue **Management:** Treat seizures, give oxygen, monitor for development of posthemorrhagic ventricular dilation Germinal matrix hemorrhage; grade I. A coronal sonographic image of a 4-day-old premature infant shows bilateral echogenic germinal matrix hemorrhages (*arrows*) adjacent to the frontal horns. (Reproduced with permission from Robert G. Wells, Diagnostic Imaging of Infants and Children; by The McGraw-Hill 2013.)
Additional Considerations	**Complications:** Include cerebral palsy, intellectual disability, and posthemorrhagic ventricular dilation. The latter may require repeat lumbar punctures and temporary or permanent ventricular drainage devices.

Neurocutaneous Disorders

CASE 42	Tuberous Sclerosis Complex (TSC)

A 7-month-old boy is brought for evaluation of brief episodes of arm twitching that occur multiple times every day. He is unable to sit up independently and has a rash on the lower back with a leathery texture. On exam he has a holosystolic, high-pitched "blowing" murmur heard loudest at the apex and radiating toward the axilla. During the exam, the child suddenly flexes his arms multiple times.

Conditions with Similar Presentations	**Sturge-Weber syndrome** (encephalotrigeminal angiomatosis): Is another neurocutaneous disorder which can present with seizures. It is a non-inherited developmental anomaly of neural crest cell derivatives that affects small blood vessels. It presents with a classic triad of (1) port-wine stain (nevus flammeus, see image), (2) capillary-venous malformations, particularly in the meninges, and (3) glaucoma. Patients commonly develop seizures. 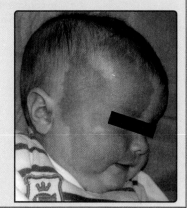 **Neonatal tetanus:** An infant may present with spasms, difficulty feeding, and hypertonicity with trismus, clenched hands, and dorsiflexed feet. Infection is more likely to occur through cord contamination during an unsanitary delivery in an unimmunized mother. There are no cutaneous lesions. Extensive right facial capillary malformation involving the ophthalmic and maxillary branches of the trigeminal nerve in a 6-month-old girl with Sturge-Weber syndrome. (Reproduced with permission from Kang S, Amagai M, Bruckner AL, et al., eds. Fitzpatrick's Dermatology. 9th ed. New York: McGraw Hill; 2019.)
Initial Diagnostic Tests	• Clinical diagnosis and genetic testing— genetic testing for *TSC1* or *TSC2* gene mutations • Check EEG, ECG, echocardiogram • Check MRI abdomen and brain to evaluate for additional masses

Next Steps in Management	• Treat seizures
	  • Infantile spasms: vigabatrin with or without ACTH
	  • Focal seizures: oxcarbazepine or carbamazepine
	• Tumor surveillance via MRI of the brain and kidneys
	• Serial echocardiography
	• Patients should undergo EEG and neuropsychiatric testing, as neurocognitive disorders such as autism spectrum disorder are associated with TSC

Discussion	TSC is the most common genetic cause of infantile spasm and is an autosomal dominant multi-organ disease and one of several neurocutaneous disorders. It is caused by mutations in one of two tumor suppressor genes: *TSC1* gene on chromosome 9 (encodes hamartin) or the *TSC2* gene on chromosome 16 (encodes tuberin). These mutations result in the growth of hamartomas (benign growths made up of abnormal cells and tissues) in various organs throughout the body. Associated tumors include subependymal nodules and rhabdomyomas; the latter usually regress after birth. **History:** • 1- to 2-second seizures where the baby thrusts out his arm or bends forward with stiff extremities • Intellectual disabilities • Autistic behavior **Physical Exam:** Patients have numerous mucocutaneous manifestations • Dermatologic findings include facial angiofibroma (image A), shagreen patches (image B), and hypomelanotic macules ("ash leaf spots," image C). • Other findings include fibrous plaques, ungual or intraoral fibromas, retinal hamartomas, dental pits • Cardiac exam may be normal or reveal a murmur due to rhabdomyomas or coarctation of the aorta 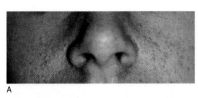 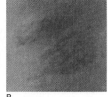 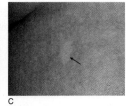 A B C A and B, Reproduced with permission from Gregg T. Lueder, Pediatric Practice: Ophthalmology; by The McGraw-Hill 2011. (From Paul R. Carney, James D. Geyer, Pediatric Practice: Neurology. Copyright 2010 by The McGraw-Hill. FIGURE 22-2. ISBN 9780071489256., C, Reproduced with permission from Wolff K, Goldsmith LA, Katz SI, Gilchrest BA, Paller AS, Lefferell DJ. Fitzpatrick's Dermatology in General Medicine. 7th ed. New York: McGraw-Hill; 2008.)

CASE 42 | Tuberous Sclerosis Complex (TSC) *(continued)*

Discussion	**Diagnostics:** • Clinical diagnosis and genetic testing for *TSC1* or *TSC2* gene mutations. • Supportive diagnostics include neuroimaging (e.g., CT or MRI) to identify hamartomas (figure, panel A) and calcified subependymal nodules (panel B) • MRI of the abdomen or renal US to identify renal angiomyolipomas • ECG and echocardiogram to evaluate for aortic disease, valvular disease, and cardiac rhabdomyomas • Detailed ocular and dermatologic exam. • Can consider EEG monitoring in patients with ongoing seizure activity. Infantile spasms are an epileptic encephalopathy syndrome characterized by a unique chaotic EEG pattern known as hypsarrhythmia.

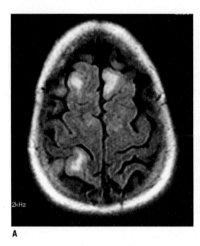
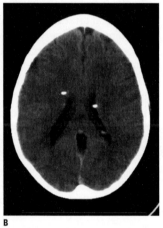

A   B

Tuberous sclerosis. A. MRI showing multiple hamartomas. B. Subependymal nodules are demonstrated on CT, where their calcific nature has led them to be termed "brain stones." (Reproduced with permission from Ropper AH, Samuels MA, Klein JP, et al., eds. Adams and Victor's Principles of Neurology. 11th ed. New York: McGraw Hill; 2019.)

Management:
• The choice of antiepileptic drugs is based on the seizure type.
  • First-line for infantile spasms and TSC is vigabatrin or corticotropin.
  • Focal seizures are treated with oxcarbazepine or carbamazepine
• Patients should undergo frequent surveillance of new lesions with imaging of the brain, heart, kidneys, and lungs.
• If brain tumors are identified, surgical resection can be considered as well as medical treatment with mTOR inhibitors (everolimus).
• A multidisciplinary team is required for management of the tumors or physical findings associated with TSC
• Patients may also require special education services and psychiatric treatment.

Neurocutaneous Disorders

Neurocutaneous Disorder	Gene Mutation and Inheritance	Neurologic Features	Other Features	Additional Considerations
Neurofibromatosis type 1	Neurofibromin protein on chromosome 17 AD, variable expressivity with complete penetrance	Cutaneous neurofibromas (benign peripheral nerve sheath tumors), intellectual disability, optic glioma	Café-au-lait spots, axillary/inguinal freckling, meningioma and associated seizures, Lisch nodules (iris hamartomas), pheochromocytoma, kyphoscoliosis	Likely to present in teens. Diagnose via MRI of the CNS, auditory testing, ophthalmologic exam, and dermatologic exam. Obtain family history.
Neurofibromatosis type 2	Merlin/schwannomin on chromosome 22 AD	Bilateral vestibular schwannoma (acoustic neuroma), meningioma, ependymoma	Juvenile cataracts, skin nodules, café-au-lait spots	

Neurocutaneous Disorders

Neurocutaneous Disorder	Gene Mutation and Inheritance	Neurologic Features	Other Features	Additional Considerations
von Hippel-Lindau disease (VHL)	Deletion on chromosome 3p for protein pVHL AD	Hemangioblastomas in the cerebellum or spine	Ocular hemangioblastoma, bilateral renal cell carcinoma, pheochromocytoma	
Tuberous sclerosis	*TSC1*: hamartin on chromosome 9. *TSC2*: tuberin on chromosome 16 AD, variable expressivity	Subependymal nodules, subependymal giant cell astrocytomas, CNS hamartomas and associated seizures, intellectual disability	Angiofibromas, ash-leaf spots, cardiac rhabdomyoma, renal angiomyolipoma, periungual fibromas, sebaceous adenomas in distribution over nose and cheeks, shagreen patches (rough papule)	May present as infantile spasms. Obtain MRI of brain, echocardiogram, MRI abdomen, and EEG. Treat infantile spasms with vigabatrin, second line ACTH.
Sturge-Weber	Activating mutation of *GNAQ* Non-hereditary, somatic mosaicism	Leptomeningeal angioma and associated seizures, hemiparesis	Nevus flammeus (unilateral port-wine stain), episcleral hemangioma resulting in glaucoma	Intracranial calcifications may form "tram-lines."

Abbreviation: AD, autosomal dominant.

Seizures

CASE 43	Childhood Absence Epilepsy (CAE)

A 7-year-old girl with no prior medical history is brought for evaluation of episodic staring off into space. Her spells last 5–10 seconds and occur several times throughout the day. She has had a recent decline in school performance over the last 8–10 months. During the mental status exam, the child stops mid-sentence and stares with blinking and right-hand picking movements, lasting 10 seconds. After the spell is over, she immediately finishes her sentence.

Conditions with Similar Presentations	**Juvenile myoclonic epilepsy (JME):** Is a form of idiopathic generalized epilepsy that presents most commonly in the ages of 8–28. The clinical hallmark is myoclonic seizures, which are quick motor jerks of the upper extremities and head that occur most often in the mornings shortly after awakening and with intact consciousness. Patients may also have generalized tonic-clonic seizures and rarely absence seizures. EEG is characterized by 4–6 hertz generalized poly-spike and slow wave discharges. Seizures in JME are often exacerbated by alcohol consumption and sleep deprivation. Unlike CAE, JME does not completely disappear with age and requires lifelong anti-seizure medication.
	Non-epileptic staring spells: Children may have staring spells in association with ADHD, intellectual disability, or autism spectrum disorder. These spells are readily broken by vocal interruption or tactile stimulation and are not associated with automatisms.
	Focal seizures with impaired awareness (previously known as complex partial seizures): Also manifest as staring and may have automatisms (lip smacking, chewing, repeating words or phrases). These last longer than absence seizures (minutes vs. seconds) and, unlike CAE, have a post-ictal state of confusion and tiredness and are not precipitated by hyperventilation.
Initial Diagnostic Tests	• Check EEG • Consider bedside hyperventilation (seizures can be brought on by 3-minute hyperventilation in 90% of cases)

CASE 43 | Childhood Absence Epilepsy (CAE) *(continued)*

Next Steps in Management	Treat with ethosuximide
Discussion	CAE is a generalized nonconvulsive epilepsy syndrome in childhood that manifests as sudden non-motor seizures characterized by staring spells and behavior arrest, which are called absence seizures (there is loss of consciousness without loss of body tone). Patients may have tens to hundreds of seizures a day. Onset occurs between the ages of 4 and 10 with a slight female predominance. Most outgrow their seizures by puberty, however there is a slight increased risk of developing adult epilepsy. **History/Physical Exam:** • Staring spells lasting less than a minute • Immediate recovery of consciousness with no memory of event and no post-ictal state. • There may be automatisms (e.g., eye fluttering, lip smacking, unilateral picking) • Decline in school grades • There may be a family history of seizures • Interictally, exam is normal • Certain medications such as carbamazepine and phenytoin can worsen absence epilepsy. • Rarely, patients can have generalized tonic-clonic seizures. **Diagnostics:** • History is highly suggestive • Routine scalp EEG shows 2.5–5 Hz spike-wave discharges diffusely throughout the brain. • Bedside hyperventilation for 3 minutes triggers similar staring spells. **Management:** • Ethosuximide is the drug of choice; alternatives include valproic acid and lamotrigine. • Avoid antiepileptic drugs that can exacerbate absence seizures, which are carbamazepine, phenytoin, and gabapentin. • Over 90% of patients will spontaneously resolve after puberty.

CASE 44 | Febrile Seizures

A 4-year-old boy diagnosed with roseola infantum 2 days ago is brought in by his parents after an episode of convulsions of his arms and legs that lasted about 5 minutes approximately 1 hour ago. During the episode, the patient's eyes rolled back and he turned blue. Prior to the episode his temperature was 104°F. After it, he was lethargic. He is currently back to normal mentation. Vitals are temperature 103.6°F, pulse 140 bpm, and BP 140/90 mmHg. There is a mild "slapped cheek" malar rash bilaterally. Patient's father reports having a similar seizure-like episode during an illness in his infancy.

Conditions with Similar Presentations	**Meningitis or encephalitis:** Such infections may also present with fever, seizures, and altered mental status but the latter will not spontaneously return to normal. If the patient is older than 12 months of age, meningeal signs may be observed such as neck rigidity, Brudzinski sign, and Kernig sign. Meningococcal meningitis may have a petechial rash. **Breath-holding spell:** Patient would have cessation of breathing usually in response to fear or pain, which may result in loss of consciousness. These spells are not associated with fever.
Initial Diagnostic Tests	Clinical diagnosis: identify the underlying cause of the fever, as directed by findings on history and physical examination.
Next Steps in Management	• Febrile seizures are self-limiting. • Antipyretics and treat underlying cause of fever

CASE 44 | Febrile Seizures (continued)

Discussion	Febrile seizures are a common pediatric neurologic condition and develop in children 6 months to 6 years of life. They present as convulsions in the setting of a high fever (>40°C or 104°F) but can also be seen at lower temperatures. Most commonly the fever is from a viral infection, less commonly a recent immunization. They are classified as simple or complex. Simple febrile seizures last less than 15 minutes and do not recur within 24 hours. Complex febrile seizures last longer than 15 minutes or recur within 24 hours. Patients with complex febrile seizures are more likely to experience nonfebrile seizures in the future. There may be a family history, and there is a slightly higher prevalence in boys. The prognosis of patients who experience simple febrile seizures is good. They are not associated with developmental delay. There is a slight increased risk for future epilepsy. The risk for recurrence of seizures is highest within 1 year of the first seizure.
	History/Physical Exam:
	• Assess length of seizure.
	• Height of temperature correlates with probability of febrile seizure diagnosis
	• Febrile seizures are associated with a brief postictal state with quick return of mental status to baseline.
	• Evaluate for underlying cause of fever, including source of infection (e.g. petechial rash, erythematous pharynx, bulging tympanic membrane)
	• Assess for meningeal signs such as neck rigidity, Brudzinski sign, and Kernig sign.
	Diagnostics:
	Testing may be done to identify the underlying cause of the fever, as directed by findings on history and physical examination.
	• Infants less than 6 months of age should have a sepsis workup (CBC, urinalysis, blood culture, urine culture, and CSF analysis and culture).
	• Otherwise, a first-time febrile seizure does not require any further investigations.
	Consider:
	• If failure to have spontaneous full recovery of mental status: check for electrolyte abnormalities with serum sodium.
	• If a complex seizure: EEG and MRI
	• If concern for CNS infection and/or patient presents with headache, neck pain, or photophobia: lumbar puncture
	Management:
	• Antipyretics can be provided to treat the fever, though aspirin should be avoided due to concern for Reyes syndrome.
	• Identify and treat any underlying condition contributing to the fever, such as meningitis or encephalitis.
	• Provide parental education regarding febrile seizures.

Mini-Case

Case	Key Findings
Breath-Holding Spells (BHS)	**Hx:** A 3-year-old girl starts crying after her mother takes a toy away from her. She cries and then holds her breath. Suddenly the child turns blue and falls to the floor.
	PE: During a cyanotic breath-holding spell, limpness and cyanosis is characteristic. There may be generalized clonic activity or seizures if prolonged.
	During a pallid breath-holding spell, bradycardia, diaphoresis, and bladder incontinence may be seen.
	Diagnostics: Breath-holding spells are diagnosed clinically.
	Management:
	• Consider CBC and ferritin to assess for iron deficiency.
	• If lab results are unremarkable, provide reassurance.

Mini-Case *(continued)*

Breath-Holding Spells (BHS)	**Discussion:** The exact cause of BHS is unknown. It is postulated that dysregulation of the autonomic nervous system contributes to BHS. Iron deficiency seems to contribute to this dysregulation and is more commonly seen in children with BHS. Iron is an essential component for catecholamine metabolism and therefore iron deficiency may impact the autonomic nervous system. BHS are most commonly seen between 6 months and 2 years of age. Family history of BHS is a risk factor. BHS most commonly resolve by age 5 and complications are not seen. The two types of BHS are cyanotic or pallid, with around 80% characterized as cyanotic: • **Cyanotic BHS** are often triggered by frustration or a temper tantrum followed by forced expiration and breath-holding with loss of consciousness and sudden limpness. • **Pallid BHS** are typically triggered by fear or pain and are associated with breath-holding, loss of consciousness, and pallor.

PEDIATRIC HEMATOLOGY

Hematologic disorders in the pediatric population are due to quantitative or qualitative abnormalities of the blood cells. Hematologic disorders have characteristic clinical presentations related to the specific affected blood component. These manifestations are not diagnostic of the cause of the disorder.

Condition	Associated Symptoms and Signs
Anemia	Pallor, fatigue
Polycythemia	Irritability, cyanosis, seizures
Neutropenia	Fever, pharyngitis, lymphadenopathy
Thrombocytopenia	Petechiae, ecchymosis, hemorrhage, epistaxis

Anemia

Anemia in the pediatric population is defined as a hemoglobin value below the age-specific range. During pregnancy, RBC production is driven by erythropoietin. At the time of delivery, the combination of decreased erythropoietin and the shortened life cycle of the RBC (fetal RBCs have a 60-day life cycle compared to 120 days of older children and adults) leads to a decrease in hemoglobin concentration. This physiologic anemia reaches its lowest point by 6–8 weeks post-gestation. During this normal part of development, hemoglobin may drop as low as 9.5 g/dL. The infant should be asymptomatic, and no intervention is required. After this nadir, the hemoglobin starts to increase again to normal childhood levels.

CASE 45	Iron Deficiency Anemia (IDA)	
A 12-month-old girl presents with irritability and poor feeding. She was born at 34 weeks and has been provided cow's milk since the age of 6 months. On exam, patient is irritable and has pale mucous membranes. CBC shows: Hemoglobin: 7 g/dL and mean corpuscular volume: 63 fl		
Conditions with Similar Presentations	**Thalassemia:** Also is a microcytic anemia. In contrast to IDA, all the cells will be of similar size, so the RDW is normal. Hemoglobin electrophoresis will help determine the exact thalassemia present. **Sideroblastic anemias:** Also cause microcytic anemia and are due to defects in heme synthesis that are congenital or acquired. Acquired causes include drugs (isoniazid, chloramphenicol, linezolid), copper deficiency, and zinc toxicity. Ringed sideroblasts are seen in the bone marrow. Lead poisoning gives a similar picture, and patients may have other symptoms such as abdominal pain and learning disabilities, and diagnosis can be made by finding elevated blood lead levels.	
Initial Diagnostic Tests	Check CBC with serum iron, TIBC, and ferritin	
Next Steps in Management	Oral iron supplementation, or IM/IV iron supplementation if GI absorption issue	

CASE 45 | Iron Deficiency Anemia (IDA) *(continued)*

Discussion	Iron deficiency is the most common cause of anemia in children, with the highest prevalence in children less than 5 years of age. Maternal iron stores maintain adequate iron levels in infants for 3–6 months. However, the majority of maternal-fetal iron transfer occurs during the third trimester of pregnancy, so maternal iron deficiency during pregnancy and premature birth both increase the risk of iron deficiency in the infant. In infants and children undergoing normal growth (for the synthesis of hemoglobin and myoglobin), 30% of daily iron needs must come from the diet in order to account for the increased iron demand. Dietary deficiencies are the primary cause of IDA in infancy and early childhood. Unmodified cow's milk increases intestinal blood loss in infants compared with formula or breast feeding. This is due to a subclinical proctocolitis. Additionally, excessive ingestion of cow's milk in young children is an important risk factor for iron deficiency due to the low concentration of iron, as well as the fact that cow milk caseins bind iron with high affinity, inhibiting the absorption of the already low Fe content in cow's milk.
	History: The most important screening test for IDA in infants is a dietary history. The child may present with fatigue, dyspnea, tachycardia, angina, syncope, and pica; however, if the anemia develops slowly, patients are generally asymptomatic.
	Physical Exam: Glossitis, conjunctival pallor, cheilosis (corners of the mouth become inflamed), koilonychia ("spoon nails").
	Diagnostics: • Confirm Diagnosis: CBC showing microcytic hypochromic anemia with a low serum ferritin and iron, and high TIBC and transferrin. Consider checking: • Reticulocyte count • The Mentzer index (MCV/RBC count) can be helpful in differentiating IDA vs. thalassemia. If the index is <13, this is more indicative of thalassemia, while if >13, this is more indicative of IDA.
	Management: • Replace iron orally until normal and for at least 4–6 months to replenish stores. • If oral supplementation is insufficient, use intramuscular or IV iron. IV iron is useful in achieving a sustained Hb response, reducing the need for future packed RBC transfusions. • Limit cow's milk ingestion. Encourage exclusive breastfeeding for the first 6 months of life.
Additional Considerations	**Screening:** Screen for IDA with Hb level in all infants 9–12 months per CDC recommendations **Complications:** Oral supplementation with iron sulfate may lead to nausea, constipation, diarrhea, abdominal pain, and black stools. IV iron dextran is associated with a small risk for anaphylaxis. Also note that antacids may interfere with iron absorption.

Type of Anemia	Etiologies and Associations	Treatments
Microcytic anemia MCV <80	*Iron deficiency* Inadequate dietary intake, excess cow's milk consumption, malabsorption	Fe supplementation
	Thalassemia Hereditary	Blood transfusions or donor stem cell transplant

	Sideroblastic anemia
	   Hereditary
	   Lead poisoning
	Old buildings, paint chips
		Treat cause, if lead poisoning give chelation therapies (succimer, EDTA, and dimercaprol)

Type of Anemia	Etiologies and Associations	Treatments
Megaloblastic anemia MCV >100	*Folate deficiency* Goat milk as sole source of milk, Hx of intestinal resection	Folate supplementation, replace dietary goat milk
	B12 deficiency Vegan diets, goat milk	B12 and Fe supplementation
	Orotic aciduria Decreased UMP synthase for pyrimidine synthesis pathway (Note: Ornithine transcarbamylase deficiency also causes orotic aciduria, but without megaloblastic anemia)	Administration of uridine monophosphate (UMP) or uridine triacetate (which is converted to UMP)
	Homocystinuria *Deficiency in cystathionine synthetase*	Vitamins B6, B9, and B12
Normocytic anemia MCV 80–100	**Hemolytic**	
	Sickle cell disease	RBC transfusions, possible stem cell transplant
	G6PD deficiency	Supportive care after episodes and avoidance of triggers
	Hereditary spherocytosis	RBC transfusions, folic acid administration, full or partial splenectomy, cholecystectomy
	Pyruvate kinase deficiency	RBC transfusions if severe anemia, splenectomy
	Microangiopathic hemolytic anemia	Plasma exchange, treat cause
	Non-hemolytic	
	Aplastic anemia	If severe, immunosuppression or bone marrow transplant
	Iron deficiency anemia (initially normocytic)	Iron supplementation
	Anemia of chronic inflammation	Treat underlying disease

Bleeding Disorders

Bleeding disorders can often be distinguished based on the age of presentation (birth vs. later in life) as well as subtle differences in labs that suggest different effects on the coagulation cascade. Please refer to Hematology and Oncology Chapter for additional cases.

	Hemophilia A	Hemophilia B	Hemophilia C
Inheritance	X-linked recessive	X-linked recessive	Autosomal recessive
Pathophysiology	Deficiency in factor VIII	Deficiency in factor IX	Deficiency in factor XI
Presentation	Hemophilia A and B present similarly: easy bruising or spontaneous hematoma formation, recurrent epistaxis, hemarthrosis, excessive bleeding following small procedures Female carriers may show mild symptoms		Similar to hemophilia A and B, but less likely to present with deep tissue bleed
Treatment	Administration of factor VII or desmopressin, which promotes release of von Willebrand factor (vWF) to elevate factor VIII concentration	Administration of factor IX	Administration of factor XI

CASE 46 | Hemophilia A

An 11-year-old boy presents with pain and swelling of his right knee after falling on the playground. He has a history of easy bruising with minor trauma. He also has two maternal uncles with a similar history of recurrent bleeding and bruising, but his sisters do not have any bleeding problems. He has a large knee effusion with overlying bruising.

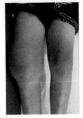

Reproduced with permission from Lichtman MA, Shafer MS, Felgar RE, Wang N, Lichtman's Atlas of Hematology 2016; by McGraw-Hill 2017.

Conditions with Similar Presentations	**Hemophilia B:** Is also an X-linked inherited bleeding disorder but can be distinguished by low factor IX levels. It is much less common than hemophilia A, but its clinical presentation is identical.
	Hemophilia C: Is an autosomal dominant or recessive disorder involving factor XI. It is the least common hemophilia. The vast majority of patients do not have abnormal bleeding, but if they do, it is similar to the other hemophilias.
	Acquired hemophilia: Occurs in patients who develop a factor VIII, IX, or XI inhibitor, usually in setting of malignancy or autoimmune condition. It is often found in elderly patients with a new history of bleeding.
	von Willebrand disease: Can also present with ↓factor VIII. However, VWF antigen would be low and ristocetin cofactor assay would be abnormal.
	Vitamin K deficiency: Can also present as a coagulation defect; however, would have a normal bleeding time and decreased activity of factors II, VII, IX, X, protein C, and protein S.
Initial Diagnostic Testing	• Check factor VIII and PTT (↓ factor VIII level and ↑PTT) • Consider checking CBC, coags, other factor levels (IX, XI, VWF antigen and activity), mixing study to detect antibodies, and genetic testing
Next Steps in Management	Factor VIII replacement therapy
Discussion	Hemophilia A (80% of hemophilias) is an inherited bleeding disorder characterized by spontaneous bleeding and/or bruising due to a mutation in the factor VIII gene on chromosome X, leading to a deficiency of factor VIII.
	History/Physical Exam: • Clinical presentation is variable and dependent on the severity of factor deficiency. • Most common manifestation is hemarthrosis, either spontaneous or traumatic. • Hematomas and mucocutaneous bleeding (oral cavity, epistaxis) can occur. • May have family history of bleeding disorders. X-linked recessive disease (much more common in men). Daughters of one affected parent can be asymptomatic carriers.
	Diagnostics: • Check coagulation studies and levels of factor VIII, IX, XI, VWF antigen and activity • Factor VIII levels will be low in hemophilia A • PTT will be prolonged with a normal PT • Other factors will be normal • Mixing study (combining the patient's plasma with normal plasma) corrects the ↑PTT and suggests a factor deficiency. If it does not correct, this is evidence of an antibody to factor VIII. • Genetic testing will confirm the causative mutation.
	Management: Bleeding severity is based on factor levels and establishes the clinical phenotype. • Patients who have active bleeding should receive recombinant factor VIII replacement. • Patients with severe hemophilia (factor VIII level <1%) should receive prophylaxis with regular factor replacement to reduce bleeding events. • Patients with mild hemophilia (factor VIII level >5%) may be treated with desmopressin (DDAVP) only if it has previously worked. • Patients should avoid NSAIDs to minimize concomitant platelet dysfunction.

CASE 46 | Hemophilia A (continued)

Additional Considerations	**Screening:** Hemophilia testing is not a routine part of newborn screening, but noninvasive prenatal testing to determine fetal sex when either parent is a carrier is recommended, as males are more commonly affected. Further invasive genetic testing is individualized.
	Complications: Life-threatening bleeding, including intracerebral hemorrhage and joint damage from recurrent hemarthroses.
	Surgical Considerations: Patients undergoing elective surgery should have factor levels monitored and should receive factor replacement before/after surgery to maintain factor levels within target range.

CASE 47 | von Willebrand Disease, Type 1

A 13-year-old girl presents with prolonged and heavy menstrual cycles since undergoing menarche. She also notices bleeding gums with brushing her teeth. Her father and brother have a history of recurrent nosebleeds. CBC shows that her platelet count, PT/INR, and PTT are normal. Bleeding time is prolonged.

Conditions with Similar Presentations	**Hemophilia A/B:** Also present with increased bleeding but are much more likely to present in men, as inheritance is X-linked recessive. Patients will have spontaneous bleeding events, and labs will demonstrate ↑PTT and ↓factor VIII or ↓factor IX levels.
	Bernard-Soulier syndrome: Is a disorder of platelet adhesion caused by absent GPIb on platelets. Absence of GPIb results in the inability of VWF to bind to platelets and thus platelets are unable to effectively adhere to exposed collagen to promote clotting. It presents with increased bleeding, however would have thrombocytopenia and normal levels of VWF and factor VIII.
	Glanzmann thrombasthenia: Is a disorder of platelet aggregation due to low glycoprotein IIb/IIIa. It also presents with increased bleeding but platelets, VWF and factor VIII levels, and ristocetin cofactor assay would all be normal.
Initial Diagnostic Testing	• Check factor VIII level and VWF antigen platelet-dependent VWF activity tests (e.g., Ristocetin assay) (↓ VWF, ↓ factor VIII levels)
	• Consider CBC (platelets), coags, bleeding time, other factor levels and checking VWF multimer assay
Next Steps in Management	• Pharmacological treatment with desmopressin for mild to moderate bleeding
	• VWF concentrates can be used for more severe bleeding
Discussion	VWF is a glycoprotein made by endothelial cells and megakaryocytes that enhances platelet adhesion and aggregation. It is also a carrier of factor VIII, increasing its circulating half-life. von Willebrand disease is a bleeding disorder characterized by a qualitative or quantitative defect in VWF. It is autosomal dominant, the most common inherited bleeding disorder, and affects all ethnicities and genders. Women are more frequently diagnosed than men due to mild disease becoming apparent with menstruation.
	History/Physical Exam:
	• Usually asymptomatic; no easy bruising or spontaneous bleeding
	• Prolonged bleeding after a hemostatic challenge (teeth brushing, dental work, surgery). Women may present with heavy menstrual cycles
	• Family history of disease may also be present
	• Physical exam may reveal mucosal bleeding
	Diagnostics:
	• Confirm diagnosis with VWF antigen platelet-dependent VWF activity tests (e.g., Ristocetin cofactor assay) and factor VIII: Reveals poor platelet aggregation and ↓ VWF, ↓ factor VIII levels
	• ↑Bleeding time
	• PTT mildly elevated
	• VWF multimer assay is a second-line confirmatory test
	Management: The goal of treatment is often to stop bleeding or provide prophylaxis for surgery.
	• Mild disease or preparing for surgery: Desmopressin (DDAVP), which increases release of VWF from the endothelium
	• Severe bleeding: VWF/factor VIII complex
	• Avoid aspirin/NSAIDs and platelet function inhibitors as these can worsen bleeding
Additional Considerations	**Acquired von Willebrand disease:** Is a disorder caused by reduced levels of VWF secondary to specific conditions or medications. Common causes include hematologic diseases and cardiac abnormalities such as aortic stenosis. The clinical presentation is similar in that patients experience bleeding from mucosal sites.

PEDIATRIC ONCOLOGY

Leukemia is the most common cancer in children and teens. The classic presenting symptoms in children (fever, pallor, and bruising) are secondary to infiltration of the bone marrow by cancer cells. The particular type of leukemia can be diagnosed based on findings on the peripheral smear or bone marrow aspirate.

Solid tumors in children are often identified during palpation of the mass on physical examination during a physician visit or when incidentally found by a parent while dressing or bathing the child. For solid tumors, a biopsy should be obtained to determine the cause of the mass.

CASE 48 | Acute Lymphoblastic Leukemia (ALL)

A 3-year-old child with Down syndrome is brought to the ED for evaluation of fever, lethargy, and bleeding gums. On exam, she is febrile, tachycardic, pale, has cervical lymphadenopathy and hepatosplenomegaly and petechiae on her extremities. Labs show hemoglobin 8.0 g/dL; WBC 62,000/mm³ with numerous large cells; platelets 16,000/mm³; absolute neutrophil count 700/mm³. Bone marrow aspirate and biopsy shows 90% lymphoid blasts.

Conditions with Similar Presentations	**Lymphoma:** Can present with similar bulky lymphadenopathy, but the presence of hyperleukocytosis and blasts makes ALL more likely. **EBV infection** (infectious mononucleosis): Can cause a lymphomononuclear leukocytosis (often with atypical lymphocytes) but presents with prodromal symptoms, (headache, malaise, fever) and characteristic exam findings such as tonsillitis/pharyngitis and tender posterior cervical lymphadenopathy. **Juvenile idiopathic arthritis:** Presents with leukocytosis, reactive thrombocytosis, and lymphadenopathy, but patients have a characteristic cyclical fever, arthralgias, and salmon-colored rash.
Initial Diagnostic Tests	• CBC with differential • Peripheral blood smear • Bone marrow aspirate/biopsy
Next Steps in Management	Chemotherapy

Discussion	ALL is the most common malignancy in children. Although less common in adults, adults have a worse prognosis. ALL is subclassified based on immunophenotype: B-cell ALL represents 85% of childhood cases, and T-cell ALL represents 15%. Similar to other acute leukemias, it has an insidious onset, with symptoms developing within days to weeks, and is the result of unregulated clonal proliferation of a lymphoid precursor cell (blast). Genetic alterations lead to abnormal granulopoiesis. Peripheral blood and bone marrow have >20% lymphoblasts.
	
	ALL is associated with radiation exposure, Down syndrome, neurofibromatosis type 1, Bloom syndrome, and ataxia-telangiectasia.
	
	History:
	• Signs/symptoms related to extent of bone marrow infiltration and pancytopenia (fatigue, dyspnea, fever, bleeding), leukostasis (vision changes, headache, AMS, chest pain, SOB/DOE, cranial nerve palsies)
	• Like other leukemias, ALL can present as an oncologic emergency (e.g., leukostasis, tumor lysis syndrome, or febrile neutropenia)
	
	Physical Exam:
	• Lymphadenopathy and/or a mediastinal mass (classically associated with T-ALL)
	• Hepatomegaly and splenomegaly are signs of extramedullary disease
	• More likely than myeloid leukemias to present with leukemic involvement in the CNS
	
	Diagnostics:
	• Bone marrow aspirate and biopsy: >20% lymphoblasts.
	• Nuclear staining is positive for terminal deoxynucleotidyltransferase (TdT), a marker of pre-T and pre-B cells.
	• B-cell ALL is positive for CD10, CD19, and CD20.
	• T-cell ALL is positive for CD2, CD3, CD4, CD5, and CD7.
	• Prognosis:
	  • t(9;22) Philadelphia (ph) chromosome translocation (seen in 4% of cases) confers a poor prognosis
	  • t(12;21) translocation (seen in 25%) confers a better prognosis

CASE 48 | Acute Lymphoblastic Leukemia (ALL) *(continued)*

Discussion	**Management:** • Chemotherapy including vincristine, prednisone, asparaginase +/− anthracycline • Consider stem cell transplant if indicated
Additional Considerations	**Complications:** ALL-associated adenopathy may compress the trachea or superior vena cava and cause the superior vena caval (SVC) syndrome presenting with facial and neck swelling with cyanosis. • ALL may infiltrate the CNS and testes • **Leukostasis** is a result of hyperleukocytosis (WBC >50,000–100,000/mm³) and can result in respiratory failure, ACS, and stroke.

CASE 49 | Retinoblastoma

A 2-year-old boy is referred to the ophthalmologist because the right pupil appears white on examination. Vital signs are normal. On physical examination he has right-sided strabismus, leukocoria (white pupil), nystagmus, bulging of the eyeball, and decreased visual acuity.

Conditions with Similar Presentations	**Retinopathy of prematurity:** More common in premature infants. Due to abnormal blood vessel growth in the retina. Retinal exam will show the abnormal blood vessels, which is not seen in retinoblastoma. **Congenital cataracts:** Clouding of the lens of the eye. Presents with poor vision. Absence of red reflex is noted on examination of the eyes.
Initial Diagnostic Testing	Check fundoscopic examination and genetic testing for mutation in the *Rb* gene
Next Steps in Management	Often multimodal and individualized: Local and systemic chemotherapy, cryotherapy, laser photoablation, radiotherapy, and enucleation (rare)

Discussion	Retinoblastoma is a cancer of the retina caused by a mutation in the *RB1* tumor suppressor gene. Both familial and de novo cases can occur. If a person inherits one functional and one dysfunctional allele, as in hereditary retinoblastoma, the remaining functional allele can protect against tumor formation unless a somatic mutation acts as a "second hit." Those with hereditary retinoblastoma develop it earlier and are much more likely to have bilateral disease. Most children are diagnosed before 5 years of age.
	
	History: Patient presents with leukocoria (white pupil), often first noticed in photographs. May also present with strabismus. There may be a family history of retinoblastoma.
	
	Physical Exam: May have strabismus, leukocoria, nystagmus, decreased visual acuity, bulging of eyeball (proptosis).
	
	As the retinoblastoma tumor grows, leukocoria (white pupil) develops. (Reproduced with permission from Mark W. Kline, Rudolph's Pediatrics, 23e; by McGraw-Hill 2018.)
	
	Diagnostics:
	Confirm with:
	• Fundoscopic examination under anesthesia reveals a chalky, off-white retinal mass with a soft, friable consistency. Lens appears normal.
	• Molecular genetic testing for *RB1* mutation.
	Consider:
	• MRI of the orbits and brain.
	• Do NOT biopsy—risk of tumor seeding.
	
	Management:
	• Treatment decisions are based on unilateral or bilateral disease, the potential to preserve vision, and tumor staging, and generally includes one or more of the following:
	  • Focal therapy (photocoagulation or cryotherapy)
	  • Chemotherapy (systemic or intra-arterial)
	  • Radiation therapy (external beam radiation or brachytherapy)
	  • Enucleation
	  • Myeloablation with stem cell rescue (for extracranial metastatic disease)

CASE 49 | Retinoblastoma *(continued)*

Additional Considerations	**Screening:** Children with a family history of retinoblastoma should undergo either clinical or genetic screening.
	Complications: Children with hereditary retinoblastoma are at risk of developing other cancers, most commonly osteosarcoma. The increased risk of osteosarcoma is due to the inactivation of the *RB1* gene and the use of radiation to treat the retinoblastoma (as sarcomas tend to show up in bone areas within the radiation field).

Abdominal Mass

Comparison Chart for Neuroblastoma & Nephroblastoma

	Neuroblastoma	Nephroblastoma Wilm's Tumor
Age	1-2 years; 90% by 5 years	<2 years old is a favorable prognostic; > 4 years old is an adverse prognostic; 1% present as adults
Cause	Embryonal neuroectoderm tumor arising from neural crest progenitors; majority in medulla of adrenal gland	Embryonal malignancy of the kidney with persistence of nephrogenic blastemal cells
Location	Adrenal medulla, paraspinal ganglia, retroperitoneal; in metastasis, orbits can be involved-"raccoon eyes" or skin involvement with blue nodules "blueberry muffin syndrome"	Kidney; can extend to renal vein, vena cava, and R atrium
Presentation	Abdominal mass (65%); Chest (20%)-may present with respiratory distress, dysphagia; Neck (5%)- may present with Horner's syndrome; Pelvis (5%)-may cause constipation, difficulty urinating	Abdominal mass; abdominal pain, hematuria, fever, hypertension; varicocele on the right may indicate inferior vena cava thrombosis or occlusion of the right spermatic vein by lower part of the tumor
Diagnosis	Urinary catecholamines: vanillylmandelic acid (VMA), homovanillic acid (HVA) CT scan to define spinal involvement Bone scan and bone marrow biopsy to define metastasis MIBG (meta-iodobenzylguanidine) radionuclide scan	Ultrasound to define location, tumor size, origin, vascular involvement CT scan of abdomen to examine contralateral kidney and liver Ct chest to detect pulmonary metastasis
Findings which impact prognosis	Stage of the disease, child's age at diagnosis (younger is better), tumor histology, tumor grade, *MYCN* gene amplification, chromosomal 11q status, tumor cell ploidy	Stage of disease; tumor histology
Treatment	Stages I or II- localized with no metastasis, no crossing of midline, no contralateral node involvement- can be treated with surgical resection Stages III or IV- (disseminated disease, crosses midline) chemotherapy and radiation are initial treatments	Stages I or II- localized to kidney and surrounding soft tissue and can be completely surgically excised Stage III- extends to nearby blood vessels, lymph nodes but not outside the abdomen- chemotherapy before kidney excision Stage IV- spread to lungs, liver, bone, brain or lymph nodes outside the abdomen- chemotherapy before kidney excision Stage V- involves both kidneys- chemotherapy before resection of both kidneys
Survival	5-year survival, 82% Low-risk neuroblastoma- >95% High risk-most have *MYCN* gene overexpression- 50% survival	5-year survival, 93% Histology with diffuse anaplasia, has 30-85% survival depending on stage

CASE 50 | Neuroblastoma

A 2-year-old girl presents to the ED with a decrease in appetite, fatigue, and weight loss for the past 2 weeks. Father states that she has also been experiencing constipation and started vomiting 1 day ago. On examination, the child is lethargic and pale. She is noted to have periorbital discoloration with proptosis. On abdominal exam, she has an irregularly shaped, large abdominal mass that crosses the midline in the right upper quadrant.

Conditions with Similar Presentations	**Wilms' tumor:** Also presents as an abdominal mass. While neuroblastoma is most commonly seen under the age of 2, Wilms' tumor is seen in ages 2–5. It is associated with hypertension and hematuria.
	Rhabdomyosarcoma: Most common malignant soft tissue sarcoma in children. Can also present with an abdominal mass with constipation. Imaging will show a mass arising from the reproductive system (e.g., bladder, uterus, or vagina)
	Hepatoblastoma: liver mass typically in child <4 years
Initial Diagnostic Tests	• Check catecholamine metabolites in serum and/or urine (homovanillic acid ($\uparrow$), vanillylmandelic acid ($\uparrow$)) • Imaging (US, CT, and/or MRI) and biopsy of involved areas
Next Steps in Management	Treatment may involve surgery, radiation, and chemotherapy, dependent on tumor metastases and patient condition
Discussion	Neuroblastoma is the most common extracranial solid tumor in children and is a malignant tumor that usually presents in children under 5 years of age, and most often seen in those <2 years of age. Neuroblastoma arises from neural crest cells, which form several tissues throughout the body including the sympathetic ganglia and adrenal medulla. It is associated with amplification of the proto-oncogene *N-myc*. The tumor can originate anywhere in the sympathetic nervous system, the most common site being the adrenal gland, but also may develop in the neck, chest, abdomen, or spine. **History:** Due to the various locations of the tumor, a variety of symptoms and presentations possible, including: • Abdominal mass, often noticed by caregiver • Fever, night sweats, weight loss, anorexia, bone/joint pain • UTI from obstructing abdominal mass • Back pain or weakness due to spinal cord compression from tumors in paravertebral ganglia • Possible hypertension, diarrhea and other symptoms related to catecholamine release • Infiltration of the bone marrow resulting in anemia and pallor **Physical Exam:** • Firm, irregular abdominal mass, crosses the midline • Opsoclonus-myoclonus syndrome: rapid eye movements and rhythmic jerking of the trunk or extremities – known as "dancing eyes and dancing feet" • Possible hypertension, ataxia • Periorbital ecchymoses (raccoon eyes) due to orbital metastases • Horner syndrome (site of origin in the cervical paravertebral sympathetic chain): ptosis, miosis and anhidrosis **Diagnostics:** • US, CT, and/or MRI: adrenal mass that does cross the midline • MIBG (meta-iodobenzylguanidine) nuclear scan can be done to help confirm presence of neuroendocrine tumors • May see elevations in catecholamine metabolites (e.g., urine homovanillic acid, vanillylmandelic acid) • Biopsy confirms diagnosis: histology will show small round blue/purple cells, Homer-Wright rosettes, positive stain for bombesin and neuron-specific enolase (NSE) Confirm Diagnosis: • Elevated urine and serum vanillylmandelic acid and homovanillic acid • MRI of the abdomen to assess the extent of the tumor • Biopsy of tissue shows small round, blue cells Consider: • CBC with differential—low blood cell counts may suggest bone marrow involvement • MIBG scan for staging and to confirm presence of neuroendocrine tumor

CASE 50 | Neuroblastoma *(continued)*

Discussion	**Management:** • Localized disease can be treated with surgery. Localized lesions have a good prognosis for long-term survival • Intermediate/high-risk disease should be treated with surgery and chemotherapy • Prognosis is worse for patients older than 18 months of age
Additional Considerations	Neuroblastoma is accompanied by syndromes such as neurofibromatosis type I and **Beckwith-Wiedemann** syndrome. This latter syndrome is associated with increased risk of embryonal tumors such as neuroblastoma, Wilms' tumor, and hepatoblastoma.

CASE 51 | Wilms' Tumor (Nephroblastoma)

A 3-year-old boy is brought to clinic for evaluation of right abdominal swelling for the past month. His temperature is 37.1°C, pulse is 100/min, respirations are 20/min, blood pressure is 90/65 mmHg, and SpO_2 is 99% on room air. On exam, there is a large, nontender mass in his right flank that does not cross the midline.

Conditions with Similar Presentations	**Neuroblastoma:** Often presents with lesions in multiple organs, usually starts in the adrenal glands and may cross the midline. **Multicystic dysplastic kidney:** Usually detected on prenatal ultrasound but if presents postnatally, very similarly on exam and requires imaging to differentiate from Wilms' tumor. **Autosomal recessive polycystic kidney disease (ARPKD):** Flank masses are bilateral. ARPKD is usually detected perinatally and infants may have Potter facies (pseudoepicanthus, recessed chin, posteriorly rotated, flattened ears, and flattened nose) or pulmonary hypoplasia from oligohydramnios in utero.
Initial Diagnostic Tests	• Check imaging (renal ultrasound, abdominal/pelvic CT) • Consider checking: CBC, creatinine, transaminases, urinalysis, chest CT and tumor biopsy
Next Steps in Management	• Radical nephrectomy • Adjuvant chemotherapy

Discussion	Wilms' tumor is the most common renal tumor of childhood, usually in children ages 2–4 years old and slightly more common in girls. Other risk factors include horseshoe kidney and persistence of renal cysts beyond adulthood. Predisposing syndromes include:
	• Beckwith-Wiedemann syndrome
	• Denys-Drash syndrome
	• WAGR (see below)
	• Neurofibromatosis type 1 (NF1)
	• Bloom syndrome
	Wilms' tumor is usually sporadic but can be hereditary in 10–15% of cases. Loss of function of Wilms tumor suppressor genes *WT1* or *WT2* on chromosome 11, necessary for normal genitourinary development, can result in Wilms' tumor. It is derived from embryonal origin and may occur as part of a syndrome or an isolated finding.
	History:
	Parents or children may describe:
	• Asymptomatic abdominal mass (most common)
	• Abdominal pain, fever, and hematuria (present in about 25–30% of children)
	• Fatigue, decreased appetite, and weight loss
	There may be a family history of Wilms' tumor or accompanying syndrome.
	Physical Exam:
	• Often well-appearing
	• Unilateral, nontender abdominal mass
	• Features consistent with predisposing syndromes:
	  • **Beckwith-Wiedemann:** hemihyperplasia, macroglossia, cleft palate, prominent eyes with infraorbital creases, visceromegaly
	  • **Denys-Drash syndrome:** gonadal dysgenesis
	  • **WAGR syndrome:** **W**ilms tumor **A**niridia, **G**enitourinary abnormalities, intellectual **R**etardation
	  • **Neurofibromatosis type 1:** neurofibromas, café au lait spots, Lisch nodules
	  • **Bloom syndrome**: developmental delay, growth delay, hypopigmentation, facial anomalies, high-pitched voice

CASE 51 | Wilms' Tumor (Nephroblastoma) *(continued)*

| Discussion | **Diagnostics:**

Imaging:
• Renal ultrasound shows an abdominal mass originating from the kidney
• CT abdomen reveals preserved renal parenchyma wrapping around the mass as it grows out from the kidney ("claw sign")
• Chest CT or CXR is recommended to evaluate lung metastases

Histology:
• Unless there is disseminated disease, biopsy is generally not needed, as tissue can be collected at the time of tumor resection

Labs:
• CBC may show anemia or thrombocytosis
• UA may show microscopic hematuria
• Creatinine to assess renal function
• Transaminases and alkaline phosphatase to assess for liver metastases

Management:

Surgical management:
• Tumor resection and staging
• Often involves partial or radical nephrectomy
• Regional lymph node sampling
Neo/adjuvant chemotherapy:
• Given before or after nephrectomy depending on protocol

Radiation:
• Generally used postoperatively in patients with greater recurrence risk

Genetic testing:
• Recommended for patients with known or suspected Wilms' tumor predisposition syndrome and their families |
CT scan of a patient with a Wilms' tumor demonstrating the characteristic "claw sign" of preserved renal parenchyma *(arrow)*. (Reproduced with permission from Lisa B. Zaoutis, Vincent W. Chiang, Comprehensive Pediatric Hospital Medicine, 2e. by McGraw-Hill 2018.) |
| Additional Considerations | **Screening:** After treatment, screening for recurrence includes abdominal ultrasound every 3 months for up to 3–6 years depending on patient characteristics.
Complications: Metastases, ESRD. |

16
Psychiatry

Lead Authors: Christy Ky, MD; Sean M. Blitzstein, MD
Contributors: Maya Cloyd, MD; Dillon Sharp, MD; Kathryn Cushing, MD; Joseph R. Geraghty, MD, PhD

INTRODUCTION

While the practice of psychiatry requires extensive interaction with a patient in order to make a diagnosis, Psychiatry questions on Step 2 CK will include enough relevant information for you to determine a diagnosis or a plan of action. Psychiatric disorders often appear similar at first glance, so utilize the patient demographics and timeline of how and when their symptoms present in order to narrow your differential diagnoses. The duration of symptoms is often key for differentiating between various disorders within a given group (e.g., schizophreniform disorder vs. schizophrenia). Remember that there is no specific psychiatry section on Step 2 CK; always make sure to differentiate primary psychiatric processes from other medical etiologies or drug side effects that may manifest as psychiatric symptoms, and to consider a psychiatric diagnosis, particularly somatic symptom disorders, when symptoms do not align.

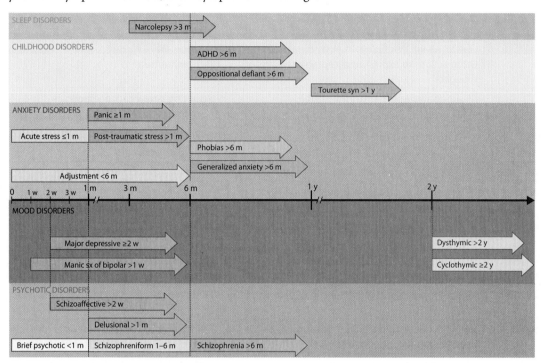

Symptom duration diagnostic criteria for common psychiatric conditions (w, week; m, month; y, year). (Reproduced with permission Le T, Bhushan V. et al. from First Aid for the USMLE Step 1 2019. New York: McGraw Hill; 2019.)

History

In addition to eliciting the chief concern, past medical and family history, medication and substance use history, explore patients' psychosocial history and support system and level of functioning. Inquire about stressors, neurovegetative symptoms (e.g., appetite, sleep, ability to concentrate, energy level), and psychotic symptoms (e.g., visual or auditory hallucinations).

Physical and Mental Status Exam

In addition to a general physical exam, it is important to assess the following components of the mental status exam:

- Appearance/behavior/impulse control
- Mood/affect and speech
- Thought process and content
- Perceptual disturbances
- Cognition/sensorium
- Memory and fund of knowledge
- Judgment and insight

Diagnostics

The Diagnostic and Statistical Manual of Mental Disorders (DSM-5) is used in the diagnosis of psychiatric disorders. It describes key criteria, clinical features, timelines, and specifiers pertaining to the vast majority of psychiatric diagnoses.

The DSM-5 criteria are used throughout this chapter. Although there is a lot of nuance in psychiatry in practice, the DSM-5 provides a framework for practitioners to follow and should be kept in mind to guide thinking in Step 2 CK. Diagnoses will generally align closely with DSM-5 criteria.

EGO DEFENSES

Ego defenses are psychological processes that can be conscious or unconscious and help an individual to cope/deal with undesired feelings such as aggression, fear, or anxiety. These defenses can be sorted into "immature" and "mature" categories, with the vast majority being "immature." Mature defenses include Sublimation, Altruism, Suppression, and Humor (remember, "Mature adults wear a 'SASH'").

Immature Defenses

Defense	Description	Example
Acting out	Using actions to express unacceptable feelings or thoughts	Temper tantrum
Denial	Avoiding awareness of painful reality	Rejecting a new cancer diagnosis
Displacement	Shifting emotions to another person or object	Yelling at a friend after being reprimanded at work
Dissociation	Separating from self (personality, memory, consciousness) to avoid emotional stress	A patient goes into a trance after disclosing significant trauma
Fixation	Remaining at a more immature level of development	Adult still collects stuffed animals
Idealization	Having extremely positive thoughts and ignoring negative ones	A person brags about their new partner, while ignoring any flaws
Identification	Modeling behavior after another person who is more powerful	An abused child later abuses his own children
Intellectualization	Using intellectual processes to emotionally distance oneself from a stressful situation	A patient with a brain tumor focuses only on rates of survival from surgery
Isolation of affect	Removing emotional responses from ideas and events	Describing a mugging with no emotional response
Passive aggression	Indirectly showing opposition in response to the needs/expectations of others	Employee shows up to work later after his boss requests he show up on time
Projection	Attributing one's unacceptable internal feelings, thoughts, or characteristics to an external source	A woman cheating on her partner accuses them of being unfaithful
Rationalization	Justifying behavior or thoughts by logical reasoning	After being rejected from a job, saying the job wasn't ideal anyway
Reaction formation	Adopting behaviors or feelings that are the opposite of true emotions	A boy is rude and insulting to the girl he has a crush on
Regression	Returning to an earlier stage of development	A previously toilet-trained child starts wetting the bed again after a move to a new home
Repression	Eliminating an idea or feeling from conscious awareness	A child does not recall abuse from her parent
Splitting	Believing that people are all good or all bad—common in borderline personality disorder	A patient states the medical student is terrific, but the resident is insensitive

Mature Defenses

Defense	Description	Example
Sublimation	Turning an unacceptable impulse into an acceptable channel	A woman channels her anger towards her partner to do well in a tennis match
Altruism	Using generosity to alleviate negative feelings	Someone with low self-esteem volunteers at a local charity every weekend
Suppression	Intentionally withholding from conscious awareness	Choosing not to worry about a big exam until test day
Humor	Expressing amusement to an adverse situation or feeling	A nervous medical student jokes about an upcoming practical exam

CHILD AND ADOLESCENT PSYCHIATRY

Childhood psychiatric disorders are often first brought to attention by problematic behavior at home or school, concerning temperaments or difficulties with social interactions or school. Many diseases appear early and remain throughout childhood. The goal of treatment is to address the problematic symptoms such that the child is able to interact well at home and at school. In addition to the child psychiatrist, the multidisciplinary team may include therapists, speech-language pathologists, occupational therapists, physical therapists, social workers, teachers, tutors, and 1:1 paraprofessionals. It is worth noting that many psychiatric disorders (e.g., major depressive disorder [MDD], generalized anxiety disorder [GAD]) not typically associated with children may initially present in childhood, but they may present differently than their adult counterparts. Children have more limited emotional expressivity, thus these disorders may manifest as somatic symptoms or increased emotional reactivity.

CASE 1 | Attention-Deficit/Hyperactivity Disorder (ADHD)

A 16-year-old girl is referred for psychiatric evaluation as she is finding it hard to concentrate at school. Per school evaluation, her teachers have noticed her "spacing out" in class and not following assignment directions correctly. She denies having challenges reading, low mood, or anxiety. She does endorse stress in not being able to keep up with assignments. Her mother adds that the patient was a very active child at home and would struggle in some elementary school classes, but now has many incomplete projects around the house (half-done paintings and knitting projects). Exam reveals circumstantial and rapid speech.

Conditions with Similar Presentations	**Specific learning disorders:** Involve difficulty in the acquisition of core academic skills; patients should first undergo a comprehensive examination to rule out medical conditions (e.g., a hearing and vision test), as well as formal educational testing to determine specific areas of need.
Initial Diagnostic Tests	• Clinical diagnosis • Consider: Neuropsychiatric testing, Vanderbilt Assessment Scale
Next Steps in Management	Stimulants (e.g., methylphenidate, amphetamines) and behavioral therapy
Discussion	ADHD is more common in boys. The diagnosis of ADHD involves the following: • Inattentive, and/or hyperactive/impulsive symptoms in two or more settings (typically home and school), for ≥6 months, with symptoms having been present before age 12 • If the patient is >12 years but had symptoms prior, this is sufficient for diagnosis Symptoms/Signs: • Inattention: Careless mistakes, impaired attention, lack of follow-through in work, avoidance of tasks that take mental effort, distractibility, and forgetfulness • Hyperactivity/impulsivity: Fidgetiness, restlessness, circumstantial speech (excessive irrelevant details), difficulty waiting turns, blurting out answers, interrupting others, and difficulty remaining seated • Some symptoms, especially those related to inattention, may persist into adulthood **Management:** • First line are stimulants in combination with behavioral therapy (e.g., positive reinforcement). Stimulants are quite effective and well tolerated when used as prescribed. • Second-line, non-stimulant options include atomoxetine and alpha-2 adrenergic agonists (e.g., clonidine and guanfacine). These can be considered in individuals with a history of substance use disorder. • For children <5 years old: Behavioral therapy involving parent management training is recommended before medications.

CASE 2 | Tourette Disorder

A 10-year-old boy presents to the pediatrician's office for a routine visit. Upon entry into the exam room, the patient is noticed to blink excessively. He also shrugs his shoulder and clears his throat repeatedly throughout the interview. His mother reports that he has been having these symptoms regularly for the past 2 years, and that they are often worse when he is stressed. The patient is embarrassed about these symptoms but "cannot control the urges." The rest of his physical exam, including neurological exam, is unremarkable.

Conditions with Similar Presentations	**Persistent motor or vocal tic disorders:** Have either (but not both) motor or vocal tics. **Provisional tic disorder:** Have motor and/or vocal tics present for <1 year. **Autism spectrum disorder** or **Rett syndrome:** May present with motor stereotypies which may be confused with motor tics.
Initial Diagnostic Steps	Clinical Diagnosis (videos or direct observation of movements are helpful)

CASE 2 | Tourette Disorder (continued)

Next Steps and Management	• Psychoeducation and behavioral interventions • If tics are severe, consider VMAT2 inhibitors (e.g., tetrabenazine), antipsychotics, or alpha-2 agonists
Discussion	Tourette disorder or syndrome is a neurologic disorder most commonly seen in male children (<18 years old). To receive the diagnosis of Tourette disorder, tics should be present for >1 year, must have started before age 18, and must not be due to another medical or psychiatric condition. • It is often associated with comorbid OCD and/or ADHD. • Severity of tics are often exacerbated by psychosocial stressors, anxiety, and fatigue. • Symptoms/signs: Multiple motor (e.g., blinking, hand raising, grimacing) and one or more vocal (e.g., grunting, throat clearing, coprolalia). Coprolalia is utterance of profanity and is rare. **Management:** • Psychoeducation and behavioral interventions such as habit reversal training (patients taught to substitute alternative, voluntary movements for the tic[s]). • If tics are severe or interfere with social and academic function, consider pharmacotherapy with VMAT2 inhibitors (e.g., tetrabenazine). • Can also consider antipsychotics or alpha-2 agonists (e.g., guanfacine or clonidine). Alpha-2 agonists are especially helpful with comorbid ADHD.

CASE 3 | Autism Spectrum Disorder (ASD)

A 6-year-old girl is brought into clinic by her mom per the request of the patient's first-grade teacher. In school, she is meticulous about organizing her folders in her desk and interacts minimally with her peers. She is sitting in the office playing with a stuffed dinosaur, and her mom comments "she will only play with this one toy" and never any others. Her mom mentions that she loves dinosaurs and has memorized facts about various species but will only talk about dinosaurs. On exam, she does not make eye contact with you, and during the physical exam, she cracks her knuckles every time you or her mother touch her. She speaks fluently, although minimally. The remainder of her physical exam is unremarkable.

Conditions with Similar Presentations	**Intellectual disabilities (ID):** Characterized by general delays across developmental domains, whereas ASD is characterized by deficits in social communication. **Specific learning disorders:** Refer to problems in one domain of either reading, writing, or math. **Rett syndrome:** Presents exclusively in females within the first few years of life due to MECP2 mutation on the X chromosome. Typically appears as developmental slowing at or after 5 months of age, which may include gross motor and speech difficulties. It is most easily distinguished from ASD by the presence of a *regression* in function that can occur suddenly. Stereotypical hand movements (e.g., hand wringing) may appear during this regression period and persist.
Initial Diagnostic Tests	• Clinical Diagnosis • Consider: Vision and hearing testing, lead levels to rule out other causes
Next Steps in Management	Special education and behavioral management
Discussion	ASD involves persistent impairment in socialization, communication, and restricted activities/ interests beginning at an early age. Girls often are diagnosed later in childhood than boys, and clinical presentation may be more subtle. Patients with high-functioning autism may go undetected throughout childhood, only to be recognized with increased social and emotional demands as they grow older. • Regarding social interaction, patients usually fail to develop or seek out peer relationships and lack social reciprocity with impaired use of nonverbal communication. • They tend to have problems with communication, including language delays, poor eye contact, and trouble initiating and maintaining conversations. • They may have difficulty in understanding sarcasm or humor and interpret statements literally. • Patients with ASD have restricted and repetitive patterns of activities (i.e., inflexible routines with insistence on sameness), behaviors (e.g., rocking, hand flapping, spinning), and perseverative interests (e.g., the patient being obsessed with dinosaurs and not showing interest in other topics). • ASD may be associated with abnormal EEG findings and seizures. • Language and intellectual impairment in ASD can be quite variable, in some patients severe enough to remain nonverbal. **Management:** • Special education and behavioral management with a multidisciplinary approach to target the core symptoms of ASD. • Risperidone and aripiprazole are FDA approved to address autism-related irritability and aggression.

CASE 4 | Fragile X Syndrome/Intellectual Disability

A 6-year-old boy is brought to clinic for evaluation due to academic difficulties. He has a difficult time reading in class, performing multi-step tasks, and has a hard time making friends. Developmental history is significant for not speaking until the age of 3. Physical exam is notable for a long, narrow face, large forehead, prominent chin, and protruding ears (as shown in the figure below). His parents note that they often have to tell him to stop biting his fingers.

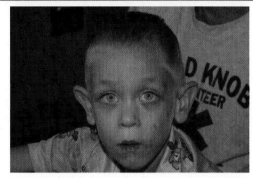

Many men with fragile-X syndrome show common characteristic facial features. (Reproduced with permission from Schaefer GB, Thompson JN. Medical Genetics: An Integrated Approach. New York: McGraw Hill; 2013.)

Conditions with Similar Presentations	**Intellectual disabilities due to other causes:** Can be distinguished by history, exam, and/or genetic testing. **ASD:** Is characterized by deficits in social communication that significantly impair the patient, whereas ID is characterized by general delays across developmental domains. **Specific learning disorders:** Refer to problems in one specific domain of either reading, writing, or math.
Initial Diagnostic Tests	• Confirm diagnosis with comprehensive evaluation, including clinical and standardized assessment of intellectual and adaptive functioning • Consider: Genetic testing for *FMR1* gene
Next Steps in Management	Early intervention, special education, and behavioral therapy to improve level of function, social skills, academic skills, and to decrease negative behavior
Discussion	More broadly, intellectual disability (ID) is characterized by deficits in intellectual function (e.g., learning, reasoning, abstract thinking, and judgment) and adaptive functioning (e.g., communication and social skills). • It is more frequent in boys. • There are several different causes for intellectual disability. Genetic causes include Fragile X Syndrome (FXS), Down syndrome, phenylketonuria, and Prader-Willi syndrome. • Prenatal causes include alcohol and illicit substance use and TORCHeS infections (Toxoplasmosis, Rubella, CMV, HIV, HSV, Syphilis). • Perinatal risk factors include prematurity, anorexia, hyperbilirubinemia, and meningitis. **FXS** is the most common inherited cause of intellectual disability worldwide. • It is X-linked dominant and caused by unstable trinucleotide (CGG) repeats within the *FMR1* gene. This results in low or absent levels of the corresponding fragile X mental retardation protein (FMRP). • Patients may also have joint hypermobility and macro-orchidism, as well as self-injuring or aggressive behaviors. • Some patients may also have ID, and FXS may have several overlapping features with ASD, so comprehensive evaluation and testing is warranted.

CASE 5 | Conduct Disorder

A 12-year-old boy is brought into clinic by his mother who is concerned about his aggressive behavior. He has been suspended from school three times over the last 2 years due to truancy, defacing school property, and most recently releasing the class's pet guinea pig into the snow outside. When asked why he did this to the guinea pig, he shrugs and says he wanted to watch it freeze to death.

Conditions with Similar Presentations	**Antisocial personality disorder:** Conduct disorder may progress to this disorder in adulthood. Diagnosis of conduct disorder is given only to those under the age of 18. **Oppositional defiant disorder:** Involves defiant behavior specifically towards authority figures, but it lacks the violation of societal norms that characterize conduct disorder. **Disruptive mood dysregulation disorder (DMDD):** Characterized as severe, chronic, recurrent angry outbursts, irritability, or sad mood out of proportion to the situation. Outbursts occur in more than one setting and interfere with home, school, or friendships. Usually occurs in children between 6 and 18 years of age. Symptoms occur for at least 12 months, and symptom-free periods may not exceed three months in a 1-year period.
Initial Diagnostic Tests	• Clinical Diagnosis • Consider: Urine drug screen

CASE 5 | Conduct Disorder *(continued)*

Next Steps in Management	Cognitive behavior therapy (CBT) and/or family therapy
Discussion	Conduct disorder usually presents in middle childhood to adolescence (must be diagnosed before age 18), is more commonly seen in males, and can progress to antisocial personality disorder. • It consists of a repetitive or persistent pattern of behavior in which the basic rights of others or societal norms or rules are violated. • Behaviors may be aggressive (e.g., animal cruelty, rape, bullying, destruction of property) or nonaggressive (e.g., deceitfulness, theft, truancy). • A urine toxicology screen may be helpful in ruling out substance use disorders. **Management:** • Individual CBT and/or family therapy. • Comorbid disorders should be treated as appropriate. • In some cases, mood stabilizers or antipsychotic medications may be used.

Anxiety Disorder Mini-Case	
Separation Anxiety Disorder	**Hx:** A 7-year-old boy is brought to clinic for evaluation due to behavioral difficulties in school. Since beginning the first-grade last fall, he has been unfocused on school and preoccupied by the absence of his parents. He insists daily that the teacher call his parents to ensure that they are "ok." He consistently complains of stomachaches or headaches to his parents when it is time to leave for school. At home he enjoys playing with his parents and siblings, but often leaves his room at night to climb into his parents' bed. The family moved into a new house last summer after a tree fell through their living room. The parents sustained minor injuries, but the patient was unharmed. **Diagnostic:** Clinical Diagnosis **Management:** • First-line treatment is psychotherapy (CBT). • For older children with significant impairment, selective serotonin reuptake inhibitors (SSRIs) may be considered. **Discussion:** Separation anxiety disorder involves severe patient worry regarding leaving their attachment figures (usually parents). Children often report physical symptoms to avoid going to school and refuse to go on play dates or sleepovers, or to sleep in another room. Onset may follow a traumatic event where the attachment figures are put in danger.

PSYCHOSIS

Psychosis refers to a dysfunctional perception of reality. Psychosis can be seen in many psychiatric illnesses, including psychotic disorders, mood disorders, substance use disorders, neurocognitive disorders, or other medical conditions such as delirium.

The foundation of psychosis is a combination of the following symptoms: delusions, hallucinations, disorganized speech, and disorganized behavior. Hallucinations due to a psychiatric etiology tend to be auditory or visual, while other types of hallucinations may make you think of other causes (e.g., tactile hallucinations due to substance intoxication or alcohol withdrawal).

If psychosis is present, it is important to identify the length of symptoms, the severity of symptoms, and whether the symptoms are caused by another condition (such as delirium or drug intoxication) as this will help define the diagnosis. Information such as age of onset, associated physical symptoms, and family history may also be helpful to refine the diagnosis.

Timeline	<1 month	1–6 months	>6 months
Diagnosis	Brief psychotic disorder	Schizophreniform disorder	Schizophrenia

Psychosis is often treated with a first- or second-generation (typical vs atypical respectively) antipsychotic. Generally, second-generation antipsychotics (serotonin-dopamine antagonists) are first-line due to better tolerability, although they have a higher risk of metabolic side effects than first-generation antipsychotics. First-generation antipsychotics (dopamine receptor antagonists) have an increased risk of extrapyramidal symptoms (see the table below) compared to second-generation antipsychotics. These symptoms can be distressing to patients and should be addressed by additional medications to manage the symptoms, a decrease in medication, or a switch in medication. Tardive dyskinesia is a late-onset extrapyramidal symptom that can be debilitating and non-reversible.

Antipsychotic Medications

Medications	Mechanism	Side Effects/Contraindications	Additional Considerations
Low-potency typical antipsychotics (chlorpromazine, thioridazine)	Block dopamine D_2 receptors	More anticholinergic and antiadrenergic effects (confusion, sedation, orthostasis, constipation) Chlorpromazine—corneal deposits Thioridazine—retinal deposits	Second- or third-line for psychotic disorders
High-potency typical antipsychotics (fluphenazine, haloperidol)	Block dopamine D_2 receptors	More extrapyramidal symptoms (EPS, including acute dystonia, akathisia, parkinsonism, and tardive dyskinesia with prolonged use) Also more likely to cause neuroleptic malignant syndrome	Second-line for psychotic disorders
Atypical antipsychotics (aripiprazole, clozapine, olanzapine, lurasidone, quetiapine, risperidone, ziprasidone)	Most block dopamine D_2 receptors; have varied effects on $5\text{-}HT_2$ and other receptors Aripiprazole is a partial dopamine antagonist	More anticholinergic and metabolic effects Less likely to cause EPS; however, still possible Clozapine—agranulocytosis Olanzapine—greater risk of weight gain, diabetes Quetiapine—lowest risk of EPS Risperidone—greater risk of hyperprolactinemia (amenorrhea, galactorrhea, gynecomastia) Ziprasidone—greater risk of QT interval prolongation	First-line for psychotic disorders Clozapine is the most effective, but is third-line due to risk of agranulocytosis and requirement for weekly CBC at first Olanzapine—avoid in obese and diabetic patients Ziprasidone—avoid in patients with conduction delay

CASE 6 | Schizophrenia

A 30-year-old man presents to the emergency department (ED) in police custody after the patient's father called 911 due to the patient's attempt to break into his parents' home. He punched through a window, resulting in several stitches. Psychiatry was consulted because of his disorganized speech and behavior. The patient states he punched the window in order to protect his mom from demonic possession. He was warned by "a prophet" who speaks only to him. Eight months ago, he had a previous run-in with police authority when a local church's mass was interrupted by his running to the altar and declaring himself "the tenth coming of Christ." On mental status exam, his hair is long and matted and he has Latin words written in ink covering his arms and legs. His thoughts are disorganized with thought blocking, and he asks that no electronics be in the room, as the government has been monitoring him.

Conditions with Similar Presentations	History-taking and collateral information can be used to confirm the time course and rule out a primary mood disorder (e.g., MDD with psychotic features, bipolar I) or other primary psychotic disorder based on diagnostic criteria. **Brief psychotic disorder:** Characterized by a period of 1 day to 1 month of one or more symptoms of: delusions, hallucinations, disorganized speech +/-, grossly disorganized or catatonic behavior, with full return of premorbid functioning. May be triggered by an acute stressful or traumatic event. **Schizophreniform disorder:** Characterized by presence of symptoms for 1–6 months. May or may not involve functional decline. **Delusional disorder:** Requires the presence of one or more delusions for ≥1 month without meeting criteria for schizophrenia and not attributable to effects of substance use or another medical condition or mental disorder. The delusions may be associated with hallucinations that are related to the delusional theme. There is not usually a significant mood component, functioning is not markedly impaired, and behavior is not obviously bizarre outside of the delusional theme. Examples of common subtypes of delusions include persecutory (e.g., they are being targeted, poisoned, or harassed), grandiose (e.g., they have great talents or special powers), jealous (e.g., partner is unfaithful, spends significant time trying to prove it), and others. Psychosis can also be a common complication of other diseases, such as **Parkinson's disease (PD)**. In PD, psychosis may occur in patients with advanced disease who are treated with dopamine agonists (e.g., pramipexole) or dopamine precursors (e.g., levodopa-carbidopa). Initial management includes dose reduction or medication substitution; however, this may result in worsening of PD symptoms. Therefore, clinicians may consider adding a second-generation antipsychotic such as quetiapine that have low potency for D_2 receptor antagonism.

CASE 6 | Schizophrenia (continued)

Initial Diagnostic Tests	• Clinical Diagnosis • Consider: Rule out other medical causes of psychosis with CBC, BMP, TSH, blood alcohol level (BAL), urine toxicology, head CT
Next Steps in Management	• Admit to the psychiatric unit for further evaluation and safety • Start an antipsychotic medication
Discussion	Schizophrenia is a lifelong illness present in <1% of the general population, with initial onset usually in young adulthood (late teens up to mid-thirties). To meet the DSM-5 diagnostic criteria for schizophrenia, the patient must have two or more of the following symptoms present for a significant portion of time during a 1-month period: 1. Delusions 2. Hallucinations 3. Disorganized speech 4. Grossly disorganized or catatonic behavior 5. Negative symptoms At least one symptom must be either delusions, hallucinations, or disorganized speech. The symptoms must cause significant disturbance in occupational or social functioning, and some symptoms must be present for at least 6 months (may include a prodromal or residual period). • Although patients with schizophrenia often present with positive symptoms (delusions, hallucinations, disorganization), many also suffer from **negative symptoms**, characterized by flat affect, poverty of speech and/or thought, anhedonia, amotivation, apathy, and lack of self-care. Whereas positive symptoms are treated successfully with antipsychotics, negative symptoms are more difficult to treat. • Patients should also be evaluated to rule out substance use or other medical causes of psychosis, particularly if psychosis develops acutely in a patient with no prior history and normal physical examination. Stimulants (e.g., cocaine, amphetamine) are especially noted to cause psychotic symptoms. **Management:** • Atypical (second-generation) antipsychotics are first-line, but have higher risk of metabolic syndrome (hyperglycemia, diabetes mellitus, dyslipidemia, weight gain). Examples include aripiprazole, quetiapine, risperidone, olanzapine, and clozapine. • Typical (first-generation) antipsychotics are second-line and have higher risk of extrapyramidal symptoms and tardive dyskinesia. Examples include chlorpromazine, thioridazine, haloperidol, and fluphenazine. No studies have demonstrated superior efficacy in typical vs. atypical antipsychotics, except for clozapine (see below). • The most efficacious antipsychotic is the atypical antipsychotic clozapine. It is considered the gold standard for treatment-resistant schizophrenia. However, it carries a risk of agranulocytosis and requires weekly blood draws initially; it is therefore a third-line medication. • Non-pharmacological treatment is also helpful as adjunctive therapy and can include CBT, family therapy, and social skills training.
Additional Considerations	**Pediatric Considerations: Pediatric (early-onset) schizophrenia** occurs prior to age 18 and may result in a more severe course of illness. Patients often have a prodromal phase (lasting weeks to years) which can involve academic decline, social withdrawal, and more. Patients experience hallucinations more commonly than delusions, and children/adolescents may even name their hallucinations similar to an imaginary friend; however, they also experience functional decline and clear deviations from baseline or prior behaviors.

CASE 7 | Schizoaffective Disorder

A 22-year-old woman presents to the ED after her roommate called emergency medical services (EMS) upon finding a hand-written suicide note. Her roommate says the patient has been very isolative for the past month. The patient is tearful and admits she has failed multiple classes, had suicidal thoughts, and made plans to step in front of a train. She reports that for over 2 months she has been hearing a female voice similar to that of her teaching assistant (TA), telling her to "end it all." She believes her TA is intentionally failing her because the TA is interested in the patient's boyfriend. The patient states that 4 months ago, her boyfriend brought her coffee to class and the next day the TA asked her to redo an incomplete assignment. On mental status exam, her affect is constricted and she appears to be responding to internal stimuli (will suddenly say "the due date is next week, not this week").

CASE 7 | Schizoaffective Disorder *(continued)*

Conditions with Similar Presentations	Schizoaffective disorder, depressed type can easily be confused for **schizophrenia** or **MDD with psychotic features**. To differentiate between these, you must determine what the primary disorder is based on the history, length, and timing of mood and psychotic symptoms from the patient and collateral sources when available. In schizoaffective disorder, *psychosis is present outside of mood symptoms*. In MDD with psychotic features, psychosis occurs only in the presence of mood symptoms, and mood symptoms are present outside of psychotic symptoms.
Initial Diagnostic Tests	• Clinical Diagnosis • Consider: Rule out reversible medical causes with CBC, BMP, TSH, BAL, urine toxicology, head CT
Next Steps in Management	• Admit to the psychiatric unit for further evaluation and safety • Start an antipsychotic medication • Consider additional treatment for the mood component (e.g., SSRI for depression, lithium for mania)
Discussion	Schizoaffective disorder has about one-third the prevalence of schizophrenia, with typical onset in early adulthood. Similar to schizophrenia, schizoaffective disorder has a significant lifetime risk for suicide. The diagnostic criteria of schizoaffective disorder require all three of the following: 1. uninterrupted period of illness during which there is a major mood episode (major depressive or manic) along with symptoms of schizophrenia; 2. delusions or hallucinations for 2 or more weeks without major mood episodes; and 3. symptoms of major mood disorder are present for the majority of the total duration of illness. **Management:** • Start antipsychotic, similar considerations as in schizophrenia. • Depending on present mood symptoms, consider addition of antidepressant or mood stabilizer.

Mini-Case

Extrapyramidal Side Effects (EPS)	**Hx:** A 20-year-old man with schizophrenia presents with concern of hand tremor and difficulty moving his arms for the last few days. He recently switched medications from aripiprazole to risperidone a few weeks ago. Exam is notable for flat affect, rigidity in his arms bilaterally, resting tremor, and slow gait. **Diagnostics:** Clinical Diagnosis **Management:** • Start benztropine • If symptoms are intolerable, consider reducing the dose or stopping the offending medication and switching to a different one. **Discussion:** The patient has developed drug-induced parkinsonism after changing antipsychotics. This typically develops within days to weeks after starting or increasing the dose of the offending medication. EPS symptoms occur due to dopamine blockade in the nigrostriatal pathway.

Extrapyramidal Side Effects of Antipsychotic Medications

Disorder	Symptoms	Onset	Treatment
Dystonia	Painful spasm/contractions of muscles (e.g., eyes [oculogyric crisis], neck [torticollis], tongue)	Hours to days	Benztropine, diphenhydramine
Akathisia	Restlessness, inability to sit still (pacing, rocking)	Days to months	Propranolol, lorazepam benztropine
Parkinsonism	Bradykinesia, resting tremor, rigidity	Days to months	Benztropine
Tardive dyskinesia	Abnormal involuntary hyperkinetic movements, commonly orofacial (e.g., lip smacking, grimacing, tongue protrusion) but can also affect trunk and limbs; usually irreversible	Months to years	Reduce, taper, or cross-taper (switch) antipsychotic VMAT2 inhibitors: Valbenazine, deutetrabenazine (expensive)

Other Side Effects of Antipsychotic Medications

Hyperprolactinemia	Galactorrhea, gynecomastia, decreased libido, amenorrhea, erectile dysfunction
Antihistaminic, adrenergic, muscarinic (HAM) effects	Antihistaminic: weight gain, sedation
	Anti-alpha 1 adrenergic: cardiac abnormalities, orthostatic hypotension
	Anti-muscarinic/Anticholinergic: dry mouth, tachycardia, constipation, urinary retention, blurred vision, increased risk of acute-angle glaucoma
Neuroleptic malignant syndrome (NMS)	Rare medical emergency characterized by fever, tremor, autonomic instability (labile HTN, tachycardia, sweating), rigidity, elevated CPK, tremor, delirium.
	Treatment: Discontinue medication and supportive care (e.g., IV fluids, cooling blanket).
Miscellaneous	Lower seizure threshold, rashes, jaundice.

MOOD DISORDERS

Mood disorders primarily consist of disturbances in mood, resulting in mania, depression, or both. Manic symptoms not caused by another medical condition or substance are seen primarily in the bipolar disorders and classified as mania or hypomania, depending on their severity. Depression not caused by another medical condition or substance is seen primarily in the depressive (e.g., MDD) and bipolar disorders. Treatment for mood disorders often includes a combination of medications and psychotherapy (e.g., CBT). CBT involves teaching patients how to recognize negative thought patterns and retrain their responses to these thoughts. Both therapy and pharmacotherapy are effective individually, but more so when used in combination. Mood disorders can present with psychotic features, and it is important to differentiate a primary mood disorder from a primary psychotic disorder by tracking the presence of psychotic symptoms over time. Psychotic symptoms in the absence of mood disturbance indicate a primary psychotic disorder.

CASE 8	Bipolar I Disorder
A 27-year-old woman presents to the ED after her husband found her scrubbing the bathroom floor at 3 in the morning. The patient states she is hosting the Queen of England tomorrow for dinner and wants her home to be impeccable. Her husband was recently out of town for a week and upon his return found the refrigerator filled with ornate desserts and a new refrigerator in the garage full of expensive meats and cheeses. Before he left, he had noticed she was up in the middle of the night furiously typing on her computer. When questioned, the patient said she was going to host a big surprise dinner party this week. On mental status exam, she is rapidly folding paper towels into elaborate shapes and has pressured speech.	

Conditions with Similar Presentations	**Bipolar II disorder:** Diagnosis requires at least one episode of hypomania in addition to one episode of major depression. A hypomanic episode consists of manic symptoms for several days without psychotic symptoms or significantly impaired functioning and does not require hospitalization. In fact, patients may have somewhat increased function from baseline or minimal decrease in function. Patients experiencing a hypomanic episode are often able to continue work or school, although their current mood and productivity are different from baseline.
	Cyclothymic disorder: Diagnosis requires ≥2 years (1 year in children) of fluctuating hypomanic symptoms and depressive symptoms (that do not meet criteria for a major depressive episode).
	Borderline personality disorder: Also has periods of unstable mood that may resemble a hypomanic or depressive episode; however, mood lability in borderline personality disorder is persistent and pervasive, and the episodes are much shorter, often only lasting hours or days, as compared to hypomanic (≥4 days), manic (≥7 days), or depressive (≥2 weeks) episodes.
Initial Diagnostic Tests	• Clinical Diagnosis • Consider: Rule out other medical causes of mood disorder with CBC, BMP, TSH, BAL, urine toxicology, head CT
Next Steps in Management	• Assess for immediate danger to self or others (suicidal or homicidal ideation). Hospitalize if present. • Treat with a mood stabilizer such as lithium or valproate. • If a patient has psychotic features (as in this case), consider addition of an antipsychotic.

CASE 8 | Bipolar I Disorder (continued)

Discussion	Bipolar I disorder is a chronic disorder characterized by recurrent episodes of mania and/or depression. Patients may first present in a major depressive episode, and it is important to conduct a careful history to determine if the patient has had previous manic symptoms. In bipolar I, the patient must exhibit a manic episode that is not due to substance use or other medical or psychiatric conditions. An additional depressive episode is NOT necessary to diagnose bipolar I if the patient has already exhibited a manic episode. Psychotic symptoms (e.g., hallucinations, delusions) are only seen with bipolar I disorder. A manic episode requiring a psychiatric hospitalization automatically qualifies as bipolar I, as opposed to bipolar II. Definition of a manic episode includes elevated/irritable mood for >1 week and three (if elevated mood) or four (if only irritable mood) of the following: 1. Inflated self-esteem 2. Decreased need for sleep 3. Pressured speech 4. Flight of ideas 5. Distractibility 6. Increase in goal-directed activity or psychomotor agitation 7. Excessive involvement in risky activities Symptoms are severe enough to interfere with occupation or social functioning, result in hospitalization, or display psychotic symptoms A useful mnemonic for diagnosing a manic episode is "**DIGFAST**": **D**istractibility, **I**mpulsivity/indiscretion, **G**randiosity, **F**light of ideas, **A**ctivity/agitation (increased), **S**leep (decreased), **T**alkativeness A patient is considered to be "rapid cycling" if they experience greater than or equal to four mood episodes per year. **Management:** • Acute treatment of mania (e.g., lithium, valproate, carbamazepine, and second-generation antipsychotics) and depression (e.g., quetiapine, lurasidone). • Maintenance therapy (e.g., lithium, valproate, carbamazepine, lamotrigine). • Antidepressant monotherapy (used for treatment of unipolar depression) should be avoided in such patients, as this may trigger a manic episode.
Additional Considerations	**Obstetric considerations:** Medications to treat bipolar disorder such as valproate and carbamazepine are highly teratogenic (increased risk of neural tube defects). Pregnant patients or those contemplating pregnancy should be switched to alternative medications such as lamotrigine or quetiapine. Though lithium has a low risk of Ebstein anomaly, it should not be started; however, if a patient is already on lithium, responding well, and wishes to continue, they should be monitored closely throughout pregnancy. **Inpatient Considerations:** Admit patients to psychiatric ward if they are an immediate danger to self or others (suicidal or homicidal ideation), involuntarily if required.

Mood Stabilizers

Medications	Mechanism	Side Effects/Contraindications	Additional Considerations
Lithium	Modulates reuptake of serotonin and norepinephrine and inhibits secondary messengers	**Acute toxicity:** GI symptoms (e.g., nausea, vomiting, diarrhea). **Chronic toxicity:** Neurologic symptoms (e.g., tremor, ataxia, confusion, seizures), hypothyroidism, renal injury, nephrogenic diabetes insipidus. Often seen with dehydration or medications (e.g., thiazides, ACE inhibitors, NSAIDs, tetracyclines). Teratogenic (Ebstein anomaly—risk is low).	First-line for acute mania and maintenance in bipolar disorder. Renally cleared, narrow therapeutic index—monitor closely in patients taking NSAIDs, ACE inhibitors, diuretics, or with impaired renal function.

Mood Stabilizers (*Continued*)

Medications	Mechanism	Side Effects/Contraindications	Additional Considerations
Lamotrigine	Selectively binds and inhibits voltage-gated Na$^+$ channels and release of glutamate	Mild to serious rashes including Stevens-Johnson syndrome, toxic epidermal necrolysis, and drug reaction with eosinophilia and systemic symptoms (DRESS). Should discontinue at first sign of rash.	Anticonvulsant, found to be beneficial in acute treatment of bipolar depression and bipolar maintenance.
Carbamazepine	Na$^+$ channel blocker	GI symptoms (e.g., nausea, vomiting, diarrhea), rash, hyponatremia, aplastic anemia, and agranulocytosis. Teratogenic (neural tube defects). Avoid in pregnancy.	Anticonvulsant, first-line for trigeminal neuralgia. Can be used in acute treatment of mania as monotherapy. Monitor CBCs and transaminases.
Valproic acid (valproate, divalproex sodium)	Na$^+$ channel blocker and increases GABA concentrations. Mechanism in regard to treating bipolar disorder is unknown	Sedation, weight gain, alopecia, tremor, pancreatitis, GI distress, hepatotoxicity, thrombocytopenia. Teratogenic (neural tube defects). Avoid in pregnancy.	Anticonvulsant. Monitor CBCs and transaminases.

CASE 9 | Major Depressive Disorder (MDD)

A 53-year-old man presents to clinic reporting fatigue for 5 weeks. He endorses sleeping 12–14 hours a day. He recently started to work from home, where he has been logging into all his conference calls from his bed. He used to enjoy going into work and talking to his co-workers, but lately hasn't had the energy to go. He is worried he will be fired because his boss called his work quality "sloppy." He feels guilty that he is letting down his team at work. He has lost 10 pounds since his last visit 2 months ago because he is not interested in eating. On exam, he has quiet speech and walks very slowly when moving from the chair to the exam table.

Conditions with Similar Presentations	**Persistent depressive disorder (dysthymia):** Consists of chronic depression most of the time (no more than 2 months without symptoms) for at least 2 years, associated with at least two of the following: poor concentration, feelings of hopelessness, insomnia/hypersomnia, appetite changes, low energy, and low self-esteem. The individual may have major depressive episodes or meet the criteria for major depression continuously.
	Grief/bereavement: A normal process that people go through which can include hearing the voice of a loved one or wishing they died instead of the loved one. Symptoms tend to occur intermittently but become less persistent and intense over time. This becomes more concerning if they continue to have a significant degree of impairment >12 months after the death of the loved one. This impairment would include one of the following: persistent yearning/longing for the deceased, intense sorrow/emotional pain, preoccupation with the deceased, or preoccupation with the circumstances of the death, in addition to significant symptoms of mood and distress relating to the death of the loved one.
	Seasonal affective disorder (SAD): A subset of MDD called MDD with seasonal patterns. Patients have symptoms of MDD in particular seasons (most often winter). Patients commonly have atypical features. Treatment involves bright light therapy ± antidepressants.
	Bipolar disorder: If a patient demonstrated previous manic or hypomanic episodes, the diagnosis would be bipolar I or II, respectively, rather than MDD, and it is important to AVOID antidepressant monotherapy as this could trigger mania in these patients.
Initial Diagnostic Tests	• Clinical Diagnosis • Consider: Rule out medical causes of depression with CBC, BMP, TSH, BAL, urine toxicology, vitamin D
Next Steps in Management	• Assess for immediate danger to self or others (suicidal or homicidal ideation) • Start SSRIs and/or CBT

CASE 9 | Major Depressive Disorder (MDD) *(continued)*

Discussion	The diagnosis of MDD requires a 2-week period of at least five of the following, with at least one of the symptoms being one of the first two:
	1. Depressed mood
	2. Diminished interest or pleasure (anhedonia)
	3. Appetite change/significant weight loss or weight gain
	4. Insomnia
	5. Psychomotor agitation/retardation
	6. Fatigue/low energy
	7. Worthlessness/guilt
	8. Recurrent thoughts of death
	9. Reduced concentration or indecisiveness
	Patients cannot have a history of mania or hypomania, and the symptoms cannot be caused by substance use or another medical condition.
	The mnemonic "**SIG E CAPS**" is often used to help remember these symptoms: **S**leep disturbance, loss of **I**nterest, **G**uilt, **E**nergy loss, **C**oncentration problems, **A**ppetite changes, **P**sychomotor retardation, **S**uicidal ideation
	• Screening for MDD can be done using the **patient health questionnaire** (PHQ)-2 or PHQ-9. Symptoms may be associated with grief or bereavement or other difficult life circumstances, but if the criteria above are met, MDD is still the diagnosis.
	• Subtypes of MDD include:
	• **Melancholic features**—insomnia, anhedonia, lack of mood reactivity (does not respond to positive events), weight loss.
	• **Atypical features**—Mood reactivity (responds to positive events), hypersomnia, increased appetite, weight gain, leaden paralysis, hypersensitive to rejection.
	• **Psychotic features**—delusions, disorganized speech or behavior, and/or hallucinations. (In this case, a thorough history to characterize timing of mood and psychotic symptoms is essential for diagnostic clarity.)
	Management:
	• First-line treatment of MDD is with psychotherapy (CBT) and/or SSRIs.
	• Second-line treatments include SNRIs, bupropion, and mirtazapine.
	• MAOIs and TCAs are no longer in common use.
	• Electroconvulsive therapy (ECT) should be considered for severe cases where rapid treatment is indicated (e.g., imminent suicide risk).
Additional Considerations	Patients with severe or debilitating medical conditions (e.g., myocardial infarction, ALS, stroke, cancer) commonly develop depression, which can result in decreased adherence to medical treatment, worse quality of life, delayed recovery, and increased mortality. It is important to screen for MDD in these patients.
	Pediatric Considerations: Depression in children often presents with somatic symptoms, including stomach aches or headaches. In adolescents, depression can be suggested by decline in school performance, increased irritability and argumentative behaviors, and social withdrawal from peers.

CASE 10 | Suicide Risk Assessment

A 29-year-old man presents to his local veteran's hospital after being honorably discharged from the military, in which he served two tours in Afghanistan. He states that he has been feeling depressed for the last 2 months and has lost multiple close friends during the war. His longtime girlfriend recently broke up with him and he feels as though he has "nothing to live for." He has daily thoughts of ending his life and he recently bought a firearm.

Initial Diagnostic Tests	• Clinical Diagnosis • Consider: Assessing for signs of overdose
Next Steps in Management	• Immediate inpatient hospitalization and if warranted, initiate medical stabilization (treatment of self-inflicted injuries and/or drug ingestions) • Once safety and stabilization ensured, treat underlying psychiatric comorbid conditions (e.g., depression, anxiety, posttraumatic stress disorder [PTSD])

CASE 10 | Suicide Risk Assessment *(continued)*

Discussion	A suicide risk assessment should be performed on all patients with suicidal ideation. It is imperative to also evaluate their intent and plan. The mnemonic "**SAD PERSONS**" can be used to remember suicide risk factors: • **S**ex (women have more attempts, but men are more likely to die by suicide) • **A**ge (young adults and older adults are more at risk) • **D**epression or hopelessness • **P**revious attempt • **E**thanol or other drug abuse • **R**ational thinking loss • **S**eparated/divorced/widowed • **O**rganized plan or serious attempt • **N**o social supports • **S**tated future intent/Sickness or injury Of these, previous suicide attempt(s) represents the major risk factor. The most common cause of suicide in adults is with a firearm, while for adolescents and young adults it is drug overdose. When assessing suicide risk, it is important to identify any protective factors that exist against completing suicide. These include parenthood, pregnancy, participation in religious activities, social support, and a sense of connection with family. **Management:** • Hospitalize (involuntarily if needed) patients with suicidal ideation, a stated plan, and intent. • Patients with suicidal ideation who lack intent or plan and have social support can be considered for outpatient treatment aimed at addressing modifiable risk factors (e.g., underlying depression, pain) with close follow-up. • Reducing access to potential means of completing suicide such as lethal medications or firearms is also helpful.
Additional Considerations	**Pediatric Consideration:** Suicide is one of the leading causes of death in patients between 10 and 24 years old. There is also a risk of **suicide contagion**, a phenomenon whereby exposure to suicide or suicidal behaviors (e.g., family, peers, through media portrayals) increases the risk of suicide in others, especially adolescents and young adults. **Medical Aid in Dying** (also known as physician-assisted suicide): A physician helps competent patients faced with end-of-life suffering to voluntarily end their lives by providing information and/or medications to die by suicide. While legal in some states and countries, it remains highly controversial. See Chapter 1 for more information.

CASE 11 | MDD with Catatonic Features

A 28-year-old woman with no significant past medical history is brought into the ED by her roommate, after 1 week of "odd behavior." The roommate states that the parents of the woman recently passed away. She has been mute, not eating or drinking, sitting still in one spot, and staring at the wall. On exam, patient does not talk and does not move from fixed position on the exam bed. When testing for rigidity, the patient has mild resistance. When positioning her arms in the air, they remain in fixed position until moved back to her side by the examiner.

Initial Diagnostic Tests	• Clinical Diagnosis • Consider: Rule out other medical causes with CBC, BMP, TSH, BAL, urine toxicology, and head imaging • Assess CK level for rhabdomyolysis, albumin for malnourishment
Next Steps in Management	Benzodiazepines or ECT

CASE 11 | MDD with Catatonic Features *(continued)*

Discussion	**Catatonia** is a psychomotor syndrome, usually reflective of a patient with another underlying psychiatric or medical disorder. It is important to recognize that it is a syndrome and not a diagnosis. Some features of catatonia include mutism, catalepsy (muscle rigidity and fixed posturing), bizarre posturing, and negativism (opposition or no response to instructions). There are three subtypes:
	1. **Stuporous catatonia:** Mutism, immobility, negativism, posturing, rigidity.
	2. **Excited catatonia:** Excitement, hyperactivity, agitation, verbigeration (constant repetition of meaningless words/phrases), delirium.
	3. **Malignant catatonia:** Acute onset of fever, autonomic instability (tachycardia, tachypnea, hyper/hypotension, diaphoresis), delirium. Malignant catatonia is a medical emergency and requires ICU-level care.
	Management:
	• Non-malignant catatonia should be treated with benzodiazepines and, if unresponsive, ECT.
	• Malignant catatonia is an emergency and should be treated with ECT.
	• In both cases, an underlying disorder should be treated as soon as it is identified.
	• ECT does not have any absolute contraindications, but additional caution should be considered in those with space-occupying brain lesions, recent CVA, unstable brain aneurysms, severe cardiovascular disease, and/or a recent MI.
	• Avoid dopamine-blocking drugs, as they can make catatonia worse.
	• Consider compression socks and anticoagulation for DVT and PE prophylaxis/treatment.
	• The underlying psychiatric disorder (e.g., bipolar, schizophrenia) will likely need to be treated after the catatonia resolves and may include restarting an antipsychotic medication.

Classes of Antidepressant Medications

Medications	Mechanism	Side Effects/Contraindications	Additional Considerations
Selective serotonin reuptake inhibitors (SSRIs)—citalopram, escitalopram, fluoxetine, fluvoxamine, paroxetine, sertraline	Serotonin reuptake inhibition, which increases levels of serotonin within the synapse. Long-term use also increases production of neuroprotective proteins such as brain-derived neurotrophic factor (BDNF).	*Acute:* GI disturbance (nausea, diarrhea, etc.), increased anxiety, dizziness, insomnia, or sedation. These symptoms usually occur in the first 1–2 weeks and resolve with time. *Chronic:* Sexual dysfunction, weight gain (especially paroxetine), SIADH, QTc prolongation (citalopram, escitalopram). Discontinuation syndrome—abrupt cessation can cause flu-like symptoms, anxiety, insomnia, nausea, sensory disturbances. Usually mild and resolves in 1–2 weeks. Avoid by tapering the medication or using one with a long half-life (e.g., fluoxetine). Serotonin syndrome—mental status changes, autonomic dysfunction, and neuromuscular hyperactivity most often in patients taking multiple serotonergic medications (e.g., SSRI, SNRI, TCAs, MAOIs, linezolid, etc.) or with serotonergic drugs of abuse such as ecstasy (MDMA).	Adequate trial of SSRIs is ~6 weeks at a therapeutic dose. First-line for treatment of MDD and persistent depressive disorder, also for some anxiety disorders (e.g., GAD, panic disorder, and OCD). SSRIs may increase risk of suicidality in younger (18–24 years old) patients during initial weeks of treatment.

Classes of Antidepressant Medications (*Continued*)

Medications	Mechanism	Side Effects/Contraindications	Additional Considerations
Serotonin-norepinephrine reuptake inhibitors (SNRIs)—duloxetine, venlafaxine	Serotonin and norepinephrine reuptake inhibition increasing levels of both in the synapse.	Similar to SSRIs, with the addition of hypertension. Can lead to serotonin syndrome.	In addition to use in disorders covered by SSRI, can be used to treat neuropathic pain and fibromyalgia.
Tricyclic antidepressants (TCAs)—amitriptyline, nortriptyline, imipramine, desipramine, clomipramine, doxepin, amoxapine	Serotonin and norepinephrine reuptake inhibition increasing levels of both in the synapse.	Acute toxicity: Hyperthermia, tachycardia, hypotension, and respiratory depression. Can be lethal in overdose. Antihistamine properties—sedation, weight gain. Anti-adrenergic (alpha-1) properties—orthostatic hypotension, ECG changes, arrhythmias, dizziness. Anticholinergic (antimuscarinic) properties—dry mucous membranes, constipation, urinary retention, blurred vision, dilated pupils, flushing. Prolonged QRS and ventricular arrhythmias. Can lead to serotonin syndrome.	Not first-line due to side effect profile. TCAs are rarely used in the treatment of depression, anxiety, and OCD. They are also used to treat migraines, chronic neuropathic pain, insomnia, and enuresis (imipramine).
Monoamine oxidase inhibitors (MAOIs)—tranylcypromine, phenelzine, isocarboxazid, selegiline	Irreversibly inhibit MAO, preventing the inactivation of biogenic amines including norepinephrine, serotonin, dopamine, and tyramine.	Hypertensive crisis risk when eating tyramine-rich foods (e.g., wine, cheese, fava beans, cured meats) or using sympathomimetics (the "cheese effect"). Can lead to serotonin syndrome.	Not used first- or second-line, but can be useful in treating atypical depression or refractory panic disorder. Wait 2 weeks (2-week washout) after switching between serotonergic medications (e.g., SSRI to MAOI)
Bupropion	Norepinephrine and dopamine reuptake inhibition increasing levels of both in the synapse.	Compared to SSRIs, lacks sexual side effects and is weight neutral. CNS activating side effects (e.g., tachycardia, insomnia, anxiety). Contraindicated in patients with epilepsy or active eating disorders (e.g., bulimia or anorexia nervosa) due to the increased risk of seizures.	Atypical antidepressant, also used for smoking cessation.
Mirtazapine	Alpha-2 antagonist, 5-HT$_2$ and 5-HT$_3$ antagonist, H$_1$ antagonist.	Drowsiness, increased appetite and weight gain, dry mouth, agranulocytosis (rare).	Atypical antidepressant, useful in MDD, particularly those with poor sleep and appetite. More sedating in *lower* doses. Clinically, often used in palliative care patients due to a favorable side-effect profile.
Trazodone	5-HT$_{2A}$, alpha-1, H$_1$ antagonist.	Sedation, nausea, postural hypotension, arrhythmias, priapism.	Atypical antidepressant, rarely used in MDD. Used most often for insomnia due to sedative effects.

POSTPARTUM DISORDERS

Postpartum mood disturbances are common but underrecognized. The hormonal changes and fluctuations that occur during and after childbirth, along with the stressors of having a newborn, may affect mental health. Also see Obstetrics and Gynecology Chapter.

Most women with symptoms will have **postpartum blues**, which describes a depressed affect that starts shortly after delivery and resolves within 1–2 weeks (this is not considered a psychiatric diagnosis).

Postpartum depression is defined by symptoms within 4 weeks of delivering a child that are severe enough to meet criteria for a major depressive episode (clinically significant symptoms lasting greater than 2 weeks).

Postpartum psychosis is much rarer; however, it can be dangerous to the patient and infant and should be considered a medical emergency. Patients with a history of mood disorder or psychotic disorder are most susceptible to this disease.

For patients who are taking psychotropic medications and become pregnant, it is important that discussion between patient and psychiatrist occur to discuss risks and benefits of continuing medications during and after pregnancy.

CASE 12	Postpartum Psychosis
A 25-year-old woman, her husband, and their 1-week-old child present to the pediatrics clinic for the baby's first outpatient well-child check. The mother is wearing a long winter coat with flip flops and her hair is markedly disheveled. The husband asks to speak to the pediatrician alone, noting that his wife has not been sleeping and is obsessively trying to feed the baby. He saw her trying to mix protein powder into the baby's formula, but he was able to quickly intervene. She said that the baby is wasting away to nothing because of the parasite that crawled in through the belly button. When confronted, she starts crying saying she's "a bad mom for not being able to protect the baby from parasites." Her past psychiatric history is notable for bulimia nervosa 5 years ago for which she had a brief stay in an eating disorders unit. She appears paranoid and is fixated on having the pediatrician treating the baby's parasite.	

Conditions with Similar Presentations	**Postpartum thyroiditis:** May follow delivery and can result in hyperthyroidism followed by hypothyroidism. In rare cases, this may result in frank psychosis.
Initial Diagnostic Tests	• Clinical Diagnosis • Consider: Rule out other medical causes of psychosis with CBC, BMP, TSH, BAL, urine toxicology, head CT
Next Steps in Management	• Ensure infant safety; the baby must not be left alone with the mother • Admit patient to the inpatient psychiatry ward and start antipsychotics.
Discussion	Postpartum psychosis is a rare psychiatric emergency but necessitates quick identification and intervention. Although relatively uncommon, this disorder increases the risk for suicide and infanticide. • Symptom onset is often rapid and includes hallucinations, delusions, bizarre behavior, and/or disorganization, and often relate to the infant (e.g., infant is sick, possessed, in danger). • Patients often have a prior psychiatric illness, and the symptoms may present in those who stop psychiatric medications during pregnancy. However, it can occur in women without previously diagnosed disorders. • Patients should be admitted, evaluated, and treated for any primary psychiatric disorders including bipolar I (most common etiology), schizophrenia, or schizoaffective disorder.

ANXIETY, OBSESSIVE-COMPULSIVE SPECTRUM, AND POST-TRAUMATIC DISORDERS

Fear and anxiety are normal and useful emotions. The former serves as a response to imminent danger, and the latter as preparation for an anticipated danger. Anxiety disorders occur when these emotions become excessive or last for extended periods, leading to behavioral disturbances that interfere with functioning. These disorders may be referred to as **ego-dystonic** conditions, which patients find distressing and at odds with their ideal self-concept (e.g., obsessive-compulsive disorder). Anxiety disorders are best treated with SSRIs/SNRIs and/or cognitive-behavioral therapy (CBT). It is important for physicians to take contextual and cultural factors into account while assessing whether the duration or level of anxiety is inappropriate.

CASE 13 | Panic Disorder

A 27-year-old man presents to clinic with episodic sharp chest pain. The first time it happened was a month ago, when he was returning home after work on the bus. He had sharp pain in the center of his chest, felt his heart pounding, and was unable to breathe. He describes having tunnel vision and feeling the bus was closing in around him. The symptoms lasted about 10 minutes, and he has had two similar events since. One happened while waiting in line for coffee and another while shopping in a grocery store. He has started taking a car to work to avoid the bus, making his coffee at home, and getting his groceries delivered in an attempt to avoid these episodes from happening again. He fears having an episode at work and is considering changing jobs so that he can work remotely.

Conditions with Similar Presentations	**Acute coronary syndrome, pulmonary embolism** and other such medical conditions are often ruled out with a thorough history and physical exam but should be considered. **Agoraphobia:** Is often seen with panic disorder and involves fear of certain places or situations where it may be difficult to escape or leave. Patients may be uncomfortable leaving their home, using certain modes of transportation, being within confined or enclosed spaces, and in severe cases may refuse to leave their home. **Substance/medication-induced anxiety disorder:** Is diagnosed instead of panic disorder if symptoms are due to intoxication with or withdrawal from a substance. It is important to differentiate this condition from someone with panic disorder who uses substances for self-medication.
Initial Diagnostic Tests	• Clinical Diagnosis, should rule out other causes • Consider: CBC, BMP, TSH, ECG, CXR, cardiac stress test to rule out other medical conditions prior to diagnosis
Next Steps in Management	• SSRI and/or cognitive behavioral therapy (CBT) • Anxiety medications (e.g., benzodiazepines) as needed, can be considered for the short term
Discussion	Diagnosis of panic disorder requires an abrupt, recurrent, and intense fear/discomfort that peaks within minutes and has four or more symptoms including: palpitations/tachycardia, sweating, trembling, SOB/smothering sensation, chest pain, nausea, dizzy/lightheaded, hot/cold chills, paresthesias, derealization/depersonalization, fear of losing control, or fear of dying. • There must be worry about further panic attacks or maladaptive behavioral changes related to attacks (avoidance behaviors) for at least 1 month. • Panic attacks are characteristically unprovoked ("out of the blue") but can also be triggered by known events or stimuli. • Symptoms may be so concerning that medical care is sought. • Important to screen for other psychiatric disorders, as panic disorder is often associated with other anxiety and mood disorders. In panic disorder, however, most of the attacks are unexpected and/or unprovoked. • Risk factors for panic disorder include a history of sexual/physical abuse, smoking, recent onset of stressors, and respiratory problems (asthma).

CASE 14 | Specific Phobia

An 18-year-old woman presents to clinic for her meningococcal vaccine prior to leaving for college. Her mother had made and canceled the appointment several times in the last 6 months, as the patient is "deathly afraid of needles." The patient hasn't received any of her recommended vaccinations since she was 6 years old. She avoids interacting with medical professionals in general as just the thought of needles causes her to feel anxious and short of breath.

Conditions with Similar Presentations	**Somatic symptom disorder:** Fixated on one or more somatic symptoms (e.g., stomach cramps), preoccupation is more enduring and less episodic, and results in increased utilization of health care services. **Illness anxiety disorder:** Patients experience high anxiety about their health (e.g., worried they have cancer) without the presence of somatic symptoms.
Initial Diagnostic Tests	Clinical Diagnosis
Next Steps in Management	Exposure therapy and consider PRN short-acting benzodiazepines

CASE 14 | Specific Phobia *(continued)*

Discussion	Specific phobia is an extreme, persistent fear and anxiety about a specific object or event (the stimulus) that is out of proportion to the actual danger it poses. The stimulus almost always provokes immediate fear and is actively avoided or endured with great distress. Onset of a phobia begins in childhood and is more common in women. Patients often practice avoidance behaviors which can lead to social and/or occupational impairment (e.g., missing sibling's wedding due to fear of flying).
	• The phobia is generally persistent and lasts ≥6 months
	• Common examples of specific phobias include fear of flying, spiders, snakes, heights, blood, needles
	• Approximately 75% of patients who have a phobia typically have more than one fear
	Phobias sometimes develop after a traumatic event (e.g., plane crash), but can also occur without this history.
	Management:
	• Exposure therapy, a form of CBT, can help decrease the patient's fear response. Treatment involves exposing the patient gradually to the stimulus in increasing amounts.
	• Patients become habituated to the stimulus over time, leading to the extinction of their fear response (a process known as systematic desensitization).
	• PRN short-acting benzodiazepines (e.g., alprazolam) can also be used short-term for a known, planned exposure (e.g., a flight).

CASE 15 | Generalized Anxiety Disorder (GAD)

A 24-year-old law student presents to clinic for persistent neck pain for several months. She states her neck pain prevents her from sleeping at night. She spends most of the day on the computer studying for the bar exam that she will be taking in 6 months. At night she mostly watches the news while in bed to distract herself from her neck pain and to keep up with world events. On further questioning she admits that she is also worried that her girlfriend will break up with her. She notes her girlfriend gets frustrated with her over-analyzing conversations she has had with friends and professors. She also has difficulty concentrating in class and recalls being extremely anxious before taking her LSAT exam. She states she is "just a highly motivated person," but admits to being more anxious for the past year as her law school course load has increased. Physical exam is normal and on mental status exam, she is restless, pacing the room, and her speech is moderately rapid but logical.

Conditions with Similar Presentations	**Panic disorder:** May have multiple somatic symptoms that may overlap but have unprovoked panic attacks and fear of further attacks as described above.
	Social anxiety disorder: Also known as social phobia, involves uncontrollable, excessive worry of embarrassment in social situations.
	Social anxiety disorder, performance only: As above but limited to public speaking/performances. Patient is otherwise unaffected in social situations.
Initial Diagnostic Tests	• Clinical Diagnosis
	• Consider: TSH, urine toxicology to rule out other conditions
Next Steps in Management	SSRI and/or CBT.
Discussion	GAD involves uncontrollable, excessive worry regarding multiple issues in one's life, lasting for ≥6 months. Patients have three or more of the following symptoms including restlessness, irritability, sleep disturbance, difficulty concentrating, fatigue, and muscle tension (e.g., neck pain as described in the above case). Women are more likely affected than men.
	• Many patients with GAD also have additional somatic symptoms such as sweating, nausea, diarrhea, headache, and trembling.
	• Symptoms typically have a fluctuating yet chronic course, and cause social, academic, and/or occupational impairment.
	Management:
	• CBT and/or pharmacotherapy with options including SSRIs, SNRIs, and/or buspirone.
	• Medication is usually chosen based on side effect profile and patient history.
	• Benzodiazepines are considered second-line due to risk of abuse and addiction.
Additional Considerations	**Pediatric Considerations:** GAD in children and adolescents often presents with prominent somatic symptoms (e.g., stomachache, headache) and a need for perfectionism or order. Patients may be easily distracted, worry excessively about academic performance, or even refuse to go to school.

CASE 16 | Obsessive-Compulsive Disorder (OCD)

A 40-year-old woman self-presents to clinic with concern of a respiratory infection. She states she has had a cough for the last year and believes the cause is "bad air." Throughout the examination she clears her throat consecutively in sets of three. When asked about her home environment, the patient states that she has an industrial-grade air purifier in each room of her house, and that she vacuums and dusts her entire house each morning before leaving for work. Despite these efforts the patient is frustrated that her condition remains unimproved and recognizes that her belief in "bad air" may be flawed. "It may be all in my head, but I can't help but try to stay safe if it's not." She asks if you can write her a doctor's note for her boss, who has become increasingly upset at the patient's tardiness to work, because he "does not understand." The physical exam is unremarkable.

Conditions with Similar Presentations	**Obsessive-compulsive personality disorder (OCPD):** Symptoms are *ego-syntonic*, meaning patients are not bothered by their compulsions. In contrast, those with OCD are considered *ego-dystonic*, meaning the patient is distressed or frustrated by the obsessions but performs the compulsions anyway. Those with OCPD are preoccupied with perfectionism, order, and rules, and may have an unhealthy focus on their work. Counterintuitively, this may interfere with the completion of tasks, as the patient continues to work until it is done to their exact liking (i.e., "perfect is the enemy of the good").
	Hoarding disorder: A patient has accumulated so many possessions that it clutters their living space and may affect them socially or occupationally or create a hazardous environment. This behavior arises from the stress that accompanies discarding an item, regardless of value.
	Trichotillomania: Recurrent pulling out of one's own hair, commonly on the scalp/face, causing significant distress. Patients have attempted to stop or decrease the hair pulling without success.
Initial Diagnostic Tests	Clinical Diagnosis
Next Steps in Management	CBT and SSRIs
Discussion	OCD is characterized by obsessions and/or compulsions that are time-consuming, distressing, and impairing. • **Obsessions** are recurrent, intrusive, undesired thoughts that increase anxiety. Examples of obsessions include fear of contamination, not turning off a stove or locking a door, objects facing a certain way, or even unwelcome violent or sexual urges or images. • **Compulsions** are repetitive behaviors or mental rituals performed in order to relieve the anxiety caused by the obsession, which may increase when a patient resists acting on them. Examples of compulsions include repetitive handwashing, cleaning objects, repeated counting, checking stoves or locks, arranging objects to all be in a certain order, or silently repeating a prayer or phrase. **Management:** • A combination of CBT and medications (SSRIs are first-line, clomipramine is typically second-line) is the most effective. • An important component of CBT involves exposure and response prevention (ERP), whereby the patient is repeatedly exposed to the object or thought that promotes their obsession and then prevented from performing the corresponding compulsion in a controlled environment.
Additional Considerations	**Pregnant or postpartum women** are at increased risk for OCD, with obsessions and compulsions often relating to the health and safety of the fetus or newborn baby.

CASE 17 | Posttraumatic Stress Disorder (PTSD)

A 23-year-old woman presents to clinic with nightmares for the past 6 months. She shares that her nightmares typically involve an ex-partner who had assaulted her on multiple occasions. When she passes by his apartment complex on her drive home from work, she often has vivid memories of his abuse. Because of this, she now takes an alternative route home that is much longer. She states she feels safe, as she has a restraining order against him, but continues to have trouble sleeping. She frequently awakens at night and has recurrent nightmares several times per week. Additionally, she notes when a coworker came from behind her and tapped her on the shoulder, she overreacted by jumping back and shrieking. On further questioning, she becomes tearful, stating she is worried about her ex-partner as he too had endured severe trauma and she was the only one helping him. She describes feeling guilty for leaving him unsupported.

CASE 17 | Posttraumatic Stress Disorder (PTSD) *(continued)*

Conditions with Similar Presentations	**Acute stress disorder:** Similar symptoms to PTSD, but the symptoms are present for ≥3 days and ≤1 month. Early intervention with trauma-focused CBT can help prevent progression to PTSD.
	GAD: PTSD can be distinguished from anxiety disorders by the presence of a traumatic event, nightmares/flashbacks, and hypervigilance following an identifiable traumatic event. Contents of intrusive thoughts, flashbacks, and nightmares pertain specifically to the traumatic event, rather than worries in GAD which focus on multiple areas of life.
	Adjustment disorder: Involves response to a specific stressful event/situation. Mood and behavioral symptoms must occur within 3 months of the onset of an identifiable stressor and not persist more than 6 months after the stressor has resolved. If symptoms persist past 6 months, consider evaluating for MDD or GAD. Symptoms must cause marked distress that is out of proportion to the stressor, or the patient must have a significant impairment in functioning. The patient must not meet the criteria for a major depressive episode or GAD, as one of these diagnoses would preclude an adjustment disorder diagnosis. Symptoms of adjustment disorder can include depression, anxiety, and/or disturbance of conduct, and are treated with supportive psychotherapy.
Initial Diagnostic Tests	Clinical Diagnosis
Next Steps in Management	• CBT and SSRI/SNRI • Prazosin for nightmares
Discussion	Risk factors for PTSD include military service, intimate partner violence, sexual trauma, child abuse, medical illness or physical injury, and displacement from one's home due to conflict (e.g., refugees). PTSD diagnosis requires an exposure to a perceived or actually life-threatening, traumatic event, as well as six additional symptoms from the following clusters of symptoms: 1. Intrusions (distressing memories, dreams/nightmares, flashbacks) 2. Avoidance (avoiding memories or triggers for the memories) 3. Negative mood/thinking (negative thoughts, distortions, negative mood, guilt, shame, diminished interest or participation, detachment) 4. Alteration in arousal (irritability, recklessness, hypervigilance, concentration or sleep issues, exaggerated startle) In addition, symptoms must be disturbing, not attributed to substance use or another condition, and be present for >1 month. **Management:** • A combination of CBT and pharmacotherapy, specifically an SSRI/SNRI, is most effective. • CBT should focus on emotional processing of trauma, including recognizing maladaptive thought patterns and developing appropriate responses. • For PTSD-related nightmares, add prazosin as adjunctive pharmacotherapy.

Anxiolytic Medications Beyond SSRIs and SNRIs

Medications	Mechanism	Side Effects/Contraindications	Additional Considerations
Benzodiazepines (e.g., alprazolam, clonazepam, diazepam, lorazepam, chlordiazepoxide, midazolam)	GABA$_A$ receptor agonists	Sedation, confusion, respiratory depression (especially concerning in elderly patients), addiction and abuse potential Paradoxical agitation shortly after initial dose is rare but important to recognize Can also lead to potentially life-threatening withdrawal (i.e., seizures), especially with shorter-acting benzodiazepines (e.g., alprazolam)	Avoid in patients at risk of delirium Also used in acutely agitated or aggressive patients for sedation and in alcohol withdrawal Flumazenil (benzodiazepine antagonist) can be used in acute overdose but may precipitate withdrawal
Buspirone	5-HT$_{1A}$ receptor partial agonist	Headache, nausea, dizziness	Unlike other anxiolytics, there is no concern for abuse potential, sedation, does not interact with alcohol, and does not lead to withdrawal

See SSRIs and SNRIs above under "Mood Disorders" section for more information.

AMNESIA, DISSOCIATION, AND DELIRIUM

Amnesia

Amnesia is a loss of memory. Amnestic disorders do not present with other cognitive problems or change in consciousness and are not caused by another medical condition. In diagnosing and treating memory disorders, it is important to assess for and to treat reversible causes (e.g., vitamin deficiencies, endocrine disorders, or chronic infection such as neurosyphilis).

Dissociation

Dissociation involves feelings of detachment and estrangement from the self. This often arises suddenly and may be temporary in duration. This is not due to another underlying medical condition, but usually related to a stressful life event. Dissociation may occur in dissociative amnesia, dissociative identity disorder, depersonalization disorder, and PTSD.

Delirium

Delirium is commonly encountered on inpatient medical and surgical wards. This condition is characterized by a waxing and waning level of consciousness. Delirium is always a result of another medical condition, such as infection, ischemia, medications, or metabolic disturbance. Hyperactive delirious patients are usually easy to identify as they may be yelling, agitated, combative, or otherwise disruptive. The hypoactive delirious patient is more commonly seen but harder to recognize, as they are withdrawn and have subtle disorientation. Delirium is by definition reversible, but it may take months to fully resolve.

CASE 18	Wernicke-Korsakoff Syndrome
\multicolumn{2}{l}{A 58-year-old man presents to the ED in police custody after being found on the ground at a bus station. He says he was "sleeping off a drink" before he went home. When asked his address, he provides the address of a local grocery store. When told that this is not a residential address, he becomes irate and tries to storm out of the ED. The patient is markedly thin and has an ataxic gait. Blood alcohol level is 0.8 and urine drug screening is negative.}
Conditions with Similar Presentations	Patients with **dementia** may present similarly, although Wernicke-Korsakoff should be suspected in those with history of alcohol abuse and thiamine deficiency. Consider age of onset and pattern of symptom development to differentiate between different subtypes of dementia. **Acute intoxication:** Would have higher BAL levels.
Initial Diagnostic Tests	• Clinical diagnosis (see Discussion) • Low blood thiamine; may be normal if recent ingestion or administration • Check: BAL and drug screen to rule out acute intoxication • Consider: CBC, CMP to assess for other complications of chronic alcohol use
Next Steps in Management	• IV thiamine supplementation • Alcohol cessation, and referral to a rehabilitation program • Closely monitor for and treat alcohol withdrawal
Discussion	**Wernicke encephalopathy** categorizes the early stages of this syndrome and is characterized by confusion (encephalopathy), ophthalmoplegia, and cerebellar ataxia. It is the result of **thiamine (vitamin B1) deficiency**. The most common cause is chronic alcohol use; however, it can also be seen in patients with prolonged malnutrition of other causes (e.g., anorexia nervosa). It is associated with necrosis and atrophy of the mammillary bodies and periventricular hemorrhage. This can progress to **Korsakoff syndrome**, a chronic irreversible amnestic syndrome characterized by impaired antegrade memory, personality changes, and confabulation (unconsciously making up answers when memory has failed—patients often do not realize they are making things up and may believe it to be true). Even with thiamine repletion, it is reversible in only about 20% of patients. Therefore, early recognition of Wernicke encephalopathy and resulting IV thiamine supplementation is important. Some patients may present with Korsakoff syndrome without a prior known episode of Wernicke encephalopathy. Neuropathological findings in Korsakoff syndrome include damage to the anterior and medial thalamus as well as the corpus callosum. **Diagnostics:** • Clinical diagnosis of Wernicke encephalopathy can be made with any two of the following criteria (Caine criteria) and approaches 100% sensitivity in persons with alcohol use disorder and absence of hepatic encephalopathy: 1. Nutritional deficiency 2. Oculomotor abnormalities

CASE 18 | Wernicke-Korsakoff Syndrome *(continued)*

Discussion	3. Cerebellar dysfunction
	4. Altered mental status or memory impairment
	• Thiamine level may be low but can be falsely elevated if recently ingested or administered.
	• If done, MRI brain may show mamillary body atrophy.
	• Additional tests:
	  • Check BAL (may be elevated) and urine toxicology screen to rule out acute intoxication.
	  • CBC (macrocytosis with or without megaloblastic anemia), CMP (elevated AST/ALT) to assess for other complications of chronic alcohol use.

Additional Considerations	When a patient provides an incorrect address or is guarded about their living situation, empathically inquire if the patient has stable housing. A patient may falsely be labeled as "confused," when they may actually be guarded or noncommittal about identification or residence (may be due to houselessness or being undocumented, among many other reasons).

CASE 19 | Dissociative Identity Disorder (DID)

A 38-year-old man is brought by his husband to clinic for evaluation of bizarre behavior. The husband reports that the patient has no significant past medical history or family history that he is aware of as the patient is estranged from his parents, who were physically abusive while the patient was growing up. The husband recently accompanied the patient to his high-school reunion last weekend and noted that he acted very differently and was more subdued compared to his usual personable and outgoing self. He referred to himself by a different name and treated his partner as though he didn't know him. He became quite frustrated with his husband and stated that he never met him before. On exam, the patient is timid, speaks in a very formal manner, and is not oriented to person or place.

Conditions with Similar Presentations	**Dissociative amnesia:** Patient cannot remember basic personal information, often due to a stressful or traumatic event. In DID, the patient has more than one distinct identity, asking to be referred to by a different name rather than simply forgetting one's name. **Depersonalization/derealization disorder:** Involves one or both symptoms of depersonalization (feeling detached from oneself as if watching one's life as a movie) and/or derealization (experiencing surroundings as unreal, as if in a dream) despite intact reality testing.
Initial Diagnostic Tests	• Clinical Diagnosis • Consider: Rule out other causes including substance use and other medical/psychiatric conditions
Next Steps to Management	• Psychotherapy is the treatment of choice. • Goals include maintenance of safety, stabilization, identity integration, and symptom reduction by working directly with traumatic memories. • Pharmacotherapy can be used to treat any comorbid conditions (e.g., MDD, PTSD).
Discussion	DID is characterized by a disruption of identity manifested by at least two distinct personality states dominating at different times, associated with extensive memory lapses in autobiographical information, daily occurrences, or traumatic events, which causes significant distress or impairment in functioning. This is not due to the effects of a substance or medication. It is often associated with past childhood trauma and has high rates of co-occurring psychiatric disorders, including borderline personality disorder, PTSD, and major depression. The personality states may be associated with prior trauma (e.g., patient acts as a fearful, crying child).

CASE 20 | Delirium

An 84-year-old woman is on day four of an inpatient admission after a complicated repair of a hip fracture. She was going to be discharged today, but overnight nursing reported the patient has been trying to pull out her IVs. On exam, she is somewhat cooperative, appears confused, and states that her overnight nurse was trying to harm her. Her vital signs and oxygenation are normal. She has no focal neurologic deficits or other abnormal findings on physical exam. Prior to hospitalization, she was living independently at home.

Conditions with Similar Presentations	**Normal aging:** Age-related declines include slowness in thinking and difficulty with attention and multitasking. Changes are subtle, and occur over months to years, not days. **Mild neurocognitive disorder:** A decline in one cognitive domain that is greater than expected. There is no substantial interference with daily life. **Dementia:** A decline in one or more cognitive domains (learning, memory, executive function, attention, perceptual-motor, or social cognition) with onset over months to years. Similar to delirium, orientation and memory may be impaired but hallucinations are less common, especially in the early stages. Symptoms demonstrate less fluctuation than in delirium.

CASE 20 | Delirium *(continued)*

Initial Diagnostic Tests	• Clinical Diagnosis • Identify and treat underlying cause(s) • Review medications and check CBC, CMP, TSH, UA, urine and blood cultures, ECG, chest x-ray, and oxygenation level
Next Steps in Management	• Treat the underlying cause of the delirium (e.g., infection, fecal impaction, ACS) • Consider pre-existing dementia that may be exacerbated by unfamiliar environment (sundowning). • Discontinue any medications that may cause or contribute to delirium, such as benzodiazepines or overly sedating pain medications. • Frequently reorient the patient to their surroundings, re-establish sleep-wake cycle, mobilize and stimulate the patient. • Avoid restraints (unless needed as a last resort to protect patient or others).
Discussion	This patient's presentation is consistent with delirium, given the sudden change in baseline cognition with waxing and waning mental status that is worse at night (sundowning). Diagnostic criteria include: 1. Disturbance of attention and awareness. 2. Develops over a short time period, fluctuates throughout the day, and is a change from baseline. 3. Additional disturbance in another area of cognition such as memory, orientation, language. 4. These disturbances are not better explained by another neurocognitive or medical condition. 5. Disturbances do not occur in setting of severely reduced level of arousal or coma 6. There should also be some evidence of an underlying cause. Delirium is associated with increased morbidity and mortality and can present as hyperactive or hypoactive delirium. This case illustrates hyperactive delirium. Delirium is more common in patients with underlying dementia, previous stroke, and in the post-operative setting.

FACTITIOUS AND SOMATIC DISORDERS

Factitious and somatic disorders may be divided into those where symptoms are conscious (malingering, factitious disorder) vs. unconscious (somatic symptom disorder, illness anxiety disorder, conversion disorder). If symptoms are intentionally produced, determine whether their motivations are conscious (malingering) or unconscious (factitious disorder).

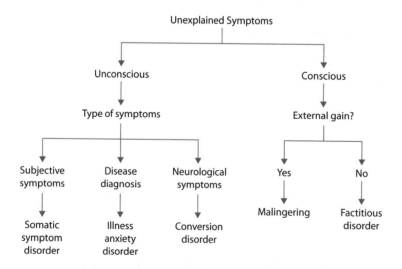

CASE 21 | Factitious Disorder

A 22-year-old woman with a history of repeated hospitalizations in childhood for acute lymphoblastic leukemia (now in remission for many years) presents to the ED via EMS with tachycardia, rash, and difficulty breathing. EMS had given her one dose of IM epinephrine en route to treat anaphylaxis. In the ED, she is given an additional dose of IM epinephrine with good response.
As the patient is stabilizing, the team calls the patient's nursing school roommate who is the patient's emergency contact. The roommate says the patient has a history of a severe peanut allergy and has had episodes of anaphylaxis requiring trips to the ED twice in the last 3 months. The roommate notes that there is an open jar of peanut butter on the patient's nightstand and that the previous admissions were also due to a "similar story." Laboratory studies are unremarkable.

CASE 21 | Factitious Disorder *(continued)*

Conditions with Similar Presentations	**Malingering:** Symptoms are falsified or exaggerated for secondary gain.
Initial Diagnostic Tests	• Clinical Diagnosis • Exclude/rule out medical etiologies of symptoms
Next Steps in Management	• Address the test results and diagnosis in a non-judgmental, non-threatening manner • Consider psychotherapy
Discussion	Factitious disorder (also known as Münchausen syndrome) is characterized by falsification of physical or psychological signs or symptoms, or induction of injury or disease, associated with identified deception, without clear external rewards. The motivation is to assume the sick role and is not due to another mental disorder. Incidence is higher among health care workers and in women. Repeated and long-term hospitalizations are common. This diagnosis should also be considered when faced with an unusual presentation of a common disorder (e.g., a skin abscess that grows enteric bacteria rather than the usual *S. aureus* or *S. pyogenes*). Patients often have a history of previous and/or repeated hospitalizations or illness, or a history of childhood physical or sexual abuse.
Additional Considerations	Factitious disorder can further be categorized as **"imposed on self"** when the patients falsified symptoms or illness are their own, or **"imposed on another"** (or Münchausen syndrome by proxy) when the patient is intentionally producing symptoms or illness on someone else under their care (e.g., one's children). Imposing illness onto a child is considered abuse and should be immediately reported.

CASE 22 | Malingering

A 32-year-old man presents with lower back pain after lifting something heavy for his job. He describes the pain as a 10/10 and that "it hurts all over." The patient is accompanied by his 3-year-old daughter, whom he lifts during the visit with no visible sensation of pain. On physical exam, he screams in pain during palpation of the upper, middle, and lower back. Straight leg test is negative. Spinal imaging is unremarkable. He then asks if paperwork can be signed stating that he cannot report to work for the next 2 weeks.

Conditions with Similar Presentations	**Factitious disorder:** Symptoms or illness is intentionally produced as the patient desires to assume the sick role rather than for an external reward or secondary gain.
Initial Diagnostic Tests	• Clinical Diagnosis • Exclude/rule out medical etiologies of symptoms
Next Steps to Management	• Avoid direct confrontation or accusing the patient of feigning their illness. • Try indirect approach such as offering scientific reasoning as to why their symptoms are not aligning with presentation, at a level appropriate to their medical literacy. • Encourage psychotherapy, but these patients are not often amenable. • Prognosis is poor as they often become defensive, angry, and abruptly leave the health care setting.
Discussion	Malingering is not considered a mental illness. Malingering patients are conscious of a secondary gain or external reward (e.g., avoiding police, monetary compensation, leave from work or school, narcotics, receiving room and board). Symptoms are either not present or extremely over-exaggerated. Malingering is more common in men and should be suspected in any patient who is inconsistent in reporting, does not cooperate with the interview, refuses a complete examination or workup, discusses impending legal proceedings, or has a history of antisocial personality disorder. There is often a history of seeking care from multiple different physicians and institutions. • Malingering may be related to a single incident or a repeated pattern of behaviors. • Patients may undergo a prolonged hospital stay or workup, and symptoms often improve once their secondary gain is obtained.

CASE 23 | Functional Neurological Symptom Disorder (Conversion Disorder)

A 27-year-old woman presents to clinic with 3 months of right-hand weakness, numbness, and tingling. She herself is not concerned, but her partner recommended she seek medical attention. She notes all fingers other than her thumb are affected. She has previously been evaluated by several neurologists and has undergone cervical MRI and EMG which were normal. On physical exam, her second through fifth digits are weak on abduction and flexion. When given a pencil to hold, it falls from her hand. Otherwise, her neurological exam is unremarkable. When leaving the appointment, she was able to successfully pull the door open with her right hand.

Conditions with Similar Presentations	**Somatic symptom disorder:** Patients present with one or more physical symptoms lasting ≥6 months and are not intentionally producing or faking their symptoms. These patients often seek treatment from multiple providers and undergo extensive workup and treatment regimens. They experience significant distress from the physical symptoms and have excessive thoughts and behaviors related to the symptoms. Symptoms may also worsen under stress. When treating a patient with somatic symptom disorder, negative test results should be delivered in a supportive manner, followed by regularly scheduled visits with the same provider while minimizing further unnecessary workup or treatments.
	Illness anxiety disorder: Patients are worried and have a high level of anxiety for ≥6 months related to either having or acquiring a serious medical illness. Patients usually lack physical symptoms, or they are very mild in nature, but they remain unconvinced by negative exam and laboratory findings. This often results in increased health care utilization.
Initial Diagnostic Tests	Clinical diagnosis
Next Steps in Management	• Validate the patient's experience of symptoms • Treat with a multidisciplinary approach including reassurance, education, physical therapy, cognitive behavioral therapy, antidepressants if appropriate (for comorbid MDD), and exercise.
Discussion	Functional neurological symptom disorder (conversion disorder) is classified by abnormal neurological symptoms that are: 1. Not consistent with a recognized neurological condition or neuroanatomic distribution 2. Cause significant distress and impairment in social or occupational function or warrant medical evaluation (e.g., sensorimotor changes in the above patient) 3. Are not better explained by another medical or mental disorder Common symptoms experienced by patients include sensory loss or paresthesias, weakness, paralysis, blindness, and seizures. Functional refers to the symptoms resulting from a failure of the functioning of the nervous system, as opposed to a structural lesion or pathology. Functional neurological symptom occurs more often in women, and patients are typically in adolescence or early adulthood. Psychological factors are not required for diagnosis but are often associated with this disorder and include depression and anxiety. This disorder should be considered when neurological symptoms are incompatible with known disease or neuroanatomic distribution or are inconsistent throughout the examination. Patients may display "la belle indifference," whereby they act surprisingly calm and unconcerned about their symptoms despite the potential severity. Symptoms often resolve or improve but may recur and be chronic.

EATING DISORDERS

Eating disorders can develop at any age, and are more frequent in females. It is important to distinguish an eating disorder from people who engage in intense/odd diets or exercise regimens but do not have a diagnosable eating disorder. Like many other psychiatric illnesses, eating disorders must include a component of psychological disturbance (i.e., the condition causes significant physical or psychological distress). Anorexia nervosa can be confused with bulimia nervosa. Anorexia by definition requires a significantly low body weight (often BMI <18.5 kg/m^2), whereas other eating disorders do not. Bulimia is characterized by binge eating episodes with any compensatory behavior, whether purging, exercise, fasting, or laxatives.

CASE 24 | Bulimia Nervosa

A 26-year-old woman presents for constipation and bloating for the past 6 months. She feels nauseous after eating meals and only has a bowel movement once a week. She takes over-the-counter laxatives in order to have a bowel movement. She denies restricting her food intake; however, after further questioning she shyly admits to eating a quart of ice cream and several other desserts two to three times per week. She has been doing this intermittently for the past 8 months and describes feeling out of control during these times. Her vitals are stable except for orthostatic hypotension. Her BMI is 20 kg/m². On physical exam, she has several dental fillings, bilaterally enlarged salivary glands (sialadenosis) and abrasions on the dorsum of her right hand. When palpating the abdomen, she demonstrates voluntary guarding.

Conditions with Similar Presentations	**Anorexia nervosa:** Differs from bulimia nervosa in that the patient's BMI is <18.5 even if the patient presents with frequent purging. **Binge-eating disorder:** Characterized by recurrent episodes of binge eating (eating an excessive amount of food in a 2-hour period associated with a lack of control), with at least three of the following behaviors: 1. Eating very rapidly 2. Eating until uncomfortably full 3. Eating large amounts when not hungry 4. Eating alone due to embarrassment 5. Feeling disgusted, depressed, or guilty after eating The binge eating occurs at least weekly for 3 months, causes severe distress, and does not occur exclusively during the course of anorexia or bulimia. Patients do not perform compensatory behaviors such as vomiting and often have elevated BMI. Treatment encompasses a multi-modal approach, with CBT or interpersonal psychotherapy, a strict diet/exercise program coordinated by a dietician, and potentially an SSRI.

Initial Diagnostic Tests	• Clinical Diagnosis
	• Check: BMP to evaluate for electrolyte abnormalities
	  • Those inducing vomiting often have a hypochloremic hypokalemic metabolic alkalosis.
	  • Those abusing laxatives may have metabolic acidosis.
	  • Patients may also have hypernatremia, signs of dehydration (including elevated BUN and signs of AKI).
	• Consider checking: CBC, transaminases, TSH, pregnancy test
	• Amylase may be elevated (salivary gland origin)

Next Steps in Management	Nutritional education, CBT, and an SSRI (fluoxetine)
Discussion	Bulimia nervosa is an eating disorder that involves binge eating in addition to compensatory behaviors to prevent weight gain. Patients may somaticize their symptoms and not be forthcoming with their body-image concerns. Diagnostic criteria include: 1. Recurrent episodes of binge eating, characterized by eating a large amount of food within a discrete period of time and a sense of lack of control over eating during the episode 2. Recurrent attempts to compensate for overeating and prevent weight gain (e.g., laxative abuse, vomiting, diuretics, fasting, or excessive exercise) at least once a week for 3 months. 3. Perception of self-worth is excessively influenced by body weight and shape. 4. Does not occur exclusively during an episode of anorexia nervosa. Psychiatric comorbidities such as MDD or GAD are common. Recurrent vomiting also results in several characteristic findings on exam, including parotid gland hypertrophy, salivary gland enlargement (sialadenosis), dental caries, callouses and abrasions on the back of the hands (Russell sign), and pharyngeal erythema. Voluntary guarding may be an indication of being self-conscious about the appearance of their abdomen. Prognosis is better than that for anorexia, although there is an elevated suicide risk.
Additional Considerations	It is important to remember to avoid the antidepressant bupropion in patients with any active eating disorder due to potential adverse effect of lowering the patient's seizure threshold.

CASE 25 | Anorexia Nervosa

A 19-year-old woman presents accompanied by her mother, who is concerned about the patient's weight. She is a dancer and is fixated on losing weight for an upcoming performance. She feels like she is still "too fat." Her mother reports she eats very little throughout the day and does aerobics for 2 hours a day in addition to dance practice. She reports not having a period in several months. Her vitals are notable for orthostatic hypotension, HR 55, and BMI 15. On physical exam, she is wearing a sweater even though it is warm outside.

Conditions with Similar Presentations	**Bulimia:** Patients often maintain a normal body weight or may be overweight.

Initial Diagnostic Tests	• Clinical Diagnosis
	• Check: BMP to evaluate for electrolyte abnormalities and AKI.
	  • Those inducing vomiting often have a hypochloremic hypokalemic metabolic alkalosis.
	  • Those abusing laxatives may have metabolic acidosis.
	  • Patients may also have hypernatremia, signs of dehydration (including elevated BUN and signs of AKI).
	• Consider checking: CBC, transaminases, TSH, pregnancy test, ECG, DEXA scan. Amylase may be elevated, salivary gland origin.

Next Steps in Management	• Hospitalize if severely underweight, significant electrolyte abnormalities, AKI, or vital sign instability • If not requiring hospitalization, consider starting an antidepressant with weight gain–promoting effect (e.g., mirtazapine, paroxetine), behavioral therapy, family therapy, and supervised eating disorder programs • Avoid bupropion due to decreased seizure threshold.
Discussion	Diagnosis is made when there is the following: 1. Restriction of energy intake relative to requirements leading to significantly low body weight 2. Intense fear of gaining weight or becoming fat, or persistent behaviors that prevent weight gain 3. Disturbed body image, undue influence of weight or shape on self-evaluation, or denial of the seriousness of the current low body weight • Patients may eat in binges, but this is followed by purging, laxatives, excessive exercise, and/or diuretic use. • Clinical features include amenorrhea, electrolyte abnormalities, arrhythmias, cardiac arrest, lanugo (fine body hair), osteoporosis. • Mortality is relatively high due to starvation, suicide, or electrolyte disturbance.
Additional Considerations	Monitor for **refeeding syndrome** as patient begins to increase intake—hypophosphatemia, hypokalemia, and hypomagnesemia can become dangerous and may require ICU-level monitoring. Fluids, electrolytes, renal function, and cardiac function should be carefully monitored.

IMPULSE CONTROL DISORDERS

Difficulties with impulse control are a symptom of many psychiatric disorders. The impulse control disorders discussed in this section are defined by dysregulation of emotional (e.g., intermittent explosive disorder) and/or behavioral (e.g., pyromania) self-control such that patients violate the rights of others or clash with societal norms. Since it is not unusual for most individuals to make impulsive decisions on occasion (especially when accounting for age and context), the frequency, persistence, and pervasiveness across situations, as well as the subsequent impairment, of these behaviors must be examined before reaching a diagnosis. These disorders start to emerge in childhood or adolescence and are often comorbid with ADHD, substance use disorders, and each other. Most (with the exception of kleptomania) are significantly more common in males. Treating impulse control disorders can be difficult, as patients may have little desire to change their behaviors. Although limited, treatment options include SSRIs and CBT.

Impulse Control Disorder Mini-Cases

Intermittent Explosive Disorder	**Hx:** A 19-year-old man presents with low mood and guilt. He reports episodes associated with destruction of household property and injuries to himself and sometimes others. Episodes occur once or twice every 2–3 days. He denies substance use.
	Diagnostics: Clinical Diagnosis
	Management: Consider treatment with an SSRI, mood stabilizer, or propranolol. Group therapy or family therapy may be helpful.
	Discussion: This is more common in men than women. Episodes of explosive behavior often resolve spontaneously. Patients typically feel remorseful for their behavior.

Impulse Control Disorder Mini-Cases *(continued)*

Pyromania	**Hx:** A 21-year-old man is brought in for evaluation after being caught setting a fire in a vacant building. He reports a fascination with fire throughout his life and has intentionally set multiple fires. He denies criminal intent. **Diagnostics:** Clinical Diagnosis **Management:** Consider treatment with an SSRI or CBT. Patients may need supervision and monitoring. **Discussion:** This is more common in men than women.
Kleptomania	**Hx:** A 20-year-old woman reports stealing behaviors since the age of 14. She will steal different items of no significant monetary value when presented with the opportunity and without premeditation. She describes overwhelming tension and difficulty resisting these impulses. She feels some shame and guilt about these behaviors and was recently fired from her last workplace after being found responsible for thefts of paperclips and pens. **Diagnostics:** Clinical Diagnosis **Management:** Consider treatment with an SSRI. CBT may be helpful. **Discussion:** This is more common in women than men. Symptoms may increase in times of stress. Kleptomania is associated with comorbid mood disorders, OCD, and eating disorders.

GENDER DYSPHORIA, SEXUAL DYSFUNCTION, AND PARAPHILIC DISORDERS

Sex refers to a person's biological status, based on appearance of external genitalia and sex chromosomes. *Gender* refers to a person's sense of oneself as a man, woman, or other, and may or may not align with the patient's sex or their assigned gender at birth. *Sexual orientation* is based on a person's sexual and romantic attraction.

Stages of the sexual response cycle include desire, excitement/arousal, orgasm, and resolution. Sexual dysfunction is a problem that can occur in any phase of a sexual response cycle. Sexual dysfunction involving any of these phases can cause clinically significant distress. The dysfunction cannot be better explained by nonsexual psychiatric disorder, a side effect of substance/medication, and/or another medical disorder.

Paraphilic disorders can be described as intense, recurrent, persistent desires to engage in unusual sexual activities and/or preoccupation with unusual sexual urges or fantasies lasting for at least 6 months. For diagnosis, these urges or fantasies must be acted upon with a non-consenting person and/or lead to significant distress or impaired functioning. Paraphilic disorders are often difficult to treat, but physicians can consider psychotherapy. Although controversial, the physician in rare cases can consider offering the patient options to reduce sexual drive, including anti-androgens, SSRIs, long-acting gonadotropin-releasing hormones, or naltrexone.

CASE 26 | Gender Dysphoria

A 16-year-old who was assigned male at birth presents for an adolescent medicine visit. Pronouns are she/her or they/them. She feels that she was born in the "wrong body," which has been causing a great deal of distress. She has felt this way ever since early childhood and has always felt she was female, based on her interests, feelings, and reactions to life events. She presents to clinic inquiring about hormone treatment to transition.

Conditions with Similar Presentations	**Gender nonconformity:** Individuals may not conform to the gender they were assigned at birth and instead desire to express their gender differently. Gender nonconformity in and of itself is not a psychiatric disorder.
Initial Diagnostic Tests	Clinical Diagnosis
Next Steps in Management	• Multidisciplinary therapy and family involvement for younger patients, including assessment of safety • Hormone replacement therapy if patient desires
Discussion	Gender dysphoria was previously referred to as gender identity disorder. Gender dysphoria is characterized by persistent incongruence between the sexual anatomy at birth and gender identity lasting ≥6 months, which is distressing to the individual. Of note, not all people who identify differently than their gender assigned at birth meet diagnostic criteria for gender dysphoria. It is important to not pathologize a patient's gender identity and to understand that gender can evolve over time. According to the DSM-5, patients must exhibit two or more of the following in addition to significant distress or impaired functioning:

CASE 26 | Gender Dysphoria *(continued)*

Discussion	1. Marked incongruence between one's experienced gender and sex characteristics 2. Strong desire to be rid of one's sex characteristics 3. Strong desire for sex characteristics of the other gender 4. Strong desire to be of the other gender 5. Strong conviction that one has the typical feelings/reactions of the other gender **Management:** • Multidisciplinary therapy and family involvement for younger patients, including assessment of safety. • Ensuring the patient has social support can be very helpful if the patient is distressed by the dissonance between their body and their gender identity. • If patients wish, they can initiate hormone replacement therapy. • Surgical sex reassignment is an option after 1 year in the desired gender role and after 1 year of continuous hormone therapy.
Additional Considerations	It is important to note the cultural context of **gender identity,** or a person's internal sense of being female, male, a combination of male and female, or neither male nor female. While gender is often reported as a binary variable (i.e., man or woman), in reality, gender exists across a continuum. A person who chooses to express a gender different from societal norms is referred to as gender nonconforming. While this may lead to distress due to lack of societal acceptance, gender dysphoria is diagnosed only when this distress is persistent and meets the DSM-5 criteria above. Health care providers providing multidisciplinary gender identity–affirming care and empathic support toward patients and families will help improve patient care.

CASE 27 | Erectile Disorder

A 26-year-old man presents to clinic for a routine checkup. During the interview he notes concerns regarding his sexual function. For the last 6 months the patient has been unable to achieve or maintain an erection when engaging in sexual activity with his girlfriend. The patient reports that his libido is unchanged, he is able to masturbate and ejaculate without issue, and occasionally wakes up with an erection. The patient reports stress at work and within the relationship and is anxious his symptoms will exacerbate stress within the latter. The patient's medical history, vitals, and physical exam (including genital exam) are unremarkable.

Conditions with Similar Presentations	**Substance/medication-induced sexual dysfunction:** Variability in achieving an erection may be caused by substance/medication use and will subsequently resolve with discontinuation of the substance/medication. **Another medical condition:** Organic causes include diabetes, hypertension, chronic kidney disease, neurologic disease (e.g., spinal cord injury), endocrine abnormalities (e.g., hypogonadism), or medication side effects.
Initial Diagnostic Tests	• Clinical Diagnosis • Rule out other medical causes of male sexual dysfunction
Next Steps in Management	• Individual or couples psychotherapy • Medications or devices as second-line
Discussion	Erectile dysfunction, or erectile disorder, is defined as marked difficulty obtaining and/or maintaining an erection during sexual activity and/or a decrease in erectile rigidity. Erectile disorder can be divided into generalized and situational (e.g., only with a particular partner, in a certain place), as well as lifelong (since the beginning of sexual activity) or acquired (after a period of normal functioning). These symptoms must have lasted for approximately 6 months and cause significant distress to the patient. In addition to a thorough medical history and workup, the presence of normal erections outside of sexual intercourse (e.g., nocturnal erections) decreases the likelihood of an underlying medical cause. Psychiatric comorbidities often include MDD and anxiety disorders. **Management:** • Once primary erectile dysfunction has been established, individual or couples' psychotherapy is the initial approach in addition to treating underlying mood or anxiety disorders, if present. • Medications such as PDE-5 inhibitors or physical instruments such as vacuum devices or constrictive rings may also be considered. • Surgical treatment with a penile prosthesis should be reserved as a last resort.
Additional Considerations	• Erectile disorder can be comorbid with other sexual disorders (e.g., premature ejaculation, hypoactive sexual desire disorder). • If treating a comorbid psychiatric disorder, keep in mind the negative sexual side effects of medications.

Paraphilic/Fetishistic Disorders in the DSM-5

Name	Description
Pedophilic Disorder	Recurrent and intense sexual arousal urges, fantasies, or behaviors involving prepubescent children (13 or younger). The patient is at least 16 years old and at least 5 years older than the child they are aroused by.
Voyeuristic Disorder	Repeated intense arousal by observing an unsuspecting person who is naked, undressing, or engaging in sexual activity. Individuals experience distress or become less able to function
Exhibitionistic Disorder	Recurrent urge to expose one's genitals to an unsuspecting person. Requires action of these urges toward a nonconsenting person and/or significant distress.
Frotteuristic disorder	Touching or rubbing against a nonconsenting individual
Sexual masochism disorder	Undergoing humiliation, bondage, or suffering from others
Sexual sadism disorder	Inflicting humiliation, bondage, or suffering on others
Fetishistic disorder	Using nonliving objects or having a highly specific focus on nongenital body parts
Transvestic disorder	Engaging in sexually arousing cross-dressing

SUBSTANCE USE

Substance use disorders affect people of all ages from all walks of life. As substance use can induce symptoms of other psychiatric illnesses (e.g., mood disorder, psychosis), it is essential to obtain a thorough history when considering these diagnoses. Individuals with other psychiatric disorders may use substances in order to help cope with their distressing symptoms. The 11 criteria for substance use (regardless of the specific substance) disorders include:

1. Taking the substance in larger amounts or for longer than intended
2. Not being able to cut down or stop using the substance
3. Spending significant time using or obtaining the substance
4. Urges or cravings to use
5. Neglecting responsibilities at work, school, or home because of substance use
6. Continuing to use despite causing problems in relationships
7. Social isolation
8. Using substances again and again even if dangerous
9. Continued use despite physical or psychotic problems
10. Needing more of a substance to get desired effect (tolerance)
11. Development of withdrawal symptoms that are alleviated by taking more of a substance

To meet the criteria for substance use disorder, the patient must have 2 of the 11 criteria within a 1-year period.

CASE 28	Alcohol Use Disorder (AUD)
A 40-year-old man with hypertension and alcohol use disorder presents to the ED with his wife, who requests he be admitted for detoxification. The patient states he is drinking 750 mL of vodka daily. His last drink was 1 hour prior to arrival, and he has been drinking in large amounts on and off for the last 20 years. He wishes to become abstinent and mentions that last time he tried to stop "cold turkey" 2 years ago, he had seizures. On exam, he is slurring his words and is unable to stand without support and has hepatomegaly.	
Conditions with Similar Presentations	**Non-pathological alcohol use:** Individuals may consume alcohol and become intoxicated without developing AUD. Recommended limits are <14 drinks/week or <4/occasion for males, <7 drinks/week or <3/occasion in females, and any drinks for pregnant people.
	Sedative, hypnotic, or anxiolytic use disorder: Individuals may present similarly to those with alcohol intoxication. It is important to note that this condition can co-occur with AUD. High doses of sedatives, hypnotics, or anxiolytics can be lethal, especially when mixed with alcohol.

CASE 28 | Alcohol Use Disorder (AUD) *(continued)*

Initial Diagnostic Tests	• Clinical Diagnosis • Check: Blood alcohol concentration (BAC) or BAL to assess for current intoxication • Consider: Urine toxicology screen, CMP, thiamine level
Next Steps in Management	Treat acute withdrawal with benzodiazepines, nutritional and volume support, thiamine, and folate.

Discussion	AUD, like other substance use disorders, requires 2 of the 11 above criteria within a 1-year period. It is a common chronic disease with the influence of genetic and environmental factors. Alcohol increases activation at the gamma-aminobutyric acid type A (GABAA) receptor. Chronic use results in downregulation of GABAA receptors. The sudden decrease in GABAA stimulation from the lack of alcohol results in withdrawal symptoms.
	
	History: Obtain a detailed alcohol use history to see if patient meets the criteria for a substance use disorder.
	
	Initial screening tools include alcohol use disorder identification test (AUDIT) and CAGE questionnaires.
	CAGE questionnaire:
	   C—Cutting down: "Do you feel you should cut down on your drinking?"
	   A—Annoyance at criticism: "Do you feel annoyed by others criticizing your drinking?"
	   G—Guilt: "Do you ever feel guilty about your drinking?"
	   E—Eye-Opener: "Do you ever need a drink first thing in the morning?"
	"Yes" answers for two or more questions are clinically significant.
	• **Alcohol intoxication:** Symptoms include mood elevation, decreased anxiety, slurred speech, impaired judgment, ataxia, emotional lability, memory blackouts, comas, and respiratory depression. BAC greater than 0.20 mg/dL (USA legal limit = 0.08) is likely to result in severe symptoms, except in those who have developed significant tolerance.
	• **Alcohol withdrawal:** Symptoms typically begin with anxiety and tremor within 6–8 hours, hallucinations within 8–12 hours, seizures at 24–48 hours, and potentially fatal delirium tremens (DTs) within 3–5 days.
	
	Physical Exam: May have postural action tremor, abnormal vital signs (decreased in intoxication, elevated in withdrawal), stigmata of liver disease (e.g., palmar erythema, telangiectasias, hepatomegaly).
	
	Diagnostics: Clinical diagnosis based on detailed history.
	• BAC or BAL can be used to assess current intoxication
	• Transaminases: elevated ALT and AST; AST is characteristically $>2 \times$ ALT
	• CBC shows macrocytosis, may show megaloblastic anemia
	• Vitamin B1 (thiamine), B6, B9 (folate), B12 and iron levels may be low
	
	For chronic management, consider:
	• Gamma-glutamyl transferase (GGT) and/or carbohydrate-deficient transferrin (CDT) at high levels indicate heavy drinking. Both return to normal within days/weeks of abstinence and therefore may be useful in monitoring abstinence.
	• Urine ethyl glucuronide (EtG), a direct metabolite of ethanol, may be used to monitor recent alcohol use 48–72 hours after last drink.
	
	Management:
	Acute withdrawal management:
	• Treat symptoms with benzodiazepines using fixed schedule or symptom-triggered treatment based on symptom score (e.g., Clinical Institute Withdrawal Assessment or CIWA).
	• Fluids, thiamine (before glucose), folate, and nutritional support.
	Chronic AUD treatment:
	• Determine what stages of change the person is in: precontemplation, contemplation, preparation, action, maintenance, relapse.
	• Treat with combination of non-pharmacologic therapy and pharmacotherapy.
	• Non-pharmacologic therapy includes individual psychotherapy (e.g., motivational interviewing, CBT), group therapy, mutual help groups (e.g., 12-step programs), and residential treatment programs.
	• Pharmacotherapy includes naltrexone, topiramate, acamprosate, disulfiram, and gabapentin.

CASE 28 | Alcohol Use Disorder (AUD) (continued)

Additional Considerations	**Complications:** • **Alcoholic hallucinosis:** 12–24 hours after last drink, may have auditory, visual, or tactile hallucinations. • **Delirium tremens (DTs):** Disturbance in cognition from alcohol withdrawal that occurs 48–96 hours after last drink and is associated with autonomic abnormalities and has a mortality up to 20% if untreated. A key feature of DTs is the presence of delirium (hallucinations, agitation, disorientation) and autonomic instability (hyperadrenergic state: elevated heart rate and blood pressure). Treat with benzodiazepines, IV fluids, thiamine and other vitamins, and nutritional support. • **Seizures:** Withdrawal seizures are generalized tonic-clonic seizures that occur within 12–24 hours after the last drink. They are single or, if more than one, occur over a several-hour period. Recurrences longer than that, or status epilepticus, warrant investigations for other causes of seizures. **Pregnancy Complication:** Fetal alcohol syndrome. **Additional Complications:** Include Wernicke encephalopathy, Korsakoff psychosis, gastritis, ulcers, varices, Mallory-Weiss tears, GI bleed, pancreatitis, liver disease (alcoholic hepatitis, cirrhosis), peripheral neuropathy, anemia (deficiency of folate, thiamine, and/or iron), cardiomyopathy, and pneumonia.

CASE 29 | Cocaine Intoxication

A 26-year-old man presents to the ED at 2 A.M. with concerns of bugs crawling underneath his skin. He reports that this sensation started 30 minutes ago after leaving his friend's house. He is pacing the room, sweating, rubbing his arms in an apparent response to internal stimuli, and has dilated pupils. His arms are unremarkable other than superficial excoriations. Vital signs are notable for a heart rate of 120 bpm and blood pressure of 150/93 mmHg. He has a postural action tremor when arms are outstretched. Urine drug screen is positive for cocaine and cannabis. When presented with the urine drug screen results, he reluctantly admits he "snorted" (i.e., nasally insufflated) a substance his friend had prepared.

Conditions with Similar Presentations	An **acute psychotic episode, amphetamine intoxication, or PCP intoxication** may present similarly, with tactile hallucinations and evidence of increased sympathetic tone.
Initial Diagnostic Tests	Urine drug screen
Next Steps in Management	• Supportive care • For mild to moderate agitation, benzodiazepines • For severe agitation, haloperidol
Discussion	Signs and symptoms of cocaine intoxication include increased sympathetic tone manifesting as euphoria, pupillary dilation, paranoia, psychomotor agitation, angina, hypertension palpitations, and hallucinations. A patient who uses cocaine regularly may experience a withdrawal "crash" with signs and symptoms of decreased sympathetic tone, including depressed mood, low energy, constricted pupils, increased sleep, and increased appetite. Withdrawal is not life threatening and treatment is supportive. Similar to alcohol (above), acute cocaine intoxication does not necessarily represent a **stimulant use disorder**. That diagnosis is appropriate when a patient uses cocaine in a pattern leading to significant impairment or distress within a 12-month period. Like AUD, this disorder is characterized by use of cocaine in larger amounts or in longer periods than intended; a desire or failed efforts to cut back; excessive time, energy, or money spent to obtain cocaine; cravings; tolerance; and recurrent use despite life disruptions.
Additional Considerations	Cocaine intoxication presents with some symptoms of psychosis, such as illusions and hallucinations; however, these symptoms resolve as the intoxication wanes (1–2 hours). If, however, psychotic symptoms persist past acute intoxication, consider **cocaine-induced psychosis**, which may present similarly to a primary psychotic disorder. **Complications:** Cocaine's vasoconstrictive effects (alpha-agonism) can lead to myocardial infarction or cerebrovascular accident; therefore, vitals must be monitored carefully in the acute setting. Repeated use of cocaine via nasal insufflation can lead to nasal septal and/or sinus perforation, requiring additional medical or surgical treatment.

CASE 30 | Opioid Intoxication

A 45-year-old woman presents to a community health clinic with a request for clean needles and HIV testing. She injects heroin multiple times daily and states that she has shared a needle with a friend who recently tested positive for HIV. On examination, the patient is slurring her words, has pinpoint pupils, and is lethargic. Near the end of the exam the patient struggles to stay awake but remains arousable to voice. Vital signs are notable for a respiratory rate of 10/min. Physical exam is notable for puncture wounds at various stages of healing in the feet, legs, groin, and arms.

Conditions with Similar Presentations	**Sedative, hypnotic, or anxiolytic intoxication or severe alcohol intoxication** may present similarly with altered mental status and somnolence.
Initial Diagnostic Tests	• Urine drug screen • Rapid reversal of symptoms following naloxone (an opioid antagonist) administration is indicative of opioid intoxication
Next Steps in Management	Give naloxone.
Discussion	As with other substance use disorders, **opioid use disorder** (OUD) is defined by a pattern leading to significant impairment or distress within a 12-month period. An important distinction from other use disorders is that patients may be prescribed opioids for medical treatment; taking opioids as prescribed does not constitute a disorder. Rather, prolonged use of opioids with no legitimate medical purpose, or in significant excess of what is warranted for a particular medical condition, is indicative of a use disorder. **Opioid intoxication:** Signs and symptoms include euphoria, slurred speech, sedation, respiratory and CNS depression, pupillary constriction, and constipation. **Opioid withdrawal:** Symptoms include depressed mood, sweating, piloerection, rhinorrhea, lacrimation, yawning, and diarrhea. While withdrawal symptoms can be severe, they are not life threatening. **Management:** **Acute intoxication:** The most worrying symptom is respiratory depression, which may lead to coma or death. • Naloxone (may require more than one dose) should be used to reverse the intoxication • Ensure airway, breathing, and circulation ("ABCs") **Withdrawal symptoms:** • Ondansetron or promethazine for nausea • Loperamide for diarrhea • Dicyclomine for abdominal cramps • Full opioid agonist (methadone) or partial agonist (buprenorphine) will help to alleviate symptoms (they may not completely alleviate withdrawal symptoms in patients with significant use) **Long-term pharmacotherapy:** • Daily oral methadone (full agonist) or buprenorphine-naloxone (partial agonist and antagonist) • Psychotherapy (CBT) therapy, group therapy, and mutual support groups (e.g., Narcotics Anonymous) • As heroin is being "cut" (i.e., mixed) with more powerful opioids, such as fentanyl, unbeknownst to the heroin user, offering fentanyl testing kits as part of a harm reduction model of care can help to prevent these overdoses
Additional Considerations	**Screening:** Test for diseases easily spread through shared needles, such as HIV and hepatitis. **Complications:** HIV, hepatitis, and other infections, including endocarditis, abscess, or local injection site wounds.

Presentation and Treatment of Substance Intoxication and Withdrawal

Drug	Intoxication Signs and Symptoms	Acute Toxicity Management	Withdrawal Symptoms	Long-Term Pharmacotherapy*
Alcohol	Mood elevation, decreased anxiety, slurred speech, impaired judgment, ataxia, emotional lability, memory blackouts, coma, respiratory depression	Supportive care with fluid and electrolyte repletion, airway assessment, lateral positioning to avoid aspiration Sedation (e.g., haloperidol) if agitated Gastric lavage ("stomach pump") in severe intoxication (i.e., >1 g/L blood alcohol concentration) and charcoal if within 2 hours of consumption	Anxiety, insomnia, tremor, tachycardia, hypertension, fever, seizures, hallucinations, delirium **Delirium tremens**—most severe alcohol withdrawal syndrome that usually begins within 72 hours of last drink Symptoms include hallucinations, tremor, autonomic instability, and life-threatening seizures	Naltrexone, topiramate, acamprosate, disulfiram, gabapentin Thiamine, folic acid, etc., for nutritional repletion
Nicotine	Restlessness, suppressed appetite	Supportive care	Irritability, anxiety, increased appetite	Nicotine replacement therapy (NRT, e.g., patch, gum, lozenges), bupropion (with or without NRT), varenicline
Cannabis	Euphoria, impaired coordination, impaired judgment, paranoia, conjunctival injection, dry mouth, increased appetite	Supportive Consider benzodiazepines if severely anxious or agitated	Irritability, anxiety, decreased appetite	
Benzodiazepines	Mood elevation, decreased anxiety, slurred speech, ataxia, sedation, respiratory depression	Supportive Flumazenil may be used in overdose, but should be used with caution in those with chronic use due to risk of precipitating a seizure	Anxiety, depression, insomnia, irritability Seizures in severe cases	Benzodiazepine taper
Opioids	Euphoria, respiratory depression, CNS depression, pupillary constriction, constipation	Address airway, breathing, and circulation Naloxone for overdose	Depression, sweating, piloerection, rhinorrhea, lacrimation, yawning, diarrhea	Buprenorphine-Naloxone, methadone
Amphetamines (e.g., methylphenidate, methamphetamine/ "crystal meth," MDMA/ Ecstasy/"Molly")	Euphoria, pupillary dilation, sweating, bruxism, dry mouth, pruritis, paranoia, increased energy, insomnia	Supportive care for mild-moderate intoxication For severe toxicity consider benzodiazepines and antipsychotics for agitation and psychosis Fluids for hypotension, tachycardia, or suspected rhabdomyolysis Additional antihypertensives after benzodiazepines if patient remains hypertensive Cooling for patients with hyperthermia	Depression, lethargy, sleep disturbances, pupillary constriction	

Presentation and Treatment of Substance Intoxication and Withdrawal (*Continued*)

Drug	Intoxication Signs and Symptoms	Acute Toxicity Management	Withdrawal Symptoms	Long-Term Pharmacotherapy*
Cocaine	Euphoria, pupillary dilation, paranoia, psychomotor agitation, angina, autonomic instability, hallucinations Cocaine's vasoconstrictive effects can lead to myocardial infarction or cerebrovascular accident	Similar to amphetamines (above) Beware of beta-blockade in cocaine toxicity due to risk of unopposed alpha stimulation (use combined alpha/beta blockade instead)	Depression, lethargy, sleep disturbances, pupillary constriction	
Phencyclidine (PCP/ "angel dust")	Aggressiveness, psychomotor agitation, impulsivity, hallucinations, tachycardia, hypertension, muscle rigidity, high pain tolerance, rotary nystagmus	Address airway, breathing, and circulation Benzodiazepines and antipsychotics for agitation and psychosis Fluids for rhabdomyolysis Restraints if needed to prevent harm to self or others		
Hallucinogens (e.g., psilocybin/"magic mushrooms," mescaline, lysergic acid diethylamide/ LSD/"acid")	Hallucinations, perceptual changes, depersonalization, pupillary dilation	Supportive care and reassurance with "talking down" the patient Benzodiazepines and antipsychotics for severe cases only	No withdrawal syndrome May lead to "flashbacks" later in life due to reabsorption of compound stored in lipids	

Note: Treatment of all substance use disorders can be aided by individual or group therapy, as well as support groups such as Alcoholics Anonymous or Narcotics Anonymous.

PERSONALITY DISORDERS

Personality disorders are defined by persistent patterns of behavior that deviate from expectations of that individual's culture and are manifested by disturbances in cognition, affect, interpersonal relationships, and impulse control. These conditions usually manifest in adolescence and early adulthood and affect multiple areas of a person's life (e.g., work, school, romantic relationships).

Personality disorders are **ego-syntonic**, which means that the beliefs and thought patterns from these disorders are in line with the patient's self-image and often do not produce personal distress (thereby leading to lack of insight); they are fundamental to the patient's personality and in line with their values. This makes personality disorders difficult to treat, as physicians often have difficulty convincing patients that they have a problem. In contrast, **ego-dystonic** disorders (e.g., OCD) are distressing to the patient, so they are more likely to be interested in treatment. As in most other psychiatric disorders, the diagnosis requires that the symptoms lead to clinically significant distress or impairment in social, occupational, or interpersonal functioning. The mainstay of treatment for most personality disorders is psychotherapy.

These disorders are grouped into clusters, which are often remembered with the mnemonic: weird (Cluster A), wild (Cluster B), and worried (Cluster C).

- **Cluster A** (weird): These individuals appear odd and eccentric. They have difficulty forming meaningful relationships but lack overt psychosis. There is a genetic association with schizophrenia. The specific personality disorders are:
  - Paranoid
  - Schizoid
  - Schizotypal

- **Cluster B** (wild): These individuals appear dramatic, emotional, or erratic. There is a genetic association with substance use and mood disorders. The specific personality disorders are:
  - Antisocial
  - Borderline
  - Histrionic
  - Narcissistic
- **Cluster C** (worried): These individuals appear anxious and fearful. There is a genetic association with anxiety disorders. The specific personality disorders are:
  - Avoidant
  - Obsessive-compulsive
  - Dependent

Personality Disorder Mini-Cases

Paranoid Personality Disorder	**Hx:** A 24-year-old man presents to the ED after assaulting a coworker. He is certain his partner is having an affair with this coworker, as she came home smelling like a man's perfume which was similar to his. When the nurse asks for his partner's contact information, the patient gets defensive and states, "Why do you need to know? Are you trying to find something wrong so you can charge my insurance?" **Diagnostics:** Clinical diagnosis characterized by the presence of at least four of the following: 1. Suspects that others are trying to harm them 2. Preoccupied with loyalty 3. Reluctant to confide in others due to fear 4. Interprets benign comments as threats 5. Bears grudges 6. Perceives attacks on character that are not apparent to others and is quick to counterattack 7. Has recurrent suspicions regarding fidelity of sexual partner **Management:** Psychotherapy; consider low-dose antipsychotics if overt psychosis or agitation are present **Discussion:** Characterized by pervasive distrust and suspiciousness, reluctance to confide in others, misinterpretation of comments as threats or attacks on character, and suspicions regarding fidelity of partner. By definition, someone does not have paranoid personality disorder if they are diagnosed with schizophrenia, bipolar disorder, or depression with psychotic features. This condition is not characterized by hallucinations.
Schizoid Personality Disorder	**Hx:** A 40-year-old computer programmer presents for her work physical. She has been living in her parent's basement and spends 20 hours a day there. She has never had an intimate partner, has no close friends, and no desire to make any. She only responds back to questions with one or two words. **Diagnostics:** Clinical diagnosis characterized by detachment from others, restricted expression of emotions, and the presence of at least four of the following: 1. No desire for close relationships 2. Proclivity for solitary activities 3. Low interest in sexual experiences with others 4. Takes pleasure in few activities 5. Lacks close friends 6. Appears indifferent to praise 7. Shows flat affect or detachment **Management:** Psychotherapy (typically lack insight) **Discussion:** Characterized by lack of desire for close relationships, preference for solitary activities, few close friends, restricted emotions, flat affect, and lack of sexual interest. Schizoid personality disorder cannot be diagnosed in the presence of schizophrenia or a mood disorder with psychotic features. Depression should be ruled out.

Personality Disorder Mini-Cases (*continued*)

Schizotypal Personality Disorder	**Hx:** An 18-year-old woman presents for her adolescent medicine appointment. She is wearing a witch outfit with a pink bottle in her hand. When the physician asks what is in the pink bottle, she replies "fairies like to drink this." She does not have close friends and gets nervous around others, although she wishes she were able to make friends. She denies auditory or visual hallucinations. **Diagnostics:** Clinical diagnosis characterized by interpersonal deficits as well as eccentric behavior and at least five of the following: 1. Ideas of reference (over-reading significance into everyday events) 2. Odd beliefs or magical thinking 3. Unusual perceptual experiences, including bodily illusions 4. Odd thinking and speech 5. Suspiciousness or paranoid ideation 6. Inappropriate or constricted affect 7. Behavior or appearance that is odd, eccentric, or peculiar 8. Lack of close friends 9. Excessive social anxiety **Management:** Psychotherapy; consider low-dose antipsychotics if significant perceptual disturbances present **Discussion:** Characterized by ideas of reference (over-reading significance in everyday events); magical thinking (belief that thoughts or ideas can influence events in the world, superstition, clairvoyance, etc.); odd or eccentric behaviors, beliefs, and appearance; suspiciousness or paranoia; lack of close relationships; social anxiety; metaphorical or idiosyncratic (using normal words or phrases in unusual ways) speech. Patients may have perceptual disturbances; however, overt hallucinations or persistent delusions are not present.
Antisocial Personality Disorder	**Hx:** A 24-year-old man presents to urgent care following a physical encounter with a neighbor which resulted in his neighbor requiring urgent hospitalization. He states that the neighbor "looked at [him] too many times" and "deserves what he got." This is his third time he has presented after a fight. When he was 15, he spent the night in jail after assaulting a peer, which he happily discusses. **Diagnostics:** Clinical diagnosis characterized by disregard for others, violations of the rights of others, and at least three of the following: 1. Failure to conform to legal norms 2. Deceitfulness or manipulating others 3. Impulsivity 4. Irritability and recklessness, physical fights 5. Reckless disregard for safety of others 6. Irresponsibility or inconsistent work behavior 7. Lack of remorse **Management:** Psychotherapy (generally ineffective); consider pharmacotherapy to treat underlying anxiety or depression **Discussion:** Characterized by illegal activity, deceit and manipulation of others, impulsivity, recklessness, irritability, disregard for the safety and rights of others, irresponsibility, and lack of remorse for actions. It is only diagnosed in adults but requires evidence of conduct disorder during adolescence. For the diagnosis, patients must be at least 18 years old (if younger, consider conduct disorder).
Borderline Personality Disorder	**Hx:** A 24-year-old woman calls her psychiatrist for a telehealth visit. She states that she got into another fight with her partner and threatens to cut her own wrists. She starts crying, saying "no one ever likes me except you—you are such a good doctor!" **Diagnostics:** Clinical diagnosis characterized by unstable interpersonal relationships, unstable sense of self, and at least five of the following: 1. Frantic efforts to avoid real or imagined abandonment 2. Pattern of unstable or intense relationships 3. Unstable self-image

Personality Disorder Mini-Cases *(continued)*

Borderline Personality Disorder	4. Impulsivity—spending, sex, substances, etc. 5. Recurrent suicidal threats or self-harm 6. Marked mood reactivity 7. Chronic feelings of emptiness 8. Inappropriate or intense anger 9. Transient, stress-related paranoid ideation or dissociative symptoms **Management:** Dialectical behavioral therapy (DBT) is the treatment of choice; consider low-dose antipsychotics, SSRIs, or mood stabilizers **Discussion:** Characterized by patterns of unstable or intense relationships, extreme efforts to avoid abandonment, impulsivity, mood reactivity, splitting (viewing others and themselves as completely good or completely bad), feelings of emptiness, intense or inappropriate anger, and transient paranoia or dissociation related to stress. In part driven by their impulsivity, patients may engage in reckless and/or suicidal behaviors including self-injury. Patients commonly have a history of childhood trauma. DBT is a form of CBT, which incorporates mindfulness and emotion regulation and was developed specifically for patients with BPD.
Histrionic Personality Disorder	**Hx:** A 46-year-old woman presents for a routine exam. On exam, she is wearing revealing clothing and jumps up dramatically, yelling that the stethoscope is "too cold!" At the end of the visit, she starts tearing up and says that no doctor has ever been so attentive to her. **Diagnostics:** Clinical diagnosis characterized by attention-seeking behavior, excessively emotional behavior, inappropriate sexuality or intimacy, and at least five of the following: 1. Uncomfortable when not center of attention 2. Inappropriately sexual or provocative 3. Rapidly shifting and shallow emotions 4. Uses physical appearance to draw attention 5. Speech is excessively impressionistic (not detailed) 6. Theatrical or exaggerated emotions 7. Suggestible 8. Overestimates intimacy of relationships **Management:** Psychotherapy **Discussion:** Characterized by theatrical, exaggerated, and/or rapidly-shifting emotions and communication style; discomfort when not center of attention; inappropriate provocative or sexual behaviors; use of physical appearance for attention; and overestimation of intimacy of relationships.
Narcissistic Personality Disorder	**Hx:** A 43-year-old man is seen in clinic after making a scene in the waiting room when being asked to wait 10 minutes for his appointment. He explains that he has a "very important job" and should not have to wait at all with "regular people in the waiting room." He explains that he is constantly needed at his work and that his coworkers are jealous of his superiority. **Diagnostics:** Clinical diagnosis characterized by at least five of the following: 1. Grandiose sense of self-importance 2. Preoccupied with fantasies of unlimited success/power/intelligence 3. Believes they are special and should have only special peers 4. Requires excessive admiration 5. Sense of entitlement 6. Interpersonally exploitative 7. Lacks empathy 8. Envious of others or believes others are envious 9. Arrogant or haughty **Management:** Psychotherapy; consider antidepressants for comorbid depressive or anxiety disorders **Discussion:** Characterized by sense of entitlement, self-importance, feeling special, lack of empathy/emotional coldness, arrogance, and fantasies of unlimited success/power/intelligence. These patients may be successful, but the underlying motivation is receiving attention, praise, and recognition. They often have relationship difficulties and may be demanding when seeking medical care.

Personality Disorder Mini-Cases *(continued)*

Avoidant Personality Disorder	**Hx:** A 19-year-old girl presents to the adolescent medicine clinic. When the nurse asked about her plans for an upcoming school dance, she quickly makes an excuse as to why she was not going. She states that she is worried that her peers would not like her dress and does not want to be embarrassed. **Diagnostics:** Clinical diagnosis characterized by a desire for social contact but fear of rejection and at least four of the following: 1. Avoids occupational activities requiring interpersonal contact 2. Unwilling to get involved with people unless certain will be liked 3. Restraint in intimate relationships due to fear or shame or ridicule 4. Preoccupied with being criticized in social situations 5. Inhibited in interpersonal situations due to feelings of inadequacy 6. Views self as inept/unappealing/inferior 7. Unusually reluctant to take personal risks due to fear of embarrassment **Management:** Psychotherapy (CBT, social skills training); consider antidepressants or anxiolytics for comorbid disorders **Discussion:** Characterized by avoidance of activities requiring interpersonal contact; restraint in intimate relationships due to fear of shame, embarrassment, or judgment of others; preoccupation with criticism in social situations; inhibition in interpersonal situations; and poor self-image. Patients may have challenges interacting with peers or coworkers and may turn down opportunities for advancement.
Dependent Personality Disorder	**Hx:** A 30-year-old man presents to urgent care after falling from a ladder. He lives with his parents and states that he came in because they told him to. He recently moved in with them after a breakup with his partner. He calls his parents three times during the appointment to ask many trivial questions, including help to fill out forms in the clinic. The patient is timid and when asked about how he fell off the ladder, he asks, "will you be mad at me if I told you the truth?" **Diagnostics:** Clinical diagnosis characterized by at least five of the following: 1. Difficulty making everyday decisions without excessive reassurance 2. Needs others to assume responsibility for major areas of life 3. Difficulty expressing disagreement with others due to fear of loss of support 4. Difficulty initiating projects due to lack of confidence 5. Goes to excessive lengths to obtain support from others 6. Feels uncomfortable or helpless when alone 7. Urgently seeks another relationship as a source of care when a close relationship ends 8. Unrealistically preoccupied with fears of being left to take care of themselves **Management:** Psychotherapy **Discussion:** Characterized by difficulty making daily decisions without reassurance, need for others to assume responsibility for major areas of life, feeling uncomfortable or helpless when alone, and seeking a new relationship as source for care when another close relationship ends. Patients are usually submissive, fear separation, and may have mood or anxiety symptoms in response to changes in relationships due to feelings of inadequacy.
Obsessive Compulsive Personality Disorder (OCPD)	**Hx:** A 24-year-old medical student presents for a routine clinic visit. She has been having insomnia after staying up all night trying to perfect her physical exam maneuvers for an upcoming exam. She has been disciplined for turning multiple assignments in late because she needs things to be perfect before it is turned in. She complains about a recent clinical evaluation which said she should work on her ability to delegate tasks to other members of the team. **Diagnostics:** Clinical diagnosis characterized by at least four of the following: 1. Preoccupation with details/rules/order to the extent that the major point of the activity is lost 2. Perfectionism that interferes with task completion 3. Excessive devotion to work at the expense of leisure activities and relationships 4. Over-conscientiousness or inflexibility in matters of morality, ethics, or values 5. Inability to discard worthless objects 6. Reluctance to delegate tasks

Personality Disorder Mini-Cases *(continued)*

Obsessive Compulsive Personality Disorder (OCPD)	7. Miserly spending attitude 8. Rigidness and stubbornness **Management:** Psychotherapy **Discussion:** Characterized by preoccupation with rules/details to the point that the point of the activity is lost, perfectionism that interferes with task completion, and excessive devotion to work. Patients are often controlling and excessively preoccupied with order, schedules, rules, and details. They may have difficulty working with others who fail to reach their standards of perfection. Compared to OCD, behaviors are pervasive (i.e., not related to specific obsessions/compulsions) and may not cause distress to the patient (i.e., ego-syntonic).

PSYCHOPHARMACOLOGIC EMERGENCIES

Psychiatric medications can have potentially dangerous side effects when taken incorrectly, in excess, or due to drug-drug interactions. This may result in hemodynamic instability and can be life-threatening. The first step in caring for these patients is assessing and supporting vital signs, including providing basic resuscitation. After the patient is stable, the offending medication(s) should be identified through careful history-taking, medication reconciliation, and physical exam. The offending medication(s) should be immediately discontinued and further intervention via antidote, other stabilizing medication, or procedures (e.g., gastric lavage, endoscopy) should be performed if indicated. After the patient is medically stable, consider whether further psychiatric hospitalization is warranted to ensure patient safety. It is essential to evaluate whether continuing the medication(s) is appropriate and safe, especially if intentional overdose is a risk.

CASE 31 | Neuroleptic Malignant Syndrome (NMS)

A 40-year-old man on the inpatient psychiatry floor admitted for acute psychosis is brought to the attention of the resident on duty after nursing staff noted abnormal vital signs this morning. He appears confused, and on physical exam is diaphoretic with generalized, lead-pipe muscle rigidity. His vital signs are significant for a temperature of 104°F, pulse of 112/min, respirations of 32/min, and blood pressure of 150/96 mmHg. On presentation to the ED 2 days ago, he was given several doses of IM haloperidol after attempting to assault nursing staff.

Conditions with Similar Presentations	**Malignant hyperthermia:** Also presents with rigidity and myoglobinuria, but malignant hyperthermia occurs with use of volatile anesthetics (e.g., fluranes, halothane) or succinylcholine rather than after administration of antipsychotics. Symptoms most often develop during induction of anesthesia or during maintenance. Both NMS and malignant hyperthermia will present with metabolic acidosis, but malignant hyperthermia will have significant hypercarbia unlike NMS.
	Serotonin syndrome: Also presents with hyperthermia, hypertension, diaphoresis, and confusion but has GI complaints of nausea, vomiting, and diarrhea. Unlike the serotonin syndrome, NMS has the characteristic lead-pipe rigidity and significantly elevated creatine kinase. Serotonin syndrome is instead characterized by clonus, hyperreflexia, and tremor. NMS typically occurs from antipsychotics, while serotonin syndrome occurs from a number of serotonergic drugs, particularly in combination. Serotonin syndrome often has a more rapid onset and offset compared to NMS.
	Malignant catatonia: Shares the same signs and symptoms of hyperthermia and rigidity, but malignant catatonia usually has a prodrome of weeks of psychosis and agitation. It also has more motor phenomena, such as dystonia, waxy flexibility, and repetitive movements.
Initial Diagnostic Tests	• Clinical Diagnosis • Check CK • Consider CBC, CMP
Next Steps in Management	• Discontinue causative agent (in this case, haloperidol) • Transfer to the ICU for supportive measures (IV fluids) • Sedation with benzodiazepines and muscle relaxation with dantrolene can be added if needed.
Discussion	NMS is a rare, potentially life-threatening condition that is associated with the use of medications including antipsychotics and antiemetics. It is more common with high-potency, first-generation antipsychotics (e.g., haloperidol), but can be seen with any antipsychotic medication. The syndrome is characterized by changes in mental status with reduced or fluctuating level of consciousness (often one of the earliest signs), generalized lead-pipe rigidity, rhabdomyolysis and myoglobinuria, hyperthermia, and autonomic dysfunction (tachycardia, elevated or labile blood pressure, and tachypnea).

CASE 31 | Neuroleptic Malignant Syndrome (NMS) *(continued)*

Discussion	**Diagnostics:**
	• Clinical diagnosis
	• CK is elevated to >1000 international units/L
	• CBC shows leukocytosis
	• CMP (ALT and AST are elevated, and metabolic acidosis)
	• Although not indicated, if performed, MRI, CT, and CSF analysis are normal.
	Management:
	• The offending medication should be discontinued immediately Typically requires ICU-level care
	• IV hydration and cooling measures to prevent rhabdomyolysis and AKI
	• If the patient does not show improvement, additional treatment may include benzodiazepines and dantrolene followed by the addition of bromocriptine or amantadine in more severe cases.
	• After symptoms resolve, patients may cautiously be restarted on antipsychotics if clinically indicated, although they have a higher risk of developing NMS again.

CASE 32 | Serotonin Syndrome

A 48-year-old woman with diabetes, MDD, and motion sickness presents to the ED with nausea and vomiting. She took her daily sertraline for her MDD and duloxetine for her diabetic nerve pain this morning. She adds that she has been taking several doses of her as-needed ondansetron consistently for the past week because she was on a weeklong road trip touring colleges with her daughter. Typically, ondansetron helps with her motion sickness and nausea, however, this morning her nausea was worse and she vomited several times. On physical exam, she is febrile to 38.3°C, pulse is 115/min, and blood pressure is 164/96 mmHg. She is diaphoretic, agitated, her pupils are dilated, and she has myoclonus and her reflexes are 4+ in all four extremities with bilateral Babinski signs

Conditions with Similar Presentations	Consider **NMS or malignant hyperthermia** as above.
Initial Diagnostic Tests	• Clinical Diagnosis • CK is elevated • CBC shows leukocytosis, and, if severe, BMP shows an anion gap acidosis from (lactic acidosis +/− AKI). • Urinalysis may show myoglobinuria (+ blood but no RBCs)
Next Steps in Management	• Stop all serotonergic agents and start IV fluids • Benzodiazepines for sedation. • Consider cyproheptadine.
Discussion	Serotonin syndrome is associated with increased serotoninergic activity in the CNS caused either by an interaction between multiple serotonergic drugs (in this case, a combination of the SSRI sertraline, the SNRI duloxetine, and the anti-emetic ondansetron, the latter being a 5-HT$_3$ receptor antagonist) or intentional overdose of a serotonergic medication. Potential medications with serotonergic effects include SSRIs, SNRIs, TCAs, MAOIs, ondansetron, dextromethorphan, linezolid, and the drug MDMA (ecstasy). Patients on SSRIs who are being switched to a different serotonergic medication should undergo a 2-week washout period (longer for fluoxetine, given its longer half-life). The syndrome is characterized by a triad of:
	1. Altered mental status—confusion, restlessness, agitation, delirium
	2. Autonomic dysfunction—hyperthermia, vomiting, diarrhea, diaphoresis, hypertension, tachycardia
	3. Neuromuscular hyperactivity (especially in lower extremities)—myoclonus, hyperreflexia, tremor, bilateral Babinski sign, rigidity
	Management:
	• All serotonergic agents should be discontinued, and supportive measures, including IV hydration and cooling measures, initiated to normalize vital signs.
	• Benzodiazepines may be used for sedation.
	• If refractory to these measures, consider the serotonin antagonist cyproheptadine.
	• If the patient was previously stable on a psychiatric regimen that included serotonergic drugs, a single agent may be restarted cautiously.
	• A risk-benefit analysis should be done by the provider when restarting or starting a combination of serotonergic drugs.

CASE 33 | Lithium Toxicity

A 60-year-old woman with hypertension and past psychiatric history of bipolar I disorder presents with confusion and lethargy. Her bipolar disorder has been well controlled with lithium. On exam, she is somnolent but arousable. There is a bin next to her containing a significant volume of non-bilious vomitus. Vital signs reveal orthostatic hypotension. She was recently started on hydrochlorothiazide for newly diagnosed hypertension, and she has otherwise been taking her psychiatric medications as prescribed. On exam, she has bilateral hand tremors and ataxia.

Conditions with Similar Presentations	If patients are also on other medications for mental health (SSRIs, antipsychotics) early stages of **serotonin syndrome and/or malignant neuroleptic syndrome** should be considered. However, lithium toxicity does not produce hyperthermia or muscle rigidity.
Initial Diagnostic Tests	• Clinical diagnoisis confirmed with elevated serum lithium level • Check BMP, urinalysis, and toxicology screen to assess baseline and rule out other causes
Next Steps in Management	• Treat with IV fluids and, if necessary, hemodialysis to remove lithium.
Discussion	Lithium is used as a treatment for various psychiatric conditions, most notably for acute mania and maintenance therapy in bipolar disorder. It has a narrow therapeutic index, with toxicity occurring at levels >1.5 mEq/L. Lithium is excreted almost entirely by the kidneys, so volume depletion, renal impairment, and drugs that alter renal function (e.g., NSAIDs, ACE inhibitors, or thiazide diuretics) can cause an increase in lithium reabsorption, resulting in toxicity. Toxicity can be divided into acute and chronic adverse effects. In acute toxicity, patients present with GI disturbances including nausea, vomiting, and diarrhea. Over time, lithium toxicity can lead to development of neurologic symptoms including confusion, lethargy, ataxia, coarse tremors/fasciculations, hyperreflexia, or seizures.

CASE 34 | Tricyclic Antidepressant (TCA) Toxicity

A 24-year-old woman with MDD and borderline personality disorder is found unresponsive at home by her sister with an empty pill bottle next to her. En route to the hospital, she has a generalized tonic-clonic seizure. Upon arrival to the ED, her temperature is 38.8°C (102°F), pulse is 110/minute, respirations are 7/min, and her blood pressure is 78/46 mmHg. Her skin is warm and flushed, mucus membranes are dry, and pupils are dilated. ECG shows prolonged QRS at 110 msec. Her sister brought the empty pill bottle of amitriptyline which was refilled two days ago.

Conditions with Similar Presentations	**Other intoxications:** Decreased mental status can be seen after ingestion of benzodiazepines, ethanol, opioids, anti-epileptic drugs, or from poisoning with carbon monoxide or cyanide. Seizures can be induced by sympathomimetic drugs (cocaine, amphetamines). Anticholinergic manifestations (dry mouth, flushing, dilated pupils) can occur with antihistamines, antiarrhythmics (procainamide, quinidine), and antipsychotics (notably clozapine).
Initial Diagnostic Tests	• Clinical diagnosis • Check CBC, BMP, ECG, urine and blood toxicology tests and alcohol level to rule out other causes and establish a baseline
Next Steps in Management	• Treat with sodium bicarbonate to prevent arrhythmias. • IV fluids for hypotension • Benzodiazepines for seizure prevention.
Discussion	TCAs are rarely used in the treatment of depression, anxiety, and OCD, but are used to treat migraines and neuropathic pain. TCAs work by inhibition of reuptake of both norepinephrine and serotonin but are not used as first- or second-line agents due to high rates of and potentially dangerous adverse effects. Many of the side effects relate to antihistaminic, antiadrenergic, and antimuscarinic effects of these medications. Examples of TCAs include the tertiary amines amitriptyline, imipramine, clomipramine, and doxepin as well as their metabolites, the secondary amines including nortriptyline and desipramine. TCA toxicity can acutely manifest with vital sign abnormalities such as hyperthermia, tachycardia, hypotension, and hypopnea. Central and peripheral anticholinergic effects cause dilated pupils, flushing, dry mucus membranes, urinary retention, and ileus. Patients may also exhibit CNS effects, including decreased level of consciousness, agitation, tremors, ataxia, seizures, and coma. Other complications include prolonged QRS and ventricular arrhythmias. An overdose of TCAs can be lethal.

17
Neurology

Lead Authors: Yasaman Kianirad, MD; Jared Davis, MD; Joseph R. Geraghty, MD, PhD
Contributors: Philip B. Ostrov, MD; Ethan Harris, MD; Helena Xeros, MD; Zachary Taub, MD

INTRODUCTION

The clinical application of neuroscience is relevant to a wide array of medical specialties. This chapter will focus on clinical neurology and related disciplines such as neurological surgery. We will also highlight important areas of overlap with the practice of psychiatry, primary care, ophthalmology, otolaryngology, orthopedics, and other medical disciplines discussed in further detail in other chapters.

When approaching a neurologic patient or USMLE-style vignette, it is important to ask yourself several questions:

Where? One of the most important aspects of neurology is the **localization** of lesions throughout the nervous system. This can be broadly divided into the central nervous system (CNS) and peripheral nervous system (PNS). The CNS includes the brain, spinal cord, and associated structures, while the PNS refers to peripheral nerves (including cranial nerves), the neuromuscular junction (NMJ), the autonomic nervous system, and specialized areas of neurons within other organ systems such as the enteric nervous system. Depending on the location of injury, different symptoms will manifest. For example, damage to upper motor neurons (UMN) in the lateral corticospinal tract (i.e., part of the CNS) descending within the spinal cord will result in classic UMN symptoms of spastic paralysis, hypertonicity, hyperreflexia, and the development of pathologic reflexes such as the Babinski or Hoffman sign. In contrast, a PNS lesion to lower motor neurons (LMNs) within spinal or peripheral nerves will result in classic LMN symptoms of flaccid paralysis, hypotonicity, hyporeflexia, fasciculations, and more pronounced atrophy. Recognizing these different patterns will aid you in arriving at the correct diagnosis.

When? A second, equally important component to consider when obtaining the history and performing the physical examination in a patient with neurologic disease is the **time course**. Various neurologic conditions such as seizures, stroke, trauma, and some infections present in the hyperacute or acute setting, often with relatively sudden onset. Timely diagnosis and treatment are critical for these patients. Other patients have a much more gradual, prolonged disease course; for example those suffering from chronic neurodegenerative diseases such as Parkinson's or Alzheimer's disease. The accompanying figure highlights various neurologic diseases based on time course.

Hyperacute (Over seconds to minutes)	Acute (Over hours to days)	Subacute (Over weeks to months)	Chronic (Over years)
Vascular Ischemic stroke Intracerebral hemorrhage Subarachnoid hemorrhage	Venous sinus thrombosis	Chronic subdural hematoma Vascular malformation	
Seizure	**Infection** Bacterial meningitis Cerebral or epidural abscess Viral meningitis Viral encephalitis	Fungal meningitis Tuberculous meningitis Tuberculosis of the spine Progressive multifocal leukoencephalopathy	HTLV-1 HIV/AIDS
Migraine			
		Syphilis	
Trauma	**Inflammatory/Demyelinating** Guillain-Barré Syndrome Acute disseminated encephalomyelitis Flare of multiple sclerosis Transverse myelitis Optic neuritis	CIDP Paraneoplastic syndromes	Primary/secondary progressive multiple sclerosis
		Neoplasm Malignant	Benign
			Neurodegenerative Dementia Parkinson's disease
Metabolic Hypoglycemia Hyperglycemia Acute intermittent porphyria	Uremic encephalopathy Hepatic encephalopathy	Vitamin B12 deficiency	
Medications/drugs/toxins Acute intoxication (e.g., alcohol, cocaine) Acute withdrawal (e.g., alcohol, benzodiazepines) Acute dystonic reaction (e.g., metoclopramide)	Antibiotic-induced encephalopathy	Drug-induced neuropathy Tardive dyskinesia Drug-induced parkinsonism	

Schematic showing differential diagnosis of neurologic disease by time course. (Reproduced with permission from Berkowitz AL. Clinical Neurology and Neuroanatomy: A Localization-Based Approach. 2nd ed. New York: McGraw Hill; 2022.)

Who? Several neurological conditions present in fairly **typical patient populations**, and remembering this can help you identify which conditions should appear at the top of your differential diagnosis. In a 20- to 40-year-old woman presenting with new-onset focal neurologic deficits, multiple sclerosis (MS) may be high on your differential. In an older patient with cardiovascular risk factors presenting with new-onset focal neurologic deficits, ischemic or hemorrhagic stroke is more likely. In elderly patients who present with gradual-onset memory loss, consider neurodegenerative diseases such as Alzheimer's disease or vascular dementia.

How? Finally, it is helpful to consider the **underlying pathophysiology** that gives rise to a particular neurological condition. In many cases, understanding the pathophysiology may also aid in identifying the appropriate diagnostics and management. For example, knowledge that MS is an autoimmune condition of the CNS can help explain why cerebrospinal fluid labs positive for IgG or oligoclonal bands can aid in the diagnosis. Further, knowledge that myasthenia gravis involves auto-antibodies against the nicotinic acetylcholine receptor in the NMJ helps explain why repeated muscle contraction leads to worsening of symptoms as the decreased number of acetylcholine receptors get saturated.

HEADACHE

In approaching a patient with a headache, identifying key patterns and clinical features will help categorize headaches into primary or secondary causes.

Primary headaches

- Are common and occur when the head pain is the main problem and not a symptom of an underlying condition
- Pain can be severe, but are not typically not life-threatening.
  - As the brain parenchyma itself lacks pain receptors, the pain is typically related to surrounding pain-sensitive structures including dura, nerves, blood vessels, and muscles.

Secondary headaches

- Caused by underlying conditions that may occur acutely and be life-threatening emergencies
- Causes include space-occupying lesions (e.g., tumors, hematomas, hydrocephalus), severe acute hypertension, traumatic injury, and infection (e.g., meningitis, encephalitis).
  - Space-occupying lesions cause increased intracranial pressure (ICP), which can result in papilledema, nausea and vomiting, impaired consciousness, and Cushing triad (widened pulse pressure, bradycardia, and irregular respirations).

Differential Diagnosis for Primary vs. Secondary Headaches

Primary Headache	Secondary Headache				
• Migraine with or without aura • Tension-type headache • Trigeminal autonomic cephalalgias (cluster headache)	*Infections* • Meningitis • Encephalitis • Brain abscess	*Vascular* • Intracranial bleeding (subarachnoid hemorrhage, epidural/subdural hematoma) • Vascular malformation (e.g., arteriovenous malformation, cavernoma) • Vasculitis (giant cell arteritis, polyarteritis nodosa) • Cerebral venous sinus thrombosis • Severe acute hypertension (Hypertensive emergency)	*Space-occupying lesions* • Tumor • Hydrocephalus	*Referred pain* • Facial pain (e.g., trigeminal neuralgia) • Eyes glaucoma, optic neuritis) • Ears • Nose • Sinuses (rhinosinusitis) • Oral cavity (including teeth) • Neck (e.g., nasopharyngeal carcinoma)	*Other* • Dehydration • Medication-overuse headache (e.g., acetaminophen) • Trauma (contusion, concussion) • Idiopathic intracranial hypertension (pseudotumor cerebri) • Substance use or withdrawal (e.g., caffeine withdrawal) • Cerebral hypoxia (e.g., carbon monoxide poisoning) • Hypercapnia • Hypoglycemia • Chiari malformations • Obstructive sleep apnea (OSA) • Generalized anxiety disorder (GAD) • Pheochromocytoma • Pituitary apoplexy

History

Assess location, frequency, quality, triggers, when the patient experiences headaches (e.g., some headaches occur more in the morning and may be related to increased ICP), and if they are positional in nature, such as worsening when lying flat and improved when upright (also related to ICP), and it is critical to rule out any red flags that may require further workup for potentially life-threatening causes.

Red Flag Signs and Symptoms for Secondary Headache: 2SNOOP4

Mnemonic	Red Flag	Differential Diagnosis
S	Systemic symptoms—fever, weight loss, rash, hypertension	Meningitis, encephalitis, vasculitis, pheochromocytoma
S	Secondary risk factors—cancer, chemotherapy, HIV, or other immunocompromised status, pregnancy	Brain tumor, meningitis, encephalitis, opportunistic infections, eclampsia
N	Neurological deficits—loss of consciousness, seizures, weakness, sensory changes	Ischemic or hemorrhagic stroke, brain tumor, vascular malformation, abscess
O	Onset (sudden)—"Thunderclap" headache beginning abruptly (seconds or minutes)	Subarachnoid hemorrhage, vascular malformation, pituitary apoplexy
O	Patients >50 years of age	Giant cell arteritis, brain tumor
P	Prior headaches—different from prior headaches or a change in the pattern of the headache (e.g., increasing frequency or severity)	Medication-overuse headache, brain tumor, subdural hematoma
P	Papilledema—sign of elevated ICP	Brain tumor, hematoma, hydrocephalus, idiopathic intracranial hypertension, meningitis
P	Precipitated by Valsalva maneuver (coughing, sexual activity, exercise).	Brain tumor, hematoma, hydrocephalus, idiopathic intracranial hypertension, meningitis, Chiari malformation, posterior fossa malformations
P	Postural—worse with certain positions such as lying down (elevated ICP) or standing up (low ICP), or bending over (sphenoid sinusitis)	Brain tumor, hematoma, hydrocephalus, idiopathic intracranial hypertension, meningitis, sphenoid sinusitis

CASE 1 | Migraine with Aura

A 19-year-old woman with no significant past medical history presents to clinic for evaluation of recurring headaches. For the past few years, she has had multiple episodes of severe, pulsating headaches that typically go away after several hours. The headaches are often preceded by some distortions in her vision that she describes as "flickering colors." Her current headache has been present for the past 2 days and is making it difficult for her to study for her final exams. It is accompanied by nausea and photophobia, and two doses of ibuprofen have provided only minimal relief. Her only other medication is a combined oral contraceptive pill which she takes daily. Her vital signs are within normal limits. Fundoscopic and neurologic exams are unremarkable.

Conditions with Similar Presentations	**Cluster headache:** Sharp, severe, unilateral orbital, supraorbital, and/or temporal pain lasting minutes to hours associated with ipsilateral autonomic signs (e.g., rhinorrhea, lacrimation).
	Tension-type headache: Squeezing, band-like pressure around the head usually lasting less than a day and not incapacitating.
	Medication-overuse headache (MOH): Daily headache occurring in patients with frequent use of abortive headache medications (e.g., acetaminophen, NSAIDs, triptans, opioids). Management of MOH involves slowly tapering off analgesic use.
Initial Diagnostic Tests	Clinical diagnosis
Next Steps in Management	• Acute therapy for headaches: NSAIDs (higher dose or stronger (i.e., ketorolac)), acetaminophen, or sumatriptan • Switch to non-estrogen-containing contraception, as estrogen-containing products are contraindicated in patients with migraine with an aura (see below). • Encourage lifestyle modifications (e.g., sleep hygiene, avoiding dehydration and triggers) • If migraines continue, consider preventive therapy

CASE 1 | Migraine with Aura *(continued)*

Discussion	Migraines are the most common reason for patients to seek outpatient care of a headache. The underlying pathophysiology involves activation of the trigeminovascular system with release of vasoactive peptides involved in pain signaling, including calcitonin gene-related peptide (CGRP). Activation of the trigeminovascular system causes peripheral sensitization of neurons innervating dural blood vessels, which explains the pounding pain. Preceding cortical spreading depolarizations across brain regions are responsible for the aura. They present between 18 and 44 years of age and tend to run in families. Prior to puberty, there is similar incidence amongst males and females; however, after puberty, migraines are more common in women. **History:** • Risk factors and triggers: Genetics, changes in lifestyle, stress, sleep deprivation, dehydration, or menses can precipitate or exacerbate headaches. • Symptoms: **POUND** mnemonic: **P**ulsatile/throbbing character, **O**ne-day duration, **U**nilateral, **N**ausea, and **D**isability (unable to perform normal activities). • Approximately one-third may have an aura that precedes the migraine headache. **Auras** may be visual (most common): (e.g., visual loss or scintillating scotomas ("flickering colors")), sensory (numbness, paresthesias), motor (weakness), or auditory (sounds, hearing loss) abnormalities. Rarely may have hemiplegia. • May last several hours or as long as a few days (4–72 hours) and may have accompanying nausea, vomiting, photophobia, or phonophobia. • May improve with going into a dark room or avoiding lights and sounds **Physical Exam:** Normal; may have photophobia **Diagnostic:** Clinical diagnosis No additional tests or imaging are required unless there are concerning features for a secondary headache. **Management:** Acute therapy • First-line: NSAIDs, triptans (e.g., sumatriptan), and ergot alkaloids (dihydroergotamine) • Triptans are serotonin 5-HT$_{1B/1D}$ receptor agonists that decrease neuroinflammation and levels of CGRP • Antiemetics may also provide symptomatic relief Preventive therapy • Consider in patients who have frequent (>4/month) or long-lasting (>12 hr) headaches, headaches that interfere with daily activities, or who have not had relief with abortive therapies • Options include daily regimens of anticonvulsants (topiramate, valproic acid), tricyclic antidepressants (amitriptyline, nortriptyline), beta-blockers (propranolol), calcium channel blockers (verapamil), antidepressants, and neurotoxins (onabotulinum toxin) • Recently, monoclonal antibody medications against CGRP (fremanezumab, galcanezumab) or its receptor (erenumab) have been approved by the FDA for prophylactic therapy.
Additional Considerations	**Women with migraine with aura** are at increased risk of thrombotic events such as ischemic stroke, likely related to cyclic changes in estrogen. This risk is further increased in women taking estrogen-containing contraceptives. Therefore, this patient should be switched to a different form of contraception that does not contain estrogen. **Pediatric Considerations:** While most cases of migraine are unilateral, some can occur bilaterally, especially in children. Children may also experience autonomic symptoms including sweating, conjunctival injection, tearing, and nasal congestion/rhinorrhea.

CASE 2 | Idiopathic Intracranial Hypertension (IIH)

A 24-year-old woman with severe acne presents with daily headaches for the last 2 months. They are primarily located in the front of her head and last all day. They are worse when she wakes up, or if she sneezes or lays down for too long. Over-the-counter analgesics have not helped. The headaches are associated with occasional nausea and ringing in her ears, and she notes that her vision has gotten worse over the last few weeks. Her only medications are doxycycline and isotretinoin for her acne, and combined oral contraceptive pills (OCPs). Vital signs are within normal limits. Her BMI is 38 kg/m². Her funduscopic exam demonstrates bilateral swelling of the optic disc and an enlarging blind spot with decreased visual acuity. On testing of her extraocular muscles, there is decreased abduction bilaterally. The remainder of her exam is unremarkable.

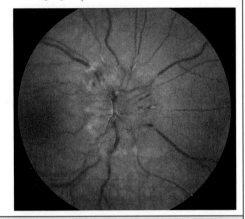

Papilledema (optic disc edema from raised intracranial pressure). This young woman developed acute papilledema, with hemorrhages and cotton-wool spots, as a rare side effect of treatment with tetracycline for acne. (Reproduced with permission from Loscalzo J, Fauci AS, Kasper DL, et al, eds. Harrison's Principles of Internal Medicine. 21st ed. New York: McGraw Hill; 2022.)

Conditions with Similar Presentations	**Space-occupying lesions:** Such as tumors can also increase ICP and cause similar fundoscopic and visual test findings; however, patients are typically older and present with additional focal neurological deficits. **Cavernous sinus thrombosis (CVST):** Occurs more commonly in prothrombotic states and causes a unilateral (rather than bilateral) abducens nerve (CN VI) palsy. Symptoms typically present more acutely, and other neurologic findings, including proptosis and additional cranial nerve palsies (i.e., CNs III, IV, and/or V), may occur.
Initial Diagnostic Tests	• Confirm diagnosis with lumbar puncture (LP) to evaluate opening pressure • Consider: Brain imaging to rule out space-occupying masses
Next Steps in Management	• Acetazolamide • Weight loss • Discontinue medications that increase risk for IIH
Discussion	Idiopathic intracranial hypertension (IIH), formerly known as pseudotumor cerebri, is a disorder characterized by increased intracranial pressure with no specific cause on neuroimaging or other evaluations. The underlying pathophysiology is largely unknown, although may involve a mismatch between the production and outflow of cerebrospinal fluid (CSF). **History:** • Risk factors: Young, obese women of reproductive age, medications (e.g., tetracyclines, OCPs, vitamin A (including isotretinoin), and the synthetic androgen danazol ["TOAD"]) • Symptoms: Headaches are generalized, worse in the morning and with Valsalva maneuvers that increase ICP. May have vision loss due to pressure on the optic nerve, and may also have pulsatile tinnitus. **Physical Exam:** • Possible elevated BMI. May have decreased visual acuity and papilledema on fundoscopic exam. • Compression of the abducens nerve bilaterally may occur, resulting in a lateral rectus muscle palsy with impaired abduction and/or esotropia (eye turned inward) **Diagnostics:** • Confirm diagnosis with LP: opening pressure (>25 cm H$_2$O). Other CSF labs are normal • Brain imaging often normal in IIH (may show an empty sella turcica sign as excess CSF disrupts the tissue). • Consider MRI of brain and orbit to rule out any space-occupying lesions that might otherwise explain elevated ICP. • Consider neuroimaging prior to LP, particularly if papilledema present, as space-occupying lesions can lead to risk of herniation during LP.

CASE 2 | Idiopathic Intracranial Hypertension (IIH) *(continued)*

Discussion	**Management:** • Patients may show temporary improvement in their symptoms from LP due to removal of some CSF. If so, repeat therapeutic LPs may continue to be of benefit. • Weight loss if increased BMI. • Acetazolamide (a carbonic anhydrase inhibitor) is first-line to acutely lower ICP—full effect may take hours to days. • If symptoms continue, can consider adding furosemide. • Medications that increase risk for IIH should be discontinued or alternatives should be sought (in this patient, consider switching her isotretinoin [vitamin A], doxycycline, and/or oral contraceptive).
Additional Considerations	**Complications:** If IIH is not controlled, it can lead to pressure on the optic nerve, resulting in permanent blindness or permanent damage to other cranial nerves such as the abducens nerve. **Surgical Considerations:** If the patient's symptoms are refractory to medical management and lifestyle modifications or vision loss are progressing, surgical intervention is indicated. Options include **optic nerve sheath fenestration** to decompress pressure on the optic nerve or placement of a **ventriculoperitoneal shunt (VPS)** to divert CSF into the peritoneal cavity, whereby it can be reabsorbed. While patients are awaiting surgery, consider serial LPs or short-term dose of corticosteroids.

CASE 3 | Aneurysmal Subarachnoid Hemorrhage (SAH)

A 38-year-old woman with hypertension is brought to the emergency department (ED) for evaluation of loss of consciousness after a severe headache. Patient's partner notes that the headache began "out of nowhere" while they were cleaning the house, and the patient stated it was the worst headache of her life. Her partner called 911 after the patient briefly lost consciousness and vomited. One day prior, she had mentioned a minor headache, but this resolved with NSAIDs. Her mother had polycystic kidney disease and died suddenly 15 years ago. The patient does not smoke, drink alcohol, or use other substances. On exam, her vital signs are temperature 37.9°C, BP 156/98 mmHg, PR 98/min, RR 18/min. The patient requires stimulation to open her eyes and briefly follows commands when aroused. Her pupils are equal, round, and reactive to light. She has bilateral papilledema.

Conditions with Similar Presentations	**Acute ischemic stroke:** Does not have headache unless there is hemorrhagic conversion. Presents with sudden-onset focal neurological deficit(s) that may include weakness or slurred speech. Patients are typically older with multiple cardiovascular risk factors. **Intracerebral hemorrhage (ICH):** Can also present with sudden-onset, severe headache, but depending on the location within brain parenchyma will also be accompanied by localizing neurological deficits. **Meningitis:** Presents with headache, neck stiffness, fever, and does not lead to sudden loss of consciousness.
Initial Diagnostic Tests	• Non-contrast head CT to demonstrate the bleeding • If CT is negative but clinical suspicion remains high, LP
Next Steps in Management	• Assess and monitor ABCs in the intensive care unit (ICU) • Optimize blood pressure and consider seizure prophylaxis • Angiography to find and treat source of SAH
Discussion	SAH is a life-threatening emergency, accounts for approximately 5% of all strokes, and has considerable morbidity and mortality. The majority of spontaneous, non-traumatic SAH cases are caused by rupture of saccular (berry) aneurysms (abnormal balloon-like dilations in cerebral arteries), most commonly at branch points in the anterior circulation of the circle of Willis (such as the anterior communicating artery). SAH is more common in women and younger adults compared to acute ischemic stroke. **History/Physical Exam:** • Risk factors include hypertension, tobacco use, family history of aneurysms, extracellular matrix disorders (e.g., Ehlers-Danlos syndrome, Marfan syndrome), autosomal dominant polycystic kidney disease (ADPKD), cocaine use. • Classically, presents suddenly as "the **worst headache of my life**" or thunderclap headache of variable location. This may be preceded by prodromal headaches due to sentinel bleeds prior to full rupture of the aneurysm. • Depending on the amount of bleed, patients may experience nausea, vomiting, focal neurologic deficits, photophobia, low-grade fever, neck stiffness (irritation of meninges from RBC products), seizures, or coma.

CASE 3 | Aneurysmal Subarachnoid Hemorrhage (SAH) *(continued)*

Discussion	**Diagnostics:**

Diagnostics:
- Urgent non-contrast head CT to evaluate for subarachnoid blood, observable by hyperintensities within CSF-containing areas such as the basal cistern (see figure) or sulci. There may also be evidence of hemorrhage extending into the ventricles (i.e., intraventricular hemorrhage).
- If CT is negative or inconclusive, LP should be performed and will show xanthrochromia (yellowish discoloration due to presence of bilirubin from breakdown of RBCs), elevated RBC, and increased opening pressure.

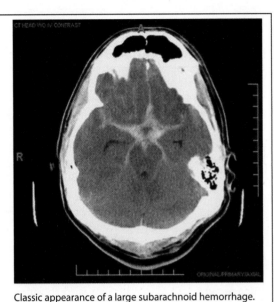

Classic appearance of a large subarachnoid hemorrhage. Notice the hemorrhage pattern fills the cerebrospinal fluid spaces at the base of the brain and around the brainstem. (Reproduced with permission from Doherty GM, ed. Current Diagnosis & Treatment: Surgery. 15th ed. New York: McGraw Hill; 2020.)

Management:
- Acutely, the greatest risk is from aneurysmal re-bleeding.
- The patient should be admitted to the ICU and monitored due to risk of elevated ICP leading to brain herniation.
- During the acute setting, optimize blood pressure (nimodipine) and consider the need for seizure prophylaxis (levetiracetam)
- Subacutely, the greatest risk related to the development of delayed cerebral vasospasm and/or ischemia classically develops 5–7 days after SAH. These result from irritative effects of RBC breakdown products and subsequent inflammation affecting blood vessels and the brain parenchyma. During this period, permissive hypertension is used to prevent delayed cerebral ischemia.
- The calcium channel blocker nimodipine is the only FDA-approved medication shown to be effective in helping prevent these deleterious complications of SAH.
- Source of SAH should be confirmed by angiography to identify cerebral aneurysms or other vascular malformations and treated

Additional Considerations	**Surgical Considerations:** Once aneurysmal SAH is confirmed, the priority should be securement of the aneurysm with clipping or coiling. **Microsurgical clipping** involves open surgery with craniotomy, whereby the brain is retracted, the aneurysm is visualized, and a small titanium clip is placed across the neck of the aneurysm. Alternatively, **endovascular coiling** is a less invasive approach that involves a catheter inserted through the femoral artery, passed into the lumen of the aneurysm under image guidance, and a pro-thrombotic coil is deployed to induce thrombosis of the aneurysm and seal it off.

To treat hydrocephalus in SAH, neurosurgeons can implant a temporary **external ventricular drain (EVD)** to divert CSF and decrease blood within the CSF.

Complications: Hydrocephalus is a common complication of SAH and can be caused by disrupted outflow of CSF due to RBC and platelet aggregation at the arachnoid granulations (communicating hydrocephalus) or formation of larger clots within the ventricular system in the setting of SAH with concomitant intraventricular hemorrhage (non-communicating, or obstructive hydrocephalus). CSF is produced by the choroid plexus and flows from the lateral ventricles, through the interventricular foramen of Monro into the third ventricle, enters the cerebral aqueduct of Sylvius, and drains into the fourth ventricle, whereby it can enter the spinal canal caudally, or exit via the foramina of Magendie and Luschka into the subarachnoid space surrounding the brain and spinal cord. Obstructive hydrocephalus interferes with normal CSF flow out of the ventricular system. Non-communicating hydrocephalus occurs due to overproduction of CSF (i.e., a choroid plexus papilloma) or decreased reabsorption of CSF at the level of the arachnoid granulations (i.e., in SAH or secondary to scarring from meningitis).

CASE 4 | Chiari I Malformation with Syringomyelia

An 18-year-old man with mild scoliosis presents for a routine physical prior to attending college. On review of systems, he notes increasing headaches over the past few years, which he initially ignored but now are accompanied by occasional dizziness. His headache is dull, rated 5/10, mostly located over his occipital region, and sometimes involves his neck as well. Physical activity seems to worsen his symptoms, and when laughing or coughing, he sometimes feels dizzy and loses his balance. The headaches last for 5–10 days now. He has no history of trauma and reports no nausea or vomiting. Over-the-counter analgesics have provided no relief. His vital signs are unremarkable. On physical exam, he has nystagmus in multiple directions and has decreased sensation to temperature and pinprick in both upper extremities and upper back. His upper extremity strength is 4/5 bilaterally with 1+ triceps and brachioradialis reflexes. Neurologic examination of his lower extremities is normal.

Conditions with Similar Presentations	**Multiple sclerosis (MS):** Patients with MS can have multiple neurologic deficits, but usually separated in space and time. It affects women more than men in a 2:1 ratio, usually in the 25- to 45-year-old age range. Imaging reveals diagnostic plaques on MRI. **Migraine:** Headache uncommonly can be located in the occipital region, but is described as pounding/throbbing and lasts <72 hours. If with an aura, there may be extremity symptoms but they are usual "positive" phenomena (tingling, warmth) instead of "negative" phenomena as seen in this case.
Initial Diagnostic Tests	MRI brain and spine
Next Steps in Management	• Symptomatic treatment for headache • Surgical intervention for other symptoms if not tolerable
Discussion	Chiari malformations are a group of congenital disorders caused by abnormal development of the cerebellum within the posterior fossa. Chiari I malformation is the most common subtype and involves protrusion of the cerebellar tonsils 5–10 mm through the foramen magnum and into the spinal canal without herniation of other cerebellar structures. Most are asymptomatic and are discovered incidentally on imaging. If patients develop symptoms, these typically present in adolescence or young adulthood with paroxysmal or dull occipital headache and/or neck pain. Headache may also be associated with dizziness, cerebellar dysfunction (nystagmus, ataxia), cranial nerve neuropathy, and/or brainstem compression. Symptoms worsen with physical activity or Valsalva maneuvers (straining, laughing, coughing, sneezing) due to increased intracranial pressure exerted on the cerebellar tonsils. Up to one-third of patients also have **syringomyelia**, characterized by the formation of a cyst-like syrinx within the spinal canal that gradually expands, leading to disruption of nearby structures such as the spinothalamic tract crossing in the anterior white commissure (diminished pain and temperature sensation in a "cape-like" distribution, as seen in this patient) or LMNs in the ventral horn (LMN signs including weakness, hypotonicity, hyporeflexia). Congenital syringomyelia associated with Chiari I malformation is most commonly found in the cervical spine. 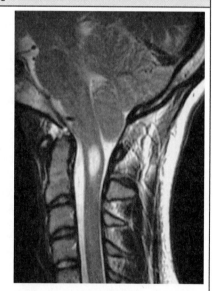 Chiari-type type I malformation and developmental syringomyelia. T2-weighted MRI of the low-lying cerebellar tonsils below the foramen magnum and behind the upper cervical cord and the syrinx cavity in the upper cord. (Reproduced with permission from Ropper AH, Samuels MA, Klein JP, et al, eds. Adams and Victor's Principles of Neurology. 11th ed. New York: McGraw Hill; 2019.) **History:** If symptomatic, onset in young adulthood, double vision, "dizziness" (ataxia), hoarseness, and dysarthria (cranial nerve injury), occipital/nuchal headache, upper extremity weakness, and loss of sensation. **Physical Exam:** Nystagmus, gait ataxia, action tremor of upper extremities. Arm reflexes decreased due to LMN compression and leg reflexes increased due to UMN compression. Decreased pain and temperature sensation in upper extremities.

CASE 4 | Chiari I Malformation with Syringomyelia *(continued)*

Discussion	**Diagnostics:** MRI is diagnostic • MRI brain and spine (both cervical and thoracic spine) to image the low-lying cerebellar tonsils extending below the level of the foramen magnum and into the vertebral canal • Up to one-third of patients will also have syringomyelia, most commonly involving the cervical spine (see figure). **Management:** Conservative treatment is usually preferred, although patients with progressive neurological symptoms should be referred to neurosurgery to be considered for decompression.
Additional Considerations	**Pediatric Considerations: Chiari II malformation** is much more severe and presents much earlier, during infancy or early childhood, due to downward herniation of both the cerebellar tonsils and vermis. It may also be detected prenatally with imaging. Herniation of these structures can result in compression of the brainstem (dysphagia, weakness, stridor, respiratory compromise) and the cerebral aqueduct (obstructive hydrocephalus). Chiari II malformations are almost always associated with lumbosacral or thoracic **myelomeningocele** caused by incomplete closure of the neural tube during neurodevelopment.

Mini-Cases

Cluster Headache	**Hx:** Severe sharp, piercing, unilateral headache; retro-orbital pain; occurs in clusters with periods of remission in between. More common in men and patients who smoke. Unlike migraine, patients tend to stay active during pain (i.e., pacing around room). **PE:** Autonomic symptoms including ipsilateral conjunctival injection, Horner syndrome (miosis, ptosis, anhidrosis), rhinorrhea, lacrimation. Neurologic and ophthalmologic exams are otherwise normal. **Diagnostics:** Clinical diagnosis **Management:** • 100% oxygen can confirm diagnosis and be used for acute therapy • Additional acute therapy includes triptans (e.g., sumatriptan) • Patient should be advised to quit smoking • Consider preventive therapy with verapamil **Discussion:** Cluster headache is a primary headache and part of a range of conditions termed trigeminal autonomic cephalalgias (TACs) whereby head pain is accompanied by autonomic symptoms. Cluster headaches are characterized by severe, unilateral, periorbital headache occurring in clusters with several episodes each day for 6–12 weeks followed by a period of remission (up to 12 months or longer). Individual headaches typically last 30 minutes to 3 hours.
Tension-Type Headache	**Hx:** Mild to moderate dull, squeezing, or pressure-like pain, usually bilateral ("band-like"), and does not impair functioning (unlike migraine and cluster). More common in women 30–40 years old. Often related to increased stress and may occur more often at the end of the day. Can be episodic (usually lasts <1 day but can last up to 1 week) or chronic (continuous, waxes and wanes throughout day). **PE:** Lacks autonomic symptoms but may have head, neck, or shoulder tenderness due to muscle tension. Otherwise, exam is normal. **Diagnostics:** Clinical diagnosis. **Management:** • Lifestyle modifications including proper sleep hygiene, exercise, meditation, proper posture. • First-line acute therapy includes NSAIDs or acetaminophen (± caffeine). • If frequent and/or disabling, can consider prophylaxis with tricyclic antidepressants (TCAs) such as amitriptyline or nortriptyline. • Cognitive behavioral therapy (CBT) may also be helpful for stress-reduction techniques. **Discussion:** Tension headache is the most common form of primary headache. It is often precipitated by stress, sleep deprivation, dehydration, hunger, over-exertion, or caffeine withdrawal. Headache classically starts in afternoon, especially after long or stressful day. Pain often occurs in temporal or occipital regions without accompanying nausea or visual symptoms.

Mini-Cases *(continued)*

Intracerebral Hemorrhage (ICH)	**Hx:** Sudden onset of a neurologic deficit and headache due to increased intracranial pressure pushing on sensory fibers of the meninges. Elevated ICP may also lead to nausea, vomiting, blurry vision, altered mental status, and possibly seizures. Usually have a history of hypertension.

PE: Variable depending on size and location of bleed, but patient may be lethargic or obtunded, may have focal weakness or deficits related to location of bleed, upper motor neuron signs (e.g., hyperreflexia, Babinski, Hoffman), and papilledema. If brain herniation occurs, patient may have decerebrate posturing. May have Cushing triad if severe.

Diagnostics:
- Urgent non-contrast head CT shows hyperdense lesion within brain parenchyma (see figure).
- Defer LP due to risk of herniation in setting of elevated ICP due to a mass lesion (in this case, the hematoma).

Management:
- Assess and monitor ABCs with low threshold for intubation and ventilation.
- Control BP with IV antihypertensives such as nicardipine or labetalol (goal systolic 140–160 mmHg).
- Reverse any anticoagulation if patient is on heparin or warfarin.
- Admit to ICU and consult neurosurgery for further management of ICP and potential surgical intervention.
- In the meantime, temporary measures to lower ICP can be used including elevation of the head of the bed, hyperventilation, and osmotic therapy (e.g., hypertonic saline, mannitol).

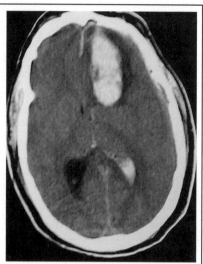

A non-contrast head CT demonstrating a large frontal intracerebral hemorrhage. Blood is also noted in the posterior horn of the left lateral ventricle. (Reproduced with permission from Stone CK, Humphries RL, eds. Current Diagnosis & Treatment: Emergency Medicine. 8th ed. New York: McGraw Hill; 2017.)

Discussion: ICH is the most common form of hemorrhagic stroke, accounting for 10–15% of all strokes, and is associated with high morbidity and mortality. Patients are typically more acutely ill compared to patients with acute ischemic stroke, and degree of severity is based on hemorrhage size, location, etiology, and underlying comorbidities. Patients may present with a range of neurological deficits depending on the location of the intraparenchymal bleed but will also show signs of elevated ICP (headache, nausea, vomiting, papilledema, and Cushing triad of increased pulse pressure, bradycardia, and irregular respirations). Common etiologies of ICH include poorly controlled hypertension (including hypertensive urgency or emergency), cerebral amyloid angiopathy, or vascular malformations.

Arteriovenous malformations (AVMs) are abnormal, direct anastomoses between arteries and veins without a capillary bed in between. This high-pressure system can promote spontaneous bleeding. Most are congenital and can be seen with genetic syndromes including **hereditary hemorrhagic telangiectasia (HHT)**. Patients are typically younger adults (<40 years old) who present with recurrent headache, seizure, or focal neurological deficits due to either SAH or more commonly intracerebral hemorrhage (ICH).

Surgical Considerations: Patients with ICH and concomitant obstructive hydrocephalus may undergo placement of an EVD for CSF diversion. Surgical hematoma decompression is indicated in severe cases, although decision to perform depends on the size, location, time since onset, clinical status of the patient, and risk of herniation. In general, decompression is performed more often for cerebellar hemorrhage compared to supratentorial hemorrhage, especially if the patient has a large bleed (>3 cm) with neurologic or radiologic evidence of brainstem compression.

TRAUMATIC BRAIN INJURY AND NEUROCRITICAL CARE

Traumatic brain injury (TBI) is a major cause of disability worldwide and can affect patients at any age. Etiologies of TBI can generally be broken down into blunt, penetrating, and blast forces, each creating vastly different patterns of injury. In addition to direct trauma to the skull and brain parenchyma, secondary injury is also common in TBI. Secondary injury includes contrecoup lesions produced opposite to the inciting force as the brain accelerates into the cranial vault, and axonal injury from the same acceleration forces causing neuronal shear stress. Also commonly accompanying severe TBI are substantial cellular catabolism, excitotoxicity, inflammation, and ischemia, all of which can worsen cerebral edema and lead to elevations in ICP and herniation.

With regard to intracranial pressure, it is helpful to consider the three main components that are inside the cranium: (1) the brain parenchyma, (2) the cerebrospinal fluid, and (3) blood. Because the skull is a rigid structure, excess volume in the brain will result in mass effect created against all of these components. Therefore, elevated ICP can compress ventricular spaces, decrease blood supply, or herniate the brain in severe cases. ICP is directly measured invasively, typically by an EVD which operates under fluid dynamics and is capable of performing CSF diversion (drainage), or by fiberoptic catheter (bolt) measurement in the white matter. Normal ICP ranges from 5–20 mmHg in adults, and when this pressure elevates, it starts to decrease the amount of blood able to perfuse the brain. Mathematically this is represented as CPP (cerebral perfusion pressure) = MAP (mean arterial pressure) – ICP, where ICP and MAP are kept in balance to maintain adequate CPP. This has formed the standard paradigm for managing elevated intracranial pressure in the neuro-ICU.

Findings in Patients with Increased Intracranial Pressure

Finding	Description
Headache	Stretching of pain receptors in meninges, often worse in the morning, when lying down (postural), or with Valsalva maneuvers (coughing, straining).
Papilledema	Optic disc swelling due to excess pressure on the optic nerve; vision may be preserved (initially) or impaired (atrophy of the optic nerve) with prolonged elevation.
Nausea/Vomiting	Increased pressure and/or decreased perfusion on chemoreceptor trigger zones within the medulla, stretching of meninges, mass effect on the diencephalon and brainstem.
Altered Mental Status	Increased pressure and/or decreased cerebral perfusion of arousal pathways (e.g., ascending reticular activating system) leads to neuronal dysfunction with loss of consciousness.
Cushing Triad	Triad of (1) systolic hypertension with increased pulse pressure, (2) bradycardia, and (3) decreased, irregular, or abnormal respiration. Pulse slows to increase diastolic filling time and increase stroke volume and raise systolic BP in an attempt to maintain cerebral perfusion in spite of increased intracranial pressure. Decreased respirations are due to pressure on the respiratory center in the upper brainstem (medulla and pons).
Other findings	Pulsatile tinnitus, cranial nerve palsies (e.g., CN III, IV, and VI commonly), bulging fontanelles (infants), diffuse hypertonia, loss of conjugate gaze.

When approaching a patient with a TBI (or any other brain injury), it is first important to assess level of consciousness, gauged by eye opening, whether spontaneous, requiring stimulation, or not occurring in a comatose state. Orientation should be assessed, if feasible, to person, place, and time. This may be possible in intubated and severely injured patients, often via yes or no questions. Patients with neurologic injury and altered consciousness may be described as confused, lethargic/drowsy, obtunded (aroused by non-painful stimuli), stuporous (aroused only with repeated, painful stimulation), or comatose (no motor response, although may have reflexes and abnormal posturing). However, there is no uniform or standardized terminology, and it is best to be descriptive about altered mental status (e.g., "when asking her to wake up, she opens her eyes but drifts and becomes unconscious in a minute").

A common objective scale used to assess patients' level of consciousness is the Glasgow Coma Scale (GCS), which assesses eye opening (1–4), verbal response (1–5), and motor response (1–5) and is graded from 3–14. A lower GCS indicates a lower level of consciousness, and usually correlates with increased severity of brain injury. Patients with a score ≤8 can be characterized as having severe TBI and may be in danger of airway protection. Any patient with TBI should also be assessed for the presence of cervical spine injury (may be a fracture or ligamentous in nature) that can destabilize the cervical spine. These patients must have cervical collars placed to prevent cord injury or reduce the risk of exacerbation.

CASE 5 | Concussion

A 17-year-old man with no past medical history presents to urgent care following a head injury during football practice which occurred 1 hour ago. He was running when he was tackled by a teammate, fell to the ground, and hit his head while wearing a helmet. He did not lose consciousness, but immediately afterward, felt dizzy and disoriented, although this improved within 20 minutes after the injury. He also experienced some nausea and a headache-predominantly over the area where his head hit the ground. His vital signs are within normal limits and on exam, the patient is alert and oriented to person, place, and time. His GCS is 15, and he has no visible injuries or hematomas to his skull. The remainder of his physical exam, including a detailed neurologic exam, is unremarkable.

Conditions with Similar Presentations	**Subdural or epidural hematoma:** Consider in patients with worsening headache, nausea, or vomiting; seizures; prolonged loss of consciousness or altered mental status; or focal neurologic deficits on exam. Contusion and traumatic SAH can also present in the same manner, and depending on the location may not produce alteration of consciousness nor focal neurologic deficits.
	Exertional heat stroke: More common in hot and humid weather with prolonged exercise, but would have elevated temperature ≥40°C with CNS dysfunction, often with tachycardia, hypotension, profuse sweating, muscle cramps, and signs of dehydration.
Initial Diagnostic Tests	• Clinical diagnosis • After ensuring stabilization, if indicated, evaluate with non-contrast head CT • Consider CT cervical spine to rule out spine injury
Next Steps in Management	• Assess and address ABCs (airway, breathing, circulation) • Check for spinal injury and stabilize patient • If stable and mild, closely monitor for 24 hours for any neurologic change (may be done at home). • Further evaluation warranted if new headache, emesis, focal neurologic deficit, altered mental status, or fluid drainage from nose or ear.
Discussion	Concussion is defined as a direct blow to the head, face, or neck that causes transient impairment in neurologic function before resolving spontaneously and with no evidence of intracranial injury on exam or imaging. It is one manifestation of a mild TBI, and is associated with amnesia (may be anterograde and/or retrograde) related to the trauma. Direct blunt impact to the head rapidly rotates the brain and brainstem, which can cause axonal shearing, neuronal depolarization, decreased cerebral blood flow, and regional ischemia. There may or may not be loss of consciousness and/or seizure. The severity of the TBI is further characterized by GCS, with "severe" constituting a GCS ≤8. The reason for this distinction among direct brain injuries is the neurologic prognosis and long-term sequelae, such as epilepsy. Patients with poor GCS without overt structural pathology should have ICP monitoring and further imaging modalities. Diffuse axonal injury can cause substantial dysfunction and may not appear on CT, so MRI is the modality of choice. **History:** Risk factors include contact sports (football, boxing, ice hockey), military service (particularly blast forces), motor vehicle accidents (MVA), predisposition for falls (e.g., elderly patients), and alcohol use. Symptoms: Direct blow to the head with associated amnesia. May have brief loss of consciousness, seizure, headache, confusion, disorientation, inattention, abnormal speech, dizziness, gait abnormalities, nausea and vomiting, or emotional lability. Presence of atypical signs, such as focal neurological findings, seizure, persistent altered mentation, prolonged loss of consciousness, or depressed skull injury, should raise suspicion for a more severe form of TBI. **Physical Exam:** Usually normal and GCS >13 **Diagnostics:** • Clinical diagnosis when there is a trauma-induced alteration in mental status that may or may not involve loss of consciousness, especially in the setting of padded low-impact head trauma, essentially from mild acceleration from a standing position. • If atypical signs are present (e.g., focal neurologic deficits, worsening mental status, signs of skull fracture), or higher impact trauma occurred, and/or there is increased concern for parenchymal injury, a non-contrast head CT should be obtained. • Criteria for obtaining CT head (New Orleans rules): headache, emesis, age ≥60, drug intoxication, persistent anterograde amnesia, or seizure. Also image in GCS <13 • Also consider CT cervical spine to rule out spine injury.

CASE 5 | Concussion *(continued)*

Discussion	**Management:** • At the scene assess and address ABCs, guard against neck injury, and obtain an evaluation from a health care provider (sports doctor on the field or transport to the ED). • Assess for need of imaging and further hospital and ICP monitoring (e.g., if GCS <8). • The patient should be closely monitored for 24 hours for any neurologic change. In stable patients with mild concussion this can be done at home by family. • If no further symptoms arise, gradual return to play after 1 week is allowed, starting with light aerobic exercise before progressing to contact sports. • Screen time should be limited and school accommodations may be necessary. • Patient should return to medical care if new headache, emesis, focal neurologic deficit, altered mental status, or fluid drainage from nose or ear occur concerning for CSF leak.
Additional Considerations	**Complications:** Patients with concussion may also develop a **post-concussive syndrome** within hours or days after the initial injury characterized by prolongation of initial symptoms. Risk of post-concussive syndrome is highest with multiple concussions or TBIs, as well as in those who return to play prematurely. In addition to symptoms of headache and vertigo, post-concussive patients may have sleep disturbances, altered mood, difficulty concentrating, or periods of amnesia. Symptoms typically resolve, but can take weeks to months. Multiple, repeated concussions (minor TBI) accumulated over several years can lead to **chronic traumatic encephalopathy (CTE)**. It is typically seen in patients with a history of multiple sports- or combat-related concussions, which result in cumulative cognitive impairments, psychologic symptoms (behavioral abnormalities, personality change, depression, suicidality), and speech and Parkinsonian-like gait abnormalities. Neuropathology involves common features of Alzheimer's dementia, including neuronal degeneration and the accumulation of hyperphosphorylated tau.

CASE 6 | Epidural Hematoma (EDH)

A 23-year-old woman is involved in a MVA in which her head strikes against the window and she loses consciousness. She is awake and conversing normally when the paramedics arrive; however, she has mild weakness over the right side, and has a GCS of 15. She is taken to a local hospital where it is noted that she has soft tissue swelling over the left frontoparietal region on her scalp but no signs of skull depression, fracture, or laceration. She has 4/5 strength in the right upper extremity and right lower extremity, and the remainder of the neurologic exam is normal. Prior to further workup, her neurologic status declines, her GCS worsens to 8, and she has a large and poorly responsive pupil on the left and a left gaze deviation.

| Conditions with Similar Presentations | **Subdural hematoma (SDH):** Consider in patients with closed-head injury which requires high impact in younger patients, but can occur with low impact in older adults, especially those taking anticoagulants. It is an injury associated with "shaken baby syndrome." It is characterized by rupture of bridging veins within the dural membrane leading to venous hemorrhage that is slowly progressive. It is a concave-shaped extra-axial hyperdensity, since it is bound superiorly by the rigid dura, and laterally and inferiorly by the dural invaginations—falx cerebri medially and the tentorium cerebelli inferiorly. While SDH can traverse large portions of a single hemisphere, it cannot cross midline or cross between the anterior and posterior fossa. Definitive treatment can range from conservative to surgical depending on radiographic size, presence of mass effect, and clinical symptoms. Surgical evacuation is done by burr holes for small SDH, and by craniotomy for larger and more severe SDH (ideally within 2–4 hours of onset of neurological deterioration).

Traumatic subarachnoid hemorrhage: Also considered in patients with closed-head injury that can occur with a wide variety of impact levels. In contrast to aneurysmal SAH, traumatic SAH is almost exclusively venous, making it less severe and less likely to produce hydrocephalus and elevations in ICP. Venous blood in the SAH space also carries much less risk of developing vasospasm than arterial blood, for reasons that are not well understood. | 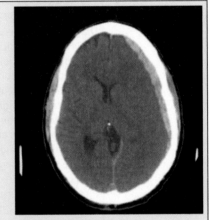
Head CT demonstrating a left frontotemporoparietal acute subdural hematoma with mass effect and mild midline shift. Subdural hematomas do not respect suture lines and are typically crescent shaped. (Reproduced with permission from Hall JB, Schmidt GA, Kress JP, eds. Hall, Schmidt, and Wood's Principles of Critical Care. 4th ed. New York: McGraw Hill; 2015.) |

CASE 6 | Epidural Hematoma (EDH) *(continued)*

Conditions with Similar Presentations	**Traumatic contusion:** This is not generally a specific category of traumatic injury, but is often used to refer to the entire conglomerate of parenchymal injuries to the brain, during a closed-head injury. The principal contusion is typically created by accelerating forces of the brain against the inside of the skull. Contusions often occur with or without a concomitant SDH and/or SAH and/or traumatic ICH, and any and all can occur at a point where the brain accelerated into the cranial vault during the injury. They may occur directly where the strike occurred (coup) or in the opposing side of the brain (contrecoup) where the brain accelerates in the opposing direction as a result of high-impact head acceleration and deceleration upon striking. Contusions are notorious for causing significant secondary injury, including mass effect, edema, axonal injury, ischemia, inflammation, and elevations in ICP. Treatment is centered around supportive measures for secondary injury and elevations in ICP. Multifocal TBI lesions often cannot be evacuated; however, surgery may be indicated to remove portions of the skull (decompression— bifrontal or hemicranial) to allow for progression of edema that is externally oriented, rather than herniating the brain downward.
Initial Diagnostic Tests	Urgent non-contrast head CT
Next Steps in Management	• Assess and address ABCs and assess and stabilize spine • Frequent neuro examinations and reverse any coagulopathies • ICP monitoring and pressure-lowering treatments if needed • Neurosurgical consultation for operative intervention

Discussion	EDH is an acute traumatic process that is more common in younger patients, usually due to high-impact closed-head injury. The pathophysiology is damage to branches of the middle meningeal artery, producing arterial hemorrhage in the epidural space. Overall prognosis is good as long as operative intervention, when indicated, is performed either before or with minimal development of secondary injury.
	
	History: Classically presents with a "lucid interval" with either minimal or no blood present at the time of the injury, but with rapid decline over minutes to hours as the arterial blood accumulates and causes mass effect.
	
	Physical Exam: May initially be normal or have mild neurologic deficit but then worsening mental status and focal deficits.
	
	Diagnostics: CT head
	• EDH radiographically forms a convex extra-axial hyperdense shape (see image) since it is under higher pressure and occur outside of the dural membrane.
	• Despite EDH occurring in the epidural space, the calvarial sutures form a tight adhesion between the dura and the periosteum of the interior skull. Therefore, EDH is bound by calvarial sutures and cannot cross midline, limited by the sagittal suture. However, it may cross in the frontal lobe where there is no midsagittal suture.
	
	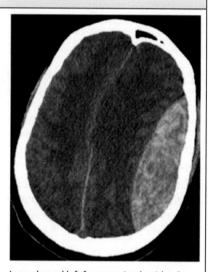
	Lens-shaped left frontoparietal epidural hematoma with an overlying skull fracture. (Reproduced with permission from Elsayes KM, A. Oldham SAA, eds. Introduction to Diagnostic Radiology. New York: McGraw Hill; 2014.)
	
	Management:
	• EDH is a type of TBI following similar guidelines to ICH regarding initial and supportive measures.
	• Address ABCs and stabilize patient
	• Cervical collar placement and spine imaging should be performed in most high-impact TBI situations, especially if the patient presents unconscious
	• Any coagulopathy should be immediately reversed and addressed
	• Depending on the size of the hematoma, ICP monitoring and control measures such as hyperventilation and osmotic therapy may be required, along with emergent neurosurgical consultation for operative intervention.
	  • Hypotension should be addressed to a systolic level of >110, per the Brain Trauma Foundation. No specific values exist for hypertension, although applying ICH guidelines of systolic pressure goal <160 is reasonable.
	  • If ICP monitoring is placed, CPP goals of 60–70 should be followed based on the formula CPP = MAP-ICP.
	  • Consider surgical evacuation if indicated (see below).

CASE 6 | Epidural Hematoma (EDH) *(continued)*

Additional Considerations	**Complications:** Common with many high-impact TBI is secondary axonal injury, usually from acceleration and shear forces. When neuronal damage involves sympathetic pathways, particularly in the brainstem, patients can develop a syndrome associated by episodic sympathetic storming. This manifests as hypertension, tachypnea, tachycardia, diaphoresis, and sometimes pyramidal or extrapyramidal abnormal movements. This syndrome is known as **paroxysmal sympathetic hyperactivity**, and is debilitating and difficult to treat. Treatment is principally pharmacologic, with agents tailored to blunt sympathetic tone, although newer ultrasound and other neurophysiologic techniques are under investigation.
	Post-traumatic epilepsy is another significant burden after TBI, and the risk is generally stratified by severity. Mild TBI carries a small increased risk of 1.5%, with no significantly increased risk demonstrated after 5 years. However, moderate TBI has a risk up to 5%, and severe TBI has a 17–24% risk of developing epilepsy.
	Surgical Considerations: Symptomatic (e.g., focal neurologic deficits) patients or those with signs and symptoms of increased intracranial pressure should undergo emergent **craniotomy** and **hematoma evacuation** due to risk of secondary brain herniation. Craniotomy involves an opening made in the skull which exposes the brain and allows for intracranial access. A piece of skull (bone flap) is removed and replaced at the end of the surgery. If the bone flap is not replaced, this is known as a craniectomy.

Herniation syndromes are a group of conditions whereby brain tissue herniates in response to mass effect. As the brain is contained within the fixed skull, there are several subtypes of herniations based on areas where brain tissue can move against rigid dural folds (see example b in accompanying image). In all cases, herniation can lead to compression of the brain tissue itself, but secondary injury occurs with compression of nearby cranial nerves and/or vasculature. If not quickly treated, these conditions can be fatal. Types of herniation syndromes include:

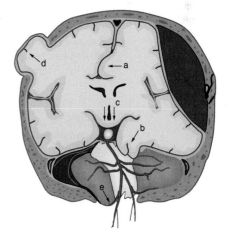

Herniation syndromes. a. Subfalcine; b. uncal; c. central transtentorial; d. external; e. cerebellotonsilar. (Reproduced with permission from Knoop KJ, Stack LB, Storrow AB, et al. The Atlas of Emergency Medicine. 5th ed. New York, NY: McGraw Hill; 2021.)

- **Subfalcine herniation** (a): occurs when the cingulate gyrus herniates under the falx cerebri, resulting in compression of the contralateral cerebral hemisphere. This can compress the anterior cerebral artery, resulting in hemiparesis predominantly affecting the lower extremities.

- **Uncal herniation** (b): occurs when a portion of the medial temporal lobe herniates through the tentorial notch separating the supratentorial and infratentorial structures.

- **Central transtentorial herniation** (c): involves downward displacement of brain tissue through the tentorium cerebelli (as opposed to across the tentorium as seen with uncal herniation). This can result in downward displacement of the brainstem, which can result in focal deficits, loss of consciousness, and death.

- **External or transcalvarial herniation** (d): occurs when there is a defect in the skull (e.g., from skull fracture or craniotomy) and can lead to focal neurological deficits from the affecting brain tissue.

- **Cerebellotonsillar herniation** (e): occurs when the cerebellar tonsils herniate through the foramen magnum. This can lead to compression of vital brainstem structures, often resulting in cardiorespiratory arrest and death.

Traumatic Brain Injury Mini-Case

Uncal (Transtentorial) Herniation	**Hx/PE**: Risk factors: Trauma, hemorrhage, infection, or tumor-causing mass effect and increased intracranial pressure (ICP) resulting in secondary damage from the brain being displaced across rigid structures.
	Symptoms and Signs: Patients have reduced level of consciousness and may have signs of elevated ICP, including headache, nausea, or vomiting, and Cushing triad.
	Classically a triad of (1) fixed, dilated pupil due to ipsilateral compression of the oculomotor nerve, (2) contralateral homonymous hemianopia due to compression and subsequent ischemia of the ipsilateral posterior cerebral artery, and (3) contralateral or ipsilateral weakness or paralysis due to compression of the cerebral peduncle and midbrain.
	Diagnostics • CT head or brain MRI will demonstrate midline shift with herniation of the uncus (part of the medial temporal lobe), and compression of nearby structures. • Patients commonly have a mass lesion from trauma, hemorrhage, infection, or tumor, as well as effacement of cerebral sulci and cisterns.
	Management • Acute stabilization (e.g., ABCDE approach, see Surgery chapter section on Trauma for more details) should be prioritized, and may involve airway management with intubation, mechanical ventilation, and/or hemodynamic support • Primary goals are to maintain adequate cerebral perfusion and to prevent secondary or delayed brain injury • Management depends on underlying etiology (e.g., hematoma evacuation for subdural hematoma, resection for tumor) • ICP should be monitored and measures done to reduce intracranial pressure, with head of the bed elevated to 30 degrees, avoiding neck flexion and rotation, short-term hyperventilation. and hyperosmolar therapy with IV hypertonic saline or mannitol • In severe cases, patient may require CSF diversion (i.e., with EVD), sedation (with propofol, benzodiazepines, or barbiturates), and/or decompressive craniectomy
	Discussion: Uncal or transtentorial herniation occurs when a portion of the medial temporal lobe herniates through the tentorial notch separating the supratentorial and infratentorial structures. Within this region, the oculomotor nerve is commonly affected, resulting in palsy with an ipsilateral "blown" pupil, since the parasympathetic fibers innervating the pupil travel around the periphery of the nerve. Compression of the ipsilateral pilocytic astrocytoma (PCA) in the same region can result in a contralateral homonymous hemianopia. Compression of the midbrain can result in decreased level of consciousness (affecting the ascending reticular activating system) as well as contralateral hemiplegia (affecting the descending ipsilateral corticospinal tract). In some cases, compression can result in damage to the contralateral midbrain against the tentorium, leading to ipsilateral hemiplegia (affecting the contralateral corticospinal tract). This is known as the Kernohan phenomenon, and is considered a false-localizing sign since the hemiplegia will be ipsilateral to the structural lesion (normally it would be expected to be contralateral).

WEAKNESS

Weakness is a common neurological concern and determining the location and acuity of weakness helps narrow the differential diagnosis. Non-neurological weakness is most often a generalized weakness due to medical conditions such as electrolyte abnormalities, infection, anemia, thyroid disease, or depression. Neurological weakness can be further delineated into central or peripheral origin. The CNS includes the primary motor cortex and the first-order motor neurons (upper motor neurons, UMNs) that descend inferiorly through the brainstem and spinal cord within motor pathways (including the corticospinal tract) to synapse on alpha motor neurons within the brainstem or spinal cord. The PNS begins in the anterior horns of the spinal cord, as the axons of these lower motor neurons (LMNs) leave the spinal cord, forming spinal nerve roots, motor nerves, and ultimately synapsing at the NMJ. Keep in mind that patients with functional neurological (conversion) disorder can also report weakness as their primary concern, and organic causes should be ruled out before making this diagnosis.

In addition to anatomical localization, careful attention should be paid to associated signs and symptoms that localize injury to UMNs vs. LMNs.

Upper vs. Lower Motor Neuron Signs

Sign (s)	UMN Injury	LMN Injury
Weakness	Yes	Yes
Atrophy	No (with time mild disuse atrophy)	Yes (usually severe)
Fasciculations (muscle twitching)	No	Yes
Fibrillations (on EMG)	None	Present
Tone	Increased (spastic, clasp knife)	Decreased, flaccid
Reflexes	Increased	Decreased/Absent
Clonus	May be present	Absent
Babinski sign (upgoing toes)	Present	Absent

There are several descending motor pathways within the CNS. Control of motor function begins in the primary motor cortex, which is somatotopically organized as shown in the motor homunculus (see image) which hangs by its toes. The most clinically significant descending motor pathway is the **lateral corticospinal tract**, which begins with pyramidal Betz cells in the primary motor cortex. Axons from these neurons enter the corona radiata and travel inferiorly through the posterior limb of the internal capsule. Damage to fibers within this relatively small structure can affect the contralateral face, arm, and leg. Axons continue traveling, and approximately 85% of the fibers cross to the opposite side within the pyramidal decussation before entering the lateral white matter of the spinal cord, forming the lateral corticospinal tract. The remaining fibers continue ipsilaterally and form the anterior corticospinal tract. Because the majority of fibers cross in the pyramidal decussation, injury to UMNs above this point (e.g., following an infarction of the middle cerebral artery territory) will result in weakness in the contralateral limbs.

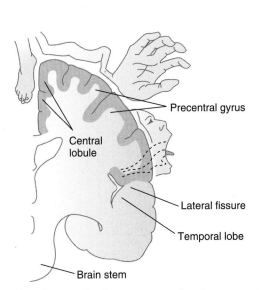

Motor homunculus drawn on a coronal section through the precentral gyrus. The location of cortical control of various body parts is shown. (Reproduced with permission from Waxman SG. Clinical Neuroanatomy. 29th ed. New York: McGraw Hill; 2020.)

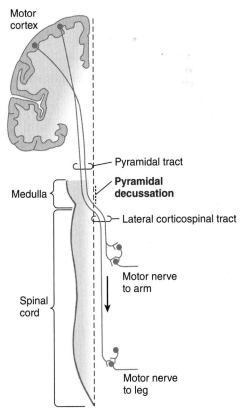

Different trades decussate at different levels. Pyramidal tract. (Reproduced with permission from Waxman SG. Clinical Neuroanatomy. 29th ed. New York: McGraw Hill; 2020.)

Differential Diagnoses: Central vs. Peripheral Causes of Weakness

Central Nervous System	Peripheral Nervous System

Central Nervous System

Brain

Vascular
- Ischemic stroke
- Hemorrhagic stroke
- Arteriovenous malformation (AVM)
- Arteriovenous fistula (AVF)
- Cerebral venous sinus thrombosis (CVST)
- Cerebral cavernous malformation (CCM)
- Vasculitis

Neoplastic
- Primary brain tumor
- Brain metastases
- CNS lymphoma

Infectious
- Abscess
- Meningitis
- Encephalitis

Inflammatory/Autoimmune
- Autoimmune encephalitis
- Multiple sclerosis
- Neuromyelitis optica spectrum

Metabolic
- Hypoxia
- Hypoglycemia
- Hyponatremia/Hypernatremia

Other
- Migraine (hemiplegic)
- Post-ictal (Todd's paralysis)
- Degenerative (Primary lateral sclerosis)

Spinal cord (i.e., descending motor pathways)

Vascular
- Spinal infarction
- Spinal AVM or AVF

Compression
- Spondylosis
- Disc herniation
- Epidural hematoma
- Conus medullaris syndrome

Metabolic
- Vitamin B12 deficiency
- Copper deficiency

Neoplastic
- Primary tumor
- Spinal metastases

Degenerative
- Amyotrophic lateral sclerosis (ALS)
- Primary lateral sclerosis (PLS)

Peripheral Nervous System

Anterior horn cells/motor nerve root

- ALS
- Poliovirus
- Multifocal motor neuropathy
- WNV
- Spinal muscular atrophy (SMA)
- Radiculopathy

Spinal nerve root

- Radiculitis
- AVF
- ALS
- Cauda equina syndrome

Plexus

- Traumatic or inflammatory plexopathy (often involving lumbar or brachial plexus)

Peripheral nerve

Compressive
- Wrist drop (radial nerve)
- Foot drop (peroneal nerve)
- Sciatica (sciatic nerve)

Inflammatory
- Acute (Guillain-Barre syndrome or acute inflammatory demyelinating polyneuropathy)
- Chronic (chronic inflammatory demyelinating polyneuropathy)

Infectious
- HSV
- Lyme disease
- EBV
- Leprosy
- Diphtheria

Toxic-Metabolic
- Tetrodotoxin
- Vitamin deficiencies
- Diabetic neuropathy
- Inherited
- Charcot-Marie-Tooth

Neuromuscular junction

Toxic-Metabolic
- Botulinum toxin (botulism)
- Tubocurarine (curare)
- Organophosphate poisoning
- Nerve gas (sarin)
- Hypermagnesemia

Inflammatory/Autoimmune
- Myasthenia gravis
- Lambert-Eaton myasthenic syndrome

Differential Diagnoses: Central vs. Peripheral Causes of Weakness

Central Nervous System	Peripheral Nervous System
Spinal cord (i.e., descending motor pathways) (Cont.)	**Muscle**
Infectious	*Infectious*
Syphilis (tabes dorsalis)	Myositis
Herpes zoster	*Inflammatory*
HTLV-1	Polymyositis
Tuberculosis	Dermatomyositis
HIV	Rhabdomyolysis
West Nile Virus (WNV)	*Degenerative*
Fungal infection	Inclusion body myositis (IBM)
Other	*Toxic-Metabolic*
Trauma	Hypercalcemia/hypocalcemia
Demyelinating disease (multiple sclerosis)	Hypokalemia
Hereditary (hereditary spastic paraplegia)	Critical illness myopathy
Radiation-induced myelopathy	Tetanus toxin
Inflammatory (Sjögren syndrome)	*Medications*
	Statins
	Steroids
	Colchicine
	Inherited
	Muscular dystrophy (Duchenne, Becker, myotonic)
	Neuromyotonia and myotonia
	Glycogen storage disorders
	Mitochondrial disorders

CASE 7 | Acute Ischemic Stroke

A 65-year-old right-handed man with type 2 diabetes mellitus, hyperlipidemia, and hypertension was brought to the ED by his wife with left-sided weakness. She reports that he was in his normal health just 1 hour ago but that after she returned from the store, he had these symptoms and she called 911. His current medications include metformin, atorvastatin, and amlodipine. His wife reports no recent trauma, surgery, or bleeding. Upon arrival to the ED, the patient is afebrile, BP 165/105, PR 95, RR 18, SpO2 100% on room air. His BMI is 38 kg/m². On exam, his speech is effortful with slurring. He has a left-sided facial droop, left arm weakness, and moderate sensory loss over the left arm and face. He is able to move his right arm and both legs. On visual field testing, he is unable to identify objects in his left visual field. When asked to draw a clock, all the numbers are written on the right side only.

Conditions with Similar Presentations	**Intracerebral hemorrhage:** Refers to bleeding into the brain parenchyma and also presents with acute neurologic deficits similar to an ischemic stroke. However, intracerebral hemorrhages commonly present with mass effect and may worsen as time progresses, and CT will demonstrate a hyperdensity due to acute hemorrhage.
	Transient ischemic attack (TIA) is differentiated from stroke by imaging. TIA is a transient episode of neurologic dysfunction due to ischemia WITHOUT acute infarction (i.e., no evidence on neuroimaging). TIAs are associated with carotid artery stenosis and risk for ischemic strokes increase as the stenosis progresses. Incidence of stroke is highest in the first 48 hours following TIA, and therefore patients should undergo urgent evaluation with brain imaging (CT or MRI) and imaging of carotid arteries (US, MRA CT angiogram).
Initial Diagnostic Tests	• Non-contrast head CT to rule out hemorrhagic stroke. • If the non-contrast CT is negative for hemorrhage, consider CT with contrast or MRI brain with or without contrast to further evaluate areas of ischemia and infarction.
Next Steps in Management	• If the patient's "last known normal" was within 4.5 hours, they should receive an IV tissue plasminogen activator (tPA) (alteplase or tenecteplase). • Consider mechanical thrombectomy for large vessel occlusion within the anterior circulation • Once the initial stroke is treated, secondary prevention of future strokes with antiplatelet therapy (aspirin and/or clopidogrel) and control of risk factors including blood pressure, hyperlipidemia, diabetes, smoking, and obesity. • Attempts should be made to identify the underlying etiology of the stroke, such as large-vessel atherosclerosis or cardioembolic source.

CASE 7 | Acute Ischemic Stroke *(continued)*

Discussion	Ischemic strokes account for more than 75% of all strokes. Etiology can broadly be characterized in three ways: 1) *Embolic* – an embolus from a thrombus elsewhere occludes a cerebral artery or its branches. Emboli may be multiple and involve several vascular territories and have an abrupt onset of symptoms that are maximal at onset. 2) *Thrombotic* - commonly due to atherosclerosis and/or plaque rupture in which a thrombus forms within a vessel which suddenly reduces blood flow, similar to acute coronary syndrome. These patients may have symptoms that fluctuate with periods of improvement, a phenomenon known as stuttering progression. 3) *Global cerebral ischemia* - due to hypoperfusion that causes damage most notably in the watershed areas. **History:** Modifiable risk factors include hypertension, diabetes mellitus, atrial fibrillation, hyperlipidemia, tobacco use, sedentary lifestyle, poor diet, kidney disease, obstructive sleep apnea, heavy alcohol intake, and poor diet. Nonmodifiable stroke risk factors include age, male sex, and underlying genetic susceptibility. Symptoms: Patients present with acute neurologic deficits related to the area of the infarct. **Physical Exam:** A new focal neurologic deficit will be noted. In addition to a comprehensive neurological exam, can calculate the NIH Stroke Scale (NIHSS) score, which assesses for neurological deficits on a 0-42 scale, with higher numbers reflecting worse stroke severity. The exam can also be used to localize the lesion to particular cerebral vessels (see table below) which is coined "vascular territory". MCA infarcts of the dominant hemisphere can result in damage to Broca's area (left frontal lobe), leading to an expressive aphasia with impaired fluency. Damage to the non-dominant hemisphere (this patient) results in hemineglect (right parietal lobe), whereby they are unaware and unconcerned (anosognosia) about the left side of his body and visual field. They may not recognize the left side as "their own" limbs. This can be confirmed with abnormal clock drawing as in this case. Sometimes when you tell them to raise their left arm, they will instead lift the right one. **Diagnostics:** • It is important to immediately recognize the signs and symptoms of stroke so that imaging and treatment can be performed as soon as possible ("Time is brain"). • After obtaining a focused history (last known normal, prior stroke/TIA, trauma, surgery, and current medications) quickly assess vital signs and check blood glucose. • A stat non-contrast head CT is performed to rule out hemorrhage, which would appear as a hyperdense lesion on non-contrast CT, and would be an immediate contraindication to thrombolytics. • Ischemic stroke can be quite variable on non-contrast CT, and may be isodense or hypodense, and is commonly not seen during the very acute stages. There may be subtle findings like effacement of the gray-white junction due to cytotoxic edema. • If non-contrast head CT is negative for hemorrhage, thrombolysis should not be delayed if the patient is a candidate (see treatment below). • Further imaging steps may involve a CT perfusion study and brain MRI, which is designed to evaluate for the presence of a tissue penumbra (at-risk tissue not yet infarcted, which is determined by perfusion imaging) that may be amenable to interventional reperfusion. • CT perfusion allows for identification of the central core of the ischemic infarct (irreversible neuronal loss) and the surrounding penumbra (potentially reversible ischemia). • Brain MRI, especially diffusion-weighted imaging (DWI) should also be performed to identify areas of core ischemia and is more sensitive for the detection of acute stroke compared to CT. DWI detects abnormalities in water movement within the brain, and restricted diffusion of water molecules due to acute infarcts can appear as hyperintensities within minutes or hours following a stroke. Acute infarction on DWI can also be confirmed by looking at the apparent diffusion coefficient (ADC) map, which would show a corresponding area of hypointensity where DWI shows hyperintensity (see image). Depending on these neuroimaging findings, patients can also be considered for angiography.

CASE 7 | Acute Ischemic Stroke *(continued)*

Discussion	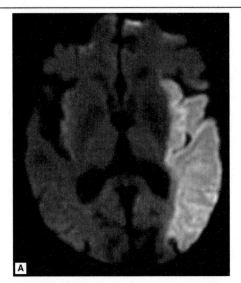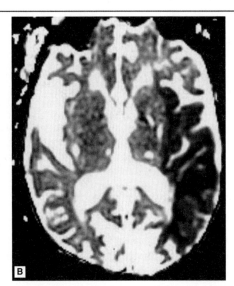

Diffusion-weighted imaging (DWI) and apparent diffusion coefficient (ADC) MRI in acute ischemic stroke. Axial DWI (A) and ADC (B) demonstrate diffusion restriction in the territory of the left MCA. (Reproduced with permission from Berkowitz AL. Clinical Neurology and Neuroanatomy: A Localization-Based Approach. 2nd ed. New York: McGraw Hill; 2022.)

Management:
- A stroke code should be called to facilitate immediate non-contrast CT and possible medical and procedural intervention.
- The first step is to identify whether the patient is a candidate for IV tPA.
  - Patients eligible for tPA are ≥18 years old, who have a new-onset neurologic deficit with time of symptom onset within 4.5 hours (3 hours is used in select populations such as age > 80 years, NIHSS >25).
  - Absolute contraindications to tPA include presence or history of intracranial hemorrhage (e.g. ICH, SAH) on CT; recent neurosurgery, head trauma, or stroke within the past 3 months; uncontrolled hypertension (SBP >185 mmHg or DBP >110 mmHg); known AVM, neoplasm, or aneurysm; active internal bleeding; suspected or confirmed endocarditis; abnormal blood glucose <50 mg/dL; or known bleeding diathesis (platelets <100,000/mm³, received heparin within 48 hrs with elevated aPTT, current use of oral anticoagulants with INR >1.7, or current use of direct thrombin or factor Xa inhibitors).
- If eligible for tPA, it should be given as soon as possible.
- If the patient has a large vessel occlusion within the anterior circulation, they should also be considered for mechanical thrombectomy regardless of whether tPA was given or not. Mechanical thrombectomy as well as intra-arterial thrombolysis can be performed in an extended time window past 4.5 hours (and up to 24 hours in select cases).
- During the acute period, permissive hypertension (<220/120 mmHg if tPA not given, <185/110 if tPA was given) is allowed to promote adequate brain perfusion.
- Once the initial acute ischemic stroke has been stabilized and treated, the next steps in management involve identification of the underlying etiology of the stroke as well as secondary stroke prevention.
- To identify the underlying etiology, patients undergo vascular imaging (e.g., CT angiography of the head and neck, carotid ultrasound) and echocardiography and ECG (for cardioembolic source).
- All patients should be started on low-dose aspirin and a statin.
- Certain patients (e.g., those with mild-moderate noncardioembolic stroke, or those with large vessel disease) may also be candidates for transient use of dual-antiplatelet therapy (DAPT) with aspirin plus an additional antiplatelet agent such as clopidogrel or ticagrelor to further decrease risk of future stroke.
- Vascular risk factors (including hypertension, hyperlipidemia, diabetes, obesity, heart disease, smoking) should be assessed and controlled through lifestyle modifications as well as medical management. |

CASE 7 | Acute Ischemic Stroke *(continued)*

Additional Considerations	**Strokes occurring in young patients (e.g., age <50 years)** should result in additional workup including for hypercoagulable state, carotid artery dissection, substance use (e.g., cocaine), and patent foramen ovale (PFO). PFO is a risk factor for paradoxical emboli originating in the venous system that traverse the PFO and enter the cerebral arterial system.
	Atrial fibrillation is the most common cause of cardioembolic stroke. Use the CHA_2DS_2-VASc score for risk assessment to determine need for anticoagulation. The CHA_2DS_2-VASc score is a point-based system and includes *C*ongestive heart failure (1 point), *H*ypertension (1 point), *A*ge ≥75 (2 points), *D*iabetes mellitus (1 point), prior *S*troke or TIA (2 points), *V*ascular disease such as prior MI or PAD (1 point), *A*ge 65-74 (1 point), and female *S*ex (1 point). Oral anticoagulation with warfarin or direct oral anticoagulants (DOACs) such as direct factor Xa inhibitors (e.g., apixaban) or direct thrombin inhibitors (e.g., dabigatran) should be used in high-risk patients, defined as men with score ≥2 or women with score ≥3.

When evaluating a patient with acute ischemic stroke, it is important to be able to localize the lesion based on history and neurological exam. Exam findings inconsistent with neuroimaging should prompt further imaging and work up. Localization relates to the major brain structure supplied by major cerebral blood vessels, either within the anterior (derived from internal carotid artery) or posterior circulation (derived from the vertebral arteries) and the circle of Willis.

Circle of Willis and principal arteries of the brainstem, as seen from below. (Reproduced with permission from Waxman SG. Clinical Neuroanatomy. 29th ed. New York: McGraw Hill; 2020.)

Key Findings Based on Affected Vascular Territory in Stroke

Blood Vessel	Key Findings
Anterior cerebral artery (ACA)	Infarct of medial motor and sensory cortices resulting in contralateral lower limb paralysis and sensory loss ± urinary incontinence. A rare syndrome of akinetic mutism and abulia can result from bilateral ACA strokes.
Middle cerebral artery (MCA)	Infarct of lateral motor and sensory cortices resulting in contralateral facial and upper limb paralysis and sensory loss, aphasia (dominant hemisphere, affecting Wernicke or Broca area), hemineglect (non-dominant hemisphere). Temporal lobe involvement can affect Meyer's loop of visual fibers, resulting in partial field cut ("pie in the sky" quadrantanopia),
Lenticulostriate artery	Often present as lacunar infarcts within the striatum or internal capsule: • **Pure motor stroke**—contralateral hemiparesis affecting face, arm, AND leg • **Ataxic hemiparesis**—contralateral hemiparesis (legs > arms) with ataxia • **Dysarthria (clumsy hand syndrome)**—dysarthria, contralateral hand weakness or "clumsiness" (i.e., with writing) • **Pure sensory stroke**—contralateral numbness affecting face, arm, AND leg ± thalamic pain syndrome • **Mixed sensorimotor stroke**—contralateral hemiparesis and numbness affecting face, arm, AND leg All of these have absence of cortical signs (aphasia, neglect, visual field loss).
Posterior cerebral artery	Infarct of occipital lobe resulting in contralateral homonymous hemianopsia, often with macular sparing.

Key Findings Based on Affected Vascular Territory in Stroke

Blood Vessel	Key Findings
Anterior spinal artery	Results in the **medial medullary syndrome** with: • Contralateral upper and lower limb paralysis (corticospinal tract) • Decreased contralateral proprioception (medial lemniscus • Ipsilateral tongue deviation (caudal medulla, hypoglossal nerve • In severe cases, a locked-in syndrome This syndrome can also be seen with vertebral artery infarctions.
Posterior inferior cerebellar artery (PICA)	Results in the **lateral medullary (Wallenberg) syndrome** with: 1. Dysphagia, hoarseness, hiccups, decreased gag reflex (nucleus ambiguus—*specific to this condition*) 2. Vomiting, vertigo, nystagmus (vestibular nuclei) 3. Decreased contralateral body pain and temperature sensation (lateral spinothalamic tract) 4. Decreased ipsilateral face pain and temperature sensation (spinal trigeminal nucleus) 5. Ipsilateral Horner syndrome (descending sympathetic fibers) 6. Ipsilateral ataxia, dysmetria (inferior cerebellar peduncle and spinocerebellar tract) This syndrome can also be seen with vertebral artery infarctions.
Anterior inferior cerebellar artery (AICA)	Results in the **lateral pontine syndrome** with: 1. Ipsilateral full facial paralysis with decreased lacrimation, salivation, and taste from anterior 2/3 of tongue (facial nucleus—*specific to this condition*) 2. Vomiting, vertigo, nystagmus (vestibular nuclei) 3. Decreased contralateral body pain and temperature sensation (lateral spinothalamic tract) 4. Decreased ipsilateral face pain and temperature sensation (spinal trigeminal nucleus) 5. Ipsilateral Horner syndrome (sympathetic fibers) 6. Ipsilateral ataxia, dysmetria (inferior and middle cerebellar peduncles) 7. Ipsilateral sensorineural deafness, vertigo (labyrinthine artery)
Basilar artery (and pontine branches)	Results in the **locked-in syndrome**, with: 1. Preserved consciousness (reticular activating system spared) 2. Quadriplegia (corticospinal tracts) 3. Loss of voluntary facial, mouth, and tongue movement (corticobulbar tracts) 4. Loss of horizontal but not vertical eye movements (ocular cranial nerve nuclei, paramedian pontine reticular formation)

CASE 8 | Myasthenia Gravis

A 32-year-old woman with no past medical history presents with blurred vision for the past 2 months. She recently delivered a healthy baby boy 1 year ago via spontaneous vaginal delivery without any complications. She works as an office manager and notes that when she gets home at the end of the day, her eyelids droop and her speech is occasionally slurred. She has been feeling fatigued for several months and has noticed that she becomes short of breath more easily. Vitals are within normal limits. On exam, she has bilateral ptosis, binocular double vision upon sustained upgaze, and weakness in her eye closure, cheek puff, tongue protrusion, and neck flexion. Sensory exam is normal and deep tendon reflexes are intact. Gait is normal.

| Conditions with Similar Presentations | **Lambert-Eaton myasthenic syndrome:** Presents with weakness that, unlike myasthenia gravis, improves with repeated use. The weakness is predominantly in proximal muscles and impacts the legs in particular. Autonomic symptoms (dry mouth, erectile dysfunction) are common. Antibodies to the presynaptic voltage–gated calcium channel inhibit the ability of calcium entry, resulting in a decrease in the release of acetylcholine. Acetylcholinesterase inhibitor administration does little to improve the symptoms. Lambert-Eaton myasthenic syndrome is commonly a paraneoplastic syndrome associated with small-cell lung cancer.

Botulism: Occurs due to ingestion or cutaneous exposure to botulinum exotoxin produced by *Clostridium botulinum*, which inhibits release of acetylcholine from neurons at the NMJ. Patients typically present with symmetric, descending weakness, often starting with ocular and bulbar muscles, autonomic dysfunction, and ultimately can lead to respiratory compromise. |

CASE 8 | Myasthenia Gravis *(continued)*

Initial Diagnostic Tests	• Check edrophonium test and/or ice pack test • Confirm with detection of antibodies to acetylcholine receptor (AChR) or against muscle-specific kinase (MUSK). • Also check chest CT to evaluate for thymoma
Next Steps in Management	• Treat with pyridostigmine (acetylcholinesterase inhibitor). • IV immunoglobulin (IVIG) and plasmapheresis for acute/serious symptoms • Glucocorticoids for ocular myasthenia gravis or chronic maintenance therapy after acute exacerbation is treated • Thymectomy if thymoma identified
Discussion	Myasthenia gravis is an autoimmune condition and the most common disorder affecting the NMJ, characterized by the formation of autoantibodies against the nicotinic acetylcholine receptor found on skeletal muscle cells. Some patients with myasthenia gravis have thymic hyperplasia or a thymoma, likely due to an autoimmune response to thymic epitopes on myoid cells similar to those seen in the NMJ. **History/Physical Exam:** More common in women of reproductive age, although can be seen in men, typically >50 years old. • It presents with fluctuating, fatigable weakness, better in the morning and worse toward the end of the day, or following exercise. • Weakness commonly affects ocular and facial muscles (resulting in ptosis, diplopia, dysphagia, dysarthria), although can also affect proximal limb muscles (commonly the upper extremity resulting in difficulty lifting arms). A more generalized form involves bulbar, limb, neck, and/or respiratory muscles and presents with fatigability of chewing and swallowing, slurred speech, shortness of breath, and proximal limb weakness. • **Myasthenic crisis** is a severe exacerbation of myasthenia gravis resulting in respiratory failure with hypoxemia and/or hypercapnia, often triggered by physiologic or pathologic stress or certain medications (especially those interfering with the NMJ, such as rocuronium). **Diagnostics:** • At the bedside, the ice pack test can be performed: An ice pack placed on the ptotic lid will raise it at least 2 mm (the cold decreases the activity of acetylcholinesterase). • The edrophonium test involves use of the short-acting acetylcholinesterase inhibitor edrophonium, which results in transient improvement in ptosis and can be useful diagnostically. • Diagnosis should be confirmed with detection of positive autoantibodies against acetylcholine receptor or against muscle-specific kinase (MUSK). Serum testing for acetylcholine receptor (AChR) antibodies is positive in 80–90%. If not present, test for anti-muscle specific tyrosine kinase (MUSK), which will be present about 50% of the time. MUSK is an enzyme that facilitates construction of the acetylcholinesterase receptors at the NMJ. • Chest CT should be performed to evaluate for thymoma and thymic hyperplasia. Up to 50% of patients with a thymoma have concomitant myasthenia gravis. Conversely, roughly 10% of patients with myasthenia gravis have a thymoma or thymic hyperplasia. • EMG may show normal response to single stimulation; however, with repetitive stimulation, there will be decreased (fatigable) response. **Management:** • The goal of treatment is to increase available acetylcholine in the NMJ cleft. The use of the acetylcholinesterase inhibitor pyridostigmine is first-line because it has the longest half-life and duration of action and does not cross the blood-brain barrier. • All patients with exacerbation of myasthenia gravis should also receive IVIG or plasmapheresis. • Patients with thymic hyperplasia or thymoma should have complete thymectomy, which can be curative. • Chronic treatment of myasthenia gravis following treatment of acute exacerbation includes glucocorticoids. • Glucocorticoids should also be considered in patients with ocular myasthenia gravis, but generally are used as chronic therapy (glucocorticoids in acute setting can worsen symptoms). • Those who do not sufficiently improve with pyridostigmine and glucocorticoids should receive additional immunotherapy with azathioprine or mycophenolate. If needed, rituximab or eculizumab can be added.
Additional Considerations	**Obstetric Considerations:** Pregnant women with myasthenia gravis may continue taking acetylcholinesterase inhibitors during pregnancy. If the pregnant patient develops preeclampsia, magnesium sulfate may be contraindicated because it can acutely exacerbate symptoms of myasthenia gravis, resulting in a severe myasthenic crisis. Seizure prophylaxis should instead be performed with levetiracetam or another agent with favorable pregnancy data.

CASE 9 | Bell's (Peripheral Facial Nerve) Palsy

A 48-year-old man presents with sudden onset of right facial weakness. In the morning, he noticed droopiness in the right corner of his mouth. By the end of the day, he could not raise his right eyebrow. The following morning, he woke up with dry eyes and increased sensitivity to sound in the right ear. He has a history of mouth sores that resurface periodically. Vital signs are within normal limits. Upon exam, he has decreased ability to keep his right eye closed, and cheek weakness, and he is unable to raise the corner of his mouth on the right side. No rashes or lesions were noted in the ear or mouth or on the skin. Sensation is intact in the upper and lower extremities, and strength is 5/5 bilaterally.

Conditions with Similar Presentations	**Central facial nerve palsy:** Due to a UMN lesion (e.g., pontine infarct) presents similarly to Bell's palsy (peripheral facial nerve palsy) with lower facial muscles affected; however, patients will be able to frown and close their eyelids, as the upper face is spared due to bilateral central innervation. Central palsy will also cause symptoms contralateral to the affected nerve.
	Hemifacial spasm: Presents with episodic muscle twitching of the face rather than sudden-onset palsy.
	Diabetic cranial neuropathy: Can present as an isolated focal neuropathy but would occur gradually and patients would have other symptoms concerning for diabetes (e.g., retinopathy, nephropathy, or lower extremity neuropathy). Cranial nerves III, IV, and VI are involved more often than VII.
	Herpes zoster oticus (Ramsay Hunt syndrome) results from reactivation of the varicella-zoster virus along cranial nerves VII and/or VIII. It causes a vesicular rash in the external auditory canal in addition to features seen in Bell's palsy (unilateral facial palsy, loss of taste sensation, and ear pain). It should be treated with acyclovir or valacyclovir and prednisone; otherwise, hearing loss and/or facial paralysis can be permanent.
Initial Diagnostic Tests	• Clinical diagnosis • If diagnosis uncertain, consider ruling out other causes (see below)
Next Steps in Management	• Eye protection (lubricants, patch at night) and prednisone • Valacyclovir can be used if severe
Discussion	Bell's palsy is a clinical syndrome that describes acute peripheral facial nerve palsy of unknown cause. A herpes simplex virus–mediated inflammatory mechanism has been proposed as a controversial etiology. Herpes zoster virus (varicella-zoster virus [VZV]) is also commonly associated with Bell's palsy. Ischemia of the facial nerve has also been suggested, especially in patients with diabetes. Before diagnosis of idiopathic facial nerve palsy, other causes such as Lyme disease and sarcoidosis should be ruled out. Patients typically present with progressive unilateral facial paralysis over several hours. The exact mechanism is not known, but symptoms presumably occur due to inflammation of the facial nerve. Symptoms may progress over days to weeks.
	History/Physical Exam: • Characteristic features include facial droop and inability to close the eye. • It is frequently accompanied by sensory, autonomic, and taste symptoms due to the multifunctional aspects of the facial nerve. These include decreased tears/dry eye, hyperacusis, and loss of taste sensation over the anterior two-thirds of the tongue. • On exam, patients will have unilateral facial weakness with involvement of forehead muscles. Decreased ability to keep eye closed when asked to do so and vertical traction placed on the upper eyelid. Flattened nasolabial fold and inability to raise the corner of the mouth. • Most patients show gradual recovery of function
	Diagnostics: • Clinical diagnosis in those with typical history and examination consistent with Bell's palsy. • Consider serologic testing for Lyme disease in endemic areas and MRI brain with and without contrast to rule out central/structural pathologies and HBA1c to assess for diabetes mellitus.
	Management: Treatment of Bell's palsy has been controversial. • All patients should be treated with eye protection (lubricants, patch at night) • In general, early treatment with oral glucocorticoids is recommended, and optimal treatment should begin within 3 days of symptom onset. • The addition of antivirals to glucocorticoids is beneficial, especially in those with severe facial palsy.
Additional Considerations	**Complications:** After episodes of Bell's palsy, nerve regrowth and reinnervation can occur imperfectly and erratically, and patients may suffer from chronic **synkinesias** (involuntary movements) when they contract facial muscles.

CASE 10 | Guillain-Barré Syndrome (GBS)

A 30-year-old man with no past medical history presents to urgent care with his partner, who reports that the patient has become increasingly weak over the past week, which has resulted in difficulty walking. Two weeks ago, the patient had severe nausea and diarrhea with occasional blood, and abdominal cramps that have since resolved. He reports mild back pain and paresthesias in his feet bilaterally. He has taken acetaminophen without relief. His vital signs are notable for orthostatic hypotension, but otherwise his vitals are stable. On exam, he is unable to raise his legs while lying in the bed, although his upper extremities are normal. Patellar and ankle reflexes are absent bilaterally. There is mild decreased sensation to light touch and pinprick bilaterally up to the level of the knee.

Conditions with Similar Presentations	**Chronic inflammatory demyelinating polyneuropathy (CIDP):** Can be considered in patients with recurrent episodes, since GBS is a monophasic illness. CIDP symptoms in contrary can develop over 8 weeks or longer (vs. GBS and other forms of acute inflammatory demyelinating polyneuropathies). Similar to GBS, patients may have predominant motor symptoms although can also have sensory abnormalities. Treatment involves corticosteroids, IVIG, plasma exchange, and immunosuppressive medications. **Transverse myelitis:** Occurs due to inflammation within one or more contiguous segments of the spinal cord, and can occur following recent infections (e.g., gastrointestinal or upper respiratory tract infection). However, the most common etiology of transverse myelitis is part of a demyelinating syndrome such as MS or NMO. Patients can have motor deficits, with UMN signs, autonomic dysfunction, and sensory abnormalities (often a distinct sensory level). Spinal MRI will show enhancement of the cord segments without compression. CSF will show increased WBCs due to ongoing inflammatory response.
Initial Diagnostic Tests	• Clinical diagnosis. • Consider LP, EMG, and imaging for supportive data
Next Steps in Management	• If signs of respiratory distress (low forced vital capacity, low SpO2) admit to ICU for monitoring. • IVIG or plasma exchange
Discussion	GBS is the most common cause of acute inflammatory demyelinating polyneuropathy (AIDP) and is characterized by acute demyelination of peripheral nerves, resulting in an ascending flaccid paralysis. Gastroenteritis from *Campylobacter jejuni* is the most common etiology, caused by molecular mimicry between bacterial antigens and those found on peripheral nerve axons and myelin. Respiratory pathogens implicated include *Haemophilus influenzae* and *Mycoplasma pneumoniae*. Other potential predisposing events include HIV, CMV, EBV, Zika virus, and (rarely) influenza and COVID vaccination. Most patients show complete recovery; however, up to 15% may have permanent deficits, as subsequent axonal loss may accompany demyelination. **History/Physical Exam:** • Patients present with progressive ascending weakness and lower extremity sensory loss occurring over a period of days after a preceding infection, involving the GI or respiratory tract. • Predominant motor symptoms due to peripheral nerve demyelination, ascending symmetric weakness and LMN signs (hypotonia, decreased or absent reflexes). • Patients may also have distal sensory abnormalities, including paresthesias as well as back or extremity pain. • GBS is typically progressive over 1–2 weeks, and ascending weakness can be life-threatening if respiratory muscles become involved. • On exam, patients will have decreased symmetric strength, especially in the lower extremities with hypotonia and decreased/absent reflexes. Symmetric distal sensory loss in lower extremities. **Diagnostics:** • Diagnosis is primarily clinical • LP with CSF analysis showing *cytoalbuminologic dissociation* (elevated CSF protein with normal cell count) is characteristic, although elevated protein may not be observed until 1–2 weeks after symptom onset. • Nerve conduction studies and EMG have very limited utility in demonstrating neuropathy acutely. May show early subtle evidence of decreased motor nerve conduction velocity and symmetric axonal demyelinating neuropathy- but may take weeks to be abnormal. • MRI of the neuraxis is typically normal; however, MRI spine may show mild enhancement of the intrathecal spinal nerve roots and the cauda equina **Management:** • Monitor for autonomic and respiratory dysfunction (forced vital capacity and negative inspiratory force) with low threshold for intubation and mechanical ventilation in ICU • IVIG or plasma exchange can hasten recovery if initiated early on in the disease course

CASE 10 | Guillain-Barré Syndrome (GBS) *(continued)*

Additional Considerations	**Miller-Fisher syndrome** is a subtype of GBS that presents with a triad of (1) ophthalmoplegia, (2) ataxia, and (3) areflexia. It is caused by autoantibodies formed against the peripheral nerve ganglioside GQ1b, which is expressed in high levels in cranial nerves III, IV, and VI (resulting in ophthalmoplegia). Similar to GBS, patients will have albuminocytologic dissociation on CSF analysis. Anti-GQ1b antibodies are present. Anti-GQ1b antibodies are also associated with rare GBS subtype **Bickerstaff's brainstem encephalitis**, which can be severely debilitating. Subtype treatment is also IVIG or plasmapheresis.

CASE 11 | Amyotrophic Lateral Sclerosis (ALS)

A 65-year-old right-handed man presents to his primary care physician with hand weakness, particularly worse in his right hand. His wife reports he has become increasingly clumsy over the past year, often dropping objects, and now has difficulty buttoning his shirts. For the past 3 weeks, he has also had difficulty climbing stairs. He denies any pain, numbness, tingling, or changes in his bowel or bladder function. Vital signs are within normal limits. On exam, he is alert and oriented to person, place, and time and able to recall 3/3 objects at 5 minutes. He has asymmetric muscle atrophy in distal hand muscles bilaterally, more pronounced on the right. Fasciculations are observed in the upper extremities. Strength is decreased in his right-hand intrinsic muscles, biceps, and deltoid as well as during left arm abduction, and during bilateral hip flexion. Reflexes are 3+ in his upper extremities. Sensation and cerebellar function are intact.

Conditions with Similar Presentations	There is a spectrum of degenerative weakness syndromes which includes primary lateral sclerosis (PLS), ALS, and progressive muscular atrophy (PMA).
	PLS: Predominantly affects UMNs, and typically begins in the lower extremities although can progress to involve the upper extremity and bulbar muscles. Patients commonly report involuntary muscle spasms, spasticity, difficulty walking or maintaining balance, and cramps, often relying on assistive devices to walk. It typically has a better prognosis compared to ALS and PMA.
	PMA: Predominantly affects LMNs, resulting in muscle weakness, atrophy, and fasciculations, without UMN signs. PMA has a better prognosis than ALS, but typically worse than PLS.
	Poliomyelitis: Asymmetric weakness typically starts in one limb and can progress to quadriplegia and respiratory failure within days. Unlike ALS, patients have only LMN signs such as hypotonia, flaccid paralysis, fasciculations, hyporeflexia, and muscle atrophy. It is caused by the poliovirus, which is largely eradicated, with Afghanistan and Pakistan being the only two endemic countries. About 90–95% of patients infected with poliovirus are asymptomatic or have flu-like symptoms and only 0.1% of patients infected develop paralysis. Legs are more commonly affected than arms, and proximal muscle groups are more affected than distal groups. About two-thirds of patients develop residual weakness. Some patients may develop post-polio syndrome decades after initial onset, likely due to premature aging of the remaining motor neurons.
	West Nile virus: can also present with motor neuron disease, similar to polio. However, in contrast to poliovirus, West Nile commonly presents with CNS infectious sequelae, such as meningoencephalitis, altered consciousness, and fever/chills, stiff neck, headache.
Initial Diagnostic Tests	Clinical diagnosis supported by EMG findings of LMN disease (fibrillations and fasciculations)
Next Steps in Management	• Riluzole (PO) or edaravone (IV) may help slow disease • Otherwise, treatment is supportive
Discussion	ALS is a progressive motor neurodegenerative disease that affects both UMNs and LMNs in the anterior horn of the spinal cord, brainstem, and motor cortex. Ninety percent of ALS is sporadic, and only 10% is familial. Of the familial cases, mutations may be observed in the *C9ORF72* gene or superoxide dismutase (*SOD1*) gene, with autosomal dominant inheritance. Sporadic ALS affects men more than women and may be increased in army veterans and athletes. The most common cause of death is respiratory failure as motor nerve degeneration involves the diaphragm and other accessory muscles of respiration, resulting in diaphragmatic paralysis. Death typically occurs within 3–5 years of diagnosis.

CASE 11 | Amyotrophic Lateral Sclerosis (ALS) *(continued)*

Discussion	**History/ Physical Exam:**
	• Can present at any age, with peak incidence in the sixth to seventh decades of life (earlier in familial cases).
	• ALS is progressive in nature, and symptoms do not tend to fluctuate.
	• Patients commonly present with asymmetric limb weakness with UMN and LMN signs in one limb.
	• UMN signs include hypertonia, spasticity, hyperreflexia, and presence of pathologic reflexes (Babinski and Hoffman signs)
	• LMN signs include atrophy, hypotonia, hyporeflexia, and fasciculations (often first noted in the tongue)
	• Muscle weakness begins focally, usually in the limbs, and spreads to involve contiguous regions.
	• A common presenting sign is weakness in the hands with hypothenar and thenar atrophy and weakness (dropping objects, handwriting)
	• Approximately 20% of patients may present with bulbar symptoms with degeneration of motor cranial nerves, such as dysarthria or dysphagia (bulbar-onset ALS), which is associated with more rapid progression of disease
	• Patients do **not** have deficits in sensory modalities or autonomic dysfunction
	
	Diagnostics:
	• Primarily a clinical diagnosis based on presence of progressive **UMN and LMN signs**; however, further studies should be ordered to rule out other causes
	• Electromyography (EMG) findings often herald the diagnosis by demonstrating motor neuronopathy with widespread denervation (fasciculations (often first observed in the tongue) or fibrillations), particularly in areas that would otherwise be unexpected (i.e., thoracic distribution, not typically caused by compressive neuropathy or radiculopathy)
	• MRI of affected spine region may be unremarkable or may show atrophy within the anterior horns
	• Patients may have a mildly increased creatinine kinase
	• Nerve conduction studies are normal, as nerves can still carry action potentials to the muscle
	
	Management:
	• Riluzole (PO) or edaravone (IV) may help slow disease
	  • Riluzole, which slows progression of ALS by limiting glutamate excitotoxicity and subsequent neuronal disruption
	  • Edavarone is a free radical scavenger that has neuroprotective effects
	• Multidisciplinary approach and discussion of goals for care
	  • Serial assessment of dysphagia and pulmonary function, and management with speech therapy, nutrition, physical therapy, occupational therapy, social workers, and potentially home care and hospice
	  • Supportive therapy, including assisted ventilation (e.g., noninvasive positive-pressure ventilation) and addressing feeding needs
	• Mainstays of acute therapy: Monitor forced vital capacity and negative inspiratory force with low threshold for intubation and mechanical ventilation with admission to the ICU. Patients should receive IVIG or plasma exchange. Glucocorticoids are not helpful
	• If prolongation of life is pursued, tracheostomy and gastrostomy support measures may be placed pre-emptively to avoid emergent need.

CASE 12 | Anterior Cord Syndrome

A 32-year-old man with sickle cell disease presents to the ED 30 minutes after a witnessed fall in which he experienced a profound loss of motor strength. There was no preceding trauma. On exam, the patient is alert, oriented, and his mental status exam is unremarkable. The patient has 0/5 strength in bilateral upper and lower extremities and bilateral biceps, triceps, brachioradialis, patellar, and Achilles tendons are areflexic. Pinprick sensation is absent below C4 dermatome. Proprioception, vibration, and light touch are normal bilaterally throughout the extremities.

Conditions with Similar Presentations	**Central cord syndrome:** Typically caused by slow-growing lesions (e.g., syringomyelia or intermedullary tumors) or by hyperextension injury in patients with chronic cervical spondylosis. This disorder primarily affects the ventral commissure, the medial aspect of the corticospinal tract, and the anterior horn white matter. This will cause pain and temperature loss at and around the level of injury, but not above or below. Further, upper extremity weakness tends to be worse than lower extremity.

CASE 12 | Anterior Cord Syndrome *(continued)*

Conditions with Similar Presentations	**Posterior cord syndrome:** Primarily caused by MS, tabes dorsalis (neurosyphilis), Friedrich ataxia, subacute combined degeneration (B12 deficiency), tumors, cervical spondylotic myelopathy, and atlantoaxial subluxation. Patients will have severe gait ataxia due to proprioception loss, and some paresthesias. Proprioception and vibration are primarily affected, and there can be some motor weakness if the corticospinal tracts are involved. Descending autonomic tracts can be affected, leading to bladder incontinence.
Initial Diagnostic Tests	CT angiography of aorta and MRI of spinal cord
Next Steps in Management	Determine and treat the specific etiology of the infarction
Discussion	The anterior spinal artery (ASA) provides blood flow to the anterior two-thirds of the spine. Therefore, occlusion or hypoperfusion of the ASA will cause anterior spinal cord infarction (see figure). The ASA originates from both vertebral arteries and receives collaterals from the aorta, the largest of which is the *artery of Adamkiewicz*. This is why the CT angiogram is the initial diagnostic test. Spontaneous spinal cord infarction is exceedingly rare due to the extent of collateral blood flow. A thrombus in the artery of Adamkiewicz can cause anterior cord syndrome as well. Schematic of spinal cord lesions. A. Anterior cord syndrome. B. Central cord syndrome. C. Posterior cord syndrome. (Reproduced with permission from Aminoff M, Greenberg D, Simon R: Clinical Neurology, 9th ed. New York: McGraw-Hill Education; 2015.) **History/Physical Exam:** Acute onset of quadriplegia. • Causes include: Aortic surgeries, radiation, tumors, disc herniation, vertebral burst fractures, or occlusive etiologies (e.g., sickle cell disease, polycythemia, decompression sickness, atherosclerosis, embolism, and vasculitis). • Early presentation of anterior cord syndrome will include areflexia (spinal shock), and UMN signs (hyperreflexia) will eventually develop over days to weeks. • It takes 2–3 spinal segments for the second-order neurons of the spinothalamic tract to decussate across the anterior commissure, so pain and temperature sensation will be affected a couple of segments below the topmost level of spinal cord infarction. • Most cases affect bilateral anterior cord, but in the case of unilateral cord infarction, contralateral pain and temperature is lost below the lesion.

CASE 12 | Anterior Cord Syndrome *(continued)*

Discussion	**Diagnostics:** • CT angiogram is necessary to evaluate whether an aortic dissection or aneurysm is the cause. • A spinal MRI should be performed to image the anterior cord infarction and provide a better view of the extent of damage. **Management:** • Next steps depend on the specific etiology of the infarction. • Antithrombotics, radiation, surgery, antibiotics, anti-inflammatories, and other medication may be used to resolve the underlying issue. • Infectious and/or inflammatory aortitis has been implicated, most notably by *Salmonella* spp. • The patient may also have urinary retention, so Foley catheter placement may be warranted. • The process of recovery is often limited and requires intense physical therapy once the underlying etiology is addressed.

CASE 13 | Myotonic Dystrophy

A 21-year-old man with no significant past medical history presents with months of progressive weakness of hands and feet, and drooping eyes. He has also noted a receding hairline and atrophy of skeletal muscles, including distal extremities and face. He mentions that his father had similar symptoms, but they started in his 30s. His vital signs are unremarkable except for mild tachypnea. On physical exam, the patient has a long and narrow face with mild ptosis. When prompted to grip the examiner's fingers firmly and let go rapidly, relaxation of the fingers is delayed. Forearm and hand intrinsic muscles are 3/5 strength, foot dorsiflexors are 4/5, but the remainder of the motor exam is 5/5. Reflexes are 2+ throughout and gait is intact.

Conditions with Similar Presentations	**Duchenne and Becker muscular dystrophies:** Are the two other most common inherited muscular dystrophies. Both are X-linked recessive deletions of the dystrophin gene (Xp21). Normal dystrophin protects the sarcolemmal membrane from degradation by intracellular proteases. In its absence, there is muscle necrosis and increased calcium influx. Duchenne usually begins at ages 2–3 years and Becker presents over a later and wider range from age 5 to age 60. In addition to progressive weakness, cardiomyopathy is a key finding, as is calf pseudohypertrophy, with associated Gowers sign where when the patient is asked to sit on the floor and then stand, they will "tripod" with their arms first, push up with their arms, place arms on their knees, and push up to an erect posture. Patients with Duchenne usually live up to 30 years, while patients with Becker may live up to age 70, with heart failure as the leading cause of mortality in both.
Initial Diagnostic Tests	Clinical diagnosis, confirmed with genetic testing
Next Steps in Management	• Physical therapy and membrane-stabilizing drugs (e.g., mexiletine, phenytoin). • Screen for and treat associated abnormalities
Discussion	Myotonic dystrophy is an autosomal dominant disease with variable penetrance that presents with myotonia and progressive muscle weakness in all three major muscle groups: smooth, skeletal, and cardiac. Genetic defects lead to abnormal accumulation of non-translated RNA sequences. These accumulate in the nucleus and interfere with expression of other gene expression. Interference with the muscle chloride channel leads to myotonia. Interference with the insulin receptor leads to hyperinsulinemia. Interference with cardiac troponin T leads to arrhythmias and cardiomyopathy. Other manifestations are frontal balding in men, cataracts, infertility, hypothyroidism, and cognitive impairment. There are two types of myotonic dystrophy: the more common *DM1* (chromosome 19q13.3, resulting in CTG repeats) and the milder *DM2* (chromosome 3q21.3, resulting in CCTG repeats). Similar to Huntington disease, *DM1* severity and age of onset is correlated with the CTG repeat size. The spectrum of disease severity from mild to severe is: *DM2*, mild *DM1*, classic *DM1*, childhood *DM1*, and congenital *DM1*. Because of the involvement of cardiac and respiratory muscles, lifespan is reduced, with death often occurring in the fifth to sixth decade of life secondary to cardiac or respiratory failure.

CASE 13 | Myotonic Dystrophy *(continued)*

Discussion	**History:** Progressive muscle weakness in distal extremities and face. May have associated baldness (in men), endocrine symptoms (e.g., glucose intolerance, hypothyroid, hypogonadism), symptoms of heart failure, cardiac conduction abnormalities, cataracts (blurred vision). Later on, patients can develop dysphagia, dysarthria, and respiratory muscle involvement. A major clue will be a positive family history given the autosomal dominant inheritance pattern. Some patients may also have muscle pain.
	Physical Exam: Diffuse hypotonia and weakness, especially involving the muscles of the face, neck, forearm, and distal extremities. Patients may have ptosis, lid lag, temporal wasting, flat affect, and limb muscle atrophy. Reflexes unchanged until late in diseases. Another specific finding includes grip myotonia, or the inability to release a person's hand after a handshake due to delayed muscle relaxation.
	Diagnostics:
	• Clinical diagnosis confirmed by genetic testing for abnormal *DM1* and *DM2* genes showing expanded CTG repeats in the dystrophia myotonica protein kinase (*DMPK*) gene or CCTG repeats in the *ZNF9* (*CNBP*) gene.
	• Screen for associated abnormalities with slit lamp examination for cataracts, ECG for cardiac conduction abnormalities, and CMP/CBC.
	• EMG is not necessary for diagnosis, but specific myotonia features may be present.
	Management:
	• Multidisciplinary team including neurology, psychiatry, occupational and physical therapy.
	• Orthotics for foot drop or gait instability. Later on, patients may need walker or wheelchair for ambulation.
	• Membrane-stabilizing drugs (e.g., mexiletine, phenytoin) slow progression and can help treat myotonia.
	• For muscle pain, can consider NSAIDs, mexiletine, gabapentin, tricyclic antidepressants, and low-dose glucocorticoids.
	• Treat any other ophthalmologic, cardiac, respiratory, or GI symptoms as needed.

CASE 14 | Multiple Sclerosis (MS)

A 27-year-old woman presents to the ED with slowly progressive difficulty in speaking for the past 5 days. Four months ago, she also had an episode of slowly progressive left-sided arm weakness that lasted for 2 weeks and subsequently resolved by the time she was able to see her primary care physician. Her vital signs are within normal limits. On exam, her pupils are equally reactive, and her extraocular muscles are intact. She has right-sided facial weakness. Her strength is 4/5 in her left arm and 5/5 throughout the remainder of her extremities. Sensation is intact bilaterally. When she flexes her neck, she experiences shooting pain that radiates into both arms. Her left biceps reflex is 3+; the remaining reflexes and her gait are normal. A non-contrast CT head is negative for hemorrhage and shows no signs of edema or grey-white junction effacement.

Conditions with Similar Presentations	**Neuromyelitis optica (NMO) spectrum disorders:** Another autoimmune CNS demyelinating disorder that exclusively affects the optic nerve and spinal cord, but usually not the brain. Presentation includes symptoms of optic neuritis and transverse myelitis. It is caused by IgG autoantibodies against the aquaporin-4 (AQP4) proteins found in astrocytes.
	Acute ischemic stroke: A negative head CT, in an otherwise healthy young woman is unlikely to be an ischemic stroke. However, MRI will be helpful to delineate both.
Initial Diagnostic Tests	• Two separate episodes of neurologic deficits occurring in different regions at different times (MacDonald criteria).
	• Check MRI with and without contrast
Next Steps in Management	• High-dose glucocorticoids (e.g., methylprednisolone) for acute flares
	• Followed by long-term disease-modifying therapy.

CASE 14 | Multiple Sclerosis (MS) *(continued)*

Discussion	MS is the most common autoimmune inflammatory disease of the CNS that results in multifocal areas of demyelination *disseminated across space and time*. It is caused by autoimmune destruction of oligodendrocytes, the myelin-producing cells of the CNS, with relative early preservation of axons. This subsequently leads to astroglial scarring and the formation of white matter plaques, most commonly observed in highly myelinated areas of the CNS. There are several forms of MS, but the most common is relapsing-remitting MS, which involves waxing and waning of multifocal areas of demyelination resulting in symptoms that partially or completely resolve due to prolonged ability to remyelinate, before new lesions develop. Eventually, these remyelination pathways can become exhausted, and the disease is then called secondary progressive MS. A small number of patients present with primary progressive MS, which does not have periods of remission, is much less responsive to disease-modifying drugs, and carries a poor prognosis. Disease-modifying drugs have a diverse range of mechanisms of action that are beyond the scope of this book but often help reduce activation of B or T lymphocytes and therefore autoimmune destruction of myelin and oligodendrocytes.
	
	History/Physical Exam:
	• Risk factors: MS is more common in women, especially those under age 50, as well as individuals who live further from the equator. Additional risk factors include vitamin D deficiency and prior exposure to Epstein-Barr virus (EBV).
	• There are numerous potential presenting signs and symptoms of MS, depending on the area of demyelination. This can include weakness (UMN signs including paraparesis, spasticity, hypertonia, hyperreflexia), sensory symptoms (numbness, paresthesias), and bowel or bladder dysfunction.
	• **Lhermitte sign** is an "electrical" shooting pain in the neck that radiates into both arms by tapping or flexing the neck (seen in the case above).
	• Patients may also demonstrate the **Uhthoff phenomenon**, whereby elevated external temperature (e.g., hot weather, exercise, shower) results in temporary worsening of symptoms as nerve impulses are preferentially slowed in demyelinated nerves.
	• Patients commonly have ophthalmologic presentations, the two most common being internuclear ophthalmoplegia (INO) and optic neuritis.
	  • INO involves demyelination of the medial longitudinal fasciculus (MLF), which is when the pathway for horizontal gaze to stimulate the contralateral oculomotor (CN III) nerve for adduction of the contralateral eye becomes impaired. The ipsilateral abducens (CN VI) nerve that abducts the ipsilateral eye does *not* travel through the MLF and therefore is *not* affected.
	  • Optic neuritis involves demyelination of the optic nerve, which can lead to sudden unilateral ocular pain with central scotoma, decreased visual acuity, poor color saturation imaging, and a relative afferent pupillary defect on exam.
	• Finally, patients may also have nonspecific symptoms including fatigue, sleep disturbances, and cognitive impairment.
	
	Diagnostics:
	• Two separate episodes of neurologic deficits occurring in different regions at different times (MacDonald criteria). Most commonly visual (decreased and/or double vision).
	• MRI with and without contrast is the preferred imaging modality and should be considered throughout the neuraxis.
	  • A common finding on brain MRI is periventricular plaques ("Dawson's fingers" termed by their appearance on sagittal MRI), or T2 hyperintensities near the corpus callosum.
	  • Spinal cord MRI will reveal focal T2 hyperintensities, depending on regions affected.
	  • Active demyelinating lesions (suggestive of an acute flare) will show enhancement with gadolinium contrast, while chronic lesions do not enhance.

CASE 14 | Multiple Sclerosis (MS) *(continued)*

Discussion

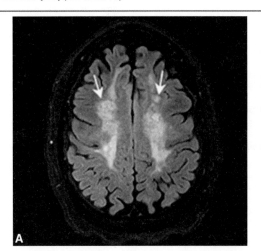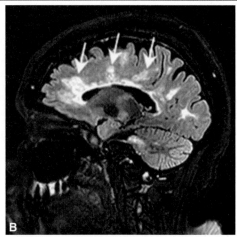

Magnetic resonance cranial images from a woman with multiple sclerosis. A. T2-weighted axial image shows bright signal abnormalities in white matter (*arrows*), typical for multiple sclerosis. B. Sagittal T2-FLAIR image shows periventricular hyperintense lesions (Dawson's fingers; *arrows*) representative of demyelination in multiple sclerosis. (Reproduced with permission from Cunningham FG Leveno KL, et al, eds. Williams Obstetrics. 26th ed. New York: McGraw Hill; 2022.)

- LP can be performed to rule out other causes.
  - The classic LP finding consists of a significantly elevated population of immunoglobulins targeting a few antigens (oligoclonal) as opposed to a single motif (monoclonal). These occur in high concentration within the CSF, and diluted in the serum, which is known as the presence of **oligoclonal bands**.
  - CSF shows the presence of oligoclonal bands, increased IgG index, and the presence of myelin basic protein (due to destruction of myelin).
  - CSF leukocyte count may be normal or slightly elevated, with a lymphocytic predominance.
  - Patients can be tested for AQP4 antibodies (for NMO) and other autoantibodies to rule out potential differential diagnoses.

Management: Treatment of MS is generally divided into the treatment of acute exacerbations/relapses and long-term treatment with disease-modifying therapy to prevent exacerbations and slow the progression of disease.
- Treat acute exacerbation with high-dose glucocorticoids (e.g., IV methylprednisolone for 5 days).
- Patients who are refractory to glucocorticoid treatment can be considered for alternative approaches, including ACTH, IVIG, or plasma exchange.
- To slow progression and reduce relapses, treat with disease-modifying therapy (e.g., beta-interferons, dimethyl fumarate, glatiramer acetate, mitoxantrone, teriflunomide, fingolimod, ozanimod, ponesimod, siponimod, cladribine, alemtuzumab, natalizumab, ocrelizumab).
  - Ocrelizumab has been shown to slow progression in primary progressive MS.
  - Natalizumab, has been associated with activation of JC virus and progressive multifocal leukoencephalopathy (PML). This a rare but serious complication of immunosuppression
  - Assess response to treatment with periodic MRI.
- Additional symptom management includes:
  - Baclofen for spasticity
  - Antimuscarinic agents (e.g., oxybutynin) for bladder dysfunction
  - TCAs or anticonvulsants for pain and seizures
  - Patients with low vitamin D should be provided with supplementation.
- Multidisciplinary support includes: physical, occupational, speech, and behavioral therapy. Patients may eventually require assistive devices for ambulation.

SENSORY ABNORMALITIES

Sensation is broadly divided into somatic, special, and visceral sensory input. Somatic input involves sensory receptors on afferent nerves predominant in the skin and mucosal membranes that convey sensations of touch, pain, temperature, vibration, and proprioception. Special input involves the special senses of vision, hearing, taste, and smell. Finally, visceral sensory input relates to receptors on the visceral organs which are used to sense mechanical and chemical changes (e.g., distension, visceral pain, nausea, hunger).

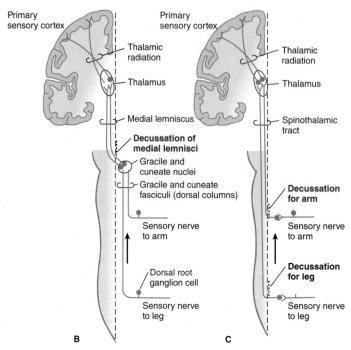

Different trades decussate at different levels. B. Dorsal column–medial meniscus pathway. C. Spinothalamic tract. (Reproduced with permission from Waxman SG. Clinical Neuroanatomy. 29th ed. New York: McGraw Hill; 2020.)

In this section, we will focus mainly on somatic sensation, which is generally conveyed from the periphery to the brain in two main pathways:

1. **Dorsal column-medial lemniscus pathway**—proprioception, vibration, and fine discriminative touch.

    a. First-order neuron with cell body in the dorsal root ganglia has one process that extends along spinal nerves to the periphery (forms dermatomes) and the other process which enters the dorsal root entry zone of the spinal cord.

    b. Sensation is arranged somatotopically with the medial fasciculus gracilis (sensation from legs and lower trunk) and lateral fasciculus cuneatus (sensation from arms, upper trunk, and neck).

    c. Ascends in the dorsal columns and synapses onto second-order neurons within the caudal medulla in the nucleus gracilis or cuneatus. Axons of these second-order neurons then decussate within the medulla and form the medial lemniscus, which ascends contralaterally.

    d. The medial lemniscus synapses within the ventral posterior lateral (VPL) nucleus of the thalamus, whereby third-order neurons then project through the posterior limb of the internal capsule and go to the primary somatosensory cortex.

2. **Anterolateral pathways** (particularly the **spinothalamic tract**)—pain, temperature, and crude touch.

    e. First-order neurons with cell bodies in dorsal root ganglia have one process that extends along spinal nerves to the periphery (forms dermatomes) and the other which enters the dorsal root entry zone. However, compared to the dorsal column pathway, these neurons immediately synapse within the dorsal horn (although some ascend a few segments in Lissauer's tract).

    f. Second-order neurons then decussate within the spinal cord anterior commissure and ascend contralaterally in the anterolateral white matter, although this decussation takes a few spinal cord segments to occur.

    g. Axons of second-order neurons ascend contralaterally and ultimately synapse with third-order neurons, also located within the VPL nucleus of the thalamus, which then project to the primary somatosensory cortex.

Deficits in somatosensory pathways may often present with a distinct "sensory level" due to the corresponding affected spinal nerve or cord region. Therefore, it is helpful to know dermatomal distributions and trace sensory deficits to a particular spinal cord level on your physical exam (see figure). Deficits in special sensations such as hearing and vision are discussed later in this chapter.

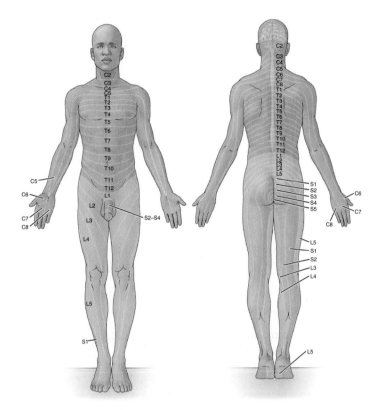

Schematic of dermatomes. (Reproduced with permission from Martin JH. Neuroanatomy: Text and Atlas. 4th ed. New York, NY: McGraw Hill; 2012.)

CASE 15 | Complex Regional Pain Syndrome (CPRS)

A 43-year-old woman presents with severe, stabbing pain in her right arm for the past 3 weeks. She had carpal tunnel release earlier this year complicated by a hematoma and has since had intermittent periods of debilitating pain. She notices decreased ability to detect temperature and increased sweating from her right forearm to her palm. Her left arm is normal. Her only other medical condition is generalized anxiety disorder. Vital signs are within normal limits. On exam, her right hand is swollen and erythematous. She has tenderness to gentle palpation of the right forearm and first to third digits, part of the fourth but not the fifth. Passive and active range are limited in her right hand, and she has decreased strength in the distribution of the median nerve. The rest of her exam is normal.

Conditions with Similar Presentations	**Peripheral neuropathy:** Can also present in pain, although pain is often described as burning or shooting pain that may radiate along the course of a nerve. Patients may have distal sensory loss and/or motor dysfunction. Common causes include diabetes mellitus, chronic alcohol use, HIV, vasculitis, or certain medications (e.g., chemotherapeutic agents such as vincristine). It is usually bilateral and symmetric.
	Compartment syndrome: A surgical emergency caused by increased tissue pressure within a compartment in a limb that compresses vessels and nerves, resulting in ischemia and neuropathy. Patients have severe burning pain, paresthesia, numbness, and late-stage compartment syndrome can result in acute limb ischemia with the six P's of pallor, pain, paresthesia, pulselessness, poikilothermia, and paralysis.

CASE 15 | Complex Regional Pain Syndrome (CPRS) *(continued)*

Initial Diagnostic Tests	Clinical diagnosis
Next Steps in Management	• Physical and occupational therapy • Pain management
Discussion	CRPS, previously known as reflex sympathetic dystrophy, is a neuropathic pain disorder characterized by severe pain that is excessive in duration and/or severity compared to the inciting event. **History/Physical Exam:** • More commonly presents in women between the fourth and fifth decade of life. May occur spontaneously but more common after trauma, or in association with medical conditions such as carpal tunnel syndrome or psychiatric conditions such as anxiety or depression. • Signs and symptoms: Unilateral increased pain in an extremity associated with abnormalities of temperature sensation and increased sweating. May be a prior history of trauma/surgery in the area. • Upper extremities are more commonly affected due to increased number of autonomic nerve fibers. There is increased sensation with noxious stimuli (hyperalgesia) or stimuli that would not normally cause pain (allodynia), autonomic symptoms (hypo/hyperthermia), motor symptoms (decreased range of motion, tremors), edema, and/or hypo/hyperhidrosis. **Diagnostics:** • CPRS is a clinical diagnosis and does not require imaging or EMG. • If ordered, x-ray may show patchy, generalized demineralization or underlying pathology (i.e., from carpal tunnel syndrome) that increases risk of CPRS. **Management:** • First-line treatment involves exercise and desensitization techniques with physical and occupational therapy in addition to patient education. • Any comorbid psychiatric conditions should also be treated. • Pain management includes NSAIDs, antineuropathic medications (e.g., gabapentin, pregabalin, amitriptyline), and topical lidocaine or capsaicin.

Sensory Abnormality Mini-Cases

Cases	Key Findings
Brown-Séquard Syndrome	**Hx:** History of trauma (blunt or penetrating), severe disc herniation, spinal hematomas, transverse myelitis, tumors, or vertebral artery dissection. **PE:** Ipsilateral flaccid paralysis at the level of the lesion, ipsilateral loss of vibration, proprioception, and light touch below the level of the lesion, and contralateral loss of pain, temperature, and crude touch below the lesion. **Diagnostics:** MRI of the spine showing hyperintensity of the entire side of the spinal cord, along with possible bony damage in the area likely secondary to trauma. **Management:** Supportive care and physical therapy. **Discussion:** Brown-Séquard syndrome is caused by hemisection of the spinal cord with resultant motor and sensory loss in a characteristic pattern. Damage to anterior horn cells leads to ipsilateral LMN signs; damage to the dorsal column leads to ipsilateral loss of vibration, proprioception, and light touch; and damage to the spinothalamic tract leads to contralateral loss of pain, temperature, and crude touch. If the lesion occurs above the level of T1, damage to the oculosympathetic pathway may result in an ipsilateral Horner syndrome.	 Loss of all sensation Impaired pain and temperature sensation Impaired proprioception, vibration, 2-point discrimination, and joint and position sensation Brown–Séquard syndrome with lesion at left tenth thoracic level (motor deficits not shown). (Reproduced with permission from Waxman SG. Clinical Neuroanatomy. 29th ed. New York: McGraw Hill; 2020.)

Sensory Abnormality Mini-Cases *(continued)*

Brown-Séquard Syndrome	Spinal cord injury can also result in **neurogenic shock**, a form of distributive shock associated with loss of sympathetic tone resulting in unopposed parasympathetic tone driven by the vagus nerve. This results in systemic vasodilation, resulting in decreased systemic venous resistance (afterload), central venous pressures (preload), and cardiac output. Most commonly occurs following injury to the cervical spine.

Trigeminal Neuralgia	**Hx:** Patient with paroxysmal attacks of severe, unilateral stabbing and shock-like facial pain in the distribution of the trigeminal nerve (CN V) lasting from seconds to 2 minutes and is triggered by innocuous stimuli (brushing teeth, chewing, talking, light touch).
	
	PE: Pain attack may be triggered by light touch to trigger zones. During an episode there may be facial muscle spasm.
	
	Diagnostics: Diagnostic criteria consist of:
	1. Recurrent paroxysms of unilateral facial pain in distribution of trigeminal nerve.
	2. Pain lasts from seconds to minutes AND severe AND quality is electric chock-like, shooting, stabbing, or sharp.
	3. Pain is precipitated by innocuous stimuli.
	  • Consider MRI/MRA to assess for structural or neurodegenerative causes.
	  • Trigeminal reflex testing can be obtained if patient cannot have MRI.
	
	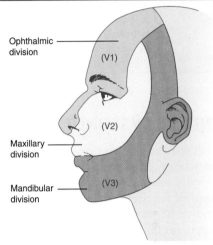
	Sensory distribution of nerve V. (Reproduced with permission from Waxman SG. Clinical Neuroanatomy. 29th ed. New York: McGraw Hill; 2020.)
	
	Management:
	• First-line treatment is carbamazepine or oxcarbazepine.
	• If medical therapy fails, consider neurosurgical microvascular decompression.
	
	Discussion: Trigeminal neuralgia involves abnormalities of the CN V root secondary to neurovascular compression, MS, space-occupying lesions, or is idiopathic. The pain most often occurs in the distribution of V_2 (cheeks to nasal cavity) and V_3 (jawline). Most often unilateral; if bilateral and in a young women, should evaluate for MS.
	
	Facial pain due to painful trigeminal neuropathy can also occur with an **acute herpes zoster** infection or post infection, which is often associated with more continuous pain and history of unilateral dermatomal distribution of vesicles on an erythematous base.

Diabetic Neuropathy	**Hx:** Patient with diabetes mellitus and numbness and paresthesias in a symmetrical stocking-and-glove distribution. **PE:** Loss of vibratory and proprioception sensation with hyporeflexia in distal upper and lower extremities. Sensory ataxia and motor weakness observed later in disease course. Nontender ulcers and joint deformity (Charcot joint) can also be observed. **Diagnostics:** • Clinical diagnosis • Consider ruling out other causes: ethanol, HIV, HCV, medications (e.g., isoniazid, nitrofurantoin, cisplatin), nutritional deficiencies (e.g., B12/folate, B1, B6), autoimmune (TSH, free T4), malignancies (serum protein electrophoresis) and paraneoplastic. • Consider EMG and NCV **Management:** • Tight glucose control • Education on appropriate foot care to prevent cutaneous and bony injury • Symptomatic treatment includes antineuropathic medications (e.g., gabapentin, pregabalin, amitriptyline)

Sensory Abnormality Mini-Cases *(continued)*

Diabetic Neuropathy	**Discussion:** Diabetic peripheral neuropathy presents as a slowly progressive distal symmetric polyneuropathy, which is a larger fiber length–dependent neuropathy. Patients are at higher risk for falls, ulcers, and amputations. Small fiber neuropathy is less common, and is characterized by painful paresthesia and burning sensations in the bilateral feet with preservation of proprioception, vibratory sensation, and deep tendon reflexes. Small-fiber neuropathic pain can be treated with several antidepressant, anti-seizure medications, and topical analgesics. Small fiber neuropathy is often associated with autonomic neuropathy and dysfunction (tachycardia, bradycardia, orthostatic hypotension, gastroparesis, neurogenic bladder, impotence). Other less common forms of diabetic neuropathy include peripheral and cranial mononeuropathies, including CN III ischemic neuropathy. Patient should also be evaluated for diabetic retinopathy.

COGNITIVE DYSFUNCTION

Cognition is a broad term that encompasses higher-order functioning and processing, including memory, learning, problem solving, executive function, judgment, perception, comprehension, attention, and production of language. Cognitive dysfunction occurs when a patient is operating below their baseline in any one of these areas, often leading to diminished functional status. Cognitive dysfunction also presents as a uniquely difficult area to assess, as the range of neurodiversity in the world is vast and more difficult to evaluate with the standard exam, but that is exactly what mental status examination sets out to accomplish.

Mental status is the first element tested in the neurological exam because it dictates the patient's ability to participate in the rest of the exam. The clinical evaluation of patients with cognitive symptoms begins with a thorough clinical history and examinations. It is important to obtain collateral information from family members and close friends, since patient recall or insight may be limited. Determining the level of functional impairment (i.e., the impact of cognitive decline on instrumental and basic daily activities) is critical for disease staging and appropriate counseling.

Mild cognitive impairment (MCI) is defined as cognitive impairment that does not interfere with activities of daily living, is not severe enough to classify the patient as demented, and patient retains general cognitive function. When cognitive decline interferes with independent function, patients meet criteria for major neurocognitive disorder or **dementia**. The term "delirium" is synonymous with encephalopathy or acute confusional state. The causes of delirium are many, and delirium can coexist with other causes of cerebral dysfunction, such as dementia or stroke, thus making diagnosis potentially challenging. The presence or absence of other neurological symptoms, as well as the time course of onset, help differentiate delirium from other disorders of mental status. It is also important to screen all patients for depression, which can present with dementia-like symptoms, especially in elderly patients ("pseudodementia").

The first goal of the clinical evaluation is to rule out potentially *reversible* causes of cognitive decline by reviewing medical comorbidities, medication and substance use, and environmental exposure. **Neurodegenerative disease** like Alzheimer's disease, dementia with Lewy bodies, and others typically have an insidious onset, are characterized by slow gradual progression, and are *irreversible*. Thus, an acute or subacute change in mental status should raise concern for a nondegenerative process.

CASE 16 | Alzheimer's Disease (AD)

A 73-year-old woman presents to clinic with her spouse for routine examination. The patient does not report any health issues, but her spouse mentions that the patient has been having some difficulty with chores around the house for the past year. The spouse observed the patient on multiple occasions leave dinner in the oven well past burning until the smoke alarm went off. The patient also has been forgetting to water her plants, which has caused some of them to die despite her professed love for gardening and planting. Last week, the patient returned home after driving around for 1 hour on her way to the grocery store but having difficulty remembering the directions of the 5-minute drive. On exam, the patient is alert and oriented to person, place, and time. She can only remember one out of three words at 5 minutes and has difficulty with counting serial sevens. Her Montreal Cognitive Assessment (MoCA) performed in the room is 19/30. All other aspects of the physical exam are unremarkable.

CASE 16 | Alzheimer's Disease (AD) *(continued)*

Conditions with Similar Presentations	**Delirium:** Acute disturbance in cognition, perceptions, alertness, and/or attention, typically with fluctuating symptoms. Patients with underlying dementia are at increased risk. Common causes include adverse effects of medications (e.g., anticholinergics), infections, electrolyte disturbances (sodium, calcium), pain, alcohol or benzodiazepine withdrawal.
	Frontotemporal dementia: Presents with earlier personality changes compared to AD, including compulsive or impulsive behaviors, disinhibition, impaired judgment, aggression, or apathy. This is later followed by memory impairments. On neuroimaging, atrophy of the frontal and temporal lobes. Patients may have aphasia due to involvement of Broca's and/or Wernicke's areas.
	Dementia with Lewy bodies (DLB): Common cause of dementia that is characterized by fluctuating cognition in addition to parkinsonism (tremor, rigidity, bradykinesia, postural instability), visual hallucinations, and REM sleep behavior disorder. Early cognitive dysfunction typically involves visuospatial ability and attention, with memory affected later in disease course. These patients also display extreme sensitivity to antipsychotics, which can worsen their underlying parkinsonism and cause autonomic dysfunction.
Initial Diagnostic Tests	• Clinical diagnosis. Screening tests: MoCA, Mini Mental Status Exam (MMSE), and mini-cognitive assessments. • Check TSH, B12, folate, RPR, ammonia, transaminases, depression screening to rule out reversible causes of cognitive dysfunction. • Neuropsychiatric testing to further characterize the extent of cognitive dysfunction.
Next Steps in Management	• Ensure patient and family buy-in for patient safety • Initial treatment is with cholinesterase inhibitors, and add NMDA receptor antagonist for moderate to severe disease.
Discussion	AD is the most common cause of dementia or major neurocognitive disorder worldwide. The majority of cases are sporadic, with symptoms beginning after the age of 65. Less than 10% of cases are attributed to familial causes, typically with mutations in amyloid precursor protein (APP), presenilin-1, or presenilin-2. The hallmark pathological findings include extracellular deposition of amyloid beta leading to diffuse neuritic plaques (Aβ or senile plaques, panel A) and intracellular hyperphosphorylated tau protein accumulation causing neurofibrillary tangles ("tau tangles," panel B in figure). 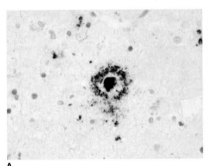 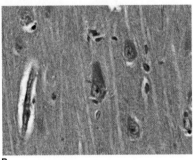 A. Senile plaque. A brown-staining senile plaque with a central core of beta-amyloid protein is in the cerebral cortex of a patient with Alzheimer's disease. B. Neurofibrillary tangle (NFT). A bright red, elongated NFT partially fills the cell body of a large neuron (center of field) in the cerebral cortex of a patient with Alzheimer's disease. (Reproduced with permission from Reisner H. Pathology: A Modern Case Study. 2nd ed. New York: McGraw Hill; 2020.) **History:** • Risk factors: advancing age, family history, hypertension, dyslipidemia, type 2 diabetes mellitus, cerebrovascular disease, Down syndrome (associated with early-onset AD as APP is on chromosome 21), and the apolipoprotein E (ApoE) *e4* haplotype. • Presentation: Slow, insidious progressive disease. The first symptom is typically memory loss, described as declarative episodic memory impairment (memory of events occurring in time and place). Often the patients themselves will not identify cognitive changes, as forgetfulness is a normal sign of aging, but family and friends of the patients will observe changes that exceed the paradigm of "forgetfulness" that cause functional impairment. • Gradual decline in executive function and judgment, problem solving, language, and spatial orientation. • Semantic memory deficits (memory for facts and concepts) develop later.

CASE 16 | Alzheimer's Disease (AD) *(continued)*

Discussion	**Physical Exam:**
	On exam, patients may have decreased scores on MoCA, MMSE, or mini-cognitive screening assessments, although this may vary based on the extent of the disease. Otherwise, neurologic exam is initially normal.
	Diagnostics:
	• Clinical diagnosis, with definitive diagnosis only available via histopathological studies of the brain at autopsy.
	• Patients should undergo testing to rule out reversible causes of cognitive dysfunction (TSH, B12, folate, RPR, ammonia, transaminases, depression screening).
	• Screening tests available include the MoCA, Mini Mental Status Exam (MMSE), and mini-cognitive assessments.
	• Neuropsychiatric testing is often used to further characterize the extent of cognitive dysfunction.
	• While not required, MRI of the brain would show diffuse cortical atrophy, although early on may be more pronounced in the hippocampus and temporal lobes.
	Management:
	• First and foremost, family discussions must be had to ensure patient's safety, whether it is safeguarding against stovetop fires, having someone available to drive the patient places, handling finances, or medication administration.
	• Advance directives and instrumental activities of daily living planning should be done early while patient has whatever decision-making capabilities and lucidity remain.
	• For medical therapy, patients with mild to moderate AD should receive cholinesterase inhibitors (donepezil, rivastigmine, galantamine). Cholinesterase inhibitors can slow progression as cholinergic neurons (particularly in the nucleus basalis of Meynert) tend to degenerate preferentially within the forebrain; however, there is no reversal or cure of disease.
	• For those with moderate to severe dementia, the NMDA receptor antagonist memantine should be added. These medications can decrease rate of decline, likely by reducing the degree of neuronal excitotoxicity.

CASE 17 | Normal Pressure Hydrocephalus (NPH)

An 82-year-old woman presents to the ED with her son, who brought her in following a witnessed fall. She did not hit her head, has some bruising on her right upper arm, and only endorses some mild pain in her right thigh. She says she has had to urgently go to the bathroom recently and while she was walking to the bathroom, she fell. She felt very unsteady on her feet. Her son mentioned she fell 2 weeks ago and she had urinated on herself. She has not had any headaches or changes in vision. She does not use tobacco, alcohol, or other substances. On exam, the patient is alert and oriented to person, place, and year but did not know the exact date. She can remember two of three words in 5 minutes. She has a bruise on her right upper arm and thigh, with mild point tenderness. She has full range of motion and strength is appropriate for her age. She walks with a wide-based gait. She had difficulty answering questions because she seemed distracted. All other aspects of the physical exam were unremarkable.

Conditions with Similar Presentations	**Wernicke encephalopathy:** Caused by chronic thiamine (vitamin B1) deficiency, presents with similar ataxia, dementia, and behavioral changes, including inattentiveness and apathy. However, the patients will also have oculomotor dysfunction (ophthalmoplegia), an important distinguishing factor from NPH. Thiamine deficiency is most commonly caused by chronic alcoholism or malnutrition, so identifying the patient's drinking history will help rule in Wernicke encephalopathy. Thiamine blood levels may be low but the best test is erythrocyte thiamine transketolase activity (ETKA) before and after the addition of thiamine pyrophosphate (TPP).
	Toxic-metabolic encephalopathy: Acute, reversible cause of cognitive dysfunction that encompasses delirium and is defined as global cerebral dysfunction. Some common causes include sepsis, liver disease, and renal disease as well as sodium, calcium, or glucose imbalances. This process occurs much more rapidly than either NPH or Wernicke encephalopathy and will have unremarkable imaging.

CASE 17 | Normal Pressure Hydrocephalus (NPH) *(continued)*

Initial Diagnostic Tests	• Check MRI and LP • Confirm with improved symptoms following CSF removal
Next Steps in Management	• Serial high-volume LPs to remove CSF • Consider ventriculoperitoneal shunt (VPS)
Discussion	NPH is a much less common cause of dementia than AD. The most common cause is idiopathic, and while there are several proposed etiologies, the true mechanism is unknown. Secondary causes of NPH are impaired absorption of CSF due to prior intraventricular or subarachnoid hemorrhage, meningitis with scarring of arachnoid granulations, or periventricular ischemias.

History:

• Symptoms present slowly over months or years with a classic triad of (1) gait ataxia, (2) urinary incontinence, and (3) dementia, which can be remembered as "wobbly, wet, and wacky."

• Gait impairment is usually the first symptom and may appear as a magnetic gait, whereby the patient's feet seem stuck to the floor. The patient will express difficulty with walking and feeling unbalanced, that can progress to falls.

• Urinary incontinence (particularly urge incontinence) presents early as well, and the combination of these symptoms can lead to falls on the way to the bathroom.

• Dementia and cognitive dysfunction present later, and patients are noted to be inattentive, apathetic, and have decreased concentration and executive functioning.

Physical Exam: Abnormal "magnetic" broad-based gait. May have abnormal mental status exam.

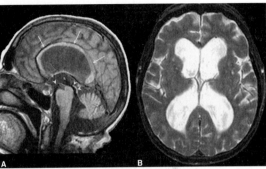

Normal pressure hydrocephalus. A. Sagittal T1-weighted MRI demonstrates dilation of the lateral ventricle and stretching of the corpus callosum (*arrows*), depression of the floor of the third ventricle (*single arrowhead*), and enlargement of the aqueduct (*double arrowheads*). Note the diffuse dilation of the lateral, third, and fourth ventricles with a patent aqueduct, typical of communicating hydrocephalus. B. Axial T2-weighted MRIs demonstrate dilation of the lateral ventricles. This patient underwent successful ventriculoperitoneal shunting. (Reproduced with permission from Loscalzo J, Fauci AS, Kasper DL, et al, eds. Harrison's Principles of Internal Medicine. 21st ed. New York: McGraw Hill; 2022.)

Diagnostics:

• MRI will show evidence of hydrocephalus, with dilation of ventricles and stretching of the corpus callosum (see image).

• Intracranial pressure on LP will be normal (<20 mmHg). Gait improvement 30–60 minutes after removal of 30–50 mL of CSF is confirmatory.

• Rule out other causes of cognitive dysfunction and ataxia with labs (TSH, B12, thiamine RPR).

Management:

In patients that improve after LP, ventriculoperitoneal shunt (VPS) placement should be considered as early as possible in the disease.

Cognitive Dysfunction Mini Cases

| Vascular Dementia | **Key History:**
• Risk factors similar to other atherosclerotic conditions: HTN, HL, CAD, PAD, DM, h/o CVA/TIA, tobacco use.
• Gradual or abrupt progressive decline in cognitive and functional abilities.

Physical Exam:
• Abnormal mini-cognitive screen or MMSE.
• May have changes in orientation
• Neuropsychiatric accompaniments may include depression, abulia, psychoses, and delusions
• Pseudobulbar affect (inappropriate crying or laughing) may occur
• Prior strokes may manifest as aphasia, gait disturbances, motor or sensory deficits

Diagnostics:
• CT head: Will show multiple small areas of prior hypodense infarction and can also rule out acute bleed
• MRI brain (T2 FLAIR, DWI imaging): Will show old infarcts with cortical atrophy and white matter hyperintensities (see image)

Management:
• Supervision of taking medications that will prevent future infarcts (e.g., antihypertensives, statins, and aspirin and/or clopidogrel).
• Functional status: Assess if patient needs assistance with ADLs or if additional care is needed (caregivers, assisted-living)
• Medications: Depending on degree of progression, cholinesterase inhibitors (donepezil or galantamine) may be used

Discussion:

Caused by infarction in either large or small arteries within the brain. Patients with large artery infarctions present in a stepwise fashion, with patients having abrupt changes in functional status that are often irreversible. Patients with small artery infarctions can also have a more gradual declining course which may be challenging to differentiate from other forms of progressive dementia such as AD. | 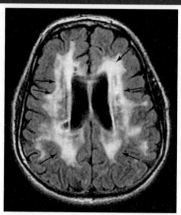
Diffuse white matter disease. Axial fluid-attenuated inversion recovery (FLAIR) magnetic resonance image through the lateral ventricles reveals multiple areas of hyperintensity (*arrows*) involving the periventricular white matter as well as the corona radiata and striatum. Although seen in some individuals with normal cognition, this appearance is more pronounced in patients with dementia of a vascular etiology. (Reproduced with permission from Jameson JL, Fauci AS, Kasper DL, et al, eds. Harrison's Principles of Internal Medicine. 20th ed. New York, NY: McGraw Hill; 2019.) |
| Progressive Multifocal Leukoencephalopathy (PML) | **Hx:**
• Seen in patients with severe immunosuppression (e.g., AIDS, leukemia, organ transplant recipients, certain immunomodulatory medications such as natalizumab).
• Presents with decline in mental status, change in vision, and difficulty with balance and gait, possible focal weakness or loss in sensation.

PE:
• Abnormal mental status and decrease in orientation
• Focal motor and sensory deficits may be seen
• Ataxia
• Decreased visual acuity

Diagnostics:
• CT with contrast or MRI brain: Multifocal white matter lesions/hyperintensities without mass effect or surrounding edema that are non-enhancing with contrast.
• LP: CSF analysis with PCR will be positive for JC virus (sensitivity of ~95%). WBC elevated but <20 and protein elevated but <100. |

Cognitive Dysfunction Mini Cases *(continued)*

Progressive Multifocal Leukoencephalopathy (PML)	**Management:** • PML has no specific treatment • Survival is improved if the cause of the immunosuppression is removed or treated **Discussion:** • PML is a life-threatening neurological disorder caused by reactivation of the JC virus (a polyomavirus typically acquired early in life, with most individuals remaining asymptomatic). This virus injures the myelin-producing oligodendroglial cells in the CNS, leading to demyelination, neuronal dysfunction. • Malignancy, specifically lymphoproliferative and myeloproliferative disease, is the most common predisposing condition to PML.
Creutzfeldt-Jakob Disease (CJD)	**History/Physical Exam:** • Often seen in younger patients than expected for onset of dementia (e.g., age 40s–60s) • Rapidly progressive decline in memory cognition, orientation and behavioral changes. • Increased startle responses and startle myoclonus (an involuntary muscle spasm that is often triggered by a benign stimulus) • May have hallucinations, change in gait • UMN signs: Hyperreflexia, spasticity, Babinski, and Hoffman signs • Cerebellar signs: Nystagmus, ataxia • Basal ganglia involvement: Dystonia, parkinsonism • Focal motor and sensory deficits **Diagnostics:** • Diagnosis is clinical, based on rapid onset of symptoms at a younger age • MRI shows hyperintensities in the cortex and corpus striatum caudate head and putamen Abnormal intensity also seen in superior frontal gyrus, superior parietal lobule, cingulate gyrus, and insular cortex • EEG shows periodic sharp-wave complexes • CSF detection of 14-3-3 protein has a 90% sensitivity and an 80% specificity • Definitive diagnosis made on autopsy showing spongiform degeneration of cortex **Management:** • Palliative management, with attention to counseling, social services, and hospice evaluation • Benzodiazepines may be used for myoclonus **Discussion:** • Most common prion disease but still exceedingly rare (one to two cases per million per year) • Abnormally folded proteins induce similar conformational changes in other proteins, resulting in accumulation of neurotoxic proteins throughout the CNS that lead to diffuse, rapid neurodegeneration • 90% of cases are sporadic, and 10% are genetic, with rare cases being iatrogenic (contact with infected neural or ocular tissue), or from contact with contaminated beef (variant CJD, extremely rare) • Incubation period is >10 years. Median survival is <12 months after diagnosis.

MOVEMENT DISORDERS

Movement disorders comprise a group of conditions that cause abnormal involuntary movements or postures, slowness, or difficulty initiating movement. They are not the result of weakness, spasticity, or sensory disturbances. These disorders result from problems of the subcortical systems involved in movement planning, execution, and coordination. Movement disorders are divided into hypokinetic and hyperkinetic.

Parkinsonism

Parkinsonism is the most common type of *hypokinetic* movement disorder. Parkinsonism is a clinical syndrome and not a specific diagnostic entity. It is characterized by the presence of two out of three features: bradykinesia, rigidity, and tremor. Postural instability is common but not a cardinal manifestation of parkinsonism. Parkinsonism can be caused by a number of entities. Secondary parkinsonism should always be excluded prior to the diagnosis of Parkinson disease (PD). The most common cause of secondary parkinsonism is medications, such as dopamine receptors blockers (e.g., haloperidol, metoclopramide) or dopamine-depleting agents (e.g., reserpine, tetrabenazine). Other causes include trauma, vascular insult, and toxins (e.g., MPTP, manganese, CO). Once secondary causes of parkinsonism have been excluded, idiopathic PD (IPD) is the most common cause, responsible for 75% of cases of parkinsonism seen.

The various *hyperkinetic* movement disorders include chorea, dystonia, myoclonus, and tics, but tremor is the most common.

Tremor

Tremor is a rhythmic, involuntary oscillation of a body part. It is described clinically by the location where it develops (hand, feet, head, chin, and/or voice) and the situation which brings it out the most (action, postural, or at rest).

Chorea

Chorea is characterized by unpredictable, irregular, brief, dance-like movements that tend to flow from one body part to the next.

Dystonia

Dystonia is a syndrome characterized by sustained, but not fixed, muscle contractions that cause twisting, repetitive movements resulting in abnormal postures. Dystonia is classified by age of onset, location, and etiology. The exact pathway resulting in dystonia has not been elucidated. While the main manifestations are motor, there may be a sensory component, as illustrated clinically by the geste antagoniste (or sensory trick) present in many (but not all) patients with dystonia, whereby a physical gesture or position (e.g., touching one's face) can temporarily reduce dystonia. This can also be confirmed by imaging studies showing changes in the sensory cortex in dystonic patients.

Myoclonus

Myoclonus refers to sudden, brief, shock-like movements. These movements may be "positive" or "negative." Positive myoclonus results in contraction of a muscle or multiple muscles. In asterixis, or negative myoclonus, there is a brief loss of muscle tone resulting in a flapping-type motion. Myoclonus can be classified several ways including by cause and by origin (e.g., cortical vs. brainstem vs. spinal). One of the most common causes of generalized myoclonus is toxic-metabolic.

CASE 18	Parkinson's Disease (PD)

A 74-year-old left-handed man with hypertension presents with a tremor of his right hand for the past 3 years. The tremor was initially intermittent and over the past year is now always present at rest. He also reports difficulty walking, with a recent fall at home that did not result in any injury. His hypertension is well-controlled on lisinopril. He has no history of trauma, substance use, toxin exposure, or medications with adverse neurologic reactions. His vital signs are stable. On exam, he speaks very softly and he has a right-hand "pill rolling" tremor at rest with right wrist rigidity. When asked to walk from one side of the room to the other, he has difficulty rising from the chair and has a narrow-based gait. He takes small steps and does not swing his arms. When asked to turn around he does so gradually, as if he is standing on a pedestal.

Conditions with Similar Presentations	**Dementia with Lewy bodies (DLB):** May have parkinsonian features, but is characterized by cognitive deficits, hallucinations, and fluctuations in mental status. Other features include sleep disorders and autonomic dysfunction (orthostasis, bladder incontinency). As seen in PD, pathology shows intracellular Lewy bodies (positive for alpha-synuclein) throughout the cortex.
	Essential tremor: Is usually limited to particular regions of the body (i.e., just hands, head), whereas PD affects the whole body and has a characteristic gait. Essential tremor is a high-frequency action tremor that is observed with movement and/or sustained anti-gravity posture (e.g., outstretched arms), and relieved by rest, which is the opposite of the resting tremor seen in PD. Tremor decreases with ethanol ingestion. Patients can be treated with propranolol (beta-blocker) or primidone (anticonvulsant).
Initial Diagnostic Tests	Clinical diagnosis requiring evidence of bradykinesia (slowness in movement) with at least one of the following: rigidity or resting tremor.
Next Steps in Management	Initiate treatment with levodopa-carbidopa

CASE 18 | Parkinson's Disease (PD) *(continued)*

Discussion	PD is a neurodegenerative disease characterized by loss of dopaminergic neurons within the substantia nigra pars compacta. The substantia nigra plays an important role in the nigrostriatal pathway to the basal ganglia, where it is involved in the initiation of movement, and loss of these neurons results in motor dysfunction. Loss of dopaminergic neurons results in a classic depigmentation of the substantia nigra pars compacta, which can be observed on gross specimens of the brain (left brain in panel A compared to normal brain on the right). The pathologic hallmark of PD is the presence of Lewy bodies, which are intracytoplasmic inclusions composed of misfolded alpha-synuclein protein (panel B).

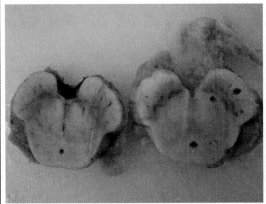 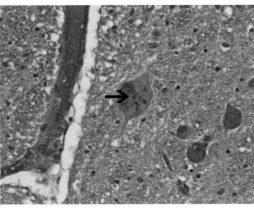

A   B

A, B. (Reproduced with permission from Kemp WL, Burns DK, Travis Brown TG. Pathology: The Big Picture. New York, NY: McGraw Hill; 2008.)

Symptoms of PD commonly manifest past middle age (60s). It is very common and affects 1% of individuals above the age of 60. The disease is typically idiopathic in origin, but a hereditary cause has been linked to some early-onset cases. Additional presentations of parkinsonism related to involvement of the basal ganglia may be due to vascular etiology (subcortical infarcts), drug-induced (neuroleptics), or toxin-induced (MPTP contaminants in synthetic opioids or manganese).

History: PD has both motor and non-motor symptoms.

Motor symptoms:
- The cardinal symptoms can be remembered by the mnemonic "TRAP": resting *T*remor, *R*igidity, *A*kinesia/ Bradykinesia, and *P*ostural instability.
- **Tremor:** A resting tremor often initially starts in one hand and eventually will progresses to the other, and can be described as a "pill-rolling tremor," where the thumb rolls over the medial aspect of the second digit.
- **Rigidity:** Manifests as resistance to passive movement and can be uniform ("lead pipe rigidity") or oscillate throughout the movement ("cogwheel rigidity").
- **Akinesia/Bradykinesia:** Difficulty initiating movements. It is the most common and disabling symptom. Upper extremity concerns are ineffective dextrous movements and trouble buttoning clothes and tying shoelaces. Lower extremity concerns are difficulty rising from a chair or getting out of a car. They notice they are taking smaller steps.
- **Postural instability:** Is not required for the diagnosis, but presents as a sense of imbalance, stooped posture, and frequent falls. The latter is related to bradykinesia. Rapid adjustments of leg position required during normal walking are slowed by the bradykinesia and patients cannot "catch their balance."

Non-motor symptoms:
- Loss of smell (anosmia)
- Autonomic dysfunction symptoms: Orthostasis, constipation, dysphagia, urinary frequency and urge incontinence, and erectile dysfunction
- Mood disorders: Anxiety, depression, abulia
- Sleep disorders: Insomnia, daytime drowsiness with sleep attacks, restless leg syndrome
- Later in the course, one-third of patients may develop cognitive dysfunction **(Parkinson disease dementia)**, with executive and visuospatial dysfunction and visual hallucinations
- Skin: Seborrheic dermatitis and melanoma are more common

CASE 18 | Parkinson's Disease (PD) *(continued)*

Discussion	**Physical Exam:** • Resting tremor in hands (most common) legs, feet, lips, tongue. Tremor decreases with action. • Bradykinesia (finger tapping and rapid alternative movement with amplitude and speed decrement). • Rigidity of extremities. • Lack of facial expression ("masked face") and decreased blinking due to bradykinesia of facial muscles. • Micrographia (small handwriting). • Hypophonia. • Stooped posture. • Gait abnormalities: Shuffling gait of many small steps that speeds up as the person walks (festinating gait). Gait is narrow based. When asked to turn around, patient does so as if turning on a pedestal. Reduced or lack of arm swing **Diagnostics:** Clinical diagnosis of bradykinesia plus at least one: tremor or rigidity. • No other diagnostic tests or images required unless concern for other causes of symptoms. **Management:** Treatment options are based on increasing dopaminergic tone or decreasing cholinergic tone within the basal ganglia. A detailed table of PD medications is provided in the table below. Here is a brief outline of when they are used: • Levodopa/carbidopa: First-line, especially for older patients. • Dopamine agonists (ropinirole, pramipexole). Alternate first-line, especially for young patients, who will be most likely to experience adverse motor effects after 5–10 years of levodopa/carbidopa. • MAO inhibitors (selegiline, rasagiline, safinamide): Initial treatment for mild disease in young patients. • COMT inhibitors (entacapone, tolcapone, opicapone): Adjunct to levodopa/carbidopa if adverse motor events occur. • Muscarinic antagonists (benztropine, trihexyphenidyl): Used to reduce tremor • Amantadine: Initial therapy in young patients or added to levodopa/carbidopa to treat dyskinesia when they occur.
Additional Considerations	**Surgical Considerations:** Once complications of therapy have arisen that cannot be adequately addressed with further medical management, stereotactic brain surgery (deep brain stimulation of the subthalamic nucleus or globus pallidus) can be considered.

Medications Used for Parkinson's Disease

Medications	Mechanism	Adverse Effects and Contraindications	Additional Considerations
Levodopa-carbidopa	Composed of L-DOPA and carbidopa. Carbidopa inhibits DOPA decarboxylase, reducing peripheral conversion of L-DOPA to dopamine to reduce peripheral side effects.	Nausea, hallucinations, confusion, agitation, postural hypotension. Over 5–10 years increased risk of on/off phenomenon, dyskinesias and dystonias.	First-line treatment for PD. 50% or more patients develop motor fluctuations and dyskinesia after 5–10 years (e.g., on/off phenomenon).
Ropinirole, pramipexole	Dopamine agonists.	Peripheral toxicity: Nausea, postural hypotension Central toxicity: Decreased impulse control, hallucinations, confusion	Alternate first-line therapy, especially in younger patients.
Selegiline, rasagiline, safinamide	Inhibits MAO-B enzyme involved in the central metabolism of dopamine. Blocks free radical formation.	May increase levodopa side effects.	Used as monotherapy in patients with mild disease or as an adjunct therapy to levodopa in patients with motor fluctuation.
Entacapone, tolcapone, opicapone	Inhibits COMT enzyme involved in central and peripheral metabolism of dopamine.	May increase levodopa side effects.	Used as an adjunct to levodopa.
Benztropine, trihexyphenidyl	Muscarinic antagonists.	Constipation, urinary difficulty, blurry vision.	Use in patients for reduction of tremor.
Amantadine	Increases dopamine release, inhibits dopamine reuptake, stimulate dopamine receptors, anticholinergic.	Depression or anxiety, blurry vision, dizziness, lightheadedness, hypotension.	Used in mild disease in young patients. Used in combination with levodopa to reduce levodopa-induced dyskinesias.

CASE 19 | Essential Tremor (ET)

A 60-year-old woman presents to the clinic with a tremor that affects her hands when she writes and when she holds eating utensils. This began in her teenage years, but it has not bothered her until the prior year. Her father and paternal grandfather had a similar tremor. On examination, she alert and oriented, her gait is normal, and there is no tremor at rest. The tremor is noticeable with finger-nose-finger maneuver and worsens considerably as she approaches her nose. Postural tremor with outstretched arms is also observed.

Conditions with Similar Presentations	**Enhanced physiologic tremor:** Postural action tremor of the hands that is an exaggeration of the 10–12 Hz tremor present in everyone. Unlike essential tremor, not seen with goal-directed action (e.g., finger-to-nose testing). **Metabolic or endocrine derangements:** Hyperthyroidism, hepatic encephalopathy, hypoglycemia, pheochromocytoma. **Drug-induced action tremor:** Thyroid drugs, corticosteroids, lithium, B2-adrenergic receptor agonists, SSRIs, valproic acid.
Initial Diagnostic Tests	• Clinical diagnosis • Would review medications and evaluate for any contributing metabolic or endocrine etiologies
Next Steps in Management	• Consider medicine if significant disability from the tremor • Propranolol and primidone are first line
Discussion	ET is the most frequent neurologic disease that causes tremor occurring in 1–5% of the general population. There is a strong genetic predisposition (50% of patients report positive family history) but a single genetic cause has not been identified. There is a bimodal age of onset, typically beginning in the second or sixth decade. The pathophysiology of ET is unknown, as well as the neurochemical basis of the disease. Dysfunction of the cerebellar thalamic connections has been implicated. Structurally, the brain is normal. **History:** • Tremor that increases with goal-directed and/or postural action • Improvement of tremor with alcohol • Family history of tremor **Physical Exam:** • Postural and kinetic action tremor, mostly involving upper extremities. • Brought on by finger-nose-finger, spiral drawing, pouring water between two cups to elicit tremor. **Diagnostics:** • Clinical diagnosis. • If the features are asymmetric, associated with other neurological findings or features of secondary tremor disorders, further workup such as serum ceruloplasmin level or MRI brain should be considered. **Management:** • Medication should be considered when the patient has occupational or social disability resulting from tremor. • First-line therapies: Propranolol or primidone. • Other agents include gabapentin, topiramate, and sometimes clozapine. • In pharmacotherapy-resistant cases in which the tremor is disabling, deep brain stimulation to the ventral intermediate nucleus of the thalamus (VIM) is effective.

CASE 20 | Huntington Disease

A 35-year-old woman presents for evaluation of recent depressed mood and changes in behavior, including aggression. She also has thoughts of self-harm but denies having a plan or intent to do so. She is having difficulty keeping her hands still and sometimes will raise her arms involuntarily. Her mother also had these "tremors" (as labeled by the patient) that started in her late 40s, and she ended her own life at age 54, about 4 years ago. On physical exam, the patient has depressed mood and affect and is short with her answers. Throughout the encounter, she wrings her hands and her arms occasionally extend and/or abduct spontaneously, though she is trying to hold them still.

Conditions with Similar Presentations	**Syndenham chorea:** Chorea associated with rheumatic fever. Patients will not have the behavioral disturbances and dementia associated with Huntington disease.

CASE 20 | Huntington Disease *(continued)*

Initial Diagnostic Tests	• Check MRI or CT brain • Confirm with genetic testing
Next Steps in Management	Symptomatic treatment with anti-dopaminergic agents (e.g., atypical antipsychotics or tetrabenazine, a VMAT2 inhibitor).
Discussion	Huntington disease is an autosomal dominant hyperkinetic movement disorder characterized by chorea, behavioral disturbances, and dementia. Chorea comes from the Latin and Greek roots "to dance." The pathophysiology is caused by expansion of the trinucleotide CAG repeats on chromosome 4 of the *HTT* gene, leading to a "gain of function" toxicity that results in chorea and behavioral disturbances. Symptoms typically manifest between ages 20 and 50. Patients often have a family history, and parents may have had later onset or less severe disease. This is due to a phenomenon known as **genetic anticipation**, whereby the number of trinucleotide repeats expands in subsequent generations, resulting in earlier onset and more severe disease in offspring. **History:** • Early onset of behavioral or neuropsychiatric symptoms, which can include aggression, depression, suicidal ideation • Involuntary dance-like movements interfering with daily activities • Family history of similar symptoms **Physical Exam:** • Behavioral or neuropsychiatric symptoms often precede movement disturbances. • Hypotonia with hyperreflexia can be seen in early disease. • Chorea is a rapid, irregular, involuntary jerky movement that moves randomly from one body part to another in an unpredictable manner. As chorea worsens, may cause dysphagia and dysarthria. • Patients who have earlier onset may also have eye saccade dysfunction. **C** Huntington disease. Coronal FLAIR image demonstrates bilateral symmetric abnormal high signal in the caudate and putamen. (Reproduced with permission from Loscalzo J, Fauci AS, Kasper DL, et al, eds. Harrison's Principles of Internal Medicine. 21st ed. New York: McGraw Hill; 2022.) **Diagnostics:** • MRI or CT brain shows atrophy of the caudate and putamen, with flattening of the head of the caudate near the lateral ventricle. • Genetic testing shows trinucleotide CAG repeats on chromosome 4 in the *huntingtin* (*HTT*) gene. **Management:** • Symptomatic treatment with vesicular monoamine transport type 2 inhibitors (tetrabenazine or deuterobenzene) that presynaptically decrease dopamine release. • If needed, add antipsychotics (e.g., risperidone, olanzapine, aripiprazole) that are dopamine receptor antagonists. • Psychiatric care should be given, as there is a high association between Huntington disease and suicide.
Additional Considerations	Lifespan is reduced, with cause of death usually due to complications of immobility, such as severe cachexia/malnutrition and/or aspiration pneumonia.

Movement Disorder Mini-Cases

Cases	Key Findings
Wilson Disease (Hepatolenticular Degeneration)	**Hx:** • Trouble concentrating • Changes in mood or behavior • "Wing-beating" tremor **PE:** • Dysarthria, gait ataxia, dystonia. Tremor is classically proximal and high amplitude, giving the appearance of "wing beating" when the arms are abducted and elbows flexed. It may involve other locations and be worse with intention or antigravity posturing. • May have parkinsonian gait and rigidity. • Hepatomegaly. • Slit-lamp exam revealing fine brown dust-like ring around the upper and lower edge of the limbus of the cornea (Kayser-Fleischer rings). This is due to excess copper deposition. **Diagnostics:** • Reduced serum ceruloplasmin • 24-hour urine shows increased copper • MRI brain shows increased signal on T2-weighted images in the caudate, putamen, midbrain, and thalamus **Management:** • Treat with D-penicillamine or trientine dihydrochloride in addition to zinc supplement and low-copper diet. • In patients with severe liver disease, liver transplant is indicated and is also curative. **Discussion:** Wilson disease (hepatolenticular degeneration) is an autosomal recessive disorder of copper metabolism resulting from mutations in hepatocyte copper-transporting P-type ATPase (*ATP7B* gene on chromosome 13). Defects in this ATPase enzyme lead to inability to bind copper to apoceruloplasmin and create ceruloplasmin. Ceruloplasmin is necessary to excrete copper from the liver into bile. This leads to copper accumulation that manifests in three organs: liver, brain, and cornea. Diagnosis is usually made between ages 5 and 35. Liver disease may be asymptomatic, or symptomatic in the form of acute liver failure (5%) or cirrhosis. Neurologic manifestations are diverse, including psychiatric, behavioral, and movement disorders.
Restless Leg Syndrome (RLS)	**Hx:** • Irresistible urge to move legs while at rest, and dysesthesia (crawling/itching feelings), most often at night. Sensation is uncomfortable not painful. • Symptoms are relieved by movement, and recur when movement stops. • May have sleep disturbances either directly or indirectly related to leg movements, including daytime somnolence, irritability, and depressed mood. • Symptoms may be exacerbated by first-generation antihistamines and dopamine antagonists (i.e., antipsychotics) **PE:** Often normal, although some patients may have signs of neuropathy on exam. **Diagnostics:** • Clinical diagnosis based on history and timing of symptoms • Additional studies to identify the source of RLS, as may be associated with iron deficiency, renal failure, neuropathy, spinal cord pathology, pregnancy, MS, and possibly PD **Management:** • Depending on the severity of disease, lifestyle modifications may relieve symptoms—including avoidance of aggravating factors, mental stimulation, regular exercise, improved sleep hygiene, and smoking/alcohol cessation. • Reduction of associated conditions can alleviate symptoms, such as iron supplementation if the patient is deficient, or hemodialysis in patients with end-stage renal disease. • For more severe, persistent disease that interrupts sleep, gabapentin, or dopamine agonists such as pramipexole or ropinirole are first-line treatments. **Discussion:** RLS is characterized as a sleep disorder due to the circadian nature of its symptom presentation. RLS may be associated with involuntary, jerking movements of the legs during sleep, called periodic limb movements of sleep (PLMS). A similar sleep disorder, periodic limb movement disorder (PLMD), is characterized by PLMS plus significant sleep disturbances and/or impaired daytime functioning, but RLS is absent.

Movement Disorder Mini-Cases *(continued)*

Parkinson-Plus Syndrome (PPS)	**Hx/PE:** • Patients present with typical signs of parkinsonism—bradykinesia plus either tremor or rigidity—*plus* additional symptoms, depending on the subclass of PPS (see table below). **Diagnostics:** • Clinical diagnosis • One very important distinguishing feature is that all of PPS diseases have little to no improvement with levodopa-carbidopa, whereas patients with PD will show symptomatic improvement **Management:** • Varies by disease, but the focus will be away from levodopa treatment (see table). **Discussion:** • PPS is defined by an overlap of classic symptoms seen in PD, but with additional symptoms that gradually manifest. • Because of the significant overlap between these syndromes and PD, the syndromes may be identified late, and the prognosis can be poor. • Multidisciplinary interventions, support groups, and medication have varying levels of success, depending on the subtype of PPS.

Parkinson Plus Syndromes (PPS)

	Multiple System Atrophy (MSA)	**Progressive Supranuclear Palsy (PSP)**	**Corticobasal Degeneration (CBD)**
Onset	~55 years (younger than PD)	~65 years (older than PD)	~62 years
Unique Clinical Characteristics	• Dysautonomia (postural hypotension, decreased sweating, bladder control issues, erectile dysfunction) • Ataxia • Dysphagia • Neurological involvement including cerebellar, pyramidal, and LMN signs • Bulbar dysfunction and laryngeal stridor • REM sleep behavior disorder • Restless leg syndrome	• Postural instability and falls; stiff, broad-based gait with knees and trunk extended • Impulsivity leads to lurching and staggering • Oculomotor findings (vertical gaze palsy, ophthalmoplegia) • Frontal lobe deficits • Bradykinesia with marked micrographia • "Surprised" facial look due to dystonia • Pyramidal signs (hyperreflexia, +Babinski) • Spastic dysarthria, dysphonia, and dysphagia • Behavioral abnormalities • Pseudobulbar palsy • Insomnia	• Asymmetric limb akinesia, extreme rigidity, dystonia, focal myoclonus, apraxia, and alien limb • Cortical dysfunction (cognitive impairment, behavioral changes, aphasia, depression) • Significant motor and gait involvement • Dysarthria and apraxia of speech • Oculomotor dysfunction
Diagnosis	Clinical: MRI may show atrophy in putamen, pons, and middle cerebellar peduncles	Clinical: MRI may show predominant midbrain atrophy	Clinical: MRI may show asymmetric cortical atrophy later in the disease, as well as atrophy of the corpus callosum, frontal lobes, basal ganglia, and brainstem

Parkinson Plus Syndromes (PPS)

	Multiple System Atrophy (MSA)	Progressive Supranuclear Palsy (PSP)	Corticobasal Degeneration (CBD)
Treatment and Management	Symptomatic, including physical therapy, fludrocortisone for orthostatic hypotension, and ENT and sleep medicine referrals for stridor and REM sleep behavior disorder	• No drugs modify disease or provide symptomatic relief • Nonpharmacologic interventions include dieticians, speech therapists, PT/OT, and assistive walking devices • Palliative care may be required shortly after diagnosis	• No disease-modifying or symptom-relieving drugs • Palliative and safety measures are emphasized • Therapy should be included, as depression is common
Additional Considerations	Disease progression over 1–18 years, with median death from MSA onset 6–10 years	• Most common PPS • Disease progression is rapid • Patients become dependent within 4 years, and death usually occurs within 6–9 years	• Heterogeneous disease so prognosis is variable • Death occurs on average between 6 and 8 years after diagnosis, most commonly from complications of immobility or dysphagia (e.g., sepsis, pneumonia)

ATAXIA

Ataxia is a neurological sign of inaccurate or uncoordinated volitional movements. It results from disease of the cerebellum (cerebellar ataxia) or defects in proprioception or the vestibular system (sensory ataxias). Similar to the cerebrum, the cerebellum consists of two hemispheres with cortex, deep white matter, and deep gray matter. The deep gray matter includes several deep cerebellar nuclei, from lateral to medial: dentate nucleus, emboliform nucleus, globose nucleus, and fastigial nucleus. Injury to the midline cerebellum vs. the cerebellar hemispheres can result in different clinical features. The midline cerebellum includes the vermis, fastigial and interposed (globus and emboliform) nuclei, the vestibulocerebellum (including the flocculus and nodulus), and the paravermis or intermediate zone. These structures are important in vestibular function, motor execution, eye movements, balance, and coordination of the lower extremities. Dysfunction of the midline cerebellum can therefore result in imbalance, truncal ataxia, titubation (involuntary wavering and instability of head, neck, and/or trunk), lower-limb dysmetria, vertigo, nystagmus, or saccadic intrusions (irregular bursts of rapid eye movements). Meanwhile, the cerebellar hemispheres regulate motor planning and coordination of complex tasks, with damage to one hemisphere resulting in *ipsilateral* deficits, including dysmetria, limb ataxia, intension tremor, dysdiadochokinesis (incoordination when performing rapid alternating movements), and ataxic dysarthria (alternating loudness and fluctuating pitch in voice). Dysmetria is classified as an intention tremor, with repeated undershooting and/or overshooting of corrective movements as the affected limb approaches a target, often demonstrated with the "finger-nose" and "heel-shin" tests.

Ataxia can be categorized as primary or secondary. Primary ataxia is often genetic and typically progresses slowly over time; primary ataxias include the spinocerebellar ataxias, ataxia-telangiectasia, and Friedreich ataxia. Secondary ataxias usually require urgent evaluation. Ataxia associated with intoxication may occur with exposure to alcohol, anticonvulsants, antihistamines, and benzodiazepines. Other causes of acute ataxia include cerebellitis, encephalitis, metabolic disorders, Wilson disease, and thiamine deficiency. Acute focal cerebellar lesions (due to stroke, tumor, and demyelination), may present with acute ataxia, and neuroimaging is often indicated. These may be accompanied by other signs localizable to the posterior fossa such as headache, emesis, and cranial nerve palsies.

CASE 21 | Tabes Dorsalis (Neurosyphilis)

A 57-year-old man presents for evaluation of loss of balance resulting in occasional falls. He has not suffered any trauma from the falls but is worried that his balance has progressively worsened over the past several years. He also reports brief shooting pain sensations in his legs bilaterally on occasion, which are not relieved with NSAIDs. He has had episodes of bladder incontinence at least once per week for the past several months. His wife reports that he is more confused and seems to lose his balance easily. He was treated for a sore on his penis 20 years ago. His vital signs are normal. On exam, his pupils constrict when focusing on near objects but do not constrict with bright light. He has loss of proprioception in his feet bilaterally and decreased patellar and Achilles reflexes. His strength is 5/5 bilaterally in both upper and lower extremities. When standing with his eyes closed and heels together, he sways and cannot maintain his balance.

Conditions with Similar Presentations	**Diabetic neuropathy:** Is a great mimicker, as it can attack various parts of the nervous system and present in numerous ways including peripheral neuropathy leading to loss of proprioception. Most commonly, it presents as neuropathic pain in the lower extremities with decreased sensation in the distal lower extremities. It does not present with confusion.
	Subacute combined degeneration (SCD): Is a neurologic manifestation of vitamin B12 deficiency characterized by demyelination of the spinocerebellar tracts, lateral corticospinal tracts, and dorsal columns of the spinal cord. Patients present with loss of proprioception, vibration, and fine touch (dorsal columns), UMN signs (lateral corticospinal tracts), ataxia (spinocerebellar tracts), numbness, lancinating pains, and paresthesias (peripheral nerves). Vitamin B12 deficiency can present in patients on a strict vegetarian diet or patients with a history of pernicious anemia, inflammatory bowel disease, bariatric surgery, or chronic use of metformin or proton pump inhibitors. Vitamin B12 deficiency results in a macrocytic, megaloblastic anemia.
Initial Diagnostic Tests	• Serum nontreponemal tests (RPR or VDRL) • Serum treponemal testing with fluorescent treponemal antibody absorption (FTA-ABS) to detect prior syphilis if RPR/VDRL negative or confirm syphilis if RPR/VDRL positive • If neurologic and ocular symptoms are present, LP for CSF-VDRL • Consider: Test for HIV, serum vitamin B12, and HBA1c
Next Steps in Management	• IV penicillin G, for 10–14 days. • Repeat CSF studies in 3–6 months to confirm successful treatment.
Discussion	Tabes dorsalis is a complication of tertiary syphilis and a form of late neurosyphilis, typically developing decades following initial infection with the spirochete *Treponema pallidum*. Neurosyphilis is more common in men than women. Initial exposure to *T. pallidum* results in primary syphilis, with a painless chancre on the genitals. If untreated, secondary syphilis can develop as the bacteria enter the blood, resulting in constitutional symptoms, maculopapular rash, and generalized lymphadenopathy. If untreated, patients progress to latent syphilis, which can progress to tertiary syphilis in approximately one-third of patients. Tertiary syphilis commonly affects the cardiovascular and nervous systems (neurosyphilis) or causes painless local tissue destruction elsewhere (gummatous syphilis). Tabes dorsalis is one of several potential manifestations of neurosyphilis, and involves destruction of the dorsal columns and dorsal nerve roots of the spinal cord. **History:** • Risk factors for syphilis include HIV, high-risk sexual activity, drug use, and limited access to health care. **Physical Exam:** • Destruction of the dorsal columns results in sensory ataxia with impaired sense of proprioception and vibration. • Positive Romberg test on exam. • Reduced deep tendon reflexes and diminished sensation of pain and temperature. • Argyll Robertson pupil: Pupil is able to constrict with accommodation (i.e., focusing on near objects) but does not react to light. • Wide-based "tabetic gait": feet will slap the ground heavily. • Other features include development of sudden lancinating pains which travel down the spine, extremities, or ocular nerves (the latter may result in lacrimation), progressive dementia, general paresis, as well as hearing or vision loss.

CASE 21 | Tabes Dorsalis (Neurosyphilis) *(continued)*

Discussion	**Diagnostics:**
	• Patients should be screened with nontreponemal serum tests (RPR/VDRL). Nonreactive in ~33%
	• Also check serum treponemal testing with fluorescent treponemal antibody absorption (FTA-ABS) to detect prior syphilis if RPR/VDRL negative or confirm syphilis if RPR/VDRL positive.
	• Patients with neurologic, ocular, or otologic manifestations should undergo LP for CSF testing for the presence of *T pallidum* (CSF-VDRL). Do not check for FTA-ABS because this is an IgG antibody that crosses the blood-brain barrier. CSF may have mildly elevated protein and leukocytes.
	Management:
	• Treatment is with high-dose intravenous penicillin G for 10–14 days.
	• If there is a non-anaphylactic penicillin allergy, patients can alternatively be treated with IV ceftriaxone for 10–14 days.
	• If there is anaphylaxis to penicillin, patients should be desensitized, then treated with it.
Additional Considerations	**Complications:**
	Neurosyphilis can generally be divided into early and late neurosyphilis. Early manifestations include meningitis, uveitis, optic neuritis, hearing loss, or **meningovascular syphilis**, which presents with signs of meningitis and ischemic stroke, often involving vasculitis of the middle cerebral artery. Late manifestations include tabes dorsalis and general paresis. **General paresis** has multiple manifestations that have PARESIS as a mnemonic:
	Personality changes
	Affect changes
	Reflexes increased
	Eye findings (Argyll Robertson pupil)
	Sensorium changes
	Intellectual decline
	Speech defects
	Pediatric Considerations: Congenital syphilis occurs secondary to vertical transmission across the placenta of *T. pallidum*. Newborns are typically asymptomatic at birth but may develop symptoms weeks to months later. Early manifestations include persistent rhinorrhea ("snuffles"), maculopapular rash, long bone abnormalities, hepatosplenomegaly, and growth restriction. Later manifestations include sensorineural hearing loss, keratitis, and dysmorphic features including notched (Hutchinson) teeth, anterior bowing of the tibia ("saber shins"), and saddle nose deformity. All pregnant women should be screened for syphilis at the initial prenatal visit to prevent these potentially devastating consequences to the developing fetus.

Ataxia Mini-Cases

Cases	Key Findings
Wernicke Encephalopathy	**Hx:**
	• History of chronic alcohol use (even if not currently intoxicated), hyperemesis gravidarum, or chronic malnutrition (e.g., anorexia nervosa, poor absorption following bariatric surgery).
	PE:
	• Wernicke encephalopathy characterized by a triad of:
	• Confusion, altered mental status, or encephalopathy
	• Ataxia with wide-based gait
	• Ophthalmoplegia with horizontal nystagmus and conjugate gaze palsies
	Diagnostics:
	• Clinical diagnosis confirmed by resolution of symptoms after administration of thiamine.
	• Thiamine levels may or may not be low and do not necessarily reflect CNS levels. A more accurate test is measurement of erythrocyte thiamine transketolase activity (ETKA) before and after the addition of thiamine pyrophosphate (TPP). However, this may not be available at all labs.
	• MRI findings may include petechial hemorrhage or atrophy in the mammillary bodies, but also in hypothalamus, medial thalamus, and periaqueductal gray matter.

Ataxia Mini-Cases *(continued)*

Wernicke Encephalopathy	**Management:** • High-dose IV thiamine can result in resolution of some or all of symptoms. Patients should NOT receive glucose or dextrose prior to thiamine, as this can cause acute exacerbation of neuropsychiatric symptoms and result in coma or death. • Underlying causes of Wernicke encephalopathy should also be addressed. For example, patients with chronic alcohol use should be monitored for withdrawal and be referred for long-term therapy. **Discussion:** • Thiamine (vitamin B1) is a cofactor for enzymes involved in energy metabolism (transketolase, alpha-ketoglutarate dehydrogenase, and pyruvate dehydrogenase pyruvate dehydrogenase) and is required in high concentrations by tissues with high metabolism and glucose intake such as the brain. • Deficiency in thiamine can result in Wernicke encephalopathy, which is a partially reversible condition if treated. However, if untreated, it can eventually progress to **Wernicke-Korsakoff syndrome**, where in addition to Wernicke encephalopathy, the patient also develops **Korsakoff psychosis**, an irreversible condition characterized by confabulation, amnesia, and personality changes.
Friedreich Ataxia	**Hx:** • Young adult presents with progressive dysarthria and incoordination of gait and limbs. • May have additional history of impaired glucose tolerance or cardiac arrhythmias. **PE:** • Loss of deep tendon reflexes • Loss of position and vibratory sense (dorsal column degeneration) • Gait unsteadiness with wide base gait • Four-limb ataxia • Motor weakness, cerebellar dysarthria, dysphagia • Reduced visual acuity and abnormal eye movements • Skeletal abnormalities including kyphoscoliosis and foot abnormalities such as pes cavus (high-arched foot), hammer toes, and intrinsic muscle atrophy **Diagnostics:** • Clinical diagnosis with genetic testing for confirmation. • MRI of brain and spinal cord recommended for exclusion of other causes. **Management:** • Supportive with multidisciplinary team including neurology, cardiology, orthopedics, endocrinology, psychology, and supportive therapy/counseling. • Requires yearly cardiovascular examination after initial cardiac evaluation. **Discussion:** • Friedreich ataxia is an autosomal recessive hereditary ataxia due to expansion of trinucleotide repeat (GAA) within the frataxin gene located on chromosome 9. Frataxin gene encodes for a mitochondrial protein, which is highly expressed in neurological, cardiac, and endocrine tissues. • Often presents in adolescence but can also present in early childhood or early/late adulthood • Cardiac manifestations (arrhythmia, hypertrophic cardiomyopathy, myocardial fibrosis, heart failure) are the leading cause of death, with the mean age of death being age 30–40. • Associated with diabetes due to pancreatic involvement. Can also be associated with autonomic dysfunction (bladder dysfunction).
Alcoholic Cerebellar Degeneration	**Hx:** • History of heavy alcohol use for >10 years' duration • Will present with unsteadiness, change in gait, and blurry or double vision over weeks to months **PE:** • Wide-based lurching gait, truncal ataxia, lower limb incoordination (inability to tandem walk, abnormal knee-to-shin testing) • Nystagmus, diplopia • Preserved upper extremity coordination (normal finger-to-nose testing) • Mild dysarthria, muscle hypotonia with pendular knee reflex (>4 persistent swings of limb after eliciting deep tendon reflexes) • Postural tremor (late-stage)

Ataxia Mini-Cases *(continued)*

Alcoholic Cerebellar Degeneration	**Diagnostics:** • Clinical diagnosis • MRI/CT for exclusion of other causes and will show prominent atrophy of the midline cerebellar structures (vermis) **Management:** • Supportive care with alcohol cessation and nutritional supplement for prevention of further worsening • Alcohol cessation may be associated with mild improvement in symptoms • Patients may require ambulatory assistance devices **Discussion:** • Alcoholic cerebellar degeneration is a chronic cerebellar syndrome caused by degeneration of the Purkinje cells within the cerebellar vermis • Degeneration occurs likely due to a combination of nutritional deficiencies and direct neurotoxicity from alcohol and its metabolites

SEIZURES

Seizures are clinical expressions of abnormal, hypersynchronous firing of neurons in the brain and are classified based on their onset/initial manifestation. They can be focal (originating in one part of the brain) or generalized (originating throughout the entire brain simultaneously).

Focal (previously called partial) **seizures** are classified based on:

- Level of awareness into focal aware (intact consciousness, previously called simple partial seizure) or focal with impaired awareness (altered consciousness, previously called complex partial seizure) and/or
- Presence or absence of motor symptoms.
  - Patients with motor seizures may also have automatisms, which are repetitive, stereotype actions, often involving the hands or mouth (e.g., lip smacking, picking, rubbing hands, chewing movements, and repeating words) that may precede or occur during a seizure (i.e., focal seizure with impaired awareness).
  - Non-motor manifestations may include behavioral arrest, abnormal sensations or emotions, intense feelings of déjà vu, or autonomic changes (e.g., flushing, sweating, epigastric fullness).
- Focal-onset seizures can spread and evolve to bilateral tonic-clonic seizures (previously referred to as secondary generalization or Jacksonian seizures).

Generalized seizures are classified based on having motor or non-motor manifestations.

- Motor manifestations include tonic (flexion or extension), clonic (rhythmic jerking), myoclonic (arrhythmic jerking), and tonic-clonic ("grand mal") seizures.
- Non-motor seizures are usually behavior arrest seizures but include atonic seizures (drop seizures) and absence seizures.

Further classifications include the following:

- Acute symptomatic seizure is one that occurs after an acute systemic (e.g., hypoxia, hypoglycemia) or brain insult (e.g., stroke, encephalitis, trauma).
- Unprovoked seizures are those that occur without a known cause or due to a known brain lesion or brain disorder.
- Remote symptomatic seizures are those seen in patients with known brain lesion or brain disorder after a long period of time.

Any seizure may be followed by a post-ictal state, during which the patient may be confused, somnolent, or have neurologic deficits, including paralysis or aphasia.

Epilepsy

Epilepsy is a chronic condition characterized by unprovoked seizures (two or more >24 hours apart, or one unprovoked seizure, with a probability of >60% of having a second seizure over the next 10 years). Epilepsy can be classified as focal, generalized, rare combined generalized and focal epilepsy syndromes such as Lennox-Gastaut epilepsy syndrome (LGS), and idiopathic epilepsy. There are also numerous epilepsy syndromes that often begin in childhood, some of which may be due to underlying genetic mutations in ion channels or neurotransmitters.

CASE 22 | Focal Seizure with Impaired Awareness

A 29-year-old woman with no past medical history presents to urgent care with her partner following an "odd spell" while sitting at a restaurant just a few hours ago. As soon as they sat down, she started smacking her lips repeatedly, and this was followed by rapid twitching in her right arm. After several seconds, her eyes began to deviate to the left and she was nonresponsive for about 1 minute. She has had events like this happen in the past and is tired and confused afterward before returning to baseline. Her vital signs are normal. She appears a little tired but is alert and oriented with no neurologic deficits.

Conditions with Similar Presentations	**Psychogenic nonepileptic seizure (PNES):** Previously called "pseudoseizures," can present similar to true epileptic seizures; however, there is no abnormal neuronal activity. Can be differentiated by the presence of complex, purposeful movements; out-of-phase (asynchronous) limb movements; closed eyes; side-to-side head shaking ("saying no"); audible, sensible, or word vocalizations (vs. ictal cries, which are often unintelligible), starting and stopping movements, lack of autonomic symptoms, and a lack of a postictal state. The patient may awaken and reorient quickly or even during the event, in contrast to a seizure. Unlike epilepsy, the episodes may be different each time. Patients commonly have psychiatric comorbidities and may have a history of physical or sexual abuse. However, it is important to keep in mind that patients may have PNES on top of true epilepsy, and as such patients should undergo video EEG monitoring to differentiate. EEG in PNES will be normal. **Febrile seizures:** Are generalized seizures that occur in young infants and children with temperatures >40°C (104°F). These are most commonly associated with viral infections or recent immunizations. Patients may exhibit a limited or absent postictal phase altogether. This disorder is typically self-limiting with resolution of the underlying etiology. Simple febrile seizures do not require additional workup but do slightly increase the risk for development of latent epilepsy. Complex febrile seizures (focal onset, lasting >15 minutes, or >1 seizure in 24 hours) may require EEG and additional investigations. Lorazepam is the first-line acute treatment if actively seizing in the health care setting. Otherwise, supportive care alone is recommended.
Initial Diagnostic Tests	• Clinical diagnosis confirmed with EEG • Check neuroimaging, CBC, serum Na and glucose, blood alcohol level, and urine toxicology screen to rule out potential causes of provoked seizures
Next Steps in Management	Initiate treatment with anti-seizure drugs (ASDs)
Discussion	This patient is experiencing focal motor seizures with impaired awareness (formerly known as complex partial seizures). Given the presence of spontaneous, recurrent, unprovoked seizures, this patient has focal epilepsy. The most common cause of focal epilepsy is temporal lobe epilepsy. **History/Physical:** • Risk factors: Generally divided into five categories: Genetic (e.g., Dravet syndrome), encephalopathy (e.g., Lennox-Gastaut syndrome, infantile spasms), structural (e.g., trauma, ischemia, hemorrhage, tumor, cortical malformations, hippocampal sclerosis), infectious (e.g., meningitis, encephalitis, neurocysticercosis), immune (e.g., autoimmune encephalitis), and idiopathic • Patients may have history of premature birth, history of seizures in childhood (including febrile seizures), prior TBI or CNS infection, prior neurosurgery, and/or a family history of epilepsy • In focal seizures with impaired awareness, patients often appear awake and aware; however, they do not interact appropriately with the environment, often described as a blank or absent stare • Patients commonly engage in automatisms (e.g., lip smacking in this patient) • Some patients may also experience an aura prior to the overt seizure. Auras may manifest with abnormal sensations, including epigastric fullness, feeling as if one is falling, olfactory hallucinations, or intense feelings of fear or déjà vu, among others. Following a seizure, the patient may enter a postictal state characterized by confusion, disorientation, and decreased consciousness • Some patients may develop postictal paralysis (also known as Todd's paralysis), with weakness or paralysis lasting minutes to hours following the seizure • In patients with known epilepsy on treatment, the most common reason for a seizure is medication nonadherence

CASE 22 | Focal Seizure with Impaired Awareness *(continued)*

Discussion	**Diagnostics:** Obtain EEG and brain imaging.
	• If epileptiform activity (i.e., spikes, sharp waves, or seizures) is seen on EEG and/or a lesion is noted on MRI, this increases the risk of a second seizure and thus warrants anti-seizure medication.
	• A normal EEG is seen in a minority of patients with epilepsy but repeat sleep EEG will usually be abnormal.
	• Brain MRI with and without contrast may be able to identify potential lesions, especially in the temporal lobe, including reduced hippocampal volume in the temporal lobe with increased T2 signal, suggesting medial temporal sclerosis (one of the most common causes of epilepsy in adulthood).
	• Consider complete blood count, comprehensive metabolic panel, blood alcohol level, and urine toxicology screen to rule out other causes.
	Management:
	• For spontaneous and recurrent episodes, start ASDs (see table below). The specific type of ASD chosen depends on the type of seizure, side effect profile, and comorbidities. Potential options in this case are sodium channel blockers such as phenytoin, carbamazepine, or oxcarbazepine, which are often first-line agents for focal seizures.
	• Avoidance of risk factors that lower seizure threshold and promote recurrence.
	• Patients should be assessed for whether they drive or operate heavy machinery. Patients with seizures that affect consciousness in some way should not drive, although specifics vary based on state laws and guidelines. Regulations vary by state, but typically, patients must be seizure-free for 6 months to a year prior to return to driving.
	• It is reasonable *not* to initiate ASD therapy after a first unprovoked seizure without a high likelihood of recurrence.
Additional Considerations	**Surgical Considerations:** Up to one-third of patients remain refractory to medical management of epilepsy. Surgical options are lobectomy, resection of the epileptic focus, or ablation, deep brain stimulation, or vagus nerve stimulation.
	Obstetric Considerations:
	• **Eclampsia** is an obstetric emergency involving the presence of new-onset tonic-clonic seizures and pre-eclampsia that can occur during pregnancy or during the postpartum period. Pre-eclampsia is defined as new-onset elevated blood pressure (SBP ≥140 or DBP ≥90) and proteinuria or signs of end-organ damage. Treatment involves immediate delivery with removal of the placenta. Patients should also receive magnesium sulfate and antihypertensives if blood pressure is severely elevated.
	• It is also important to consider the potential **teratogenic effects of ASDs** on the developing fetus in women of reproductive age who may become pregnant. For example, valproic acid can lead to neural tube defects and in utero exposure to phenytoin can lead to fetal hydantoin syndrome. Women of reproductive age with epilepsy should be counseled on taking prenatal vitamins and high-dose (e.g., 4 mg daily) folic acid.

CASE 23 | Status Epilepticus

A 61-year-old man with epilepsy since childhood is brought in by ambulance to the ED with generalized tonic-clonic seizure. His son accompanies him and states that he was sitting at home when he lost consciousness, became stiff, and then began violently jerking his arms and legs. The son immediately called 911, and by the time EMS arrived, the patient had been seizing for 12 minutes. He was administered bag-mask ventilation in the field, had two peripheral IVs inserted, and was administered IV lorazepam, which resulted in cessation of his seizure. Upon arrival to the ED, his vital signs are normal and glucose is normal. The patient is lethargic and responds to verbal stimuli. He appears confused and is oriented to person only. He has no focal neurologic deficits. His son mentions that the patient has recently stopped taking his anti-seizure medication as he had not had a seizure in 5 years.

Conditions with Similar Presentations	**Generalized tonic-clonic (GTC) seizures:** Present similarly; however, they typically last <5 minutes.

CASE 23 | Status Epilepticus *(continued)*

Initial Diagnostic Tests	Clinical diagnosis. Once stable, should undergo non-contrast head CT and MRI brain and continuous video EEG monitoring.
Next Steps in Management	Stabilize the patient (ABCs), administer IV benzodiazepines (e.g., lorazepam), and load with additional ASD to prevent seizure recurrence (e.g., phenytoin).
Discussion	Status epilepticus is a neurological and medical emergency defined as continuous seizures lasting ≥5 minutes, or more than one seizure without full recovery in between events. Incidence follows a U-shaped distribution, with highest incidence in children <1 year old and a second high incidence in adults >60 years old. Convulsive status epilepticus is the most severe form, causing neuronal dysfunction with a higher risk of systemic derangements, including rhabdomyolysis, arrhythmia, asystole, aspiration, or apnea. Patients can also develop non-convulsive status epilepticus (NCSE), which involves ongoing seizure activity (often detected on EEG) without convulsions. NCSE is particularly common in critically ill patients and may result in mental status changes that may be hard to detect. Mortality rate is up to 20% in patients with status epilepticus, and therefore it should be recognized and treated immediately, including prior to arrival at the hospital if possible.

History/Physical:
- Occurs in approximately 30% of patients with epilepsy, especially in patients who miss or skip doses of their anti-seizure medication. Other risk factors are similar to those for seizures and epilepsy in general (discussed in the previous case) and include anything that can lower a patient's seizure threshold.
- A focused evaluation should be performed, including assessment of respiratory and cardiovascular status, with particular attention paid to airway safety and protection, breathing, and circulation. A rapid neurological exam should be performed, including assessment for head trauma and signs of meningitis.

Diagnostics:
- Given high risk of brain injury, status epilepticus is a clinical diagnosis and causes should be investigated AFTER seizure activity has been stopped (see management below).
- Typical workup includes continuous video EEG, neuroimaging with non-contrast CT and/or MRI with and without contrast to evaluate for structural abnormalities, and LP can be considered if no explanation is readily apparent.
- Additional labs should be ordered including CBC, CMP, ASD levels (to ensure within therapeutic window), and urine toxicology studies.
- Patients should be admitted for continuous monitoring of heart rate and rhythm, breathing, and pulse oximetry, with frequent clinical assessments including neurological examination.

Management:
- IV benzodiazepines (e.g., lorazepam, diazepam) should be given ASAP and patients may require additional doses.
- Patients should also be given ASDs to prevent recurrence of seizure (e.g., phenytoin, levetiracetam, valproic acid).
- If status epilepticus is refractory to these measures, can consider further augmentation with anesthetics/sedatives including pentobarbital, phenobarbital, or propofol.

Seizure Mini-Case

Case	Key Findings
Childhood Absence Epilepsy (CAE)	See Pediatrics Chapter
Juvenile Myoclonic Epilepsy (JME)	**Hx/PE:** • Typical onset is between the ages of 8 and 28. • The patient or patient's family will report quick motor jerks typically of the upper extremities and head (myoclonic seizures) that occur most often in the mornings shortly after awakening and with intact consciousness. May report dropping things in the morning. • Patients may also have concurrent generalized tonic-clonic seizures and/or a history of absence seizures in earlier childhood. **Diagnostics:** EEG is characterized by 2- to 4-Hz generalized spike and slow wave discharges, and commonly faster 4- to 6-Hz.. **Management:** • Valproic acid is the most effective medication, but caution must be used in young women of reproductive age that could become pregnant. Lamotrigine and levetiracetam are alternatives in this situation. • Patients should be counseled to avoid triggers, including alcohol consumption and sleep deprivation. **Discussion:** JME is a form of idiopathic generalized epilepsy that presents most commonly in otherwise healthy adolescents or young adults. A classic scenario is a college student who has been staying up late and/or drinking alcohol who develops generalized myoclonus (both sleep deprivation and alcohol can lower seizure threshold). JME generally progresses to chronic epilepsy.
Tuberous Sclerosis Complex (TSC)	See Pediatrics Chapter

Common Anti-Seizure Medications, Mechanisms, and Side Effects

Epilepsy therapy

	PARTIAL (FOCAL)[†]	1° GENERALIZED TONIC-CLONIC	1° GENERALIZED ABSENCE	STATUS EPILEPTICUS	MECHANISM	ADVERSE EFFECTS	NOTES
Benzodiazepines				** ✓	↑ $GABA_A$ action	Sedation, tolerance, dependence, respiratory depression	Also for eclampsia seizures (1st line is $MgSO_4$)
Carbamazepine	✓				Blocks Na^+ channels	Diplopia, ataxia, blood dyscrasias (agranulocytosis, aplastic anemia), liver toxicity, teratogenesis (cleft lip/palate, spina bifia), induction of cytochrome P-450, SIADH, SJS	1st line for trigeminal neuralgia
Ethosuximide			* ✓		Blocks thalamic T-type Ca^{2+} channels	EFGHIJ—Ethosuximide causes Fatigue, GI distress, Headache, Itching (and urticaria), SJS	Sucks ('Sux') to have silent (absence) seizures
Gabapentin	✓				Primarily inhibits high-voltage-activated Ca^{2+} channels; designed as GABA analog	Sedation, ataxia	Also used for peripheral neuropathy, postherpetic neuralgia

Common Anti-Seizure Medications, Mechanisms, and Side Effects *(Continued)*

Epilepsy therapy	PARTIAL (FOCAL)[†]	1° GENERALIZED TONIC-CLONIC	1° GENERALIZED ABSENCE	STATUS EPILEPTICUS	MECHANISM	ADVERSE EFFECTS	NOTES
Lamotrigine	✓	✓	✓		Blocks voltage-gated Na⁺ channels, inhibits the release of glutamate	SJS (must be titrated slowly), hemophagocytic lymphohistiocytosis (black box warning)	
Levetiracetam	✓	✓			SV2A receptor blocker; may modulate GABA and glutamate release, inhibit voltage-gated Ca^{2+} channels	Neuropsychiatric symptoms (eg, personality change), fatigue, drowsiness, headache	
Phenobarbital	✓	✓		*** ✓	↑ $GABA_A$ action	Sedation, tolerance, dependence, induction of cytochrome P-450, cardiorespiratory depression	1st line in neonates ("pheno*baby*tal")
Phenytoin, fosphenytoin	✓	* ✓			Blocks Na⁺ channels; zero-order kinetics	PHENYTOIN: cytochrome P-450 induction, Pseudolymphoma, Hirsutism, Enlarged gums, Nystagmus, Yellow-brown skin, Teratogenicity (fetal hydantoin syndrome), Osteopenia, Inhibited folate absorption, Neuropathy. Rare: SJS, DRESS syndrome, drug-induced lupus. Toxicity leads to diplopia, ataxia, sedation.	
Topiramate	✓	✓			Blocks Na⁺ channels, ↑ GABA action	Sedation, slow cognition, kidney stones, skinny (weight loss), sight threatened (glaucoma), speech (word-finding) difficulties	Also used for migraine prophylaxis
Valproate	✓	* ✓	✓		↑ Na⁺ channel inactivation, ↑ GABA concentration by inhibiting GABA transaminase	VALPPROaTTE: Vomiting, Alopecia, Liver damage (hepatotoxic), Pancreatitis, P-450 inhibition, Rash, Obesity (weight gain), Tremor, Teratogenesis (neural tube defects). Epigastric pain (GI distress).	Also used for myoclonic seizures, bipolar disorder, migraine prophylaxis
Vigabatrin	✓				↑ GABA. Irreversible GABA transaminase inhibitor	Permanent visual loss (black box warning)	Vision loss with GABA transaminase inhibitor

* = Common use, ** = 1st line for acute, *** = 1st line for recurrent seizure prophylaxis.

[†] Includes partial simple/complex and 2° generalized seizures.

Reproduced, with permission, from Le T, et al. First Aid for the USMLE Step 1 2022. New York : McGraw Hill; 2022.

NECK AND BACK PAIN

The spinal cord is a CNS structure that arises from the inferior medulla of the brainstem above the C1 vertebra and runs in the spinal canal to terminate at the L1–L2 level of the lumbar spine. It is covered in the meninges, which are contiguous with the meninges of the brain. Although the spine ends at the level of L1–L2, the arachnoid and dura continue to the S2 vertebral level. The subarachnoid space is clinically relevant as the site from which CSF can be collected in a LP without risk to the spinal cord if performed at the L3–L4 or L4–L5 level. The spinal cord is divided longitudinally into the cervical, thoracic, and lumbar regions, with the sacral spinal cord region that represents the very lower aspect of the spinal cord referred to as the conus medullaris. The neuroanatomy of the spinal cord is somatotopically and segmentally organized, with tracts and pathways that transmit sensory information from organs and peripheral receptors to the brain and motor information from the brain to internal and peripheral effector organs. Pairs of sensory and motor nerve roots emerge at distinct spinal levels throughout the length of the cord. Sensory nerve roots emerge dorsally from the cord, and motor nerve roots emerge ventrally before they meet to form mixed motor and sensory spinal nerves. The nerve roots are numbered C1 through C8 when they arise from the cervical cord and T1 through T12 when they arise from the thoracic cord. The lumbar L1 nerve roots emerge just below the T12 nerve roots. The lowermost nerve roots (lumbar, L2–L5; sacral, S1–S5; and the coccygeal nerve) fan out distally from the lower cord and are referred to as the cauda equina (Latin for horse's tail).

Here, we briefly discuss common causes of neck and back pain as it relates to spinal cord pathology. However, it is important to note that neck and back pain are common chief concerns treated by a diverse array of medical specialists. For additional information, see Rheumatology and Musculoskeletal Disorders Chapter.

Neck Pain Mini-Case

Cervical Radiculopathies	**Hx:** Adult with neck pain radiating down affected shoulder, arm, and hand with possible upper extremity or hand weakness.
	PE: Physical findings with sensory, strength, and reflex deficits dependent on affected cervical nerve root. Please see the table below with cervical nerve root and associated physical exam findings.
	Diagnostics: • Check EMG • MRI and CT can be used to confirm compression of nerve root.
	Management: • Multimodal supportive approach is recommended • Nonoperative therapies include: cervical collars, traction, physical therapy • Medications for neuropathic pain and selective nerve blocks
	Discussion: Cervical and lumbar radiculopathies are associated with pain, paresthesias, and motor deficits within the distribution of a nerve root. Common etiologies include structural lesions such as herniated discs, arthritic bone spurs, spondylosis, and mass lesions. Thoracic radiculopathies are very rare.
	Differential Diagnosis: Most common diagnoses to consider include plexopathy, proximal neuropathy, and entrapment neuropathy. Others to consider include orthopedic conditions and muscle spasms.

Clinical Manifestations of Cervical Radiculopathies

Root	Area of Pain	Sensory Deficits	Motor Deficits	Reflex Deficits
C3–C4	Superior shoulders, paraspinal muscles	Neck	Diaphragm, neck (infrahyoid, nuchal muscles)	N/A
C5	Neck, shoulders, anterior arm	Shoulder	Shoulder/Back (deltoid, supraspinatus, infraspinatus, rhomboids), biceps, brachioradialis	Biceps, brachioradialis
C6	Neck, shoulders, anterior arm	Hand (thumb, second digit), radial forearm	Shoulder/back (deltoid, supraspinatus, infraspinatus, rhomboids), biceps, brachioradialis hand/wrist (pronator teres, flexor carpi radialis, extensor carpi radialis)	Biceps, brachioradialis
C7	Neck, shoulders, forearm	Third digit	Triceps, wrist (pronator teres, flexor carpi radialis, extensor carpi radialis)	Triceps
C8	Neck shoulders, forearm	Fourth and fifth digit, hypothenar eminence	Intrinsic hand, finger extensors/flexors	None
T1	Neck, shoulders, ulnar arm	Ulnar arm	Intrinsic hand	None

*Detailed description of lumbar radiculopathies is provided in the Rheumatology and Musculoskeletal Disorders Chapter and is also important to know for neurology exams!

CASE 24 | Cauda Equina Syndrome (CES)

A 38-year-old man with a history of herniated lumbar disk and laminectomy presents with back pain and lower extremity weakness. Lower back pain got worse yesterday and now radiates down both of his legs. The pain was not relieved with ibuprofen or acetaminophen. This morning he awoke to numbness and weakness of both his feet and was unable to walk without support. He also had new-onset urinary hesitancy and dribbling of urine. He has no previous episodes of weakness or sensory loss and reports no recent injuries. Patient had a herniated lumbar disc and laminectomy 2 years earlier due to a skiing injury. Vital signs are normal. Physical exam demonstrates motor weakness of bilateral plantar flexion with absent bilateral patellar reflex, impaired sensation to soft touch within the scrotum, perianal area and bilateral feet, and reduced anal sphincter tone.

Conditions with Similar Presentations	Additional conditions that should be considered include peripheral nerve damage and lumbosacral plexopathy. **Conus medullaris syndrome:** Occurs with compression or lesions of the terminal spinal cord at L1–L2 (i.e., the conus medullaris). Presents with predominant UMN symptoms due to disruption of tracts within the lumbosacral spinal cord. Patients present with severe back pain, motor weakness, and saddle anesthesia that is usually symmetric (vs. patchy, asymmetric pattern seen in CES). Etiology includes disc herniation, spinal fracture, and spinal tumors. Diagnosis with MRI with and without contrast. Once confirmed, will require urgent neurosurgical consultation and decompressive surgery.
Initial Diagnostic Tests	Urgent MRI with and without contrast of the lumbosacral spine.
Next Steps in Management	Consult neurosurgery for surgical decompression
Discussion	CES occurs when there is dysfunction of multiple (two or more) lumbar and sacral nerve roots of the cauda equina. Dysfunction is secondary to compression of the cauda equina, which can be caused by multiple etiologies. Most common cause is a massive herniated disc. Other causes include spinal cord lesion/tumors, spinal cord infections/inflammation (epidural abscess), spinal stenosis, injuries to lower back, postoperative complication, and spinal anesthesia complication. **History:** Patient will report progressive lower back radicular pain with one or more of the following symptoms: • Motor weakness in affected myotomes • Patchy sensory loss in affected dermatomes, including **saddle anesthesia**, which is impaired sensation in buttocks, perineum, and/or perianal area • Rectal sphincter, bladder, and erectile dysfunction **Physical Exam:** • Will demonstrate motor deficit (predominant LMN symptoms compared to conus medullaris syndrome), absent knee/ankle reflexes, sensory loss including saddle anesthesia, and bladder/rectal sphincter weakness/paralysis. • Patients will commonly have a positive straight-leg raise test. **Diagnostics:** • Emergent MRI with and without contrast of lumbosacral spinal cord which will demonstrate gadolinium enhancement of the affected nerve roots as well as the associated etiology (in this case, may see herniated disc extending into the body of S2-S4 with central canal stenosis and compression of the cauda equina). **Management:** • Requires urgent neurosurgical consultation for decompression surgery within 24-48 hours with doses of dexamethasone. • After decompression, patient will require rehabilitation to regain neurological function.

CASE 25 | Spinal Epidural Abscess

A 37-year-old man with history of IV heroin use and upper extremity cellulitis presents with severe upper back pain and new-onset weakness. The pain began 3 weeks prior and has gradually worsened in severity and is associated with low-grade fevers and fatigue. Over the last week, he developed progressive upper and lower extremity weakness and worsening urinary incontinence. He has been having trouble moving his arms and legs and had to be brought in by his friend. Temperature is 39°C, PR 102 bpm, RR 17 bpm, BP 100/60 mmHg O2 99% on room air. On physical exam, an erythematous, edematous, tender furuncle is found on his left forearm. He has extreme point tenderness at the C3-C5 spinal level. On neurological exam, he is quadriparetic with hyperreflexia in the biceps, knees, and ankles bilaterally with a positive Babinski reflex. He has decreased rectal tone and loss of bilateral fine touch, vibration, pain, and temperature sensation from C5 and below.

CASE 25 | Spinal Epidural Abscess *(continued)*

Conditions with Similar Presentations	Presentation is consistent with spinal cord compression, which can be also caused by disc herniation, malignancy or metastatic disease, epidermal hematoma (EDH), and injury (e.g., MVA). More progressive symptoms can also be associated with degenerative joint disease.
	Spinal EDH: Occurs most often as a complication of a spinal procedure, including neuraxial anesthesia, LP, or spinal surgery, and can lead to spinal cord compression symptoms caused by venous bleeding. This includes slowly progressive localized back pain with point tenderness, radicular pain, and UMN and sensory abnormalities. If it is a complication of a LP can be associated with symptoms of cauda equina symptoms. Risk factors include anti-thrombotic medications, coagulopathies, and spinal abnormalities. This requires emergent MRI of spine with and without contrast, which will demonstrate EDH which will evolve overtime. Spinal EDH is a neurosurgical emergency and requires emergent neurosurgical consult for urgent evacuation/decompression and laminectomy.
Initial Diagnostic Tests	• Emergent MRI with and without contrast. • Drain and culture furuncle and send blood cultures.
Next Steps in Management	• Urgent neurosurgical consultation for drainage • Broad-spectrum IV antibiotics
Discussion	Spinal epidural abscess is a rare infection of the epidural space that can cause compression of the spinal cord leading to paralysis. Most often occurs due to hematological spread from distant infections, such as cellulitis or continuously from vertebral discitis or osteomyelitis. The most common organism is *Staphylococcus aureus* followed by streptococci, anaerobic organisms, and gram-negative bacilli.

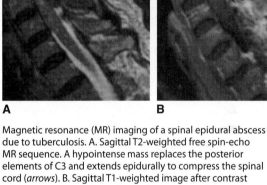

Magnetic resonance (MR) imaging of a spinal epidural abscess due to tuberculosis. A. Sagittal T2-weighted free spin-echo MR sequence. A hypointense mass replaces the posterior elements of C3 and extends epidurally to compress the spinal cord (*arrows*). B. Sagittal T1-weighted image after contrast administration reveals a diffuse enhancement of the epidural process (*arrows*) with extension into the epidural space. (Reproduced with permission from Loscalzo J, Fauci AS, Kasper DL, et al, eds. Harrison's Principles of Internal Medicine. 21st ed. New York: McGraw Hill; 2022.)

History/Physical:
- Risk factors include intravenous drug use, any remote infection sites, spine injury/abnormality, spinal surgery/procedure, and other comorbidities (DM, alcohol use disorder, HIV infection, and renal disease).
- Classic triad is fever, severe localized back pain, and neurological deficits, although this triad will only occur in the minority of cases. Most often patient will present with severe localized back pain with radicular shooting pain and neurological manifestations, including weakness and sensory abnormalities depending on level of spinal cord affected.
- Severe point tenderness over affected spinal cord region.
- If associated with neurological abnormalities can include UMN signs with sensory and autonomic abnormalities.

Diagnostics:
- Emergent MRI with and without contrast is required and will demonstrate enhancement with epidural collection and surrounding inflammation.
- Blood culture and aspirate culture should be done to determine organism and narrow antibiotic regiment as indicated.

Management:
- This is a neurological and neurosurgical emergency and requires aspiration or surgical evacuation/decompression.
- Empiric broad-spectrum IV antibiotics started immediately and modified based on culture results. Treatment duration is 4–6 weeks total.

CASE 25 | Spinal Epidural Abscess *(continued)*

Additional Considerations	**Complications: Autonomic dysreflexia:** A life-threatening complication of a spinal cord injury. As a result, the spinal cord is not able to activate compensatory parasympathetic response following the activation of the sympathetic nervous system by a noxious stimulus. Above the lesion, both the initial sympathetic and compensatory parasympathetic response will occur. Below the lesion, there will be no compensatory parasympathetic response, leading to unregulated sympathetic response which is associated with severe hypertension and hypertensive urgency/emergency. Management includes quick reduction of blood pressure through orthostatic blood pressure reduction (sitting patient in upright position) or medication treatment of hypertension. The noxious stimuli should also be removed as quickly as possible.

TUMORS OF THE NERVOUS SYSTEM

Brain tumors present with many neurologic symptoms, most commonly headache, seizures, focal neurologic deficits, hydrocephalus, and other sequelae related to mass effect. Headache is almost never the only symptom. Neurologic findings depend on size, location, pathophysiology, and rate of growth. Patients with progressive symptoms and/or systemic side effects more likely have a faster-growing tumor (malignant) as opposed to a more indolent progression (benign). Though most brain tumors are from metastases (lung, breast, kidney), there are >30 different kinds of primary CNS tumors. Primary CNS tumors very rarely metastasize. Brain tumors are the second most common cause of pediatric cancer after leukemia, accounting for approximately 20% of all cases of pediatric cancer. Most pediatric brain tumors are primary tumors and arise infratentorially. Craniopharyngioma is a common exception, which is supratentorial.

Adult Brain Tumors and Associated Findings

Diagnosis	Key Findings
Meningioma (benign)	• Most common benign CNS tumor in adults (rarely malignant) • Arise from meningothelial cells from the arachnoid layer of the meninges • Extra-axial (outside the brain parenchyma) • May have estrogen receptors, so more common in women • Homogenously (diffuse) enhancing lesions contiguous with meninges often containing a radiographic "dural tail" feature
Primary CNS lymphoma (malignant)	• Ring-enhancing solitary lesion on CT • Associated with HIV or other cell-mediated immunosuppression
Glioblastoma multiforme (malignant)	• Most common primary brain tumor in adults (age 50–60) • Tumor crosses the corpus callosum ("butterfly glioma") • High-grade malignancy arising from astrocytes • Strong heterogeneous enhancement and commonly bilateral and/or multifocal • Prognosis is poor, median survival ~1 year

Brain Tumors Associated with Genetic Condition

Diagnosis	Genetic Condition	Key Findings
Schwannoma (benign)	Neurofibromatosis type 2 (bilateral)	• Benign tumor involving cranial and spinal nerves (CN VII tumors result in tinnitus and hearing loss) • Arise from Schwann cells producing myelin sheath around axons
Ependymoma (malignant)	Neurofibromatosis type 1	• Arise in fourth ventricle from ependymal cells, which are ciliated epithelial cells lining the ventricles in the brain and spinal canal • Notorious for causing communicating hydrocephalus • Poor prognosis
Hemangioblastoma (malignant)	Von-Hippel Lindau disease	• Most commonly located in the cerebellum • Arises from hemangioblasts, which are precursor cells to erythrocytes and vascular endothelial cells • Produces erythropoietin resulting in secondary polycythemia

Pediatric Brain Tumors and Associated Findings

Diagnosis	Key Findings
Pilocytic astrocytoma (benign)	• Most common primary brain tumor in children • Appears cystic with solid components on CT • Insidious with often cystic morphology, arising from glial cells and commonly located in the cerebellum
Craniopharyngioma (benign)	• Benign suprasellar neoplasm arising from embryonic tissue in the sellar region near the pituitary gland, referred to as Rathke's pouch (oral ectoderm). • Derived from the ectoderm • Can cause bitemporal hemianopsia • Can compress pituitary, leading to pituitary insufficiency
Medulloblastoma (malignant)	• Arise in cerebellum from cerebellar neural progenitor cells • Can cause vast cerebellar dysfunction, including truncal and appendicular ataxia • Can cause obstructive hydrocephalus • Poor prognosis

CASE 26 | Meningioma

A 70-year-old woman with hypertension, type 2 diabetes mellitus, and ischemic stroke 1 month ago, presents for follow-up. She has been taking her medications and her speech has normalized. She is concerned about an incidental brain mass that was seen on the CT scan last month. Patient has no postural headaches, nausea, vomiting, changes in vision, lightheadedness, dizziness, abnormal movements, or other neurological deficits. There is no family history of brain tumors. Vital signs are within normal limits. Fundoscopic exam demonstrates no papilledema. No neurological deficits noted on exam. Previous non-contrast CT scan demonstrated an extra-axial well-circumscribed, hyperdense 2.5-cm mass in the parasagittal region.

Conditions with Similar Presentations	Rarely, other **primary brain tumors** can be incidentally found on brain imaging for an asymptomatic patient, including low-grade gliomas and pituitary adenomas. Dural **metastasis** should also be considered based on the patient's history.
Initial Diagnostic Tests	• MRI with contrast
Next Steps in Management	• Observation for small (≤3 cm), asymptomatic tumors • Surgical resection for symptomatic or enlarging tumors

Discussion	Meningioma is a common, almost always benign, slow-growing CNS tumor that is derived from arachnoid cells in the meninges. It is extra axial and occurs along the surfaces of the brain and spinal cord in the cerebral convexities, parasagittal region, parasellar region, and spinal canal. It is more common in women by a 2:1 ratio. Peak occurrence is 60–70 years of age.
	
	History/Physical Exam:
	• Risk Factors: Neurofibromatosis type II, previous radiation, breast cancer
	• Symptoms: Often asymptomatic; tumor found incidentally on brain imaging
	• Most are slow growing, and the progression of symptoms is gradual. If large, or depending on the region, may have focal neurological deficits, seizures, headaches, and associated nausea and vomiting
	
	Diagnostics:
	• MRI with contrast is the imaging modality of choice for diagnosis
	  • Extra-axial, well-circumscribed, homogenously enhancing lesion often with a dural tail.
	• Biopsy for definitive diagnosis
	  • Histology: monomorphic cells with oval nuclei and psammoma bodies.
		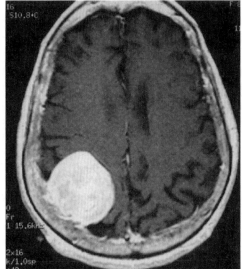
		Meningioma. Axial T1-weighted magnetic resonance imaging scan after gadolinium contrast administration shows a right frontoparietal, well-circumscribed meningioma that enhances intensely and homogeneously with contrast. This tumor grows from the meningeal covering of the brain and will typically compress but not invade into the brain tissue. (Reproduced with permission from Brust JCM, ed. Current Diagnosis & Treatment: Neurology. 3th ed. New York, NY: McGraw Hill; 2019.)

CASE 26 | Meningioma *(continued)*

Discussion	**Management:** Management is dependent on the size and symptoms of the meningioma.
	Small (≤3 cm), benign, asymptomatic tumor
	• Serial MRI for surveillance for enlargement
	• Surgical resection
	• If the mass enlarges or becomes symptomatic
	• May consider earlier in asymptomatic healthy younger patients with the expectation that tumor progression will eventually necessitate intervention
	Large (>3 cm) or symptomatic benign tumors
	• Complete surgical resection
	• Radiation therapy is an alternative option if unable to perform surgery
	Malignant meningioma
	• Surgical resection with radiation therapy is required
Additional Considerations	Meningiomas are associated with **neurofibromatosis type 2**, which is an autosomal dominant mutation in the NF2 gene leading to the characteristic syndrome of bilateral vestibular schwannomas, meningiomas, spinal tumors, cataracts, peripheral neuropathies, and cutaneous tumors.

CASE 27 | Glioblastoma Multiforme (Grade IV Astrocytoma)

A 58-year-old previously healthy man is brought into the clinic following a generalized tonic-clonic seizure. He reports progressive headache for the past several months. He is unable to describe the precise location but does note they worsen with coughing or when lying down. His vital signs are normal and he is alert and oriented to person, place, and time. He has mild left-sided asymmetry of the lower face, with strength 4/5 in the left arm and 5/5 in the right arm. Lower extremity motor function is normal bilaterally.

Conditions with Similar Presentations	**Ischemic or hemorrhagic stroke:** Can also present with weakness, facial asymmetry, headache, and/or seizure; however, symptoms would develop acutely.
	Primary CNS lymphoma: Can also present with headache, confusion, lethargy, seizure, and focal neurological deficits; however, patients are typically immunocompromised. Brain MRI with contrast will show a solitary, irregular, ring-enhancing lesion with edema.
	Oligodendroglioma: Slow-growing, rare tumor, most often located within the frontal lobes and derived from neoplastic oligodendrocytes. Clinical manifestations may vary but include headache, personality changes, and seizures. Imaging commonly shows a contrast-enhancing mass with characteristic calcifications and biopsy shows "fried egg" appearance of cells.
Initial Diagnostic Tests	CT with contrast or MRI brain with and without contrast.
Next Steps in Management	Surgical resection followed by chemotherapy and adjuvant radiation.
Discussion	Glioblastoma multiforme (GBM) is a high-grade (grade IV) astrocytoma and is the most common primary malignant brain tumor in adults. The tumor is derived from poorly differentiated, neoplastic astrocytes. It generally occurs in patients over the age of 50 and is slightly more common in men. Patients often have no family history; however, in rare cases may be associated with genetic syndromes including Li-Fraumeni syndrome or Lynch syndrome.
	History/Physical Exam:
	• Risk Factors: Previous exposure to ionizing radiation (e.g., treatment for childhood brain tumor or leukemia).
	• Symptoms: Occur due to mass effect or increased intracranial pressure and may include headache (never by itself), seizure, altered mental status, or focal neurologic deficits including weakness, visual symptoms, and language deficits. Involvement of the frontal lobes can lead to abnormal behaviors or changes in personality.
	Diagnostics: Imaging and biopsy are necessary to make a definitive diagnosis.
	• Head CT with contrast or MRI brain with and without contrast (preferred).
	• GBMs often have rim enhancement with central clearing due to necrosis. The heterogeneously enhancing mass may extend across the corpus callosum, sometimes referred to as a "butterfly mass."
	• MRI findings are as shown.

CASE 27 | Glioblastoma Multiforme (Grade IV Astrocytoma) *(continued)*

Discussion	

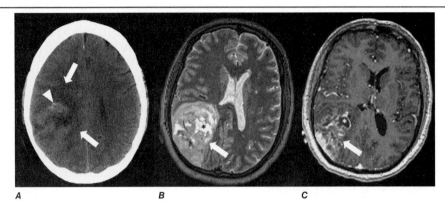

Glioblastoma multiforme. Axial nonenhanced CT (A) shows an ill-defined lesion in the right cerebral hemisphere (*arrows*). Internal hyperdensities represent hemorrhagic foci (*arrowheads*). Axial T2-weighted (B) and postcontrast T1-weighted (C) MRI demonstrate a peripherally enhancing right parietal lesion (arrows), with necrosis (*). (Reproduced with permission from Loscalzo J, Fauci AS, Kasper DL, et al, eds. Harrison's Principles of Internal Medicine. 21st ed. New York: McGraw Hill; 2022.)

- Biopsy should be done for definitive diagnosis.
  - Tissue will show glial fibrillary acidic protein (GFAP), a known marker of astrocytes, and show pleomorphic, poorly differentiated cells in a "pseudopalisading pattern" with central necrosis and hemorrhage.
  - Molecular testing may reveal several gene mutations which can help differentiate between low- and high-grade astrocytomas; however, there is considerable heterogeneity of tumor genetic profiles.

Management:
- Multimodal treatment with surgical resection followed by chemotherapy and adjuvant radiation therapy are used.
- The standard chemotherapy regimen typically lasts for more than 6 months.
  - The alkylating agent temozolomide is used as it is lipophilic, readily crosses the blood-brain barrier, and is available orally.
- Patients should undergo frequent surveillance during and after treatment with repeat MRI.
- Patients typically have a poor prognosis even with standard treatment due to high rate of recurrence and overall poor survival, which can range between 1.5 and 2 years.

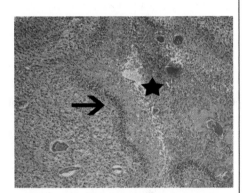

The distinction between the various grades of infiltrating astrocytic neoplasms is based upon four histologic features: nuclear pleomorphism, mitotic figures, endothelial proliferation, and necrosis. GBMs, by definition, contain at least three of these four histologic features. In this section, the necrosis is apparent (*star*). As is characteristic for GBMs, this tumor has palisading of neoplastic cells at the edge of the necrosis (*arrow*). Hematoxylin and eosin, 100×. (Reproduced with permission from Kemp WL, Burns DK, Travis Brown TG. Pathology: The Big Picture. New York, NY: McGraw Hill; 2008.)

CASE 28 | Pilocytic Astrocytoma (PCA)

An 8-year-old previously healthy boy presents to urgent care for evaluation of persistent headaches for the past 3 weeks. His mother states that he has had to miss school on several occasions. The headaches typically occur in the morning and are associated with some nausea and occasional vomiting. Per mom, there were no complications at birth and he has met all developmental milestones and has been doing well in school. Vital signs are within normal limits. On ophthalmologic exam, there is swelling of the optic discs bilaterally and he has difficulty with abduction of his right and left eye (abducens nerve palsy). His neurologic exam is significant for dysmetria on finger-nose test and a wide-based gait. Strength is 5/5 in the upper and lower extremities and sensation is intact to light touch and pinprick bilaterally.

CASE 28 | Pilocytic Astrocytoma (PCA) *(continued)*

Conditions with Similar Presentations	**Ependymoma:** Arises from ependymal cells that line the ventricles, most commonly within the fourth ventricle. More common in early childhood but can occur at any age, with a slight male predominance. Can result in hydrocephalus with signs and symptoms of elevated intracranial pressure, seizures, and focal neurologic deficits. MRI will show prominent gadolinium enhancement, although definitive diagnosis requires biopsy, which demonstrates perivascular pseudorosettes.
	Medulloblastoma: Most common malignant pediatric brain tumor derived from primitive neuroectoderm and most commonly found in the cerebellum. Also, more common in male children. Can invade the nearby fourth ventricle, resulting in hydrocephalus. Patients typically have morning headaches, nausea, vomiting, and difficulty with coordination and balance. Diagnosis is by imaging (including the entire neuraxis due to risk of drop metastases) and biopsy, with histology showing poorly differentiated, small, round, blue cells.
Initial Diagnostic Tests	Brain MRI with contrast
Next Steps in Management	Dexamethasone (to control edema) and surgical resection
Discussion	PCA is the most common benign brain tumor in childhood. Median age of diagnosis is 8 years. It is a slow-growing, usually well-circumscribed tumor that arises from astrocytes, and is most commonly located within the posterior fossa (especially the cerebellum); however, they can appear anywhere in the CNS. Most occur sporadically although there is an association with neurofibromatosis type 1, with tumors commonly occurring within the optic pathway.

History/Physical Exam:

Signs and symptoms: Related to mass effect within the posterior fossa and increased intracranial pressure.
- Subacute or chronic hydrocephalus can lead to increased intracranial pressure, resulting in morning headaches, nausea, vomiting, papilledema, and/or abducens nerve
- When located in the hypothalamus, PCAs can interfere with neuroendocrine signaling
- When located within the optic pathway, PCAs can lead to optic nerve atrophy or vision defects including bitemporal hemianopsia
- Mass effect can disrupt normal cerebellar functions. If the cerebellar hemispheres are involved, patients will develop dysmetria, peripheral ataxia, and nystagmus. If the cerebellar vermis is involved, patients may have truncal ataxia, titubation, and a broad-based gait

Diagnostics:
- Brain MRI with contrast: will reveal a well-demarcated, T2-hyperintense mass with an enhancing mural nodule, often surrounded by a cyst most often within the posterior fossa near the cerebellum.

Pilocytic astrocytoma. Axial T2-weighted and T1-weighted postgadolinium images (A, B) show a cystic lesion with peripheral enhancement and an enhancing solid component located in the posterior fossa (*arrows*). These findings are suggestive of a pilocytic astrocytoma. Note that the lesion exerts mass effect on the fourth ventricle, which is compressed (*curved arrows*). (Reproduced with permission from Loscalzo J, Fauci AS, Kasper DL, et al, eds. Harrison's Principles of Internal Medicine. 21st ed. New York: McGraw Hill; 2022.)

CASE 28 | Pilocytic Astrocytoma (PCA) *(continued)*

Discussion	• Definitive diagnosis by biopsy which will reveal GFAP+ neoplastic cells with hairlike projections and Rosenthal fibers (see image).

Management:
- Complete surgical resection can result in cure.
- Chemotherapy and radiation often not required if complete resection is achieved.
- Patients with hydrocephalus may require CSF diversion with an external ventricular drain or ventriculoperitoneal shunt.
- Prognosis is favorable, with a 10-year survival rate of 95% with complete resection. Recurrence is rare, although can occur with subtotal resection.

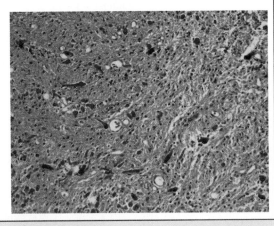

Rosenthal fibers. The thick, irregular, eosinophilic structures scattered throughout this image are Rosenthal fibers. Rosenthal fibers are associated with pilocytic astrocytomas and a number of other indolent CNS neoplasms, but can also be seen at the edge of chronic non-neoplastic processes. In this regard, Rosenthal fibers indicate slow growth, which is consistent with pilocytic astrocytomas. Hematoxylin and eosin, 200×. (Reproduced with permission from Kemp WL, Burns DK, Travis Brown TG. Pathology: The Big Picture. New York, NY: McGraw Hill; 2008.)

Additional Considerations	**Complications:** Risk of herniation, death if untreated

Brain Tumor Mini-Cases

Craniopharyngioma	**Hx:**

Hx:
- Occurs in children or older adults
- Symptoms: May be asymptomatic or have progressive headaches, visual defects; compression of pituitary may cause hypopituitarism (weight gain, fatigue, swelling, weakness, urinary frequency (loss of ADH); symptoms of hypoglycemia

PE:
- Possible findings include papilledema (increased ICP), signs of hypopituitarism (orthostatic hypotension (loss of ACTH); delayed reflexes.
- Visual field testing may reveal bitemporal hemianopsia due to the tumor arising in the suprasellar region (near the pituitary gland) and compressing the optic chiasm.

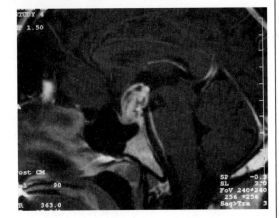

Contrast-enhanced sagittal magnetic resonance imaging showing suprasellar craniopharyngioma. (Reproduced with permission from Riordan-Eva P, Augsburger JJ, eds. Vaughan & Asbury's General Ophthalmology. 19th ed. New York: McGraw Hill; 2018.)

Diagnostics:
- CT will reveal a suprasellar mass with cysts and calcification.
- MRI with contrast demonstrates a solid tumor with cystic features and fluid of intermediate intensity.
- Labs: Evaluation of pituitary hormone function (TSH, Free T4, cortisol, IGF-1). Serum sodium, serum osmolality, and urine specific gravity to test for central diabetes insipidus.
- Diagnosis is confirmed with histology showing cholesterol crystals in a "motor oil"–like fluid within the tumor.

Brain Tumor Mini-Cases *(continued)*

Craniopharyngioma	**Management:** • Surgical resection via transsphenoidal approach is the definitive therapy • If complete resection is not possible, it is typically followed with radiation therapy **Discussion:** Craniopharyngiomas are the most common benign supratentorial lesion in children, although occur in a bimodal distribution and therefore can also be seen in older adults. They are extra-axial, developing from embryonic surface oral ectodermal remnants that form Rathke's pouch. For this reason, patients can present with symptoms of increased intracranial pressure (e.g., headache, visual disturbances, pituitary dysfunction) from mass effect. Other findings may include signs of hypopituitarism (hypothyroidism, adrenal insufficiency, growth hormone deficiency). Prognosis is better in younger individuals.
Brain Metastases	**Hx:** • Patients present with symptoms due to mass effect and surrounding edema, most commonly headaches (especially in the morning and/or when lying down), seizures, and focal neurological deficits (i.e., hemiparesis). Some patients may occasionally present with stroke from metastasis or invasion of vasculature. Patients may have a known primary tumor, although in some patients, brain metastases may be the presenting manifestation. **PE:** Depending on location, patients may have localizing deficits (i.e., hemiparesis) and changes in vision. **Diagnostics:** • Patients with underlying primary tumors who develop above symptoms should undergo urgent neuroimaging (preferably MRI brain with contrast). MRI will reveal well-circumscribed, ring-enhancing lesions (usually multiple), commonly located at the gray–white matter junction. Masses often have surrounding vasogenic edema. 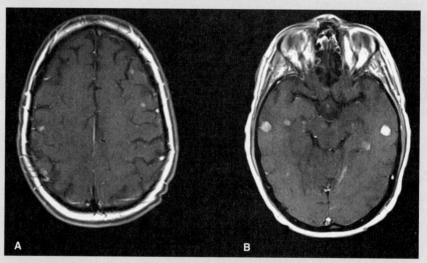 Cerebral metastases. Axial T1-weighted postcontrast MRI images demonstrating multiple small enhancing lesions at the gray–white junction in a patient with breast cancer. (Reproduced with permission from Berkowitz AL. Clinical Neurology and Neuroanatomy: A Localization-Based Approach. 2nd ed. New York: McGraw Hill; 2022.) • If primary tumor source is unknown, body imaging with chest x-ray, CT chest, CT abdomen and pelvis, and/or PET should be performed to evaluate for a primary site. • Brain biopsy may be necessary in some cases, and histopathology will be consistent with the underlying primary source of the tumor (e.g., breast cancer).

Brain Tumor Mini-Cases *(continued)*

Brain Metastases	**Management:** • Treatment is based on the tumor type, extent of the disease, and size and number of metastases, but should be started as soon as possible to limit further disease progression. • Those with multiple brain metastases are typically treated with whole-brain radiation therapy, although surgical resection may be performed for symptomatic relief. • Those with single or limited number of metastases often undergo surgery, stereotactic radiosurgery, and/or chemotherapy. • The mainstay of treatment is brain radiation and treatment of the underlying primary tumor. • Patients may also be prescribed corticosteroids to control ICP and edema as well as anti-seizure medications. • Prognosis is poor with multifocal brain metastatic disease. Patients may consider clinical trials or palliative therapy. **Discussion:** Brain metastases are the most common intracranial tumors in adults. The most common causes include lung cancer, breast cancer, melanoma, colorectal cancer, and renal cell carcinoma. Because they occur via hematogenous spread, lesions occur within the cerebral hemispheres at the gray–white matter junction, where cerebral blood vessels decrease in size, resulting in trapping of tumor cells. Patients may have a known primary tumor (e.g., small cell carcinoma in the lung); however, in some cases, neurological symptoms due to metastases may be the reason the patient seeks medical attention.

HEARING LOSS

Hearing loss has a wide variety of etiologies, from benign to malignant, but can broadly be categorized into three main groups: conductive, sensorineural, and mixed (conductive + sensorineural).

Conductive hearing loss is the inability of sound waves to reach the inner ear via conduction. Most commonly, conductive hearing loss is caused by cerumen impaction, trauma (e.g., tympanic membrane perforation), cholesteatoma, and otosclerosis. Sensorineural hearing loss affects nerve conduction and subsequent connection to the brain. Inner ear structures are most commonly affected, such as the cochlea, vestibulocochlear nerve (CN VIII), internal auditory canal, or brain structures such as the inferior olive or medial geniculate nucleus. Common sensorineural disorders include presbycusis (physiologic age-related hearing loss), Meniere disease, ototoxic substances (e.g., aminoglycosides, loop diuretics, platinum-based chemotherapy, heavy metals), and tumors (e.g., acoustic neuromas). Congenital malformation is a cause of all three types of hearing loss.

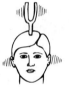
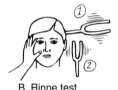

A. Weber test   B. Rinne test

Tests of hearing perception and conduction. A. Weber test: The vibrating tuning fork is on the midline of the skull. Lateralization of the sound to one ear indicates a conductive loss on that side, or a perceptive loss on the other side. B. Rinne test: The handle of the tuning fork is first placed against the mastoid process then near the external ear. Each time the patient indicates when the sound ceases. Normally, duration of air conduction is twice that of bone conduction. (Reproduced with permission from Suneja M, Szot JF, LeBlond RF, Brown DD. DeGowin's Diagnostic Examination. 11th ed. New York: McGraw Hill; 2020.)

Evaluation of hearing loss includes eliciting a history including the time course, medications, any recent illnesses, and associated symptoms, especially pain and vertigo. Examination of the ear with otoscope and Weber and Rinne tests will help localize the hearing loss and determine whether the cause is of conductive or sensorineural origin. Further audiology and speech testing can be conducted if the initial workup is non-confirmatory. CT imaging can be helpful in cases of cholesteatoma or otosclerosis.

Treatment depends on the etiology of the hearing loss. For congenital hearing loss and presbycusis, hearing aids, cochlear implants, or other assistive listening devices may be used. Surgery is an option for intracranial tumors, tympanic membrane rupture, cholesteatoma, and otosclerosis. Tympanoplasty, mastoidectomy, and ossicular chain reconstruction are the respective procedures. For infection-related hearing loss, treat the underlying cause with appropriate antibiotics.

CASE 29 | Otosclerosis

A 27-year-old woman presents with progressive hearing loss, tinnitus, and occasional spells of vertigo, where she feels the room spinning causing her to feel nauseous and needs to sit down. These symptoms started 12 months ago and have been worsening to the point where she is having difficulty hearing people speaking to her and is unable to swim because she feels too dizzy. She has no ear pain, recent illnesses, or history of aminoglycoside treatment. She states her paternal uncle needed hearing aids in his early 40s but is unsure of anyone else in her family who had hearing issues. On exam, the patient has decreased hearing of whispered voice in both ears, although worse in her left ear. Otoscopic exam shows normal tympanic membrane appearance. Weber test localizes to the left ear and Rinne test shows bone conduction greater than air conduction in both ears. Dix-Hallpike maneuver does not provoke a new episode of vertigo.

Conditions with Similar Presentations	**Cholesteatoma:** Middle ear disorder due to growth of desquamated, stratified, squamous epithelium. It eventually erodes the ossicular chain, mastoid, and external auditory canal. This often occurs after tympanic membrane trauma. It can lead to sensorineural hearing loss, lateral sinus thrombosis, brain abscess, sepsis, or facial paralysis. Treatment is a tympanomastoidectomy. **Chronic otitis media:** Otitis media is one of the most common infections of children. Recurrent or undertreated otitis media can lead to cholesteatoma and mastoiditis in adults. This will present with middle ear pain and changes to the tympanic membrane able to be visualized with otoscopy. Treatment is antibiotics and imaging to evaluate the extent of damage. **Tympanic membrane perforation:** Can be caused by either of the above conditions, or by trauma (e.g., barotrauma, foreign body trauma, temporal bone fractures, or self-inflicted trauma from a cotton-tipped swab). These will cause sharp severe ear pain, with audiosensitivity in the affected ear. Most acute perforations heal on their own, but the ear should be examined to ensure skin is not trapped under the tympanic membrane, which could lead to cholesteatoma formation.
Initial Diagnostic Tests	Clinical diagnosis; consider pneumoscopy and/or tone audiometry
Next Steps in Management	Hearing amplification (i.e., hearing aids) or surgery

Discussion	Otosclerosis is a conductive hearing disorder caused by a bony overgrowth of the footplate of the stapes. Abnormal bone overgrowth causes the stapes to become stiff and fixed and sclerotic, preventing the normal conduction of sounds to vibratory waves within the middle ear.
	
	History:
	• Risk factors: Viral infection (e.g., measles), family history (genetic causes follow an autosomal dominant pattern, but penetrance is so variable that true inheritance pattern is inconclusive).
	• Symptoms: Painless, progressive conductive hearing loss, often bilateral.
	
	Physical Exam:
	• Whispered voice test and tuning forks can evaluate the extent of hearing loss.
	• The Weber and Rinne tests will confirm the conductive hearing loss origin.
	  • The Weber test will make the sound more prominent in the ear most affected by conductive hearing loss when the tuning fork is placed on the forehead (in this case, the patient's left ear).
	  • The Rinne test will show that bone conduction of sound is more prominent than air conduction of sound when the tuning fork is placed on the mastoid bone.
	
	Diagnostics: Clinical based on the physical exam findings and absence of additional symptoms that would suggest more concerning pathology (e.g., CNS tumor, posterior circulation stroke).
	
	Management: Beyond hearing amplification devices, replacement of the stapes bone with prosthesis can be performed. If advanced otosclerosis, cochlear implant may be most beneficial.

High-Yield Causes of Sensorineural Hearing Loss

Diagnosis	Features
Presbycusis	Gradual sensorineural hearing loss that is age-related and occurs in elderly patients. It starts with reduced hearing of higher frequency sounds and may continue to progress. Consider the age of the patient when diagnosing presbycusis, as it is a diagnosis of exclusion.
Meniere disease	A triad of episodic vertigo, tinnitus, and hearing loss. It is caused by endolymphatic hydrops of the labyrinthine system of the inner ear and usually presents between 20 and 40 years of age. If children present with Meniere disease, it is often due to congenital malformation. The disease is relapsing-remitting, where goals of treatment are supportive, aimed at enhancing patient quality of life.

High-Yield Causes of Sensorineural Hearing Loss

Diagnosis	Features
Acoustic neuroma	Schwann cell tumors that arise from CN VIII. They most commonly occur in adults, but if found in a child, are most likely associated with neurofibromatosis type 2. They are associated with childhood exposure to low-dose radiation. Imaging will confirm the tumor and treatment is surgical resection.
Drug ototoxicity	Ototoxicity is triggered by prolonged treatment with the antibiotic in question. The drugs are associated with cochlear and vestibular toxicity, leading to the presenting symptoms of hearing loss and disequilibrium. There is a strong association with aminoglycoside use and nephrotoxicity as well, so extreme caution should be considered in patients who need antibiotic treatment and have either acute or chronic kidney disease. Other drugs and substances known to cause ototoxicity and sensorineural hearing loss include loop diuretics (e.g., furosemide), platinum-based chemotherapy agents (e.g., cisplatin, carboplatin), some NSAIDS, cocaine, and heavy metals. Hearing may recover following discontinuation of the offending agent, but in cases of irreversible hearing loss, hearing aids may be required.

DIZZINESS AND VERTIGO

Dizziness is a common chief concern that is often challenging to interpret because it is used to describe a wide range of symptoms that a patient may experience. The word "dizzy" means different things to different people, so patients should be asked to use a different word. They will usually choose one of the following:

1. **Lightheadedness.** The patient states they feel like they are going to faint. The differential is the same as for syncope.
2. **Sensation of motion.** The patient states they and/or the room is moving or spinning. The differential is that of vertigo.
3. **Unsteadiness of gait.** The patient states they are off balance and/or cannot tell where their feet are. The differential is that of ataxia.
4. **None of the above.** The patient has difficulty categorizing their concern in the ways stated above. The differential includes psychogenic causes (depression, anxiety, conversion reactions).

Syncope is transient loss of consciousness due to cerebral hypoperfusion and may be preceded by episodes of "dizziness" or may occur suddenly without warning. For additional syncope cases, see Cardiovascular Chapter.

Differential Diagnosis for Syncope and Pre-Syncope

Type of Syncope	Examples and Key Findings
Reflex	• **Vasovagal:** Syncope is brought on by a trigger (e.g., emotional stress, anxiety, pain, heat, prolonged standing, claustrophobia) with prodrome (e.g., nausea, sweating, warmth, dizziness, diaphoresis). The trigger causes an initial increase in sympathetic tone which increases cardiac contractility, which is sensed by tension-sensitive C-fibers in the myocardium that are vagal afferents. In predisposed individuals, stimulating these fibers leads to an exaggerated increased vagal tone with resultant bradycardia, vasodilation, and hypotension, leading to a transient loss of consciousness. These can be managed with preventive physical counterpressure maneuvers (leg crossing and tensing of lower extremity, clenched fist with tensing of upper extremity) during prodrome to help improve venous return, cardiac output, and BP. • **Situational:** Syncope with micturition, defecation, swallowing, or coughing. • **Carotid sinus hypersensitivity:** See case below.
Orthostatic	• Syncope is triggered by changing to an upright position. • Caused by medications that are vasodilators (alpha-1 blockers, anti-hypertensives), or inotropic/chronotropic blockers (beta blockers), hypovolemia, and/or autonomic dysfunction (advanced age, diabetes, PD).
Cardiac	• **Left ventricular outflow obstruction** (aortic stenosis, hypertrophic cardiomyopathy): Syncope occurs with exertion. Will have systolic ejection murmur • **Arrhythmia** (ventricle tachycardia): No prodrome prior to syncope. May have history of CAD, cardiomyopathy, MI, QT-interval prolongation. • **Conduction impairment** (sick sinus syndrome, advanced AV block): Diagnostic ECG abnormalities.

Vertigo is the false perception of motion of either oneself (subjective vertigo) or the surroundings (objective vertigo). The most common terminology associated with vertigo is a "room-spinning" sensation. Vertigo indicates a vestibular, inner ear, brainstem, or cerebellar pathology. If the patient expresses symptoms that are consistent with vertigo, the next step is to distinguish if it is due to a peripheral or central cause.

Peripheral vertigo is due to pathology within the vestibular apparatus of the inner ear (utricle, saccule, or semicircular canals) or the vestibular nerve. In peripheral vertigo, symptoms are intermittent or positional, and can often be stopped by visual fixation. Associated symptoms can include hearing loss, tinnitus, unsteadiness, or nausea/vomiting. Peripheral vertigo can be associated with a non-torsional, unidirectional nystagmus which is fatigable, short in duration, and suppressed by visual fixation.

In contrast, central vertigo is associated with pathology within the brainstem nuclei, cerebellum, or central vestibular pathways, including ischemic stroke. Central vertigo requires urgent evaluation. The symptoms are non-positional and do not improve with visual fixation. Patients commonly have additional neurological deficits including facial droops, dysarthria, and gait impairment. Central nystagmus is non-fatiguing, longer in duration, and is torsional or vertical.

Key steps within the physical exam for distinguishing between peripheral and central vertigo include orthostatic blood pressure measurement, full neurological examination, nystagmus assessment, and the Dix-Hallpike physical exam maneuver (The patient begins upright in a seated position. The examiner turns the patient's head 45 degrees to the right or left and, while supporting the patient's head, lowers them to a supine position so that the head is hanging over the edge of the bed. The head should be extended backward by about 20 degrees. The eyes are observed for rhythmic oscillatory horizontal or vertical involuntary eye movements (nystagmus). The maneuver should be performed on both sides and is considered positive if nystagmus is detected.

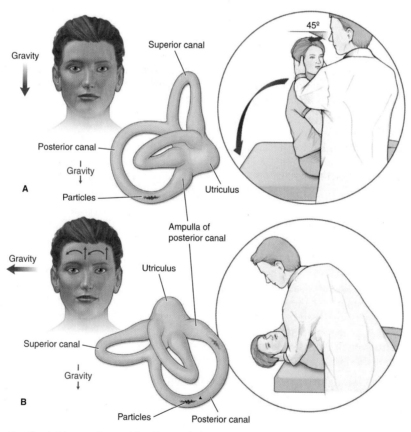

Dix-Hallpike test. A. For testing the right posterior semicircular canal, the patient sits on the examination table and turns his or her head to the right 45 degrees. This places the posterior semicircular canal in the sagittal plane. The examiner stands facing the patient on the patient's right side or behind the patient. B. The patient is then moved by the examiner from the seated to the supine position with the head slightly hanging over the edge of the table. The right ear is down and the chin is pointing slightly up. The eyes are observed for the characteristic geotropic nystagmus. (Reproduced with permission from Lalwani AK, ed. Current Diagnosis & Treatment in Otolaryngology—Head & Neck Surgery. 4th ed. New York: McGraw Hill; 2020.)

CASE 30 | Benign Positional Paroxysmal Vertigo (BPPV)

A 32 -year-old woman with no significant past medical history presents with dizziness for the last month. She reports intermittent 30-second episodes that are described as a sensation of the "room-spinning." They occur when the patient is getting out of bed in the morning or when she turns her head to the right, and are associated with nausea. She has no hearing loss, tinnitus, or focal neurological deficits. Vital signs, including orthostatics, are normal. Cardiac and neurological exams are normal. Horizontal nystagmus is noted, and the patient reports both vertigo and nausea when the Dix-Hallpike maneuver is performed on the right side but not on the left.

Conditions with Similar Presentations	**Meniere disease:** Disorder of the inner ear due to increased pressure in the endolymphatic system. It is characterized by a triad of vertigo, sensorineural hearing loss, and tinnitus. Management is restriction of potential triggers: sodium, monosodium glutamate (MSG), caffeine, nicotine, and alcohol. Manage vertigo with antihistamines, benzodiazepines, and/or antiemetics.
	Vestibular neuritis/labyrinthitis: Acute-onset severe vertigo with head motion intolerance and gait unsteadiness which is presumed to occur from viral infections. Vestibular neuritis lacks auditory symptoms, while labyrinthitis often has tinnitus, sensation of ear fullness, and/or hearing loss. Management includes corticosteroids if given less than 72 hours after symptom onset, and acute symptomatic relief as needed. Resolves spontaneously in weeks to months.
	Central vertigo: Due to vertebrobasilar artery disease. Patient may have cardiovascular risk factors and/or signs or symptoms consistent with a stroke/TIA.
Initial Diagnostic Tests	Clinical diagnosis that is confirmed with a positive Dix-Hallpike maneuver
Next Steps in Management	Particle repositioning maneuvers (Epley, Semont)
Discussion	BBPV is the most common cause of peripheral vertigo (about half of cases). It is caused by displacement of canaliths (calcium debris) within the semicircular canals. The debris is from loose otoconia (calcium carbonate crystals) that originate within the utricle. The semicircular canals are responsible for detection of angular acceleration of the head; therefore, if canaliths obstruct the normal movement of endolymph, it may result in the sensation of spinning with movements of the head. The most common location affected is the posterior semicircular canal, and the condition is most often idiopathic although may be associated with prior trauma.
	History/Physical Exam: BPPV is more common in women, and prevalence increases with age. Patients will present with brief (often <1 minute), episodic vertigo episodes with nystagmus triggered by specific changes in head position which often improve with visual fixation. Patients do not have hearing loss or other neurologic complaints.
	Diagnostics: • Positive Dix-Hallpike maneuver, which will induce vertigo and horizontal nystagmus when the head is turned toward the affected side. • Additional testing is not indicated, but if performed, audiometry and imaging would be normal.
	Management: • Particle repositioning maneuvers (Epley, Semont), should be repeated at home over the course of days until symptoms subside. • Medications are not recommended unless severity and frequency of episodes is high. For patients who experience nausea and vomiting during the repositioning maneuvers, antihistamines can be given prior to them. • Persistent vertigo or nystagmus that is not purely horizontal or torsional after head movement should raise concerns for central vertigo due to CNS lesion or stroke. Next steps would be urgent brain imaging.

CASE 31 | Carotid Sinus Hypersensitivity/Carotid Sinus Syndrome

A 70-year-old man with hypertension presents with recurrent episodes of dizziness and lightheadedness. Patient reports five episodes over the last month, and the most recent resulted in a brief episode of loss of consciousness which lasted <30 seconds. Episodes occurred in the morning while he was shaving. Episodes do not occur with exertion. Patient has no nausea, vomiting, changes in vision, or other neurological deficits. Denies tongue biting, lip smacking, abnormal movements, or incontinence. Vital signs including orthostatics are normal. Cardiac and neurologic exams are normal.

Conditions with Similar Presentations	There are three major categories of syncope or loss of consciousness due to acute drops in cerebral perfusion: **reflex/vasovagal**, **orthostatic**, and **cardiac syncope** (see table above). **Seizure:** Typically unilateral or prolonged abnormal limb movements, tongue biting, incontinence, lip smacking, or prolonged confusion after an event.
Initial Diagnostic Tests	• Carotid sinus massage • Also check ECG, Holter and/or event monitor
Next Steps in Management	Permanent pacemaker
Discussion	Dizziness and lightheadedness are common symptoms of pre-syncope that may lead to brief loss of consciousness (syncope). Carotid sinus hypersensitivity (CSH) is a common cause of syncope in which overly sensitive baroreceptors trigger an exaggerated vagal response. Hypersensitive carotid sinus baroreceptors, located at carotid bifurcation, are triggered by minimal tactile stimuli which stimulates the parasympathetic nervous system leading to sinus bradycardia, hypotension, and presyncope or syncope due to an acute drop in cerebral perfusion. **History/Physical Exam:** • CSH is more common in elderly men with underlying vascular risk factors, especially a history of atherosclerotic disease. Other risk factors include prior neck surgery and neck irradiation. • Patients will report sudden episodes of dizziness, lightheadedness, and/or syncope that occur with minimal tactile stimulus of the carotid sinus (e.g., shaving, rubbing of a shirt collar while dressing, turning the head). **Diagnostics:** • Clinical diagnosis when presyncope or syncope occur after a clear trigger. CSH is confirmed with a positive carotid massage test. • Carotid massage test is positive when the carotid vessel is massaged for 5–10 seconds and results in a greater than 3-second ventricular pause and greater than 50-mmHg drop in systolic blood pressure. If symptoms are reproduced during the carotid massage test, the diagnosis is carotid sinus syndrome (CSS) • Carotid massage test can be aided by the tilt table test. • If there is uncertain diagnosis based on history, consider additional testing, including ECG, echocardiogram, neuroimaging, and EEG for seizure rule out. **Management:** Placement of permanent pacemaker; consider driving restrictions.

18
Ophthalmology

Lead Author: Amy Y. Lin, MD
Contributors: Eitan A. Katz, MD; Joseph R. Geraghty, MD, PhD

Ophthalmology is the subspecialty of medicine that deals with medical and surgical management of eye disorders. In this section, we will review some eye-related chief concerns and common and/or important ophthalmic diagnoses that may be encountered in a primary care clinic or emergency department.

Aqueous humor:

- Produced in the ciliary body
- Flows between the iris and lens into the anterior chamber, where it is mostly reabsorbed at the iridocorneal angle through the trabecular meshwork into the canal of Schlemm
- Dysregulation of its production, flow, or drainage can result in elevated intraocular pressure (IOP) and cause glaucoma

Three main layers of the eye:

1. **Sclera**—the white, nontransparent structure that is continuous with the cornea in the front of the eye
2. **Uvea**—includes the iris, ciliary body, and choroid
3. **Retina**—the innermost layer, composed of rod and cone photoreceptors, retinal ganglion cells with axons giving rise to the optic nerve, and other cell types involved in converting light signals to electrochemical signals

The retina is part of the central nervous system and an extension of the diencephalon of the developing brain. As such, the eye serves as a unique window into various neurologic disorders. These include neurologic injuries resulting in increased intracranial pressure (which will manifest as papilledema), demyelinating disorders (which may present as optic neuritis, gaze palsies, and internuclear ophthalmoplegia), or injuries to cranial nerves involved in extraocular muscles, corneal sensation, or autonomic innervation (CN III, IV, V1, or VI).

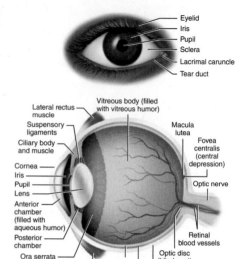

Anatomy of the eye. The eye has three aspects: the anterior segment, the posterior segment, and the surrounding tissues. The anterior segment includes the conjunctiva, sclera, cornea, iris, ciliary body, and crystalline lens. The posterior segment includes the vitreous humor, retina, choroid, and optic nerve. The eyelids, extraocular muscles, and lacrimal drainage system are other important structures relevant to eye anatomy. (Reproduced with permission from Huppert LA, Dyster TG. eds. Huppert's Notes: Pathophysiology and Clinical Pearls for Internal Medicine. New York: McGraw Hill; 2021.)

As with any specialty of medicine, the history is a key component to formulating and narrowing the differential diagnosis. A good general physical and neurologic exam and a thorough ophthalmic exam can provide additional clues to the diagnosis.

Eye exam:

- Inspect conjunctiva/sclera, eyelids, pupils, cornea, and lens bilaterally.
- Check visual acuity, extraocular movements (see figure), pupillary reaction (light and accommodation) and visual fields.
- Perform fundoscopic exam (check optic disc, cup, retina, and retinal vessels).

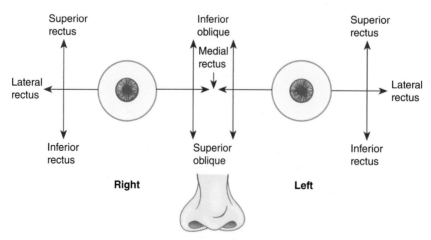

Diagram of eye muscle action. (Reproduced with permission from Waxman SG. eds. Clinical Neuroanatomy, 29e. New York: McGraw Hill; 2020.)

When assessing changes in vision, both eyes must be assessed.

- Vison is documented using denotation based on Latin terminology: OS for the left eye, OD for the right eye, and OU for both eyes.
- Visual acuity is measured at a 20-foot distance, with 20/20 vision indicating that a patient can clearly see objects that are normally visible from 20 feet away.
- Higher denominators indicate worse vision. For example, 20/40 vision indicates that, at a distance of 20 feet, the patient can see objects that others can see from 40 feet.

The ophthalmologist's basic tool is the **slit lamp** microscope, which allows observation of any of the three layers of the eye. The ophthalmoscope (or fundoscope) allows for visualization of the retina, including the macula, optic disc, and blood supply. Additional tools/techniques commonly used by ophthalmologists include tonometry, gonioscopy, and pachymetry.

Tonometry is used to measure the IOP within the eye (typical IOP is 10–21 mmHg).

- Used to diagnose glaucoma in the setting of ocular trauma, and after eye surgeries.

Gonioscopy involves evaluation of the anterior chamber angle to assess for abnormalities in the intraocular drainage of aqueous humor at the iridocorneal angle.

- Used in evaluation of glaucoma (narrowing of the iridocorneal angle can result in decreased outflow of aqueous humor and resulting increase in IOP).

Pachymetry is used to measure the thickness of the cornea.

EYE REDNESS

Eye redness is a common presenting concern with a large differential diagnosis, including inflammatory or infectious conditions of ocular or periocular tissues (e.g., conjunctivitis, keratitis, episcleritis, scleritis, uveitis, blepharitis, dacryocystitis, endophthalmitis), mechanical trauma (e.g., abrasion, foreign body), chemical trauma (e.g., acid or alkali burn), subconjunctival hemorrhage, contact lens overwear, and angle closure glaucoma. Some symptoms may be helpful in narrowing down the differential diagnosis of red eye (see table). It is important to distinguish causes of eye redness that require urgent or emergent referral to an ophthalmologist for treatment.

Symptom	Cause(s)
Itching	Allergy
Burning	Lid disorders, dry eye
Foreign body sensation	Foreign body, corneal abrasion
Deep intense pain	Scleritis, iritis, acute glaucoma
Photophobia	Corneal abrasion, iritis, acute glaucoma
Halo vision	Corneal edema

Comparison of Different Types of Conjunctivitis

Feature	Bacterial Conjunctivitis	Viral Conjunctivitis	Allergic Conjunctivitis
Unilateral or bilateral	Unilateral or bilateral	Starts unilateral and becomes bilateral	Bilateral
Discharge	Purulent	Watery	Watery with stringy white mucus
Associated conditions	Secondary infection in patients after viral conjunctivitis	History of upper respiratory infection (URI) or exposure to someone with URI symptoms	Hay fever, asthma, eczema
Associated signs/ symptoms		Sore throat, fever, other URI symptoms Preauricular (parotid) lymphadenopathy	Itching eyelid and conjunctival edema (chemosis)
Common causes	*Staphylococcus, Streptococcus, Haemophilus*	Adenovirus	Contact allergy from drugs, chemicals, cosmetics, pollen

CASE 1 | Neonatal Gonococcal Conjunctivitis

A 3-day-old neonate is brought in emergency by her mother for evaluation of bilateral red eyes. Her mother had a history of gonorrhea and had a home birth. Examination of the neonate shows intense hyperemia with bilateral purulent discharge. Patient is in considerable distress and is resistant to examination.

Conditions with Similar Presentations	**Chlamydia conjunctivitis:** Has a longer incubation period and presents at 7–14 days post birth with mild edema, hyperemia, tearing, and mostly mucoid discharge. Diagnosed via immunoassay, PCR, or DNA-hybridization probe showing basophilic intracytoplasmic inclusion bodies in conjunctival epithelial cells, polymorphonuclear leukocytes, or lymphocytes on Giemsa stain. **Viral conjunctivitis:** May have typical herpetic vesicles on eyelid margins. **Chemical conjunctivitis:** Due to use of silver nitrate drops in the eyes at birth. Rarely seen now that erythromycin is used. Typically lasts no more than 24–36 hours. Treatment is supportive with eye lubricant.
Initial Diagnostic Tests	Check conjunctival scrapings for Gram and Giemsa stain.
Next Steps in Management	• Hospitalize patient and irrigate eye • Treat with IM ceftriaxone and oral erythromycin (for possible chlamydial conjunctivitis)
Discussion	Conjunctivitis in the first month of life (ophthalmia neonatorum) can be caused by bacterial, viral, or chemical agents. Infection typically occurs through direct contact with genital secretions as the newborn exits the birth canal. Pathogens can also ascend to the uterus and fetus, especially with prolonged rupture of membranes. It is more common in areas with higher rates of STIs and poorer public health. Worldwide prevalence ranges from 0.1–10%. Consider in infants whose mothers were not screened during pregnancy, have risk factors for STIs, limited prenatal care, or lack of postpartum prophylaxis with erythromycin. **History and Physical Exam:** • Presents within 2–5 days post birth with varying hyperemia, copious discharge, and rapid corneal involvement • May have preauricular lymphadenopathy **Diagnostics:** • Confirm diagnosis with Gram stain showing gram–negative intracellular diplococci and/or NAAT testing • Can consider checking conjunctival cultures with blood and chocolate agars **Management:** • Saline irrigation to remove discharge • Hospitalize to evaluate for disseminated infection • Treat with ceftriaxone IM (preferred) or IV • Should also treat for chlamydial infection with oral erythromycin • Treat mother and sexual partner with ceftriaxone and doxycycline for 7 days
Additional Considerations	**Prophylaxis:** Erythromycin ointment **Complications:** If not treated early can lead to corneal opacification, perforation, endophthalmitis, and loss of the eye. Some systemic complications can also arise, such as pneumonia from chlamydia conjunctivitis or meningitis and sepsis from gonococcal conjunctivitis.

CASE 2 | Bacterial Conjunctivitis

A 12-year-old boy presents with right eye redness and burning for 1–2 days. He was brought in for evaluation today as his eye was crusted shut this morning. Exam shows intense redness of the right eye (hyperemia) with a large amount of purulent discharge and crusting along the eyelids. His vital signs are normal and there are no other significant findings on physical exam.

Conditions with Similar Presentations	**Allergic conjunctivitis, viral conjunctivitis** (see table): Discharge is more watery in these conditions. **Systemic conditions/diseases:** Conjunctivitis can also be seen in other systemic diseases (e.g., psoriasis, rosacea, reactive arthritis, Kawasaki disease, measles) or spread from other infected areas (e.g., streptococcal pharyngitis). These would all have additional findings other than the eye findings.
Initial Diagnostic Tests	• Clinical diagnosis • If severe, recurrent, or not responsive to therapy, conjunctival culture and Gram stain to determine the exact pathogen and specific therapies.

CASE 2 | Bacterial Conjunctivitis *(continued)*

Next Steps in Management	Topical antibiotics for 5–7 days (e.g., trimethoprim/polymyxin B or fluoroquinolone drops four times daily).

Discussion	Bacterial conjunctivitis is more common in children; adults are more likely to have viral conjunctivitis. Bacterial conjunctivitis may occur as a secondary infection in patients after viral conjunctivitis. Infection of the conjunctiva occurs from direct contact with the pathogen. Most common pathogens are *Streptococcus pneumoniae*, viridans Streptococci, *Haemophilus influenzae*, and *Staphylococcus aureus*. If onset is hyperacute (<24 hours), suspect *Neisseria gonorrhoeae*. Gonococcal conjunctivitis is a sexually transmitted infection.
	
	History: Eye redness, foreign body sensation, purulent discharge, worse in the morning with eye "stuck shut"
	
	Physical Exam: Purulent discharge (see image)
	
	Diagnostics: Diagnosis is made clinically
	• If gonococcal infection is suspected, NAAT testing and/or Gram stain and culture on chocolate agar or Thayer-Martin media
	
	Management:
	• Nongonococcal:
	  • Most cases resolve in 2–7 days without treatment
	  • Empiric treatment can be initiated with polymyxin B-trimethoprim, aminoglycoside *or* fluoroquinolone drops, *or* bacitracin *or* ciprofloxacin ointment 4–6 times per day for 5–7 days
	  • Refer to ophthalmologist if no significant clinical improvement in 3 days
	• Gonococcal:
	  • Examine the entire cornea for ulcers and perforations
	  • Systemic treatment with intramuscular ceftriaxone and treat for chlamydia (see Case 1)

CASE 3 | Viral Keratitis (Herpes Simplex Virus)

A 37-year-old woman presents with left eye pain, redness, light sensitivity, and discharge. She suffers from cold sores on and off in the past but has never had this happen to her and does not use contact lenses. Exam of the left eye shows hyperemia and decreased visual acuity compared to the right. Vital signs are normal.

Conditions with Similar Presentations	**Bacterial keratitis:** Presents with acute eye pain, redness, with opacification of the cornea. Often occurs in the setting of improper or prolonged contact lens use but can also occur from trauma or foreign bodies. Common pathogens include *Staphylococcus aureus*, *Pseudomonas aeruginosa*, and *Serratia marcescens*. Can result in a central, round ulcer with mucopurulent discharge. Treatment involves removal of contact lens and treatment with topical broad-spectrum antibiotics. **Herpes zoster ophthalmicus:** Occurs due to reactivation of the varicella zoster virus (VZV) within the V1 distribution of the trigeminal nerve. Typically occurs in immunocompromised or elderly patients and may have systemic symptoms, sensation of burning or tingling, and then a unilateral vesicular rash within the distribution of V1. Can lead to keratitis, ulceration, with loss of vision. Treat with acyclovir or its prodrugs (valacyclovir, famciclovir). **Corneal abrasions:** Common eye injury due to minor trauma or foreign body (e.g., debris, contact lens) that disrupts the corneal epithelium, resulting in eye pain, redness, photophobia, lacrimation. Fluorescein staining will show staining of basement membrane. Treat by irrigating the eye to remove debris, removing any visible foreign bodies, topical antibiotics (e.g., erythromycin ointment, polymyxin B/trimethoprim drops or fluoroquinolone drops). If from contact lenses, coverage of *Pseudomonas* with topical ciprofloxacin is required.
Initial Diagnostic Tests	• Obtain slit lamp exam • Consider scrapings of cornea or skin lesion (edge of corneal ulcer) for Giemsa stain, viral PCR
Next Steps in Management	• Oral acyclovir or valacyclovir is commonly prescribed • Topical treatment is an option as well.

CASE 3 | Viral Keratitis (Herpes Simplex Virus) *(continued)*

Discussion	HSV infection is common in humans, and recurrent infections occur in about one-third of the world's population. HSV-1 causes infections typically above the waist, but both HSV-1 and HSV-2 can lead to keratitis. The virus spreads from infected skin and mucosa to sensory nerve axons where it lies dormant; reactivation of this latent infection can occur due to fever, stress, or trauma. Most primary exposures occur early in life, but developing countries have later onset of primary infection. Increased risk of infection in immunocompromised patients (e.g., HIV) in which case may occur bilaterally.	 Herpes simplex keratitis. Epithelial dendrites seen after fluorescein staining. (Used with permission from The University of Iowa and EyeRounds.org.)
	History: • Primary infection: Vesicular rash with associated conjunctivitis • Recurrent keratitis: Foreign-body sensation, redness, pain, photosensitivity, and blurred vision	
	Physical Exam: Mild hyperemia and classic dendriform lesion described below	
	Diagnostics: Diagnosed clinically with history and slit lamp exam • Slit lamp exam with fluorescein staining shows a thin, linear, branching epithelial ulceration with club-shaped terminal bulbs • Can do corneal scrapings to look for multinucleated giant cells and intranuclear inclusions • PCR for HSV is confirmatory	
	Management: • Although many physicians prescribe oral agents, topical treatment was shown to be just as effective. • Options include PO acyclovir, valacyclovir, or famciclovir, trifluridine eye drops, vidarabine ointment. If no resolution in 1–2 weeks, consider a different source of infection.	
Additional Considerations	**Complications:** Neurotrophic keratopathy (loss of corneal sensation) can occur because of infection. Scarring of cornea as a complication of corneal stromal involvement. **Surgical Considerations:** Corneal transplant can be done in patients with visually significant scarring. **Other Considerations:** Topical corticosteroids are contraindicated.	

Red Eye Mini-Cases

Cases	Key Findings
Chemical Burn	**Hx:** History of chemical splash to eye(s). The chemical may be acid, alkali, or neutral. Ask if the patient was wearing eye protection. **PE:** The pH of the eye is not within physiologic range (7.0–7.3). Conjunctival and corneal epithelial defects and ulcers. Possible involvement of surrounding skin. Foreign bodies or particles of caustic material may be present in the conjunctival fornices. **Diagnostics:** Clinical diagnosis. Check pH of the eye. **Management:** Immediate irrigation with water, saline, or lactated Ringers for at least 20 minutes until pH returns to physiologic range.

Red Eye Mini-Cases (*continued*)

Chemical Burn	**Discussion:** Chemical injury is an ophthalmic emergency that requires immediate intervention. It is important to elicit information about the time of injury, specific type of chemical, whether the patient was wearing eye protection, time from exposure until irrigation was started, and duration, amount, and type of irrigation. Acid burns generally cause damage by denaturing and precipitating proteins, which act as a barrier to prevent further penetration into the tissue. Alkali burns can cause more extensive damage because they are able to penetrate tissues more rapidly. The damaged tissues then secrete proteolytic enzymes that lead to further damage.
Subconjunctival Hemorrhage	**Hx:** Bright red eye with normal vision and no pain. May be preceded by coughing or straining (e.g., Valsalva maneuver). Patients may be on antiplatelet or anticoagulant medications. **PE:** Blood underneath the conjunctiva (see image). No pus or purulence. **Diagnostics:** Clinical diagnosis. **Management:** Reassurance. No treatment required. Blood will clear in 2–4 weeks. **Discussion:** Subconjunctival hemorrhage is a common, benign condition caused by rupture of small blood vessels within the conjunctiva, often from minor trauma or increased venous pressure (e.g., following Valsalva maneuvers). Sometimes there is no cause identified. No treatment is required unless there was a more severe traumatic blow to the eye, in which case the patient should be evaluated by ophthalmology. Traumatic hyphema (yellow arrow) and associated subconjunctival hemorrhage (white arrows). (Reproduced with permission from Paul Riordan-Eva, James J. Augsburger, Vaughan & Asbury's General Ophthalmology, 19e. McGraw-Hill 2018.)

VISION LOSS

Vision loss is a reduction in visual acuity or visual field, affecting over 1 billion people worldwide. Ninety percent of vision loss is preventable or treatable and is caused by uncorrected refractive errors or cataract. Other leading causes of vision loss include age-related macular degeneration, diabetic retinopathy (DR), and glaucoma. In children, the most common cause of vision impairment is amblyopia.

Vision loss may be acute- or gradual-onset, monocular or binocular, transient (lasting <24 hours) or persistent (lasting at least 24 hours) and affect central or peripheral vision. A careful history that characterizes the nature of the visual disturbance, associated ocular, neurologic or systemic symptoms, and past ocular and medical history, followed by ophthalmic, neurologic, and general physical exam can help narrow down the differential diagnosis.

Many causes of monocular acute vision loss are urgent or emergent, including acute angle closure glaucoma, retinal detachment, central retinal artery occlusion, ischemic optic neuropathy, giant cell arteritis, and optic neuritis. These entities are important to identify so that the vision loss can be mitigated.

Key Findings and Acute Vision Loss Differential Diagnoses

Acute Vision Loss and Key Associated Findings	Diagnoses
Pain	Acute angle closure glaucoma, optic neuritis, giant cell arteritis (headache), chorioretinitis, scleritis
Painless	Central retinal artery occlusion, retinal detachment
Associated neurologic symptoms	Optic neuritis
History of trauma	Retinal detachment
Systemic symptoms	Giant cell arteritis, central retinal artery occlusion
History of high myopia	Retinal detachment
History of high hyperopia	Acute angle closure glaucoma

Visual field defects may be monocular or binocular, depending on the location of the lesion along the visual pathway. Lesions at various points along the pathway from the optic nerve to the occipital lobe can result in a multitude of visual field defects. Understanding the visual field defects can help localize the neuroanatomic location of the insult (see figure).

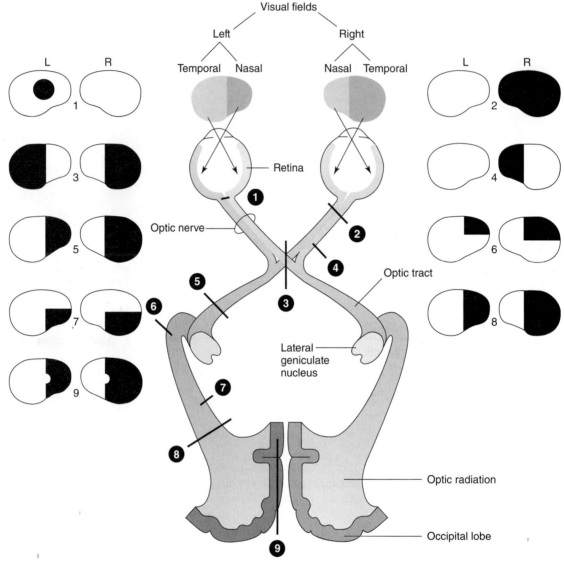

Common visual field defects and their anatomic bases. 1. Central scotoma caused by inflammation of the optic disk (optic neuritis) or optic nerve (retrobulbar neuritis). 2. Total blindness of the right eye from a complete lesion of the right optic nerve. 3. Bitemporal hemianopsia caused by pressure exerted on the optic chiasm by a pituitary tumor. 4. Right nasal hemianopsia caused by a perichiasmal lesion (e.g., calcified internal carotid artery). 5. Right homonymous hemianopsia from a lesion of the left optic tract. 6. Right homonymous superior quadrantanopia caused by partial involvement of the optic radiation by a lesion in the left temporal lobe (Meyer loop). 7. Right homonymous inferior quadrantanopia caused by partial involvement of the optic radiation by a lesion in the left parietal lobe. 8. Right homonymous hemianopsia from a complete lesion of the left optic radiation. (A similar defect may also result from lesion 9.) 9. Right homonymous hemianopsia (with macular sparing) resulting from posterior cerebral artery occlusion. Defects are shown in black. (Reproduced with permission from Greenberg DA, Aminoff MJ, Simon RP: Clinical Neurology, 11th ed. New York, NY: McGraw Hill; 2021.)

As signals are conveyed along the optic nerve, the fibers from the nasal retina (portraying vision from the temporal field) in each eye decussate at the level of the optic chiasm, ensuring that the entire left or right visual field ends up in a single lateral geniculate nucleus of the thalamus on the contralateral side. Generally, lesions before the level of the optic chiasm result in unilateral or monocular visual field defects, while lesions at or past the level of the optic chiasm result in bilateral visual field defects. As signals are then conveyed from the lateral geniculate nucleus to the primary visual cortex along the optic radiations, they are further separated into superior and inferior visual fields. When an image finally converges on the primary visual cortex, it is upside-down and left-right reversed. The optic chiasm located anatomically in the suprasellar region, just rostral to the sella turcica housing the pituitary gland, is the most common location for a lesion in **bitemporal hemianopsia**.

CASE 4 | Bitemporal Hemianopsia

A 33-year-old man presents for evaluation after getting into a motor vehicle accident. He reports that he was blindsided at a stop sign by a car "that was not there." The car was going very slowly, and minimal damage was done, but he is concerned that he didn't see the vehicle. Review of systems is notable for recent intermittent dull headaches. He notes that he and his wife have been having difficulty conceiving for the last 2 years. They do have an 8-year-old child together. On exam, his visual acuity is normal, but he has a temporal field defect on confrontational visual fields.

Conditions with Similar Presentations	Lesions to the lateral aspect of the optic chiasm (i.e., from **ICA aneurysm**) may result in an ipsilateral nasal hemianopsia. Glioma of optic nerve involving the optic chiasm can also lead to vision loss. **Craniopharyngioma:** Is a rare type of benign brain tumor that may present with bitemporal inferior temporal quadrantanopsia or bitemporal hemianopsia. MRI or computed tomography (CT) imaging will show a mass with cysts and calcified components. Visual field loss due to **retrochiasmal lesions** are less common, and can occur from vascular abnormalities (e.g., stroke, hemorrhage) or compressive lesions (tumors).
Initial Diagnostic Tests	• Visual field testing with perimetry (see below) • Also check serum prolactin levels • If perimetry confirms bitemporal hemianopsia, obtain MRI to locate the exact location and nature of the lesion.
Next Steps in Management	• Treat with bromocriptine or cabergoline for prolactin-secreting adenomas • Surgical resection for neoplastic lesions or if medical therapy fails
Discussion	The optic chiasm is the most common location for a lesion resulting in **bitemporal hemianopsia**. Pituitary tumors such as a **prolactinoma** (as in this case) can compress the medial optic chiasm, causing loss of temporal visual fields in both eyes or resulting in headaches from mass effect. Nasal visual fields are initially unaffected, as the fibers from the temporal hemiretina do not cross in the optic chiasm and remain ipsilateral. Pituitary adenomas can be described as functional (i.e., they secrete hormones such as prolactin, growth hormone, ACTH) or non-functional (i.e., they do not secrete hormones but can still cause symptoms of mass effect). Although rare in childhood, pituitary tumors may occur at any age in adults, and may enlarge during pregnancy. Craniopharyngiomas are common in children and have a second incidence peak in adulthood 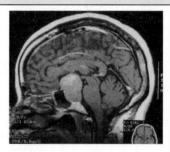 Pituitary adenoma. Sagittal T1-weighted magnetic resonance imaging scan after gadolinium contrast enhancement demonstrates a very large tumor arising from the sella. (Reproduced with permission John C.M. Brust, CURRENT Diagnosis & Treatment: Neurology, 3e. New York: McGraw Hill; 2019.) **History/Physical Exam:** • Nonsecreting pituitary adenomas typically just cause vision loss/visual field defect • Pituitary adenomas that actively secrete hormones may have systemic findings based on hormone secreted (see Chapter 9) **Diagnostics:** • Perimetry with either Humphrey visual field (HVF) or Goldmann visual field (GVF) testing to determine the extent of visual field loss and if the lesion crosses the midline • Once confirmed, MRI can locate and help determine the nature of the lesion (see image) • Check serum prolactin levels and other hormones to identify whether defect is caused by a hormone secreting pituitary adenoma **Management:** • Treat prolactin-secreting adenomas with bromocriptine or cabergoline (helps reduce the size), surgical resection if medical therapy fails • Neoplastic and other hormone-secreting tumors usually require surgical excision
Additional Considerations	**Complications: Pituitary apoplexy** is a life-threatening, acute hemorrhage or infarction of an enlarging pituitary tumor, thought to be caused by compression of blood supply. Patients develop symptoms of severe headache, nausea, altered consciousness, diplopia, and bitemporal hemianopsia. Expansion of the tumor and hemorrhage into the cavernous sinuses can lead to motility disorders of the extraocular muscles. Patients also develop hypopituitarism, which can lead to loss of ACTH and acute adrenal insufficiency. Treatment involves volume resuscitation, IV corticosteroids, and potentially neurosurgical resection of the tumor. **Surgical Considerations:** Transsphenoidal approach or craniectomy for lesions requiring resection.

CASE 5 | Diabetic Retinopathy (DR)

A 57-year-old woman with a 20-year history of poorly controlled diabetes mellitus (DM) presents with progressively worsening vision over the past several months. Exam of the retina shows hard yellow exudates, microaneurysms, and dot-blot hemorrhages diffusely.

Conditions with Similar Presentations	**Central retinal vein occlusion (CRVO):** Presents with sudden onset, unilateral vision loss, and on exam has a swollen optic disc and dilated and tortuous veins without hard exudates.

Hypertensive retinopathy: Can be progressive, with gradual vision loss due to systemic HTN resulting in decreased perfusion at multiple levels of the retina. It progress through three phases: vasoconstrictive (arteriole constriction), sclerotic (further narrowing), and exudative (disruption of blood-brain barrier and leakage). Exam findings vary depending on the severity of the disease. Flame-shaped hemorrhages, arteriolar narrowing (copper or silver wire appearance), hard exudates, cotton wool spots, and edema are seen in severe cases (see image). Treatment is focused on systemic blood pressure control.

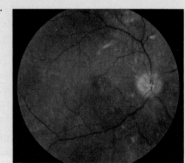

Hypertensive retinopathy with blurred optic disc, scattered hemorrhages, cotton-wool spots (nerve fiber layer infarcts), and foveal exudate in a 62-year-old man with chronic renal failure and a systolic blood pressure of 220. (Reproduced with permission Joseph Loscalzo, Anthony Fauci, Dennis Kasper, Stephen Hauser, Dan Longo, J. Larry Jameson, Harrison's Principles of Internal Medicine, 21e. New York: McGraw Hill; 2022.)

Initial Diagnostic Tests	• Dilated fundoscopic exam
Next Steps in Management	• Optimize blood glucose control and treat significant findings with laser photocoagulation • May also consider intravitreal anti-vascular endothelial growth factor (VEGF) medications (i.e., bevacizumab) if macular edema is present
Discussion	Roughly one-third of patients with DM are estimated to have DR, and risk increases with longer duration of DM. Hyperglycemia for prolonged periods of time leads to endothelial and pericyte damage, which leads to occluded capillaries and decreased retinal perfusion. This leads to vascular abnormalities, serum leakage, and edema. Ischemic retinal tissue releases VEGF, leading to retinal neovascularization and further edema. These new vessels are fragile and can rupture, leading to vitreous hemorrhage. DR can be broken down into nonproliferative (NPDR) and proliferative (PDR). In NPDR there is no development of extraretinal vascular tissue, whereas PDR develops after retinal neovascularization. Diabetic macular edema (DME) can occur at any stage and results in swelling of the central retina.

History:
• Occurs in setting of poorly controlled sugars and nonadherence with diabetic medications
• Patients may present with decreased visual acuity

PE: Fundoscopic exam findings:
• NPDR
  • Microaneurysms
  • Intraretinal hemorrhages
  • Cotton-wool spots
  • Dilation and beading of retinal veins
• PDR
  • Neovascularization of extraretinal tissue (iris, angle, optic disc, etc.)
  • Vitreous hemorrhage
• DME
  • Retinal thickening close to foveal center
  • Hard exudates close to foveal center

Diagnostics: Clinical diagnosis confirmed with fundoscopic exam
• Dilated fundus exam to confirm and stage severity
• Consider optical coherence tomography angiography (OCTA) and fluorescein angiography to view retinal vessels and assess for perfusion abnormalities, foveal ischemia, microaneurysms, and neovascularization

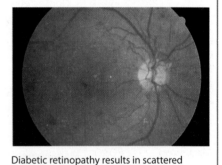

Diabetic retinopathy results in scattered hemorrhages, yellow exudates, and neovascularization. This patient has neovascular vessels proliferating from the optic disc, requiring urgent panretinal laser photocoagulation. (Reproduced with permission Joseph Loscalzo, Anthony Fauci, Dennis Kasper, Stephen Hauser, Dan Longo, J. Larry Jameson, Harrison's Principles of Internal Medicine, 21e. New York: McGraw Hill; 2022.)

CASE 5 | Diabetic Retinopathy (DR) *(continued)*

Discussion	**Management:**
	• NPDR
	  • Control of blood glucose level and continue monitoring for DME
	  • Use of anti-VEGF therapy in those without DME is currently being studied
	• PDR
	  • Intravitreal anti-VEGF or laser ablation of ischemic retina or DME

Additional Considerations	**Screening:** Dilated fundus exam annually upon diagnosis in type 2 and 5 years after diagnosis in type 1. Pregnant patients should be screened after conception and early in first trimester, and then every 3–12 months if no findings, or every 1–3 months if severe NPDR. **Complications:** Vitreous hemorrhage, retinal detachment, blindness. **Surgical Considerations:** Panretinal photocoagulation (PRP) is used to control neovascularization in PDR.

CASE 6 | Primary Open-Angle Glaucoma (POAG)

A 68-year-old woman with hypertension notes progressively worsening vision in both eyes over the past 2 years. She does not use alcohol, tobacco, or any other substances. She wears corrective lenses for nearsightedness. On exam, visual acuity is decreased without pain, and confrontational visual field testing elicits a superior visual field defect in both eyes. Funduscopic exam shows an increased cup–disc ratio with enlargement of the optic cup (see image).

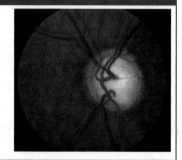

Reproduced with permission Joseph Loscalzo, Anthony Fauci, Dennis Kasper, Stephen Hauser, Dan Longo, J. Larry Jameson, Harrison's Principles of Internal Medicine, 21e. New York: McGraw Hill; 2022.

Conditions with Similar Presentations	**Compressive lesion of optic nerve:** Tumors involving the optic nerve or chiasm can also lead to visual loss; however, often this will be monocular or if involving both eyes, could present as a bitemporal hemianopsia if the optic chiasm is involved. Patients may also have other symptoms of mass effect due to the lesion. **Ischemic optic neuropathy:** Can be arteritic (AION) or non-arteritic (NAION), involving damage to the optic nerve due to disruption of blood supply, with or without inflammation. Vision loss is typically more rapid (minutes to days) and can involve one or both eyes. **Toxic or nutritional optic neuropathy:** Occurs in setting of toxins (e.g., alcohol, lead, medications [e.g., ethambutol, amiodarone]) or malnutrition. Patients have painless, bilateral, symmetric vision loss with thinning of retinal nerve fibers, decreased visual acuity. The optic disc early on may be normal or swollen.
Initial Diagnostic Tests	• Confirm diagnosis by checking IOP with tonometry • Also check visual field testing (perimetry), gonioscopy to assess for angle-closure, and consider pachymetry to assess corneal thickness
Next Steps in Management	• Goal is to reduce pressure to normal, and first-line treatment is with topical prostaglandins (e.g., latanoprost) • Other options include topical alpha-agonists (e.g., brimonidine), topical beta-blockers (e.g., timolol), topical cholinomimetics (e.g., pilocarpine, less common), and topical carbonic anhydrase inhibitors (e.g., dorzolamide)
Discussion	POAG is defined as a progressive optic neuropathy leading to visual field defects and often accompanied by increased IOP (normal IOP is 10–21 mmHg). The exact pathophysiology is not fully understood, but increased IOP is thought to compress either the retinal blood supply to the optic nerve or lead to compression of retinal ganglion cells. POAG has the highest prevalence in Black patients, followed by those of Hispanic ethnicity. Risk factors include increased IOP, DM, older age, thinner corneas, high myopia, and genetic predispositions. **History:** • Asymptomatic early on, with gradual vision loss (peripheral vision often affected first). • May describe tripping on objects or near-miss car accidents. **Physical Exam:** • May have visual field defects (usually occurs late in the disease). • Funduscopic exam will show an increased cup–disc ratio with enlargement of the optic cup. The optic nerve head is usually round and oval-shaped with a central cup; the ratio of vertical cup–disc diameter ranges between 0.1 and 0.4, with larger cup–disc ratios signaling potential glaucomatous damage.

CASE 6 | Primary Open-Angle Glaucoma (POAG) *(continued)*

Discussion	**Diagnostics:** • IOP is typically elevated (normal range 10–21 mmHg) and optical coherence tomography (OCT) with measurement of retinal nerve fiber layer (RNFL) thickness allows for objective measurement of damage to the optic nerve as well as the ability to detect progression of the disease. • Visual field testing with perimetry monitors the pattern of visual field loss and aids in grading glaucoma severity. **Management:** The pharmacologic treatment for POAG can be broken up into agents that promote aqueous humor outflow (topical prostaglandin analogues [most commonly used] and cholinergic agonist) and those that reduce the production of aqueous humor (beta-blockers, alpha-2-agonists and carbonic anhydrase inhibitors) (see table).
Additional Considerations	**Complications:** End-stage POAG causes irreversible blindness. **Surgical Considerations:** Many surgeries are done to get patients off pharmacologic treatment. • Laser trabeculoplasty increases outflow of aqueous humor through the trabecular meshwork and has been shown to be effective when done early in disease course. • Tube shunt surgery and trabeculoplasty are typically reserved for when other therapies are ineffective, and minimally invasive glaucoma surgeries (MIGS) are trialed initially.

Medications Used to Treat Primary Open-Angle Glaucoma

Medications	Mechanism	Side Effects/Contraindications	Additional Considerations
Prostaglandin analogues (latanoprost, travoprost)	Increases uveoscleral outflow of aqueous humor	Flulike symptoms, headache, increased pigmentation of iris and lashes, blurred vision, conjunctival hyperemia	Maximum effect may take up to 6 weeks
Beta-blockers (timolol)	Decreases aqueous humor production	Blurred vision, irritation, aggravation of myasthenia gravis, bradycardia, heart block, bronchospasm	May be less effective with concurrent use of systemic beta-blockers
Alpha-agonists (brimonidine)	Decreases aqueous humor production	Headache, fatigue, hypotension, insomnia, depression, syncope, dizziness, anxiety, blurred vision, foreign-body sensation, eyelid edema, dryness, miosis	Should not be used in younger population
Carbonic anhydrase inhibitors (dorzolamide, brinzolamide)	Decreases aqueous humor production	Side effects of topical carbonic anhydrase inhibitors are minimal and include transient stinging and bitter taste in the mouth. Occasionally, oral agents may be used for acute or refractory cases, but may have additional side effects	Even though administered topically, it may be absorbed systemically and cause adverse reactions
Cholinergic agonists (pilocarpine)	Increases trabecular outflow of aqueous humor	Headache/brow ache and accommodative spasm (difficulty changing focus between distance and near objects), keratitis, miosis, cataract, potential for angle-closure, increased salivation and secretions, abdominal cramps	More effective in people with a lighter iris

CASE 7 | Acute Angle-Closure Glaucoma (AACG)

A 53-year-old woman with hypertension presents with intense headache and blurred vision in the left eye that occurred while she was watching a movie. She wears corrective lenses for farsightedness. On exam, she has a mid-dilated, sluggish, and irregularly shaped left pupil with conjunctival hyperemia. Funduscopic exam shows increased cup–disc ratio in the left eye.

Conditions with Similar Presentations	**Traumatic (hemolytic) glaucoma:** Occurs after trauma or intraocular bleeding with RBCs in the anterior chamber (hyphema) or obstruction of the trabecular network by macrophages ingesting RBCs. **Cluster headache:** Presents with unilateral periorbital/temporal sharp pain associated with ptosis, miosis (not mid-dilated), lacrimation, rhinorrhea, and conjunctival injection. **Retrobulbar hemorrhage:** Occurs after trauma and would not be associated with pupillary abnormalities.
Initial Diagnostic Tests	• Gonioscopy, IOP measurement (tonometry) • Consider slit-lamp exam

CASE 7 | Acute Angle-Closure Glaucoma (AACG) *(continued)*

Next Steps in Management	• Give as many pressure-lowering drops as possible • Recheck pressure and visual acuity after 1 hour • If no improvement, repeat drops and give IV acetazolamide or mannitol • Definitive treatment is laser peripheral iridotomy
Discussion	AACG is the result of a blockage of aqueous humor outflow through the trabecular meshwork resulting in suddenly increased IOP and damage to the cornea. In primary AACG, the iris blocks the outflow of the aqueous humor (see figure) leading to increased IOP which can cause corneal edema and damage to the optic nerve. AACG is more common in eyes that have a narrow anterior chamber angle recess, anterior iris insertion, and hyperopia (shorter eye and farsightedness). It also increases with and has a genetic component. AACG has the highest prevalence in Asian populations. Risk factors include increased age, female sex and known family history. An attack can be precipitated by mydriatics, anticholinergics (including decongestant medications), lens accommodation such as reading (thickens the lens), or dim lighting (pupillary dilation). 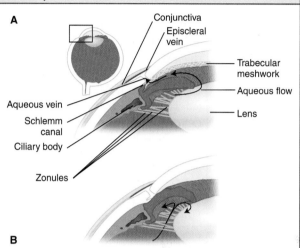 **A.** Normal flow of aqueous from ciliary body, through the pupil, and out through the trabecular meshwork and Schlemm canal located in the anterior chamber angle. **B.** Angle-closure glaucoma with pupillary block. Iris leaflet bows forward, blocking the chamber angle and prohibiting aqueous outflow. Meanwhile, aqueous production continues, and intraocular pressure rises. (Reproduced with permission from Tintinalli JE, Ma O, Yealy DM, Meckler GD, Stapczynski J, Cline DM, Thomas SH. eds. Tintinalli's Emergency Medicine: A Comprehensive Study Guide, 9e. New York: McGraw Hill; 2020.) **History:** Patients have intense eye pain, blurred vision, halos around lights, headache, and nausea/vomiting. **Physical Exam:** Affected eye with fixed, non-reactive, mid-dilated pupil with a cloudy cornea due to edema. In addition, they have congested conjunctival and episcleral vessels leading to an erythematous conjunctiva. IOP is increased and eyeball is firm to palpation. **Diagnostics:** • Gonioscopy is the gold standard and allows the measurement of the angle. In addition to visualization of a closed angle, patients will also have acutely increased IOP and corneal edema. Gonioscopy should be repeated after the IOP is reduced to document the angle has opened. • Also perform slit-lamp examination to assess damage to cornea and iris anatomy, as well as funduscopic exam to look for any retinal arterial damage or optic nerve cupping. • If secondary causes are suspected, a B-scan ultrasound may be helpful. **Management:** • Definitive treatment of AACG is laser peripheral iridotomy (LPI), which creates a hole in the iris to relieve the pupillary block. • In mild cases, the iris can be pulled away from the trabecular meshwork by inducing miosis through use of cholinergic agents such as pilocarpine. • Most patients are treated with other IOP-lowering agents such as topical prostaglandin analogues (e.g., latanoprost), beta-blockers (e.g., timolol), alpha 2-agonists (e.g., brimonidine), and carbonic anhydrase inhibitors (e.g., acetazolamide). • Hyperosmotic agents can be used if needed. • Serial gonioscopy is important to be sure that the angle has reopened. • If the other eye is found to have similar anatomy leading to increased risk, an LPI is performed to decrease the chance of that eye going into angle-closure.
Additional Considerations	**Complications:** If not treated early can lead to irreversible optic nerve damage and blindness. **Surgical Considerations:** LPI is the standard surgical procedure to relieve AACG. However, lensectomy is another possible treatment option.

CASE 8 | Giant Cell Arteritis (GCA)

An 85-year-old woman presents with decreased vision over the past day and associated headache on the right side. She also reports pain in her jaw while eating, shoulder achiness and weakness when brushing her hair, and feeling feverish. She has a temperature of 101°F and tenderness over her right temporal scalp. Vision in the right eye is decreased as compared to the left, and there is decreased color vision and a relative afferent pupillary defect on the right. Fundoscopy reveals a swollen pale disc on the right. IOP is normal.

Conditions with Similar Presentations	**Optic neuritis:** Can also present with monocular vision loss and pain; however, typically the pain is involving the eye. Patients are afebrile and do not have jaw claudication or tenderness to palpation over the temporal artery. **Glaucoma:** Can present with decreased vision and temporal headache but would not have jaw claudication, fever. IOP is usually elevated, and the optic disc shows increased cupping but not swelling or pallor. **Central retinal artery occlusion (CRAO):** Sudden, painless, and complete vision loss in one eye and a cherry-red spot on the macula. **CRVO:** Sudden, painless, and variable vision loss in one eye, and funduscopic exam will show dilated and tortuous veins with hemorrhages throughout the retina ("blood-and-thunder" appearance). **Non-arteritic ischemic optic neuropathy (NAION):** May have progressive vision loss and is not associated with any systemic symptoms, and inflammatory markers are normal. **Amaurosis fugax:** Transient vision loss due to retinal ischemia from microscopic emboli usually from carotid artery. This is a TIA. Vision usually returns in minutes, and ocular examination is unremarkable. Requires assessment of carotid artery occlusion.
Initial Diagnostic Tests	• Check erythrocyte sedimentation rate (ESR), C-reactive protein (CRP) • Confirm diagnosis with temporal artery biopsy
Next Steps in Management	Immediately start high-dose IV methylprednisolone (1 g/day for the first 3–5 days).
Discussion	GCA (previously called temporal arteritis but can involve other arteries) is a granulomatous vasculitis affecting medium and large arteries. Occlusion of the short ciliary arteries from inflammation or thrombosis can cause pain and vision loss. Occurs in adults over the age of 50, and risk increases greatly with age. Women are at higher risk as well as those of Northern European and Scandinavian descent. Up to 50% of patients can also have polymyalgia rheumatica (PMR)—involving the proximal shoulders and hips (presenting with muscle aches and morning stiffness). **History and Physical Exam:** Headache and scalp tenderness are common. Jaw claudication is a very specific symptom to GCA. Generalized symptoms such as malaise, fever, and anorexia can occur. Some patients may have a "cord-like" temporal artery that can be palpated on exam. Exam can show diplopia or decreased vision in one or both eyes. On funduscopic exam, the optic nerve head is edematous and "chalky-white" and can result in visual disturbances that lead to **anterior ischemic optic neuropathy (AION),** which can result in permanent visual loss. Other large vessel involvement beyond the temporal artery can also result in development of aortic aneurysms in some cases. 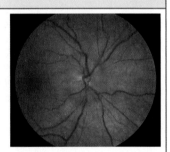 Anterior ischemic optic neuropathy from temporal arteritis in a 64-year-old woman with acute disc swelling, splinter hemorrhages, visual loss, and an erythrocyte sedimentation rate of 60 mm/h. (Reproduced with permission Joseph Loscalzo, Anthony Fauci, Dennis Kasper, Stephen Hauser, Dan Longo, J. Larry Jameson, Harrison's Principles of Internal Medicine, 21e. New York: McGraw Hill; 2022.) **Diagnostics:** • Elevated ESR (typically >50 mm/h) and CRP (may be more specific) • Gold standard for diagnosis is temporal artery biopsy showing inflammation with giant cells and loss of the internal elastic lamina. False negatives can occur, and if suspicion is still high, another biopsy of the contralateral temporal artery should be performed. **Management:** Treatment should be initiated immediately with high-dose IV steroids (1 g/day) and slowly tapered over 12 months. Oral prednisone 1 mg/kg/day can be used in suspected GCA with no vision loss. If left untreated, the contralateral eye will be affected within a few weeks. The affected eye usually does not regain vision. Temporal artery biopsy in giant cell arteritis. This temporal artery biopsy demonstrates a panmural infiltration of mononuclear cells and lymphocytes that are particularly seen in the media and adventitia. Scattered giant cells are also present. (Reproduced with permission Joseph Loscalzo, Anthony Fauci, Dennis Kasper, Stephen Hauser, Dan Longo, J. Larry Jameson, Harrison's Principles of Internal Medicine, 21e. New York: McGraw Hill; 2022.) 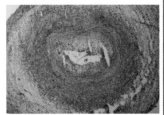

Acute Vision Loss Mini-Cases

Cases	Key Findings
Central Retinal Artery Occlusion (CRAO)	**Hx:** Sudden, painless, and complete vision loss in one eye. **PE:** Markedly reduced visual acuity (if there is a patent cilioretinal artery, the macula might still have some blood flow with less severe visual impairment). Funduscopic exam shows a cherry-red spot on the macula. **Diagnostics:** Clinical diagnosis **Management:** • There is no proven therapy, although methods to recover vision may include anterior chamber paracentesis and ocular massage • Patients should be started on aspirin, statin, and/or anticoagulation **Discussion:** Vision loss in one eye due to embolism (from common or internal carotid artery or cardiac source) or thrombosis. Vision loss typically is irreversible after about 90 minutes. Central retinal artery occlusion in a 78-year-old man reducing acuity to counting fingers in the right eye. Note the splinter hemorrhage on the optic disc and the slightly milky appearance to the macula with a cherry-red fovea. (Reproduced with permission Joseph Loscalzo, Anthony Fauci, Dennis Kasper, Stephen Hauser, Dan Longo, J. Larry Jameson, Harrison's Principles of Internal Medicine, 21e. New York: McGraw Hill; 2022.)
Central Retinal Vein Occlusion (CRVO)	**Hx:** Sudden, painless, and variable vision loss in one eye that is typically less severe than CRAO. **PE:** Varies based on severity, but funduscopic exam will show dilated and tortuous veins with hemorrhages throughout the retina, often described as a "blood-and-thunder" appearance. **Diagnostics:** Clinical diagnosis **Management:** • Patients need to be followed closely for neovascularization of the iris, angle, and disc, as well as vitreous hemorrhage and macular edema • Intravitreal injection of anti-VEGF for macular edema is an effective therapy that can help recover some visual acuity • Treat underlying risk factors **Discussion:** Vision loss due to thrombosis of the central retinal vein can lead to both nonischemic (mild) or ischemic (severe) disease. HTN, DM, HLD, and open-angle glaucoma are all risk factors. Central retinal vein occlusion can produce massive retinal hemorrhage ("blood and thunder"), ischemia, and vision loss. (Reproduced with permission Joseph Loscalzo, Anthony Fauci, Dennis Kasper, Stephen Hauser, Dan Longo, J. Larry Jameson, Harrison's Principles of Internal Medicine, 21e. New York: McGraw Hill; 2022.)
Non-Arteritic Ischemic Optic Neuropathy (NAION)	**Hx:** Vision loss can be progressive before stabilizing, and is not associated with any systemic symptoms. **PE:** Less severe loss of visual acuity compared to GCA, visual field loss in the horizontal half of the visual field ("altitudinal"), and optic nerve head edema initially, progressing to atrophy in 6–8 weeks. **Diagnostics:** Clinical diagnosis; should rule out other causes. Contrast MRI is useful to rule out optic neuritis or intracranial mass. Inflammatory markers are normal. **Management:** No proven therapy exists. Some patients may recover some visual acuity within 6 months. **Discussion:** Most common cause of ischemic optic neuropathy, due to interruption of microvascular circulation from overcrowding of the optic nerve head ("disc at risk") or vasculopathies (DM, HTN, HLD, OSA). Fellow eye involvement is infrequent at about 15% in 5 years.
Retinal Detachment (RD)	**Hx:** Symptoms: Flashes of light, floaters, and/or a curtain coming over the field of vision. May have peripheral or central vision loss Risk factors: History of high myopia (nearsightedness) **PE:** Separation of the retina from the retinal pigment epithelium (RPE) can be seen with folds of retinal tissue (see image)

Acute Vision Loss Mini-Cases (*continued*)

Retinal Detachment (RD)	In rhegmatogenous RD, a retinal break is also present. An associated posterior vitreous detachment can be seen sometimes with pigmented vitreous cells and a ring of white, fibroglial tissue (Weiss ring) over the optic disc. **Diagnostics:** Indirect ophthalmoscopy with scleral depression to look in the peripheral retina. If there are media opacities, a B-scan ultrasound can be performed. **Management:** Bed rest until surgical repair can be performed (laser photocoagulation, cryotherapy, pneumatic retinopexy, vitrectomy, and scleral buckle). **Discussion:** There are three forms of RD. • Rhegmatogenous: A retinal break leads to fluid accumulation separating the retina from the RPE • Exudative: May have many etiologies such as neoplastic, inflammatory, or vascular • Tractional: Fibrocellular bands in the vitreous contract and pull the retina with them.	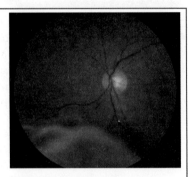 Retinal detachment appears as an elevated sheet of retinal tissue with folds. In this patient, the fovea was spared, so acuity was normal, but an inferior detachment produced a superior scotoma. (Reproduced with permission Joseph Loscalzo, Anthony Fauci, Dennis Kasper, Stephen Hauser, Dan Longo, J. Larry Jameson, Harrison's Principles of Internal Medicine, 21e. New York: McGraw Hill; 2022.)
Toxoplasma Chorioretinitis	**Hx:** Asymptomatic or may present with blurred vision, floaters, eye redness and/or photophobia. There may be a history of handling or eating raw meat (e.g., pork, lamb, venison) or exposure to cat feces. **PE:** Yellow or white retinal lesion adjacent to an old pigmented chorioretinal scar, accompanied by moderate to severe vitreous inflammation ("headlight in the fog" appearance). **Diagnostics:** • Clinical diagnosis with fundoscopic exam as seen in image • PCR testing of aqueous or vitreous is sensitive and specific • Serology for anti-toxoplasma IgG or IgM may have limited value because of high prevalence of seropositivity in the population **Management:** • Triple therapy with pyrimethamine, folinic acid, and sulfadiazine • Pyrimethamine may cause bone marrow suppression, so CBC must be checked weekly to monitor • Prednisone may be added at least 24 hours after initiating antimicrobial therapy **Discussion:** White retinal lesions of toxoplasma chorioretinitis may also be seen in patients with CMV or HSV retinitis. However, patients with CMV retinitis would most likely be immunosuppressed and those with HSV retinitis may have a clinical history of HSV with characteristic skin findings.	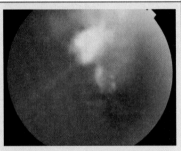 Toxoplasmosis: active chorioretinitis adjacent to scarring from previous lesion. (Reproduced with permission Paul Riordan-Eva, James J. Augsburger, Vaughan & Asbury's General Ophthalmology, 19e. New York: McGraw Hill; 2018.)
Neuromyelitis Optica (NMO)	**Hx:** • Decreased visual acuity that worsens over days; associated pain on eye movement may also be present • Uthoff phenomenon: Vision blurs as body temperature rises • May also describe loss of color vision and flashes of light • May present with acute transverse myelitis **PE:** May have the following findings: • Decreased visual acuity and visual field defects • Relative afferent pupillary defect on swinging flashlight test if unilateral • Pain on extraocular movement **Diagnostics:** • T2-weighted MRI showing hyperintensity of the optic nerve • MRI showing transverse myelitis (intramedullary lesion greater than two contiguous elements) • Aquaporin-4 IgG antibody is elevated in the serum **Management:** Prognosis is typically worse than in multiple sclerosis (MS). Therapy is directed at immunosuppression through high-dose IV corticosteroids, plasma exchange, and/or IVIG depending on response. **Discussion:** Optic neuritis refers to any inflammation of the optic nerve and can occur in a variety of infectious or autoimmune disorders. NMO is one of the acute inflammatory demyelinating optic neuritis disorders including MS and myelin oligodendrocyte glycoprotein G-associated disorder (MOG).	

Chronic Vision Loss Mini-Cases

Cases	Key Findings
Refractive Errors	**Hx:** Decreased vision when not wearing corrective lenses. Distant objects are blurry and near objects are clear (**myopia**). Distant objects are clear and near objects are blurry (**hyperopia**). Near objects that are blurry become clearer when held farther away (**presbyopia**). May report eye strain. **NORMAL VISION MYOPIC VISION HYPEROPIC VISION** 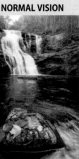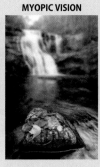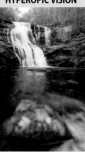 A visual graphic of a patient's view (visual images) of specific refractive errors. (Reproduced with permission Matthew L. Boulton, Robert B. Wallace, Maxcy-Rosenau-Last Public Health & Preventive Medicine, 16e. New York: McGraw Hill; 2022.) **PE:** Decreased uncorrected visual acuity improves with pinhole testing, glasses, or contact lenses. **Diagnostics:** Uncorrected visual acuity and refraction. **Management:** Glasses or contact lenses. Consider refractive surgery. For presbyopia, bifocal glasses or reading glasses. **Discussion:** Refractive error is failure of the eye to focus images sharply on the retina, causing blurred vision. There are four main types of refractive error: myopia, hyperopia, astigmatism, and presbyopia. **A. Normal vision (emmetropia)**  **B. Myopia** **Myopia correction** 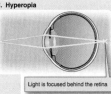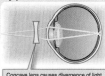 Light is focused in front of the retina Concave lens causes divergence of light before it enters the long eyeball **C. Hyperopia** **Hyperopia correction** 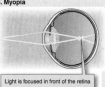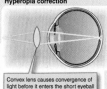 Light is focused behind the retina Convex lens causes convergence of light before it enters the short eyeball Myopia (nearsightedness) and hyperopia (farsightedness). **A.** The normal eye focuses light from a distant point on the retina with the ciliary muscles relaxed. **B.** Myopia results when the eyeballs are longer than normal, causing light to be focused on a point in front of the retina. Myopia can be corrected using eyeglasses with a concave lens. **C.** Hyperopia results when the eyeballs are shorter than normal, causing light to be focused behind the retina. Hyperopia can be corrected using eyeglasses with a convex lens. (Reproduced with permission from Kibble JD. eds. The Big Picture Physiology: Medical Course & Step 1 Review, 2e. New York: McGraw Hill; 2020.) • **Myopia**, also known as nearsightedness, occurs when the eye is too long or the cornea is curved too steeply, which results in the image being focused in front of the retina. This is corrected with a concave lens. • **Hyperopia**, also known as farsightedness, occurs when the eye is too short or the cornea is too flat, which results in the image being focused behind the retina. This is corrected with a convex lens. • **Astigmatism** occurs when the corneal or lens curvature is not spherical, which results in light rays of different orientations to focus on different points. This is corrected with a cylindrical lens. • **Presbyopia** is a normal aging change in the eye when the lens is unable to change shape to focus on near objects. This is corrected with a convex lens when viewing near objects (reading glasses or bifocals).

Chronic Vision Loss Mini-Cases (*continued*)

Age-Related Macular Degeneration (AMD)	**Hx:** Gradual loss of central vision. May report distortion of straight lines that appear wavy Risk factors: Advanced age, family history, smoking, obesity, hypertension, hypercholesterolemia, hyperopia, and blue eyes **PE:** **Nonexudative (dry):** Macular drusen deposits, RPE atrophy, clumps of pigment in peripheral retina **Exudative (wet):** subretinal fluid and choroidal neovascularization **Diagnostics:** • Amsler grid testing to identify early distortion of straight lines, central scotoma, and metamorphopsia • When concerned about exudative AMD, should perform intravenous fluorescein angiography (IVFA) and OCT macula **Management:** Nonexudative (dry): Focus is on reducing the risk of progression to advanced AMD through vitamin supplements containing vitamin C, vitamin E, beta-carotene, zinc, and cupric oxide. If exudative (wet) AMD has developed, perform intravitreal anti-VEGF or photodynamic therapy (PDT) for subfoveal choroidal neovascularization. **Discussion:** AMD is a leading cause of blindness in developed countries worldwide and presents with progressive loss of central vision. Differential should always be in mind with central vision loss without pain.	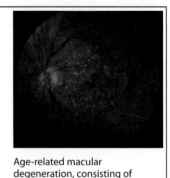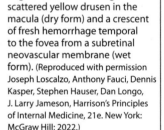 Age-related macular degeneration, consisting of scattered yellow drusen in the macula (dry form) and a crescent of fresh hemorrhage temporal to the fovea from a subretinal neovascular membrane (wet form). (Reproduced with permission Joseph Loscalzo, Anthony Fauci, Dennis Kasper, Stephen Hauser, Dan Longo, J. Larry Jameson, Harrison's Principles of Internal Medicine, 21e. New York: McGraw Hill; 2022.)
Cataracts	**Hx:** Progressive vision loss including glare from lights at night and some reduced color vision **PE:** Opacification of the lens **Diagnostics:** Clinical diagnosis. Determine whether cataract is responsible for vision loss and if surgical removal will improve vision. **Management:** Surgical removal is the only treatment but is not urgent unless there is a secondary complication (glaucoma). **Discussion:** Cataracts are a normal part of aging as the lens epithelial cells differentiate throughout life and form new lens fibers, which infoliate into the lens over time. These eventually may form protein aggregates, which lead to opacity within the lens and scatter light. Cataracts can also be secondary (e.g., from corticosteroid use, diabetes, disorders of galactose metabolism, trisomies, congenital infections [e.g., rubella], Marfan syndrome, Alport syndrome, myotonic dystrophy, neurofibromatosis type 2, trauma, uveitis). Cataract surgery can rarely result in **postoperative endophthalmitis** within 7 days of surgery due to exposure of the aqueous and vitreous humor to natural flora of the conjunctiva during surgery. Patients may have discharge, purulence, and layering of white blood cells in the anterior chamber (hypopyon). Treatment involves intravitreal injection of antibiotics ± vitrectomy.	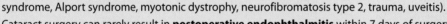 Mature age-related cataract viewed through a dilated pupil. (Reproduced with permission Paul Riordan-Eva, James J. Augsburger, Vaughan & Asbury's General Ophthalmology, 19e. New York: McGraw Hill; 2018.)
Amblyopia	**Hx/PE:** May report "lazy eye" and have an eye that turns inward or outward (strabismus), eyes that appear to not work together, or poor depth perception. Risk factors: Premature birth, small size at birth, family history, and developmental disabilities. **PE:** • May squint, shut one eye, or tilt head • May have ocular misalignment (strabismus), difference in the amount of refractive error between the eyes or obstruction of vision (e.g., from cataract or droopy eyelid [ptosis]) **Diagnostics:** Clinical diagnosis Ophthalmic exam: Including cover-uncover and alternate-cover tests for strabismus, retinoscopy for refractive error and to rule out cataracts, and dilated fundus exam for optic nerve or retinal pathologies	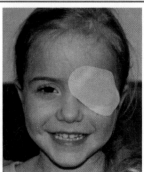 Reproduced with permission Gregg T. Lueder, Pediatric Practice: Ophthalmology. New York: McGraw Hill; 2011.

Chronic Vision Loss Mini-Cases (*continued*)

Amblyopia	**Management:**
	• Amblyopia is managed by forcing the "weaker" eye to work more actively. This is typically done by patching the better-seeing eye (see image).
	• Glasses or contact lenses are used to correct amblyopia caused by refractive error.
	• Surgery, if the cause of amblyopia is droopy eyelids or cataract.
	Discussion: Amblyopia is also called lazy eye because the vision in one eye does not develop normally and the other eye becomes "stronger." Reduced vision in one eye is caused by abnormal visual development early in life. It usually develops from birth to age 7 years, and rarely can affect both eyes. It can be caused by strabismus (when the eyes are misaligned), differences in refractive error between the two eyes, or visual deprivation, such as from cataract or eyelid ptosis (drooping). Any one of these can result in the brain ignoring the input from the "weaker" eye.

MOTILITY AND PUPIL ABNORMALITIES

Extraocular motility is controlled through three cranial nerves (oculomotor [III], trochlear [IV], and abducens [VI]), while the pupil is controlled through CN III and autonomic signaling. Lesions along the supranuclear, internuclear, and infranuclear pathways lead to motility disorders. The internuclear pathway is the medial longitudinal fasciculus which connects CN VI and the contralateral CN III. Supranuclear pathways are above the CN nuclei, and lesions at this point affect both eyes in the same way. Infranuclear pathways are after the CN nuclei, and lesions at this point affect each eye differently. Motility disorders typically produce binocular diplopia, which can be very uncomfortable and disorienting for patients. It is important to do a thorough physical exam and assess changes in diplopia with different gazes as well as head tilting.

On the other hand, pupillary abnormalities are not always noticed by patients, and are typically easier to spot in those with lighter-colored irises. A thorough pupillary exam is essential to localize the lesion so an underlying cause can be determined.

CASE 9	Horner Syndrome

A 67-year-old woman presents for evaluation of right eyelid droopiness. Her vision has not changed. She also reports 15 pounds unintentional weight loss and worsening cough over the past 3 months. She has a 40-pack-year history of smoking cigarettes. Exam is notable for mild ptosis on the right and anisocoria with a larger pupil on the left that worsens in dim light. She has some right-sided facial flushing, lymphadenopathy in the right supraclavicular region, and wheezing over the right upper lobe.

Conditions with Similar Presentations	**Oculomotor nerve (CN III) palsy:** Can involve the pupil and result in a dilated or "blown" pupil, especially when compressed (e.g., with an aneurysm of the posterior communicating artery). There will also be complete ptosis as CN III innervates the levator palpebrae superioris muscle, which raises the eyelid. However, CN III palsy would also have impairment of extraocular movements and would not present with anhidrosis or facial flushing. The pulmonary symptoms in this patient are more suggestive of a neoplastic process that disrupts sympathetic pathways.
	Argyll Robertson pupil: Seen in tertiary syphilis due to infection with the spirochete Treponema pallidum. Bilateral pupils are small and poorly reactive to light. However, the near reflex pathway is intact, so accommodation is intact and the pupil constricts when looking from distant to near objects. Patients may have other manifestations of neurosyphilis including general paresis and tabes dorsalis.
Initial Diagnostic Tests	• Compare pupil sizes in light and dark (if anisocoria is greater in light, suggests abnormality is on the side of the larger pupil).
	• Evaluate for a relative afferent pupillary defect (RAPD) using swinging flashlight test.
	• Check extraocular motility, ptosis, and pupillary margin under slit lamp.
	• Consider: Use cocaine 10% or apraclonidine (0.5% or 1%) drops in both eyes if suspecting Horner syndrome. Topical cocaine will result in anisocoria ≥1 mm, while apraclonidine will reverse the anisocoria.
	• CT chest to evaluate for superior pulmonary sulcus (Pancoast) tumor
	• MRI of the brain and neck to evaluate for lesions along the sympathetic chain (can also do MRA or carotid Doppler to look for carotid artery dissection)
Next Steps in Management	Treat underlying cause

CASE 9 | Horner Syndrome *(continued)*

Discussion	**Anisocoria** is an asymmetry between the diameters of the two pupils. The pupils can still react normally to light, signaling physiologic anisocoria or a problem with the sympathetic chain. One cause of anisocoria is Horner syndrome, involving a lesion anywhere along the oculosympathetic pathway. Lesions can be central (first-order), preganglionic (second-order), or postganglionic (third-order).

Discussion *(continued)*

Central lesions (e.g., stroke, MS, cervical cord trauma, syringomyelia) can injure first-order neurons originating in the hypothalamus, descending through the pons, lateral medulla, and spinal cord down to the level of C8–T2 (the ciliospinal center of Budge-Waller). These lesions are often associated with other focal neurological deficits depending on the exact location of injury.

- Second-order neurons then ascend toward the head and neck in the paravertebral cervical sympathetic chain, pass through the stellate and middle cervical ganglia, passing very close to the brachial plexus and apex of the lung, before synapsing within the superior cervical ganglion at the level of C3–C4. **Horner syndrome** is most often acquired due to secondary causes (examples listed above) but can also be hereditary. **Pancoast tumors** (as in this case) in the apex of the lung, cervical ribs, brachial plexus injuries, or surgeries in this region (e.g., thyroidectomy) can compress the sympathetic chain at this point.
- Third-order neurons then continue from the superior cervical ganglion as postganglionic fibers continuing within the wall of the carotid vessels and cavernous sinus, eventually joining the nasociliary branch of CN V1 within the cranium. ICA dissection and cavernous sinus lesions can disrupt third-order neurons and result in Horner syndrome. In children, birth trauma can also result in Horner syndrome.

History: Patients may be unaware of abnormalities, although some may describe photophobia, difficulty focusing with near or far objects, a recent change in medication, droopy eyelid, headache, neck or facial pain.

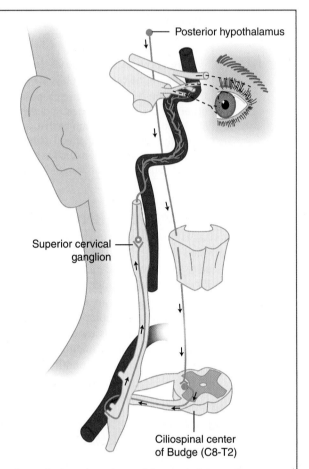

Sympathetic nerve pathway of the eye. An interruption anywhere along this pathway can cause Horner syndrome. (Reproduced with permission from Tintinalli JE, Ma O, Yealy DM, Meckler GD, Stapczynski J, Cline DM, Thomas SH. eds. Tintinalli's Emergency Medicine: A Comprehensive Study Guide, 9e. New York: McGraw Hill; 2020.)

Labels on figure: Posterior hypothalamus; Superior cervical ganglion; Ciliospinal center of Budge (C8-T2)

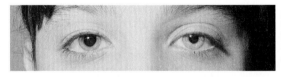

Congenital Horner syndrome. Ptosis, miosis, and heterochromia. Lighter colored iris is on the affected left side. (Reproduced with permission Maya Bunik, William W. Hay, Myron J. Levin, Mark J. Abzug, Current Diagnosis & Treatment: Pediatrics, 26e. New York: McGraw Hill; 2022.)

CASE 9 | Horner Syndrome *(continued)*

Discussion	**Physical Exam:** The classic triad of signs on exam includes ipsilateral: 1. *Miosis*—constricted pupil resulting in anisocoria due to damage to the innervation of pupillary dilator muscles. Patients may also have a dilation lag. 2. *Ptosis (partial)*—from sympathetic innervation of the superior tarsal muscle (Mueller muscle), which keeps the eyelid raised once the levator palpebrae superioris (innervated by CN III) originally elevates it. Patients also have lower lid reverse ptosis (resulting in a partially elevated lower lid). 3. *Anhidrosis*—decreased sweat resulting in facial flushing; degree of anhidrosis depends on level of lesion, with central or pre-ganglionic lesions resulting in anhidrosis of the ipsilateral face and neck and post-ganglionic lesions resulting in ipsilateral anhidrosis of the forehead only. Another potential feature is iris heterochromia, or a difference in the pigmentation of the iris, which is more common in patients with congenital Horner syndrome. **Diagnostics:** Pharmacological testing can be used to confirm Horner syndrome. • Administration of apraclonidine drops in both eyes will reverse the anisocoria in the affected eye. Apraclonidine is a weak alpha 1-agonist, and the affected pupillary dilator muscle will dilate more than the unaffected eye. This change may not be observed immediately following the injury but can develop within 2–5 days. • Administration of cocaine drops in both eyes will also result in anisocoria that is ≥1 mm in the affected eye. Cocaine blocks norepinephrine reuptake in sympathetic nerve terminals, but since the sympathetic pathway is dysfunctional, there is no effect in the affected eye and it remains miotic. • Patients should also undergo screening for suspected causes of Horner syndrome, including CT chest if there is suspicion for Pancoast tumor (as in this patient with smoking history presenting with cough and unintentional weight loss). • Patients with suspicion for carotid dissection can undergo MR angiography or carotid Doppler ultrasound. **Management:** Identify and treat the underlying cause of the Horner syndrome. For example, in a patient with confirmed Pancoast tumor on chest CT, induction chemotherapy and surgical resection may be an option. For patients with suspected carotid dissection or aneurysm, neurosurgery or vascular surgery should be consulted urgently.

Pupil Abnormalities Mini-Cases

Cause	Key Findings
Afferent Pupillary Defect (Marcus Gunn Pupil)	**Hx:** Asymptomatic or have symptoms related to the underlying cause of optic nerve or retinal disease **PE:** With the swinging flashlight test, pupils of both eyes constrict when light stimulus is shone into the normal eye; pupils of both eyes dilate when light stimulus is rapidly swung to the abnormal eye **Diagnostics:** Swinging flashlight test **Management:** Treat the underlying disease **Discussion:** Under normal circumstances, the pupil should constrict when exposed to bright light (direct pupillary light reflex). Signals are conveyed by the optic nerve (CN II), which sends some fibers to the parasympathetic Edinger-Westphal nucleus in the midbrain. Output from the Edinger-Westphal nucleus occurs via the oculomotor nerve (CN III) bilaterally, resulting in both the direct reflex and a consensual light reflex in the other eye. Marcus Gunn pupils involve disruption of the afferent limb of the pupillary light reflex. Any disorder that affects the optic nerve can lead to an afferent pupillary defect (APD), including optic neuritis (i.e., in MS or neuromyelitis optica), ischemic optic neuropathy (arteritic or non-arteritic), and optic nerve tumors (e.g., glioma, meningioma). APD may also be seen in patients with severe retinal disease, such as ischemic retinal disease (e.g., central retinal vein occlusion, central retinal artery occlusion, severe DR), ocular ischemic syndrome, and retinal detachment. In the swinging flashlight test, when the flashlight is initially shown in each eye, there is constriction; however, when rapidly swinging back and forth from the unaffected to the affected eye, the affected eye will dilate rather than constrict when light is shown into it, due to impaired afferent signaling.

CASE 10 | Internuclear Ophthalmoplegia (INO)

A 31-year-old woman presents with a change in vision for the past 3 days. She says that it looks like things are "doubled, side-by-side." This has never happened to her before, and she doesn't have any other symptoms. When she is reading up close the blurriness seems to go away. However, when she's in a hot shower she finds the blurriness gets worse. On exam, she has limited adduction of the left eye. Right eye exam is normal. There is no ptosis, and repeated movement of the eye does not change her abnormal findings. Pupils are equal and reactive to light. Neurologic exam is otherwise normal.

Conditions with Similar Presentations	**CN III palsy:** Although this can cause limited adduction (due to loss of innervation to the medial rectus) there is usually weakness of the other muscles innervated (superior rectus, inferior rectus and inferior oblique) that causes additional abnormalities in extraocular motion. In addition, pupillary abnormality (mydriasis) may be seen.
Conditions with Similar Presentations	**Ocular myasthenia gravis:** Autoimmune disorder involving autoantibodies against the nicotinic acetylcholine receptor (AChR) or muscle-specific receptor tyrosine kinase (MuSK) that commonly involves the levator palpebrae superioris, orbicularis oculi, and/or extraocular muscles. Patients may present with ptosis, diplopia, or impaired extraocular movement (e.g., impaired adduction as in this case). This patient lacks ptosis, and symptoms are not fluctuating or fatigable as would be expected in ocular myasthenia gravis.
Initial Diagnostic Tests	• Confirm diagnosis with MRI brain with and without contrast to look for white matter lesion or stroke (for younger woman stroke is less likely) • Consider: Prism alternate cover test to assess degree of diplopia; forced duction test to distinguish paretic from restrictive cause
Next Steps in Management	Treat MS if white matter lesions typical of MS are found (see Neurology Chapter).
Discussion	Extraocular motility consists of a complex interaction of six different muscles within the orbit. These six muscles are innervated by cranial nerve III (oculomotor), IV (trochlear), and VI (abducens). CN IV innervates the superior oblique, CN VI innervates the lateral rectus, and CN III provides innervation to the other four (inferior rectus, medial rectus, superior rectus, and inferior oblique). Damage to these nerves along the pathway from the brainstem to the orbit can result in misalignment of the eyes and binocular diplopia. This is a case of internuclear ophthalmoplegia (aka internuclear ophthalmoparesis), which is due to a lesion in the medial longitudinal fasciculus (MLF), a highly myelinated tract within the brainstem responsible for rapid communication and coordination between the medial rectus (innervated by CN III) and the lateral rectus (innervated by CN VI) muscles. Lesions to the MLF disrupt communication between CN VI and CN III resulting in limited or slowed adduction of the eye ipsilateral to the lesion and abducting nystagmus of the contralateral eye. Most likely in a younger patient this is caused through demyelinating disease such as MS. INO is the most common eye abnormality in MS and may be bilateral. **History:** • Abnormality in vision most commonly described as double vision when looking to the side (incomitant diplopia) • Double vision goes away when one eye is closed (binocular diplopia) • Images most commonly look stacked side-by-side (horizontal diplopia) but may be on top of each other (vertical diplopia) • May have known diagnosis of MS **Physical Exam:** • Movement of eyes should be assessed in all fields of gaze—patients will have impaired adduction on conjugate gaze in the affected eye as well as an abducting nystagmus in the unaffected eye • Other special tests can help determine if the misalignment is the same in all directions of gaze (comitant) or changes (incomitant) **Diagnostics:** MRI of the brain can be useful to assess for ischemic insult leading to cranial nerve palsies or any other lesions

CASE 10 | Internuclear Ophthalmoplegia (INO) *(continued)*

Discussion	
	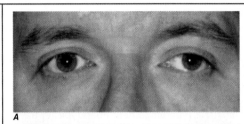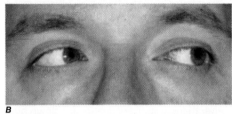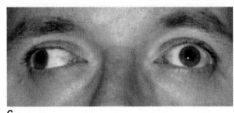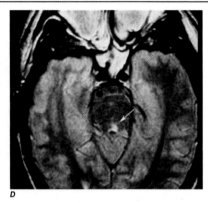 Left internuclear ophthalmoplegia (INO). **A.** In primary position of gaze, the eyes appear normal. **B.** Horizontal gaze to the left is intact. **C.** On attempted horizontal gaze to the right, the left eye fails to adduct. In mildly affected patients, the eye may adduct partially or more slowly than normal. Nystagmus is usually present in the abducted eye. **D.** T2-weighted axial magnetic resonance image through the pons showing a demyelinating plaque in the left medial longitudinal fasciculus (*arrow*). (**A-D,** Reproduced with permission Joseph Loscalzo, Anthony Fauci, Dennis Kasper, Stephen Hauser, Dan Longo, J. Larry Jameson, Harrison's Principles of Internal Medicine, 21e. New York: McGraw Hill; 2022.) **Management:** • Manage the underlying condition that led to motility disorder (e.g., diabetes, MS). • Can prescribe prisms for glasses to help correct double vision.

CASE 11 | Cranial Nerve III (Oculomotor) Palsy

A 62-year-old man with hypertension presents with an inability to open his right eye and double vision when he manually opens it. He also had sudden onset of a headache at the time he noticed this problem. Exam shows complete ptosis of the right eyelid and limited extraocular movements (adduction, supraduction, and infraduction) but preserved abduction of the right eye. He also has a fixed and dilated pupil on the right. Left eye has intact extraocular movement and normally reactive pupil.

Conditions with Similar Presentations	**Cavernous sinus lesions:** May also result in dysfunction of CN III; however, there are additional manifestations including impairment of CN IV or VI, the V1 division of CN V, or oculosympathetic fibers (which results in Horner syndrome). The cavernous sinus. The cavernous sinus and associated structures. **A.** Relationship to skull and brain. **B.** The cavernous sinus wraps around the pituitary. Several important structures run through the cavernous sinus: the internal carotid artery; the oculomotor, trochlear, and abducens nerves; and the ophthalmic branch of the trigeminal nerve and trigeminal ganglion. (Reproduced with permission from Waxman SG. eds. Clinical Neuroanatomy, 29e. New York: McGraw Hill; 2020.)
Initial Diagnostic Tests	Confirm diagnosis with CT angiography
Next Steps in Management	CT angiography to identify an aneurysm and immediate referral to neurosurgery for potential intervention (clipping/coiling).

CASE 11 | Cranial Nerve III (Oculomotor) Palsy *(continued)*

Discussion	The oculomotor nerve innervates four of the extraocular muscles (medial, superior, and inferior recti; inferior oblique) the levator palpebrae superioris, and the pupillary sphincter through parasympathetic innervation. Loss of partial aspects of CN III is more common than complete palsy. Oculomotor nerve palsy can occur from lesions anywhere along the neuroanatomical course of CN III, originating within the oculomotor nucleus at the level of the superior colliculus in the midbrain to the extraocular muscles within the orbit.
	There are many different causes for a CN III palsy, but the most common is microvascular disease (such as diabetes). Other causes include a posterior communicating artery aneurysm or a mass lesion in the cavernous sinus (thrombosis or neoplasm). Within CN III, parasympathetic fibers typically travel within the periphery of the nerve while more somatic motor fibers travel centrally. Therefore, microvascular disease that tends to most affect the center of the nerve typically spares the pupils due to the peripherally running parasympathetic fibers. Pupillary involvement is common in a posterior communicating artery aneurysm due to the proximity of the pupillomotor fibers, which can be compressed.
	Microvascular disease increases risk of any CN palsy, and typically occurs later in life.
	History: Diplopia, photophobia, ptosis
	Physical Exam: Eye position is "down and out" with ptosis. Divided into pupil-sparing and non-pupil-sparing subtypes depending on whether there is pupillary dilation (a "blown pupil"). Blown pupil is more suggestive of compressive lesions, although can be seen in later stages of microvascular disease due to long-standing hypertension or diabetes.
	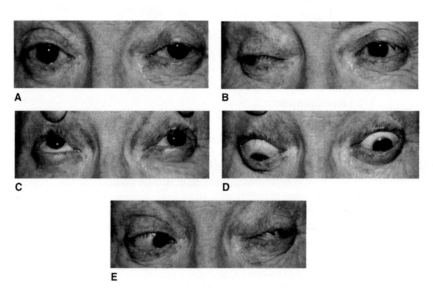
	Left partial third nerve palsy with ptosis **(A)**, reduced adduction **(B)**, reduced elevation **(C)**, and reduced depression **(D)** but normal abduction **(E)** of the left eye. (Reproduced with permission Maxine A. Papadakis, Stephen J. McPhee, Michael W. Rabow, Kenneth R. McQuaid, Current Medical Diagnosis & Treatment 2022. New York: McGraw Hill; 2022.)
	Diagnostics: • CN III palsies accompanied by other neurological deficits should undergo neuroimaging and/or lumbar puncture. • Isolated CN III palsies without additional neurologic signs or symptoms should also have neuroimaging performed. • CT or MR angiogram to rule out aneurysm should be performed on an emergent basis, especially in patients with a blown pupil.
	Management: Treat the underlying disorder. • Patients with an identified aneurysm on CT or MR angiogram should be referred to neurosurgery for microvascular clipping or endovascular coiling to prevent aneurysm rupture. • In patients with ischemic causes of CN III palsy, control of underlying risk factors should be done (e.g., improved glycemic control, antihypertensives).

CASE 11 | Cranial Nerve III (Oculomotor) Palsy *(continued)*

Additional Considerations	**CN IV palsy**—The trochlear nerve (CN IV) is the smallest cranial nerve and the only cranial nerve to originate from the dorsal surface of the brainstem, where it exits the midbrain at the level of the inferior colliculus. The fibers of CN IV innervate the superior oblique muscle, which is responsible for depression, abduction, and intorsion of the eye.

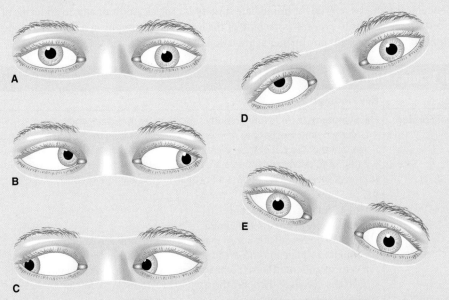

Schematic of right fourth nerve palsy. The right eye appears higher at baseline due to impaired depression **(A)**. Depression of the eye is most impaired when looking away from the side of the affected eye, placing the affected eye in the adducted position **(B)**, with less deficit when looking toward the affected side (affected eye abducted) **(C)**. When the head is tilted toward the side of the affected eye, the affected eye cannot intort as it normally would, leading to increased disconjugate gaze **(D)**. When the head tilts away from the affected side, the eyes are aligned since extorsion is preserved **(E)**. (Reproduced with permission from Aminoff M, Greenberg D, Simon R: Clinical Neurology, 9th ed. New York, NY: McGraw-Hill Education; 2015.)

Patients with CN IV palsy will report diplopia that worsens when tilting the head toward the affected eye, looking away from the affected eye, or looking down (i.e., reading, walking down stairs). While the most common cause of isolated CN IV palsy is congenital, the nerve can also be injured through microvascular disease or trauma. A mass lesion in the cavernous sinus can affect this nerve as well. With congenital CN IV palsy, it is often mistaken for torticollis due to the head tilt.

CN VI palsy—The abducens nerve (CN VI) is a thin nerve with the longest intracranial course and originates in the pons near the floor of the fourth ventricle and exits the brainstem at the junction of the pons and medulla. It also travels within the cavernous sinus in close association with the cavernous portion of the ICA.

CN VI controls the lateral rectus muscle and injury will lead to an inability to abduct the affected eye. Because of its long course and proximity to the fourth ventricle, it is susceptible to stretching and crushing in the setting of increased intracranial pressure (e.g., hydrocephalus, hemorrhage, malignancy). This may lead to bilateral CN VI palsy. Palsy can also occur due to vasculopathy (diabetic neuropathy) or a cavernous sinus mass lesion.

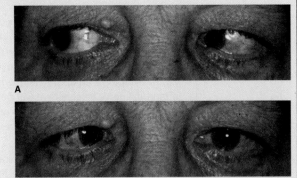

Sixth nerve palsy. Left sixth nerve palsy looking right **(A)** and looking left **(B)**. (Reproduced with permission Maxine A. Papadakis, Stephen J. McPhee, Michael W. Rabow, Kenneth R. McQuaid, Current Medical Diagnosis & Treatment 2022. New York: McGraw Hill; 2022.)

OCULAR TRAUMA

The eyes are exposed to a high level of environmental stress and thus traumatic damage to the ocular structures is common. As the foremost superficial tissue of the eye, the cornea has remarkable regenerative capabilities, but other tissues are less fortunate. Trauma to the eye can occur in an isolated fashion such as with a corneal foreign body or in the setting of a more generalized injury (i.e., blunt head trauma leading to orbital floor fracture). It is important to recognize the more emergent cases of ocular trauma, as referral for immediate surgery is crucial. Additionally, in all forms of ocular trauma it is important to take certain safeguards to prevent worsening of the injury. For example, in a ruptured globe the exam should be deferred, and a shield placed to prevent any further aggravation of the injury.

Ocular Trauma Mini-Cases

Cases	Key Findings
Corneal Foreign Body	**Hx:** Symptoms include foreign body sensation, tearing, pain, and redness • Determine the mechanism of injury (e.g., metal striking metal, use of power tools or weed-whackers) • Ask whether the patient was wearing safety glasses • Attempt to determine the size, shape, velocity, force, and composition of the object • Always keep in mind the possibility of an intraocular foreign body **PE:** • Visual acuity may be affected • Corneal foreign body and infiltrate • If foreign body contains iron, it may oxidize and form a "rust ring" • Conjunctival injection and eyelid edema may be present • If vertically oriented linear corneal abrasions are seen, look for a foreign body under the upper eyelid • Evert the eyelids and inspect the conjunctival fornices for foreign bodies **Diagnostics:** Clinical diagnosis • Consider CT orbit or ultrasound if there is concern for intraocular or intraorbital foreign body • Avoid MRI if possibility of metallic foreign body **Management:** • Remove the foreign body and as much of a rust ring (if present) as possible via slit lamp exam after applying topical anesthetic to the eye • Treat with topical antibiotics • Consider topical NSAID drops or oral medications, such as acetaminophen, NSAIDs, or narcotics for pain control **Discussion:** Ocular foreign bodies are a common form of ocular trauma. Determining the type of material is important for assessing the risk of infection or complication. Organic or vegetable materials are associated with a higher rate of infection. Metallic materials are likely to cause a rust ring. Inert material (e.g., glass, ceramic) tend to be nonreactive and have less risk of an inflammatory response. Mechanisms of injury that are higher risk for penetrating the eye include grinding, hammering, metal shaving, machine yard work, and exposure to explosives.
Orbital Floor Fracture	**Hx:** Blunt trauma to the eye/orbit. Ask about the mechanism of trauma, if they have double vision, numbness to the face (infraorbital nerve injury), and vision loss. **PE:** A full examination of facial structures should be performed to assess the extent of injury. • May have diplopia on upgaze or downgaze, or enophthalmos • Infraorbital nerve involvement will create numbness in cheek, upper lip, and upper gingiva • Palpation of inferior orbital rim may reveal stepoff • Orbital or lid emphysema may be present and worsen with nose blowing **Diagnostics:** CT scan of orbit to examine the size of the fracture, herniation of orbital contents into the sinuses, entrapped extraocular muscle, and distinguish from other types of fractures including medial or lateral wall fractures, orbito-zygomatic fractures, and LeFort fractures. **Management:** • Initial treatment includes nasal decongestants, ice packs to the eyelids, and avoidance of nose blowing • Consider broad spectrum oral antibiotics for patients with history of chronic sinusitis, diabetes, or other immunocompromised states • Consider oral corticosteroids to reduce swelling Coronal computed tomography scan of orbits showing right orbital floor fracture (*arrows*). (Reproduced with permission Paul Riordan-Eva, James J. Augsburger, Vaughan & Asbury's General Ophthalmology, 19e. New York: McGraw Hill; 2018.)

Ocular Trauma Mini-Cases (*continued*)

Orbital Floor Fracture	• Surgical repair should be done immediately (within 24–48 hours) if there is muscle entrapment with oculocardiac reflex symptoms (bradycardia, heart block, nausea, vomiting or syncope) • Consider surgical repair within 1–2 weeks for persistent symptomatic diplopia in primary or downgaze that does not improve, or for large orbital floor fractures with enophthalmos or inferior displacement of the eye (hypoglobus) **Discussion:** Orbital floor fractures (aka "blowout" fractures) occur secondary to an explosive increase in intraorbital pressure. Common mechanisms include falls, high-velocity ball-related sports, interpersonal violence, and traffic accidents. In addition to evaluating for facial injury, it is important to check pupils and color vision for evidence of traumatic optic neuropathy, and examine the eye for injury, including rupture, hyphema, and lens dislocation. Fractures in pediatric patients differ from those in adults because their bones are more pliable. As a result, when the bone breaks, orbital tissues herniate through the fracture site and the bone snaps back into place like a "trap door," causing entrapment of the inferior rectus muscle and perimuscular soft tissue.
Ruptured Globe	**Hx:** History of trauma, fall, or sharp object entering the globe. **PE:** • Visual acuity is decreased • May have full-thickness scleral or corneal laceration, severe subconjunctival hemorrhage (especially involving 360 degrees of bulbar conjunctiva, often bullous), a deep or shallow AC compared to the fellow eye, a peaked or irregular pupil, lens material or vitreous in the anterior chamber, foreign body tract, or new opacity in the lens • Intraocular contents may be outside of the globe • May have blood in the anterior chamber (hyphema) and periorbital ecchymosis. **Diagnostics:** CT scan of orbit and brain to rule out intraocular foreign body **Management:** • Once a ruptured globe is diagnosed, further examination should be deferred to prevent inadvertent pressure on the globe and further extrusion of intraocular contents, and a hard shield should be placed over the eye. • Admit to hospital for emergent evaluation/treatment by an ophthalmologist. • Administer systemic antibiotics, tetanus shot, antiemetics, and pain medication. **Discussion:** Ruptured globe is an ophthalmic emergency. Trauma to one eye can lead to **sympathetic ophthalmia**, an autoimmune reaction whereby T lymphocytes are exposed to antigens in the eye that are normally sequestered from the adaptive immune system. These T cells may then react against antigens in both the injured and uninjured eye, resulting in further inflammation, erythema, and impaired vision. 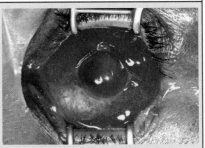 Massive hemorrhagic chemosis following severe blunt ocular trauma. A globe rupture in the superonasal quadrant was confirmed by surgical exploration. (Reproduced with permission Paul Riordan-Eva, James J. Augsburger, Vaughan & Asbury's General Ophthalmology, 19e. New York: McGraw Hill; 2018.)
Retrobulbar Hemorrhage (Orbital Compartment Syndrome)	**Hx:** Trauma or surgery to the eyelids or orbit. History of anticoagulation. Patients may report pain and decreased vision. **PE:** • May have vision loss and afferent pupillary defect • Proptosis, eyelids are tense ("rock-hard"), with limited movement of the eye, resistance to retropulsion of the globe, and increased intraocular pressure • May have periorbital ecchymosis • Extraocular motion may be impaired due to compression of cranial nerves and/or extraocular muscles **Diagnostics:** Clinical diagnosis **Management:** Immediate orbital decompression with lateral canthotomy and cantholysis (separation of lower lid from its insertion into the canthus at the lateral aspect of the lid). **Discussion:** Orbital compartment syndrome is an ophthalmic emergency. It occurs when there is a sudden rise in pressure in the orbital tissue. Because the orbit is a closed space, orbital hemorrhage from trauma can cause stretching and compression of the optic nerve and increased intraocular pressure, which can lead to ischemia to the optic nerve, globe, and retina, potentially leading to permanent vision loss.

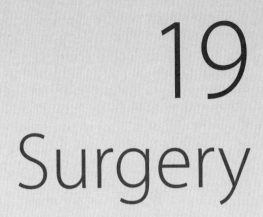

19
Surgery

Lead Authors: Amelia Bartholomew, MD; Nathaniel Koo, MD; Alejandra Perez-Tamayo, MD
Contributors: Katherine Petrovich, MD; Haley Kittle, MD; Soobin Kim, MD;
Diana Rapolti, MD; Elsa Nico, MD; Arjun Singh, MD; Mary B. Coomes, MD; Samantha Lagestee, MS;
Andrew Mudreac, MD; Adam Miller, MD; Meghana Babu, MD; Sarah Russel, MD, MPH;
Carolina Baz, MD; Alan Carneiro, PhD; Joseph R. Geraghty, MD, PhD

INTRODUCTION

While the practice of surgery is complex and comprised of many specialized branches, surgery for Step 2 CK will include characteristic cases from the areas of surgery seen most frequently in clinical practice, including: cardiothoracic, colon and rectal, transplant, trauma, pediatrics, vascular and general surgery. Additional surgical cases and pearls are covered elsewhere in this book. It is important to recognize that some cases require emergent or urgent surgical intervention, others can be elective procedures once the patient is stabilized, and finally some may not require any intervention and can just be closely observed.

PRE-OPERATIVE ASSESSMENT

Once an operation is considered as a viable therapy, the next step is to determine the pre-operative risk—which is the cumulative risk of death a patient faces in undergoing the operation. Operative risk can be considered in two broad categories: patient-related risk factors and those related to the operation. Every effort is made to reduce patient risk by optimizing their medical condition. Patient-related risk factors can be further estimated by specific risk calculators. These risk calculators help fulfill the goal of the surgical team to reduce morbidity and mortality and return patients to normal activities in a reasonable time.

Three commonly used calculators (all available online) include:

- **American Society of Anesthesia Risk Assessment Model:** Has six physical status classifications, with each class demonstrating progressively greater illness severity in the pre-operative patient. Every patient is assigned a classification before surgery on the anesthesia record.
- **American College of Surgeons National Surgical Quality Improvement Program Model (ACS NSQIP):** Four categories designed to help predict length of hospital stay, likelihood of serious complication (e.g., cardiac, pulmonary, renal), readmission or requirement for discharge to skilled care facility, and likelihood of death.
- **Revised Cardiac Risk Index (RCRI) for Pre-Operative Risk:** Can be especially helpful in identifying risk in patients >50 years old of major adverse cardiac events (MACE)—defined as death, myocardial infarction, or cardiac arrest at 30 days from noncardiac surgery.

American Society of Anesthesia (ASA) Risk Assessment Model and Classification*

Classification	Definition	Examples
ASA I	Normal, healthy	• Nonsmoker, no or minimal alcohol use
ASA II	Mild systemic disease, no significant functional limitation	• Current smoker, social alcohol drinker • Obesity (BMI 30–40) • Well-controlled diabetes or hypertension • Pregnancy
ASA III	Substantive functional limitations: one or more moderate to severe systemic diseases	• Morbid obesity (BMI ≥40) • Poorly controlled diabetes, hypertension, COPD • ESRD requiring dialysis • Remote history (>3 months) of myocardial infarction, stroke, TIA, or coronary stent • Active hepatitis, alcohol dependence • Premature infants (up to 60 weeks post-conceptional age)
ASA IV	Severe systemic disease that is a constant threat to life	• Recent history (<3 months) of myocardial infarction, stroke, TIA, or coronary stent, • Ongoing cardiac ischemia, severe cardiac valve dysfunction, or reduced ejection fraction • Shock, sepsis, DIC • Acute renal disease or failure not undergoing regular dialysis
ASA V	Survival is not expected if there is no operation	• Massive trauma • Ruptured abdominal or thoracic aneurysm • Intracranial bleed with mass effect • Multiple system organ dysfunction
ASA VI	Declared brain-dead patient undergoing organ retrieval	

Abbreviations: BMI, body mass index; COPD, coronary obstructive pulmonary disease; ESRD, end-stage renal disease; TIA, transient ischemic attack; DIC, disseminated intravascular coagulation.

*Includes six categories (I–VI) and each can be modified by adding an "E" to indicate emergent status.

The ACS NSQIP Model

Category	Description
Age	>65 Years Old
Chronic conditions	ASA Class 3, BMI <20 or recent weight loss, diabetes, hypertension, congestive heart failure, current use of tobacco within one year, severe COPD, dialysis, steroid use
Acute conditions	Hepatic decompensation with ascites within 30 days, systemic sepsis within 48 hours, ventilator dependency, disseminated cancer, acute renal failure
Poor functional status	*According to Metabolic Equivalents (MET):* Patients capable of activities requiring 10 MET have less risk than those only capable of activities requiring 1 MET. See table below.

Functional Status According to Metabolic Equivalents (MET)

MET	Able to Perform the Following Activities
1	Self-care, including dressing, eating, toilet use, walking around the house 2–3 miles per hour (mph)
4	Light housework, climbing stairs, moderate recreational activities (dancing, golf, doubles tennis), walking 4 mph
10	Participate in strenuous sports (e.g., skiing, swimming, basketball, singles tennis)

Revised Cardiac Risk index (Lee Criteria)*

Criteria	Example(s)
High-risk surgery	Intraperitoneal, intrathoracic, or supra-inguinal vascular surgery
Ischemic heart disease	History of angina, myocardial infarction, use of nitrates ECG with Q waves or a positive stress test
Congestive heart failure	Dyspnea on exertion, orthopnea, and/or paroxysmal nocturnal dyspnea; chest x-ray with pulmonary edema; bilateral rales or S3 gallop on physical exam
Cerebrovascular disease	History of transient ischemic attack or stroke
Diabetes mellitus on insulin	N/A
Serum creatinine >2 mg/dL	N/A

*The most frequently used tool to assess cardiac risk for noncardiac surgery in patients >50 years old. It identifies the above six criteria to identify patients with higher risks of major adverse cardiac events (MACE).

Additional Considerations Affecting Operative Risk

Pulmonary Disease

Post-operative pulmonary complications can occur in 5–10% of patients and can include atelectasis resulting in hypoxemia, pneumonia, bronchial plugging with pulmonary collapse, respiratory failure, acute lung injury, ARDS, and pulmonary embolism. This risk doubles in high-risk patients. Patient conditions which increase risk include:

1. *Age >65*
2. *Chronic obstructive pulmonary disease*: Patients should be treated medically to optimize condition. Those who fail to show improvement in pulmonary function tests have increased risk of respiratory failure and mortality.
3. *Congestive heart failure*
4. *Liver or renal disease*: Evidenced by albumin <3.0 g/dL or BUN >30 mg/dL.
5. *Obstructive sleep apnea*: Increases risk of pulmonary complications and risk of post-operative myocardial infarction.
6. *Surgical procedure*: Risk factors inherent to the operation include abdominal, vascular, head and neck, neurosurgery, or emergent surgery. Operations >3 hours also have increased risk of post-operative pulmonary complications.

Renal Impairment

Patients with chronic kidney disease (CKD) have increased risk of acute kidney injury (AKI), cardiac complications, and death. In general, decreased eGFR is associated with increased mortality, especially in patients with stage 4 CKD and above.

Renal impairment can also occur post-operatively, adding to post-operative risk of mortality. Post-operative AKI is more common after cardiac surgery than noncardiac surgery; risk factors include older age (>75 years), heart failure, prior myocardial infarction, peripheral vascular disease, chronic obstructive pulmonary disease requiring bronchodilator therapy, hepatic disease, emergent surgery, and high body mass index (BMI).

Management of patients with kidney disease or at risk for post-operative AKI includes the avoidance of potential nephrotoxic agents and medications perioperatively such as NSAIDs, certain antibiotics, IV contrast, low-molecular-weight heparins, diuretics, ACE inhibitors, and angiotensin II receptor blockers.

Hepatic Disease

Hepatic risk can be assessed by two instruments, the Child-Pugh and MELD scores. Whether MELD or Child-Pugh is used, recognition of the severity of liver disease is critical to identifying patients at risk for post-operative complications leading to death.

Child-Pugh Score for Classifying Cirrhosis Severity

The classic 15-point Child-Pugh score relies on the subjectivity of the physical exam to quantify the presence of ascites and encephalopathy and the degree of hypoalbuminemia and coagulopathy (INR). Class A is 5-6 points and has a 10% perioperative mortality; Class B (7-9 points) and Class C (10-15 points) have 30 and 82% perioperative mortalities, respectively, making hepatic function assessment a critical factor in deciding the merits of an operative intervention.

Criteria	Points		
	1	2	3
Ascites	Absent	Slight	Moderate or severe
Bilirubin	<2 mg/dL	2–3 mg/dL	>3 mg/dL
Albumin	>3.5 g/dL	2.8–3.5 g/dL	<2.8 g/dL
INR	<1.7	1.7-2.3	>2.3
Encephalopathy	None	Mild to moderate (Grade 1 or 2)	Severe (Grade 3 or 4)

MELD Score Prediction of 3-Month Mortality

The 40-point MELD (Model for End-Stage Liver Disease) score was developed to predict 3-month survival in patients >12 years old to prioritize transplant candidates and relies entirely on blood tests of serum bilirubin, creatinine, and INR. Most liver transplant recipients are transplanted with a MELD score of 25 or more; this score indicates a 20-30% 3-month mortality, whereas a score of 30 or more has >50% 3 month mortality. Its prediction of survival past 3 months can be inaccurate in 15–20% of patients.

Frailty and Functional Assessment

Patients with poor functional status demonstrate higher rates of post-operative complications. Identification of patient performance status pre-operatively is done by defining their abilities to carry out activities of daily living (ADLs). Defining the risk for falls can be accomplished by recording a timed get-up-and-go test: the amount of time it takes to stand up from a seated position, walk 10 feet, and return to the chair. Additional frailty assessments that would raise concern for post-operative recovery include:

- History of more than one fall in the past 6 months
- Poor nutritional status (e.g., albumin <3 mg/dL)
- Cognitive impairment (e.g., poor performance on Mini-Cog test)

For elective surgeries, management of frailty can reduce risk of mortality with a pre-rehabilitation program specifically designed to modify the patient's individual risk factors. Programs target improving physical, psychological, and nutritional status to decrease post-operative complications, improve pain control, lead to faster mobilization, and decrease hospital length of stay.

Metabolic Considerations

Patients with diabetes have increased risk of delayed extubation, cardiac and respiratory complications, nonhealing incisions, post-operative infections, and increased mortality. Factors which further increase post-operative complications in the diabetic patient include age >65 years old, hyperglycemia, and renal impairment.

Avoidance of hyper- or hypoglycemia is critically important, with target levels <180 mg/dL. Surgical stress and anesthesia promote hyperglycemia in the diabetic patient; intra-operative glucose levels >200 mg/dL or <140 mg/dL are associated with increased morbidity and mortality.

CASE 1 | Cardiac Risk Assessment

A 67-year-old man with coronary artery disease (status post three-vessel coronary artery bypass grafting 3 years ago) presents for pre-operative assessment for low anterior resection for rectal adenocarcinoma. He has well-controlled type 2 diabetes mellitus, hypertension, and hyperlipidemia. His daily medications include insulin glargine, insulin aspart, metoprolol, lisinopril, aspirin, and atorvastatin. The patient swims three to four times a week and has no anginal symptoms, orthopnea, or dyspnea. He previously smoked (30-pack years) but quit 3 years ago. A stress echocardiogram performed 1 year ago showed an ejection fraction of 55–60% with no abnormalities during exercise. On exam, BP is 150/80 mmHg, and the rest of the vital signs are normal. He has no murmurs, gallops, or rubs. Lung and abdominal exams are normal and there is no peripheral edema.

Initial Diagnostic Tests	• Assess patient's risk for a major adverse cardiac events (MACE) to determine need for further pre-operative cardiac evaluation • Obtain baseline CBC, BMP, HbA1c, ECG
Next Steps in Management	Optimize chronic conditions in perioperative period
Discussion	In evaluating a patient's perioperative risk, both the patient's risk factors and the risk of the surgery need to be considered. The Revised Cardiac Risk Index (RCRI) helps predict risk for MACE and is important in this patient, who is over 50 years old. Of the six RCRI considerations (see table above), this patient's colorectal surgery will occur intraperitoneally and therefore is high-risk surgery. Additionally, he has ischemic heart disease and diabetes requiring insulin, which add to his risk. He has no known history of CKD, and the BMP will determine baseline creatinine. He has an RCRI score of 3, and ASA Class III, which correlates to an elevated risk of MACE. In addition to the initial diagnostic tests, to help optimize his intraoperative and post-operative management, would consider the following steps to help his care: • Obtain a baseline B-type natriuretic peptide (BNP). Recommended for patients ≥65 years, those with significant cardiac disease, or if RCRI is ≥1. If BNP is elevated, will guide care team to obtain an ECG in the post-operative period and daily troponins for 2–3 days. • Consider: Cardiac stress testing or echocardiography. If he had been symptomatic or had poor functional status, could consider coronary catheterization. • Consider: Spirometry or pulmonary function testing, based on his history of 30-pack-years of tobacco use and age >65 years. • Diabetes management: Most target a range of ≤7% to reduce the risk of myocardial infarction, surgical site infection, and renal failure, which needs to be balanced with a patient's frailty and comorbidities. Blood sugars should be closely monitored in the perioperative period.

Hemostasis: Pre-Operative Management of Anticoagulation

After cardiac ischemia, bleeding is the most common cause of post-operative cardiac arrest. Understanding hemostasis and the pre-operative and operative factors that affect it is of critical importance. For major surgery, platelet count should be ≥50,000/μL while for minor surgery, it should be ≥30,000/μL.

Millions of patients are on antithrombotic medications to prevent clot formation. These medications can broadly be divided into two classes: antiplatelet and anticoagulant medications. Antiplatelet medications include aspirin and the ADP receptor antagonists (e.g., clopidogrel, prasugrel, ticagrelor). Anticoagulants include warfarin, heparins (unfractionated and low-molecular weight), and direct oral anticoagulants (DOACs). DOACs are further subdivided into two categories: (1) direct thrombin inhibitors (dabigatran), and (2) factor Xa inhibitors (e.g., rivaroxaban, apixaban, edoxaban). For details on antiplatelet and antithrombotic agents as well as reversal agents, refer to Chapter 8 (Hematology and Oncology).

For elective procedures, there is time to stop anticoagulants to reduce bleeding risk. In emergent surgery, reversal protocols should be initiated promptly and closely monitored for efficacy to prevent life-threatening hemorrhage.

CASE 2 | Pre-Operative Anticoagulation Management

A 77-year-old man with atrial fibrillation and hypertension presents for a left hip arthroplasty due to osteoarthritis. He has left hip pain when getting in and out of chairs, has trouble walking up the stairs, and pain disturbs his sleep. His daily medications include rivaroxaban, carvedilol, and naproxen. On exam, he is afebrile with pulse of 68 bpm, respirations 12 bpm, and blood pressure 142/82 mmHg. He has a noticeable limp, walks with a cane, and has decreased range of motion of the left hip. Hip X-rays show osteophyte formation, joint space narrowing with remodeling of the articular surface, and sclerosis of the subchondral bone plate.

Initial Diagnostic Tests	• Check baseline labs: CBC, coagulation factors, BMP • Check baseline ECG and CXR

CASE 2 | Pre-Operative Anticoagulation Management *(continued)*

Next Steps in Management	1. Assess patient's risk for a MACE to determine need for further pre-operative cardiac evaluation 2. Rivaroxaban should be held for 1–2 days before surgery and resumed 1–2 days after surgery, depending on surgeon's assessment of bleeding risk

Discussion	The most common indication for anti-coagulation when reviewing pre-operative conditions is atrial fibrillation; other indications include venous thromboembolism, post-operative conditions in which venous thromboembolism poses a high risk, and mechanical heart valve.
	Diagnostics:
	• CBC and coagulation studies: Although the patient is on rivaroxaban (Factor Xa inhibitor), which does not directly affect PT/INR, having a baseline is helpful for patients on anticoagulation.
	• BNP: Based on this patient's RCRI of 1 and his age, a baseline BNP will determine post-operative need for ECG and troponins.
	• ECG: To document the patient's current rhythm
	• Chest x-ray: Based on age and known atrial fibrillation, patient should undergo a baseline chest x-ray.
	Management:
	1. Assess patient's cardiac risk for MACE using the RCRI and ASA classifications to determine need for further cardiac evaluation. This patient is undergoing high-risk surgery (joint replacement) and has an RCRI of 1. His ASA class is 3 as he has functional limitations and nonlife-threatening severe disease (atrial fibrillation, hypertension), translating to an elevated risk of MACE. His age and RCRI prompt the need for a BNP level (see above). His ASA class warrants further assessment of cardiac risk, and based on his limited functional status, a pharmacological stress test would be considered.
	2. Decide when to stop the anticoagulation. Decision is made based on risk of surgery and half-life of the anticoagulant.
	3. Decide when and how to restart therapy, based on surgeon's assessment of bleeding risk.
	  • DOACS will have immediate therapeutic effects when started
	  • Bridging therapy with heparin is used for high-risk patients on warfarin, dabigatran, and edoxaban.

ANESTHESIOLOGY

Anesthesia can affect surgical outcomes in a variety of ways. Anesthetic drugs have a variety of mechanisms of action and can cause patients to experience adverse effects which impact their recovery. Rapid recognition and treatment of certain complications of anesthesia, such as malignant hyperthermia, can be lifesaving. All techniques, whether inhaled or intravenous, have four main goals, known as the "Four A's of Anesthesia:"

- *Awareness:* Reduction in level of consciousness
- *Amnesia:* Lack of memory related to the procedure
- *Analgesia:* Relief of pain and reactions to pain, including both somatic (movement or withdrawal) and autonomic (hypertension, tachycardia, sweating, tearing) reflexes
- *Akinesia:* Lack of overt movement (may require addition of neuromuscular junction blocking agents such as succinylcholine or rocuronium)

Different forms of anesthesia have different risks and benefits.

Type of Anesthesia	Mechanism and Notes	Additional Risks or Benefits
Local	Local injection, will have regional effects	May have unintended systemic effects with excessive absorption
Regional	Peripheral nerve blocks or through segmental anesthesia by spinal or epidural administration	Patient remains conscious; can lower the risk for pulmonary complications Prolonged post-operative analgesia; reduces the need for narcotics
General	May be intravenous or inhaled Often used in abdominal, neurosurgical, spine, and head and neck surgery	Can allow for complete paralysis Requires ventilatory support

Common Intravenous, Inhaled, and Local Anesthetics

Anesthetic Agent	Route	Mechanism of Action	Adverse Hemodynamic Effects	Other Notes
Propofol	IV	Potentiates GABA$_A$	Hypotension due to vasodilation, pain with intravenous administration	Lipid emulsion—has a characteristic milky white appearance avoid if peanut allergy.
Midazolam	IV	Benzodiazepine, helps opening of GABA$_A$ receptor channels	May lead to post-operative respiratory depression and hypotension	May result in transient anterograde amnesia
Etomidate	IV	GABA$_A$ agonist	Hemodynamically neutral; minimal effect on blood pressure and heart rate	May lead to transient adrenal insufficiency
Ketamine	IV	N-methyl-D-aspartate (NMDA) receptor antagonist	Sympathetic activation (e.g., hypertension, tachycardia)	Causes dissociative amnesia. May hallucinate, have vivid dreams after emergence
Sevoflurane, desflurane, isoflurane	Inhaled	Affects various ion channels including GABA$_A$, NMDA, acetylcholine, and glycine	Hypotension due to vasodilation	May cause malignant hyperthermia in susceptible patients
Lidocaine	Local	Blocks inner portion of voltage-gated sodium channels, preventing membrane depolarization and loss of initiation and propagation of action potentials	Can depress left ventricular function, especially if patient is hypovolemic. May lead to arrhythmia, hypertension, or hypotension	Contraindicated in complete heart block without pacemaker. May reduce the threshold for seizures in children, especially after opioids and anti-emetics
Bupivacaine	Local	Also blocks inner portion of voltage-gated sodium channels	Cardiovascular toxicity, arrhythmia, hypertension, or hypotension	Cardiovascular collapse has been associated in patients treated with verapamil and timolol

Common Neuromuscular Blocking Drugs Used in Anesthesiology

Anesthetic Agent	Route	Mechanism of Action	Adverse Hemodynamic Effects	Other Notes
Succinylcholine	IV	Nicotinic acetylcholine receptor agonist at neuromuscular junction, resulting in a depolarizing neuromuscular blockade	Arrhythmias, hypotension, hypertension	May cause malignant hyperthermia in susceptible patients. May cause hyperkalemia—higher risk if burns, stroke with paralysis, prolonged immobilization, or spinal cord injury. Patients with myasthenia gravis and Lambert-Eaton myasthenic syndrome may have longer-term paralysis.
Rocuronium, vecuronium	IV	Nicotinic acetylcholine receptor antagonist at the neuromuscular junction, resulting in a nondepolarizing neuromuscular blockade	Rocuronium: Faster onset of action; associated with tachycardia, hypertension, and increased cardiac index in first 5 minutes. Vecuronium: Can be associated with hypotension in first 5 minutes	Patients with myasthenia gravis and Lambert-Eaton myasthenic syndrome may have longer-term paralysis.

CASE 3 | Malignant Hyperthermia (MH)

A 30-year-old man with no past medical history was taken to the operating room for debridement and open fixation of a femur fracture after a motor vehicle accident (MVA). He was intubated and isoflurane was administered. About 15 minutes into the surgery, his temperature is increased to 40°C, pulse is 120/min, respirations are 30/min, and blood pressure is 150/120 mmHg. He is diaphoretic and his masseter muscle is rigid. An arterial blood gas shows a PO_2 70 mmHg, PCO_2 55 mmHg, and pH 7.30. His labs show K^+ 6.5 mEq/L and highly elevated creatine kinase (CK). Urinalysis shows myoglobinuria.

Conditions with Similar Presentations	**Neuroleptic malignant syndrome:** Presents similarly (i.e., hyperthermia, vital sign instability, rigidity), though also has acute mental status changes and occurs in patients taking antipsychotic medications (e.g., haloperidol). **Serotonin syndrome:** Presents with a characteristic triad of mental status changes, autonomic dysregulation, and neuromuscular hyperactivity. This occurs in patients taking medications that increase serotonin (e.g., SSRI, SNRI, MAO inhibitors, TCAs), especially when taken in combination or at high doses. **Rhabdomyolysis:** May present with hyperkalemia, elevated CK, and myoglobinuria in a patient with a crush injury, but will not present with hyperthermia or tachypnea. **Sepsis:** Presents with fever and acidosis but rigidity and increased serum CK are not seen. **Pheochromocytoma crisis:** Can manifest with hypertension, tachycardia, and hyperthermia. Rigidity and rhabdomyolysis would not be seen. **Thyrotoxicosis:** May present with hyperthermia, hypercarbia, and tachycardia but does not include muscle rigidity or rhabdomyolysis.
Initial Diagnostic Tests	• Clinical diagnosis • Check arterial or venous blood gases, BMP, ECG, CK level, urinalysis, and coagulation profile
Next Steps in Management	• Immediate cessation of triggering anesthetic agent • IV fluids and hyperventilation with 100% oxygen at 10 L/minute • Administration of dantrolene (ryanodine receptor antagonist which inhibits calcium release) • Admission to the intensive care unit (ICU)

Discussion	MH is a rare, life-threatening metabolic response to inhalational anesthetics (e.g., sevoflurane, isoflurane) alone or in combination with a depolarizing muscle relaxant such as succinylcholine. Patients younger than 19 make up 50% of the cases, with a higher incidence in men. Susceptibility to MH is inherited in an autosomal dominant pattern with variable penetrance, due to mutations in the skeletal muscle ryanodine receptors (*RYR1* gene), resulting in abnormal calcium release from the myocyte sarcoplasmic reticulum.
	
	These inhaled anesthetics trigger an uncontrolled release of calcium from the sarcoplasmic reticulum resulting in sustained contracture of skeletal muscles. Rhabdomyolysis ensues, resulting in hyperkalemia and excretion of myoglobin in the urine, which may lead to renal failure. In severe cases, the patient may develop disseminated intravascular coagulation (DIC), heart failure, and compartment syndrome in the limbs due to profound muscle swelling. If the body temperature exceeds 41°C, patient mortality is usually due to DIC.
	
	History: May have a family history of MH. The timing of signs and symptoms is highly variable but they occur during or immediately after use of volatile anesthetic agents or succinylcholine. Rarely, MH can develop during the 24 hours after surgery, typically while the patient is recovering from anesthesia.
	
	Physical Exam: Earliest signs in order of early to late occurrence are hypercarbia, tachypnea, masseter spasm, sinus tachycardia, muscle rigidity, rapidly increasing temperature (with an increase of 1–2 degrees every 5 minutes), arrhythmias (ventricular tachycardia, fibrillation, asystole), myoglobinuria (cola-colored urine).
	
	Diagnostics:
	• MH is a clinical diagnosis based on combination of hypercarbia, tachycardia, and muscle rigidity. However, additional workup is needed.
	• The patient will need frequent monitoring of:
	  • Arterial or venous blood gases: assess for respiratory and metabolic acidosis
	  • BMP: hyperkalemia may occur rapidly due to muscle breakdown and acute kidney injury in context of rhabdomyolysis
	  • CK: to detect rhabdomyolysis
	  • ECG: to assess for hyperkalemia-associated changes
	  • Urinalysis: to detect myoglobinuria
	  • Coagulation profile: to assess for the development of DIC
	• Definitive diagnosis is made by genetic testing (ryanodine receptor gene sequencing).

CASE 3 | Malignant Hyperthermia (MH) *(continued)*

Discussion	**Management:** • Immediate cessation of triggering anesthetic agent. • Procedure should be terminated or completed as quickly as possible with a nontriggering anesthetic such as opioids or a nondepolarizing muscle relaxant. • Administration of dantrolene: ryanodine receptor antagonist which inhibits calcium release. Additional dantrolene may be given to prevent recurrence within 24 hours. • Admission to the ICU for management. • For hyperthermia, cooling with ice bags in axilla and elsewhere when temperature >39°C. • Hyperventilation with 100% oxygen at 10 L/min. • Monitor urine output and administer IV fluids and possible sodium bicarbonate to prevent AKI in setting of rhabdomyolysis.

POST-OPERATIVE COMPLICATIONS

Any surgery has intrinsic risk of infection, bleeding, or injury to surrounding structures. Aseptic techniques and careful performance of surgery by skilled surgeons are the standard of care to reduce these risks. The rates of complications vary depending on the surgery and patient condition. Patients with high cardiac risks are at higher risk of post-operative cardiac events, thus the importance of risk assessments pre-operatively.

More than 60% of post-operative complications occur within the first 3 days after surgery. High-risk surgical procedures such as intraabdominal GI or vascular procedures, emergency surgery, and operative duration >2.5 hours also add risk. The goal of post-operative evaluation is to recognize and manage complications in the immediate period after surgery.

The first part of assessing patients for post-operative complications is your history. Evaluate patients for pain that is out of proportion to the procedure and whether they have passed gas or stools, voided urine, or have nausea or vomiting after the procedure. During your exam, assess vitals, pulse oximetry, line sites, drains, wounds (including the surgical incision), lungs, heart, extremities for swelling, and pulses. Other pertinent organ systems should be examined based on the surgery performed.

From a diagnostic standpoint, any changes from baseline lab values should be investigated:

• Complete blood count: Changes may suggest post-operative hemorrhage, infection, and sepsis if associated with other clinical and laboratory findings

• Renal function: Creatinine increase indicates an acute kidney injury

• Electrolyte abnormalities:

  • Hypo- or hypernatremia may result from over- or underhydration during the procedure, respectively

  • Hyperkalemia can occur from tissue injury or in the setting of an AKI

Complications that occur in the post-operative period are categorized as general complications and surgery-specific complications. General complications are grouped by organ system and are presented in the table below based on peak occurrence post-operatively.

Post-Operative Complications by System and Typical Time Ranges

Organ System	Complications	Post-Operative Day (POD)
Cardiac	Myocardial infarction	1–3
	Heart failure, atrial fibrillation	1–4
Pulmonary	Atelectasis	1–3
	Pneumonia	4–7
	Respiratory failure (failure to wean from ventilator)	1–3
Infection	Skin and soft tissue infection	1–30
	UTI	3–6
Hematology	Deep vein thrombosis	7–90
	Pulmonary embolism	7–30
Renal	Pre- or post-renal factors	1–3
	Drug toxicity	8–90

Post-Operative Complications by System and Typical Time Ranges

Organ System	Complications	Post-Operative Day (POD)
Nervous system	Stroke	1–7
	Seizures	1–3
	Cognitive impairment	1–90
	Post-operative delirium	1–90
	Peripheral nerve injury	1–90
Gastrointestinal	Post-operative ileus	1–5
	Acalculous cholecystitis	1–90
	Anastomotic leak	5–30

Cardiac Complications

Post-operative increases in sympathetic tone (i.e., tachycardia), coagulation, and inflammatory responses alter pre-existent plaque morphology predisposing to subsequent myocardial injury and infarction. Development of supraventricular arrhythmias is frequently seen.

Pulmonary Complications

Complications such as atelectasis and pneumonia are frequently seen. Failure to wean from the ventilator often occurs in critically ill patients such as those who are designated Class III ASA status or higher, have pre-operative shock, thrombocytopenia, neutrophilia, or renal insufficiency, and patients with insulin-dependent diabetics. Failure to wean from a ventilator is associated with longer hospital stays and higher mortality.

Hematologic Complications

Post-Operative Bleeding

Several different blood products can be used to address operative or post-operative bleeding. The most common cause of post-operative bleeding is thrombocytopenia. See Chapter 8 (Hematology and Oncology) for further details.

Blood Products and Considerations

Product	Clinical Considerations
Platelets	Life span: 7-10 days
	Wait 5-7 days after stopping anti-platelet therapy for elective surgery
	Platelet adhesion/aggregation can still occur in presence of heparin if vWF is present; fibrinogen needed as cofactor
Fresh frozen plasma (FFP)	Half-life: 6 hours
	Contains clotting factors/cofactors + AT-III, Protein S, Protein C
	Used to treat congenital or acquired clotting factor deficiencies
	Factors V and VIII activity present in FFP but lost in stored blood
	Immediate in action
Cryoprecipitate	Contains factors I, VIII, XIII, vW and fibronectin
	Also known as Cryoprecipitated Antihemophilic Factor
Prothrombin complex concentrate (PCC)	Prothrombin complex endogenously forms on platelets and catalyzes the formation of thrombin
	Contains factors II, VII, IX, X and protein C and S
Specific Coagulation Factors	
Factor I (Fibrinogen)	Half-life: 72-120 hours
Factor II (Prothrombin)	Half-life: 60 hours
Factor VII	Half-life: 3-6 hours
Factor X	Half-life: 30-40 hours

Venous Thromboembolism

Includes deep vein thrombosis (DVT) and pulmonary embolus (PE)—see below case

Renal Complications

Post-Operative Acute Kidney Injury (AKI)

Typically occurs within 7 days of surgery. It can be identified by an increase in serum creatinine of >0.3 mg/dL or >1.5 times increase in creatinine from baseline, or decreased urine volume of <0.5 ml/kg/h for 6 hours. It is seen more commonly after cardiac surgery. Subsequent development of CKD, cardiovascular events, and death place this complication as one which requires extreme vigilance in at-risk patients. Risk is increased in patients with age >60, pre-existing kidney dysfunction, and diabetes. Perioperatively or intra-operatively, kidney injury occurs from pre-renal factors such as hypovolemia, increased intraabdominal pressure, anesthetic-related decreased cardiac output or vasodilation, and post-renal urinary obstruction.

Post-Operative Oliguria

Oliguria is considered as <0.5 mL/kg/h, or <500 mL urine output in 24 hours. If the patient is not showing signs of hypovolemia (i.e., tachycardia, hypotension, orthostasis), the urine output can be averaged over 4 hours in order to make a more informed assessment.

Preventative Strategies

- Nephrotoxic drugs should be avoided, as their effects are often detected after the seventh post-operative day and can contribute to the longer-term complication of post-operative kidney disease. In addition, avoidance of post-operative hyperglycemia (>180 mg/dL) and perioperative hypotension (MAP <65) are important strategies to prevent this complication.
- **Maintenance fluid post-surgery:** If patients are free of nausea, they can begin an oral diet as early as 4 hours post-surgery. Once adequate oral intake is established, intravenous therapy is discontinued. If the patient is unable to maintain oral intake, maintenance fluids should be given, at a rate of 25–30 mL/kg per day using a hypotonic crystalloid instead of isotonic fluids which contain excess sodium. If the patient has significant fluid losses (i.e., high ileostomy output or vomiting), balanced isotonic crystalloid solutions can be used to replace the loss to achieve a zero fluid balance. Both fluid deficits and excessive fluid can increase post-operative complications.

Fluids	Considerations
Isotonic crystalloid	Used to replace extracellular volume deficits and GI losses. • Balanced electrolyte solutions (e.g., Lactated Ringer's solution, Plasma-Lyte): contain lactate which is converted by the liver to bicarbonate, which is helpful in addressing acidosis. • 0.9% sodium chloride: high chloride content may lead to hyperchloremic metabolic acidosis but is a good choice for correcting hyponatremia, hypochloremia, and metabolic alkalosis.
Hypotonic crystalloid	• D5 0.45% sodium chloride: can be used for maintenance IV fluid, as it supplies a modest number of calories, sufficient free water to replace insensible losses, and adequate amounts of sodium.
Hypertonic crystalloid	• 3.5% and 5% sodium chloride solutions: can be used to correct hyponatremia and are not used to restore extracellular volume deficits.
Colloids	• Albumin, dextran hetastarch, and gelatins: are not used post-surgery because they are more costly, can traverse the impaired capillary endothelium leading to pulmonary edema, and have shown no benefit over crystalloid in resuscitation of trauma, burn, or post-surgical patients. Further, they can trigger anaphylactic reactions.

Gastrointestinal Complications

Post-operative ileus is frequently seen, and anastomotic leaks are critical to recognize in patients after abdominopelvic surgeries. **Acalculous cholecystitis** can occur post-operatively in critically ill patients. Risk factors include diabetes, vasculitis, congestive heart failure, cancer, shock, or cardiac arrest. These conditions predispose to gallbladder ischemia and subsequent bacterial invasion. The diagnosis, determined by ultrasound, should be considered in a critically ill patient with sepsis and right upper quadrant pain or tenderness but may occur with no localizing signs. While cholecystectomy is the treatment of choice, a temporary percutaneous cholecystostomy tube can mitigate the condition in an unstable patient until the patient can tolerate cholecystectomy.

Neurologic Complications

The most common post-operative CNS complications include **stroke, seizures, and altered mental status**. Risk factors include vascular disease, prior transient ischemic attack (TIA) or stroke, diabetes, hypertension, smoking, and increased age.

Perioperative stroke incidence varies with type of surgery; noncardiac, nonneurological, and nonmajor vascular procedures have the lowest rate, whereas the highest rate occurs in major vascular and cardiac surgery.

- Stroke may be observed immediately upon emergence from anesthesia or may occur several days after surgery. In cardiac surgery, ischemic brain lesions can occur in up to 50% of patients and carry future risk of cognitive dysfunction.
- Seizures, either focal or generalized, can manifest as behavioral changes, altered consciousness, or tonic-clonic activity. Generalized seizures are more common after cardiac surgery or cardiac arrest. Since neuromuscular blockade anesthetics may mask seizure activity, patients at risk for seizures may benefit from EEG monitoring during surgery for rapid detection and immediate treatment to prevent cognitive impairment.
- Post-operative cognitive dysfunction can range from decrements in attention, concentration, and memory loss, loss of executive function, and loss of verbal fluency. Following cardiac surgery, cognitive dysfunction can affect 10–30% of patients; noncardiac surgery can result in slightly less rates of dysfunction identified at 1 week, with reduction to roughly 10% at 3 months.
- Post-operative delirium is most often observed after hip fracture repair and cardiac surgery and can occur in 30–60% of patients in patients >65. Post-operative delirium is associated with both short- and long-term cognitive decline and may be aggravated by deep levels of anesthesia, severe illness, and dehydration.

Peripheral nerve injury can occur due to compression, stretch ischemia, direct nerve trauma, or local anesthetic toxicity. Susceptibility is increased in patients with impaired microvascular function such as those with diabetes, hypertension, or a smoking history. Most common involvement includes:

1. **Ulnar nerve injury (C8–T1):** through direct pressure on the ulnar groove in the elbow and prolonged forearm flexion presenting with tingling or numbness along the medial 1½ digits, weakness with flexion of these digits or abduction and adduction, or "ulnar claw" on digit extension.
2. **Brachial plexus injury (C5–T1):** via compression against the clavicle during retraction of a median sternotomy, stretching by arm abduction, external rotation with posterior shoulder displacement, or direct injury by regional anesthetic block. The arm may hang by the side, pronated and medially rotated ("waiter's tip" or Erb palsy) following a C5–6 injury; a claw hand may result from a C8–T1 injury. Tourniquets or blood pressure cuffs or compression of the arm against an arm board placed too low can result in a radial nerve injury. The patient may complain of wrist drop and numbness along the posterior surface of the forearm and dorsum of the hand.
3. **Femoral nerve injury (L2–4):** can occur with compression at the pelvic brim, ischemia from aortic cross-clamp, hip arthroplasty, and lithotomy position. The patient may present with loss of sensation on the anterior thigh and medial leg, weak hip flexion, and loss of knee extension, causing problems climbing stairs and a diminished or absent patellar reflex.
4. **Superficial peroneal nerve injury (L4–S2):** can occur following lithotomy position where the nerve can be compressed by the fibular head. The patient will present with loss of dorsiflexion and eversion of the foot. Adequate padding of this area can prevent this injury.

Infectious Complications

Post-operative fever is defined as a temperature >38.0°C (>100.4°F). Common causes of post-operative fever include pneumonia, pulmonary embolism, urinary tract infection, surgical site infection, and drug fevers. A helpful mnemonic to remember causes of post-operative fever are the **"5 Ws": Wind** (pneumonia), **Water** (UTI), **Wound** (wound infection), **Walk** (DVT/PE), and **Wonder drugs** (drug fever). Many post-operative fevers spontaneously resolve or are not life-threatening.

Common Causes of Fever Based on Timing with Post-Operative Day (POD)

Immediate—POD 3	POD 3	POD 5	POD 7	POD Any
Malignant hyperthermia	Pneumonia	Thrombophlebitis	Pulmonary embolism	Drug fever
Blood products	Urinary tract infections			Wound infection
Prior trauma or infection				

Drug fever presents post-operatively with nonspecific symptoms and can be due to a variety of causes, including malignant hyperthermia, hypersensitivity, altered thermoregulation, and chemotherapy. Withdrawal from opioids, alcohol, or barbiturates can also occur >72 hours after surgery and lead to fever. Workup is primarily based on a thorough history of the addition of new medications in the absence of other potential causes of fever. Diagnosis and management are by cessation of offending drug. Administer dantrolene for treatment of malignant hyperthermia or neuroleptic malignant syndrome. Administer serotonin antagonist (e.g., cyproheptadine) for moderate-severe cases of serotonin syndrome. Treat withdrawal appropriately (see Chapter 16, Psychiatry).

A subset of febrile conditions that carry significantly higher mortalities and require timely and aggressive management include pulmonary embolism, necrotizing fasciitis, gangrene due to *Clostridium* infection, sepsis, malignant hyperthermia, serotonin syndrome, neuroleptic malignant syndrome, delirium tremens, adrenal insufficiency, and thyroid storm. While myocardial infarction is not typically thought of during the post-operative fever workup, its incidence is highest on day 0, and a post-myocardial fever can be observed in patients 2–5 days following acute myocardial infarction.

The immunodeficient post-operative patient requires a specialized head-to-toe exam for post-operative fever because of inability to manifest usual signs and symptoms. Immunodeficient patients can include patients on chronic immunosuppressants such as transplant recipients, nutritionally depleted patients (albumin <3.0 g/dL), HIV/AIDS, chemotherapy recipients, and those with frailty.

Post-Operative Complication Mini-Cases

Case	Key Findings
Myocardial Infarction	**Hx:** • Risk factors: Valvular surgery, tobacco use, history of ischemic heart disease **PE:** • May have signs of cardiogenic shock including hypotension, tachycardia, cool extremities, thready pulses • May have a new murmur **Diagnostics:** Check ECG and troponins **Management:** • Continue pre-operative beta-blockade in the perioperative period • Short-term intravenous beta-blockade in response to perioperative tachycardia can be effective in reducing cardiac ischemia **Discussion:** • Post-operative myocardial infarction carries a very high mortality and management is identical to that of acute myocardial infarction
Atrial Fibrillation	**Hx:** • Risk factors: History of ischemic heart disease or structural heart disease, increased age, tobacco use **PE:** • Irregular heart rate; possible hypotension in patients with rapid ventricular heart rate **Diagnostics:** Check ECG **Management:** • Identical to atrial fibrillation management, with goal of maintaining cardiovascular output. • Options focus on rate or rhythm control for patients who are hemodynamically stable, with cardioversion reserved for patients who are hemodynamically unstable. **Discussion:** • Can occur in response to post-surgical inflammation, increased sympathetic tone, and increase in intravascular volume occurring during post-operative fluid mobilization, stretching the atria. • Often self-limited, but carries an increased risk of stroke and hemodynamic instability.
Atelectasis	**Hx/PE:** • Risk factors: Pre-existing pulmonary disease, smoking, poor compliance with incentive spirometry, and need to lie flat (i.e., post-spinal surgery), and intrathoracic and abdominal surgery, and upper abdominal incisions that cause pain with deep breathing. • May present within POD 1–2 with tachypnea, dyspnea, hypoxemia, and bilateral crackles in the lower lung fields due to inability to clear accumulated secretions following intubation. No signs of consolidation. **Diagnostics:** Chest X-ray **Management:** • Deep breathing exercises with an incentive spirometer, early mobilization out of bed, chest physiotherapy, postural drainage, adequate hydration, and humidified air to loosen secretions • If bronchospasm is present, intermittent positive pressure breathing with bronchodilators **Discussion:** • Post-operative atelectasis is attributed to hypoventilation and decreased clearance of secretions leading to bronchial obstruction. If left untreated, it can progress to pneumonia.
Pneumonia	**Hx:** • Risk factors: Prolonged intubation post-operatively can increase risk of ventilator-associated pneumonia (VAP) due to bacterial colonization of the endotracheal tube; underlying lung disease • Presents POD 1–3, can follow atelectasis, and is more common in patients who smoke

Post-Operative Complication Mini-Cases *(continued)*

Pneumonia	**PE:** • Tachypnea and hypoxia, may have crackles, rhonchi, or decreased breath sounds, dullness to percussion in area of consolidation, along with egophony, increased fremitus **Diagnostics:** • Chest X-ray confirms a consolidation (if lobar) or diffuse infiltrates (if interstitial). • Positive sputum and/or blood cultures may help guide antibiotic therapy **Management:** • Empiric broad-spectrum antibiotics, supplemental oxygen, IV fluids

Venous Thromboembolism	**Hx:**
	• Risk factors: Age >60 years, prolonged operating time (>2 hours), and prolonged (>72 hours) post-operative immobilization, orthopedic surgeries (hip or knee replacements), personal history of malignancy, prior venous thromboemboli, or hypercoagulable states
	PE:
	• Deep vein thrombosis (DVT): Swelling or edema of extremity, calf pain, or warmth in lower extremity along deep vein system; difference in calf or thigh diameter; palpable cord, collateral superficial vein dilation
	• Pulmonary embolism: Tachypnea, tachycardia, low SpO_2, although some patients may have no pulmonary findings
	Diagnostic:
	• CT pulmonary angiography is the gold-standard diagnosis for detecting filling defects in the pulmonary vasculature. In patients who may not tolerate contrast (due to allergy or renal insufficiency), V/Q scan is an alternative.
	• Lower extremity venous duplex ultrasound to detect DVT
	Management:
	• Anticoagulation with heparin and DOACs.
	• Early ambulation out of bed, intermittent pneumatic compression, anticoagulation (e.g., low-molecular weight heparin) are preventative measures
	Discussion:
	• DVT occurs in 7% of post-operative patients.
	• VTE prophylaxis is critical!
	  • For all patients, early mobilization is important
	  • For patients at low risk, intermittent pneumatic compression and anti-embolic stockings
	  • For high-risk patients (i.e., those undergoing hip or knee surgery), pharmacoprophylaxis is added and can include either subcutaneous injection of low molecular weight heparin (LMWH) or oral factor Xa inhibitors (apixaban, rivaroxaban, edoxaban)
	  • Unfractionated heparin (UFH) should be used instead of LMWH in patients with low GFR, and fondaparinux can be used if other agents are contraindicated.
	  • Aspirin is not recommended for VTE prophylaxis.

Post-Operative Ileus (POI)	**Hx:** • Risk factors: Age >60, prolonged total surgery time, increased blood loss, and opiate use • Nausea, vomiting, abdominal pain, distention, bloating, constipation **PE:** • Decreased or slow bowel sounds, distended abdomen **Diagnostics:** • Clinical diagnosis, confirmed with abdominal x-ray (KUB) **Management:** • Avoid opioids if possible, prevent and treat hyperglycemia, and maintain euvolemia • Encourage proper nutrition (i.e., early oral diet 4 hours after surgery), and early mobilization (i.e., sitting or standing at bedside; ambulation if tolerated) **Discussion:** • Post-operative ileus (POI) or post-operative gut dysfunction (POGD) typically occurs after abdominal surgery but can occur after any surgery. While the small intestine typically recovers motility within several hours, the stomach within 24–48 hours, and the colon within 3–5 days, patients with POI or POGD have delay in recovery of gut motility >3 days. • The surgical trauma of gut manipulation can trigger an inflammatory response affecting the neural, glial, and smooth muscle cells leading to disturbances in motility. POI can delay wound healing, worsen atelectasis, and increase the incidence of pneumonia and thromboembolism. • Prevention is key! Prior to surgery, encourage smoking cessation, screen for anemia or malnutrition, maintain euvolemia, administer prophylactic antibiotics. Intraoperatively, aim for euvolemia and normothermia and avoid certain medications such as benzodiazepines and opioids if possible.

Post-Operative Complication Mini-Cases *(continued)*

Anastomotic Leaks	**Hx:** • Often occur 5–7 days after surgery, may be associated with a failure to improve post-surgery evidenced by prolonged ileus or a clinical deterioration • Risk factors include diabetes, obesity, malnutrition, smoking, and the use of drugs that impair wound healing, such as corticosteroids and immunosuppressants • Surgical risk factors include longer operative time, emergency surgery, fecal or purulent contamination of the operative field, and esophageal-gastric or rectal anastomoses **PE:** • Fever, tachycardia, increased abdominal tenderness or rebound tenderness **Diagnostics:** • CT scan of abdomen and pelvis with contrast **Management:** • Bowel rest, antibiotics, and percutaneous drainage if the leak is small • Operative revision is indicated if percutaneous drainage is likely not to be successful due to multiple fluid collections, collection >5 cm, or the patient is septic **Discussion:** • An anastomotic leak can occur at any location at which intraluminal contents leak where tissues have been surgically connected. If left unattended, they can lead to sepsis, multi-organ failure, and death.
Urinary Tract Infections	**Hx:** • Can present POD 3–5 with urinary urgency, dysuria, frequency, suprapubic or flank pain, and costovertebral angle tenderness • Risk factors: Prolonged urinary catheterization, unsterile placement or care of a urinary catheter, female sex, older age, history of diabetes, and history of previous UTIs **PE:** • Possible fever, suprapubic tenderness, or costovertebral angle tenderness **Diagnostic:** • Urinalysis: May have positive leukocyte esterase, positive urine nitrites (if due to common gram-negative bacilli) • Urine culture: The most common organisms in catheter-associated UTI are *E. coli*, *Enterococcus* spp., *Candida* spp., *P. aeruginosa*, and *Klebsiella* spp. **Management:** • To prevent development of resistant organisms, *asymptomatic* catheter-associated UTIs are not treated with antibiotics. • *Symptomatic* UTIs do require antimicrobial treatment which should be guided by susceptibility results.

Wound Healing and Surgical Site Infections

Factors that impair wound healing include advanced age, hypoxia, anemia, hypoperfusion, malnutrition, diabetes, obesity, use of steroids, and chemotherapeutic drugs. These factors may increase wound dehiscence to 30% and there is increased risk of wound infections.

Factors that can augment wound healing: Optimize nutritional status as needed, add vitamin A supplementation in the severely injured patient, and add zinc supplementation in those with known deficiency, more often seen in patients with Class 3 obesity.

Chronic wounds: A wound failing to close by 4 weeks is considered a chronic wound. More than 80% of chronic wounds occur in the setting of diabetes, venous insufficiency, or high arterial blood pressure.

Surgical Site Infections (SSIs)

SSIs can occur after any operative procedure and can compose up to 20% of all health care–associated infections. They are defined as superficial incisional, deep incisional, and organ space SSI and affect at least 5% of patients undergoing surgery.

- **Superficial incisional infection** involves only the skin and subcutaneous tissue of the incision and occurs within 30 days post-surgery.
- A **deep incisional infection** is defined as occurring within 30–90 days post-surgery involving deep soft tissues such as fascia and muscle, and may include an abscess. The most serious of these is necrotizing fasciitis, in which thrombosis of the vessels between the skin and deep layers leads to skin and fascial necrosis.
- An **organ space SSI** also can occur within 30–90 days post-surgery and involves any part of the body deeper than the fascial and muscle layers.

Avoid superficial cultures of wounds, because these contain skin flora and have poor predictive value of true pathogens. After cleansing the skin, expression of fresh purulent drainage can be used to identify the organism(s) and antibiotic susceptibilities. The most common genuses are *Streptococcus*, *Staphylococcus*, and *Enterococcus*.

Patients with hemodynamic instability, high fever, or high WBC may require imaging, such as a CT scan, to define the extent of deep space infection. Rare life-threatening wound infections, such as Group A beta-hemolytic streptococcal infections causing necrotizing fasciitis or *Clostridium* spp. causing gangrene should be considered in patients whose clinical condition is rapidly deteriorating.

Antibiotics should be chosen according to the hospital antibiogram, empirically treating for the most likely organisms and then tailoring the antibiotic regimen according to culture results. Deep infections require operative drainage or a drain placed by interventional radiology if the location of the deep infection can be accessed percutaneously.

The development of SSIs is impacted by the ASA status, oxygen delivery to the wound capillary bed, hyperglycemia, procedure duration, and the **surgical wound classification**, which describes the degree of gross contamination. Post-operative wounds are classified as clean, clean-contaminated, contaminated, or dirty-contaminated.

Surgical Wound Classification

Class	Description	Example	Antibiotics
I: Clean Wounds	No infection, minimal inflammation. Do not involve the respiratory, alimentary, genital, or urinary tract	Eye surgery. Primary closure of exploratory surgery for repair of splenic laceration after blunt trauma	Pre-operative, only if prosthetic placement is involved
II: Clean-contaminated wounds	Involves colonized respiratory, alimentary, or genitourinary tract. No unusual contamination	Cholecystectomy. Appendectomy. Lung resection. Hysterectomy. Tonsillectomy	Pre-operative
III: Contaminated wounds	Open, fresh, accidental wounds or operations with major breaks in sterile technique	Gross spillage from the gastrointestinal tract. Open traumatic wounds that are more than 12–24 hours	Pre- and post-operative
IV: Dirty-contaminated wounds	Organisms were present in the field prior to operation. Incisions where viscera are perforated, there is acute inflammation (pus), or delayed presentation of chronic or traumatic wounds	Peritonitis with gross fecal contamination. Chronic wound debridement	Therapeutic antibiotics for the infection that was present prior to surgery

CASE 4 | Necrotizing Fasciitis

A 28-year-old man is post-operative day 3 from an emergent exploratory laparotomy with hemicolectomy and ileostomy construction after a stab wound to the right lower quadrant. The patient describes excruciating abdominal pain for the last 6 hours that is not improving with pain medication, accompanied by nausea and vomiting. His temperature is 38°C, pulse 110 bpm, and blood pressure 90/50 mmHg. On exam, the patient is distressed due to the pain. There is erythema and swelling surrounding the laparotomy incision that was not present 3 hours ago and a thin, gray discharge. There is crepitus surrounding the incision.

Conditions with Similar Presentations	**Nonnecrotizing surgical site infection** (including superficial, deep, and organ space infections): Presents with erythema and discharge from the incision. However, the drainage is usually purulent, and the patient has less severe pain and lacks crepitus. The erythema may expand if the infection goes untreated but does not expand as rapidly as described above. **Acute mesenteric ischemia:** Presents with abdominal pain out of proportion to exam, in which the patient is in excruciating pain with a soft abdomen and no rebound or guarding on physical exam. It is not associated with erythema or discharge from a surgical incision and can be associated with hematochezia.
Initial Diagnostic Tests	• Can be diagnosed clinically with rapidly progressive post-op wound infection, associated with pain out of proportion to appearance of wound, crepitus, and/or bullae, sepsis • Confirmed by emergency exploratory surgery with debridement
Next Steps in Management	• Broad-spectrum antibiotics to cover MRSA, gram-positives, gram-negatives, and anaerobes • Emergent surgical debridement with removal of all tissues and structures that are necrotic • Intra-operative Gram stain and culture

CASE 4 | Necrotizing Fasciitis *(continued)*

Discussion	Necrotizing fasciitis is a rapidly progressing, life-threatening condition and constitutes a surgical emergency, with mortality approaching 25%. Misdiagnosis as an uncomplicated wound infection can lead to delay in care and increased morbidity and mortality. The most common pathogens are group A *Streptococcus*, *Staphylococcus aureus*, *Klebsiella*, *Escherichia coli*, *Bacteroides*, *Clostridium*, *Pseudomonas*, and *Prevotella*. The neurovascular bundle that supplies blood and sensory neurons to the skin runs along the top of the fascia. If organisms cause infection this deep, they can cause clotting of the arterial supply leading to necrosis of overlying skin and cause intense pain as neurons are inflamed. As this progresses and nerves die, hypoesthesia can develop. Crepitus can develop if the causative organism is gas-forming. **History:** • Severe pain out of proportion to appearance after a surgical procedure or trauma. • As infection progresses, pain may diminish due to sensory nerve destruction • Risk factors: Diabetes mellitus, peripheral vascular disease, malnutrition, age >60 years, malignancy, cirrhosis, immunocompromised, and corticosteroid therapy **Physical Exam:** • Rapidly progressive cellulitis with thin, grey, "dishwater" discharge, bullae formation, and crepitus • Skin death (necrosis) manifests as dark discoloration • Septic shock: Hypotension, tachycardia, tachypnea, and fever 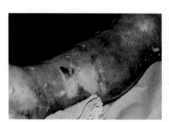 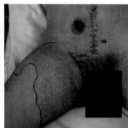 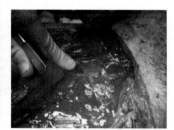 Necrotizing soft tissue infection. (A) This patient presented with hypotension due to severe late necrotizing fasciitis and myositis due to β-hemolytic streptococcal infection. The patient succumbed to his disease after 16 hours despite aggressive debridement. (B) This patient presented with spreading cellulitis and pain on motion of his right hip 2 weeks after total colectomy. Cellulitis on right anterior thigh is outlined. (C) Classic dishwater edema of tissues with necrotic fascia. (Reproduced with permission from F. Charles Brunicardi, Dana K. Andersen, Timothy R. Billiar, David L. Dunn, Lillian S. Kao, John G. Hunter, Jeffrey B. Matthews, Raphael E. Pollock, Schwartz's Principles of Surgery, 11e. Copyright 2019 McGraw-Hill Education.) **Diagnostics:** • Clinical diagnosis when severe pain out of proportion to exam, fever, edema, erythema, bullae, and necrosis. • Definitive diagnosis on tissue exam during debridement. The tissue is often de-vascularized, causing it to grossly appear gray without bleeding. • A Gram stain and culture from the site of infection taken during the debridement can help determine the causative organism(s) and guide the choice of antibiotic regimen. • Consider the following supportive tests but should not delay surgical intervention: CBC (leukocytosis or leukopenia, possible drop in hemoglobin due to hemolysis), CMP (hypocalcemia, lactic acidosis, elevated creatinine), blood culture to help determine organism(s), lactate, CK, and CRP. • Imaging may also be supportive in the diagnosis, but also should not delay surgical intervention. MRI is best suited to show soft tissue findings, but both MRI and CT may show thickening of fascia and the presence of gas. CT demonstrating extensive soft tissue gas due to necrotizing fasciitis. **Management:** • Empiric broad-spectrum antibiotics should be immediately started; vancomycin and piperacillin-tazobactam are a common combination. The antibiotics can be narrowed when the culture susceptibilities result. Antibiotics will not be fully effective until debridement has removed all identifiable dead tissue, as antibiotics cannot penetrate devascularized tissue. • Emergent surgical debridement. Timing and adequacy of the initial debridement has the biggest impact on mortality. Surgical debridement with removal of all tissues and structures that are necrotic; may include whole muscle groups or whole limbs or multiple debridements. Obtain intra-operative Gram stain and culture to guide therapy.
Additional Considerations	There are separate names for necrotizing fasciitis in specific anatomic locations: **Fournier gangrene:** Perineum/external genitalia **Ludwig angina:** Submandibular space

TRAUMA OVERVIEW

Most trauma accidents are related to MVAs, followed by self-inflicted violence and interpersonal violence. Together, these three make up >50% of all incidents. Other categories, in order of decreasing frequency, include drowning, war, falls, poisoning, and fires.

Death due to trauma is categorized based on timing:

- Immediate—within seconds to minutes, accounts for up to 50–60% of all trauma-related death and usually not survivable. Common causes include rupture of the heart or aorta, and apnea due to severe brain or spinal cord injury.
- Early—within 24 hours.
- Late—within days to weeks, often due to multiple organ dysfunction and/or sepsis.

The "**golden hour**" after trauma plays a critical role in determining survival. To prioritize injuries, the trauma patient is evaluated by a trauma team performing a rapid **primary survey**, seeking to identify and stabilize life-threatening injuries. When the patient is stabilized, a more detailed **secondary survey** is performed. Successful treatment of the trauma patient relies on rapid recognition and treatment of life-threatening injuries with restoration of perfusion to all tissues. Brain injury and hemorrhage account for most of the immediate and early deaths. Accurate identification and control of the source of bleeding is the priority after the airway is established and breathing is confirmed.

Primary Survey

When examining a trauma patient, the primary survey includes an assessment of **ABCDE** and management and stabilization of the life-threatening injuries. This is performed immediately, before performing a detailed formal history and physical exam. The **FAST** (Focused Assessment with Sonography in Trauma) exam may be performed as part of the abdominal exam and as an adjunct to the primary survey in a hemodynamically unstable patient. It is performed to evaluate for pathologic fluid in the pericardium and peritoneal cavity (Morrison's pouch [hepatorenal recess in RUQ], the hepato-diaphragmatic area, the right paracolic gutter, and the caudal edge of the left liver lobe and/or LUQ/spleno-renal fossa).

Primary Survey in Order of "ABCDE" Prioritization

Priority of Assessment	Assessment	Abnormal Findings	Potential Causes of Impairment
A- Airway maintenance with cervical spine protection	Check if conscious and able to speak with regular tone	• Unconscious (GCS ≤8) • Unable to speak, noisy breathing, accessory muscle use • Stridor with defect at sternoclavicular joint	• Compromise due to head trauma, shock • Airway trauma or obstruction, smoke injury • Posterior dislocation of clavicular head
B- Breathing and ventilation	Check for pulse oximetry, symmetrical chest movement, crepitus or chest deformity on palpation, bilateral equal breath sounds	• Tracheal deviation away from site of injury, jugular venous distention, hypotension • Jugular vein distention (may not be present if hypovolemic), absence of breath sounds on one side with dullness to percussion; hypoxia • Sucking chest wound • Paradoxical motion of the chest wall during inspiration and expiration, ribs or cartilage fracture	• Tension pneumothorax or massive hemothorax • Massive hemothorax • Open pneumothorax • Flail chest with pulmonary contusion
C- Circulation with hemorrhage control	Palpate pulses—palpable carotid or femoral pulses means SBP is at least 60 mmHg, palpable radial pulses means SBP is at least 80 mmHg	• Hypotension • Beck's triad: neck vein distention (may not be present if hypovolemic), hypotension, muffled heart tones; Kussmaul sign (increased jugular venous distention on inspiration) • Expanding hematoma with loss of distal pulses • Hypotension, diathesis of pubic symphysis or tenderness along pubic rami or sacroiliac joint(s) with blood at penile meatus	• Rule out urgent causes of hypotension (e.g., tension pneumothorax, cardiac tamponade, neurogenic shock or hemorrhage, and/or hemorrhagic shock due to external bleeding (limb with vessel laceration) or internal bleeding (e.g., retroperitoneum and pelvis are often areas of "hidden" internal bleeding) • Cardiac tamponade • Traumatic arterial disruption • Pelvic fracture; high likelihood of additional associated internal injuries

Primary Survey in Order of "ABCDE" Prioritization (*Continued*)

Priority of Assessment	Assessment	Abnormal Findings	Potential Causes of Impairment
D- Disability (neurologic status)	• Evaluate level of consciousness, pupillary reaction, lateralizing signs, spinal cord injury level • Glasgow coma scale (GCS) (scale 3–15, with 15 indicating normal function) is used to determine level of consciousness and extent of neurologic disability based on three categories: motor (6 points), verbal (5 points), and eye opening (4 points)	• GCS ≤8 • Rapidly deteriorating neurologic status with evidence of head trauma • Altered level of consciousness demands re-evaluation of oxygenation level, perfusion (e.g., life-threatening hemorrhage), and other causes such as alcohol, drugs, hypoglycemia, and seizures	• Probable severe brain injury and a high likelihood of airway loss (patient should be intubated) • Sharply increased intracranial pressure created by mass effect of intracranial hemorrhage causing herniation
E- Exposure/ **e**nvironmental control	• Disrobe patient entirely (need for speed often dictates cutting clothes off) to expose any missed or additional injuries, especially hidden in axillary or inguinal folds	• Burns, rashes, abrasions, entry or exit wounds, necrotic tissue, "hidden injuries"	• Avoid hypothermia and the "**lethal triad**" during resuscitation, which is hypothermia, coagulation, and acidosis (discussed below)

Assessment/Management—Secondary Survey

The patient is continuously monitored for any deterioration in condition which may require emergent intubation, thoracotomy, abdominal exploration, or a decompressive bone flap craniotomy. An **eFAST** exam (extended Focused Assessment with Sonography in Trauma) may be performed at this time. In addition to the areas examined in the FAST exam, the eFAST exam incorporates views of the right and left anterior hemithoraces to detect the presence of a pneumothorax. A chest X-ray is not used to confirm a pneumothorax or hemothorax in the hemodynamically unstable patient because the life-threatening nature of either of these conditions dictates definitive action without delay based on physical findings. Once the patient is stabilized, a more comprehensive evaluation of nonlife-threatening injuries is performed, which includes obtaining a more thorough history (e.g., medications, allergies, past illnesses, pregnancy status, last meal), physical exam, and other diagnostic tests.

Important Diagnoses Detected on Secondary Survey

Site	Finding	Likely Diagnosis
Head	Confusion, unable to recall events surrounding trauma	Traumatic brain injury
Cervical spine	Tenderness at any point on cervical spine or history of trauma above the clavicles	Presumed cervical spine fracture until ruled out
Thorax	• Hemoptysis, subcutaneous emphysema, tension pneumothorax; incomplete expansion of lung after chest tube placement • Hypotension, wall motion abnormality by echocardiography; infarction changes, atrial fibrillation, premature ventricular contractions on ECG • Widened mediastinum on chest X-ray	• Tracheobronchial tree injury • Blunt cardiac injury • Traumatic aortic disruption
Thoraco-abdominal	Suspected by elevated right hemidiaphragm by chest X-ray or by CT scan on left	Traumatic diaphragmatic injury
Abdominal	• Bloody gastric aspirate by nasogastric tube or retroperitoneal air on abdominal X-ray • Seatbelt sign (transverse bruising across abdomen)	• Duodenal injury • Small bowel injury

Important Diagnoses Detected on Secondary Survey

Site	Finding	Likely Diagnosis
Genitourinary	Hematuria	Anterior pelvic fracture, bladder rupture, or urethral disruption
Pelvis	Mechanical instability of the pelvic ring; open wounds of the flank, perineum, and/or rectum; vaginal blood from vaginal laceration; blood at urethral meatus	Pelvic fracture
Lower limb	Groin pain, painful hip with limited range of motion and severe pain with internal rotation; limb lies in external rotation and abduction appearing shortened	Hip fracture

Diagnostics

Labs and imaging may be helpful in evaluation of a trauma patient; however, they should not delay resuscitation and definitive operative treatment.

Diagnostic Tests for the Trauma Patient

Assessment/Tests		Helpful in Diagnosing Below Pathology
Entry to trauma unit	• Pulse oximeter ⟶	• Monitors oxygen saturation continuously
	• CBC ⟶	• Hemorrhage
	• ABG ⟶	• Acidosis, hypercarbia, hypoxia
	• Type and cross match ⟶	• Preparation for massive transfusion protocol (MTP)
	• PT/PTT, fibrinogen, D-dimer ⟶	• Detects coagulopathy (e.g., DIC)
	• Thromboelastography (TEG) ⟶	• Detects trauma-induced fibrinolysis; can be used to monitor coagulopathy during MTP
	• Blood alcohol ⟶	• Detects blood alcohol level
	• Urine drug screen ⟶	• Detects presence of toxic drugs
	• Urinalysis ⟶	• Detects hematuria as an indicator of trauma to GU system (kidneys, ureters, bladder)
	• Serum lactate ⟶	• Sensitive measure of hypoperfusion/Shock
Primary Survey		
Airway (A)	Laryngoscopy as needed to secure definitive airway	Airway is determined by asking the patient to tell their name and describe the circumstances of the trauma. Laryngoscopy may be performed to confirm ETT placement.
Breathing (B)	Can perform portable chest x-ray if patient otherwise hemodynamically stable	If hemodynamically stable, can be used to detect pneumothorax or hemothorax; confirm chest tube or endotracheal tube position if placed (Tension pneumothorax is a clinical diagnosis and one should not wait for a chest x-ray to make the diagnosis)
Circulation (C)	• Focused assessment with sonography in trauma (FAST) exam • Extended FAST (eFAST) ⟶ • Pelvic x-ray ⟶	• Diagnosis of intraabdominal bleeding and pericardial tamponade; cannot detect retroperitoneal bleeding • Extended to include both hemithoraces for pneumothorax and hemothorax • Detects pelvic fracture and need for transfusion
Disability (D)	Glasgow coma scale (GCS) maximum points = 15 Eye opening (4 points) + Verbal (5 points) + Motor (6 points) = 15	GCS 13-15: Minor brain injury GCS 9-12: Moderate brain injury GCS 3-8: Severe brain injury In patients with asymmetric neurologic findings, the best motor response predicts outcome
Exposure (E)	Imaging determined by injuries	Imaging should not interrupt resuscitation and is performed when the patient has been stabilized, usually during the secondary survey

Diagnostic Tests for the Trauma Patient (*Continued*)

Assessment/Tests	Helpful in Diagnosing Below Pathology
Secondary Survey	
Cervical spine x-rays or CT scan of neck as indicated	Used to determine cervical spine fracture in any patient with head or neck trauma or patients with multiple injuries If neurologic signs warrant a head CT to rule out intracranial bleed, then the CT scan can be extended to the neck to rule out cervical spine fracture
CT head	Detects intracranial hematoma, contusion, shift of midline (large shifts may require evacuation)
CT angiogram of suspected vascular injury	Great vessels of neck, chest, or suspected limb arterial injury
CT chest, abdomen, and pelvis	Identification of diaphragmatic rupture; liver, spleen, and/or kidney hemorrhage source; identification of pancreatic or bowel injury; genitourinary injury
Esophagram	Esophageal injury by penetrating trauma or rupture
Laryngoscopy/bronchoscopy	Evaluate injury after penetrating neck injury
Other x-rays	Evaluate possible fracture of any pain or swelling identified in limbs or elsewhere; can be used to identify bullet location or predict path of injury of penetrating trauma
Retrograde urethrogram	Identify ruptured urethra or bladder

Pediatric Considerations

Pediatric patients are smaller, thus trauma delivers more energy per body surface area than adults, leading to a higher incidence of injury in multiple organs than adults. The child's head is larger than an adult by proportion. There is a higher frequency of traumatic brain injury in children than adults, which leads more often to apnea, hypoventilation, and hypoxia instead of hypovolemia due to hemorrhagic shock. Children also have a higher cardiovascular reserve. Shock may present subtly with only tachycardia or a decrease in mentation. Because of this, familiarity with normal values of heart rate and blood pressure by age is critical.

Geriatric Considerations

- Five pre-existing conditions dramatically increase the risk of death: cirrhosis, coagulopathy, chronic obstructive pulmonary disease, ischemic heart disease, and diabetes.
- Blunt trauma is the most common mechanism of injury. Penetrating trauma is often due to gunshot wounds (GSWs) for intentional self-harm or suicide.
- Elder abuse can be recognized by:
  - Contusions on inner arms, inner thighs, scalp, ears, mastoid area, buttocks, nasal bridge, or temple
  - Periorbital ecchymoses (i.e., from being struck while wearing glasses)
  - Fractures not involving the hip, humerus, or vertebrae
  - Contact burns
  - Scalp hematomas

HEMORRHAGIC SHOCK

Hemorrhagic shock is a subtype of hypovolemic shock and is commonly encountered following trauma. Signs include hypotension, altered mental status, weak pulses, pale and cool extremities, and low urinary output. Hypotension in a trauma patient without a cervical spine injury is hemorrhagic shock until proven otherwise. Hemodynamic manifestations of hemorrhagic shock include low central venous pressure (CVP), low cardiac output (CO), and a compensatory high systemic vascular resistance (SVR).

During the primary and secondary surveys, pay attention to areas where large-volume blood loss can occur. This includes external blood loss (i.e., at the scene of the trauma), chest (each hemithorax can accommodate up to 40% of blood volume), abdomen (can accommodate entire blood volume), pelvis (can accommodate entire blood volume and may be "hidden" within retroperitoneum), and the thigh (each thigh can accommodate 1–2 L of blood).

There are four classes of hemorrhagic shock in increasing order of amount of blood loss. Common injuries that may lead to enough blood loss to cause Class III or Class IV hemorrhagic shock include rib fracture–induced lung or intercostal artery lacerations leading to a hemothorax, splenic rupture, retroperitoneal bleeding from pelvic fractures or renal trauma, bilateral femur fractures, and extensive scalp lacerations.

Key Findings that Discriminate Classes of Hemorrhagic Shock

	Class I	Class II	Class III	Class IV
Blood loss (% blood volume)	Up to 750 mL (<15%)	750–1500 mL (15–30%)	1500–2000 mL (30–40%)	>2000 mL (>40%)
Heart rate (bpm)	Normal (60–100)	**Tachycardia (100–120)**	Tachycardia (120–140)	Tachycardia (>140)
Respiratory rate (bpm)	Normal (14–20)	Tachypnea (20–30)	**Tachypnea (30–40)**	Tachypnea (>35)
Urine output (mL/hr)	>30	20–30	5–15	<5
Mental status	Slightly anxious	Anxious	Confused	**Confused/lethargic**
Fluid replacement	Crystalloid	Crystalloid	Crystalloid + blood	Crystalloid + blood

Bolded physical exam findings indicate the most significant change with each class of hemorrhagic shock

Other categories of nonhemorrhagic shock can also be encountered in the trauma unit. These are discussed in further detail in Chapter 20 (Emergency Medicine).

General principles for managing traumatic hemorrhage include:

1. **Stop the bleed**—get control of the bleeding by tourniquet or digital compression and early transfer to trauma center and/or operating room for definitive control.
2. **Gain IV access**—Place two large-bore IVs in order to administer fluids, medications, or transfusion products. Early Intra-osseus (IO) access should be considered in profound shock or difficult IV access.
3. **Start limited IV fluids**—Patient should receive 1–2 L of crystalloid (either normal saline or Lactated Ringer's solution). Given potential adverse effects associated with large-volume transfusion of crystalloids, goal should be to switch to blood products as soon as they are available.
4. **Administer blood products early**—Transfusion protocols should be followed for best practices. In the case of any initial transfusion of red blood cells (RBCs), the blood bank should be notified immediately. For situations of rapid blood loss, can give universal donor blood which is O negative (O positive can be given to men or women past childbearing age). Those with extensive blood loss may meet criteria for **massive transfusion protocol (MTP)** consisting of a 1:1:1 ratio of fresh frozen plasma, platelets, and packed RBCs. Typically, at least six units of each are given in this situation.

Massive Transfusion Protocol (MTP) Criteria and Potential Adverse Effects

Criteria	Potential Adverse Effects
MTP indicated if patients present with ≥2 of the following: 1. Penetrating trauma 2. Positive FAST exam 3. HR ≥120 bpm 4. SBP ≤90 mmHg	Lethal triad: 1. *Hypothermia*: due to transfusion of large volumes of cold or room temperature IV fluids, removal of clothes in trauma unit, diminished heat production 2. *Coagulopathy*: Hemodilution of clotting factors and thrombocytopenia 3. *Acidosis*: Anion gap metabolic acidosis due to lactate formed from organ hypoperfusion or hyperchloremic nonanion gap metabolic acidosis from large volumes of normal saline Additional adverse effects include: • *Transfusion purpura*: Donor platelets stimulate formation of anti-platelet antibodies, causing platelet destruction • *Hypocalcemia*: Citrate in blood products can chelate calcium and lead to decreased cardiac contractility

Trauma-Induced Coagulopathy

When considering massive transfusion, it is critical to assess the patient's coagulation state. Trauma resuscitation with crystalloid and blood products requires vigilant monitoring of coagulation which can be accomplished using thromboelastography (TEG), a viscoelastic assay performed to measure formation and growth of a clot. TEG allows for assessment of the function of the entire hemostasis system from coagulation to fibrinolysis and can identify what aspects of clot formation are deficient, directing the choice of blood products with greater precision.

THORACIC TRAUMA

Chest trauma is the cause of 25% of all trauma-related deaths; two-thirds of these deaths occur after the patient reaches the hospital. Injuries can be divided into two categories:

- **Penetrating injuries** such as stab wounds, gunshot wounds (GSWs), and impalements with a foreign body usually injure the peripheral lung and produce both a hemo- and pneumothorax.
- **Blunt trauma** such as a fall from a height or an MVA can lead to rib fracture, increased intrathoracic pressure, and bronchial rupture.

Knowing the mechanism of injury, patient trajectory, and if relevant, missile trajectory or weapon length and direction can be helpful when creating a differential diagnosis for possible injuries. Thoracic injuries must be identified as quickly as possible on the primary survey and corrected immediately upon discovery.

Absolute Life-Threatening Thoracic Injuries

Injury	Description	Presentation	Management
Airway obstruction (e.g., laryngeal fracture, hematoma)	Blows to thorax often accompanied by injuries to the neck which can lead to compression of the airway.	Air hunger, use of accessory muscles of respiration, stridor, expanding neck hematoma, neck crepitus.	Intubation or surgical airway (cricothyrotomy).
Tracheobronchial tree injury	Direct injury to trachea, carina, or mainstem bronchi.	Hemoptysis.	Secure airway, treat associated pneumothorax with chest tube, immediate surgical repair.
Tension pneumothorax	Air leaks out of lung, filling pleural space and forcing lung to collapse. Pressure in pleural space can push mediastinum to opposite side of injury. Increased intra-thoracic pressure collapses SVC/IVC and RA decreasing venous return and cardiac output	Rapid-onset, severe dyspnea, hemodynamic instability, tracheal shift away from injury, one-way valve in injured lung, circulatory collapse secondary to obstructive shock.	Immediate decompression via needle thoracostomy, followed by intubation and definitive tube thoracostomy.
Open pneumothorax	"Sucking" chest wound due to direct injury to chest wall with inflow of atmospheric air through defect, collapsing ipsilateral lung.	Similar findings as tension pneumothorax above.	Prompt closure using occlusive dressing taped only on three sides, with fourth side left open to allow egress of air (and prevent causing a tension pneumothorax).
Massive hemothorax	>1,500 mL of blood within one side of the chest or 200 mLs/hr output during the first 2-4 hours following chest tube placement.	Lung parenchymal or intercostal artery injury, total whiteout of lung field on CXR eFAST is more sensitive.	Immediate placement of chest tube and operative exploration.
Cardiac tamponade	Compression of heart by accumulation blood, typically from penetrating injury to the cardiac box (defined as the area of the anterior chest wall bounded by the sternal notch and clavicles superiorly, the nipples laterally, and the subcostal margin inferiorly) or cardiac rupture secondary to massive deceleration injury (e.g., motor vehicle accident or fall from a height).	Beck's triad (hypotension, distended neck veins, muffled heart sounds); pulsus paradoxus (decrease in systolic pressure ≥10 mmHg with inspiration). This triad may also occur with left-sided tension pneumothorax, but with tamponade the patient will have bilateral breath sounds present. Can also be identified on eFAST exam.	Immediate operative intervention; decompensation in clinical status can be temporarily treated by needle pericardiocentesis but the patient emergently requires thoracotomy or sternotomy for cardiac repair.

Absolute Life-Threatening Thoracic Injuries

Injury	Description	Presentation	Management
Traumatic circulatory arrest	Absence of consciousness and no pulse. Etiologies include extreme hypovolemia, hypoxia, tension pneumothorax, severe cardiac contusion, cardiac tamponade, ventricular fibrillation, and cardiac arrest.	Coma (GCS ≤8) and no pulse.	Immediate CPR with intubation, 100% oxygen, two large-bore IVs and epinephrine, ideally in an operating room. If no response, bilateral chest tubes should be placed with resuscitative thoracotomy occurring within 3 minutes of intubation.

Secondary Survey to Identify 8 Potentially Life-Threatening Thoracic Injuries

Injuries	Description	Presentation	Management
Simple pneumothorax	After blunt trauma increased intrathoracic pressure leading to bronchial rupture or parenchymal injury from rib fracture. After penetrating trauma directly injuring the lung, usually associated with a hemothorax.	Tachypnea, respiratory distress, hyperresonance to percussion, decreased or absent breath sounds; CXR with air in pleural space and no tracheal shift or shift toward the pneumothorax.	Chest tube thoracostomy unless small < 3.5 cm and asymptomatic
Hemothorax	After blunt or penetrating trauma for same reasons as described above. Can also be seen after aortic rupture, myocardial rupture, or injury to hilar structures.	CXR with fluid in pleural space and bloody fluid on thoracentesis.	Immediate drainage by tube thoracostomy followed by surgical thoracostomy if ≥1,500 mL of blood present.
Flail chest	Two or more contiguous ribs fractured in two sites, usually associated with pulmonary contusion and hypoxemia.	Paradoxical motion of chest wall, often with underlying lung contusion.	Mainly directed towards the associated hypoxia and analgesia to improve ventilatory effort.
Pulmonary contusion	"Lung bruise" resulting in accumulation of blood and inflammatory fluid in the injured lung. Most common potentially lethal chest injury.	Respiratory failure develops within first 24 hours, often not seen on initial CXR. In adults, it is often associated with flail chest or rib fractures. Children are more likely to suffer contusions without rib fractures due to their flexible chest walls and incompletely ossified ribs.	Resultant hypoxia is treated in awake patients with supplemental oxygen and judicious fluid management. Mechanical ventilation may be required if unable to maintain oxygenation.
Blunt cardiac injury (BCI)	Occurs from a massive deceleration force (i.e., from >30 to 0 mph) or direct trauma to the chest. Mechanisms of injury include motor vehicle accident (steering wheel or airbag impact to chest), a fall from 20-foot height or higher, player impact in athletics, or blast trauma. Injury can cause cardiac contusion, coronary artery dissection, and/or valvular disruption.	Chest pain, hypotension, arrhythmias (e.g., tachycardia, atrial fibrillation, right bundle-branch block, ST segment elevation), cardiac rupture (associated with sternal fracture and hemopneumothorax). Cardiac contusion can lead to ***commotio cordis***, or sudden cardiac death due to induced ventricular fibrillation from blow timed just prior to T-wave peak.	Trauma that could lead to blunt cardiac contusion requires continuous ECG monitoring for 24 hours following injury. Normal troponin and ECG effectively rules out BCI. Chest x-ray may identify a sternal fracture, which indicates an increased risk of cardiac injury. FAST ultrasound (echo) may detect abnormal cardiac wall motion but should be reserved for patients with hypotension and/or arrhythmias. Treatment is supportive and aimed at rapid defibrillation and antiarrhythmics if indicated.

Secondary Survey to Identify 8 Potentially Life-Threatening Thoracic Injuries *(Continued)*

Injuries	Description	Presentation	Management
Aortic Transection (Traumatic aortic injury or disruption)	Occurs due to high-energy rapid deceleration injuries (e.g., fall from >10 feet, high-speed MVA, aviation accident). Approximately 90% of cases are lethal at the time of injury due to uncontained rupture where mobile thoracic aorta joins the fixed aortic arch and ligamentum arteriosus. Those who arrive at hospital likely have incomplete tear or contained rupture preventing immediate exsanguination.	On CXR may see widening of the mediastinum, obliteration of the aortic knob, tracheal and esophagus (NGT) deviation to the right, depression of the left mainstem bronchus, a pleural apical cap. Associated with fractures of the first or second rib or scapula.	Control of heart rate via beta blockade with short-acting esmolol for a goal of 80 bpm and blood pressure control for a MAP 60–70 to decrease likelihood of conversion from a contained rupture to a free rupture. Direct repair of the torn segment or endovascular repair. Treatment should not be performed if the patient is hypotensive.
Traumatic diaphragmatic injury	Blunt or penetrating thoracoabdominal injuries cause sudden rise in intraabdominal pressure. Often overlooked and identified during operation for other abdominal injuries. Commonly occurs on the left side (less protected due to liver on the right side). Diaphragmatic rupture with herniation of abdominal contents is the highest cause for mortality, followed by bowel strangulation through a previously undiagnosed penetrating injury.	The stomach and colon are the most frequently herniated structures. CXR will show abdominal organs (e.g., gastric fundus) or NG tube in chest with elevated hemidiaphragm; delayed diagnosis (may be asymptomatic) if defect is small. Any penetrating injury from T4–T12 spinal level anteriorly and through L3 posteriorly should raise suspicion.	First aimed at resolving any associated pneumothorax or hemothorax. Urgent surgical repair is required because these injuries do not spontaneously heal and pose a risk of gastric or colonic strangulation.
Esophageal injury	More common with penetrating compared to blunt trauma and has high mortality if missed. If blunt injury, often occurs as a linear tear in the lower esophagus.	Penetrating trauma, subcutaneous air, may see GI contents within pleura or mediastinum. Subsequent mediastinitis and death can occur due to sepsis and respiratory failure. Patients may present with left pneumothorax or hemothorax following severe blow to lower sternum or upper abdomen with particulate matter present in chest tube.	Surgical repair can be life-saving if performed within a few hours of injury.

CASE 5 | Penetrative Chest Trauma (Pneumothorax and Cardiac Tamponade)

A 21-year-old man is brought in to the trauma unit by ambulance after suffering a stab wound to the chest. He is awake, confused, and combative. He is afebrile with BP 90/70 mmHg, HR 110/min, and RR 22/min. On primary survey, the airway is patent but breath sounds are absent on the left. A wound is noted just above the left nipple. There is no bubbling of air from the wounds, but crepitus is palpated. The neck veins are distended but the trachea is midline. Heart sounds are muffled. The abdomen is soft and nontender. No other injuries are identified. Glasgow coma scale (GCS) is 14.

Considerations	Penetrating thoracic trauma can result in injury to the chest wall, lungs, heart, great vessels, tracheobronchial tree, esophagus, or diaphragm. Asking about the type of weapon, its length, and the trajectory of the injury (i.e., was he stabbed in a downward motion or horizontal motion?) can further help identify potential targets of injury.
Initial Trauma Assessment/ Management (Primary Survey)	First assess and address ABCDEs. Given the multiple potential injuries this patient may have, prioritization of injury identification is made using the primary survey and **FAST** exam. This patient is hypotensive and likely has a tension pneumothorax and cardiac tamponade. • Treat tension pneumothorax with needle decompression and chest tube • Treat cardiac tamponade in this trauma setting with immediate pericardiocentesis while patient is being transported to the operating room, where further treatment including subxyphoid pericardial window can be performed. • IV fluid resuscitation

CASE 5 | Penetrative Chest Trauma (Pneumothorax and Cardiac Tamponade) *(continued)*

Next Steps (Secondary Survey)	• Repeat ABCDE and perform **eFAST exam** • Once patient stable, obtain more thorough history and physical exam and address/manage abnormal findings
Discussion	Penetrating thoracic trauma includes trauma from anywhere below the neck up to the abdomen including the diaphragm. Penetrating chest trauma is less common but more deadly than blunt chest trauma, and occurs most often as a result of gunshots, stabbings, motor vehicle collisions, or other accidents. Thoracic structures at risk from penetrating chest trauma include the chest wall, lungs, tracheobronchial tree, heart, aorta and thoracic vessels, esophagus, diaphragm, spinal cord, thoracic vertebrae, and the thoracic duct. **Assessment/Management:** **Primary Survey:** First assess and address ABCDEs and perform a primary survey. • *Airway:* A stab wound above the nipple (T4) to the left chest would place entry above the carina, which bifurcates at T5 at the level of the sternomanubrial junction. Potential injury to the trachea or tracheobronchial injury which could present with hemoptysis, cervical subcutaneous emphysema, tension pneumothorax, or cyanosis. This patient's airway is patent (he is able to speak); however, left chest crepitus suggests injury to the tracheobronchial tree and/or pneumothorax. • *Breathing:* Distended neck veins and absent breath sounds are signs of a tension pneumothorax. A needle decompression at the fourth or fifth intercostal space, mid-axillary line, should be followed by a chest tube in this unstable patient. A CXR is not required for this diagnosis, as it delays life-saving treatment. • *Circulation:* A pulse pressure (SBP-DBP) <30 mmHg is considered narrow and is indicative of reduced left ventricle stroke volume. In the trauma setting, the first differential diagnosis for a narrow pulse pressure is obstructive shock (e.g., pericardial tamponade, tension pneumothorax). If either of these conditions is not present or is treated successfully and the patient continues to be hypotensive, then hemorrhage must be the next consideration as the cause of shock. This patient is hypotensive and tachycardic, which indicates he is in shock. Two large-bore (14 or 16 gauge) IV catheters, one in the antecubital fossa, should be placed, and a warmed 1 L bolus of Lactated Ringer's solution is given. Resuscitation is carefully monitored using lactate and base deficit by arterial blood gas. Patients with a mild base deficit (−2 to −6 mEq/L) tend not to require blood products, whereas greater base deficits require blood products and possibly a massive transfusion protocol. • *Disability:* This patient is combative and confused, but otherwise neurologically intact. GCS is 14. Examination for head trauma possibly due to a potential fall after being stabbed must be considered. • *Exposure:* The patient's street clothes should be removed and the patient should be logrolled in order to check for wounds to the back and other locations. **Next Steps (Secondary Survey):** Prioritization is given to treatment of the life-threatening findings on primary survey first. After these are addressed, the potentially life-threatening conditions observed on the secondary survey are addressed. If shock persists after the treatment of a tension pneumothorax and cardiac tamponade, the subsequent possible causes of shock in this patient include: • Massive hemothorax. • Thoracoabdominal injury of the liver, spleen, kidney, and/or inferior vena cava. • For these reasons, an **eFAST** exam should also be performed at this juncture to identify intraabdominal hemorrhage and massive hemothorax if missed by exam on the primary survey. Other tests to consider: • **CXR:** In this unstable patient, a CXR would be obtained *after* placement of the chest tube to confirm appropriate tube location and re-inflation of the lung. • **Chest tube drainage and surgical considerations:** If the chest tube produces 1500 mL at first or if hemorrhagic drainage persists at 200 mL/h during the first 2–4 hours, the patient must be taken to the operating room for a thoracotomy to address the source of bleeding. • **Bronchoscopy:** If injury to the tracheobronchial tree is suspected, bronchoscopy should be performed in the stable patient. It is contraindicated in patients in whom cervical spine injuries are suspected and require C-Spine immobilization. • **Contrast esophagography:** Performed with water-soluble contrast to avoid mediastinitis caused by barium, this exam requires the patient to stand and may not be possible in the trauma patient. • **Thoracic CT:** May be obtained in the hemodynamically stable patient and may be used to diagnose esophageal rupture, traumatic aortic disruption, and traumatic diaphragmatic rupture. This test is selected if a patient is wearing a neck brace/requires C-spine immobilization, remains on a backboard, or is otherwise immobile, which precludes other diagnostic studies.

CASE 5 | Penetrative Chest Trauma (Pneumothorax and Cardiac Tamponade) *(continued)*

Additional Considerations	**Complications:**
	• Airway obstruction—laryngeal stenosis, injury to nerves of the vocal cords
	• Tracheobronchial disruption—associated esophageal injury, major vascular injury, cardiac injury, spinal cord injury, recurrent laryngeal nerve injury requiring permanent tracheostomy, failed surgical repair, critical airway stenosis, tracheoesophageal fistula
	• Tension pneumothorax—respiratory failure, arrhythmias, pleural effusion, empyema
	• Open pneumothorax—respiratory failure, bronchopulmonary fistula, empyema, pneumomediastinum, pneumopericardium
	• Massive hemothorax—empyema, fibrothorax
	• Cardiac tamponade—pulmonary edema, heart failure, cardiogenic shock
	• Traumatic circulatory arrest—mild neurologic injury, persistent vegetative state
	Inpatient Considerations: The trauma patient is dynamically changing. Frequent re-examinations of the patient with special attention for suspicion of life-threatening injuries are required within the first 24–48 hours.

Thoracic Trauma Mini-Case

Rib Fracture/ Flail Chest	**Hx:** A 55-year-old roofer falls from a 10-foot roof onto his left side.
	Trauma Primary Survey:
	A: Airway is intact and he can relay slipping backward off the roof. He notes pain on the left side, worse with deep breaths.
	B: There are breath sounds bilaterally but paradoxical chest wall movement is noted over the left seventh through tenth ribs.
	C: Pulse is 90 bpm and blood pressure is 110/80 mmHg.
	D: Disability assessment shows GCS of 15.
	E: Exposure of the rest of his body shows bruising on the left side of flank and a clavicle fracture.
	Secondary Survey: A fall from a height with obvious rib fractures can have additional injuries which must be identified:
	• **CXR** will show rib fractures that are single or nondisplaced or complex, in which they become displaced or misaligned. In this patient a flail chest segment is identified on exam in the area most common for rib fractures, the seventh through tenth ribs. Fractures of the first and second ribs are rare but can be associated with brachial plexus injury, head or facial trauma, and thoracic aortic injury. A flail chest injury is commonly associated with pulmonary contusion and pneumothorax, both of which can be observed on CXR.
	• **CT angiography**—If findings on CXR are consistent with a mediastinal hematoma (as described above), a thoracic aorta injury must be investigated.
	• **eFAST exam**—Lower rib fractures are more likely associated with injuries to the diaphragm, liver, or spleen. In this case, left-sided injury could indicate a splenic laceration or rupture, which can be detected by FAST exam. In addition, the eFAST exam can include visualization of a pneumo- or hemothorax.
	Management:
	• Oxygenation support: Pulmonary contusion is often associated with flail chest. Careful monitoring of O_2 saturation and treatment with supplemental oxygen is of greatest importance. Humidified oxygen should be used to help loosen secretions and aid in sputum clearance.
	• Analgesia: Should be multi-modal, starting with NSAIDs, opioids, gabapentin, regional nerve blocks, and thoracic epidural analgesia. An epidural is contraindicated in patients with concomitant spinal injuries, coagulopathy, or thoracic vertebral body fracture.
	• Operative fixation of flail segment and respiratory compromise: Rib fracture fixation is performed if there is respiratory failure requiring ventilation, significant chest wall deformity or displaced ribs, or failure to wean from mechanical ventilation, which will decrease morbidity and mortality.
	• Most rib fractures with flail chest will heal with conservative measures.
	Discussion: Rib fractures are a result of blunt trauma, usually from an MVA, fall, or blow to the chest. The number of ribs fractured correlates with the severity of the injury, and together with the age of the patient are the most important predictors of morbidity and mortality. The elderly are particularly vulnerable to morbidity and mortality, and up to one-third of elderly patients develop pneumonia. Because of decreased muscle mass and weakened diaphragm in the elderly, alterations in respiratory mechanics with rib fractures or flail chest severely compromise lung function, with subsequent hypoventilation leading to atelectasis and pneumonia. Because this sequence of events takes time, respiratory compromise does not manifest until 48–72 hours post injury.

ABDOMINAL TRAUMA

Abdominal trauma may be penetrative, blunt, or caused by a blast. Any patient with trauma to the torso from a penetrating, deceleration, or blast injury can be assumed to have injuries to the abdominal viscera, vasculature, and pelvic structures until disproven by careful workup.

Blunt abdominal trauma, usually from a motor vehicle crash, fall from a height, or a direct blow (i.e., from a steering wheel or motorcycle handlebars) can rupture organs, causing hemorrhage and contamination from intraluminal contents. Approximately half of blunt trauma injuries involve the spleen, followed by the liver and small bowel.

In **penetrating abdominal trauma**, signs of shock, peritonitis, or evisceration necessitate immediate surgical exploration. Forty percent of abdominal stab wounds involve the liver, and then, in descending frequency, small bowel, diaphragm, and colon. In contrast, GSWs are more likely to affect multiple structures, with nearly half involving injury to the small bowel and/or colon. Liver and abdominal vascular structures are involved less frequently.

Blast trauma can involve a combination of penetrating (i.e., fragments, shrapnel, projectiles), blunt (i.e., being thrown), and overpressure injuries (i.e., from the blast wave itself). Overpressure injury can affect multiple organs and tissues, including the tympanic membranes, lungs, and bowel.

In the absence of shock, peritonitis, or evisceration, penetrating abdominal trauma may be evaluated with CT of the abdomen and pelvis with contrast. In blunt abdominal trauma, signs of peritonitis prompt immediate surgical exploration. Hypotension warrants a **FAST** exam to identify potential source of hemorrhage; a CT of the abdomen and pelvis with contrast can be performed if the patient is hemodynamically stable.

An additional conceptual framework for abdominal trauma involves anatomical regions, including the peritoneal cavity, pelvis, and retroperitoneum. Retroperitoneal organs can be remembered using the **"SAD PUCKER"** mnemonic: **S**uprarenal (adrenal) gland, **A**orta/IVC, **D**uodenum (second and third part), **P**ancreas (except tail), **U**reters, **C**olon (ascending and descending), **K**idneys, **E**sophagus, and **R**ectum. Injuries to these structures may appear as free fluid in the abdomen without solid organ injury. Retroperitoneal injuries are difficult to diagnose because they may not show symptoms of peritonitis or signs of bleeding on FAST exam.

Pertinent History and Physical Exam by Type of Abdominal Trauma

Abdominal Trauma	History	Physical Exam
Motor vehicle accident (MVA) or collision (MVC)	• High vehicle speed • Impact: front, side, rear, or rollover • Type of restraint, deployment of airbags • Status of other occupants	• Inspect abdomen, lower chest, perineum, including presence of "seatbelt" contusions from seatbelts • Inspect flank, scrotum, urethral meatus, and perianal area for blood, swelling, and/or bruising • Percuss abdomen for peritoneal signs • Examine for clues of pelvic fracture including inability to void (ruptured urethra), scrotal hematoma, blood at meatus, vaginal laceration, and/or perineal hematoma
Fall from height	• Height of the fall	
Penetrating trauma	• Time of injury • Type of weapon (i.e., stabbing, gunshot wound, shrapnel, etc.) • Distance from source (shorter distance has higher kinetic energy and may cause more damage) • Number of stab or gunshot wounds • Amount of bleeding at scene • Severity and location of abdominal pain	• Examine gluteal area for penetrating trauma, as 50% of penetrating injuries to this region can have associated intraabdominal injuries
Blast	• Explosion in confined space (mines, buildings, large vehicles) have higher morbidity and mortality • Structural collapse (i.e., buildings, bridge, etc.) • Distance between victim and blast • High-order explosive produces over-pressurization shock wave (e.g., TNT, C-4, dynamite)	• Over-pressurization injury affects gas-filled structures (lungs, GI tract, and middle ear), with the most common being blast lung injury • Penetrating fragments or occult eye injuries may also be present • Fractures, traumatic amputation, traumatic brain injury • Burns

CASE 6 | Penetrating Abdominal Trauma (Gunshot Wound)

A 22-year-old man arrives to the emergency department (ED) after a gunshot wound (GSW) to the right lower abdomen. His blood pressure is 85/65 mmHg, heart rate is 135/min, and respiratory rate is 25/min. He is diaphoretic and in distress. On primary survey, he has a patent airway and equal breath sounds bilaterally. Femoral pulses are weak bilaterally and there is a single GSW in the right lower abdomen. His abdomen is rigid and diffusely tender with guarding and rebound present.

Considerations	A right lower quadrant GSW is likely to create multiple injuries which can include: • Viscera: bowel, liver • Vasculature: iliac, lumbar, and/or mesenteric vessels • Pelvic structures: pelvic bones, bladder, rectum • Retroperitoneal structures: "SAD PUCKER" (described above)
Initial Trauma Assessment/ Management (Primary Survey)	• First assess and address ABCDEs and perform a FAST scan • For hemodynamic unstable patient with signs of peritonitis (as in this case), immediate exploratory laparotomy is indicated
Next Steps (Secondary Survey)	• Continue fluid resuscitations and transfusions • Broad spectrum antibiotics to cover bowel flora • If hemodynamically stable, can first perform eFAST scan and additional tests

Discussion	A GSW to the abdomen more often than not will cause multiple injuries due to damage from the track of the missile, cavitation effect, and bullet fragmentation. This hypotensive patient with diminished pulses is hemodynamically unstable from continued bleeding most likely due to vascular injury. Additionally, peritoneal signs manifested as a rigid abdomen suggest perforation, which will need to be identified and repaired immediately with an exploratory laparotomy.
	
	Assessment/Management
	Primary Survey:
	• Airway, Breathing, and Circulation assessments on the primary survey will lead to prioritization of addressing the cause of hemorrhage and its treatment.
	• Disability assessments may also include a brief neurologic exam to determine gross neurologic deficits caused by a bullet lodging in the spine.
	• Exposure should include log-rolling the patient to define bullet wounds and to quantify the number of wounds.
	• **FAST** exam may be performed as part of the abdominal exam in a hemodynamically unstable patient.
	• The unstable patient with penetrating abdominal trauma will require immediate operative intervention. Absolute indications for operation include:
	  • Shock (hypotension or hemodynamic instability)
	  • Peritonitis (e.g., rigid abdominal wall, rebound tenderness)
	  • Evisceration of abdominal contents (bowel or omentum)
	  • Impalement
	  • Hematemesis or gross blood per rectum
	• The purpose and goals of the exploratory laparotomy are to (1) control hemorrhage, (2) control GI injuries by stopping content spillage either through primary repair or by stapling off and returning in 24 hours when the patient is more stable, and (3) minimize operating time to reduce hypothermia and effects of coagulopathy. Patients are often taken back to the OR at a later time for complete resection and anastomosis; in rare cases, stomas are created.
	
	Next Steps (Secondary Survey):
	• If the patient is hemodynamically stable, can perform eFAST scan, CT scan, and/or local exploration of the wound with serial abdominal exams.
	• Obtain trauma unit admitting labs: type and screen, CBC, coagulation studies, serum lactate, urinalysis, and ABG.
	• A radio-opaque marker should be taped to all entrance and exit wounds to identify trajectory.
	• Chest x-ray is routinely performed to identify the presence of bullet, thoraco-abdominal injury causing herniation of abdominal contents into the chest, and pneumo- or hemothorax, depending on trajectory. Findings of perforation and intraperitoneal free air include subdiaphragmatic air in upright thoracic x-ray and outlining of various peritoneal reflections between mesenteric folds on supine abdominal images.
	• Abdominal x-ray can be used to identify presence of free air and bullet location.
	• If there is pelvic pain, should also perform pelvic x-ray.
	• CT scan of the chest, abdomen, and pelvis with contrast is used to identify retroperitoneal and pelvic organ injuries which are not identified by FAST scan or physical exam. It may also identify bowel injury in asymptomatic patients but sensitivity is not high.

CASE 6 | Penetrating Abdominal Trauma (Gunshot Wound) *(continued)*

Discussion	• The most accurate method to diagnose intrabdominal injury in a stable patient with a penetrating abdominal wound is serial abdominal exams.
	• Consider laparotomy if significant internal organ injury is identified.
	• May forgo operative management, if:
	  • Hemodynamically stable
	  • CT scan shows no intraabdominal injury (to hollow viscus or major vasculature)
	  • Frequent patient reassessment can be performed over the next 24 hours, including serial abdominal exams for signs of peritonitis
	  • Rapid transport to the OR can be accomplished if concerning clinical signs develop

Additional Considerations	**Firearm injury** is a major cause of morbidity and mortality in the United States. As of 2022, firearms are the leading cause of death in children and adolescents (aged 0–19 years). Nonfatal firearm injuries are even more common. Nearly all unintentional firearm injuries in children occur at home, indicating a strong need for gun safety programs, safe handling and storage, safety devices, and possible legislation. **Complications:** • **Acute traumatic coagulopathy** ("Lethal Triad of Death"): With hypothermia, coagulopathy, and acidosis. • **Abdominal compartment syndrome** (see case below). • **Sepsis** • **Anastomotic leak:** Following bowel anastomoses, resulting in GI contents spilling into the peritoneum, often within 1 week post-operatively. Presents with abdominal pain, fever, tachycardia. Diagnosed with CT abdomen or GI series with oral contrast. Requires urgent surgical repair, and can have high morbidity and mortality.

CASE 7 | Blunt Abdominal Trauma (Splenic Injury)

A 42-year-old woman is brought to the ED as the restrained passenger of a motor vehicle collision (MVC). Per paramedics, there was extensive front-end damage to the vehicle, extrication took 45 minutes, and the driver was pronounced dead at the scene. On arrival, the patient is conscious and responsive. Her blood pressure is 85/50 mmHg and her heart rate is 105/min. Respiratory rate is 20/min and shallow but she is able to convey her name and what happened. Breath sounds are clear bilaterally. Her abdomen is slightly distended, mildly tender to palpation, without rebound or guarding. She has no obvious deformities in her extremities.

Considerations	• MVCs can cause compression and/or crushing injuries to other abdominal organs or pelvic bones. • A restrained driver can sustain seatbelt injuries: rupture of small bowel or colon, pancreatic or duodenal injury, or tear of bowel mesentery (see below).
Initial Trauma Assessment/ Management (Primary Survey)	First assess and address ABCDEs and perform a FAST ultrasound exam to identify intraabdominal cause of hemorrhage as an explanation of the hypotension.
Next Steps (Secondary Survey)	Splenic injury can be managed with observation, angiographic embolization, or surgery. • Hemodynamically stable patients should be managed nonoperatively. • Hemodynamically unstable patients should undergo exploratory laparotomy with splenectomy or splenorrhaphy (repair of spleen).
Discussion	Blunt abdominal trauma (BAT) accounts for 80% of abdominal injuries seen in the ED, and the majority of cases in the United States involve motor vehicles (e.g., collisions, pedestrians hit by vehicle). Additional cases include falls, recreational injuries, and assault. Mechanisms of injury in BAT include sudden increase in intraabdominal pressure resulting in rupture of hollow viscus structures, seatbelt compression, crush injury from anterior abdominal wall pressing against the posterior vertebral column, and deceleration injury with shearing forces injuring both solid and hollow organs (especially at points of attachment) as well as vascular tissue. The most commonly injured organs in blunt abdominal trauma are the liver and spleen, followed by the small bowel. This patient in the vignette most likely has a splenic injury resulting from BAT. Splenic injury in BAT can include contusion, hematoma (subcapsular), laceration, and rupture (see image). **History:** Prehospital history can help determine severity of injury in patients presenting with blunt abdominal trauma. If possible, it is important to obtain the following information from first responders (e.g., EMS, police): mechanism of trauma, loss of consciousness, blood loss at the scene, whether the patient was intubated at the scene or en route. In the setting of MVCs, should also assess for seatbelt use, airbag deployment, damage to vehicle, velocity, fatality at the scene, rollover, patient location within vs. outside vehicle, and steering wheel deformity.

CASE 7 | Blunt Abdominal Trauma (Splenic Injury) *(continued)*

Discussion	**Physical Exam:** Up to 20% of patients with intraabdominal injury will not have clinical findings on exam. Findings associated with intraabdominal injury may include vital sign changes (signs of shock including hypotension and tachycardia should always be presumed hemorrhagic in trauma until proven otherwise), abdominal wall contusion (e.g., seatbelt sign), abdominal distension, rebound tenderness, guarding, concomitant femur fracture. **Assessment/Management:** **Primary Survey:** • First assess and address ABCDEs. • The patient above is hemodynamically unstable due to her hypotension and tachycardia. In the setting of BAT, the next step is to evaluate for peritonitis. This patient lacks peritoneal signs, and therefore can undergo a FAST exam to identify intraabdominal cause of hemorrhage. • If the patient had peritonitis or free fluid was identified on FAST exam, the patient should go to OR for laparotomy. When evaluating for splenic injury specifically, findings on imaging may include ultrasound showing hypoechoic rim around the spleen and fluid in Morrison's pouch (between the liver and right kidney). • For hemodynamically unstable patients with peritoneal signs or positive FAST exam (i.e., free fluid), an immediate exploratory laparotomy is required with splenectomy or splenorrhaphy (repair of spleen). 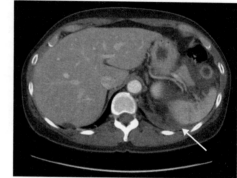Splenic laceration with linear hypodensity crossing the spleen and surrounding perisplenic hematoma (arrow). (Reproduced, with permission, from Schaefer GB, Thompson JN. Medical Genetics: An Integrated Approach. New York: McGraw Hill; 2013.) **Next Steps (Secondary Survey):** • Hemodynamically stable patients who lack peritoneal signs should undergo contrast-enhanced CT of the abdomen and pelvis • Findings suggestive of splenic injury include CXR with elevation of left hemidiaphragm, left lower lobe atelectasis, or left pleural effusion • CT abdomen pelvis may show varying grades of injury depending of severity, evidence of contrast extravasation. Pseudoaneurysm should prompt Interventional Radiology consultation for possible embolization • Splenic injury can be managed with observation, angiographic embolization with serial hemoglobin monitoring, or surgery. • Preserving the spleen reduces the possible mortality from post-splenectomy sepsis, which occurs due to the inability to adequately opsonize encapsulated bacteria (e.g., *Streptococcus pneumoniae, Haemophilus influenzae, Neisseria meningitidis*). • If patient undergoes splenectomy, they must be vaccinated against encapsulated bacteria ideally 2 weeks following surgery. • A drawback to splenic preservation can be post-traumatic delayed splenic rupture, in which the patient can present with hemorrhagic shock 48 hours or later after injury. • For those who undergo splenectomy after BAT, may develop an acute, reactive thrombocytosis that most often resolves within weeks to months.
Additional BAT Injuries	**Duodenal injury**—The duodenum can be compressed against the vertebral column, increasing the pressure, resulting in tear or rupture, typically at fixed points (e.g., ligament of Treitz or hepatoduodenal ligament). Spillage of intraluminal contents may occur into the retroperitoneum, since the second and third portions of the duodenum are retroperitoneal structures and therefore patients may lack typical signs of peritonitis. **Pancreatic duct injury**—Also due to compression against vertebral column, results in leakage of inflammatory pancreatic enzymes and fluids, presenting with upper abdominal pain, fever, nausea, and vomiting. Challenging to diagnose, as initial lipase levels are inconsistent but may increase over time and CT has low sensitivity. **Liver injury**—The liver is the most commonly injured organ across all types of abdominal trauma, especially when trauma involves the RUQ ± rib fractures. Patients present with RUQ tenderness, distended abdomen, and may have vital sign changes depending on the severity of the laceration. If bleeding cannot be controlled with packing and fluid resuscitation, the Pringle maneuver (temporary clamp placed across common bile duct, portal vein, and common hepatic artery) can help control bleeding temporarily, giving the surgeon time to identify and treat any lacerated vessels.

CASE 8 | Abdominal Compartment Syndrome (ACS)

A 34-year-old man arrives to the ED following a high-speed MVC in which he was a restrained passenger. On arrival, he is hypotensive, tachycardic, tachypneic, and has a GCS of 8. He is intubated in the ED for airway protection, and a bedside FAST exam is positive for fluid in the hepatorenal recess. The patient undergoes an exploratory laparotomy that reveals a grade IV liver laceration requiring left lobe resection and a high-grade splenic laceration requiring splenectomy. Intraoperatively, the patient receives a massive transfusion protocol consisting of 10 units each of packed red blood cells, fresh frozen plasma, and platelets. Abdominal fascia is closed with the skin left open and he is admitted to the surgical ICU on mechanical ventilator support. Eight hours later, the patient develops increasing peak airway pressures, hypotension, oliguria, and an increasing creatinine despite continued product resuscitation. On exam, his abdomen is distended, dull to percussion, and tense to palpation.

Conditions with Similar Presentations	**Mesenteric ischemia:** Due to vascular injury or hypotension from hemorrhage, especially in patients with pre-existent atherosclerosis. This can be detected at the time of laparotomy by the appearance of dusky bowel. May also manifest as hematochezia. Hypotension may occur from sepsis, in which case temperature alterations would be seen. Treatment is with vascular repair if there is vascular injury.
	Bowel obstruction: Can present with worsening abdominal distension with nausea or vomiting. Patients are unable to pass flatus or have a bowel movement. Bowel sounds are classically high pitched. The abdomen would be tympanic on percussion. Plain radiographs demonstrate intraluminal air. CT will often show a transition point at the site of the obstruction. Treatment is supportive, including intravenous fluids and decompression with a nasogastric tube.
	Toxic megacolon: Can also present with hypotension but imaging would reveal a dilated colon (>6 cm). Usually associated with fever. It is associated with inflammatory bowel disease and bowel infections, but not trauma. Fifty percent of patients require partial or colectomy.
	Ruptured abdominal aortic aneurysm: Would also present with hypotension and, depending on the site, oliguric renal failure, and/or lower extremity ischemia. Imaging would reveal paraaortic extravasated blood. Treatment is laparotomy and vascular repair.
Initial Diagnostic Tests	Measure intraabdominal pressure (IAP) using a bladder catheter
Next Steps in Management	• Sedation, analgesia, supine body position, neuromuscular blockade, and GI decompression. • If above fails, can perform decompressive laparotomy.
Discussion	Abdominal compartment syndrome (ACS) occurs when fluid within the peritoneal and retroperitoneal spaces accumulates to such a high volume that the abdominal wall can no longer stretch to accommodate the volume, which leads to rising pressures within the abdominal compartment. ACS is more common in patients who undergo MTP (>10 units in 24 hours) and receive large amounts of fluids (>5 L in 24 hours). This condition leads to compression of the renal arteries (leading to decreased glomerular blood flow) and renal veins (leading to increased resistance to filtration in the glomerulus), decreased venous return (which decreases cardiac preload and cardiac output), increased intrathoracic pressure (which leads to increased cardiac afterload and decreased cardiac output), and increased intracranial pressure (ICP). Mortality is approximately 50%, even with abdominal decompression, and can be fatal within 24 hours if not successfully treated. 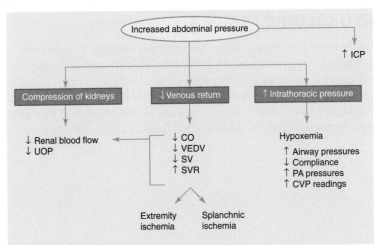Abdominal compartment syndrome is defined by the end organ sequelae of intra-abdominal hypertension. CO = cardiac output; CVP = central venous pressure; ICP = intracranial pressure; PA = pulmonary artery; SV = stroke volume; SVR = systemic vascular resistance; UOP = urine output; VEDV = ventricular end diastolic volume. (Reproduced with permission from Brunicardi F, Andersen DK, Billiar TR, Dunn DL, Kao LS, Hunter JG, Matthews JB, Pollock RE. Schwartz's Principles of Surgery, 11ed. New York: McGraw Hill; 2019.)

CASE 8 | Abdominal Compartment Syndrome (ACS) *(continued)*

Discussion	ACS is reported in 30% of patients following major abdominal trauma or surgery. The underlying process involves increased capillary permeability causing fluid to leak into the gut wall, mesentery, and retroperitoneal tissues. Originally observed following trauma, ACS can also occur following other conditions involving large volumes of resuscitation and inflammatory conditions, such as severe acute pancreatitis, major burns, ruptured aortic aneurysm, and intestinal surgery. Though a rare complication, it can be prevented by regular measurement of intraabdominal pressure in patients at risk.
	History: Risk factors include diminished abdominal wall compliance (major trauma, abdominal surgery), increased intraluminal contents (gastroparesis, ileus, volvulus), increased intraabdominal contents (acute pancreatitis, hemoperitoneum, infection, tumors), and increased capillary leak (acidosis, hypothermia). Affected patients are often diagnosed in the ICU on ventilatory support.
	Physical Exam: The classic presentation includes increased peak airway pressure, decreased urine output, a tense, distended abdomen in an extubated patient, and increased respiratory effort. The patient may be hypotensive and show signs of right heart failure (jugular venous distension, peripheral edema).
	Diagnostics: Measure IAP with a bladder catheter. Intraabdominal hypertension is defined as a sustained IAP >12 mmHg, and higher-grade ACS is associated with higher IAP and organ dysfunction. If the patient does not need immediate surgical intervention, x-ray should be done to look for free air which indicates bowel perforation.
	Management: The overall goal of ACS management is to decrease IAP and allow for improved perfusion of visceral organs. • Consider minimally invasive treatments, including increasing abdominal wall compliance via sedation, analgesia, supine body position, and neuromuscular blockade. • Evacuate intraluminal contents via decompression with tubes or endoscopy. • If less invasive treatments fail, perform decompressive laparotomy. There is no specific IAP that requires laparotomy. • Surgery is indicated when there is evidence of end-organ dysfunction. During surgery, edematous bowel often readily releases from the abdomen. Any ascites, hemorrhage, or hematoma should be evacuated. The abdomen should be left open, including fascia, and temporarily closed with vacuum-assisted devices, meshes, or zippers. • Definitive closure of fascia and skin occurs upon resolution of the cause of ACS and return to normal intraabdominal pressure, which can take several days.
Additional Considerations	**Complications:** Complications include renal failure, low cardiac output leading to bowel or extremity ischemia, respiratory distress, and increased intracranial pressure.

PELVIC AND UROLOGIC TRAUMA

Pelvic fracture can be a life-threatening injury; great force is required to disrupt the pelvic ring and consequently, pelvic fracture is often associated with other injuries. Notably, life-threatening hemorrhage occurs either from the fractured pelvic bone or the anterior-posterior pelvic venous plexus. Arterial injuries, including the superior gluteal and internal pudendal vessels, make up less than 15% of the source of bleeding and can be treated by embolization. Venous and bone sources of bleeding benefit from pelvic bone re-alignment or immobilization with a pelvic binder centered over the greater trochanters. Operative management includes external fixation and/or intraoperative packing to induce a direct tamponade effect.

Categories of Unstable Pelvic Fractures

Injury Type	Trauma Force	Common Associations	Schematic	Pelvic X-Ray
Lateral compression (70%)	Forces from the side of the pelvic (i.e., a fall)	Bladder injury, more common in elderly patients	Lateral compression fracture (arrows 1 and 2) with rupture of posterior sacroiliac ligaments (R), sacrospinous/ sacrotuberous complex (T), and rupture of pubic ramus (B). (Reproduced with permission from Tintinalli JE, Ma O, Yealy DM, Meckler GD, Stapczynski J, Cline DM, Thomas SH. Tintinalli's Emergency Medicine: A Comprehensive Study Guide, 9e. New York: McGraw Hill; 2020.)	A Reproduced with permission from Brunicardi F, Andersen DK, Billiar TR, Dunn DL, Kao LS, Hunter JG, Matthews JB, Pollock RE. Schwartz's Principles of Surgery, 11e. Copyright 2019 McGraw-Hill Education.
Anteroposterior compression (15–20%)	External rotation on the anterior pelvis	Pelvic floor structure injury, bladder injury, highest risk of urethral injury	Open-book fracture, with opening of the anterior pelvis (arrow) and rupture of the sacral ligaments. (Reproduced with permission from Tintinalli JE, Ma O, Yealy DM, Meckler GD, Stapczynski J, Cline DM, Thomas SH. Tintinalli's Emergency Medicine: A Comprehensive Study Guide, 9ed. New York: McGraw Hill; 2020.)	B Reproduced with permission from Brunicardi F, Andersen DK, Billiar TR, Dunn DL, Kao LS, Hunter JG, Matthews JB, Pollock RE. Schwartz's Principles of Surgery, 11e. Copyright 2019 McGraw-Hill Education.
Vertical shear (<15%)	Fall from a height	Highest incidence of vascular injury, hemodynamic instability, neurologic injuries (e.g., L5, S1)	Vertical shear fracture. Injury vector is delivered in a vertical plane (arrow). There is injury to the posterior (R) and anterior (A) sacroiliac ligaments and sacrospinous/ sacrotuberous (T) ligaments. (Reproduced with permission from Tintinalli JE, Ma O, Yealy DM, Meckler GD, Stapczynski J, Cline DM, Thomas SH. Tintinalli's Emergency Medicine: A Comprehensive Study Guide, 9ed. New York: McGraw Hill; 2020.)	C Reproduced with permission from Brunicardi F, Andersen DK, Billiar TR, Dunn DL, Kao LS, Hunter JG, Matthews JB, Pollock RE. Schwartz's Principles of Surgery, 11e. Copyright 2019 McGraw-Hill Education.

Urologic trauma may be associated with penetrating (e.g., high- or low-velocity projectiles, knife, blast) or blunt (e.g., motor vehicle, assault, blast) abdominal and pelvic trauma. Bladder and urethral injuries are often associated with pelvic fracture and require specific and rapid assessment.

Sites, Mechanisms, and Management of Genitourinary Trauma

Site	Mechanism	Signs	Diagnostics	Treatment
Renal	History of rapid deceleration injury Penetrating abdominal or thoracic injury	Gross or microscopic hematuria with hypotension	CT scan with and without IV contrast if hemodynamically stable	Surgical intervention needed if: 1. Hemodynamically unstable 2. Expanding/pulsatile peri-renal hematoma during operative exploration 3. Shattered kidney or renal pedicle injury or avulsion Otherwise, interventional radiology can embolize bleeding source if there is no operative indication or other injuries
Bladder	Blunt trauma (e.g., pelvic fracture) Penetrating injury to lower abdomen or perineum	Gross hematuria, abdominal tenderness, inability to void, bruising over suprapubic region, abdominal distension	If gross hematuria and pelvic fracture are present, CT cystography must be performed	Surgical intervention must be performed for: 1. Penetrating injury 2. Blunt intraperitoneal injury 3. Blunt extraperitoneal injury with pelvic fracture
Urethra	*Anterior injury* often due to sexual intercourse; associated with penile fracture *Posterior injury* often associated with pelvic fracture Urethral injuries in women are rare	Blood at external meatus, hematuria on first voided specimen, pain on urination, inability to void, blood at vaginal introitus (female pelvic fracture), blood on rectal exam with pelvic fracture (suggests rectal and/or urethral injury), penile and scrotal swelling or hematoma	Retrograde or CT urethrography with avoidance of urethral catheterization until urethra is imaged If patient is unstable, a suprapubic catheter is inserted and urethrogram can be performed later	Anterior injury treated by primary repair if associated with penile fracture or penetrating wound Posterior injury repaired in stable patients with penetrating wounds; otherwise, treated with a suprapubic cystostomy
External genitalia	Motor vehicle collision, sports, assault, 80% of cases due to blunt trauma	*Penile trauma*—typically from trauma to erect penis; sudden cracking or popping sound, pain, detumescence, swelling *Scrotal trauma*—testicular dislocation or rupture, hematocele	Penile ultrasound or MRI; exam of the perineum, rectum, and scrotum	Penile trauma—if tunica albuginea is ruptured, surgical repair is required Scrotal trauma—if dislocation, manual reposition with orchidopexy if unsuccessful; if hematocele >3 times size of opposite side testis, needs surgical removal of clot and closure of tunica albuginea

CASE 9 | Pelvic Fracture with Bladder Disruption

A 31-year-old man is brought to the ED after a ski injury where he lost control and hit a tree, straddling it. He was wearing a helmet and denies striking his head. He is not able to bear weight due to pelvic and abdominal pain following the injury. Ski patrol helped him off the mountain. On arrival, his blood pressure was 100/60 mmHg, pulse 105/min, respirations 20/min, and SpO$_2$ 99% on room air. On primary survey, airway and breathing were unremarkable. Patient had no signs of thoracic hemorrhage by chest x-ray or expanding hematomas of the limbs. Abdominal exam revealed lower abdominal and suprapubic tenderness. He also had tenderness over the pubic symphysis and blood was noted at the urethral meatus. There was no scrotal swelling, penile or peritoneal hematoma, or high-riding prostate on rectal exam. No other musculoskeletal abnormalities were identified. Neurovascular exam was normal.

Considerations	**Pelvic fracture with urethral disruption:** Pelvic fractures can lead to genitourinary injuries which may be missed. A stepwise approach is used to first define injury to the lower tract, starting with the urethra and then bladder, ureter, and kidney. Urethral disruption can present with blood at the meatus and hematuria on a first-void specimen. There may also be pain with urination or inability to void. A rectal exam may show a high-riding prostate; however, this is not a reliable predictor. Urinary extravasation can cause penile and scrotal swelling. Urethral rupture typically occurs in the posterior membranous urethra at the sphincter, where the urethra is fixed at the urogenital diaphragm and is associated with pubic rami fractures and widening of the pubic symphysis. Diagnosis is made by retrograde urethrogram.

CASE 9 | Pelvic Fracture with Bladder Disruption *(continued)*

Initial Trauma Assessment/ Management (Primary Survey)	• First assess and address ABCDEs and perform FAST exam • Immediately stabilize pelvis with a pelvic binder while undergoing resuscitation in hemodynamically unstable patient. • Consider MTP
Next Steps (Secondary Survey)	• Anteroposterior (AP) x-ray of pelvis • If there is gross hematuria, rule out urethral injury and consider CT cystogram
Discussion	High-energy pelvic fracture combined with hemodynamic instability is among the most severe of traumatic injuries, with mortality approximately 30%. Pelvic fractures are often complicated by additional musculoskeletal injuries, intrabdominal injuries (e.g., liver, small bowel, spleen, kidney), bladder or urethral injury, neurologic injury (e.g., cauda equina syndrome) and/or hemorrhage (e.g., presacral, lumbar venous plexus). Bladder rupture is a rare, often missed injury, typically occurring at the dome of the bladder where it is weakest. If the bladder is full, blunt force can lead to intraperitoneal bladder rupture. Usually, the bladder rupture occurs in the retropubic space of Retzius (between the pubic symphysis and anterior bladder wall). Suspicion of extraperitoneal bladder rupture should be high if there is widening of the symphysis pubis and sacroiliac joint and/or gross hematuria. Patients with bladder rupture can go undiagnosed for days due to minimal or no signs of acute peritonitis (compared to GI perforation). **History:** • History of high-energy trauma, inability to ambulate at accident scene, severe pelvic pain is suggestive of pelvic fracture • If blunt trauma, increased likelihood of bladder injury or rupture **Physical Exam:** • Pelvic deformity, tenderness to palpation over bony landmarks of the pelvis, diminished sensation or pulses in the lower extremities if concomitant nerve or arterial injury occurs • Flank ecchymosis may be present due to retroperitoneal hemorrhage • Presence of blood on rectal/vaginal exam suggests open pelvic fracture; proctoscopy may be required • Suprapubic tenderness, blood at urethral meatus, gross hematuria with concomitant bladder injury **Assessment/Management:** **Primary Survey:** • Assess and address ABCDEs • Pre-hospital placement of pelvic binder or patient wrapped in sheet to tamponade hemorrhage in pelvis while other sources of hemorrhage are identified and patient is resuscitated (i.e., MTP) • FAST scan can determine if the patient has hemorrhage or intraabdominal injuries that require immediate attention • If fluid is observed on the FAST scan, patient is immediately taken to the operating room for control of intraabdominal hemorrhage; the pelvic fracture and associated hemorrhage are treated with pre-peritoneal packing intra-operatively • If the FAST scan is negative and no other source of hemorrhage is observed, hemodynamic instability can be assumed to be due to the pelvic fracture • Pelvic view examining rectovesical pouch in males and the rectouterine pouch (pouch of Douglas) in females **Next Steps (Secondary Survey):** Pelvic x-ray (AP view): • Indicated in any trauma patient with abdominal, pelvic, or back pain • Bladder disruption is associated with widening of pubic symphysis *and* the sacroiliac joint • Pelvic fracture: pelvic x-ray shows widened pubic diastasis with pelvic ring disruption Retrograde urethrogram (RUG): • Indicated if any of the following are observed: blood at the meatus, hematuria in first free void, or a high-riding prostate on rectal exam • Placement of a foley in the presence of a urethral injury can extend the urethral injury and is avoided until a normal RUG is obtained • If the RUG is normal, a foley can be inserted to perform a cystogram, the next step in the workup of genitourinary trauma CT scan: • If patient is hemodynamically stable, obtain contrast-enhanced CT abdomen and pelvis to better characterize injury and identify extent of fracture, presence of ongoing pelvic bleeding, and with cystogram, bladder rupture • If gross hematuria is present, CT cystogram can be ordered to evaluate for bladder rupture once urethral injury is ruled out

CASE 9 | Pelvic Fracture with Bladder Disruption *(continued)*

Discussion	Other diagnostics: • If urethral disruption is observed, a suprapubic cystostomy tube is placed and the cystogram is performed through the suprapubic tube **Additional Management:** Pelvic fracture: • Open pelvic fractures with exposed bone or blood present on rectal or vaginal exam require broad-spectrum antibiotics and assessment of the need for tetanus prophylaxis • Unstable pelvic fractures, defined as two or more breaks in the pelvic ring with displacement, require definitive treatment with either external or internal fixation, depending on associated injuries and fracture location Bladder rupture: • Extraperitoneal rupture treated by decompression with urethral or suprapubic cystostomy catheter • Intraperitoneal rupture requires surgical repair
Additional Considerations	**Pelvic Fracture Complications:** • Hemorrhage: Most often venous, involving the presacral and lumbar venous plexus and pre-vesical veins. Hemorrhage from these vessels can extend into retroperitoneum. Less commonly arterial, involving the anterior branches of the internal iliac artery, the pudendal and obturator arteries anteriorly, and/or superior gluteal artery and lateral sacral artery posteriorly. • Changes in defecation and voiding patterns. • Sexual dysfunction. • Sitting and gait abnormalities with leg-length discrepancy. • Chronic low back and sacroiliac pain • Nerve injury of L5 and S1 at root or involving sciatic, femoral, pudendal, obturator, and/or superior gluteal nerves. • Pelvic vein thrombosis. • Bladder rupture: If unrecognized, can result in peritonitis, sepsis, ileus, stress incontinence, fistula, and stricture formation. **Pediatric Considerations:** Pelvic avulsion fractures may occur in pediatric patients. In these cases, the growth plate is still open and sudden forceful muscular contraction avulses the growth plate away from the rest of the bone. These injuries are managed conservatively. Most pediatric pelvic fractures are associated with serious injuries such as head, chest, or abdominal injury and femur or tibia fracture.

Urologic Trauma Mini-Case

Urethral Injury (Anterior vs. Posterior Injury)	**Hx:** Blunt force injury, straddle type injury, or physical or sexual assault. Patients may present with difficulty urinating, gross hematuria, or lower abdominal pain and a history of injury to the pelvis. **PE:** Blood at the urethral meatus; swelling or ecchymosis of the penis, scrotum, or perineum; abnormally positioned (high-riding) prostate may be present on rectal exam (more often in posterior urethral injury). **Diagnostics:** • RUG must be done prior to catheterization to prevent worsening of potential tear. This involves injection of contrast through the urethral meatus followed by x-ray. A positive RUG demonstrates extravasation of the contrast outside of the urethral tract. • Pelvic x-ray may also be ordered to evaluate for fractures if there is pelvic tenderness, instability, or mechanism of trauma involving lower abdomen or pelvis. • CT to evaluate kidneys, ureters, and the bladder (in contrast to the urethra). • UA may reveal hematuria on first void (not necessary for diagnosis). **Management:** Unstable patients are treated with a suprapubic cystostomy, with more extensive evaluation and treatment when hemodynamically stable. Stable patients undergo operative repair. **Discussion:** Urethral injuries are much more common in males because the urethra is longer and attached to the pubic bone (vs. shorter and not attached to the pubic bone in females). • *Anterior urethral injuries* (within penis): Straddle injury or direct blows result in anterior urethral injuries (crushing injuries) affecting the bulbous and pendulous portions of the anterior urethra. • *Posterior urethral injuries* (from penis through prostate and into the bladder): Pelvic fractures and iatrogenic causes result in posterior urethral injuries (shearing forces) affecting the prostatic and membranous portions of the urethra. **Complications:** There is a 50% incidence of erectile dysfunction after a urethral injury with pelvic fracture. Urethral trauma can also result in fibrotic narrowing in the bulbar urethra, resulting in urethral stricture with weak stream, incomplete emptying, and dysuria. Patients will have an elevated post-void residual confirmed with voiding cystourethrogram. If significant, patients may require dilation or surgery.

HEAD AND NECK TRAUMA

This section will cover trauma to the head, spine, spinal cord, and neck. For further details, please refer to Chapter 17 (Neurology) sections on traumatic brain injury, neurocritical care, and neck and back pain.

Head Trauma

Operative management of head trauma is required in four conditions:

1. **Scalp wounds** that can lead to severe hemorrhage and death
2. **Depressed skull fractures** if the degree of depression is greater than the thickness of the calvaria or if there is an open fracture
3. **Intracranial mass lesion** due to a rapidly expanding hematoma
4. **Penetrating brain injuries** in which repairs to injured vessels and evacuation of hematomas are critical

Any patient with head trauma who becomes unconscious should be evaluated for intracranial bleeding with an urgent noncontrast head CT. Intracranial bleeding can occur above or below any of the three meningeal layers that cover the brain: the dura mater, which adheres to the skull above which is the epidural space; the arachnoid mater, above which is the subdural space and below it is the subarachnoid space; and the pia mater, which is attached to the surface of the brain and above which is the subarachnoid space. Cerebrospinal fluid lies within the subarachnoid space and throughout the ventricular system. Intracranial bleeding will not cause hemorrhagic shock, as the cranium does not have enough space for sufficient blood loss; however, because the intracranial space is fixed, any increase in volume can cause an increase in ICP and increased risk for herniation and death. Patients with elevated ICP may also develop the Cushing reflex with systolic hypertension with widened pulse pressure, bradycardia, and irregular respirations.

Head trauma often results in traumatic brain injury (TBI), which can be classified as one or a combination of these four external mechanisms:

1. **Direct impact:** Head striking a windshield or a head assault with a bat.
2. **Rapid acceleration and deceleration:** Whiplash injury when the head moves rapidly forward and backward causing shearing and stretching forces on axons.
3. **Penetrating injury:** Projectiles like bullets, lower velocity objects like knives, or even bone fragments from a skull fracture driven into the brain by a depressed skull fracture.
4. **Blast injury:** Injury caused by a pressure wave generated by an explosion.

The injury caused from these external forces can result in three types of internal damage:

1. **Diffuse axonal injury:** Bundles of axons within white matter undergo shearing forces, resulting in twisting or tearing of these fibers. This can present with altered mental status and dysfunction in cognition, speech, and motor function. It is usually not detectable by imaging studies unless severe. Treatment is supportive, including physical and occupational speech therapies and cognitive training.
2. **Focal contusions (bruises):** Also known as coup (French for "blow") and contrecoup (French for "counterblow"). When the skull strikes an object, the force can be directly transferred to the underlying brain, causing a coup injury. The force applied to the brain can also cause it to shift backward, striking the opposite side of the cranium and causing a contrecoup injury. This explains why symptoms can originate from the brain opposite from the site of impact. Coup and contrecoup injuries can occur separately or together. Treatment of these injuries is supportive.
3. **Intracranial hemorrhage and hematomas:** Bleeding can occur within the cranium but external to the brain parenchyma, as in the case of subdural (40–60% of severe head trauma), epidural (1–6% of head trauma), and subarachnoid (40–50% of all head trauma) hemorrhages. Alternatively, bleeding can occur within the brain parenchyma, which includes intraparenchymal/intracerebral hemorrhage (20–30%) or intraventricular hemorrhage (<5%). Many patients have more than one type of hemorrhage. Brain hemorrhage is a serious problem and carries an overall 10–15% mortality. Operative intervention may be required depending on the size and location of the hemorrhage as well as risk of herniation. Surgical options include evacuation of hematomas via craniotomy or, in more severe cases complicated by cerebral edema, a craniectomy, where a portion of the skull bone is removed to allow for expansion of edematous brain tissue. Sources of bleeding should be identified and may also be treated surgically (i.e., surgical clipping of a ruptured berry aneurysm) or endovascularly (i.e., endovascular coiling of a ruptured aneurysm).

CASE 10 | Basilar Skull Fracture

A 54-year-old man presents to the ED after an MVA. The airbag did not deploy, and he sustained a blow to his head from the dashboard. He is conscious and answering questions appropriately. He has no blurred vision or pain with extraocular movements. On exam, vital signs are temperature 36.9°C, pulse 100/min, respiratory rate 16/min, and blood pressure 150/80 mmHg. He has a continuous runny nose and clear fluid draining from his ear. Periorbital, retroauricular, and mastoid ecchymoses are present.

Considerations	**Retrobulbar hematoma:** Blood collecting within the retrobulbar space immediately behind the globe. Can occur following trauma (especially with orbital floor fracture) or sinus or ocular surgery. Presents with proptosis, blurry vision, headache, nausea/vomiting, pain with extraocular movements, elevated intraocular pressure, and can lead to orbital compartment syndrome with complete vision loss.
Initial Trauma Assessment/ Management (Primary Survey)	First assess and address ABCDEs, with particular attention paid to potential associated cervical spine injury
Next Steps (Secondary Survey)	• Once stabilized, obtain noncontrast head CT with bone window • Consult neurosurgery for evaluation due to signs of cerebrospinal fluid leak (rhinorrhea, otorrhea) and perform frequent neurology checks

Discussion	The base of the skull is made up of the ethmoid, sphenoid, occipital, frontal, and temporal bones. Anatomically, the skull base is divided into the anterior, middle, and posterior cranial fossae, each housing distinct brain regions, vasculature, and cranial nerves (see table below). A basilar skull fracture occurs with a fracture of any of these bones at the base of the skull, most commonly the temporal bone, which can result in damage to the nearby middle meningeal artery and result in epidural hematoma.
	
	History:
	• Recent head trauma, most commonly high-energy blunt force trauma (e.g., motor vehicle or motorcycle accident)
	• Concomitant brain injury is common and can result in headache, altered mental status, nausea, vomiting, or loss of consciousness.
	• Concomitant cervical spine injury is also common
	
	Physical Exam: Look for the following exam findings suggestive of basilar skull fractures:
	• CSF rhinorrhea or otorrhea
	• Anosmia
	• Periorbital ecchymosis ('Raccoon eyes')
	• Retroauricular or mastoid ecchymosis (Battle sign)
	• Hemotypanum
	• Visual and/or oculomotor deficits
	• Facial weakness
	• Hearing loss
	
	Assessment/Management:
	Primary Survey:
	• Assess and address ABCDEs with particular attention paid to potential associated cervical spine injury
	• Avoid nasogastric tube insertion or nasopharyngeal intubation
	
	Next Steps (Secondary Survey):
	• Secondary survey should include evaluation for:
	  • Hemotympanum
	  • Cranial nerves V, VI, VII, VIII
	• Once stable, urgent noncontrast head CT with bone window is indicated to identify lines of fracture. Linear or nondisplaced fractures may be difficult to identify.
	• Additional CT findings may include intracranial air (pneumocephalus), sphenoid or frontal sinus air-fluid level, cribriform plate fracture, and hematoma.
	• If CT head is inconclusive but clinical suspicion remains high, consider MRI.
	• If concerned for CSF leak, can assess for "double-ring" sign on bedding or filter paper, where CSF will form large inner ring of pink, bloody fluid and small outer ring of clear fluid. Confirm by laboratory testing for beta-2 transferrin.
	• Bedside glucose of fluid will have glucose >30 mg/dL, while nasal secretions will not. Blood contamination may yield false-positive results.
	• Can also consider CT cisternogram, a study in which iodinated contrast is injected into the lumbar thecal sac to visualize CSF leaks.
	• Neurosurgery should be consulted to determine need for surgery.

CASE 10 | Basilar Skull Fracture *(continued)*

Discussion	**Additional Management:** • Simple linear fractures without associated neurovascular injury can be managed conservatively with closed reduction, wound care, and pain control. • Operative repair of open, displaced, or comminuted linear skull fractures, or when there is neurovascular injury or hematoma.
Additional Considerations	**Complications:** Meningitis, cranial nerve palsies, cavernous sinus thrombosis, **CSF leak** (usually resolves within 7 days). Neurosurgery is indicated if there is high-volume leak or a leak that persists for >7 days.)

Spine and Spinal Cord Trauma

Spinal injuries often accompany head injuries; 5% of patients with brain injury have a spinal injury and 25–30% of patients with a spinal injury have an associated blunt cerebrovascular injury. More than half of all spine injuries occur in the cervical spine; those who sustain a cervical spine fracture may also have a second vertebral fracture.

Movement of the cervical spine should be avoided following trauma; immediate immobilization by cervical collar and long spine backboard is required to prevent additional neurological damage from cervical spine movement. Protection by immobilization allows attention to be directed to life-threatening issues in the unstable patient, such as hypotension or respiratory dysfunction, which take priority over a spine injury.

Whether or not to perform imaging of the spine following trauma is based on stratifying patients into low- and high-risk categories. Evaluation of the cervical spine in *low-risk patients* can be accomplished without imaging. Low risk is defined by the National Emergency X-Radiography Utilization Study (NEXUS criteria) as patients who meet all of the following criteria:

1. No focal neurologic deficits
2. No posterior midline bony cervical spine tenderness
3. No altered mental status (GCS 15)
4. No evidence of intoxication
5. No painful distracting injuries which may distract the patient from noticing neck pain (e.g., long bone fractures, large degloving or crush injury, burns)

A helpful mnemonic is "**NEXUS**"—**N**euro deficit, **E**thanol/intoxication, e**X**treme distracting injury, **U**nable to provide history (altered mental status), **S**pinal tenderness. Patients who have one or more of these should undergo a CT cervical spine.

Once life-threatening injuries are addressed, imaging in *high-risk patients* should be performed in patients who meet any of the following criteria, which form part of the Canadian C-Spine Rule (CCR):

1. Age ≥65
2. Dangerous mechanism of injury, typically high-energy injuries such as:
   a. High-speed MVC (>100 km/hour or 60 miles/hour, rollover, or ejection from vehicle)
   b. Rapid deceleration injuries such as fall ≥3 ft (or ≥5 stairs)
   c. Traumatic axial loads to the head (e.g., diving)
   d. Bicycle collisions
   e. Collisions involving a motorized recreational vehicle
3. Paresthesias in any extremity

For patients with any high-risk factor, CT imaging of the cervical spine ranging from the occiput to T1 should be performed. The cervical collar cannot be removed until imaging and neurologic assessment demonstrate the absence of injury.

Spinal cord injuries (SCI) are described by the vertebral level of the injury. Further details on common forms of SCI can be found in Chapters 17 (Neurology) and 10 (Rheumatology and Musculoskeletal Disorders). These include complete SCI, Brown-Séquard syndrome, anterior cord syndrome, central cord syndrome, and posterior cord syndrome.

Neck Trauma

The neck is a small area that contains a densely packed number of critical structures which can be categorized anatomically.

1. *Respiratory system*: oropharynx, larynx, cervical trachea
2. *Vascular system*: common, internal, and external carotid arteries; vertebral arteries; internal and external jugular veins
3. *Gastrointestinal system*: oropharynx, cervical esophagus

4. *Skeletal system*: cervical vertebrae, hyoid bone
5. *Nervous system*: spinal cord, cranial nerves VII (facial), IX (glossopharyngeal), X (vagus), XI (spinal accessory), and XII (hypoglossal)
6. *Endocrine system*: thyroid and parathyroid glands
7. *Lymphatic system*: thoracic duct
8. *Immune system*: cervical extension of thymus

Inspection of neck wounds is done to confirm penetration of the platysma muscle, which would indicate potential for serious injury. Rapid surgical exploration for penetrating neck trauma is always indicated for hard signs such as active arterial bleeding, expanding hematoma, worsening vital signs indicative of shock, or signs of esophageal or tracheal injury such as hemoptysis or hematemesis. If there are no hard signs, surgical exploration versus diagnostic imaging depends on which zone of the neck is injured.

The neck is divided into three anatomic zones to aid in the initial assessment of a neck injury, with Zone III being the most superior and Zone I the most inferior (see figure and table below). Surgical access is the easiest with Zone II and the most challenging with Zone III. Zone I may cause complications related to vascular control, while Zone III injuries have high mortality due to close anatomical relation to the skull base and difficulty accessing the internal carotid artery. All zones contain the spinal cord.

It is important to remember that neck zones are not mutually exclusive and a penetrating injury at zone II does not exclude the possibility of that injury extending into other zones of the neck or traversing into the chest caudally or brain cephalad.

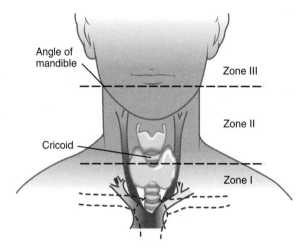

Zones of the neck. (Reproduced with permission from Doherty GM. Current Diagnosis & Treatment: Surgery, 15ed. New York: McGraw Hill; 2020.)

Zones of the Neck and Underlying Anatomic Structures

Zone	Lower Border	Upper Border	Underlying Anatomic Structures	Most Common Injuries
III	Angle of mandible	Base of skull	Oropharynx, cervical spine and cord, cranial nerves IX-XII, proximal portions of internal and external carotid arteries, vertebral arteries, parts of jugular veins	Vertebral artery, external carotid artery
II	Cricoid cartilage	Angle of mandible	Esophagus, larynx, trachea, cervical spine and cord, vagus nerve (CN X), recurrent laryngeal nerve, phrenic nerve, mid-carotid and vertebral arteries, jugular veins	Internal carotid artery, internal jugular vein, sympathetic trunk (can lead to hypotension), recurrent laryngeal nerve (hoarseness), trachea, esophagus
I	Clavicles and sternal notch	Cricoid cartilage	Thymus, thoracic duct, thyroid, lung apices, distal trachea, esophagus, cervical spine and cord, brachial plexus, great vessels, common carotid and vertebral arteries	Pneumothorax, hemothorax, common carotid artery, subclavian artery

Injuries to Zone II have a lower threshold for immediate surgical exploration as access can easily be obtained via a standard oblique cervical incision. Stable patients without hard signs may only undergo CT imaging. Zone I and III injuries are first imaged with CT angiography (CTA). If CTA does not demonstrate definitive injury in Zone I or III, catheter arteriography should be performed if there is concern for arterial injury, and triple endoscopy (laryngoscopy, esophagoscopy, and bronchoscopy) should be performed if there is concern for a tracheoesophageal injury. Zone III injuries may be accessed through oblique cervical incision; however, they may also require endovascular procedures due to difficulty accessing the internal carotid artery.

Life-threatening injury within the neck is based on two aspects: compromise of the airway and hemorrhage.

1. **Asphyxiation:** Asphyxiation occurs from an injury in Zone II, either from a direct wound to the trachea or from compression of the airway by a vascular hematoma.

2. **Hemorrhage:** Hemorrhage can occur in any of the zones. In Zone I, hemorrhage can occur intrapleurally and may require a sternotomy to repair. Zone II hemorrhage may occur in response to direct injuries to any of the vascular structures that can be accessed by a neck incision. Exsanguination from Zone III would likely involve injury to the internal carotid artery occurring at a difficult-to-reach location, often at the base of the skull.

CASE 11 | Penetrating Neck Injury (PNI)

An 18-year-old man presents with a gunshot injury to the neck. His vitals are temperature 37.0°C, blood pressure 90/60 mmHg, pulse 120/min, respirations 22/min, and SpO$_2$ 96%. Voice is muffled. Airway exam shows blood along the right neck and within the oropharynx with no clear source of bleeding. Chest wall is without injury, trachea is midline, and breath sounds are present bilaterally. There is a wound in the posterior neck at the superior trapezius inferior to the mandible and another wound at the anterior border of the sternocleidomastoid muscle superior to the cricoid cartilage. Blood is oozing from the wounds but there is no bubbling, sucking, or uncontrollable bleeding. Crepitus and edema are present along the wounds. The radial, femoral, and carotid pulses are palpable but diminished bilaterally without bruits or thrills. The patient receives IV resuscitation but remains hypotensive.

Conditions with Similar Presentations	**Superficial neck injury:** This is defined as trauma to the neck that *does not* penetrate past the platysma, making injury to vital structures within the neck unlikely. **Blunt neck trauma:** This occurs during MVAs, often secondary to shearing trauma from seatbelts, or from sports injuries. Patients are susceptible to occult cervical spine injury with this mechanism, as well as delayed presentation of laryngeal, vascular, or esophageal injuries. **Near-hanging/strangulation:** Asphyxiation secondary to compression of cervical vessels or tracheal obstruction can lead to cerebral hypoxia and subsequent neuronal death.
Initial Trauma Assessment/ Management (Primary Survey)	• Assess and address ABCDEs • Priority is in evaluating and securing the airway and evaluating the source of hypotension and tachycardia • Initiate MTP
Next Steps (Secondary Survey)	• This patient is hemodynamically unstable as noted by signs of shock, including tachycardia and hypotension despite IV fluid resuscitation. • With the "hard sign" of shock and a zone II injury, the patient will require immediate surgical exploration in the OR.
Discussion	The most common causes of a penetrating neck injury are stab wounds, followed by GSWs, self-harm, and road traffic accidents. Arterial injury is observed in 25% of penetrating neck injuries and commonly involves the carotid artery (80% of arterial injuries), vertebral artery, or both. Aerodigestive injury is detected in 20–30% of patients with penetrating neck trauma. Together, these injuries are the prevailing causes of mortality following penetrating neck injury. A penetrating neck injury is defined as trauma that penetrates past the platysma—the thin, sheet-like, superficial muscle covering the anterior and lateral neck. The patient above has an injury to neck zone II, as the sites of the gunshot wounds are between the cricoid cartilage and the angle of the mandible. **History:** • Specific information on knife width and length or angle of gunshot trajectory can be helpful in identifying suspected injuries. A trajectory medially, anterior to the sternocleidomastoid may imply injury to major vessels, trachea, or esophagus, while a lateral trajectory may be less injurious. • Dysphagia, hoarseness, bleeding from nose or mouth. **Physical:** • *Airway injury*—crepitus, stridor, or respiratory distress • *Vascular injury*—active hemorrhage from site, expanding neck hematoma, bruits, or absent radial pulse; hemiparesis may occur from carotid injury • *Esophageal injury*—may have crepitus, may also be asymptomatic with delayed presentation as a neck abscess • *Neurologic injuries*—paresis (suggestive of carotid injury with cerebral ischemia), cranial nerve deficits

CASE 11 | Penetrating Neck Injury (PNI) *(continued)*

Discussion	Assessment/Management:
	Primary Survey:
	• Assess and address ABCDEs
	• Given that he is refractory to IV fluids, blood products (MTP) should also be initiated
	• Should also consider rapid-sequence intubation (RSI) or cricothyrotomy
	• Hemodynamically **unstable** patients require immediate operative exploration without further diagnostic workup
	• Following penetrating neck trauma, "hard signs" that require immediate operative exploration are:
	• Shock
	• Pulsatile bleeding or expanding hematoma
	• Audible bruit or palpable thrill
	• Airway compromise
	• Bubbling wound
	• Stridor, hoarseness
	• Neurologic deficits
	• Hemoptysis
	• Hematemesis
	Next Steps (Secondary Survey):
	• Hemodynamically stable patients may be taken to the OR for neck exploration for Zone II injuries or may be monitored with serial exams and evaluated with CTA (CTA is 100% sensitive for a vascular injury but not as sensitive for aerodigestive injuries).
	• If there are intermediate findings on CTA for possible aerodigestive injuries, patients may need to undergo bronchoscopy, laryngoscopy, upper endoscopy, barium swallow, and/or endovascular intervention.
	• Confirmation of injury by these complementary studies leads to surgical exploration and repair.

ORTHOPEDIC TRAUMA

Orthopedic trauma is the diagnosis and treatment of fractures of bones in the torso, upper and lower extremities, and pelvis. In the trauma assessment, certain orthopedic injuries can threaten life and limb and need to be considered first:

1. Life-threatening injuries:
   a. **Hemorrhage** from a femur or pelvic fracture or traumatic amputation resulting in shock.
   b. **Crush syndrome** leading to acute rhabdomyolysis, renal failure, and/or shock.
2. Limb-threatening injuries requiring urgent operative intervention include:
   a. **Open fracture or open joint injury** (when the bone breaks through the skin): This can lead to infection and impaired healing (e.g., osteomyelitis, nonunion, malunion, post-traumatic arthritis) and requires immediate antibiotics, irrigation, and debridement of the wound.
   b. **Musculoskeletal injury with concomitant vascular injury** can occur from a traumatic severance of the vessel or from an intimal tear with partial disruption of blood flow leading to ischemia of the soft tissue. Must be repaired immediately.
   c. **Compartment syndrome:** Seen more commonly with long bone fractures of the tibia, distal radius, and supracondylar portion of the humerus. Increased pressure within a compartment impedes limb circulation and nerve function. Patients present with pain out of proportion to the injury, pain worsened with passive stretching, tense swelling, and paresthesia. Treatment is immediate fasciotomy to restore circulation to the limb.

Orthopedic fractures may be classified as open or closed and displaced or nondisplaced.

- **Open fractures** involve bone penetrating through the skin whereas **closed fractures** remain completely inside the body. Open fractures are classified by Gustilo grade to help determine management and prognosis.
- **Displaced fractures** result in a misalignment of the bone fragments. **Nondisplaced fractures** result in a preservation of proper bone alignment. As a general rule, displaced fractures often require surgical correction whereas nondisplaced fractures may be managed with reduction and cast immobilization.

Restoring anatomical alignment of the fracture that is displaced anatomically can tamponade bleeding at the site, reduce tension on vessels to restore blood supply, reduce tension on nerves to prevent neuropraxia, or reduce muscle traction to relieve soft tissue swelling. Unstable fractures result when the muscle pulls across the fracture, preventing realignment. In these cases, such as femoral shaft or neck fractures, surgical fixation is required.

Pediatric Considerations

Most children's fractures are simply reduced and immobilized because of a higher degree of bone remodeling and a faster healing process than adult bones. Fractures involving the growth plate in children may require surgical correction to prevent uneven growth.

Type of fracture depends on the mechanism of injury, loading forces, and compressive stress. Unique patterns commonly seen in pediatric patients include greenstick fracture, plastic deformity, and buckle (torus) fracture. Typical mechanisms of injury include a fall on an outstretched hand, direct blow, or MVA. A focal area of tenderness, swelling, and overlying ecchymosis of a long bone (femur, humerus, and tibia) of a child who is nonambulatory is suggestive of abuse.

Commonly Seen Pediatric Fractures Due To Trauma	
Distal tibial fractures in children often involve the growth plate, so there is an increased risk of growth arrest and limb-length discrepancy. Patients may also be at increased risk for premature osteoarthritis. Fractures in children can be classified using the **Salter-Harris (SH) fracture classification;** Type III and Type IV fractures require surgical open reduction and internal fixation.	Salter-Harris Fractures: injuries affecting the growth plate of long bones. 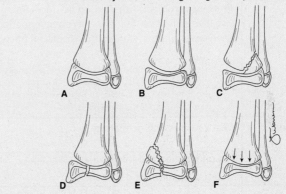 Reproduced with permission from Ziegler MM, Azizkhan RG, Allmen D, Weber TR. Operative Pediatric Surgery, 2ed. New York: McGraw Hill; 2014.
Spiral fracture of long bones is usually caused by a twisting force that produces the injury.	
• **Toddler's fracture** is a nondisplaced spiral fracture of the distal tibia in ambulatory children 9 months-4 years of age. They typically occur after a fall while children are learning to walk, resulting in a twisting injury. Children may experience pain or refuse to walk or bear weight on the affected limb. On exam, twisting of the knee or ankle may reproduce pain and there may be swelling. Diagnosis is via X-ray, although may be normal at first or may only see a hairline fracture (white arrow in figure to right). • **Greenstick fracture** is a partial thickness fracture in which cortex and periosteum are damaged on only one side of the affected bone. Pediatric patients' bones are mostly calcified cartilage (not ossified yet) which puts them at greater risk of these bending-type fractures. Vitamin D deficiency adds risk. **Plastic deformity** implies bending of the bone without necessarily breaking **Buckle (Torus) fracture** is a distal fracture in the radius or ulna often seen in children <10 years old. After a fall, patients present with pain, swelling on the distal forearm and bulging along the metaphysis from compression failure. Most heal within a few weeks without complications	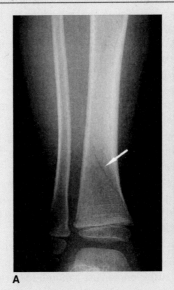 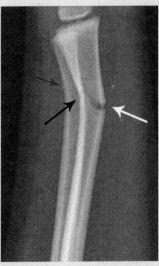 Toddler fracture. A. There is a classic spiral fracture (arrow) in this 19-month-old child. B. Greenstick fracture of radius, and torus fracture of ulna. Lateral forearm radiograph shows unicortical greenstick fracture of distal radial diametaphyseal region (white arrow), plastic deformity of dorsal cortex at the same level (thick black arrow), and small buckle fracture diametaphyseal region of ulna (thin black arrow). (Reproduced with permission from Tehranzadeh J., Basic Musculoskeletal Imaging, 2e. Copyright 2021 McGraw-Hill Education. All rights reserved.)

CASE 12 | Scaphoid Fracture

A 17-year-old girl presents with a 2-day history of left wrist pain after falling onto outstretched hands while rollerblading. Her vital signs are unremarkable. The patient has tenderness in the shallow depression in her right dorsoradial wrist (anatomic snuffbox) and over the scaphoid tubercle on her dorsal palm at the base of the thumb. Resisted pronation of the wrist also elicits pain.

Conditions with Similar Presentations	**Distal radius fractures:** Can occur from a fall on outstretched hands. Causes tenderness and swelling at the distal radius, but no anatomic snuffbox tenderness. Colles and Smith fractures are distal radius fractures named based on the direction of fracture displacement. • **Colles fracture** involves dorsal displacement with a "dinner fork deformity" and, when severe, can result in neurovascular compromise (e.g., median nerve, radial artery). • **Smith fracture**, also known as a reverse Colles fracture, involves volar or anterior displacement. **Boxer fracture:** commonly presents with lateral hand pain and tenderness to palpation over the fourth or fifth metacarpal following punching an object with a closed fist. Most fractures can be managed with immobilization. Surgery with open reduction and internal fixation reserved for open or significantly displaced fractures. 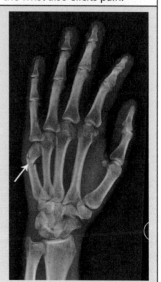 Boxer fracture. There is a dorsally angulated fracture at the fifth metacarpal neck (*arrow*). (Reproduced with permission from Tehranzadeh J. Basic Musculoskeletal Imaging, 2e. Copyright 2021 McGraw-Hill Education.)
Initial Diagnostic Tests	Wrist x-ray to confirm fracture
Next Steps in Management	• Thumb spica cast for nondisplaced fracture • Surgery for displaced fracture
Discussion	Falls onto an outstretched hand can result in several bony fractures. The wrist is formed from two bones in the forearm (radius and ulna) and eight small carpal bones in the hand. The carpal bones are divided into a proximal row and distal row. The scaphoid (navicular) is the most commonly fractured carpal bone, as it lies on the floor of the anatomic snuffbox. The anatomic snuffbox is bounded medially by the extensor pollicis longus tendon and laterally by the abductor pollicis longus and extensor pollicis brevis tendons. **History:** Often occurring following a fall onto an outstretched hand (e.g., sports activities, MVA); resulting in pain in the anatomic snuffbox is highly suspicious for scaphoid fracture. Patients may also complain of pain in the radial wrist or at the base of the thumb. **Physical Exam:** Swelling and tenderness to deep palpation in the anatomic snuffbox and over the scaphoid tubercle (near base of thumb on palmar side). Pain with resisted wrist pronation. **Diagnostics:** X-ray is diagnostic of choice (see image); however, fractures may not show for several days up to 2 weeks, especially if it is a nondisplaced fracture. In cases where scaphoid fracture is still highly suspected, perform MRI or CT. **Management:** • For nondisplaced fracture or no fracture seen on x-ray but high clinical suspicion, can use a thumb spica cast for wrist immobilization. • For displaced or unstable fractures, surgical fixation is necessary and involves open reduction and internal fixation with a screw. Patients will often undergo repeat x-ray to monitor for signs of osteonecrosis and nonunion. 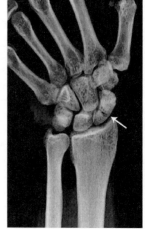 Scaphoid fracture. There is a nondisplaced fracture through the waist of the scaphoid bone (arrow). (Reproduced with permission from Tehranzadeh J. Basic Musculoskeletal Imaging, 2e. Copyright 2021 McGraw-Hill Education.)
Additional Considerations	**Complications:** Due to the blood flow to the scaphoid, which enters at the distal portion of the bone and flows proximally (retrograde flow), a fracture can disrupt blood supply to the proximal segment of the scaphoid and result in **avascular necrosis (osteonecrosis)**.

CASE 13 | Ankle Fracture

A 13-year-old boy is brought to the ED by his father after he twisted his right ankle during a soccer game. He is unable to walk on his right ankle. The patient's temperature is 37.4°C, pulse 98/min, blood pressure 124/70 mmHg, and respirations 16/min. On physical exam, there is focal tenderness over the medial malleolus most pronounced on the posterior margin. There is also swelling of the ankle.

Conditions with Similar Presentations	**Ankle sprain:** Accounts for the majority of ankle injuries, common in young athletes. Patients are able to bear weight on the ankle even though it may be painful, and x-ray of ankle will show no deformity or fractures as the ligaments are stretched or torn but bones are intact. The most common ligament involved is the anterior talofibular ligament in the lateral ankle. If uncomplicated, conservative management is recommended (rest, ice, compression, elevation) with physical therapy as needed.
Initial Diagnostic Testing	• Determine whether the patient requires imaging using the Ottawa ankle rules • Confirm diagnosis with ankle x-ray (this patient has pain in the malleolar zone with tenderness at the posterior margin and is unable to bear weight)
Next Steps in Management	Depending on x-ray results, options include immobilization with a walking boot and nonweight-bearing cast, closed reduction, or potentially surgery.

Discussion	Ankle fractures account for 5% of all pediatric fractures; they are more common in males 2:1, and usually occur between ages 8 and 15. Patients who participate in sports and have an increased BMI are at an increased risk. The mechanism of injury is either a twisting injury (rotation about a planted foot and ankle) or a result of direct trauma. While pediatric fractures are more common, they can also occur in adults.
	
	History: Acute injury (e.g., sports, trauma, nonaccidental trauma) with focal pain and/or inability to bear weight to the affected ankle.
	
	Physical Exam: Physical exam findings depend on whether the fracture is displaced. There is often focal tenderness, ecchymosis, and swelling.
	• If displacement is present, there may be deformity of the ankle
	• The location of focal tenderness may vary, but common sites include the distal fibula or tibia, the medial or lateral malleolus, the navicular, and the base of the fifth metatarsal
	
	Diagnostics:
	• The Ottawa ankle rules are used to determine the need to obtain radiographs in patients with a foot injury concerning for ankle fracture. The goal of these rules is to help reduce unnecessary imaging and promote value-based health care.
	
	{{TABLE}}
	• AP, mortise, and lateral view x-rays should be obtained to evaluate for fracture and displacement
	• If x-ray is negative but suspicion remains high, can consider CT scan
	
	Management:
	• Nonoperative:
	  • If nondisplaced fibula fracture (<2 mm) seen on imaging, then walking boot and nonweight-bearing cast is indicated
	  • If displaced Salter-Harris Class I or II fracture to the fibula or tibia is seen, then closed reduction and cast are indicated
	  • CT scan should be obtained post-reduction to assess fracture displacement and determine if further operative management is required
	• Operative:
	  • If displaced Salter-Harris Class I or II to the fibula or tibia is seen and closed reduction does not work, operative intervention is necessary
	  • If displaced Salter-Harris Class III or above, operative intervention

Additional Considerations	**Complications:** Ankle pain and degeneration; growth arrest can occur if there is a large degree of initial displacement.

Radiograph	Ottawa Rules
Ankle	Bone tenderness at the posterior edge or lateral tip of the lateral malleolus OR posterior edge of medial malleolus OR inability to bear weight both immediately and in the ED
Foot	Bone tenderness at base of the fifth metacarpal OR navicular bone OR inability to bear weight both immediately and in the ED

CASE 14 | Polytrauma with Multiple Fractures (Open and Closed)

A 26-year-old man is brought into the ED following an MVA and is reporting severe pain in his left leg and shoulder. On presentation the patient is awake and alert, has a bleeding scalp laceration approximately 5 cm long, and an obvious deformity of his left clavicle. The tibia is poking through the skin of the left lower extremity. Distal motor and sensory function in his left leg are intact, and pedal pulses are 2+. There is no tenderness or deformity in his right thigh or right lower leg. X-rays confirm a closed clavicular fracture and an open tibia fracture.

Considerations	History and physical helps guide areas which require further investigation.
Primary Survey	Assess and address ABCDEs.
Secondary Survey	• After stabilization of ABCs, examine extremities and treat open fractures with IV antibiotics, irrigation, and surgical debridement and external fixation • X-ray tender areas on exam
Discussion	Polytrauma is used to describe patients with more than one injury. An open fracture involves communication with the external environment secondary to disruption of the overlying skin and soft tissue (see image). This open communication increases the risk for osteomyelitis and infection of hardware that may be placed during surgery for fracture fixation. Bone healing is also slowed in open fractures and more often results in nonhealing, known as nonunion 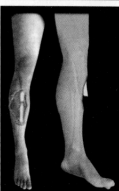 **History:** Knowing the mechanism of injury can help direct assessment. A history of smoking can impede fracture healing and increase the risk of nonunion. **Physical Exam:** The extremities should be evaluated to assess the four functional components: blood vessels, nerves, bones, and soft tissues). **Diagnostics:** • Following the primary survey, perform a thorough secondary survey to avoid missing additional fractures. • Radiographs must include the joint above and below all fractures seen on x-ray, as multiple bones may be fractured (i.e., tibia and fibula in accompanying x-ray). • Any soft tissue wounds in conjunction with a fracture constitute an open fracture. Gustillo-Anderson fracture type III open fracture. (Reproduced with permission from Brunicardi F, Andersen DK, Billiar TR, Dunn DL, Kao LS, Hunter JG, Matthews JB, Pollock RE. Schwartz's Principles of Surgery, 11e. Copyright 2019 McGraw-Hill Education.) **Management:** **Open Fracture:** • All open fractures should receive antibiotic coverage based on the Gustilo grade of fracture. Anaerobe coverage should be added if there is soil or fecal contamination. For saltwater or freshwater wounds, fluoroquinolones are added. • Operative approach includes irrigation, debridement of devitalized soft tissue, open reduction, and either internal or external fixation of the fracture. • Soft tissue coverage of the open wound is also required to prevent osteomyelitis. **Closed Fracture:** • Depending on location, there may be option for nonsurgical treatment (e.g., closed reduction followed by immobilization). • For those that require surgical management, typically this is done within 2–12 hours with intramedullary nailing as quickly as possible to reduce risk of fat embolism syndrome. 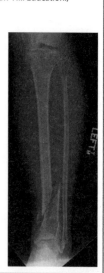 Radiograph of left tibia and fibula fracture. (Reproduced with permission from Stahel PF. Surgical Patient Safety: A Case-Based Approach. Copyright 2017 McGraw-Hill Education.)
Additional Considerations	**Complications:** Main surgical risks of open fractures include osteomyelitis, nonunion, malunion, nerve or vessel injury, thromboembolic events, and, if insufficient tissue is available for reconstruction, amputation.

CASE 15 | Femur Fracture with Fat Embolism Syndrome

A 24-year-old man presents to the ED following an MVA. He had no head injury or loss of consciousness and is endorsing severe right leg pain. On exam, blood pressure is 143/83 mmHg, pulse 89/min, respirations 20/min, and SpO_2 99% on room air. There is a notable deformity in the right mid-thigh with significant swelling. Sensation, as well as dorsalis pedis, posterior tibial, and popliteal pulses, are intact in the right lower extremity. X-ray reveals a comminuted mid-shaft femoral fracture. The patient is taken to the OR for surgical fixation. There are no surgical complications, and the patient is admitted for post-surgical management. Two days later, he suddenly develops dyspnea and his SpO_2 drops to 90% on room air. The patient appears confused and has developed a petechial rash over his chest.

Conditions with Similar Presentations	**Pulmonary embolus:** Presentation is often with similar respiratory symptoms; however, neurologic abnormalities and rash are not seen.
	Atelectasis: Hypoxia (if it occurs) would be more gradual in onset. It is not associated with neurologic abnormalities or rash.
	Pneumonia: Would expect cough, fever, and evidence of focal consolidation on lung exam and chest x-ray. It is not associated with rash.
	Congestive heart failure: Uncommon in this age group, and would not cause a rash.
Initial Diagnostic Tests	• Clinical diagnosis • Chest x-ray may show alveolar infiltrates but is not required for diagnosis since these are not always seen.
Next Steps in Management	• **Femur fracture:** Surgical fixation and early stabilization of fractures decreases the risk for fat embolism. • **Fat emboli:** Supportive treatment including oxygen and mechanical ventilation as needed.
Discussion	Femur fractures typically occur following trauma such as an MVA in younger patients or falls in older populations. The patient above has a comminuted fracture, defined as a fracture involving more than two segments of bone. Fat embolism syndrome presents with the classic triad of hypoxemia, neurologic abnormalities, and a petechial rash most commonly in the setting of trauma. It is particularly common after fracture of long bones or the pelvis, and most often presents 24–72 hours following the injury. The risk increases with the number of fractured bones. It occurs more with closed fractures than open fractures. Marrow in the bone, containing free fatty acids and hematopoietic cells, is liberated from the fracture site and results in inflammation, increased vascular permeability (capillary leak syndrome), and platelet aggregation. The fat droplets liberated from the fracture site may travel systemically to deposit in microcapillary beds in the lungs, brain, skin, and retina, leading to hypoxia, confusion, petechiae, and visual acuity changes, respectively. **History/Physical Exam:** Symptoms and signs of fat embolism occur 24–72 hours after trauma or surgery. • Vague chest pain, shortness of breath, confusion and petechial rash • May have tachycardia, hypotension and fundoscopic retinal exam may show hemorrhage. **Diagnostics:** • Fat embolism syndrome is a clinical diagnosis based on history, physical, with three major findings: petechial rash, respiratory distress, and confusion following closed or multiple fractures of the lower extremities and/or pelvis. • Consider: chest X-ray (to identify other causes of hypoxia), CBC (anemia, thrombocytopenia), metabolic panel (metabolic acidosis, elevated creatinine), ABG (Increased A-a gradient with V/Q mismatch due to impaired perfusion and normal ventilation), CT head (to evaluate altered mental status), CT chest (bilateral ground glass opacities) **Management:** • Femur fracture should be treated with open reduction and internal fixation as quickly as possible to decrease the risk for fat embolism • Treatment of fat embolism syndrome is supportive care with supplemental oxygen and mechanical ventilation as needed. Intubation may be necessary. • Prophylaxis against thromboembolism • Provision of adequate nutrition
Additional Considerations	**Other Complications of Femur Fracture:** • Hemorrhage occurs in 40%—hemorrhage can be particularly devastating to the elderly, who lack cardiac reserve • Pudendal nerve palsy from direct compression or ischemia occurs in 10% of patients following femoral shaft fracture • Femur fracture is the most common cause of thigh compartment syndrome but incidence is only 1%; however, in venous injuries accompanying femur fracture, one can also develop lower leg compartment syndrome from thrombosed or inadequate venous drainage • Other potential complications include GI bleed (2%) and TIA/stroke (1%) • Overall mortality is ~ 3%

Orthopedic Trauma Mini-Cases

Cases	Key Findings
Acute Compartment Syndrome	**Hx:** • Severe pain out of proportion to the injury in the setting of upper or lower extremity trauma (e.g., fracture), prolonged extremity compression, circumferential third-degree burns, or following revascularization of an ischemic limb. • Pain may be present with passive stretching along with paresthesias in early stages. **PE:** • Skin lesions, swelling, and some color changes may be present. • Affected compartment may feel warm, tense, and tender on palpation • Pulses may be diminished or absent, especially over time. • Neurologic function can also be impaired resulting in decreased two-point discrimination, diminished light touch sensation, and motor weakness. **Diagnostics:** • Clinical diagnosis requiring immediate treatment. • If there is uncertainty about the diagnosis, intercompartmental pressure can be measured via needle manometry: >30 mmHg confirms the diagnosis (normal pressure is 0–8 mmHg). **Management:** • Compartment syndrome is a surgical emergency which threatens the viability of the limb due to ischemia. • Fasciotomy should be performed immediately. • Pre-operative antibiotics, supplemental oxygen, removal of any restrictive casts, bandages, or dressings to release pressure, and extremity should be kept at the level of the heart to prevent hypoperfusion. Fasciotomy of the leg. (Reproduced with permission from F. Charles Brunicardi, Dana K. Andersen, Timothy R. Billiar, David L. Dunn, Lillian S. Kao, John G. Hunter, Jeffrey B. Matthews, Raphael E. Pollock, Schwartz's Principles of Surgery, 11e. Copyright 2019 McGraw-Hill Education.) **Discussion:** Acute compartment syndrome is a limb-threatening condition occurring from direct trauma to the extremity or reperfusion tissue damage following vascular injury due to excess edema within muscle. The tissues of the compartment of the limb swell but are confined by the fascia. As the pressure builds, it limits perfusion to muscle and nerves. • The classic presentation of compartment syndrome is associated with "The six P's:" Pain out of proportion to exam and on passive stretch, Paresthesia, Paralysis, Poikilothermia, Pallor, and Pulselessness. The last to occur is pulselessness. As compartment pressure increases, the first vasculature compromised is capillary perfusion followed by venous outflow, and finally arterial inflow. • Compartment syndrome most commonly is observed in the leg, although can also occur in the arm. Reproduced with permission from Brunicardi F, Andersen DK, Billiar TR, Dunn DL, Kao LS, Hunter JG, Matthews JB, Pollock RE. Schwartz's Principles of Surgery, 11ed. New York: McGraw Hill; 2019. • Within the leg, there are four compartments: anterior, lateral, deep posterior, and superficial posterior (see image). The first symptom may be numbness of the great toe due to involvement of the anterior compartment and compression of the deep peroneal nerve.
Post-Amputation Phantom Limb Pain	**Hx:** • Tingling, throbbing, sharp, pins, and needles in the limb that is no longer present due to amputation. • Pain severity can vary from patient to patient and also the timeline can vary (from months to years after the amputation), although often presents within 1 week.

Orthopedic Trauma Mini-Cases (*continued*)

Post-Amputation Phantom Limb Pain	**PE:** The goal of the physical exam is to rule out causes of pain within the residual limb such as infection, ischemia, and pressure-related wounds. • Sensory exam may be abnormal, revealing allodynia (pain to normally nonnoxious stimuli) and hyperalgesia (increased pain to normally noxious stimuli). Otherwise, physical exam is normal. **Diagnostics:** • Clinical diagnosis, although ultrasound can evaluate for and rule out post-traumatic neuromas. **Management:** There are very few treatment options for phantom limb pain that have proven to be effective. • NSAIDs and acetaminophen are the most used pharmacologic treatments. • Several medications (e.g., amitriptyline, lidocaine, gabapentin, memantine, ketamine) have been shown to be somewhat helpful. • Graded motor imagery has been reported to improve pain by redirecting brain signaling through laterality reconstruction (left-right discrimination exercises), motor imagery, and mirror therapy. **Discussion:** Phantom limb pain is the perception of pain or discomfort in a limb that is not there (post-amputation or trauma). The pain is thought to be due to a mismatch between neural pathways that have been affected, attempting to return to prior amputation state; however, multiple mechanisms are likely at play. Pain tends to resolve with wound healing, although this may take some time.

BLAST AND BURN INJURIES

Blast injuries are defined as complex physical trauma due to direct or indirect exposure to an explosion. An explosion is an extremely rapid release of energy in the form of light, heat, sound, or shock waves. Shock waves travel radially at supersonic speed. In addition to burns, commonly affected systems include hearing, vision, limbs, lung, and the brain.

Blast injuries depend on the explosive material, the distance between the explosion and the victim, and whether the victim is surrounded by protective barriers or is in a confined space. The U.S. Centers for Disease Control and Prevention (CDC) classifies blast injuries as primary, secondary, tertiary, and quaternary based on the mechanism of injury (see table below). It is especially important to remember the psychological consequences of trauma. Blast lung, presenting with dyspnea, cough, hemoptysis, or chest pain, is the most common deadly primary blast injury among initial survivors.

Classification of Blast Injuries

Classification	Description	Commonly Associated Injuries
Primary	Blast wave–induced overpressure injury with direct tissue damage from shock wave.	Air-filled organs are at highest risk: Tympanic membrane rupture, middle ear damage, blast lung (pulmonary barotrauma), concussion, GI tract perforation or hemorrhage, globe (eye) rupture
Secondary	Projectile debris and fragments either from the exploding device, additional fragments added to the device to raise lethality, or from the environment (e.g., glass, rocks).	Skin lacerations, penetrating trauma (e.g., to head, thorax, abdomen, pelvis, limbs), soft tissue injury (including traumatic amputations)
Tertiary	Rapid acceleration and deceleration of the body onto stationary objects (i.e., being thrown by the blast).	Blunt trauma, traumatic amputation, fractures, crush injury, impalement on another object
Quaternary	Miscellaneous injuries not included in primary, secondary, or tertiary categories. Typically caused by exposures resulting from the explosion, such as heat, toxins, fuel, and metals. Also includes impact on underlying medical illnesses and psychological disease.	Burns, inhalation injury (e.g., carbon monoxide, dust, hot gases), chemical exposure, radiation injury, exacerbating of underlying disease (e.g., COPD, asthma, coronary artery disease, hypertension), infection/sepsis, anxiety, depression, PTSD

Mass casualty events require rapid triaging of injuries by clinical severity. The Simple Triage and Rapid Treatment (**START**) triage system takes less than 1 minute of assessment to assign the patient into one of four color-coded categories, as shown in the table below.

START Adult Triage System for Mass Casualty Events

Category	Description
Expectant (black)	Unlikely to survive given severity of injuries, requires palliative care and pain relief
Immediate (red)	Could be helped by immediate intervention and transport, requires medical attention within minutes (up to 1 hour) for survival, often involving compromises to ABCs
Delayed (yellow)	Serious and potentially life-threatening injury, but stable enough to delay and not expected to deteriorate significantly over several hours
Minor (green)	Relatively minor injuries, status unlikely to deteriorate over several days, may be able to assist with their own care

Burn injuries can be chemical (alkaline or acidic), thermal (e.g., fire or scald burn), electrical, or due to radiation. They can be classified as first-, second-, third-, or fourth-degree based on tissue depth.

Classification of Burn Injuries

Thickness	Degree	Depth	Example	Characteristics	Healing
Superficial	First	Epidermis	Sunburn	Redness, hypersensitivity, pain, no skin sloughing; not included in total body surface area calculations	Heals spontaneously in 1 week without residual scarring; outer layer peels away from healed adjacent skin
Partial thickness (divided into superficial and deep)	Second	*Superficial*: Epidermis and superficial dermis *Deep*: Epidermis and deep dermis, sweat glands, hair follicles	*Superficial*: Hot water scald *Deep*: Hot liquid, steam, grease, flame	Red, edematous, blisters, weepy or wet, very painful	*Superficial*: Heals spontaneously within 2–3 weeks without scar *Deep*: Heels over 3–8 weeks but may have scarring (grafting may be required to minimize scarring)
Full thickness	Third	Entire epidermis and dermis, dermal appendages (e.g., sweat glands, nails, hair follicle, nerves)	Flame	Whitish, charred appearance with coagulated vessels; dry leathery skin or "eschar"; painless (loss of nerves)	May heal over months but results in severe scarring and usually requires surgery; scar contractures may occur even with skin grafting
Subdermal fat	Fourth	Entire epidermis and dermis, dermal appendages, subcutaneous tissue, fat, fascia, muscle and/or bone	Flame	Dry leathery skin or "eschar"; painless (loss of nerves)	May partially heal over months but typically requires multiple surgeries; scar contractures may occur even with skin grafting

For estimation of burn size and to calculate IV fluid requirements, the body is divided into regions whose surface areas are multiples of nine (the **"rule of nines"**): head (anterior and posterior), 9%; each arm (anterior and posterior), 9%; anterior torso, 18%; posterior torso, 18%; each leg (anterior and posterior), 18% (see figure). While this is a rough estimation, many burn centers will also adjust for differences based on age. The percentages of these regions differ in children. This rule is used for burns that are second-degree or higher.

The percentage of total body surface area (**TBSA**) burned can be calculated by adding up percentages of the affected regions. Knowing the TBSA burned is important when calculating fluid replacement as there can be a lot of fluid lost from the intravascular space, leading to hypovolemic shock. Historically, in adults and children ≥14, this has been used in the **Parkland formula** for burn resuscitation, where the estimated fluid requirements in the first 24 hours = 4 mL × TBSA × weight (kg). However, current recommendations are somewhat different (from ATLS and American Burn Association), where estimated fluid requirements in the first 24 hours = 2 mL × TBSA × body weight (kg). Ideally, half of this volume should be administered within the first 8 hours, and the remaining volume can be administered in the ensuing 16 hours.

Determining burn size by the "rule of nines." (Reproduced with permission from Feliciano DV, Mattox KL, Moore EE. Trauma, 9ed. New York: McGraw Hill; 2020.)

Inhalational Injury

History of exposure to fire in a closed space, findings of carbonaceous sputum, singed nasal hairs, or significant facial burns are suggestive. Changes in voice quality or stridor are hard signs of injury. There are three components of inhalational injury:

1. **Supraglottic:** Upper airway inflammation and edema, which may cause patient to lose airway and obscure landmarks for successful intubation. Therefore, intubate before the condition progresses.

2. **Infraglottic:** Sloughing of the epithelial lining of the airway, resulting in airway obstruction, mucus hypersecretion, inflammation, pulmonary edema, and impaired local immune defenses. Tracheobronchitis with severe wheezing may occur within hours, while acute respiratory failure secondary to a chemical pneumonitis from the products of combustion may occur later.

3. **Fire fume intoxication:** Inhalation of fire smoke results in exposure to a complex mixture of gases formed as combustion products, which can include carbon monoxide and hydrogen cyanide gas.

   a. **Carbon monoxide (CO) poisoning:** CO is a tasteless, odorless, and colorless gas formed as a byproduct of combusting organic matter. It binds to hemoglobin with 200–300 times greater affinity than oxygen, resulting in the formation of carboxyhemoglobin and compromised oxygen transport. Mild-moderate symptoms include headache, dyspnea on exertion, nausea, dizziness, altered mental status, and red-colored skin. Severe symptoms include severe headache, syncope, seizure, hallucinations, arrhythmias, and coma. Diagnosis is made by detecting an elevated percent of carboxyhemoglobin in the blood on ABG. Treatment involves high-flow oxygen, which competes with CO for hemoglobin binding. If unresponsive, consider intubation and/or hyperbaric oxygen chamber.

   b. **Hydrogen cyanide poisoning:** Can coexist with CO poisoning, especially in fires with combustion of compounds containing carbon or nitrogen (e.g., cotton, paint). Cyanide is a potent, rapid-acting poison that binds to cytochrome oxidase and inhibits mitochondrial oxidative phosphorylation and the production of ATP. This results in anaerobic metabolism and elevated lactate. Early signs include tachypnea, tachycardia, flushing, anion gap metabolic acidosis, but eventually this can lead to altered mental status, hyperreflexia, seizures, coma, hypotension, and cardiovascular collapse.

Chemical Burns

Chemical agents can cause burns in four ways: absorption through skin and mucous membranes, oral ingestion, inhalation, or a combination of these.

- *History:* Information should be sought about the specific agent, how the exposure occurred, the duration of contact, ocular involvement, and whether pre-hospital decontamination occurred.
- *Unique treatment considerations:* For chemical burns, dry chemicals should be brushed off and then continuous irrigation with large amounts of water used to dilute chemical residue. Never attempt to neutralize the chemical, due to potential generation of an exothermic reaction causing further tissue destruction.
  - **Alkali burns** result in liquefaction necrosis, which liquefies protein. This can be caused by wet cement, wax stripping agents, and anhydrous ammonia.
  - **Acid burns** lead to coagulation necrosis and protein precipitation. This can be caused by hydrochloric acid, sulfuric acid, and hydrofluoric acid
    - Hydrofluoric acid is found in many industrial settings but also in household cleaning agents. Decontamination includes removal of contaminated clothing, dilution with water, and calcium gluconate (to bind the free fluoride)
  - **Organic compounds** act as solvents on the fat in cell membranes, melting fatty tissue. This can be caused by phenols and petroleum products like gasoline.

Electrical Burns

Even if superficial tissue appears normal, electric current may still cause severe injury to deep tissues. The appearance of the contact point is not like thermal burns but instead appears blackened and dry with a hole in the skin. Cardiac arrhythmia is the most feared, immediate, and life-threatening complication. Patients may also sustain other systemic injuries that should be evaluated, including muscle necrosis, posterior shoulder dislocations, long bone fractures, and acute kidney injury.

- *History:* Information needed includes whether high- vs. low-voltage source, alternating (AC) vs. direct (DC) current and power, contact point and duration of contact, whether the patient was thrown or fell, whether there was loss of consciousness, and whether CPR was administered on the scene.
- *Important diagnostics:* ECG with 24-hour monitoring to identify cardiac arrhythmias. Continuous ECG monitoring should be maintained if arrhythmia or ectopy is identified.
- *Unique treatment considerations:* Electrical burns can cause rhabdomyolysis leading to myoglobinuria and acute kidney injury. If observed, fluids should be increased to achieve a urine output of 75–100 mL/h until the urine clears.

Radiation Burns

Injury occurs following exposure to electromagnetic waves that can ionize molecules to react with local tissue, damaging cellular DNA. There are three types of radiation injury: external without contamination, internal with contamination, or external with contamination.

- Patients with external radiation due to exposure but no contact with radionuclides are not a risk to others and no decontamination is required.
- Internal contamination can occur following inhalation, ingestion, or transdermal absorption of radioactive elements.
- If open wounds are present, decontamination is required to prevent rapid systemic absorption of radioactive elements. If radionuclide material touches external body surfaces or clothing, a hazard is created which can also affect the caregiver, and both patient and health care worker require decontamination procedures.
- While patients exposed to a radionuclide via an isolated limb are not often lethal, those who receive external total body radiation can progress to hematopoietic (0.7–10 Gy, survival is based on the magnitude of dose), GI (>10 Gy, death within 2 weeks) or neurologic syndromes (>50 Gy, death within 3 days) with mortality due to hemorrhage, infection, and cerebral edema.
- To detect radionuclide contamination, a Geiger-Mueller counter scan should be performed and patients should be considered contaminated unless there is a negative scintillation counter scan.
- Copious irrigation with water will remove most contaminants. A system for collection of the contaminated irrigation fluid is required.

CASE 16 | Burn Injury

A 59-year-old woman arrives at the ED after a house fire. She is awake but confused and disoriented, showing obvious facial burns. She complains of a severe headache and demonstrates high-pitched sounds with breathing. On exam, temperature is 38.3°C, BP 150/90 mmHg, HR 110/min, RR 26/min, and SpO$_2$ 90% on room air. She is 5 ft 5 in (1.65 m), weighs 135 lbs (61.2 kg), and has a BMI of 22.5 kg/m². She has soot at the base of her nostrils with some full-thickness burns to her face, neck, anterior aspects of torso, arms, hands, and legs.

Associated Conditions	**Inhalational injury:** Carbonaceous sputum, singed nasal hairs, facial burns, and changes in voice quality or stridor are consistent with this injury. **Carbon monoxide poisoning:** Cherry-red skin is a classic sign of CO poisoning. Patients initially present with headaches and other nonspecific constitutional symptoms.
Initial Trauma Assessment/ Management (Primary Survey)	• First address ABCDEs and protect cervical spine • Intubate and administer 100% oxygen until carboxyhemoglobin levels normalize • Insert two large-bore IVs and start IV fluids
Next Steps (Secondary Survey)	• Full history and physical examination • Monitor SpO$_2$; check CBC, BMP, PT/PTT, carboxyhemoglobin levels, lactate, urinalysis, ECG • Calculate **TBSA** • Transfer to a burn unit
Discussion	The skin provides protection from infection and injury, prevention of loss of body fluid, and regulation of body temperature. Thermal burns may occur from a flame, contact with a hot surface, or hot liquid. The most common cause of burn injuries in adults is fire while in children it is more often a scalding injury from exposure to hot water. Factors associated with the highest mortality in burn patients include age >60 years, burns >40% TBSA, and inhalational injury. Burn injuries result in release of large amounts of pro-inflammatory factors which increase vascular permeability, resulting in increased interstitial fluid ("third spacing") and insensible losses. If not addressed, this can eventually lead to hypovolemic shock. **History:** History of exposure to flames, fire, or explosion (e.g., house fire) or exposure to scalding, hot, or boiling liquids. Depending on the thickness of the burn, patients may report pain or no pain at all (see table). **Physical Exam:** Also depends on degree of burn injury as described in table above. More superficial injuries may have erythema, swelling, blisters, and tenderness. As the thickness of the burned tissue increases, the skin may appear charred, leathery, or white in appearance. Patients may also show signs of dehydration. **Assessment/Management:** **Primary Survey:** The first priority in all burn injuries should be primary survey (ABCDEs), stabilization of any identified injuries, and resuscitation with IV fluids. • *Airway maintenance with cervical spine protection*: if the patient was involved in an explosion, blast injury may have caused head and neck trauma. The patient above has signs of inhalation injury (i.e., fire in a closed space, facial burns, soot at nostrils, and stridor) and should be immediately intubated. Her decreased mental status requires imaging of the cervical spine to rule out fracture. • *Breathing and ventilation*: Following intubation, 100% oxygen should be used until carboxyhemoglobin levels are normalized. Based on this patient's history, hydroxocobalamin should be administered intravenously to prevent hemodynamic instability and cerebral edema from cyanide poisoning. Hydroxocobalamin will turn the urine dark red. • *Circulation with hemorrhage control*: The patient's blood pressure is not suggestive of hemorrhagic shock; however, continuous cardiac monitoring with pulse oximeter on an unburned extremity or ear should be initiated. Tachycardia is due to release of catecholamines, and rates >120 bpm may indicate inadequate oxygenation or unrelieved pain. Two large-bore IVs through unburned skin should be inserted. IV fluids should be given *before* calculating TBSA based on the age of the patient. Patients 14 years and older can be started on 500 mL/hr of Lactated Ringer's (LR) solution. Definitive assessment of TBSA occurs in secondary survey. Circulation compromise in a limb with a circumferential burn is suggested if there is pain, pallor, paresthesia, and, importantly, the absence of a radial or dorsalis pedis pulse by Doppler ultrasound. • *Disability and neurological deficit*: Patient was confused on admission, which suggests carbon monoxide poisoning, substance use, hypoxia, or a pre-existing medical condition. These can be investigated through the admitting trauma labs. In cases of blast injury, exam should identify gross limb deformities involving open or closed fractures. Immediate initiation of 100% oxygen is the most important treatment of CO poisoning; hyperbaric oxygen therapy (HBOT) may be considered and initiated within 6 hours in patients with neurologic deficits, unconsciousness, or cardiac ischemia.

CASE 16 | Burn Injury *(continued)*

Discussion	
	• *Exposure and environmental control*: Stop the burning process by removing all clothing, jewelry, piercings, shoes, and, in babies, diapers. If material is adherent to skin, cool the adherent material with cool water prior to removal. Remove contact lenses, which can carry adherent chemicals. Maintain core body temperature with warmed intravenous fluids.
	• *Admitting trauma labs* that should be ordered include:
	• CBC to assess hemoglobin and platelet count
	• Type and crossmatch for potential blood transfusion in preparation for burn wound debridement within 24 hours if patient is not transferred to a burn center
	• Screening for coagulopathy/DIC—PT, PTT, fibrinogen/fibrin degradation products, D-dimer, TEG (more sensitive than PT, PTT)
	• ABG may be normal in CO poisoning and only show increased carboxyhemoglobin
	• Check carboxyhemoglobin level and electrolytes to assess acid-base status
	• Serum lactate to aid in fluid resuscitation and if >4 mmol, predictive of burn sepsis
	• Urinalysis—proteinuria may indicate acute kidney injury on admission due to severe burns (>30% TBSA)
	• ECG to assess myocardial ischemia from CO poisoning
	• Ethanol and toxicology screen to investigate altered mental status
	Next Steps (Secondary Survey):
	• Obtain history of events with specific information on location of the fire, how the patient escaped, whether others were injured or killed at the scene, whether clothes caught on fire and how they were extinguished, any fuel or chemical involved (gasoline or other), and duration of smoke exposure.
	• Examine entire body, assessing for additional injuries; examine patient to determine TBSA and associated injuries:
	• Based on the "rule of nines" and the patient's full-thickness burns described above, her estimated burn size can be determined: face (4.5%) + anterior torso (18%) + both sides of her arms (9%) + both sides of her legs (9%) = 40.5%.
	• Determine depth of burn as either partial or full thickness—apply current ATLS and American Burn Association calculations for recommended volume of LR to be administered within 24 hours for any second-degree burns or higher: 2 mL × 40.5% TBSA × 61.2 kg = 4,957 mL, or approximately 5 L.
	• One-half of the total fluid volume should be administered in the first 8 hours from the time of injury and the second half in the subsequent 16 hours; however, the amount of fluid infused is adjusted according to urinary output (0.5 mL/kg/hour in adults and for young children <30 kg, 1 mL/kg/hour) and clinical response.
	• Monitor hourly vitals.
	• Insert nasogastric tube in this intubated patient.
	• Insert urinary catheter in patients with ≥20% TBSA.
	• Monitor ventilation—circumferential burns of the chest or abdomen may increase the work of breathing; escharotomy may be needed to release constriction of a circumferential chest burn.
	• Pain and anxiety management—morphine can be given for pain; benzodiazepines can be given for anxiety.
	• Image the C-spine to determine presence of fracture; if none, elevate head of bed to reduce facial and airway edema.
	• Psychosocial assessment and support for recovery.
	• Transfer to a burn unit if any of the following criteria are met: ≥10% TBSA in partial-thickness; any full-thickness burn; burns involving the face, hands, feet, genitalia, perineum, or joints; electrical or chemical burn; inhalational injury; associated traumatic injuries; or if the patient is a child.
	Additional Management: Patients with >20% TBSA demonstrate increased capillary permeability, particularly in the first 24 hours, which can lead to decreased intravascular volume. Resuscitation targets adequate perfusion using the least amount of fluid possible to avoid over-resuscitation, which can lead to compartment syndrome and acute respiratory distress. Under-resuscitation can result in shock and organ failure. Early management of the burned patient in the first few hours will affect long-term outcome and focuses on early excision and immediate coverage of the burn wounds in extensively burned patients. In general, patients with burns do not present with decompensated shock immediately after injury. If the patient presents in shock, other sources should be investigated such as hemorrhage from other injuries.
	• *Fluid management:* Monitor for electrolyte abnormalities and correct as needed: hyponatremia can result from compartmental fluid shifts, and hyperkalemia can result from the destruction of tissues and lead to cardiac conduction abnormalities.

CASE 16 | Burn Injury *(continued)*

Discussion	• *Wound management:* Local treatment of burn wounds involves cleansing, debridement, antimicrobial agents, and wound dressings. Early tangential excision of the burn eschar to viable bleeding points is performed as soon as the patient is hemodynamically stable (ideally within 24 hours post-burn) for deep partial and full-thickness burns. Skin grafting (autografting) is performed usually immediately after excision; autologous skin can be harvested for TBSA of 35% or less. • *Allografts:* For larger TBSA burns, donor sites may not be sufficient, and cadaveric cryopreserved skin or skin stored in glycerol can be used to temporarily close the wound. The temporary covering can reduce incidence of wound infection, prevent wound contracture, and decrease pain. Eventually, the allogeneic skin is rejected. Skin grafts are contraindicated if there is evidence of infection. Skin substitutes are another option for temporary coverage besides allografts.
Additional Considerations	**Burn Wound Infection:** In the first few hours after a burn the wounds are usually sterile, but by day 4–5 there is extensive bacterial colonization, hastened by the avascular nature of the burned tissue. Burn wound debridement should be done within 24 hours to prevent this. Suspect in patients with changes in their wound (e.g., color, leakage, erythema, swelling) or loss of a previously viable skin graft. Diagnosis is confirmed by a tissue biopsy with a bacterial count of ≥ 10,000 per cm squared of burn tissue. If an infection does develop, treat with antibiotics based on whether there are systemic manifestations suggestive of invasive infection. The leading cause of mortality in patients with severe burn injuries is subsequent development of **burn wound sepsis.** **Compartment Syndrome:** May occur if the eschar impedes blood flow to limb, thorax, or abdomen, and most respond by escharotomy instead of a fasciotomy to relieve pressure and restore blood flow. **Acute Kidney Injury:** May develop as a consequence of hypovolemia, hypotension, and/or associated rhabdomyolysis. Proteinuria on initial urinalyses may identify those at risk for acute kidney injury and need for early prophylactic measures such as avoidance of NSAIDs, ACEI, ARBs, and diuretics. Correct dosing of renally excreted medications and optimize intravascular volume and kidney perfusion by avoiding and rapidly treating hypovolemia, congestive cardiac failure, and sepsis. **Pediatric Considerations:** TBSA and estimated fluid requirement calculations differ in children <14 years old and infants, and corresponding guidelines and calculations should be consulted for this patient population.

GENERAL AND COLORECTAL SURGERY

General Surgery

General surgery is a central discipline of surgery involving the diagnosis, pre-operative, operative, and post-operative management of nine primary components of surgery: the alimentary tract; abdomen and its contents; breast, skin, and soft tissue; head and neck; vascular system; endocrine system; surgical oncology; comprehensive management of trauma; complete care of critically ill patients with underlying surgical conditions.

Abdominal Pain

Many conditions exist that present with abdominal pain that do not require surgery and are not classified as emergent situations. The most important method of identifying the acute abdomen is through the history. See Chapter 6 (Gastroenterology) for additional cases.

Character of abdominal pain: The abdomen has both visceral and parietal sensory networks, which sense pain differently.

Visceral pain: detected by bilateral thoracolumbar or sacral sensory afferent C fibers in the walls of hollow viscera, occurs if the hollow viscera are distended, inflamed, or ischemic; pain is organized embryologically.

- *Foregut structures,* mostly supplied by branches of the celiac trunk, include the distal end of the esophagus, stomach, duodenum, pancreas, liver, and gallbladder. and manifest as pain in the mid-epigastric region.
- *Midgut structures* supplied by branches of the superior mesenteric artery include the distal half of duodenum, jejunum, ileum, appendix, cecum, ascending colon, and proximal half of transverse colon, and manifest as pain in the periumbilical area.
- *Hindgut structures* supplied by branches of the inferior mesenteric artery include the distal half of the transverse colon, descending colon, sigmoid colon, and proximal third of the rectum, and manifest as lower abdominal or suprapubic pain.

Visceral fibers also convey hunger, thirst, and alterations in the respiratory and circulatory systems. Visceral pain, therefore, can be accompanied by autonomic responses such as sweating, pallor, nausea, GI disturbances, or vital sign changes in blood pressure, heart rate, and body temperature. The visceral peritoneum is a serous membrane that lines the internal organs inside the peritoneal space. It receives its innervation from the autonomic nervous system, including fibers from the vagus and spinal nerves. The visceral peritoneum responds to traction and pressure but not to cutting, burning, or electrostimulation.

Parietal pain is detected by both afferent C fibers and the faster, larger, A delta nerve fibers. It corresponds to the spinal nerves supplying the overlying muscle of levels T6–L1, hence pain can be localized to one of the four quadrants or the epigastric area. Helpful reference points include the umbilicus, which is supplied by T10, and the groin, supplied by L1. The parietal peritoneum is the outer layer of the peritoneum, which attaches to the abdominal and pelvic walls and is sensitive to pain, pressure, touch, friction, cutting, and temperature. It is innervated by the phrenic nerves and by the spinal and viscero-somatic nerves.

The difference in nerve supply between the inner visceral layer which wraps around the organs, and outer parietal peritoneum explains the change in pain in appendicitis or a perforated peptic ulcer. In early appendicitis, the dull pain occurs in the periumbilical area, related to stretching of the visceral peritoneum over the swollen appendix. Once inflammation involves the parietal peritoneum, the pain becomes sharp and more precisely located in the right lower quadrant. Early perforated peptic ulcer begins in the epigastrium but leaking gastric contents, as gravity forces them down along the right paracolic gutter, inflame the parietal peritoneum, leading to right lower quadrant pain.

Referred pain is believed to occur when visceral and somatic afferent innervation converge. Referred pain can present as a deep somatic pain that is often confined to the muscles but may extend superficially to the skin (see examples in figure below). Convergence of these fibers can also produce confusing pictures; for example, a patient with coronary disease and gallbladder calculi might experience more frequent attacks of angina and biliary colic due to partial overlapping of the T5 afferent pathways of the heart and gallbladder.

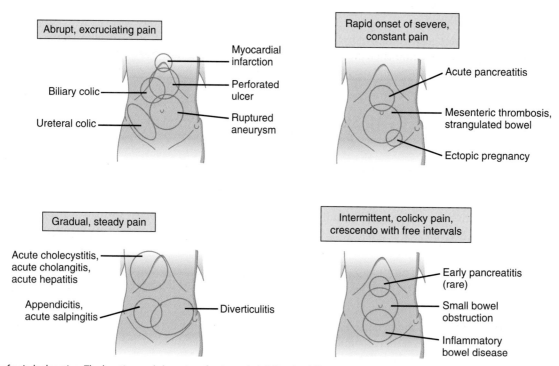

Severity of pain by location. The location and character of pain are helpful in the differential diagnosis of the acute abdomen. (Reproduced with permission from Doherty GM. Current Diagnosis & Treatment: Surgery, 15ed. New York: McGraw Hill; 2020.)

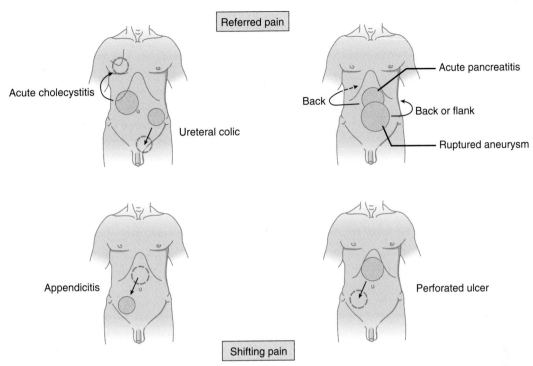

Referred pain (top) and shifting pain (bottom) in the acute abdomen. Solid circles indicate the site of maximum pain; dashed circles indicate sites of lesser pain. (Reproduced with permission from Doherty GM. Current Diagnosis & Treatment: Surgery, 15ed. New York: McGraw Hill; 2020.)

Time course of pain: Pain onset may occur within minutes, as in a ruptured aortic aneurysm or ruptured ectopic pregnancy, within 1–2 hours as observed in acute cholecystitis, acute pancreatitis, strangulated bowel, renal colic, or proximal bowel obstruction, or the pain can gradually build over time, as observed in appendicitis or diverticulitis.

Acute Abdomen

- Characterized by new-onset severe abdominal pain of less than 24 hours
- Reflects an urgent or emergent situation which demands immediate medical and surgical care
- May be caused by obstruction, infection, inflammation, or vascular occlusion

History/Physical Exam

- It is important to localize pain and inquire about characteristic features and presence of associated symptoms (e.g., fever, nausea, vomiting, hematemesis, melena, blood in stool, diarrhea, constipation).
- Concerning exam features include: fever, hypotension, tachycardia, tachypnea, absent bowel sounds, peritoneal signs (guarding, rebound tenderness). It is also important to check a rectal exam and in females a pelvic exam.
- Nonsurgical causes of acute abdomen include myocardial infarction, PE, sickle cell crisis, diabetic ketoacidosis, uremia, familial Mediterranean fever, acute intermittent porphyria.

Examples of Acute Abdomen Requiring Surgical Evaluation and Key Findings

Key Findings	Diagnoses
Acute epigastric pain, history of NSAID use or *H. pylori*, tenderness, peritoneal signs, free air on abdominal x-ray	Ruptured peptic ulcer disease
Acute chest/epigastric pain, dyspnea after violent vomiting or post EGD, free air on abdominal x-ray	Esophageal perforation (Boerhaave syndrome)
Acute RUQ pain/tenderness, positive Murphy sign, RUQ US with gallbladder wall thickening, gallstones, and pericholecystic fluid	Acute cholecystitis
RUQ pain, fevers/chills, jaundice (Charcot triad) The preceding plus mental status changes, hypotension (Reynold pentad)	Ascending cholangitis

Examples of Acute Abdomen Requiring Surgical Evaluation and Key Findings (*Continued*)

Key Findings	Diagnoses
RLQ pain, initially periumbilical pain, with positive McBurney's point sign, Rovsing's and psoas signs	Appendicitis
Severe LLQ pain, history of diverticulosis or diverticulitis, LLQ tenderness, peritoneal signs, and free air on abdominal x-ray	Ruptured sigmoid diverticulum
Severe intermittent crampy abdominal pain, vomiting, currant jelly stools, RUQ mass in children	Intussusception
Acute abdominal pain, nausea, vomiting, constipation, tender, irreducible abdominal mass	Incarcerated hernia
Acute diffuse abdominal pain, nausea, vomiting, rectal bleeding, and history of cardiac risk factors, atrial fibrillation, pain out of proportion to exam, elevated lactate	Acute mesenteric artery ischemia
Abdominal pain radiating to back; pulsatile abdominal mass and peritoneal signs	Ruptured abdominal aortic aneurysm
Acute pelvic pain, young female with adnexal tenderness, negative beta-hCG, US with enlarged ovary with decreased blood flow	Ovarian torsion
Young sexually active female, missed menses, and now with pelvic pain and adnexal tenderness, positive beta-hCG	Ectopic pregnancy
Periumbilical (Cullen sign) and flank (Turner sign) ecchymosis	Hemoperitoneum (pancreatitis, dissection)
Epigastric pain radiating to the back with history of alcohol use or gallstones or associated elevation in lipase	Acute pancreatitis

CASE 17 | Appendicitis

A 20-year-old woman presents with progressively worsening abdominal pain and nausea and vomiting for several hours. The pain started in the periumbilical area but is now in the RLQ. On physical exam, she is in moderate distress, her temperature is 38°C, BP is 100/72 mmHg, and pulse is 100/min. She has RLQ tenderness one-third of the distance from the anterior superior iliac spine and umbilicus, guarding, and rebound tenderness. She reports pain in the RLQ with palpation of LLQ and pain in the RLQ with passive extension of the right hip and active flexion of the right hip against resistance.

Conditions with Similar Presentations	**Diverticulitis:** Most commonly presents in the left colon with pain in the LLQ; however, it can present in the right colon and the RLQ if near or at the cecum. Patients are older than those with appendicitis. May also have a fever and leukocytosis similar to appendicitis.
	Inflammatory bowel disease: Can present with pain anywhere in the abdomen. Patients often have associated blood in the stool and may have history of similar presentations in the past.
	Ectopic pregnancy: Will often present with vaginal bleeding and a missed period. If the ectopic pregnancy has ruptured, the patient may be hemodynamically unstable and have peritoneal signs. Fever is not common.
	Ovarian torsion: Presents as unilateral lower quadrant pain that may be on the left or the right. It often has prodromal colicky pain that is worsened by physical activity when the ovary twists and untwists. The onset of severe, unrelenting pain indicates complete torsion and lack of blood supply. An adnexal mass may be palpable.
	Pelvic Inflammatory Disease or tuboovarian abscess: can present with RLQ pain and vaginal discharge. These patients do not usually suffer from anorexia. Vaginal exam will elicit cervical motion tenderness.
	Ureteric stones: can present with migratory abdominal pain as the stone makes it way down the ureter. Pain onset can be sudden with radiation to the flank and possibly inferiorly. There may be an association with nausea, vomiting, micro- or macrohematuria and crystals on urine analysis.
	Urinary tract infection/pyelonephritis: can present with right lower quadrant pain, high fever and costovertebral angle tenderness on exam.
Diagnostics	• Confirm diagnosis: CT scan with contrast in adults, abdominal ultrasound in children • Consider: CBC to detect leukocytosis and left shift and C-reactive protein • All females of child bearing age must have beta-hCG to rule out ectopic pregnancy
Management	• Patients should be made NPO and IV fluids started. • Empiric IV antibiotics and pain control • Appendectomy- though patients with uncomplicated, nonperforated appendicitis may be treated with IV antibiotics only.

CASE 17 | Appendicitis (continued)

Discussion	Appendicitis is caused by inflammation and infection proximal to an obstruction of the appendix by either a fecalith or lymphoid hyperplasia (children). Although the appendix was once thought to simply be a vestigial organ with primary function, it is now theorized that the appendix plays a role in maintaining the normal bacterial flora of the colon post-enteric infection.

History:
- Symptoms may be subtle at first but progressively worsen with increasing inflammation.
- Typical presentation is abdominal pain that starts in the periumbilical region (due to inflammation of the visceral peritoneum) and then migrates to the RLQ (due to inflammation of the parietal peritoneum); however, this migratory pain occurs in only about half of patients.
- Nausea and vomiting are frequent, and fever or anorexia may develop later in the course with increasing inflammation.

Physical Exam:
- Guarding and rebound tenderness may be present if the appendicitis is complicated by perforation and subsequent peritonitis.
- McBurney sign (RLQ tenderness: one-third distance from anterior superior iliac spine and umbilicus).
- Rovsing sign (pain in RLQ with palpation of LLQ), psoas sign (pain in RLQ with passive extension of the right hip and active flexion of the right hip against resistance), obturator sign (pain in the RLQ with flexion and internal rotation of the right hip), and rebound are signs of local inflammation and irritation of the peritoneum, while rigidity and diffuse abdominal pain that worsens with movement would indicate peritonitis.

Diagnostics:
- CT is the imaging modality of choice; CT shows an enlarged appendix with wall thickening and fat stranding (sign of inflammation). An appendicolith (calcified deposit) may also be seen.
- MRI or ultrasound can be used in pregnant patients, and abdominal ultrasound is typically first-line in pediatric cases to avoid radiation exposure. MRI would show a large, fluid-filled appendix.
- Patients often present with leukocytosis and a left shift, although this may not be seen early on in the disease process and is not specific.
- Beta-hCG should be routinely checked in women of child-bearing age prior to CT. Although ectopic pregnancy is on the differential at early gestational age, a positive beta-hCG does not rule out appendicitis, and ultrasound may help differentiate between the two.

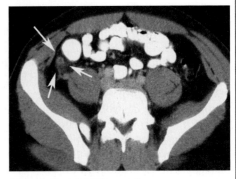

Appendicitis. Axial CT image shows hyperenhancement of the wall of the appendix and periappendiceal fat stranding (*arrows*). (Reproduced with permission from Greenberger NJ, Blumberg RS, Burakoff R. CURRENT Diagnosis & Treatment: Gastroenterology, Hepatology, & Endoscopy, 3e. Copyright 2016. McGraw-Hill Education.)

Management:
- Patients should be made NPO and IV fluids started.
- Empiric IV antibiotics (cefoxitin, cefotetan, or cefazolin and metronidazole).
- Pain control, with understanding that there is potential risk of masking peritoneal signs and increasing the chance of ruptured appendix. Pain managed with NSAIDs, acetaminophen, or opioids.
- Appendectomy (usually laparoscopic) is the most common treatment for appendicitis.
- Antibiotics alone are an effective treatment for uncomplicated, nonperforated acute appendicitis. Up to 90% of these patients will be able to avoid surgery during their hospital course. However, there is a high risk of recurrence in the following months ultimately leading to surgery |
| **Additional Considerations** | **Complications:**

Appendiceal perforation:
- If the patient is hemodynamically unstable, they should undergo immediate appendectomy.
- The patient may remain hemodynamically stable with the presence of a phlegmon or abscess. These patients may initially be treated with IV antibiotics +/- drainage by interventional radiology. Follow-up appendectomy in 6-8 weeks may be considered following clinical improvement, especially if there is concern for appendiceal neoplasm.

Obstetric Considerations: Appendicitis may have an atypical presentation during pregnancy, as the appendix is displaced by the enlarged uterus. Abdominal pain may localize to the right middle or upper quadrant or right flank as opposed to the right lower quadrant. This can result in a delayed diagnosis with increased risk of appendix rupture or intrauterine fetal demise. Appendicitis can also irritate the uterus, resulting in contractions and fetal tachycardia. |

CASE 18 | Small Bowel Obstruction (SBO)

A 50-year-old woman presents to the ED with abdominal pain, nausea, and vomiting for the past 36 hours. The abdominal pain is cramping, can be as severe as 8/10, and located mainly near the umbilicus. She has had multiple episodes of bilious, nonbloody emesis and has been unable to tolerate food. She has not passed flatus or stool since the day prior. She is relatively healthy, although did undergo open abdominal surgery for a ruptured appendix six years ago. On exam, her temperature is 37.1°C, HR 120/min, BP 125/82 mmHg, and RR 14/min. She has dry mucous membranes and has abdominal distension with a well-healed vertical incision near the umbilicus. Auscultation reveals high-pitched tinkling bowel sounds. She has mild tenderness throughout the abdomen, tympany to percussion, but there is no rebound, guarding, or rigidity. No masses or hernias are identified. Rectal examination reveals normal tone, no gross blood, no masses, and no stool in the rectal vault.

Conditions with Similar Presentations	**Gastroenteritis:** Cramping abdominal pain may be associated with nausea, vomiting, but would also have diarrhea. Exam may show poorly localized tenderness without guarding. May have history of recent travel, sick contacts, new foods, or other viral illnesses.
	Acute pancreatitis: Epigastric pain radiating to the back with tenderness in the epigastrium. It may present with localized ileus around the inflamed pancreas. X-ray may show a dilated loop of transverse colon, called the colon cut-off sign.
	Paralytic ileus: Distension with no localized tenderness. May be associated with recent surgery, narcotic use, hypokalemia.
	Large bowel obstruction: Gradually increasing abdominal pain, abdominal distension, obstipation; vomiting may be feculent.
	Ischemic or strangulated bowel: May not be distended until late in the course; severe pain; may have scant rectal bleeding.
	Intraabdominal hemorrhage: Distension associated with pallor, shock; pulsatile mass (if due to aortic aneurysm), or lower quadrant mass (if due to ectopic pregnancy); may have scant rectal bleeding.

Initial Diagnostic Tests	• Abdominal series to look for dilated loops of bowel and air-fluid levels and rule out free air in the peritoneum
	• Also check: CBC, BMP, liver transaminases, lipase
	• Consider:
	  • Abdominal and pelvic CT with oral and/or IV contrast if abdominal series is inconclusive or more information is needed
	  • Arterial blood gas, serum lactate if intestinal ischemia is suspected

Next Steps in Management	• **Adhesive SBO:** Nonoperative management—gastric decompression, bowel rest, correct electrolyte abnormalities • **Bowel obstruction with intestinal ischemia:** Urgent surgical exploration • **Malignant SBO:** See below
Discussion	Bowel obstruction occurs when the normal flow of intraluminal contents is interrupted. A SBO can be caused by an intraluminal mass (e.g., tumor) or extrinsic compression or kinking of the bowel (e.g., adhesive disease, hernia). Gas and fluid accumulate proximal to the site of obstruction, causing dilation of the bowel followed by increased motility in attempt to overcome the obstruction. This increased peristaltic activity is the cause of the characteristic colicky pain which increases to a severe peak with sudden release of pain. The small bowel distension stretches visceral peritoneum, which results in autonomic stimulation with progressive nausea and emesis. Failure to pass gas (obstipation) or stool per rectum is often caused by a complete mechanical obstruction. The most common etiology for SBO in the United States is prior abdominal surgery leading to adhesions. Hernias are the most common cause of SBO worldwide. Other common causes of small bowel obstruction include hernias with bowel incarceration and neoplasms (intrinsic or extrinsic). Less common causes include Crohn's disease, gallstone ileus, fecal impaction, intussusception (common in children), volvulus (rare), and inflammatory stricture (radiation, IBD, diverticulitis). **History:** • Most commonly presents with acute onset colicky abdominal pain, nausea, vomiting, and constipation. • History of prior pelvic or abdominal surgery (adhesive SBO) or recent surgery (ileus, functional SBO). • Severe abdominal pain is suggestive of a complicated or strangulated SBO, in which vascular perfusion is impaired. **Physical Exam:** • Fever: suggests gangrenous bowel. • Bowel sounds are initially increased and have a high-pitched, tinkling sound. However, over time intestinal motility decreases and bowel sounds diminish. In the presence of intestinal ischemia or perforated bowel, sounds may be absent. • Inspection: Distension is minimal in a proximal obstruction but more pronounced in a distal obstruction.

CASE 18 | Small Bowel Obstruction (SBO) *(continued)*

Discussion	• Percussion: Tympany near midline suggests air trapped within distended bowel loops. • Palpation: Examine for incisional, umbilical, groin, or other hernias • Guarding or rigidity is an indication of peritoneal irritation and requires urgent exploration. **Diagnostics:** • Abdominal series (upright chest radiograph to look for free air, upright abdominal radiograph to look for air-fluid levels, and supine abdominal radiograph to look for distension and dilation of bowel). Classic radiographic findings include dilated loops of bowel and air-fluid levels in the small bowel proximal to the obstruction with collapsed colon devoid of gas distal to the obstruction (see image below). • Abdominal and pelvic CT with oral and/or IV contrast if x-rays are inconclusive or additional information is needed. 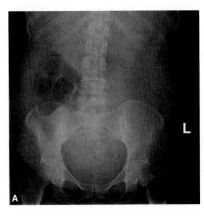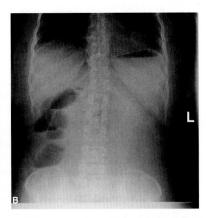 Small bowel obstruction. Plain radiographs (A) supine, which show dilated loops of small bowel in the right upper quadrant; (B) erect, which confirm the presence of air-fluid level in the loops of small bowel as well as the stomach, consistent with small bowel obstruction. (Reproduced with permission from Brunicardi F, Andersen DK, Billiar TR, Dunn DL, Kao LS, Hunter JG, Matthews JB, Pollock RE. Schwartz's Principles of Surgery, 11e. Copyright 2019 McGraw-Hill Education.) • Also check**:** CBC, CMP, serum lactate to assess degree of volume depletion. Hypochloremic, hypokalemic metabolic alkalosis (a result of repeat bouts of emesis with loss of hydrochloric acid) with elevated serum lactate and hyponatremia may indicate bowel ischemia and a complicated SBO. **Management:** • Fluid resuscitation**:** Restoration of intravascular volume and renal perfusion along with correction of electrolyte abnormalities can facilitate resolution. Significantly ill patients should receive an indwelling catheter to monitor hourly urine output. • Early placement of a nasogastric tube to evacuate air and fluid will allow for gastric decompression and a decrease in nausea, vomiting, distension, and the risk of aspiration. **Adhesive SBO:** Nonoperative management includes gastric decompression, bowel rest, correct electrolyte derangements such as hypokalemia and hypomagnesemia; nonoperative management can be effective in 70–90% of patients with adhesive small bowel obstruction in which the lumen is occluded in a single place. **Bowel obstruction with intestinal ischemia:** May occur with a closed-loop obstruction in which the intestinal lumen is occluded in two places. Fever, leukocytosis, and elevated lactic acid are indicators of gangrenous bowel and need for urgent exploration; peritoneal signs (rebound, guarding, rigidity) will develop following perforation. **Malignant SBO:** More common in elderly patients; survival is less than 6 months. Nonoperative management has high failure rate. Palliative option may include percutaneous decompressing jejunostomy. In peritoneal carcinomatosis, operative intervention provides little or no relief and often leads to prolonged hospitalization and re-obstruction; surgery is not recommended.

CASE 18 | Small Bowel Obstruction (SBO) *(continued)*

Additional Considerations	**Complications:** Include aspiration, bowel necrosis and perforation, short bowel syndrome (if excessive bowel is necrotic and requires resection), intraabdominal abscess, or surgical site infection
	Pediatric Considerations: Causes of bowel obstruction in the pediatric population differ from that in adults. In neonates, causes include congenital intestinal atresia, Hirschsprung's disease, malrotation, meconium ileus, patent vitellointestinal duct, and imperforate anus. In older children, the mnemonic "AIM" can be used: "A" includes appendicitis and adhesions, "I" includes intussusception, inguinal hernias, inflammatory bowel disease, ingested foreign body, or iatrogenic causes, and "M" includes Meckel's diverticulum and malrotation with midgut volvulus.
	Other Considerations: Following gastric bypass surgery, the most common cause of SBO is an internal hernia.

CASE 19 | Sigmoid Volvulus

An 85-year-old man with diabetes and Alzheimer's disease presents to the ED with lower abdominal pain and distention for 1 day. His caregiver reports that his last bowel movement was 48 hours ago. His temperature is 37.1°C, pulse is 90/min, respirations are 16/min, and blood pressure is 135/70 mmHg. On exam, the abdomen is distended, tender to palpation in the left lower quadrant, with decreased bowel sounds and no guarding or rigidity.

Conditions with Similar Presentations	**Small bowel obstruction:** presents with abdominal pain, distention, and constipation, but more commonly has nausea and vomiting. Focal tenderness in the left lower quadrant would not be seen. Common risk factors include abdominal surgery or hernias.
	Colonic pseudo-obstruction (Ogilvie Syndrome): Seen most often in debilitated, elderly hospitalized patients in the setting of recent surgery, severe infection, cardiovascular disease, electrolyte abnormalities, and/or medications (e.g., opioids, anticholinergics). Will also present with diffuse abdominal pain, nausea, vomiting, abdominal distention, but lacks mechanical obstruction. Patients may also continue to pass gas. Abdominal X-ray shows a diffusely dilated colon.
	Severe constipation: May present similarly with diffuse abdominal, pain, nausea, and vomiting with abdominal distension on exam; however, patients would not have focal left quadrant tenderness. Patients may also continue to pass gas.
	Rectal cancer: Most often presents with blood per rectum and/or abdominal pain. Additional symptoms can include diminished stool caliber, pain with defecation, constipation, and mucous discharge.
Initial Diagnostic Tests	• Check upright abdominal x-ray to rule out or perforation and confirm diagnosis: May see classic "coffee bean" sign • Consider: CT abdomen and pelvis with IV contrast to rule out ischemia
Next Steps in Management	• If hemodynamically stable and no imaging evidence of perforation or ischemia: flexible sigmoidoscopy for detorsion and to assess bowel viability • If hemodynamically unstable or imaging/endoscopy shows evidence of perforation or bowel ischemia: emergent resection of affected colon
Discussion	Volvulus is the twisting of the colon around its mesentery. This is caused by a redundant segment of colon twisting around its mesenteric axis causing compromised blood supply to the colon.
	Sigmoid volvulus most commonly occurs in men >70 years old. Common risk factors include diabetes, neuropsychiatric disorders, institutionalization, and chronic constipation. It rarely occurs in children; however, some risk factors in younger patients include megacolon due to Hirschsprung or Chagas disease.
	In contrast, **cecal volvulus** occurs in the second or third decade of life, can either be due to a clockwise axial rotation of the cecum alone or a counterclockwise rotation in combination with the ileum. Unlike sigmoid volvulus which can be treated via sigmoidoscopy, a cecal volvulus usually requires operative intervention.
	History: Patients present with lower abdominal pain/cramping, distention, and constipation. If there is perforation, patients have severe, sudden-onset pain. Risk factors are a history of diabetes and chronic constipation.
	Physical Exam: On exam, patients will have abdominal tenderness most severe in the LLQ, distention, tympany, and decreased bowel sounds. If there is perforation or ischemia, patients may have signs of sepsis (fever, hypotension, and tachycardic) with presence of peritoneal signs such as guarding and rigidity.

CASE 19 | Sigmoid Volvulus *(continued)*

Discussion	**Diagnostics:**
	• Initial diagnostic test is an upright abdominal x-ray to rule out perforation or obstruction. Upright abdominal x-ray: may see "coffee bean" sign (large, dilated colon in inverted U-shape pointing to the pelvis), colonic dilation with loss of haustrations, ascending and transverse colon may be dilated.
	• Consider: CT abdomen and pelvis with IV contrast to rule out ischemia and confirm diagnosis. Confirmatory imaging is with abdominal CT scan, which will show a dilated proximal colon, transition zone, and absence of air in distal colon.
	Management:
	• If hemodynamically stable and there is no imaging evidence of perforation or ischemia, flexible sigmoidoscopy should be performed immediately for detorsion, restoration of blood supply, and to assess bowel viability.
	• Following detorsion, repeat abdominal x-ray should be obtained to assess for successful reduction and absence of perforation from the procedure.
	• If hemodynamically unstable or there is imaging/endoscopic evidence of perforation or bowel, there should be emergent resection of the affected colon.
	• Recurrence of volvulus is common. An elective sigmoid resection can be considered a few days after endoscopic detorsion to prevent recurrence; for these patients it is important to decompress bowels to maximize the chance of a primary anastomosis
Additional Considerations	**Complications:** Complications of sigmoid volvulus include bowel wall perforation and ischemia.

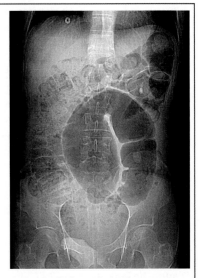

Sigmoid volvulus with the characteristic radiologic appearance of a "bent inner tube," also referred to as the "coffee bean sign." (Reproduced with permission from oscalzo J, Fauci A, Kasper D, Hauser S, Longo D, Jameson J. Harrison's Principles of Internal Medicine, 21e. Copyright 2022 McGraw-Hill Education.)

Mini-Case

Superior Mesenteric Artery (SMA) Syndrome	**Hx:** • Postprandial epigastric pain, nausea, vomiting, loss of appetite, and/or weight loss. • Symptoms usually chronic with intermittent exacerbations. • May have prior history of weight loss from other illnesses such as anorexia nervosa, cancer, or malabsorptive disorder. • Symptoms may also occur after a corrective surgery for scoliosis due to anatomical changes. **PE:** • Epigastric tenderness, distention, and/or succussion splash. • Typically underweight. **Diagnostics:** • An upper GI series will show dilation of first and second parts of the duodenum and delay in transit through the duodenum. • An abdominal ultrasound or CT can also be used to assess the aortomesenteric angle and the aortomesenteric distance. **Management:** • Initial management is conservative, with fluid and electrolyte correction, nasogastric tube, and increasing nutrition. • May improve with smaller, more frequent meals and changing positions after eating to left lateral decubitus or knee to chest. • Surgery is considered when nonoperative treatment fails, and includes duodenojejunostomy or mobilization of the duodenum and re-positioning to the right of the SMA (Strong's procedure). **Discussion:** SMA syndrome is a rare cause of GI obstruction. It is caused by the compression of the third part of the duodenum between the aorta and the SMA. It is typically seen in patients with decreased mesenteric fat due to weight loss. Corrective surgery for scoliosis is also a cause due to decreased aortomesenteric angle, and it will typically present within the first post-operative week.

CASE 20 | Acute Mesenteric Ischemia

A 70-year-old woman with diabetes, coronary artery disease, and atrial fibrillation presents with severe diffuse abdominal pain for 3 hours. She has had intermittent, cramping abdominal pain for the past several months. These episodes occur 20 minutes after meals and are associated with some nausea and occasional vomiting, and subside after 30 minutes. She has had decreased foot intake and weight loss. Medications are metformin, atorvastatin, metoprolol, and rivaroxaban, which she takes intermittently. Her temperature is 37.5°C, pulse is 100/min and irregularly irregular, respirations are 20/min, and blood pressure is 110/70 mmHg. On exam, the abdomen is soft and nontender with no guarding or rigidity, and blood is present on rectal exam.

Conditions with Similar Presentations	**Small bowel obstruction:** Presents with acute abdominal pain, distention, constipation, but would not expect history of intermittent pain after meals. **Ischemic colitis or colonic ischemia:** Patients may present with crampy abdominal pain and hematochezia. The splenic flexure and the rectosigmoid junction are areas of high risk and are referred to as watershed areas (receive dual blood supply from the most *distal* branches of two large *arteries* (i.e., SMA and IMA). In the case of severe hypoperfusion, blood supply through these end arteries becomes insufficient). Mucosal edema/hemorrhage may show thumbprint sign on imaging. **Abdominal aortic aneurysm (AAA):** Often asymptomatic unless it becomes very large or ruptures. Pain with AAA radiates to the back, and a pulsating abdominal mass may be palpated. A bedside ultrasound can be used to quickly assess for an AAA.
Initial Diagnostic Tests	• CT angiogram (CTA) of abdomen • Consider abdominal x-ray to rule out obstruction and CBC, lactate, CMP
Next Steps in Management	Exploratory laparotomy and revascularization
Discussion	**Chronic mesenteric ischemia** may progress to acute mesenteric ischemia if not treated. It is caused by atherosclerosis and involves arterial stenosis or occlusion of multiple vessels such as the superior mesenteric and inferior mesenteric arteries. Symptoms result from inadequate intestinal blood flow, especially during increased demand for blood flow after eating. Acute thrombosis, embolism, or low blood-flow states can cause **acute mesenteric ischemia**. CT with contrast or MR angiogram can identify atherosclerosis and partial or complete occlusion of vessels of the intestines: • *Celiac artery:* Supplies blood to the foregut—liver (common hepatic artery), stomach (left gastric artery), abdominal esophagus, spleen (splenic artery), and portions of the duodenum and pancreas. • *Superior mesenteric artery (SMA):* Supplies blood to the midgut—distal duodenum through much of the transverse colon and pancreas. • *Inferior mesenteric artery (IMA):* Supplies blood to the hindgut—colon from splenic flexure to upper rectum. **History/Physical Exam:** • Severe, acute abdominal pain with nonfocal or minimal findings on abdominal exam (pain out of proportion to exam) and may have "currant jelly" stools. • Risk factors include cardiac arrhythmia (atrial fibrillation), valvular heart disease, recent MI, endocarditis, heart failure (low-flow states), known atherosclerosis (coronary artery disease, TIA/stroke, peripheral arterial disease) and patients of older age. **Diagnostics:** • Metabolic acidosis and elevated lactic acid • May also have leukocytosis • Confirm with CTA or MRA of abdomen • Gold standard is angiography if other imaging nondiagnostic **Management:** • Hemodynamically unstable, critically ill patients with peritonitis and/or evidence of bowel infarction on imaging should undergo immediate **exploratory laparotomy** to determine intestinal viability. Signs of bowel viability are pink intestinal color, strong peristalsis, and a palpable mesenteric arterial pulsation. • In patients without peritonitis, immediate **revascularization** via open embolectomy (if embolus is present) with bypass graft or endovascular thrombolysis is indicated. • In addition, all patients should be started on broad-spectrum antibiotics and anticoagulation (if not actively bleeding) to reduce the risk of clot expansion.
Additional Considerations	**Complications:** Acute mesenteric ischemia is a life-threatening emergency that can lead to bowel necrosis, sepsis, and death if timely revascularization is not performed.

Hernia

Hernias are defined as an abnormal protrusion of tissue or organs through a defect in a surrounding wall. In the abdominal wall, defects can occur congenitally in the inguinal, femoral, umbilical, linea alba or lower portion of the semilunar line or they can occur iatrogenically at sites of incisions or stoma sites. Conditions that increase intra-abdominal pressure such as COPD with a chronic cough, chronic constipation, or prostatism, can worsen abdominal wall hernias. Within the abdomen, hernias can occur internally through acquired mesenteric defects, or following prior surgery like gastric bypass. While internal hernias only make up 5% of all small bowel obstructions, delay in detection due to nonspecific clinical presentation can result in over 50% mortality.

Inguinal hernia repair is the most common elective surgical procedure performed in the United States and Europe. If asymptomatic and reducible, no surgical repair is required. Surgery is required if the hernia becomes painful, **incarcerated** (when the hernia contents are not reducible), or **strangulated** (when the blood supply to the hernia contents has been compromised and the contents are at risk for or have become ischemic). Post repair, surgical complications can include short-term and long-term effects (see table).

Post-Surgical Acute Complication	Post-Surgical Late Complications
Surgical site infection	Chronic groin pain
Hematoma	Neuralgia: ilioinguinal (anterior thigh numbness), iliohypogastric (suprapubic, gluteal skin), or genitofemoral n (upper thigh, scrotum)
Urinary retention	Recurrence

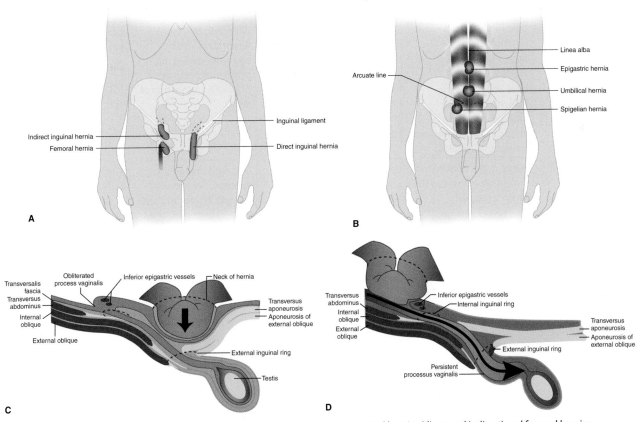

Anatomy of different types of hernias. A. Common types of groin hernias include inguinal hernias (direct and indirect) and femoral hernias. B. Anterior abdominal wall (ventral) hernias include epigastric, umbilical, and Spigelian hernias. C. Direct inguinal hernias form medial to the inferior epigastric vessels and go through the external (superficial) inguinal ring only. D. Indirect inguinal hernias form lateral to the inferior epigastric vessels and go through both the internal (deep) and external (superficial) inguinal rings. (Reproduced with permission from Tintinalli JE, Ma O, Yealy DM, Meckler GD, Stapczynski J, Cline DM, Thomas SH. Tintinalli's Emergency Medicine: A Comprehensive Study Guide, 9ed. New York: McGraw Hill; 2020.)

Presentation and Differential Diagnoses of Hernias

Hernia	Presentation	Anatomy	Pathophysiology	Differential Diagnosis
Indirect inguinal (most common type of hernia in men and women)	Bulge in groin with heaviness or dull discomfort; worse with straining, prolonged standing, or heavy lifting More common in men and on right side of body; often congenital and can occur in infants and adults	Bowel enters the internal (deep) inguinal ring lateral to the inferior epigastric vessels, goes through the inguinal canal and external (superficial) inguinal ring, into the groin. Follows pathway of testicular descent and is covered by all three layers of spermatic fascia	Failure of closure of the processus vaginalis	Hydrocele Varicocele Undescended testes Epididymitis Lipoma Hematoma Abscess Lymphadenopathy Lymphoma Femoral artery aneurysm or pseudoaneurysm
Direct inguinal	Bulge in groin with heaviness or dull discomfort; worse with straining, prolonged standing, or heavy lifting Most often occurs in older men	Protrudes through the inguinal (Hesselbach) triangle, directly through parietal peritoneum medial to the inferior epigastric vessels and lateral to the rectus abdominis. Only goes through the external (superficial) inguinal ring and is covered by external spermatic fascia only	Acquired weakness of transversalis fascia or floor of the inguinal canal, acquired with age and related to physical activity	Similar to indirect inguinal hernia above
Femoral	Bule inferior to inguinal ligament More common in women, typically later in life, and more likely to present with incarceration or strangulation compared to inguinal hernias	Sac protrudes below the inguinal ligament, through the femoral canal, bounded superiorly by the iliopubic tract and Cooper's ligament, laterally by the femoral vein, and medially by the lacunar ligament	Widening of the femoral ring due to aging, following injury, from prior pregnancy or prior inguinal hernia repair	Lymphadenopathy Ectopic testis Distended psoas bursa Hip joint effusion
Abdominal wall (ventral)	Bulge in the abdominal wall in areas besides the inguinal region Can be congenital (umbilical, epigastric), iatrogenic (incisional, port site, parastomal)	*Umbilical*: defect where umbilical structures enter abdominal wall during embryogenesis *Epigastric*: defect in linea alba superior to umbilicus *Incisional*: most common, deep to surgical scar *Spigelian*: caudal end of semilunar line at lateral edge of rectus muscle, below umbilicus *Port site*: Fascial defect from laparoscopic port site *Parastomal*: Defect through ostomy site	Depends on specific subtype. For incisional hernias, higher risk with wound infection, age, obesity, malnutrition	Tumor Rectus sheath hematoma Eventration Enlarged abdominal vessels
Internal	Vague epigastric pain, nausea, vomiting, recurrent signs and symptoms of intestinal obstruction; do not have an external bulge	Sac protrudes through any normal or abnormal peritoneal or mesenteric aperture within the confines of the peritoneal cavity.	Weak intestinal or other abdominal tissue wall, named based on tissues involved (typically involving bowel loops)	Tumor Adhesions Gallstone ileus

CASE 21 | Strangulated Inguinal Hernia

A 56-year-old man presents to the ED with severe abdominal pain for 3 hours with associated nausea and vomiting. He endorses the presence of a bulge in his right groin over the past 6 months. It is usually soft and easily pushed back in, but this morning it was hard and would not go back in. His temperature is 38.6°C, pulse 115 bpm and BP 87/59 mmHg. He is diaphoretic. The skin surrounding the right groin mass is erythematous and he has pain with palpation of the mass. There is no rebound or guarding.

Conditions with Similar Presentations	**Testicular torsion:** Most common in teenage boys. Presents with acute unilateral testicular pain, may have a high riding testicle and absent cremasteric reflex on exam. **Hydrocele:** Painless collection of fluid around the testes; some hydroceles can communicate with the peritoneal fluid or form cysts within the spermatic cord that can manifest as groin swelling which transilluminates. **Epididymitis:** Inflammation results in warm, red, swollen testes which is tender to palpation posterior to it. Elevation of the testes relieves the pain. **Lipoma of the spermatic cord:** Herniated fat that is located posterior to the internal spermatic fascia and protrudes through the internal ring lateral to the spermatic cord. It can present as a painless groin mass that does not transilluminate. **Hematoma of the groin:** Can be caused by trauma, procedures that include femoral artery canulation, or aneurysms. Treatment is elevation, ice, and compression with analgesia; aneurysms, however, must be repaired. **Lymphadenopathy:** May present as a discrete mass or masses in the groin which may be a sign of sexually transmitted infections or malignancy. **Femoral artery aneurysm or pseudoaneurysm:** Caused by atherosclerotic disease or trauma, typically presents as a pulsatile mass in the groin.
Initial Diagnostic Tests	• Clinical diagnosis • CT abdomen and pelvis with contrast will help confirm diagnosis and type of hernia • Consider: Ultrasound
Next Steps in Management	• Empiric antibiotics covering enteric bacteria • Fluid resuscitation • Emergent surgery
Discussion	Inguinal hernias can be either direct or indirect and should also be differentiated from femoral hernias (see mini-cases below). Strangulation of hernia contents occurs when the hernia is trapped in the abdominal wall defect, causing diminished venous and lymphatic flow. This causes edema of the hernia contents, which further disrupts the vasculature supplying the trapped structures. Subsequently, if the arterial flow is compromised, the contents become ischemic. Incarcerated hernias are at risk of progressing to strangulation. Other risk factors include small defects and femoral hernias. Only about 0.3–3% of groin hernias become incarcerated or strangulated each year. **History:** Patients may or may not have a known history of hernia/groin mass on presentation. However, a history of a previously reducible hernia that is now irreducible, painful, and hard are hallmarks of strangulation. Obstructive symptoms include abdominal pain, nausea, and vomiting, and are acute in onset. Further obstructive symptoms such as constipation may occur if bowel obstruction has occurred. **Physical Exam:** Strangulated hernias are irreducible, hard/edematous, and exhibit pain with palpation. Patients do not initially present with peritoneal signs, as the strangulated loop of bowel is within the hernia sac. However, patients may eventually have peritoneal signs if the bowel perforates and there is spillage of hernia contents into the abdomen. Bowel sounds may be high-pitched or decreased, depending on the level and duration of obstruction. **Diagnostics:** • Strangulated hernias can be diagnosed clinically: hard, irreducible, tender inguinal/scrotal mass on physical exam • If the diagnosis is unclear and the patient is hemodynamically stable, a CT can help confirm the diagnosis and give anatomic information for surgical planning. • Ultrasound of the groin may also visualize the hernia and may be beneficial if testicular torsion is on the differential.

CASE 21 | Strangulated Inguinal Hernia *(continued)*

Discussion	**Management:** • Patients with strangulated hernias should undergo emergent surgery. • Laparotomy or laparoscopic approach may be utilized. If the patient is exhibiting signs of infection, bowel necrosis, or perforation, mesh should not be used to repair the defect, as it may seed bacteria. A tissue repair should be used. • These patients should also be started on empiric antibiotics covering enteric bacteria. • If there are clinical signs of obstruction, an NGT should be placed.
Additional Considerations	Nonincarcerated femoral hernias should be repaired electively, as they are at higher risk for strangulation than inguinal hernias.

Uncomplicated Groin Hernia Mini-Cases

Case	Key Findings
Inguinal Hernia (Direct and Indirect)	**Hx:** Symptomatic patients present with pain that is worse with Valsalva and improves after lying down. They may report the presence of a bulge in their groin/testicles. **PE:** For men, patient should be standing during the exam. The examiner's index finger should track with the spermatic cord, starting at the lateral testicle into the inguinal canal. For women, direct palpation of the groin should be done. A soft, reducible mass in the groin can be palpated. The edges of defect may be distinguishable. **Diagnostics:** • Inguinal hernias usually can be diagnosed clinically in men but may be more difficult in women. • If the diagnosis is unclear clinically, a groin ultrasound can be performed. • Direct vs. indirect inguinal hernias cannot be reliably distinguished on exam. **Management:** • Patients can undergo elective surgical repair. • A strategy of watching and waiting may be elected if patients are asymptomatic. **Discussion:** **Direct inguinal hernias** are due to a defect in the abdominal wall medial to the inferior epigastric vessels and superior to the inguinal ligament. They are more common in middle-aged or older men and are often right sided. **Indirect inguinal hernias** protrude through the internal inguinal ring. The hernia sac therefore originates lateral to the inferior epigastric vessels and superior to the inguinal ligament. Indirect inguinal hernias are common in young boys due to a patent processus vaginalis but also manifest in adults due to increased intraabdominal pressure.
Femoral Hernia	**Hx:** Symptoms similar to inguinal hernias. Patients are more likely to be women, in contrast to inguinal hernias. **PE:** A mass may be palpated in the groin or medial thigh in the case of femoral hernia. **Diagnostics:** Diagnosis is identical to direct inguinal hernia. If ultrasound is not definitive, MRI can be considered. **Management:** Elective surgery should be offered to all patients with femoral hernias as these are at higher risk for complications including incarceration and strangulation (see case above). **Discussion:** Femoral hernias are due to a defect in the abdominal wall inferior to the inguinal ligament. As most groin hernias in women are femoral in origin, women with a hernia in the groin should undergo surgical repair.

Common Esophageal Conditions

A patient with esophageal disease will often present with dysphagia, odynophagia, and/or gastroesophageal reflux. See Chapter 6 (Gastroenterology) for additional discussion.

Esophageal Conditions	Medical and Surgical Management
GERD/reflux esophagitis	Gastroesophageal reflux disease (GERD): Most common esophageal condition and affects >20% of adults and 7–20% of the pediatric population. • Medical management includes lifestyle modifications (e.g., avoid dietary triggers, weight loss), and acid-suppressing medications (e.g., antacids, H2 blockers, proton pump inhibitors) • For patients with severe symptoms who fail medical management for GERD, surgery is used to recreate the lower esophageal sphincter (LES) by wrapping the fundus of the stomach completely (Nissen) or partially (Toupet) around the lower esophagus. • A **Nissen fundoplication** procedure is the most common procedure and is most often performed laparoscopically or robotically. Post-operative symptoms of dysphagia and bloating can occur as well as gastroparesis secondary to vagal nerve injury. • If esophagitis is not recognized early, it can progress to fibrosis and strictures that may necessitate surgical intervention. The most common treatment for strictures involves dilation of the affected esophagus via insertion of a balloon that expands in size once placed, or placement of progressively larger dilators. In the case of complex strictures, esophageal stents can be placed to further prop open fibrosed areas of the esophagus. • Serial endoscopic surveillance for Barrett esophagus (every 1–3 years) to identify dysplasia even if reflux is treated, because dysplasia must be treated with either endoscopic ablation or resection or surgical excision
Motility disorders (achalasia)	• Medical management to decrease the pressure of the lower esophageal sphincter (LES) includes calcium channel blockers, botulinum toxin injection, and/or pneumatic dilation. • If medical treatment fails, the most common surgical treatment is the **Heller myotomy**, most often performed laparoscopically. The surgeon cuts the muscle fibers of the LES to weaken it and alleviate dysphagia symptoms. • Two less invasive procedural treatments include balloon dilation and peroral endoscopic myotomy (POEM). In balloon dilation, the patient swallows a collapsed balloon that is guided via fluoroscopic x-ray imaging down to the LES. It is then gradually inflated. In POEM, a small electrical scalpel is passed through an endoscope to create cuts in the muscle layer. • Since all three of the above procedural options are essentially different techniques that aim to therapeutically destroy the LES muscle fibers, the most common complication is acid refluxing from the stomach into the esophagus. • To prevent post-operative reflux, most surgeons will simultaneously perform a Nissen fundoplication.
Diverticula	Diverticula are epithelial-lined pouches that may include all layers (true diverticulum) or a subset of layers (pseudo-diverticullum) which protrude out of the esophageal lumen • Zenker diverticulum, the most common diverticulum of the esophagus, is a pulsion diverticulum caused by increased intraluminal pressure creating an outpouching between the thyropharyngeus and cricopharyngeus muscles. Patients present with dysphagia, regurgitation of undigested food, gurgling in the throat, and fetid breath. A barium swallow confirms the diagnosis and treatment is a myotomy of the cricopharyngeus along with a diverticulectomy. • Epiphrenic diverticula are rare, pulsion-type diverticula found in the distal 10 cm of the esophagus and often associated with motility disorders. Patients present with dysphagia, retrosternal chest pain, and regurgitation. If symptoms are significant, these are also treated by myotomy and diverticulectomy. • Traction diverticula are true diverticula that can secondary to a malignancy or parabronchial secondary to TB, mediastinal granulomatosis, or histoplasmosis
Benign tumors	May cause dysphagia; the most common tumor is a leiomyoma, which occurs in the distal third of the intramural esophagus causing dysphagia, odynophagia, regurgitation, and heartburn. Barium swallow can localize the lesion, which can be biopsied via endoscopic ultrasound followed by surgical enucleation or resection.

(Continued)

Esophageal Conditions	Medical and Surgical Management
Esophageal cancer	Patients with adenocarcinoma and squamous cell carcinoma of the esophagus are managed similarly. **Esophagogastroduodenoscopy (EGD)** is used to directly visualize and biopsy lesions; transesophageal ultrasound and chest/abdominal CT are used to stage the tumor. Resection is the preferred treatment for locally invasive cancers, while unresectable cancers are managed with a combination of chemotherapy, radiation, and palliative stenting. In cases of late-presenting cancer (as is often the case with squamous cell carcinoma), resection often involves nearby structures, such as portions of the pharynx, larynx, and thyroid gland.
Hiatal Hernia	

Type	Description	Management
I	GE junction slides into chest due to weakening of the phrenoesophageal ligament	Most can be managed medically for reflux
II	Fundus herniates into chest but GE Junction does not	Types II-IV are paraesophageal. If symptomatic, these should be repaired surgically especially those with bleeding, acute obstructive symptoms (progressive chest pain, unproductive retching, epigastric distention), and gastric strangulation
III	Combination of type I & II	
IV	Giant structures other than stomach herniate into the chest	

Type I: Sliding Hernia. (Reproduced with permission from Doherty GM. Current Diagnosis & Treatment: Surgery, 15ed. New York: McGraw Hill; 2020.)

Paraesophageal hernia. (Reproduced with permission from Doherty GM. Current Diagnosis & Treatment: Surgery, 15ed. New York: McGraw Hill; 2020.)

CASE 22 | Hiatal Hernia

A 47-year-old woman presents with worsening heartburn over the past 10 years. She was diagnosed with GERD 10 years ago and started on a proton pump inhibitor (PPI) without full resolution of symptoms. She often uses antacids after large meals and prior to bedtime. Over the last 3 months she has had worsening of these symptoms, including new onset of pain in her mid-chest with swallowing. On exam, her BMI is 39 kg/m^2 and she has mild epigastric tenderness to palpation. Barium swallow study shows a 3-cm separation between the diaphragmatic hiatus and top of the mucosal stomach folds. Upper endoscopy has similar findings with the diaphragmatic indentation seen 3 cm distal to the squamocolumnar junction (z-line) with evidence of esophagitis in the lower esophagus.

Conditions with Similar Presentations	**Uncomplicated GERD:** Presents with heartburn but usually resolves with antacids, H2 blockers, or PPIs. GERD is due to an incompetent lower esophageal sphincter rather than displacement of the stomach upward. (See table above for other possibilities.)
Initial Diagnostic Tests	Confirm diagnosis with barium contrast swallow study or upper endoscopy

CASE 22 | Hiatal Hernia *(continued)*

Next Steps in Management	• Lifestyle changes • Medical management of GERD • Surgical treatment with an anti-reflux procedure if symptoms persist despite medical management with a type I hernia or if symptoms are present with types II–IV hernias
Discussion	A hiatal hernia occurs when the stomach herniates through the diaphragmatic hiatus into the thorax. Incidence is positively correlated with age and is often associated with obesity. Prevalence is difficult to determine due to the asymptomatic course in many patients. There are four types of hiatal hernias (see table above). The majority (>90%) of hiatal hernias are type I (sliding) and can be managed medically. For those patients that fail medical management, surgery can improve quality of life and improve control of symptoms.

Discussion (continued)

A hiatal hernia occurs when the stomach herniates through the diaphragmatic hiatus into the thorax. Incidence is positively correlated with age and is often associated with obesity. Prevalence is difficult to determine due to the asymptomatic course in many patients. There are four types of hiatal hernias (see table above). The majority (>90%) of hiatal hernias are type I (sliding) and can be managed medically. For those patients that fail medical management, surgery can improve quality of life and improve control of symptoms.

History: Hiatal hernias are often asymptomatic.
- May present with symptoms of gastroesophageal reflux (e.g., heartburn, dysphagia, regurgitation)
- Paraesophageal hernias (types II–IV) may present with obstructive symptoms (dysphagia, postprandial fullness), compressive symptoms (respiratory complications and recurrent pneumonia), or with reflux and/or chronic anemia

Physical Exam: The physical exam is normal.

Diagnostics:
- Hiatal hernias are usually diagnosed while working up GERD.
- Barium contrast swallow studies and upper endoscopies are the most common modalities that lead to diagnosis. Barium swallow shows the anatomy of the esophagus and stomach in relation to the thorax and diaphragm.
- In a sliding (type I) hiatal hernia, the gastroesophageal junction moves above the diaphragm alongside part of the stomach (left image below).
- In a paraesophageal hernia type II, the gastroesophageal junction remains within the abdomen; however, the gastric fundus moves into the mediastinum (right image below).
- Endoscopies can detect any esophagitis from long-standing reflux.
- Paraesophageal hernias (shown below) are sometimes incidentally discovered on plain chest radiographs as a retrocardiac air-fluid level or soft tissue opacity in the thorax.

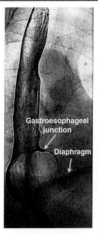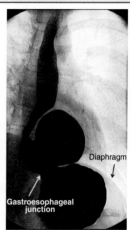

Left panel: Large sliding hiatal hernia. Right panel: Paraesophageal hernia. Note that the cardioesophageal junction remains in its normal anatomic position below the diaphragm. (Reproduced with permission from Doherty GM. Current Diagnosis & Treatment: Surgery, 15e. Copyright 2020 McGraw-Hill Education.)

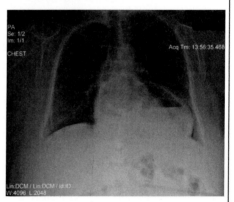

Chest radiograph in a patient with a large paraesophageal hernia. Note the air-fluid level in the chest from the herniated stomach. (Reproduced with permission from Zinner MJ, Ashley SW, Hines O. Maingot's Abdominal Operations, 13e. Copyright 2019 McGraw-Hill Education.)

Management:
- Asymptomatic type I hiatal hernia: No treatment.
- Gastroesophageal reflux symptoms:
  - Lifestyle changes including weight loss if obese, avoiding spicy/triggering foods, and sitting upright for 2–3 hours after meals
  - Medical management including PPIs (most effective), H2 blockers, and antacids
  - Surgical treatment with Nissen fundoplication if symptoms are refractory to medical management
- Asymptomatic paraoesophageal (grade II–IV) hernias can be repaired or may be monitored depending on the patient's comorbidities.
- All symptomatic paraoesophageal hernias should be repaired; approximately 14% of asymptomatic paraesophageal hernias become symptomatic each year.

CASE 22 | Hiatal Hernia *(continued)*

Additional Considerations	**Surgical Complications Following Anti-Reflux Procedures:**
	Mesh: Mesh is sometimes placed to repair the large diaphragmatic defect; occasionally, mesh migration or erosion into the esophagus or stomach can occur following repair of large hernia repairs.
	Gas-bloat symptoms: Excessive production of gas with abdominal pain.
	Recurrence: Approximately 5% will require surgical revision.

Mini-Case	
Esophageal Perforation	**Hx:**
	• Sudden-onset severe retrosternal sharp chest pain radiating to the back and worsening with swallowing.
	• Pain often begins after severe retching (Boerhaave syndrome) from overeating, bulimia, hyperemesis of pregnancy, cyclic vomiting syndrome, or alcoholic binge.
	• It can iatrogenically follow endoscopy, esophageal dilation, esophageal biopsy, or placement of endotracheal, orogastric, or oroenteric tubes.
	PE:
	• Acute distress, fever, and tachycardia may be present.
	• Crepitus may be present on chest palpation from subcutaneous emphysema. Hamman sign may be present (mediastinal crackling that is concurrent with each heartbeat while the patient is in the left lateral decubitus position).
	Diagnostics:
	• Chest x-ray: May show pneumothorax, pneumomediastinum, or pleural effusion, however these may be late findings
	• Contrast esophagram with a water-soluble agent will show extravasation of contrast if there is a large perforation. Barium should be avoided, as it can cause an inflammatory reaction after extravasation.
	• CT is considered the diagnostic of choice due to its ability to identify small leaks undetectable by contrast esophagram.
	Management:
	• Esophageal perforation is a surgical emergency if there are any signs of shock or sepsis or if the abdominal esophagus is perforated.
	• Prior to surgical management, patient should be in the ICU, initiate IV fluids, antibiotics, place NPO.
	• Operative repair is indicated for definitive treatment of esophageal perforation.
	• If there is no rupture in the abdominal esophagus and the pleural space is not involved, may manage by giving IV fluids, keeping the patient NPO (≥7 days), giving broad-spectrum antibiotics that cover aerobes and anaerobes, and careful monitoring.
	Discussion: Esophageal perforation is most commonly iatrogenic secondary to esophagogastroduodenoscopy. **Boerhaave syndrome** is a spontaneous transmural tear of the esophagus from forceful vomiting, as opposed to a **Mallory-Weiss tear**, which is a tear of only the mucosa and submucosa.
	Complications include:
	• Sepsis, mediastinitis, empyema, and mediastinal abscess
	• More than 50% of esophageal perforations are iatrogenic complications; 15% are spontaneous, ~10% are from foreign body ingestion, and another ~10% are from trauma

Biliary and Gallstone Disease

Cholecystectomy, performed for gallstone disease, is one of the most common surgical procedures performed in the United States. The most common type of gallstone is cream-colored and made of cholesterol (80%); in patients with hemolytic disease, black pigment stones, which are predominantly calcium bilirubinate, are more common. Once a patient develops symptoms there is an 80% chance of complications. Gallstones also are the most common risk for gallbladder cancer and are found in 80% of patients with gallbladder cancer.

• *Symptoms:* post-prandial pain after a fatty meal; RUQ pain or epigastric pain which persists for 15 minutes up to several hours and resolves; nausea or vomiting can be associated with the pain

• *Risk Factors:* Forties (age >40), Female, Fertile (increased risk with increased pregnancies), Fasting (prolonged fasting or total parenteral nutrition), Fats (Fatty food intolerance, obese, hyperlipidemia). Other factors include European and Native American ancestry and diabetes

• *Lab investigations of RUQ pain:* CBC, CMP, AST/ALT, ALP, lipase, lactase, pregnancy test, ultrasound of the abdomen.

Gallbladder (GB) Pathology and Treatment

Condition	Presentation	Diagnostics	Management
Cholelithiasis Stones in GB due to precipitation of cholesterol ("yellow stones") or bilirubin ("pigment stones")	May be asymptomatic or have colicky RUQ pain precipitated by consumption of fatty meal. Resolves on its own within a few hours. Afebrile, no jaundice, negative Murphy sign (gallbladder not inflamed).	*Labs:* Normal limits *RUQ US:* GB wall within normal limits. Gallstones or sludge visualized.	Pain control with NSAIDs during episode and diet modification. Elective cholecystectomy if symptomatic episodes
Cholecystitis Inflammation of the GB, 90% due to stones or sludge in GB +/− cystic duct	**Calculous cholecystitis** Steady RUQ pain that radiates to the right shoulder that does not resolve on its own. May have history of prior colicky RUQ pain. Patient may be febrile. No jaundice. Positive Murphy sign. May exhibit rebound and guarding.	*Labs:* Leukocytosis, possible elevated alkaline phosphatase and mildly elevated aminotransferases *RUQ US:* Most sensitive: Gallstones with positive sonographic Murphy sign. May also see gallbladder wall thickening and pericholecystic fluid. *HIDA (hepatobiliary iminodiacetic acid):* No radiotracer in GB	IV fluids, pain medication, antibiotics Cholecystectomy If the patient is a poor surgical candidate a percutaneous cholecystostomy tube can be placed followed by an interval cholecystectomy when stable; if no cholecystectomy is performed, there is a high incidence of recurrence
	Acalculous cholecystitis RUQ pain typically seen in hospitalized/critically ill or post-operative patients. May be febrile. No acute jaundice. Positive Murphy sign. May have rebound, guarding, and peritoneal signs.	*Labs:* Leukocytosis, elevated alkaline phosphatase, and mildly elevated aminotransferases *RUQ US:* GB wall thickening, pericholecystic fluid, absence of stones	IV fluids, pain medication, antibiotics Cholecystostomy tube if patient is too unstable for cholecystectomy Consider cholecystectomy if patient is stable or there are signs of GB perforation, gangrene, or emphysematous cholecystitis indicating emergent surgery
Choledocholithiasis Gallstone(s) in common bile duct (CBD)	RUQ pain. If complicated by gallstone pancreatitis, epigastric pain that radiates to the back. May be febrile. May be jaundiced if complicated by cholangitis. Positive Murphy sign, epigastric tenderness.	*Labs:* Leukocytosis, elevated alkaline phosphatase, GGT, and total and direct bilirubin. May have elevated lipase if complicated by pancreatitis. *RUQ US:* Dilated CBD suggests biliary obstruction *ERCP* (endoscopic retrograde cholangiopancreatography) is an invasive procedure which allows stenting or removal of stones endoscopically. *MRCP* (magnetic retrograde cholangiopancreatography) is a non-invasive imaging that can be performed for diagnosis of biliary obstruction.	IV fluids, pain management ERCP to remove stone and elective cholecystectomy

930 CHAPTER 19 SURGERY

Gallbladder (GB) Pathology and Treatment *(Continued)*

Condition	Presentation	Diagnostics	Management
Ascending cholangitis Infection of bile ducts/biliary system due to obstruction (stone, tumor, stricture)	Charcot triad (fever, RUQ pain, jaundice). If severe, patient might present with Reynold pentad (Charcot triad + shock and altered mental status). Positive Murphy's sign. May have rebound and guarding	*Labs:* Leukocytosis, elevated alkaline phosphatase, aminotransferases, and total and direct bilirubin. *RUQ US:* Bile duct dilation is observed usually with stones however benign or malignant biliary strictures can also be causative *ERCP/MRCP*	IV Fluids, pain medication, empiric antibiotics covering enteric organisms ERCP drainage and stone removal (if stone is the cause of obstruction) or stent placement (for stricture) Elective cholecystectomy if a stone is the cause of the obstruction
Gallstone pancreatitis Inflammation of pancreas due to bile reflux from stone obstruction of common bile duct, or increased pancreatic pressure from obstruction of the pancreatic duct	Epigastric pain ± radiation to back, nausea/vomiting	*Labs:* Elevated lipase *ERCP/MRCP*	ERCP (urgent if with cholangitis) + semi-elective cholecystectomy performed during same hospital admission
Gallstone ileus Bowel obstruction due to stone impaction in the ileum via biliary-enteric fistula	Intermittent diffuse abdominal pain, nausea/vomiting, fever, abdominal distension	Abdominal x-ray RUQ US, CT abdomen	Enterolithotomy +/– cholecystectomy and biliary-enteric fistula closure

CASE 23 | Cholecystitis

A 43-year-old G5P5 woman presents with RUQ pain radiating to her right shoulder for 10 hours. She is also having nausea, vomiting, and loss of appetite. She has had similar intermittent pain in the past after eating fatty meals, but this episode is more severe and constant. The pain reaches a crescendo, then suddenly releases. On exam, she is in moderate distress and her vital signs are temperature 37°C and HR 115 bpm. Her BMI is 40. She has anicteric conjunctiva, tenderness in the RUQ, inspiratory arrest with deep palpation in the RUQ (Murphy sign), guarding, and rebound tenderness.

Conditions with Similar Presentations	Cholelithiasis, choledocholithiasis, peptic ulcer disease (PUD), pancreatitis may all present acutely with upper abdominal pain, nausea, and vomiting. **Pancreatitis:** Abdominal pain is epigastric rather than RUQ, and Murphy sign is absent. The pain characteristically radiates to the back and is improved by sitting up. **Choledocholithiasis and ascending cholangitis:** May present similarly but jaundice is more likely due to common bile duct obstruction (instead of just cystic duct obstruction). Ascending cholangitis may have Charcot triad (fever, jaundice, and RUQ tenderness). **PUD:** May have hematemesis or melena but would not have Murphy sign. **Esophageal spasm:** may also present with epigastric pain, but may also have any of the following: chest pain, dysphagia, heartburn and regurgitation. **Myocardial infarction:** may also present with epigastric pain, nausea and vomiting; there may also be chest pain radiating to jaw, neck or arms and associated shortness of breath.
Diagnostics	• Obtain: RUQ ultrasound • Also check: CBC (to look for leukocytosis), CMP (specifically looking at AST, ALT, alkaline phosphatase, bilirubin) • Consider: Lipase, to rule out pancreatitis and ECG/troponins to rule out myocardial infarction
Management	• Patient should be made NPO and IV fluids started • Medications for pain control • IV antibiotics that cover gram-negative aerobes and anaerobes • Cholecystectomy

CASE 23 | Cholecystitis *(continued)*

Discussion	**Cholelithiasis** refers to the presence of biliary stones. Composition of stones varies and may include cholesterol (most common), black pigment (bilirubin), or mixed/brown (cholesterol and calcium carbonate and phosphorus salts). Acute or chronic inflammation of the gallbladder is **cholecystitis**. Stone impaction in the cystic duct (calculous cholecystitis) causes obstruction and stasis, which leads to thickening and inflammation of the gallbladder wall and allows infection to set in proximal to the obstruction in approximately 50% of cases. **History:** Patients present with RUQ pain that may radiate to the right shoulder. The pain may reach a severe crescendo then suddenly dissipate (colicky pain). There may be associated nausea/vomiting. The onset may be after the consumption of a fatty meal and is differentiated from biliary colic (transient blockage of the cystic duct) by persistence of symptoms. Risk factors include the "four Fs": female, forty (middle-aged), fertile (multiparous), and "fat." Patients may also present with a fever that is secondary to the inflammatory process and/or superimposed infection. A fever, therefore, does not necessarily indicate an infection. **Physical Exam:** On exam, patients will have pain with palpation in the RUQ and may also have rebound tenderness and guarding. There will often be a positive Murphy sign, which is inspiratory arrest with deep RUQ palpation at the costal margin when the inflamed the gallbladder moves down to the level of the examiner's hand. **Diagnostics:** • Cholecystitis is confirmed by RUQ ultrasound showing wall thickening, edema, pericholecystic fluid or a sonographic Murphy sign (Murphy sign occurring during deep RUQ ultrasound probing). Gallstones or biliary sludge may be visualized but are not necessary for diagnosis nor is their presence diagnostic. • HIDA scan may be done if ultrasound is equivocal. HIDA is excreted by hepatocytes into the bile and should normally enter the gallbladder via the cystic duct. If a cystic duct stone is present, the gallbladder will not be visualized. **Management:** • The definitive treatment of cholecystitis is cholecystectomy. Early cholecystectomy (within 7 days of presentation) is associated with better outcomes than late cholecystectomy (>7 days after presentation). • Patients are given prophylactic antibiotics at presentation to prevent or treat infection, which are discontinued post-operatively. • Intraoperative cholangiogram can be performed to rule out the presence of a stone in the common bile duct (choledocholithiasis). 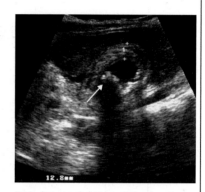 RUQ ultrasound characteristic of acute calculous cholecystitis. Note thickening of the gallbladder wall (*arrow*) and presence of stones (*bright spots*) in the gallbladder. (Reproduced with permission from Elsayes KM, Oldham SA. Introduction to Diagnostic Radiology. Copyright 2015 McGraw-Hill Education.)
Additional Considerations	**Complications:** • **Retained stone**: If intraoperative cholangiogram is not performed, there is a chance that a stone may have migrated to the common bile duct (CBD) and not be removed with the gallbladder. Patients may present with signs of pancreatitis (the gallstone causes obstruction of the pancreatic duct) and failure to see improvement of AST, ALT, alkaline phosphate, or bilirubin. • **Sphincter of Oddi dysfunction:** The sphincter of Oddi is the muscle that controls the flow of contents from the common bile duct and main pancreatic duct into the duodenum. Post-cholecystectomy, the patient will present with symptoms similar to cholelithiasis (colicky RUQ pain) despite the absence of a gallbladder with elevated AST/ALT/alkaline phosphate and mild hyperbilirubinemia. RUQ ultrasound will show bile duct dilation with no evidence of a stone. • **Ascending cholangitis** is due to an infection in the biliary tract proximal to an obstruction, typically a gallstone obstructing the common bile duct. Classical presentation is known as Charcot triad: fever, RUQ pain, jaundice. As the infection progresses and becomes more severe, patients may also develop hypotension and alterations in mental status, known as Reynolds pentad. Patients with cholangitis frequently present with a cholestatic pattern of lab abnormalities (elevated serum total and direct bilirubin and alkaline phosphatase). Abdominal ultrasound can show signs of bile duct dilation or bile duct stones. If the abdominal ultrasound is normal and ascending cholangitis is suspected, magnetic resonance cholangiopancreatography (MRCP) is performed. CT scans may also detect bile duct dilatation but are less adept at identifying bile duct stones. Treat with intravenous hydration and empiric antibiotics with activity against gram-negative enteric aerobes and anaerobes. The biliary obstruction must be removed urgently because antibiotics do not penetrate an obstructed biliary tree very well. The intervention of choice is endoscopic sphincterotomy via endoscopic retrograde cholangiopancreatography (ERCP) with stone extraction and possible stent placement. Non-surgical alternative is percutaneous drainage.

CASE 24 | Hemorrhoids

A 55-year-old man presents to clinic with blood in his stool for the past month. He feels a grape-sized mass at his anus and sees streaks of bright red blood coating his stool. He describes pain with defecation but has had no melena or weight loss. He has no family history of colorectal cancer. On exam, external hemorrhoids are noted without tenderness to palpation.

Conditions with Similar Presentations	**Anal fissures:** Dyschezia (difficulty with defecation) will be present; exam will reveal a central fissure usually in the posterior midline. If a patient continues to have anal fissures even after medical therapy, treatment options include botulinum toxin injection, fissurectomy (excision of fissure), or internal sphincterotomy (lateral incision is made in the internal sphincter to help release tension so fissure can heal). A complication of sphincterotomy is fecal incontinence.
	Rectal cancer: Can be visualized on colonoscopy. Tumors located in the upper (proximal) third of the rectum can be treated like colon cancers and resected, whereas tumors in the lower two-thirds often require an end colostomy with proctosigmoidectomy.
	Inflammatory bowel disease or other forms of colitis: Can also present with rectal bleeding but is accompanied by abdominal pain and diarrhea.
	Diverticulosis: Present in 50% of people at age 60. Predominates in left colon but right colon diverticula bleed more commonly. Rectal bleeding is painless.
	Angiodysplasia: Usually a disease with mean age in the seventh decade; may present with hematochezia (if from a lower GI source), melena (if from an upper GI source), or occult bleeding. There may be accompanying iron deficiency anemia. Most lesions are found in the cecum. Bleeding is painless.
Initial Diagnostic Testing	• Physical exam and digital rectal exam • If no hemorrhoids are detected, an anoscopy followed by a colonoscopy should be performed
Next Steps in Management	• Diet and lifestyle modification (high-fiber diet and exercise) • Medications for symptomatic relief like psyllium, topical analgesics and steroids, and sitz baths for flare-ups
Discussion	Hemorrhoids are large, dilated veins in the rectum that occur when the vasculature in the anal canal is swollen or inflamed, most commonly from straining with defecation due to constipation. **External hemorrhoids**—distal to the dentate line • Usually present with dyschezia • Arise from inferior hemorrhoidal plexus, somatic innervation • If thrombosed, there is severe pain **Internal hemorrhoids**—proximal to the dentate line • Usually present with painless hematochezia • Arise from the superior rectal plexus, visceral innervation • First degree—painless, bleeding with defecation • Second degree—protrude with defecation only • Third degree—require manual reduction after protruding • Fourth degree—permanently prolapsed **History:** • Risk factors for developing hemorrhoids include age 45–65, diarrhea, pregnancy, pelvic tumors, prolonged sitting, straining with defecation, constipation. • Symptoms: Hematochezia, pain (if external), perianal pruritis or irritation **Physical Exam:** • Hemorrhoids on examination of the anoderm, bluish elevation of the skin (seen in thrombosed external hemorrhoids, skin tags, blood on digital rectal exam (DRE) • Thrombosed hemorrhoids may be tender to palpation **Diagnostics:** • Anoscopy—indicated if hemorrhoids not detected on exam. Allows for evaluation and visualization of the anal canal and distal rectum. • Colonoscopy/flexible sigmoidoscopy—if patient is >40 years old, to rule out more proximal causes of LGI bleed. **Management:** First-line treatment • Lifestyle management—high-fiber diet, hydration, exercise, avoid straining/lingering on the toilet (reading/phone) • Medications for symptomatic relief—stool softeners (psyllium), topical analgesia, sitz baths

CASE 24 | Hemorrhoids *(continued)*

Discussion	Second-line treatment • For nonthrombosed internal hemorrhoids, options include infrared coagulation, rubber band ligation, and sclerotherapy, all of which aim to limit blood supply to the hemorrhoid, thereby shrinking it. These techniques are avoided in external hemorrhoids because severe pain can occur due to innervation below the dentate line. • External hemorrhoidectomy is an option for patients who have symptoms after medical therapy and cannot tolerate office-based procedures, or with large symptomatic external hemorrhoids, bleeding, severe pain, or thrombosis. • Thrombosis is most associated with external hemorrhoids and causes severe pain, along with a characteristic blue bulge. An option is to alleviate the pain by cutting into the hemorrhoid and removing the thrombus; however, recurrence is common.
Additional Considerations	**Complications of Hemorrhoidectomy** **Constipation**—fear of painful defecation because of pain and/or bleeding. **Post-operative bleeding**—higher-risk individuals include patients on systemic anticoagulation. **Infection**—fever, worsening pain after initial improvement, and delayed urinary retention suggest infection and may require operative intervention. **Urinary retention**—usually from irritation or blockade of pelvic nerves and pain-evoked reflexes. Advanced age, male sex, epidural and spinal anesthesia increase risk of urinary retention. **Anal stricture or stenosis**—presents as a late complication with smaller-caliber stools and pain with defecation; treated with stool softeners and fiber supplements; anoplasty if needed. **Fecal incontinence**—sphincter or associated nerves may be injured. **Chronic pain**—occurs in up to 30% long term.

BARIATRIC SURGERY

Obesity is a growing health concern in the United States, with increasing prevalence and an impact on additional comorbid conditions. Obesity is diagnosed and classified based on BMI as shown in the table below. BMI is based on population studies, and so on an individual basis will have limitations. Waist circumference and waist-to-hip ratio are also useful measurements for adiposity and risk assessment.

BMI-Based Definition of Obesity in Adults and Children

Classification	Adult BMI (kg/m²)	Pediatric BMI Percentile (age 2–19)
Underweight	<18.5	<5%
Healthy weight	18.5–24.9	5–85%
Overweight	25–29.9	85–95%
Class I obesity	30–34.9	95–120%
Class II obesity	35–39.9	120–140%
Class III obesity	40	>140%

More patients are seeking surgical management in the form of bariatric surgery. The table below highlights the indications for considering bariatric surgery, based on BMI and obesity-related comorbidities. Comorbidities that may be treated by weight loss include hypertension, type II diabetes, sleep apnea, osteoarthritis, and nonalcoholic fatty liver disease. Patients are assessed in a multimodal approach, including laboratory and exam data, nutritionist and health psychology evaluations. Additional factors are considered for adolescent patients, typically with a multidisciplinary team: family support, understanding of the condition, and decisional capacity.

Indications for Bariatric Surgery in Adults and Children

BMI (kg/m²)	Pediatric BMI Percentile	Other Requirements
30		Uncontrolled insulin-dependent type II diabetes in setting of maximal medical and lifestyle intervention
35	120–140%	One or more obesity-related comorbidities that can be treated with weight loss
40	>140%	

Bariatric surgery can be classified into three groups, based on their mechanism of weight loss: restrictive, malabsorptive, or a combination of both mechanisms.

Bariatric Surgery Procedures and Their Mechanism of Action

Mechanism	Type of Surgery	Mechanism
Restrictive	Gastric (lap) banding Sleeve gastrectomy	↓ size of stomach, leading to early satiety and ↓ calories consumed
Malabsorptive	Jejunoileal bypass	↓ absorption of nutrients and therefore calories
Combination	Roux-en-Y gastric bypass Bilio pancreatic diversion	A small gastric pouch is created by dividing the stomach, and a roux limb is used to anastomose to the gastric pouch 70% gastrectomy and biliopancreatic diversion yields stable weight loss for 10 years or more

Patients undergoing bariatric surgery should be followed by a multidisciplinary health care team including their primary care physician, a nutritionist, and their surgeon both pre- and post-operatively. They may have baseline cardiovascular disease (hypertension), pulmonary disease (sleep apnea), endocrine disease (diabetes), and may require complex care. These patients are also at high risk for nutritional deficiencies following their surgery, and should be assessed for vitamin and mineral deficiencies including iron, calcium, vitamins D, B1 (thiamine), B12, and vitamin K. Vitamin A, zinc, and copper should be assessed in patients undergoing malabsorptive procedures. It is recommended that patients take a daily multivitamin and be given supplements for any deficiencies they develop.

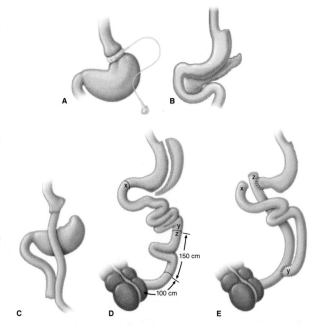

Bariatric surgical procedures. Examples of operative interventions used for surgical manipulation of the gastrointestinal tract.
A. Laparoscopic adjustable gastric banding. B. Laparoscopic sleeve gastrectomy. C. The Roux-en-Y gastric bypass. D. Biliopancreatic diversion with duodenal switch. E. Biliopancreatic diversion. (Reproduced with permission from Loscalzo J, Fauci A, Kasper D, Hauser S, Longo D, Jameson J. Harrison's Principles of Internal Medicine, 21ed. New York: McGraw Hill; 2022.)

CASE 25 | Bariatric Surgery Complications (Dumping Syndrome)

A 42-year-old woman with diabetes mellitus type 2 presents two weeks after a Roux-en-Y bypass surgery with postprandial abdominal pain, nausea, diarrhea, and lightheadedness. Abdominal pain is associated with palpitations and facial flushing. Her diet consists mostly of pasta, cereal, and sandwiches on white bread. On presentation, her temperature is 37.2°C, pulse 88 bpm, and blood pressure 124/78. Abdominal exam shows no pain with palpation, rebound, or guarding. Her laparoscopic incisions are nonerythematous with no drainage. Random blood glucose is 212 mg/dL.

Conditions with Similar Presentations	**Insulinoma and pancreatic islet cell hyperplasia:** Both present with autonomic signs consistent with hypoglycemia, including tachycardia, diaphoresis, confusion, anxiety, or tremor. Blood glucose will be low and C-peptide will be high in these conditions.
	Carcinoid syndrome: Presents with facial flushing, diarrhea, and hypotension. Additionally, it may cause bronchospasm and signs of right-sided valvular heart disease. It is due to a neuroendocrine tumor in the gut releasing excessive amounts of serotonin.
	Biliary colic: Is common in middle-aged women and presents with colicky RUQ abdominal pain after meals. However, autonomic signs and lightheadedness are not seen.
Initial Diagnostic Tests	• Diagnosis is based on clinical presentation, can be supported by oral glucose challenge test • Consider upper GI endoscopy to rule out other causes

CASE 25 | Bariatric Surgery Complications (Dumping Syndrome) *(continued)*

Next Steps in Management	Dietary modification including: • Small, frequent meals • No fluid intake with meals • Avoidance of simple sugars, consumption of meals with high complex carbohydrates and protein

Discussion	Dumping syndrome (DS) is a common complication of gastric bypass surgeries, especially when patients consume a large amount of simple carbohydrates. DS occurs due to the rapid emptying of hyperosmolar stomach contents into the small intestine, causing a fluid shift from the vasculature of the intestine into the lumen which leads to hypotension and lightheadedness. Distention of the bowel leads to pain, nausea, and autonomic dysfunction. Release of gut hormones (vasoactive intestinal polypeptide, neurotensin, and incretins) induces splanchnic vasodilation and can worsen hypotension. Bradykinin release causes flushing.
	
	DS (also termed *early dumping syndrome*) often occurs soon after surgery and resolves in the first 12 weeks. In this presentation, symptoms often occur within 30 minutes of eating. Late DS (now known as *postprandial hyperinsulinemic hypoglycemia*) may present months to years post-operatively, and symptoms occur 1–3 hours after carbohydrate-rich meals.
	
	History: Symptoms occur within 30 minutes to 3 hours after eating. Common gastrointestinal (GI) symptoms include nausea, postprandial fullness, diarrhea, and sometimes vomiting. Patients may also have palpitations/tachycardia, fatigue, dizziness, the urge to lie down, and possibly syncope.
	
	Physical Exam: During an episode there may be orthostatic hypotension, sweating, and tachycardia.
	
	Diagnostics:
	• The diagnosis of DS is clinical, based on a typical time course and set of symptoms.
	• Diagnosis can be supported by a positive oral glucose challenge
	• Consider:
	  • Hydrogen breath test post-oral glucose ingestion
	  • GI follow-through to rule out gastric pouch leak or fistula formation
	  • Upper GI endoscopy to rule out peptic ulcer disease or partial obstruction
	
	Management:
	Dietary modification is the first line of treatment.
	By decreasing the load of simple carbohydrates, the stomach contents emptied into the small intestine will not be as hyperosmolar.
	• If dietary modification is unsuccessful:
	  • Acarbose given after a carbohydrate-rich meal delays the breakdown of complex carbohydrates to monosaccharides and decreases the osmolarity of stomach contents
	  • Octreotide slows the rate of gastric emptying and inhibits the release of gut hormones and insulin
	• If both dietary restriction and medications fail for >1 year, then surgical revision may be considered, including reconstruction of the pylorus.

Additional Considerations	**Complications:** Vitamin B12 and iron deficiencies are most common.

PEDIATRIC SURGERY

Pediatric surgery is a unique subspecialty of surgery in that many of the conditions treated are congenital anomalies presenting soon after birth rather than acquired later in life. A useful approach to the differential diagnosis of pediatric abdominal pain begins by identifying the patient age group:

1. **Newborn within 24 hours of life**—concern for a surgical problem should be raised if there is a history of maternal polyhydramnios, abdominal distension, or failure to pass meconium

2. **First few days of life**

3. **Late infancy and childhood**

Certain pathologies exclusively or very commonly appear in a particular age group. For example, esophageal atresia presents immediately after the first feed, whereas hypertrophic pyloric stenosis is extremely rare before 2 weeks of life. Refer to Chapter 15 (Pediatrics) for more details.

Conditions Requiring Abdominal Surgery

Conditions Presenting with Emesis		Abdominal Wall Defects	Abdominal Tumors
Nonbilious emesis	*Bilious emesis*	Gastroschisis	Neuroblastoma
Pyloric stenosis	Malrotation with midgut volvulus	Omphalocele	Nephroblastoma
Congenital duodenal obstruction	Intussusception	Umbilical hernia	
	Meckel diverticulum	Inguinal hernia	
	Incarcerated hernia		
	Necrotizing enterocolitis		
	Hirschsprung disese		

Thoracic Anomalies that Require Surgical Intervention

1. **Congenital diaphragmatic hernia (Bochdalek and Morgagni hernia)**—Caused by a failure of fusion of the postero-lateral diaphragmatic foramina the abdominal contents enter the thoracic cavity and impede the development of the lung leading to pulmonary hypoplasia and pulmonary hypertension. Bochadalek occurs on the left posterior side and accounts for 85% of cases. Morgagni hernias are typically anterior and often do not cause symptoms. Surgery to repair the diaphragm and restore abdominal contents to the abdomen can be performed once the infant is medically stable.

2. **Esophageal atresia and TEF**—Caused by a failure of separation of the trachea from the esophagus, TEFs are characterized by a blind-ending esophagus, also known as esophageal atresia with a fistula to the trachea. Fifty percent or more are affected by other congenital anomalies including VACTERL complex (vertebral defects, anal atresia, cardiac defects, tracheoesophageal fistula, renal abnormalities, and limb abnormalities). Surgical correction includes disconnection of the fistula, closure of the hole in the trachea, and anastomosis to reconnect the two segments of esophagus.

3. **Duplication cysts: bronchogenic, esophageal, or mediastinal cyst**—These conditions can occur anywhere along the bronchial tree, with corresponding obstructive symptoms which can lead to pneumonia, chest pain, shortness of breath (bronchogenic), within the lower third of the esophagus presenting with dysphagia or chest pain (esophageal), or in the right posterior inferior mediastinum, which may cause cardiac arrhythmia, retrosternal back pain, or cyst rupture with mediastinitis. Initially appear as a mass on chest x-ray, definitively diagnosed by endoscopic ultrasound followed by resection in symptomatic patients.

CARDIOTHORACIC SURGERY

Conditions can be categorized as those involving (1) the heart and thoracic aorta, (2) the lungs, esophagus, and mediastinum, and (3) transplantation of the lung (s) and/or heart. Refer to Chapter 4 (Cardiology) for details and additional cases.

- With the continual improvement of minimally invasive procedures for cardiac disease, open cardiac surgeries that were traditionally performed for the treatment of medical conditions such as aortic stenosis and acute MI are being displaced by interventional cardiac procedures. Notably, the first-line treatment for acute ST-segment elevation myocardial infarctions (STEMI) is percutaneous cardiac intervention (PCI) in the form of angioplasty and a stent; coronary artery bypass grafting (CABG) is only indicated in left main disease, or if stenting fails or is anatomically not possible.

- Aortic valve replacement is a procedure that is performed by interventional cardiologists in the form of transcatheter aortic valve replacement (TAVR), though it was once only done by cardiac surgeons as surgical aortic valve replacement (SAVR). TAVR introduces the new valve into the heart via a catheter. This new valve fits inside the opening of the diseased native valve, negating the necessity of removing the existing valve. This gives patients who are poor surgical candidates the opportunity to undergo aortic valve replacement, leading to decreased mortality and increased quality of life. All TAVRs should be performed in centers with a cardiac surgeon on site in case there is a complication that requires surgical intervention.

Valve Replacement	Surgical Indications
Aortic stenosis	• SAD symptoms occur (syncope, angina, dyspnea [from heart failure])
Aortic insufficiency	• Symptomatic patients with severe aortic regurgitation • Asymptomatic patients with cardiomegaly or left ventricular ejection fraction (LVEF) ≤ 50% • Patients with aortic regurgitation undergoing CABG, surgery of the ascending aorta or of another valve

Valve Replacement	Surgical Indications
Mitral stenosis	• Symptomatic patients • Patients with mitral valve area <1.5 cm² may be a candidate for percutaneous balloon commissurotomy.
Mitral regurgitation (MR)	• Symptomatic (e.g., dyspnea on exertion) patients • Acute onset of MR

CASE 30 | Coronary Artery Bypass Grafting (CABG) after an NSTEMI

A 57-year-old man with diabetes, hypertension, and hyperlipidemia presents to the ED due to substernal chest pain and shortness of breath for 1 hour. The symptoms of chest pressure radiating to both arms started while he was watching television. He has nausea but no vomiting. His vitals are temperature 37.2°C, pulse 87 bpm, blood pressure 145/86, respiratory rate 22 bpm, SpO_2 96% on room air. On exam, he has equal pulses in both arms, JVP of 5 cm, nondisplaced PMI, and normal S1 and S2. ECG shows ST-segment depression in precordial leads V1–V6, and troponin I is >0.40 ng/L. The patient is diagnosed with a non-ST elevation myocardial infarction (NSTEMI) and started on a heparin drip, 325 mg aspirin, sublingual nitroglycerin, metoprolol, clopidogrel, and atorvastatin.

Conditions with Similar Presentations	**Stable angina:** Predictable chest pain or pressure brought on by exertion and relieved with rest. **Unstable angina:** New-onset angina or any change in previous angina and normal troponin I levels. **ST elevation myocardial infarction (STEMI):** As in an NSTEMI, troponin I will be elevated. However, there will be ST-segment elevation on ECG.
Initial Diagnostic Tests	Cardiac catheterization: Shows 80% stenosis in the left main coronary artery, a completely occluded proximal RCA, and an ejection fraction of 30%
Next Steps in Management	Confirm indications for CABG: • Lesions not amenable to percutaneous coronary intervention (e.g., high-complexity coronary artery disease, patients with diabetes with multivessel coronary artery disease involving the left anterior descending artery) • Life-limiting or threatening coronary artery disease on cardiac catheterization (e.g., left main coronary artery disease, MI with mechanical complications such as ventricular septal rupture, mitral valve insufficiency due to papillary muscle infarction, or free wall rupture). Continue blockers, aspirin, and statins up to the day of surgery but stop $P2Y_{12}$ inhibitors and other anticoagulants.
Discussion	Acute coronary syndrome (ACS) most commonly occurs due to rupture of a thrombotic occlusion of a coronary artery with underlying atherosclerosis. ACS can be divided into three categories: • **Unstable angina** = partial occlusion of the vessel without necrosis or infarction of the myocardium. • **NSTEMI** = subtotal occlusion of the vessel that results in necrosis and infarct in the sub-endocardium. • **STEMI** = complete occlusion of the vessel that results in a transmural infarct. See Chapter 4 (Cardiology). **History:** Patients with coronary artery disease and ACS usually present with chest pain and/or pressure brought on by exertion and relieved by rest and may have associated diaphoresis and nausea/vomiting, although elderly and female patients may present with atypical signs, such as epigastric pain. **Physical Exam:** The physical exam may be normal, or the patient might have hypoxemia, hypotension, the presence of an S3 or S4, or signs of sequelae secondary to the MI such as heart failure or new mitral regurgitation (pansystolic murmur at the apex). **Diagnostics:** • Any patient presenting with chest pain and concern for ACS should have an ECG within 10 minutes of presenting to the ED and immediate cardiac troponin assay. • If STEMI or NSTEMI, proceed to cardiac catheterization to determine if occlusive lesions can be managed by percutaneous coronary intervention (PCI) with endovascular stenting or if CABG is more appropriate (e.g., anatomy difficult to stent or L main disease). • Carotid artery duplex ultrasound should be performed if the patient has risk factors for carotid stenosis, such as age >65 years, smoking history, history of cerebrovascular disease, hypertension, or diabetes.

CASE 30 | Coronary Artery Bypass Grafting (CABG) after an NSTEMI (continued)

Discussion	**Management:** • PCI is the first-line treatment in patients diagnosed with STEMI, with CABG being indicated if PCI fails or cannot be performed. • Beta-blockers, aspirin, and statins should all be continued up to the day of surgery for patients undergoing CABG. • P2Y$_{12}$ inhibitors will be initiated in setting of ACS but will be stopped prior to surgery (depending on if emergent). • Anticoagulants should also be stopped prior to surgery. • The left internal mammary artery is the primary choice with the radial artery graft as second choice. • Dual antiplatelet therapy with aspirin and a P2Y$_{12}$ inhibitor should be initiated once deemed safe post-operatively.
Additional Considerations	**Complications:** • **Arrhythmia: Ventricular ectopy** is the most common arrhythmia and if frequent, >6–10/minute, should be treated with lidocaine bolus and subsequent continuous infusion with cardioversion if there is sustained ventricular tachycardia. Supraventricular tachycardias—atrial fibrillation and atrial flutter—should be treated with IV beta blockade, calcium channel blocker, or amiodarone to control the rate. • **Stroke** after CABG occurs in 1–2%. • **Infection:** *Sternal wound infection* presents with post-operative fever, wound erythema, and/or drainage, and is more common in the presence of obesity, diabetes, COPD, or prolonged OR time. *Sternal dehiscence* can accompany sternal wound infection and can lead to mediastinitis. This presents with fever, chest pain, and abnormal motion of the sternum when compressed laterally. • **Postpericardiotomy syndrome** occurs 2–3 weeks after surgery and presents similarly to pericarditis with chest pain and diffuse ST-segment elevations on ECG. It is an immune reaction to injured pericardium and is treated with nonsteroidal anti-inflammatory drugs. • **Heart failure:** Presents with signs and symptoms of low perfusion, including acidosis, hypothermia, acute kidney injury, pulmonary edema, and altered mental status. Decreased cardiac function may be due to a **perioperative myocardial infarction**; an ECG is required for diagnosis (troponin will already be elevated due to cardiac surgery) and an echocardiogram can help identify changes in cardiac contractility. An inotropic agent such as dobutamine can be administered; if the condition persists, an intra-aortic balloon pump can be placed for support. • **Renal failure:** Low renal perfusion during the acute cardiac event and post-operative course may lead to acute kidney injury. Avoidance of nephrotoxic drugs, maintenance of mean arterial pressure at least 65 mmHg, and maintenance of urine output of >30 mL/hr can be helpful. Progression to renal failure requiring hemodialysis is associated with mortality of >20%. • **Respiratory failure:** Prolonged intubation post-operatively can be due to many causes including pulmonary edema, pneumonia, atelectasis, mucus plugs. Vigorous pulmonary toilet and close monitoring of fluid status can improve this status. • **Bleeding:** Causes can include medications, hypothermia, transfusion reaction, and consumption of clotting factors. Diagnosis of coagulation defects is detected by thromboelastogram or, if not available, coagulation tests such as PT, PTT, and platelet count. Treatment should target normothermia, restoration of coagulation with fresh frozen plasma, platelets, or protamine to reverse heparinization as indicated by thromboelastogram. • **Cardiac tamponade:** Due to post-operative bleeding, and manifests with decreasing cardiac output, blood pressure, and urine output. Echocardiography confirms the diagnosis and emergent exploration is required. • **Death:** Overall perioperative death is greatly dependent on comorbidities and the urgency of the surgery, with aggregate rates around 1–2%.

Lung Nodules

Nonmalignant solitary pulmonary nodule: The majority of nodules seen on CXR or CT are not malignant.

• Benign: hamartoma, chondroma, lipoma, respiratory papillomatosis

• Infectious: mycobacteria, fungi, lung abscess, septic emboli, hydatid cyst

• Immune-mediated: rheumatoid arthritis, sarcoidosis, nonspecific granulomas

• Congenital: arteriovenous malformation, bronchogenic cyst, pulmonary sequestration

Malignant nodules: Most common lung malignancies, in decreasing order, are bronchogenic lung cancer, lymphoma, sarcoma, and lung metastasis. Nodules can be assigned a probability of being malignant based on presence of three main risk factors:

1. Current or past history of tobacco smoking (>20 pack/year history)
2. Age 50–80: >half of all lung cancers develop after the age of 70.
3. Nodule size
   - <6 mm has a <1% risk of cancer
   - >8 mm have a 9.7% of cancer, and any growing nodule is likely to be malignant
   - >3 cm is considered a lung mass and indicative of lung cancer until proven otherwise

Lung Cancer

Lung cancer arises from the epithelium and can be categorized as either **small-cell lung cancer (SCLC),** or **nonsmall-cell lung cancer (NSCLC)**. Also review Chapter 5 (Pulmonology).

SCLC is considered a neuroendocrine tumor and comprises roughly 15% of bronchogenic carcinomas. Cells are anaplastic and have a rapid doubling time capable of metastasizing in a short period of time. Only 30% of patients diagnosed with SCLC have limited-stage disease that can be treated by resection.

- Limited-stage disease is defined as disease limited to one hemithorax (Stage I) and may include regional lymph nodes (Stage II).
- Extensive disease includes patients with tumors involving contralateral lymph nodes (Stage III) or metastatic involvement of other tissues (Stage IV).
- Survival with treatment is stage dependent and varies from a median survival time of >5 years for Stage I and 10% for Stage IV.

NSCLC comprises >80% of all lung cancers. Surgery can provide curative resection in patients with early and local NSCLC tumors. More advanced stages of NSCLC, Stages III (tumor with contralateral nodal involvement) and IV (tumor with any metastasis), require multimodal treatment, including chemotherapy, radiotherapy, and possibly surgical resection.

CASE 31	Thoracic: Lung Adenocarcinoma
	A 68-year-old man with a 50-pack-year history and ongoing smoking is referred to pulmonary clinic after a chest x-ray performed for a cough of 3-weeks duration identified a 1.8-cm nodule in the right upper lobe. Physical exam is remarkable for an enlarged right supraclavicular lymph node.
Conditions with Similar Presentations	**Nonmalignant solitary pulmonary nodule:** The majority of nodules seen on CXR or CT are benign. **Malignant nodules:** Nodules can be assigned a probability of being malignant based on presence of risk factors, symptoms, and tumor size.
Initial Diagnostic Tests	CT chest with contrast
Next Steps in Management	Biopsy and staging with other images if needed
Discussion	Lung cancer is the most common cause of cancer death in the United States and worldwide, with tobacco as the most commonly identified risk factor (in 85–90% of cases). Smoking leads to diffuse tissue injury, which proceeds to epithelial damage characterized by mutations in oncogenes, tumor suppressor genes, gene arrangements, gene amplifications, or epigenetic changes. Other risk factors include: • Exposure to secondhand smoke. • Radiation exposure (radiation therapy to breast or chest, radon exposure at home or work, CT scans). • Air pollution. • Chronic obstructive pulmonary disease—increases risk twofold. • Family history—patients who have first-degree relatives with lung cancer have a twofold higher risk of lung cancer. • Occupational exposure to carcinogenic agents: asbestos, silica, soot, beryllium, chromium, arsenic, nickel cadmium, radon diesel fumes. These increase risk in a nonsmoker twofold, but in a smoker the risk can be nine times higher

CASE 31 | Thoracic: Lung Adenocarcinoma *(continued)*

Discussion	
	History: Up to 25% of patients are asymptomatic, with incidental finding on imaging. Nearly all patients have a smoking history.

History: Up to 25% of patients are asymptomatic, with incidental finding on imaging. Nearly all patients have a smoking history.

Centrally located, with bulky mediastinal lymphadenopathy can cause cough, chest pain, hemoptysis, weight loss, and dyspnea.

Other symptoms may occur as a result of compression of tissues: laryngeal nerve compression causing hoarseness or esophageal compression causing dysphagia.

Metastatic involvement of the brain may present as a neurologic deficit or personality change. Bone involvement may present with bone pain.

Physical Exam: Usually unremarkable, but may have finger clubbing, weakness, wheezing, signs of pneumonia, or lymphadenopathy. Right supraclavicular lymphadenopathy raises concern for malignancy related to lung or mediastinum. Paraneoplastic syndromes (see below) can precede diagnosis.

Diagnostics:
- CT with contrast of chest and upper abdomen.
- Biopsy for histology: options include bronchoscopy with transbronchial needle aspiration, endobronchial ultrasound-guided needle aspiration, endoscopic ultrasound-guided needle aspiration, transthoracic needle aspiration, and mediastinoscopy.
- Surgical biopsy can be done via open thoracotomy or video-assisted thoracoscopy (VATS) wedge resection. VATS is often preferred due to lower morbidity and shorter hospitalization. Patients leave the OR with a chest tube in place, which can be removed when there is no air leak, blood, or chyle.

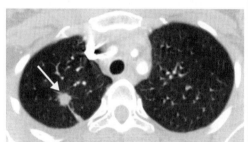

Adenocarcinoma. Axial chest CT demonstrates a right upper lobe nodule (*white arrow*) which was biopsied and found to be adenocarcinoma of the lung. The patient already had stage IV disease. (Reproduced with permission from Elsayes KM, Oldham SA. Introduction to Diagnostic Radiology. Copyright 2014 McGraw-Hill Education. All rights reserved.)

Also check: CBC, CMP, pre-operative pulmonary function tests.
- Tumor markers may also be useful, such as CEA, SCC antigen, neuron-specific enolase (NSE), cytokeratin 19 fragment (CYFRA), pro-gastrin-releasing peptide (proGRP).
  - CEA is sensitive for adenocarcinoma;
  - SCC and CYFRA for squamous cell carcinoma;
  - NSE and proGRP for small cell carcinoma.

Management:
- Decisions should be made with an interdisciplinary team including an oncologist, thoracic surgeon, and patient.
- The specifics depend on the stage of the disease and resectability.
- Resection is also guided by consideration for the patient's pulmonary function prior to resection.
  - *Pre-operative pulmonary function tests*: For resection, targets include FEV1 >1.5 L for lobectomy, >2 L for pneumonectomy, and FEV1 >80% predicted.
  - If pulmonary function tests indicate post-resection lung volume is adequate and surgical resection is feasible, a lobectomy with mediastinal lymph node dissection or sampling can be performed to define stage and need for systemic therapy with or without radiation therapy.

Complications of lobectomy:
1. Atelectasis (96%)—usually associated with poor ability to cough post-operatively, poor pain control, impaired pulmonary function, and chest wall or diaphragm dysfunction. If not treated with aggressive pulmonary physiotherapy, it can progress to pneumonia.

CASE 31 | Thoracic: Lung Adenocarcinoma *(continued)*

Discussion	2. Atrial fibrillation (10–40%) occurs most commonly on post-operative day 2 or 3 and is associated with age >70 years, right pneumonectomy, previous history of congestive heart failure, male gender, prior arrhythmia, or blood transfusions. Preventative strategies include hydration and correction of electrolyte imbalances and a short post-operative course of amiodarone and diltiazem.
	3. Prolonged air leak (7.6%)—defined as a leak lasting >7 days usually associated with emphysematous lungs, larger parenchymal resection, or inadequate drainage by thoracostomy tube.
	4. Mortality (2.6%).
	5. Additional complications, which are infrequent, include right middle lobe torsion from complete mobilization of the lung and lack of adhesions, hemorrhage, chylothorax from injury to the thoracic duct, and damage to the phrenic nerve or laryngeal nerves.
Additional Considerations	**Paraneoplastic Syndromes:** Paraneoplastic syndromes are seen with 10% of lung cancer patients; small cell lung cancer being the most common type. The two most common are hypercalcemia and SIADH. The symptoms of paraneoplastic syndromes often precede the diagnosis of lung cancer; early recognition may contribute to the detection of early-stage tumor.

Mediastinal Masses

Location in Mediastinum	Differential Diagnosis
Anterior (50% of all mediastinal masses)	"The Ts": Thymomas, teratoma, thymic cysts, thyroid masses, "terrible" lymphomas
Middle	• Most commonly lymphadenopathy • Less commonly congenital cysts (bronchogenic, pericardial, enteric cysts) • Least common are esophageal abnormalities (i.e., tumors achalasia, diverticulum, hiatal hernia, or stromal tumor) or vascular abnormalities (i.e., aortic aneurysm or dissection)
Posterior	Majority are neurogenic tumors (paraganglionomas, ganglioneuromas, Schwannomas, neurofibromas, neuroblastomas, ganglioblastomas), meningocele, neuroenteric cyst, paravertebral abnormalities (i.e., infections, malignancies, and fractures/dislocations)

CASE 32 | Thoracic: Mediastinal Mass (Thymoma)

A 35-year-old woman presents for evaluation of droopiness in the eyelids that gets worse throughout the day, fatigue, and shortness of breath. On exam, she has bilateral ptosis, binocular double vision upon sustained upward gaze, and weakness of eye closure, cheek puff, tongue protrusion, and neck flexion. Sensory exam is normal, and deep tendon reflexes are intact. Acetylcholine receptor antibodies are detected, and she is diagnosed with myasthenia gravis and started on treatment with acetylcholinesterase inhibitors. Mediastinal imaging reveals a thymoma.

Conditions with Similar Presentations	**Mediastinal masses** can be categorized by location (see above table).
	Lambert-Eaton syndrome: In contrast to myasthenia gravis, Lambert-Eaton syndrome presents with weakness that improves with repeated use and is due to antibodies against presynaptic calcium channels. The weakness is predominantly in proximal muscles and particularly involves the legs. Lambert-Eaton syndrome is a paraneoplastic syndrome associated with small-cell lung cancer.
Initial Diagnostic Tests	CT chest
Next Steps in Management	Referral to cardiothoracic surgery for consideration of thymectomy

CASE 32 | Thoracic: Lung Adenocarcinoma (continued)

Discussion	Thymomas are rare tumors originating in the epithelial cells of the thymus gland. They are slow growing, localized, and are the most common tumors of the anterior mediastinum. All thymomas have malignant potential and ability to metastasize. Thymomas may have molecular abnormalities including EGFR or IGF-1 overexpression. Additional somatic gene mutations have been identified. There are 15 histologically different neoplasms of the thymus, which can give rise to more than 20 paraneoplastic syndromes. The most common are myasthenia gravis (30–65% of patients with thymoma), hypogammaglobulinemia (Good syndrome, 5–20% of patients with thymoma), and autoimmune pure red cell aplasia (<5% of patients with thymoma). Patients with paraneoplastic disease are more likely to be diagnosed with early-stage thymoma and undergo complete surgical resection. **History:** Symptoms are often absent; one-third may present with symptoms of paraneoplastic disease. Local symptoms may include chest pain, cough, hoarseness, phrenic nerve palsy, dyspnea. **Physical Exam:** Evaluate for superior vena cava obstruction signs including facial swelling or arm swelling. Check for signs of paraneoplastic syndromes (such as motor weakness) if not already diagnosed. **Diagnostics:** • *CT chest with intravenous contrast*—can provide clinical staging of thymoma by identifying tumor size, location, and growth into vessels, pericardium, and/or lungs. Smooth tumors are indicative of thymomas, while irregular borders are consistent with thymic carcinoma. • On CT, thymomas are often well-defined round masses anterior to great vessels and heart without evidence of lymph node enlargement. 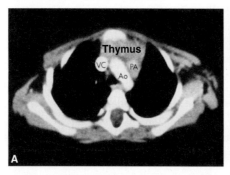 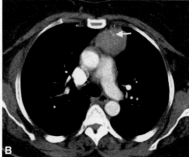 Left panel: Normal appearance of the thymus gland in childhood. Ao = aorta; PA = pulmonary artery; VC = vena cava. (Reproduced with permission from Brunicardi F, Andersen DK, Billiar TR, Dunn DL, Kao LS, Hunter JG, Matthews JB, Pollock RE. Schwartz's Principles of Surgery, 11e. Copyright 2019 McGraw-Hill Education.) Right panel: An axial CT image reveals a mass anterior to the pulmonary artery with punctuate areas of calcification (arrow) as seen in a thymoma. (Reproduced with permission from Chen MM, Pope TL, Ott DJ. Basic Radiology, 2e. Copyright 2011 McGraw-Hill Education. All rights reserved.) *Chest x-ray:* 50% can be identified on chest x-ray if they are localized within the thymic capsule and do not infiltrate. *MRI:* can distinguish between thymic hyperplasia, benign, and malignant tumors. It can also identify phrenic nerve involvement and is better than CT scan at identifying chest wall invasion. *PET scan:* fluorine F 18-fludeoxyglucose (18F-FDG) PET may be performed if thymic carcinoma is suspected. **Management:** • Medical treatment of myasthenia gravis prior to surgery • Thymectomy via a median sternotomy: minimally invasive surgery can be accomplished through a transcervical VATS or robotic approach, which may provide better visualization of the tumor than VATS. • If surgically resectable, total thymectomy is indicated. A total thymectomy includes removal of thymic gland with surrounding fatty tissue. This can be achieved via open thymectomy or VATS, which may reduce complications but with similar overall survival rates.
Additional Considerations	**Complications:** • Uncontrolled myasthenia gravis: May lead to respiratory failure during surgery. Patient should be counseled regarding myasthenic crisis in response to stress or certain drugs. • Tumor seeding: Surgical biopsy should be avoided to decrease the chances of potential tumor seeding. • Phrenic nerve injury: Can lead to severe respiratory morbidity post-operatively. • Recurrent laryngeal nerve injury: Can lead to vocal cord paralysis and hoarseness. Only the left recurrent laryngeal nerve is in the operative field. • Recurrence: Occurs 10–15% of the time, which necessitates same approach as original tumor; CT scan imaging every 6–12 months can assist in early detection.

VASCULAR SURGERY

Vascular surgery encompasses the diagnosis and treatment of arterial, venous, and lymphatic systems. This includes the aorta and its branches, the arteries of the neck, abdomen, pelvis, and extremities but not the cardiac or intracranial arteries, which are treated by cardiothoracic and neurosurgical teams, respectively.

- Clinical evaluations of the diseases of these vessels often include duplex ultrasonography to identify vascular flow patterns, and angiography through magnetic resonance imaging or CT scans to obtain whole-body perspective of the continuity of these systems.
- Once an obstruction or injury is identified, strategic approaches involve either an open approach of repair or replacement or a minimally invasive endovascular treatment (treatment is deployed from within the blood vessel by cannulating a peripheral artery such as the femoral artery and deploying a wire laden with a deployable stent or graft).
- The choice of treatment depends on anatomical considerations, technical feasibility, and the operative risk to the patient.
- Patients who suffer from arterial vascular disease may have atherosclerosis worsened by diabetes, hypertension, hyperlipidemia, and/or renal failure. These comorbidities generate high operative risk, which may move the choice of treatment more toward minimally invasive endovascular strategies instead of open operative ones.
- Endovascular approaches for the repair of an aortic aneurysm, for example, have lower 30-day mortality but higher 6-year mortality and risk of rupture requiring re-intervention.
- Endovascular stent treatment for carotid artery stenosis may be indicated in symptomatic patients for whom operative management is not feasible, such as patients who have had prior neck radiation or surgeries, have high perioperative mortality.

Acute Aortic Syndromes

Aortic dissection

- These forms of acute aortic syndromes can be anatomically classified into 3 De Bakey types:
  - *Type I* - affecting ascending, descending, and abdominal aorta
  - *Type II* - affecting the ascending aorta only
  - *Type III* - affecting the descending thoracic and abdominal aorta, beginning at the left subclavian artery.
- The Stanford Classification uses A and B with type A involving the ascending aorta (De Bakey I and II) and B involving the descending aorta (De Bakey type III).
- The conditions are diagnosed most rapidly by chest CT scan with contrast.
- In patients with chronic aortic dissection in the descending thoracic aorta or thoracoabdominal aorta with a maximal aortic diameter of 5.0 cm or more, preemptive surgical therapy should be undertaken.
- Transthoracic endovascular aneurysm repair (TEVAR) is performed by percutaneously placing a stent within the true aortic lumen to preserve perfusion and has been used for aortic aneurysmal disease type B aortic dissection, traumatic aortic transection, and penetrating aortic ulcer/intramural hematoma.
  - Complications of TEVAR include device migration, endoleak (blood finding its way around the stent and into the aneurysm), stroke due to embolization to the carotid artery, paraplegia due to spinal cord ischemia, visceral ischemia due to compromise of the celiac artery, and an inflammatory response to the graft known as the post-implantation syndrome.

Aortic Aneurysm

Indications for Surgical Aneurysm Repair

Location of Aneurysm	Size	Additional Considerations
Ascending aorta	≥4.5 cm	Marfan syndrome *with* family history of aortic dissection or bicuspid aortic valve and severe aortic stenosis or regurgitation
Ascending aorta	≥5.0 cm	Marfan syndrome *without* family history of aortic dissection or bicuspid aortic valve *with* family history of aortic dissection
Ascending aorta and aortic root	≥5.5 cm	Regardless of above
Aortic arch	≥6 cm	
Descending aorta	≥6.5 cm	
Descending aorta	<5.5 cm	If growth ≥0.5 cm/year

Rupture of the descending thoracic aortic aneurysm accounts for 30% of aortic ruptures and carries a high mortality. It requires immediate intervention, usually through an operative approach however transthoracic endovascular aneurysm repair (TEVAR) may also be an option.

CASE 33 | Carotid Artery Stenosis (CAS)

A 68-year-old woman with diabetes, hyperlipidemia, hypertension, and 30-pack-year tobacco use presents with intermittent left-sided vision loss that evolves over minutes and resolves within a few minutes. The vision loss is not associated with pain, and she describes it as "a curtain falling over the left eye." Her temperature is 37.5°C, pulse 80/min, respirations 14/min, and blood pressure 135/90 mmHg. On exam, a carotid bruit is heard on the left. Cranial nerves are intact with normal range of motion, strength, and sensation bilaterally.

Conditions with Similar Presentations	**Multiple sclerosis:** May present with vision loss due to optic neuritis but occurs over hours to days, not minutes. Also, it is painful in over 90% of patients. More common in young women of reproductive age. **Cardioembolic or hemorrhagic stroke:** Causes a permanent, not transient defect.
Initial Diagnostic Tests	Carotid duplex ultrasonography of bilateral carotid arteries
Next Steps in Management	• *Medical management* for asymptomatic patients and stenosis <70% • *Operative management* for symptomatic patients or with those with stenosis ≥70%
Discussion	CAS involves formation of an atherosclerotic plaque composed of lipoprotein and cholesterol in the carotid arteries. As the plaque grows, there is progressive narrowing of the vessel lumen. Plaque rupture and subsequent thrombosis, or embolism, can lead to stroke, or as in this case, amaurosis fugax transient vision loss due to a TIA involving the retina due to a shower of microemboli from the atheromatous plaque in the carotid artery. **History:** • Risk factors: Male sex, older age, smoking, diabetes, hyperlipidemia, hypertension, history of other atherosclerotic diseases such as peripheral artery disease and coronary artery disease. • Patients may be asymptomatic, with CAS discovered incidentally when imaging is performed for another reason. • Symptomatic patients classically present with transient, painless monocular vision loss (amaurosis fugax) or focal neurological deficits consistent with TIA or stroke. **Physical Exam:** • Physical exam may be unremarkable. • Classic signs include carotid bruit (nonspecific finding, may be present with >60% stenosis) or other manifestations of atherosclerotic disease (e.g., decreased femoral pulses, shiny lower extremities). • Patients may have motor or sensory deficits on neurological exam. **Diagnostics:** • Duplex Doppler ultrasound of bilateral carotid arteries provides degree of stenosis, velocity of flow across stenosis, and flow reversal, but is limited if the artery has calcification. Moderate stenosis is 50–69%, and severe stenosis is >70%. • Magnetic resonance angiography (MRA) or CTA if there is high clinical suspicion and results of ultrasound are indeterminate. • Patients also commonly undergo transcranial Doppler (TCD) to examine intracranial vessels downstream from the internal carotid artery, such as the middle cerebral artery. • The gold standard is cerebral angiography; however, patients are usually evaluated with more noninvasive tests, such as above. • Pre-op evaluation includes baseline CBC, coagulation studies, BUN, creatinine, ECG. Consider stress echocardiogram if the patient has new cardiac symptoms. **Management:** *Medical management:* preferred in asymptomatic patients or those with mild to moderate stenosis (<70%). It includes high-intensity statins, an antiplatelet agent (i.e., aspirin), and medical optimization of comorbid conditions (diabetes, hypertension, hyperlipidemia). Patients should be advised on smoking cessation, weight loss, healthy diet, and physical exercise when applicable.

CASE 33 | Carotid Artery Stenosis (CAS) *(continued)*

Discussion	*Operative management*: **Carotid endarterectomy** is indicated in 1. Symptomatic patients 2. Those with stenosis ≥70% 3. >50% stenosis if male greater than 75 years old or history of stroke Note that surgery is contraindicated if the carotid artery is completely occluded, severe neurologic deficits, or if patient has severe comorbidities which increase risk of post-operative mortality **Carotid artery stenting** • Performed when risk of surgery is unacceptably high such as the patient with multiple comorbidities, prior neck radiation or surgeries. • Patients need to remain on lifelong statin and aspirin and require interval monitoring of recurrent stenosis or thrombosis with carotid duplex
Additional Considerations	**Post Operative Complications of Carotid Endarterectomy** 1. Death or stroke, 3.2%—observed to be higher in patients undergoing carotid endarterectomy who are symptomatic 2. Myocardial infarction, 4% 3. Minor neurologic complications, 6.9%, observed higher in symptomatic patients 4. Wound complications, 6.0% 5. Noncardiac complications, 3.2%—ventilatory assistance, thrombosis, pulmonary embolism, GI bleeding

CASE 34 | Abdominal Aortic Aneurysm (AAA)

A 62-year-old man with hyperlipidemia, hypertension, and smoking presents to clinic with sudden-onset epigastric pain which radiates to the back. His temperature is 37.5°C, pulse is 120/min, respirations are 20/min, and blood pressure is 100/60 mmHg. On exam, the abdomen is slightly distended, tender but soft, with rebound and guarding. He has a pulsatile mass in the midline of his abdomen which is tender to palpation. Femoral pulses are palpable bilaterally.

Conditions with Similar Presentations	**Acute mesenteric ischemia:** Also presents with acute onset of abdominal pain and may have rebound and guarding. It can be due to an acute thrombosis of an atherosclerotic artery or emboli, typically from atrial fibrillation. It would not present with a pulsatile mass. **Pancreatitis:** Presents with epigastric pain that radiates to the back, but unless complicated, would not have rebound or guarding and would not have a pulsative mass.
Initial Diagnostic Tests	Abdominal ultrasound, abdominal CT with contrast if a repair is considered and patient is hemodynamically stable
Next Steps in Management	*Operative management*: Ruptured AAA (emergently), symptomatic AAA (urgently), and elective repair of unruptured AAA when size is >5.5 cm or <5.5 cm but rapidly expanding (>0.5 cm in 6 months).
Discussion	The normal aorta measures 2 cm in diameter; aneurysmal dilation is defined as 3 cm or greater. The abdominal aorta begins at the diaphragmatic hiatus (T12) and bifurcates into the right and left common iliac arteries (L4). Aneurysms typically develop below the renal arteries (level of L2) and above the common iliac arteries (level of L4). Pathophysiology involves elastin fiber disruption. Collagen is degraded by proteases and elasticity of aortic wall is lost, resulting in bleeding into a false lumen. Risk of rupture increases as the aneurysm increases in size. **History:** • Risk factors: age >60, male sex, cigarette smoking (greatest risk factor), family history, atherosclerosis, coronary artery disease, peripheral artery disease, connective tissue diseases (e.g., Marfan syndrome, Ehlers-Danlos syndrome). • Symptomatic patients will present with abdominal, back, and/or flank pain that is not associated with meals. • In severe symptomatic or ruptured cases, patients will have severe sudden-onset abdominal, flank, and/or back pain and hypovolemic shock. More distal aneurysms may have pain in the lower abdomen or groin. **Physical Exam:** • Asymptomatic patients may have an enlarged, pulsatile nontender mass or an abdominal bruit on exam, although many patients lack these findings until the aneurysm has expanded significantly or ruptures. • Symptomatic patients may have the same findings in addition to tenderness to palpation of the mass and/or umbilical or flank hematoma. The physical exam should include assessment of femoral pulses, which may be decreased in ruptured AAA.

CASE 34 | Abdominal Aortic Aneurysm (AAA) *(continued)*

Discussion	**Diagnostics:**
	• Rapid ultrasound should be performed on an unstable patient in preparation for the operating room if no known history of aneurysm; if patient is known to have AAA and becomes symptomatic, ultrasound is unnecessary and patient should go immediately to the operating room.
	• CT scan with contrast provides visualization of the aorta, visualizing thrombus, length and diameter of the aneurysm, and has replaced aortography as the study of choice in pre-operative planning if nonemergent.
	• For patients who are asymptomatic or symptomatic but hemodynamically stable, preferred imaging modality is an abdominal CT with contrast to determine the location of the aneurysm.
	
	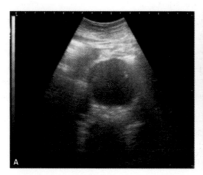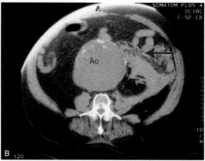
	
	A. Ultrasound image of an abdominal aortic aneurysm in the transverse plane. B. CT scan of a patient with a 12-cm abdominal aortic aneurysm. Calcification of the aortic wall is seen in the anterior aspect of the aneurysm. Evidence of hemorrhage and surrounding inflammation (*arrow*). (Reproduced with permission from Tintinalli JE, Ma O, Yealy DM, Meckler GD, Stapczynski J, Cline DM, Thomas SH. Tintinalli's Emergency Medicine: A Comprehensive Study Guide, 9e. Copyright 2020 McGraw-Hill Education.)
	
	Management: Management by vascular surgery is based on classification into asymptomatic vs. symptomatic and ruptured (hemodynamically unstable) vs. unruptured (hemodynamically stable).
	• For asymptomatic AAA, aneurysms <4 cm do not require monitoring. For AAAs 4-5.5 cm in size, monitor every 6 months with abdominal US (or with abdominal CT if location is infrarenal or juxtarenal).
	• Elective repair of asymptomatic AAA is recommended when >5.5 cm or expanding >0.5 cm in 6 months.
	• Symptomatic AAA of any size should be repaired urgently, and if the patient is hemodynamically unstable this should be done on an emergent basis.
	• Preferred approach is endovascular abdominal aortic aneurysm repair (EVAR)
	  • Complications of this procedure include endoleaks or leaking around the graft, graft migration, damage to the iliac artery during insertion of the graft, and renal failure
	• Open repair usually only if not EVAR not available or not feasible due to patient's anatomy and risk factors
	  All patients should be counseled on smoking cessation and started on aspirin and statin therapy.

Additional Considerations	**Screening:** U.S. Preventive Services Task Force (USPSTF) guidelines recommend a one-time screening with an abdominal ultrasound in all men aged 65–75 who have ever smoked (Grade B recommendation).
	Complications:
	• Cardiovascular: MI can occur in 3–16%; in elective surgeries, pre-operative revascularization would precede aortic aneurysm repair
	• Embolic stroke
	• Atheroembolic complications
	  • Foot ischemia due to atheromatous fragments or thrombosis from aortic cross-clamp
	  • Renal ischemia due to atheromatous fragments or due to hypovolemia from hemorrhage, or due to decreased blood flow from aortic cross-clamp
	  • Colonic ischemia
	  • Spinal cord ischemia
	• Aortic enteric fistula
	• Infected graft
	• Overall mortality if ruptured is >80%

CASE 35 | Peripheral Artery Disease (PAD)

A 65-year-old man with diabetes, hypertension, tobacco use, and coronary artery disease presents with exertional bilateral calf pain for nine months. The pain occurs after walking up the three steps into his house or after walking more than one block; pain resolves with rest. On exam, he has no lower extremity edema or skin rashes, but he has hair loss bilaterally up to the mid-calf circumferentially. Femoral and popliteal pulses are 2+ bilaterally, and dorsalis pedis pulses are nonpalpable bilaterally but monophasic with Doppler ultrasound.

Conditions with Similar Presentations	**Leriche syndrome:** Occurs due to aortoiliac occlusion and presents with a triad of erectile dysfunction, lower extremity claudication, and decreased femoral pulses. **Neurogenic claudication (pseudoclaudication):** Due to spinal stenosis presents with posture-dependent claudication (symptoms are increased with standing and relieved by sitting or lying down) rather than with exertion. Pulses are normal. **Thromboangiitis obliterans (Buerger disease):** Is a vasculitis presenting with nonatherosclerotic, segmental inflammation of small to medium-sized arteries and veins of the extremities. Patients are typically <45 years old and smokers who present with ischemia of the digits. **Chronic lower extremity venous disease (venous insufficiency):** Is more common than PAD, with variable presentation including lower extremity discomfort worse with prolonged standing or walking, abnormal venous dilation (e.g., telangiectasias, varicose veins), edema, dermatitis, and/or venous ulceration.
Initial Diagnostic Tests	• Pulse exam with Dopplers to assess vascular flow • Measure the ankle-brachial index (ABI). An ABI ≤0.9 is diagnostic
Next Steps in Management	• Medical optimization of comorbid conditions • Angiography with stenting or bypass indicated in cases refractory to medical treatment
Discussion	PAD is an atherosclerotic disease of the peripheral arteries, most often involving the lower extremity (femoral, popliteal, tibial, dorsalis pedis arteries) resulting in claudication and potentially limb ischemia. Intermittent claudication presents with exertional limb pain due to insufficient blood flow to muscles with activity or exercise that is relieved with rest. As PAD progresses, it can eventually lead to pain at rest, ischemia, and necrosis or gangrene of the extremity. The pathophysiology of PAD is similar to the development of coronary artery disease, and the concurrence rate is very high. Disease progression is accelerated by vascular damage from smoking, hypertension, and diabetes. **History:** • Strongest risk factors are smoking and diabetes. Other risk factors include hypertension, hyperlipidemia, and age >65 years. • The most common manifestation of PAD is claudication (leg pain on exertion, relieved with rest). Worsening disease can result in ischemic rest pain (worsened with elevation). Pain location can be correlated with the level of occlusion (e.g., buttock pain is suggestive of aortoiliac occlusion, calf pain is suggestive of superficial femoral or popliteal artery occlusion).

Physical Exam: On exam, patients will have diminished or absent distal pulses. Additional findings include shiny, hairless, and cold lower extremities. They may also have arterial ulcers (painful, necrotic, located in distal areas such as toes) that can be differentiated from venous ulcers (hemosiderin staining, weeping, located at the medial malleolus).

Diagnostics:
- Dopplers can be used to assess nonpalpable flow.
- ABI is calculated by dividing systolic BP in the ankle by systolic BP taken from the brachial artery.
- An ABI ≤0.9 is diagnostic of PAD and can be further classified based on the table below.
- Consider exercise testing if normal ABI in symptomatic patient.
- CTA or MRA is used to assess the location and severity of the occlusion and plan for revascularization. Imaging should be performed bilaterally.
- Angiogram used to be gold standard but is invasive and may be used with duplex ultrasound when considering catheter-based interventions.

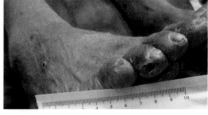

Typical appearance of extremity with PAD. Extremities that have PAD tend to have thin shiny skin, atrophied subcutaneous tissue and muscles, thick yellow nails, lack of hair, dry fissured skin, discoloration, and dependent hyperemia (termed rubor of dependency). (Reproduced with permission from Hamm RL. Text and Atlas of Wound Diagnosis and Treatment, 2e. Copyright 2019 McGraw-Hill Education.)

CASE 35 | Peripheral Artery Disease (PAD) *(continued)*

Discussion	ABI	Classification	Presentation
	<0.4	Severe, limb-threatening	Rest pain; potential for tissue loss with ulceration, ischemia, gangrene
	0.4–0.9	Mild to moderate	Intermittent claudication
	0.9–1.1	Normal	No symptoms
	>1.1	Elevated	Can be seen if arterial calficiations are present in patients with atherosclerosis because vessels are not easily compressible. Consider assessing toe-brachial index (TBI) in these patients, with TBI <0.3 indicative of severe ischemia

Management:
- Optimize treatment of underlying medical conditions such as diabetes, hypertension, hyperlipidemia, and obesity
- Advise patients on smoking cessation and exercise therapy (e.g., supervised exercise program)
- Medical therapy includes high-intensity statins, antiplatelet agents (e.g., aspirin, clopidogrel)
- Cilostazol, a phosphodiesterase III inhibitor (causes vasodilation and decreases platelet aggregation), can increase walking distance and reduce symptoms of claudication but is contraindicated in patients with left ventricular dysfunction
- For patients with lifestyle-limiting symptoms refractory to medical therapy or severe, limb-threatening PAD, revascularization is indicated
  - Percutaneous endovascular therapy involves introducing a catheter proximal to the occlusion, inflating a balloon, and stenting the previously occluded vessel lumen
  - Bypass involves using a graft (commonly the great saphenous vein) to divert blood around an obstruction (e.g., femoral popliteal bypass)
- Amputation of toes or leg may be necessary in severe refractory cases

Additional Considerations	**Complications:**
	Acute limb ischemia is a disruption of an atherosclerotic plaque with subsequent arterial thrombosis, may result in acute limb ischemia. Presents with the "six P's"—pain, pallor, paresthesia, poikilothermia, paralysis, and pulselessness. This is a surgical emergency requiring anticoagulation with heparin and revascularization with thrombolysis or thrombectomy following intraoperative angiography.
	Critical limb ischemia is a chronic complication of PAD characterized by rest pain, tissue loss, non-healing ulceration, and gangrene. While less common, acute limb ischemia can also occur in the upper extremities, most commonly secondary to cardiac thromboemboli (e.g., in setting of atrial fibrillation or valvular disease).

Lower extremity ulcers are common in patients with vascular disease. Considerations in differentiating between arterial, venous, diabetic, and pressure ulcers are (1) the location of the wound, (2) the description of the wound, and (3) the individual risk factors of the patient.

Foot Ulcer Mini-Cases

Arterial Ulcer	**Hx:** Risk factors: PAD, and other manifestations of atherosclerosis (TIA/stroke, angina, MI). Symptoms: Usually presents with pain at rest and pain with elevation of the leg (gravity-mediated decreased blood flow). **PE:** Ulcers are common over bony prominences and at the tips of the distal toes (areas furthest from blood supply). There will be a sharply demarcated, punched-out wound and little to no granulation tissue and exudate. The base of the ulcer is dry, pale, or necrotic. The surrounding skin is cool, shiny, tight, and may have alopecia and dermal atrophy (all from lack of arterial supply). Patients will have diminished or absent distal pulses (e.g., dorsalis pedis). **Diagnostics:** • Clinical diagnosis, confirmed with measuring ABI and MRA or CTA **Management:** • Proper wound care, management of arterial disease (medical optimization and therapy), revascularization for tissue healing **Discussion:** The ulcer results from ischemia; thus, this is sometimes known as an arterial insufficiency ulcer. Inadequate perfusion to the tissue results in ulceration of the skin, fat, and muscle. This can result from any arterial disease such as atherosclerosis, vasculitis, or thromboangiitis obliterans.	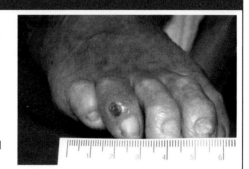 The typical arterial wound due to PAD is located on the distal digit, has a round punched-out appearance, dry-to-necrotic wound bed, and little or no granulation tissue. The wounds tend to be painful with poor healing potential without restoration of blood supply. (Reproduced with permission from Hamm RL. Text and Atlas of Wound Diagnosis and Treatment, 2e. Copyright 2019 McGraw-Hill Education.)
Venous Ulcer	**Hx:** Patients may have a history of deep vein thromboses and/or venous incompetence (e.g., telangiectasias, varicose veins). May have itchy, scaly wounds on their calves. Often painless or associated with some discomfort. **PE:** Wound often present between the knee and the ankle, most commonly above the medial or lateral malleolus or posterior calf. Will appear as an erythematous, beefy red wound with granulation tissue, weeping, and covered in yellow fibrinous tissue. There may also be eczema and scaling on the surrounding skin. Skin will be warm, with overlying hyperpigmentation, brown-blue discoloration due to hemosiderin deposition, edema, stasis dermatitis, and xerosis. Pulses will be present. **Diagnostics:** • Clinical diagnosis • Obtain venous duplex ultrasound if concern for thrombosis **Management:** Compression therapy (e.g., stockings, Unna boot), leg elevation, wound care **Discussion:** Venous ulcers occur as a result of chronic venous insufficiency—usually due to venous thrombosis or incompetent valves. Increased venous pressure leads to increased vascular permeability, release of inflammatory cells, and subsequent skin ulceration.	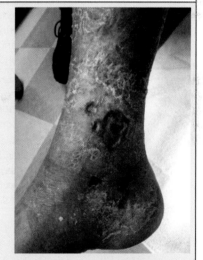 Venous ulceration located proximal to the medial malleolus. (Reproduced with permission from Brunicardi F, Andersen DK, Billiar TR, Dunn DL, Kao LS, Hunter JG, Matthews JB, Pollock RE. Schwartz's Principles of Surgery, 11e. Copyright 2019 McGraw-Hill Education.)
Diabetic (Neuropathic) Ulcer	**Hx:** Patient will have a history of long-standing diabetes mellitus, typically poorly controlled, with neuropathy and vascular insufficiency. Patient may not notice the wound is there, usually painless.

Foot Ulcer Mini-Cases *(continued)*

Diabetic (Neuropathic) Ulcer	**PE:** Commonly present on pressure points such as the plantar metatarsal heads and the heel (places the patient cannot see often and may not notice). Ulcer will be punched-out with clear borders. Foot often has hyperkeratotic callouses. May have exposed bone (diagnostic of osteomyelitis). Skin will be warm with decreased sensation and associated foot deformities. Reflexes will be absent, and pulses may be absent or present. **Diagnostics:** • Clinical diagnosis. • Underlying osteomyelitis is confirmed if bone is visible or can be probed through the wound. • MRI has the highest sensitivity for detection. • Bone biopsy should be done for culture because superficial cultures do not correlate well with the bacteria infecting the bone. **Management:** • Wound care—debridement and curettage are often necessary. • Mechanical offloading with walkers and special shoes. • Improved glycemic control • Educate patients on proper foot care including regularly inspecting feet, ensuring appropriate moisturization, and regular podiatric care. **Discussion:** Diabetic foot ulcers are a type of neuropathic ulcer caused by repeated friction, pressure, and/or trauma to the foot that the patient does not notice due to decreased sensation from peripheral neuropathy in the setting of diabetes. Neuropathy involves sensory, autonomic, and motor nerve fibers leading to lack of awareness of injury, delay in treatment, loss of appropriate arteriolar and capillary tone, decreased tissue perfusion, atrophy of small intrinsic muscles of the feet, and sometimes clawing of the toes due to MTP hyperextension. Ulcers may be secondarily infected, resulting in soft tissue infection or osteomyelitis. 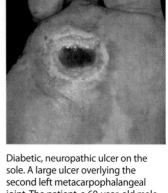 Diabetic, neuropathic ulcer on the sole. A large ulcer overlying the second left metacarpophalangeal joint. The patient, a 60-year-old male with diabetes mellitus of 25 years' duration, has significant sensory neuropathy of the feet and lower legs as well as peripheral vascular disease, which resulted in amputation of the fourth and fifth toes. (Reproduced with permission from Wolff K, Johnson R, Saavedra AP, Roh EK. Fitzpatrick's Color Atlas and Synopsis of Clinical Dermatology, 8e. Copyright 2017 McGraw-Hill Education.)
Pressure Injuries	**Hx:** Pressure injuries result from vertical pressure, friction, moisture, and shearing forces, most commonly over bony prominences in immobilized patients (e.g., bed-bound, wheelchair-bound, in the ICU or long-term nursing facility). Additional risk factors include presence of cerebrovascular disease, cardiovascular disease, fecal or urinary incontinence, diabetes, recent lower extremity fractures, and malnutrition. **PE:** Ulcer will be on a bony prominence that undergoes prolonged, constant pressure on the skin and soft tissues when patient is immobilized. The sacrum is the most common location, followed by buttocks (ischium), heel, and trochanter; less frequently injuries on the lateral malleolus and occiput. The highest incidence is observed in orthopedic patients, followed by oncology and ICU patients. Erythema, loss of skin, necrosis, draining sinus tracts, granulation tissue, and/or foul smell may be present. 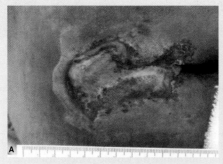 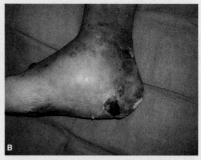 A. Moisture on skin. Moisture is one of the contributing factors to pressure ulcers, especially in the perineal and perianal areas. The changes in skin as a result of prolonged exposure include maceration, blanched color, and a papillary-like texture, as seen on the area around this sacral pressure ulcer. The drainage can be fecal, urinary, or wound moisture. In addition, the moisture can cause changes in the skin pH, especially in the case of fecal incontinence, which further weakens the skin and increases the risk of tissue damage. B. Infection. The erythema and edema surrounding the pressure ulcer on the heel indicate there is deep infection. Other signs to note are warmth, pain with weight-bearing, and drainage from the wound. For diabetic foot ulcers, erythema that extends more than 2 cm from the edge of the wound is highly correlated with infection. If the wound can be probed to bone, there is a strong probability of osteomyelitis, or infection of the underlying bone. (Reproduced with permission from Hamm RL. Text and Atlas of Wound Diagnosis and Treatment, 2e. Copyright 2019 McGraw-Hill Education.)

Foot Ulcer Mini-Cases *(continued)*

Pressure Injuries	**Diagnostics:** Clinical diagnosis **Management:** • Prevention: frequent pressure redistribution in immobilized patients, as well as use of pressure-reducing devices and proper patient positioning. • Wound care: moist environment with vacuum-assisted closure and debridement of necrotic tissue. • Optimize nutrition **Discussion:** Pressure injuries (previously known as decubitus ulcers) are the third most costly disease after cancer and cardiovascular disease, with a prevalence of 12% of hospitalized patients worldwide. Pressure causes tissue injury in a cone-shaped pattern that expands from the pressure point downward, known as a deep tissue injury. Pressure ulcers should be staged to determine severity and treatment. Stage 1 injury has not broken the skin and makes up of roughly 45% of injuries; Stage 2 transgresses epidermis and dermis and makes up 45% of injuries; Stage 3 extends into the subcutaneous fat affecting 5%; Stage 4 injuries are deep injuries involving muscle, tendon, ligaments, and bone, affecting 5%. If the depth of the injury cannot be assessed because of overlying eschar, it is called an unstageable pressure injury. For those patients with Stage 3 or 4 injuries, surgical coverage of the wound is required to reduce pain, infection, and the development of sepsis. Coverage is accomplished by raising a flap consisting of skin, subcutaneous and muscle tissues, and rotating it over the bony prominence.

Stage 1
Observable pressure-related alteration of intact skin whose indicators as compared to the adjacent or opposite area of the body may include changes in one or more of the following: skin temperature (warmth or coolness), tissue consistency (firm or boggy feel), and/or sensation (pain, itching). The ulcer appears as a defined area of persistent redness in lightly pigmented skin, whereas in darker skin tones the ulcer may appear with persistent red, blue, or purple hues.

Stage 2
Partial-thickness skin loss involving epidermis and/or dermis. The ulcer is superficial and presents clinically as an abrasion, blister, or shallow crater.

Stage 3
Full-thickness skin loss involving damage or necrosis of subcutaneous tissue that may extend down to but not through underlaying fascia. The ulcer presents clinically as a deep crater with or without undermining of adjacent tissue.

Stage 4
Full-thickness skin loss with extensive destruction, tissue necrosis, or damage to muscle, bone, or supporting structures (for example, tendon or joint capsule). Undermining and sinus tracts may also be associated with Stage 4 pressure ulcers.

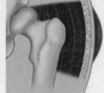
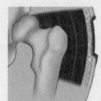
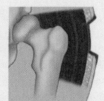
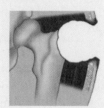

A   B   C   D

The staging system for pressure sores. (Reproduced with permission from Brunicardi F, Andersen DK, Billiar TR, Dunn DL, Kao LS, Hunter JG, Matthews JB, Pollock RE. Schwartz's Principles of Surgery, 11e. New York: McGraw Hill; 2019.)

BREAST SURGERY AND PATHOLOGY

Most breast concerns are due to benign etiologies. However, breast cancer is the most common invasive malignancy in females (affecting about one in eight patients) and the second most common cause of cancer death (after lung cancer). Refer to Obstetrics and Gynecology Chapter for additional information and cases.

The risk of breast cancer increases with age, obesity, female sex, high estrogen levels, nulliparity (or older age with first pregnancy), alcohol consumption, and family history of breast cancer, or certain mutations (e.g., *BRCA*). The risk of breast cancer can be reduced by breastfeeding.

Breast cancer can present with a hard "rock-like" mass, nipple discharge, thickening of the skin, skin erythema, or dimpling (peau d'orange). If the cancer has metastasized, patients may present with axillary lymphadenopathy and/or systemic symptoms depending on the organ involved (e.g., back pain with bone involvement, abdominal pain or jaundice with liver involvement, headache or neurological findings with brain involvement).

Diagnostic

Imaging:

- **Mammogram:**
  - Breast cancer screening: USPSTF recommends mammography every two years for women aged 50–74 while the American College of Obstetrics & Gynecology (ACOG) recommends mammography every 1–2 years for women aged 40–74
    - If increased risk (e.g., family history, *BRCA* mutation), start sooner
  - If symptomatic (i.e., mass, pathologic discharge), should perform in all women ≥30 years old as well as all men
    - Younger women (<30) have more dense breast tissue which could result in higher false-positive rates
- **Ultrasound:** performed in symptomatic patients, including women <30-years old, or for further characterization of abnormalities detected by exam or mammogram
- **MRI:** May be used for further evaluation, especially in patients with mammographically dense breasts or as an annual screening tool only in high-risk patients with significant risk factors
- Breast Imaging Reporting and Data System (BI-RADS) is a standard system used by radiologists to describe mammogram results and sorts the findings into categories 0 through 6. While you likely won't have to know or memorize this for USMLE Step 2 CK, it is helpful to know for clinical settings.

BI-RADS	Interpretation
0 (Incomplete)	May need additional tests such as mammogram with spot compression, and/or magnified views, and/or ultrasound, or may need to compare results with older mammograms.
1 (Negative)	Normal test result.
2 (Benign finding)	Negative for cancer, but may have other findings such as benign calcifications, masses, or lymph nodes.
3 (Probably benign finding)	Very low (<2%) chance of being cancer. Typically recommend follow-up with repeat imaging in 6–12 months and regularly thereafter to ensure stability (usually at least 2 years).
4 (Suspicious abnormality)	Findings may look like cancer and recommend biopsy. 4A: Low likelihood of being cancer (2–10%) 4B: Moderate likelihood of being cancer (10–50%) 4C: High likelihood of being cancer (50–95%)
5 (Highly suggestive of malignancy)	Findings have a high chance (≥95%) of being cancer, and biopsy very strongly recommended.
6 Known biopsy-proven malignancy	Used for findings on a mammogram or other imaging that have been already proven by biopsy to be cancer. Imaging may be done to monitor treatment response.

Biopsy:

- Fine needle aspiration (FNA): useful in evaluating palpable lesions and draining cysts
- Core needle biopsy: to evaluate solid lesions
- Excisional biopsy: completely removes lesion

Benign Breast Conditions

Benign breast disease can be categorized into three categories: no increased risk, mild to moderate increased risk, and high risk of breast cancer.

No Increased Risk	Mild-to-Moderate Increased Risk	High Risk
• Cysts • Epithelial hyperplasia • Duct ectasia • Nonsclerosing adenosis • Periductal fibrosis • Fat necrosis	• Intraductal papilloma and papillomatosis • Ductal hyperplasia • Sclerosing adenosis • Radial scar • Fibroadenoma • Phyllodes tumor (cystosarcoma phyllodes)—rarely malignant	• Atypical ductal hyperplasia • Atypical lobular hyperplasia • Lobular carcinoma in situ

Nipple Discharge

May be due to physiologic causes such as nipple stimulation or medication adverse reactions (e.g., antipsychotics, metoclopramide). Patients usually undergo work up to exclude hyperprolactinemia and hypothyroidism. Discharge can be categorized as bilateral or unilateral. Bilateral milky, clear, gray, yellow, brown, or green is more likely to be related to benign pathologies (e.g., physiologic, mammary duct ectasia). Unilateral and bloody or serosanguinous discharge is more often associated with malignancy. Nipple discharge in men is a common presentation of breast cancer.

Nipple Discharge Evaluation

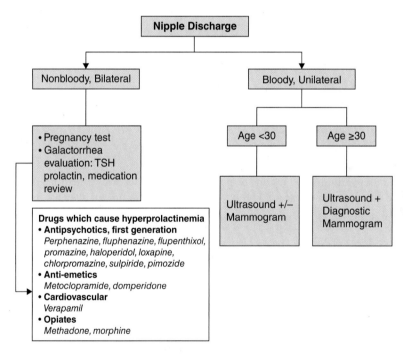

CASE 36 | Intraductal Papilloma

A 29-year-old woman with no past medical history presents with bloody discharge from her right nipple. She is not currently lactating and has no fevers or chills. She performs occasional self-breast exams and has not detected any unusual masses. She has no breast pain or recent trauma. On exam, unilateral serosanguinous discharge is expressible from the right nipple. There are no masses or skin lesions, and the breasts are otherwise symmetric.

Conditions with Similar Presentations	**Physiologic discharge:** Usually nonbloody, *bilateral* nipple discharge. May be due to nipple stimulation or medication adverse effects.
	Fibrocystic changes of the breast: May present with unilateral or bilateral serous discharge. Patients may also note intermittent changes in breast size or the presence of lumps that enlarge just before menstruation.
	Intraductal breast carcinoma: May also present with unilateral bloody nipple discharge. It may or may not be associated with a mass.

CASE 36 | Intraductal Papilloma *(continued)*

Initial Diagnostic Tests	Breast ultrasonography (ultrasound) is the initial exam for women aged 30 or younger
Next Steps in Management	Surgical excision of involved duct
Discussion	Intraductal papilloma is a benign cause of unilateral nipple discharge in the nonlactating patient. However, there may be associated malignant regions and it is therefore excised when symptomatic. Intraductal papillomas can occur at any age post-menarche but are more common in middle-aged adults. The older the patient, the more likely their nipple discharge is due to a malignant process.
	History: Usually unilateral, serous, or serosanguinous nipple discharge in middle-aged female. There may be an associated mass, but this is not typical.
	Physical Exam: Discharge can be seen on exam. There is an absence of skin changes. If a mass is present, it is often subareolar.
	Diagnostics: The diagnostic approach to unilateral or bloody nipple discharge is age-dependent due to the increased density of breast tissue in younger patients: • <30: Breast ultrasound followed is initial exam; may be followed by mammogram if suspicious • 30–39: Mammogram or ultrasound can be initial exam • > 40 (or male sex): Both mammogram and ultrasound are performed If both the mammogram and ultrasound are negative and the patient is still experiencing nipple discharge, a breast MRI can be considered.
	Management: • Surgical excision of involved duct and continue with routine breast screening. • If there is concern for malignancy, core needle biopsy and clip placement should occur prior to excision.

Breast Masses and Lesions

- *Fibrocystic changes:* Most common benign breast condition. Occurs due to exaggerated stromal tissue response to hormones and growth factors, presenting as cyclical bilateral mastalgia. May present with masses, nodularity/lumpiness with or without pain that rapidly fluctuate in size in relation to the menstrual cycle. More prevalent in pre-menopausal patients and those taking hormone therapy.

- *Breast Cysts:* Discrete, mobile, fluid-filled lesions responsive to hormones and growth factors. Simple or milk-filled are benign; bloody may be due to atypia or cancer. FNA to confirm cystic nature and alleviate pain.

- *Fibroadenoma:* Well-circumscribed, mobile mass with peak occurrence between the ages of 15 and 35. Observe most lesions.

- *Phyllodes tumor (cystosarcoma phyllodes):* Rare fibroepithelial neoplasm (rarely malignant) with a similar presentation to fibroadenoma. The mass is larger, with more rapid growth and with greater metastatic potential. On histology, this neoplasm can be differentiated by papillary projections of the stroma, lined with epithelium, and associated with hyperplasia and atypia. Treatment is wide excision or simple mastectomy for large tumors.

- *Intraductal papilloma:* A benign tumor involving the subareolar ducts causing bloody nipple discharge; treatment is excision of the duct.

- *Sclerosing adenosis and ductal hyperplasia:* No treatment required.

- *Fat necrosis:* Occurs secondary to blunt breast trauma (however, patients may not report a history trauma) resulting in saponification of damaged breast tissue. This will present as a firm, discrete mass, and will appear calcified on imaging.

- *Lactating adenoma:* The most common breast mass during pregnancy and lactation.

- *Mammary duct ectasia:* May present with retroareolar mass, dilation of subareolar ducts or bloody discharge; treat by excising area

- *Atypical hyperplasia (AH):* Increased risk of breast cancer; similar to low-grade ductal carcinoma in situ (DCIS) or lobular carcinoma in situ (LCIS). Treat with tamoxifen or aromatase inhibitor (if post-menopausal).

Palpable Breast Mass Evaluation

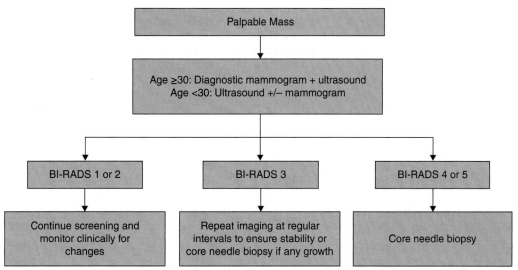

Flowchart:

Palpable Mass
↓
Age ≥30: Diagnostic mammogram + ultrasound
Age <30: Ultrasound +/– mammogram
↓
- BI-RADS 1 or 2 → Continue screening and monitor clinically for changes
- BI-RADS 3 → Repeat imaging at regular intervals to ensure stability or core needle biopsy if any growth
- BI-RADS 4 or 5 → Core needle biopsy

CASE 37	Fibroadenoma

A nulliparous 25-year-old woman presents with a left breast mass she noted a few weeks ago. She denies pain, nipple discharge, or dimpling of the skin overlying the mass. She has not noted any changes to the size of the mass since discovering it. She has no family history of breast cancer. She has been taking combination oral contraceptives since age 17. On exam there is a 2-cm, nontender, well-circumscribed, firm, rubbery, mobile mass in the lower inner quadrant of the left breast and there are no palpable lymph nodes in the axilla.

Conditions with Similar Presentations	**Fibrocystic change:** May present cyclical bilateral mastalgia and/or masses that fluctuate in size in relation to the menstrual cycle.
	Phyllodes tumor: Similar presentation to fibroadenoma but mass is larger and has papillary (leaf-like) projections of the stroma
	Fat necrosis: Occurs secondary to blunt breast trauma (however patients may not report a history trauma). Firm, discrete mass that will appear calcified on imaging.
	Breast cyst: Discrete, mobile, fluid-filled lesions responsive to hormones and growth factors.
	Breast cancer: May present with a single, nontender, immoveable firm to hard mass with ill-defined margins. Advanced findings include axillary lymphadenopathy, pain, erythema, skin dimpling, and fixation of the mass to the chest.
Initial Diagnostic Tests	• Breast ultrasound • Can confirm with biopsy
Next Steps in Management	Conservative management with yearly follow-up to monitor for growth or changes.
Discussion	Fibroadenoma is a benign slow-growing breast tumor with epithelia and stromal components which is likely influenced by hormones given its growth during pregnancy and shrinking during menopause. Most common breast lesion in women <30 years of age. Women with oral contraceptive use before the age of 20 at slightly increased risk compared to the general population.
	History/Physical Exam: Often noted on self-breast exam and does not change in size during the menstrual cycle. Usually not associated with pain, nipple discharge, skin dimpling, or enlarged lymph nodes.
	Lesion is a round, rubbery, discrete, relatively mobile mass 1–3 cm in diameter. Usually nontender and solitary (up to 20% of patients present with multiple).
	Diagnostics: • Breast ultrasound: Shows a well-circumscribed, round mass with uniform hypoechogenicity. • FNA or needle biopsy can be done to confirm the diagnosis and rule out malignancy. Fibroadenoma triad—fibromyxoid stroma, staghorn clusters, and many single bare nuclei.
	Management: • If risk of malignancy is minimal based on initial diagnostic tests and a diagnosis of fibroadenoma confirmed, patient can be conservatively managed with yearly follow-up to monitor for growth or changes. • If mass causes discomfort or is >3 cm, patient can be referred for lumpectomy.

Inflammation/Infection

- *Mastitis/cellulitis:* Infection usually in lactating females caused by *Staphylococcus* or *Streptococcus*; breast may be engorged, firm, erythematous and painful; treatment includes antibiotics, warm compresses, and may continue breast feeding.

- *Mondor disease:* Thrombophlebitis of the thoracoepigastric vein; can occur after trauma or surgery. Treat with nonsteroidal anti-inflammatory drugs.

- *Inflammatory breast cancer:* A malignant condition that can present similarly to cellulitis/abscess. If an abscess incision and drainage is required, tissues should be sent for histological analysis. Inflammatory breast cancer has a poor prognosis.

Miscellaneous

- *Gynecomastia:* Or enlarged breast tissue in male children or adults, can be caused by drugs (marijuana, estrogens, spironolactone, thiazides, diazepam, tricyclic antidepressants, phenothiazines, phenytoin), disease states (cirrhosis, renal failure, hyperthyroidism, hypogonadism), or carcinoma. A mass, especially in a male >50 years should be biopsied. In contrast, pubertal boys rarely have cancer; their gynecomastia is likely to resolve spontaneously by the age of 16 or 17.

- *Mastalgia:* Breast pain that may be cyclic (worse before menses) or noncyclic (no pattern); usually benign. Treatment includes analgesics, supportive bra, restriction of caffeine.

Malignant Breast Disease

- A new breast mass in a postmenopausal woman is breast cancer until proven otherwise. The overall median age of diagnosis is 62 years. Breast cancer–associated mortality has decreased due to increased screening leading to early detection and treatment.

- The diagnosis of breast cancer requires biopsy to determine the histology/subtype and receptor status. Premalignant (noninvasive) disease includes ductal carcinoma *in situ* (DCIS) and lobular carcinoma *in situ* (LCIS). The invasive subtypes include infiltrating ductal carcinoma, infiltrating lobular carcinoma, medullary carcinoma, and inflammatory carcinoma.

- **DCIS:** considered Stage 0 breast cancer, the malignant cells are confined to the mammary ducts. It is a precursor to invasive cancer but not all cases of DCIS progress to invasive cancer.

- **Invasive Cancer:** The majority of breast cancers (>80%) are diagnosed as invasive, growing into surrounding breast tissue. The majority of these are categorized as *invasive ductal carcinoma* (75%). The next most common is *lobular carcinoma* (10%); of these, 30-40% are bilateral. Medullary, tubular, mucinous, and cribriform types are rare with good prognosis. Inflammatory breast cancer is also rare, often presents with metastasis and has an unfavorable prognosis.

- **Molecular Subtypes:**
  - Hormone Receptor (HR) and Human Epidermal Growth Factor Receptor 2 (HER2) status of the tumor helps predict prognosis and guide therapy.
  - Approximately 20% of breast cancers express HER2 and they tend to grow more quickly.
  - Estrogen receptor (*ER*) and progesterone receptor (*PR*) status are strongly related, >75% of ER-positive tumors are also positive for PR.
  - Compared to women with ER+/PR+ tumors, women with ER+/PR-, ER-/PR+, or ER-/PR- tumors experience higher risks of mortality, which are independent of demographic and clinical tumor characteristics.

- **Genetic testing for Hereditary Breast and Ovarian Cancer (BRCA):** Hereditary factors can increase the risk of developing breast cancer at an earlier age. Multiple cancers in a family member, cancer at a young age or rare cancers suggest a hereditary risk. For example, any of the following diagnoses in a first or second-degree relative carries risk of hereditary breast cancer: relative with breast cancer age 50 or younger, bilateral breast cancer (any age), male breast cancer, history of ovarian cancer, metastatic prostate cancer, Ashkenazi descent with history of a breast, ovarian, pancreatic or prostate cancer. These patients should begin enhanced surveillance no later than 30 years old.

- **Axillary lymph nodes** receive about 85% lymphatic drainage from the breast. They should be evaluated with an ultrasound or sentinel lymph node biopsy in patients with invasive breast cancer to accurately stage the patient.

- **Tumor Staging:** is based on tumor size (T), node involvement (N), and metastasis (M). Early-stage breast cancer patients will only undergo additional diagnostic imaging if there are particular symptoms concerning for metastatic disease such as recurrent headaches, bone pain, or abdominal pain. Higher stage patients are recommended to have CT scan of the chest, abdomen, and pelvis to rule out any distant metastases, as well as an MRI of the brain if there are concerns for CNS involvement.

- **Treatment:** varies by the stage.
  - Low-stage breast cancers (>85%) are treated surgically with breast-conserving surgical excision (local excision, lumpectomy, partial mastectomy) ± radiation. Chemotherapy may be needed for high-risk patients or can be used pre-operatively to reduce tumor size prior to breast conservation surgery.
  - High-stage breast cancers are often treated with total mastectomy (entire breast including breast tissue, skin, areola, and nipple) or modified radical mastectomy (entire breast plus most axillary lymph nodes), followed by radiation and/or chemotherapy.
  - For patients with hormone receptor-positive lesions, can also use selective estrogen receptor modulators (SERMS) such as tamoxifen, aromatase inhibitors such as anastrozole, immunotherapies such as the HER2 receptor monoclonal antibody trastuzumab, or tyrosine kinase inhibitors such as lapatinib.

CASE 38	Breast Cancer (Invasive Ductal Carcinoma)
	A 44-year-old G3P2003 woman with a history of tobacco use presents for evaluation of abnormal findings on self-breast examination. She notes that there is a region on the lateral aspect of her right breast with a small mass and dimpling of the skin. She has a family history of cancer, including two maternal aunts with breast cancer diagnosed in their 40s and ovarian cancer in her maternal grandmother at age 54. On physical exam, there is a firm and fixed mass present on her right breast in the upper lateral quadrant with some overlying erythema. She has axillary lymphadenopathy and breast edema with dimpling (peau d'orange).
Conditions with Similar Presentations	Other forms of invasive carcinoma may present similarly. **Invasive lobular carcinoma:** On biopsy will show an orderly row of cells (in "single file") without duct formation or desmoplastic response. This form of breast cancer is often bilateral. **Inflammatory breast cancer:** Involves dermal lymphatic invasion. It presents with breast pain, warm, swollen, erythematous skin, exaggerated hair follicles, and peau d'orange, but lacks a palpable mass. **Paget disease of the breast:** Unusual presentation of breast cancer that may have associated palpable mass. More common presentation is itching and burning with eczematous, scaly patch on or surrounding the nipple, with some ulceration and yellow crusting/discharge.
Initial Diagnostic Tests	Diagnostic mammogram and ultrasound followed by biopsy
Next Steps in Management	Surgical and medical management dependent on stage, hormone receptor/HER2 status, and patient preferences

Discussion	Development of breast cancer involves ductal hyperproliferation, progression to carcinoma in situ, and then invasive carcinoma. Invasive breast cancer can lead to invasion of nearby pectoral muscles, deep fascia, Cooper ligaments, and overlying skin, leading to nipple retraction or a characteristic skin dimpling pattern referred to as peau d'orange ("skin of the orange"). Risk factors in women include increased age, increased estrogen exposure (e.g., nulliparity, early menarche), alcohol and/or tobacco use, family history of breast cancer, and BRCA1/BRCA2 mutations. Breast cancer in men comprises <1% of all cases. Risk factors in men include BRCA2 mutations and Klinefelter syndrome. The BRCA genes are tumor-suppressor genes involved in DNA repair, and mutations are associated with earlier onset of disease.
	
	History: Presenting symptoms include palpable breast mass, nipple or breast skin changes, breast pain, and nipple discharge. There may be presence of risk factors as noted above.
	
	Physical Exam: Inspection may reveal skin dimpling, edema, erythema, or nipple discharge. Palpable breast masses are often located in the upper outer quadrant. Axillary and supraclavicular lymphadenopathy may be present.
	
	Diagnostics:
	• For palpable breast mass:
	  • Age <30: ultrasound +/− mammogram
	  • Age ≥30: diagnostic mammogram and ultrasound
	  • MRI may be considered in patients with BRCA mutations.
	• If mammogram results are suspicious for malignancy:
	  • Confirm with core needle biopsy of mass (including tumor subtyping and hormone receptor/HER2 testing)
	  • Sentinel lymph node biopsy

CASE 38 | Breast Cancer (Invasive Ductal Carcinoma) *(continued)*

Discussion	Typical findings for a similar patient presenting with cancer may include:
	• Mammogram: with a spiculated, hyperdense lesion with microcalcifications.
	• Biopsy: a solid mass with sharp margins and small, glandular, duct-like cells in a desmoplastic stroma. Sentinel lymph node biopsy with evidence of lymph node invasion. Genetic testing confirms mutation in *BRCA1*.
	
	Management: Management is dependent on tumor stage, hormone receptor/HER2 status, and patient preferences; however, it usually involves a combination of medical and surgical management.
	• *BRCA* testing if clinically suspected based on family history
	• Surgical management and decision-making depend on tumor characteristics, patient preferences, and necessary follow-up.
	  • If there is clinical involvement of axillary lymph nodes, a sentinel lymph node biopsy can be performed concurrently. Metastasis to axillary lymph nodes is an important prognostic factor.
	  • Breast-conserving therapy includes lumpectomy (also called partial mastectomy) followed by radiation to eradicate residual disease and prevent local recurrence.
	  • Simple (total) vs. modified radical mastectomy (involves removing the entire breast and level I/II axillary lymph nodes).
	  • Mastectomy can be followed by immediate or delayed reconstruction by plastic surgery.

Additional Considerations	**Screening:** USPSTF recommends breast cancer screening with a mammogram every two years in women aged 50–74 years with average risk while ACOG recommends mammography every 1–2 years for women aged 40–74. Women with higher risk should start screening earlier. **Complications:** • Breast cancer: metastases to bone, liver, lung, brain • Axillary node dissection: nerve damage to the long thoracic nerve, leading to winged scapula • Tamoxifen: thromboembolic events, increased risk of endometrial cancer • Trastuzumab: heart failure, reversible upon discontinuation

ENDOCRINE SURGERY

Endocrine surgery is a diverse field that crosses multiple surgical specialties. Like many surgical problems, the main question is whether medical management has been maximized and/or whether surgery is first-line. Often, these tumors present with signs and symptoms associated with hypersecretion of a particular hormone. Some, however, are more indolent or do not secrete anything at all and are more likely to present with signs and symptoms associated with mass effect on nearby structures. Pituitary masses are a diverse group of neoplasms that are covered in other chapters. We will briefly review other common indications for endocrine surgery here. Refer to Chapter 9 (Endocrinology) for more details.

Thyroid Masses and Goiters

Surgery is indicated if the thyroid nodule and/or goiter is malignant or causes local symptoms. Symptoms such as dyspnea, dysphagia, and odynophagia occur from compression of surrounding structures (e.g., trachea, esophagus).

Testing:

• Obtain baseline thyroid function tests

• Evaluate for malignancy with thyroid ultrasound and FNA

• If cytology from the FNA is concerning for or diagnostic of cancer, obtain imaging to determine the extent of disease and proceed with thyroidectomy

Treatment for any differentiated thyroid cancer is surgery—either a **total thyroidectomy** or **lobectomy**. The extent of thyroid resection is determined by tumor size and node involvement. The most important complication to be aware of is **injury to the recurrent laryngeal nerve**, which will result in vocal cord paralysis. Another important consideration is the anatomy and location of the parathyroid glands and associated vascular supply. Inadvertent removal of the parathyroid glands can cause hypoparathyroidism and hypocalcemia. Parathyroids should not be removed during surgery unless compromised by thyroid malignancy.

Management after total thyroidectomy:

• Monitor for complications:

  • Obtain PTH and calcium levels (as high risk for iatrogenic hypoparathyroidism due to accidental removal of the parathyroid glands)

- Monitor for post-op stridor due to injury of the recurrent laryngeal nerve
- Following thyroid surgery, **radioiodine ablation therapy** is used to lower the chance of tumor recurrence.
- Thyroid replacement therapy is initiated to treat any resultant hypothyroidism and also to suppress pituitary TSH secretion, which can stimulate tumor growth and/or tumor recurrence.

Parathyroid Surgery

The only definitive management for hyperparathyroidism is surgical removal of parathyroid glands (parathyroidectomy). Patients may be asymptomatic but be incidentally found to have hypercalcemia on routine labs followed by an elevated PTH level, or hyperparathyroidism may be discovered after investigating causes of osteoporosis.

Primary hyperparathyroidism is an excess of parathyroid hormone being secreted from a parathyroid adenoma (85%) or multiglandular hyperplasia (15%) or a parathyroid carcinoma (1%). Indications for removal of benign causes are symptoms of hyperparathyroidism, osteoporosis (fragility fracture or DEXA scan < −2.5), decreased renal function (GFR <60), recurrent nephrolithiasis, or age <50 years old.

Secondary hyperparathyroidism arises in patients with end-stage renal disease whose parathyroid levels are elevated due to decreased serum calcium. This causes parathyroid hyperplasia and requires removal of 3.5 parathyroid glands. The remaining ½ gland is retransplanted often into either the sternocleidomastoid muscle or the arm to make it more easily accessible if further removal is needed. Intraoperative parathyroid hormone levels are measured as an immediate assessment of whether adequate tissue has been removed, taking advantage of the short half-life of parathyroid hormone (<5 minutes).

Following surgery, patients' calcium levels are closely monitored. Patients are often placed on calcium repletion and calcitriol. Some may experience "hungry bone" syndrome, in which their bones absorb much of the calcium in their blood now that elevated parathyroid hormone levels are no longer stimulating osteoclastic activity.

Endocrine Tumors of the Abdomen

Endocrine tumors of the abdomen are rare and are sometimes discovered incidentally on imaging (e.g., adrenal incidentaloma). The tumors are often named for the hormone they secrete (see below). Presenting symptoms correlate with the hormone that is being hypersecreted. Signs, symptoms, and characteristics of these tumors are summarized in the below table.

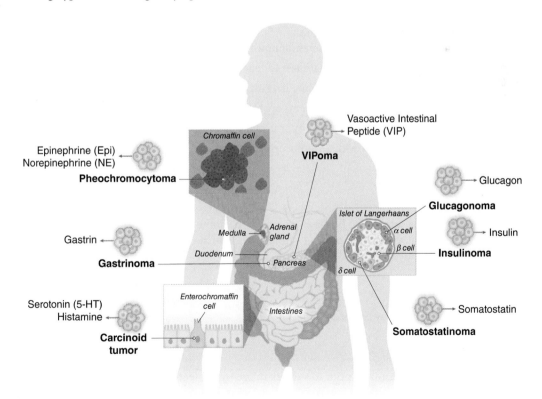

Types of Abdominal Neuroendocrine Tumors

Neuroendocrine Tumors of the Abdomen: Presentation and Treatment

Type	Signs and Symptoms
Glucagonoma	Chronic secretory diarrhea, weight loss, hyperglycemia, necrolytic migratory erythema, depression, altered mental status, venous thrombosis
Insulinoma	Episodic hypoglycemia causing altered mental status, elevated C-peptide
Somatostatinoma	Glucose intolerance, gallstones, steatorrhea, achlorhydria; decreased insulin, glucagon, gastrin, GIP, secretin, and CCK
Gastrinoma	Chronic secretory diarrhea, ulcers beyond duodenal bulb causing abdominal pain, rugal thickening with acid hypersecretion, diarrhea, elevated gastrin even after secretin administration
VIPoma	Chronic secretory diarrhea, muscle weakness and cramping
Pheochromocytoma	Hypertension (may be episodic), tachycardia, headache, diaphoresis
Carcinoid tumor	Asymptomatic if tumor limited to GI tract, as 5-HT is metabolized in liver; if symptomatic, will have pellagra, bronchospasm, chronic secretory diarrhea, cutaneous flushing, elevated 5-HIAA in urine, and right-sided valvular heart disease (elevated 5-HT stimulates fibroblast growth and causes deposits on R heart valves, MAO in lungs metabolizes 5-HT and prevents L heart damage)

Management

- For symptom relief, octreotide (a somatostatin analog) is recommended for most types of abdominal endocrine tumors to manage associated diarrhea and/or carcinoid syndrome.
- Surgical resection is indicated for definitive management of these tumors, particularly when they are large (>2 cm), the patient is young, or metastases are present.
- Smaller tumors may be hormonally inactive and less likely to be aggressive or metastatic; when necessary to remove them surgically, endoscopic approach can be used.

Adrenal Incidentaloma

- An adrenal incidentaloma is a > 1 cm mass lesion serendipitously found by radiologic examination.
- Surgical intervention (adrenalectomy) on an adrenal mass is dependent on the likelihood that it is malignant.
- Imaging characteristics that suggest malignancy include irregularity, mixed density, >4-cm diameter, or calcification.
- In addition to evaluation with CT, laboratory assessments are indicated, which include:
  - Pheochromocytoma should be ruled out with serum or urinary metanephrines and catecholamines
  - Cushing syndrome should be ruled out with 24-hour urine cortisol measurement followed by a dexamethasone suppression test

Pheochromocytomas

- Should be pre-treated with alpha-adrenergic blocker (phenoxybenzamine) and then beta-adrenergic blockade (propranolol) pre-operatively to prevent unopposed alpha-1 stimulation, which could lead to a hypertensive crisis when the tumor is manipulated intraoperatively.

Glucagonoma and Insulinoma

- Blood glucose-stabilizing therapies may be needed

Carcinoid

- Stabilize with octreotide and antihistamines prior to surgery to prevent potential carcinoid crisis perioperatively.

CASE 39 | Carcinoid Tumor

A 35-year-old woman with no significant past medical history presents with intermittent abdominal pain for 5 months. She has also had intermittent facial flushing and watery diarrhea for 2 months. Her temperature is 37°C, pulse is 105/min, respirations are 16/min, and blood pressure is 110/60 mmHg. On exam, the abdomen has mild periumbilical tenderness without rebound or guarding. Skin exam is notable for transient pink flushing in the face and upper trunk. Cardiac and respiratory exam reveals no murmurs or wheezing.

Conditions with Similar Presentations	**VIPoma:** Is a pancreatic neuroendocrine tumor that presents with a syndrome of severe watery diarrhea, hypokalemia, and achlorhydria due to excess vasoactive intestinal peptide. Although flushing may be seen, it is not characteristic and abdominal pain is usually absent. **Pheochromocytoma:** Is an adrenal neuroendocrine tumor that presents with hypertension, intermittent headache, flushing, palpitations, and diaphoresis due to excess catecholamines. **Serotonin syndrome:** May have acute-onset cramping, abdominal pain, and diarrhea, but would have a history of serotonergic drug use. **Menopause:** Occurs in women around 40 to 50 years old and would expect other symptoms (vaginal dryness, hot flashes, irregular menses) in addition to flushing.
Initial Diagnostic Tests	• Plasma or 24-hour urine 5-hydroxyindoleacetic acid (5-HIAA) • If above abnormal, then imaging with CT or MRI • Biopsy recommended for GI tumors
Next Steps in Management	• Treat with somatostatin analog (octreotide and lanreotide) • Nonmetastatic disease: surgical resection if possible, otherwise observation, chemotherapy, and/or radiation • Metastatic GI tumors: resection and somatostatin analog therapy • Avoidance of triggers
Discussion	Carcinoid tumors are of neuroendocrine origin and most commonly affect the GI tract, with 85% found in the appendix. They can also be found in the small bowel and the respiratory system. Carcinoid tumors produce an excess of amine and peptide hormones such as serotonin (most common), histamine, and substance P. Patients are often asymptomatic, as these hormones are metabolized by monoamine oxidase in the liver. When there are metastases in the liver or other distant sites, however, hepatic metabolism is bypassed and it can lead to the **carcinoid syndrome** (flushing, watery diarrhea, right-sided valvular heart disease). Of note, gastric/proximal duodenal and distal colonic/rectal carcinoids are not usually associated with carcinoid syndrome, as they arise from other cell types that produce different hormones: gastrin or somatostatin and glucagon-like peptide or pancreas polypeptide, respectively. Carcinoid tumors occur more commonly in women. They usually arise sporadically but may be associated with genetic syndromes, such as multiple endocrine neoplasia type 1 (MEN-1), von Hippel-Lindau disease, or neurofibromatosis type 1 (von Recklinghausen disease). **History:** May be asymptomatic and tumors may be discovered incidentally on imaging or endoscopy. Symptoms primarily are based on the tumor location; in the GI tract, abdominal pain may be present. If there are metastases to the liver or other distant sites, carcinoid syndrome may be present with certain triggers such as alcohol. **Physical Exam:** Tachycardia and hypotension can be present due to vasodilation. Skin flushing, abdominal tenderness, and wheezing may be observed based on the tumor location. Right-sided valvular heart disease, most commonly tricuspid regurgitation (holosystolic murmur at left lower sternal border), may be present in carcinoid syndrome. **Diagnostics:** • Check plasma or 24-hour urine 5-hydroxyindoleacetic acid (5-HIAA) which is a metabolite of serotonin • Imaging with CT or MRI to determine tumor location and assess for metastases • Biopsy recommended for GI tumors (immunohistochemistry with synaptophysin, chromogranin A, CD56) • Transthoracic echocardiogram for patients with carcinoid syndrome to evaluate for presence of right-sided valvular disease **Management:** • Management varies based on tumor location, symptoms, and presence of metastases; however, typically involves surgical resection. • Medical management includes somatostatin analogs (octreotide, lanreotide), chemotherapy, and/or radiation. • For nonmetastatic and metastatic disease, surgical resection and lymph node resection if possible. • For unresectable liver metastases, hepatic artery embolization may be attempted.

Additional Considerations	**Screening:** Screen for neuroendocrine tumors in patients with **MEN-1**, using CT, MRI, gastroscopic examinations, endoscopic ultrasound, or somatostatin receptor scintigraphy. **Complications:** Complications of abdominal carcinoid tumors include right-sided valvular disease, anemia, and pellagra. • Carcinoid heart disease can result in tricuspid and pulmonic valve regurgitation or stenosis, and if severe can lead to right heart failure. • GI bleeding from abdominal carcinoid tumors can produce anemia. • Tryptophan is a precursor for niacin and serotonin. It is consumed to make serotonin by carcinoid tumors; patients may become deficient in tryptophan and niacin and develop pellagra (diarrhea, dementia, dermatitis). • Complications may also arise due to involvement of the carcinoid tumor with nearby GI tissues or vasculature. Carcinoid tumors can produce GI obstruction through mesenteric desmoplastic reaction, in which the growing mass extends connective tissue fibers outward in a distinctive radial pattern to pull on the mesentery or nearby intestines. • Abdominal carcinoid tumors can also become entangled with major vessels, most commonly branches of the mesentery artery. This can produce local ischemia to parts of abdominal organs or increase the risk of uncontrolled bleeding during surgical resection. • Hormones released by carcinoid tumors can cause the development of vascular sclerosis.

OTOLARYNGOLOGY (EAR, NOSE, AND THROAT)

Otolaryngology, head and neck surgery, or "ear, nose, and throat" (ENT) is a surgical specialty that encompasses many structures and organ systems. Head and neck abnormalities include neoplasms, deformities, disorders, and injuries of the ears, nose, sinuses, throat, respiratory and upper alimentary systems, face, and jaws, including disorders of hearing and voice. Please review the following chapters for additional cases: Endocrinology, Pulmonology, Neurology, and Pediatrics. This section includes neoplastic and nonneoplastic masses arising in the head and/or neck, many of which may require surgical resection.

CASE 40 | Thyroglossal Duct Cyst (TGDC)

A 10-year-old boy presents with a painless fluctuant swelling in his midline neck. He has no prior history of upper respiratory infections or otitis. On exam, the child is afebrile. The neck mass is mobile, nontender, and moves upwardly when the tongue is protruded. An indirect laryngoscopy was normal.

Conditions with Similar Presentations	**Thyroid nodule or ectopic thyroid:** Imaging will help define anatomy. Obtain T3, T4, TSH, and thyroid scan to identify hot or cold areas. **Lymphadenitis:** Can occur in setting of bacterial or viral infections, but patients would have tender lymphadenopathy (e.g., cervical lymph nodes) and may have other signs of infection (e.g., fever, fatigue, pharyngitis). **Dermoid or sebaceous cyst:** Defined as a cystic malformation lined with squamous epithelium and containing keratin, they often present as soft nodular lesions with a sessile base. These cysts are found in the ovaries, testes, head and neck (scalp, orbit, nasal, cervical), or within the oral cavity (buccal, floor of mouth, tongue). These may present as painless masses, with dysphagia or dysphonia from mass effects, or may leak and cause inflammation, presenting as a tender, inflamed mass. **Lipoma:** Soft, movable, and painless, these masses can occur anywhere in the body and are located more superficially (just beneath the skin); they are more commonly found on trunk and extremities and usually appear during the ages of 40–60 years. **Branchial cleft anomalies:** Congenital anomalies arising from the first through fourth pharyngeal pouches that can form branchial cleft cysts, fistulae, or sinus tracts. The most common type arises from the second branchial cleft. They are present at birth but do not become apparent often until the first or second decade of life. Cysts will present with a neck swelling, most often as a lateral neck mass anterior to the sternocleidomastoid muscle, and do not move with protrusion of the tongue or with swallowing. Fistulae will present with swelling and discharge from a skin opening and will be tender, erythematous, often accompanied by fever.
Initial Diagnostic Tests	• Imaging (e.g., ultrasound, CT neck with contrast, MRI) to define anatomical relation between the mass and thyroid • FNA to confirm diagnoses and exclude other diagnoses

CASE 40 | Thyroglossal Duct Cyst (TGDC) *(continued)*

Next Steps in Management	Surgery to excise the thyroglossal tract
Discussion	Thyroglossal duct cysts (TGDCs) are the most common cause of midline neck masses in children and comprise 70% of all congenital neck abnormalities. In the embryo, the thyroid diverticulum descends in front of the neck and pharyngeal gut to its final position in the neck. The diverticulum is connected to the tongue by the thyroglossal duct, which opens in the tongue via the foramen cecum. When this duct fails to atrophy during embryologic development, a thyroglossal cyst forms as an open connection between the two. It may be associated with failure of the thyroid to descend during development, resulting in thyroid tissue remaining in or near the tongue (lingual thyroid) or incomplete descent (cervical thyroid). **History/Physical Exam:** Presents as a midline, fluctuant, cystic mass in the upper neck, most often in children before the age of 6 years, although can be found in adults as well. Most are asymptomatic, although can sometimes be tender. The cyst can appear anywhere along the tract of thyroid descent from the foramen cecum on the dorsal posterior one-third of the tongue to the suprasternal notch. A common location is at or just below the hyoid bone. When the tongue is protruded, the cyst will move upwardly in the neck. Palpation of the thyroid gland can be done, although can be unreliable. **Diagnostics:** • Imaging is often performed to identify potential thyroid tissue. Preferred imaging is CT neck with contrast; however, MRI and ultrasound can also be used. TGDCs are typically well circumscribed with homogeneous fluid attenuation and a thin enhancing rim. This can also help define anatomical relationship to the hyoid bone and thyroid gland for surgical planning. • FNA to confirm diagnosis and rule out other potential diagnoses (e.g., lipoma, neoplasm). Tissue will show ciliated columnar epithelial cells with immune cell infiltration, although this can be nonspecific. • Thyroid function tests are also performed to demonstrate normally functioning thyroid tissue. **Management:** Surgical removal via a transverse midline incision excising the thyroglossal tract from the base of the tongue to the foramen cecum along with the medial segment of the hyoid bone (Sistrunk procedure).

CASE 41 | Squamous Cell Carcinoma (SCC) of Head and Neck

A 52-year-old man presents for evaluation of a painless right neck mass that he first noticed 2 months ago. The mass has grown in size, is firm, and has not drained. He has no associated dyspnea, rhinorrhea, numbness, weakness, or otalgia, but he reports progressive hoarseness over the last month. He smokes one pack per day for the past 35 years and drinks six beers per day. On exam, he is afebrile. His voice is rough, but he is not stridorous. The thyroid is not enlarged. A 2-cm mass located in the upper two-thirds of the right neck along the anterior border of the sternocleidomastoid is firm and nonmobile with no associated fluctuance, erythema, or tenderness to palpation. Cranial nerves are intact, and no lesions are noted on the remaining head and neck exam. Flexible laryngoscopy identifies a pink lesion on the anterior third of the right vocal cord.

| Conditions with Similar Presentations | A new neck mass in a >40-year-old with smoking history is considered malignant (usually squamous cell carcinoma) until proven otherwise by biopsy. Other, less likely causes to be considered are:

Lymphoma: The second most common site of extra-nodal lymphomas after the GI tract is within in the oral and para-oral regions, mainly from Waldeyer's ring (e.g., tonsils, nasopharynx, base of tongue). It presents with dysphagia, dysphonia, weight loss, and painless, enlarged cervical lymph nodes. This can only be differentiated from squamous cell cancer by biopsy.

Salivary gland cancer: Tumor of the parotid or submandibular glands include a painless enlarging mass which may be associated with an ipsilateral facial nerve paralysis as the mass expands or fixation to the skin or underlying muscle. Minor salivary gland cancer can present with a submucosal mass that ulcerates. All can present with cervical lymphadenopathy. In the absence of salivary gland or intra-oral abnormalities, this diagnosis is unlikely.

Melanoma of the scalp, ear, cheek, neck: All can present with a cutaneous lesion with or without cervical lymphadenopathy. In the absence of a skin lesion, this diagnosis may be less likely.

Metastatic cancer: These constitute 1% of head and neck malignancies, with the most frequent sites of origin being breast, lung, GI tract, genitourinary tract, and uncommonly, the central nervous system. Typically, these involve cervical or supraclavicular lymphadenopathy. Lymphadenopathy of the upper two-thirds of the neck reflects a source primarily from the head and neck, while lower third reflects an infraclavicular source. An enlarged left supraclavicular lymph node (Virchow's node) usually indicates a metastasis from the GI tract but can be from the thorax or pelvic organs. |

CASE 41 | Squamous Cell Carcinoma (SCC) of Head and Neck *(continued)*

Conditions with Similar Presentations	**Goiter:** Enlargement of thyroid gland that can present with hoarseness due to enlarged thyroid compressing the trachea, dyspnea, or dysphagia. Patients may also have symptoms of hyper- or hypothyroidism. It is important to differentiate from thyroid cancer. **Reactive lymphadenopathy:** Can occur in setting of bacterial or viral infections, but patients would have tender mass within the distribution of lymph nodes (e.g., cervical lymph nodes). Patients may have other signs of infection (e.g., fever, fatigue, pharyngitis).
Initial Diagnostic Tests	• Flexible laryngoscopy with biopsy of the mass • CT and/or MRI imaging from skull base to clavicles • Consider chest CT and bone scan to identify distant metastases as well as FDG-PET/CT for further detection of unknown primary tumor
Next Steps in Management	• Grading and staging based on imaging, biopsy, and presence of metastasis. • For primary head and neck cancer, treatment involves multimodal therapy involving chemotherapy, radiation, and/or surgery.
Discussion	This patient likely has SCC of the larynx affecting the glottis (vocal cords) with metastases to lymph nodes in the right neck. SCC comprises more than 95% of laryngeal cancers. SCCs of the head and neck (HNSCC) are derived from the mucosal epithelium of the oral cavity, pharynx, or larynx. Oral cavity and larynx cancers are usually associated with alcohol and tobacco, and are collectively referred to as human papillomavirus (HPV)-negative HNSCC. In contrast, pharyngeal carcinomas can be associated with human papillomavirus infection, including strains 16 and 18, thus making these cancers more commonly HPV-positive HNSCC. HPV is associated with >70% of oropharyngeal cancers. **History:** • Risk factors: Tobacco use (smoked and smokeless), alcohol use disorder (effects are synergistic with tobacco), older age, HPV infection (oral sex), Epstein-Barr virus; males have a 3–6 times higher prevalence. • Patients may present with a painless neck mass due to a metastasis from cancer of unknown origin, but this patient also presents with associated voice changes, which is concerning for a glottic malignancy that has metastasized. • Other symptoms that could indicate a possible cancer include dyspnea, dysphagia (progressive starting with solids and moving to liquids), odynophagia, weight loss, otalgia (due to referred pain from the pharynx), and hemoptysis. **Physical Exam:** • A head and neck exam should be done with special attention to the cranial nerves. Deficit of a cranial nerve could be a sign of a cancer invading that nerve. • A thorough exam of the oral cavity should be done looking for lesions, and neck palpation should be performed in all areas looking for additional masses. **Diagnostics:** • A hoarse voice lasting more than 4 weeks should be examined endoscopically with a flexible laryngoscopy. • In addition to endoscopy, any suspicious lesion should be sampled for malignancy. • In a patient such as this, flexible laryngoscopy may show a rough, pink mass and immobility of the right true vocal cord. The immobility of the vocal cord indicates a more advanced laryngeal cancer that has invaded enough to tether the vocal cord and limit its motion. • Biopsy via FNA of the neck mass should be performed. If FNA does not yield a sufficient sample for pathology, an excisional biopsy may be necessary. • CT and/or MRI imaging from skull base to clavicles to assess local, regional extent of disease. MRI offers higher resolution of soft tissues to assess laryngeal cartilage; CT scan has fewer motion artifacts and is more readily available. • Metastatic workup as noted above: chest CT and bone scan to identify distant metastases. If primary tumor remains unknown, can perform FDG-PET/CT for further detection. Should also perform a dental exam (including a panorex x-ray involving the entire mouth), audiometry, assessment of speech and swallowing, and possibly pulmonary function tests. • For further definition of primary source, can also do endoscopy under anesthesia with biopsy (i.e., direct laryngoscopy, esophagoscopy, nasopharyngoscopy, and bronchoscopy).

CASE 41 | Squamous Cell Carcinoma (SCC) of Head and Neck *(continued)*

Discussion	**Management:**
	• Most patients with HNCC require multimodal care, including chemotherapy, radiation, and surgery.
	• For oral cavity cancers, surgery is followed by chemoradiotherapy, depending on the disease stage.
	• Larynx cancers can be treated with surgery or radiation alone.
	• For pharynx cancers, chemoradiotherapy is the primary approach.
	• In patients with HPV-negative cancers who are unable to tolerate cytotoxic chemotherapy, the monoclonal EGFR antibody cetuximab is used with radiation.
	• The immune checkpoint inhibitor pembrolizumab is the primary treatment for unresectable disease.
	• For patients with laryngeal and hypopharyngeal SCC who do not have distant metastasis, surgical removal of a portion or the entire larynx could offer a potential cure.
	  • A total laryngectomy is indicated if a partial resection would not remove the primary tumor completely or would significantly impair function.
	  • An additional indication for laryngectomy is for severe dysfunction causing aspiration, also called salvage surgery due to the treatment course of chemoradiotherapy.
	  • Finally, laryngectomy can be indicated if there is recurrence following chemoradiotherapy.

CASE 42 | Pleomorphic Adenoma

A 41-year-old woman who is otherwise healthy presents with a left-sided preauricular mass that she first noticed 4 months ago. The mass is painless and does not increase in size with eating. She has had no weight loss, trismus, facial weakness, or xerostomia. She does not use tobacco, and received all her childhood immunizations. On exam, a 2-cm mobile, nontender mass is noted in the left parotid region. No mass is present on the right. The facial nerve is intact bilaterally, and the rest of the head and neck exam is unremarkable.

Conditions with Similar Presentations	**Benign salivary gland tumors:** The second most common benign salivary gland tumor is the **Warthin tumor** (papillary cystadenoma lymphomatosum), which is most commonly found in middle-aged and elderly men with a history of smoking. Other benign tumors that can present in the parotid gland include oncocytomas, hemangiomas, and monomorphic adenomas. **Malignant salivary gland tumors:** The most common malignant neoplasm of the parotid gland is **mucoepidermoid carcinoma.** Those with prior radiation to the head or neck are at higher risk for this. This is more likely to invade the facial nerve and local lymph nodes. Other malignancies of the parotid gland include adenoid cystic carcinoma, acinic cell carcinoma, squamous cell carcinoma, and lymphoma.
Initial Diagnostic Tests	• Imaging to identify extent of tumor using CT, MRI, and/or US • FNA or US-guided core needle biopsy of the mass
Next Steps in Management	• Staging and grading of tumor followed by surgical resection. • If high-risk malignant features are present or margins are positive following initially surgery, can consider additional radiation therapy and chemotherapy.
Discussion	Salivary gland tumors can be benign or malignant, and a majority (85%) arise in the parotid gland. Most parotid gland tumors (75–80%) are benign, while those arising in the submandibular glands, sublingual glands, or minor salivary glands are more likely to be malignant. This patient has a pleomorphic adenoma, which is the most common benign salivary gland tumor. Pleomorphic adenomas are heterogenous, slow-growing tumors with mixed epithelial and myoepithelial components. They are slightly more common in women. These masses often have finger-like projections known as pseudopods that can be difficult to see, which can limit the surgeon's ability to completely resect the tumor. Consequently, pleomorphic adenomas often recur. Nonetheless, a small percentage of these tumors will transform into carcinoma ex-pleomorphic adenoma and should be removed. **History:** • Radiation may increase the risk of developing a pleomorphic adenoma, but tobacco and alcohol use do not. • Patients will often present with a firm, mobile, painless mass unilaterally. • Rarely, they will have accompanying facial nerve palsy (the facial nerve courses through the parotid gland) and may have dysphagia, dyspnea, or hoarseness if the tumor extends into the pharynx or larynx.

CASE 42 | Pleomorphic Adenoma *(continued)*

Discussion	**Physical Exam:**

Physical Exam:
- A full head and neck exam should be done with special attention to the cranial nerves, especially the facial nerve exam with attention to all main branches (frontal, zygomatic, buccal, marginal mandibular, and cervical).
- Palpate the neck to ensure there are no additional masses, which would suggest a malignancy instead with metastases to the neck.

Diagnostics:
- Initial imaging should be performed to evaluate the extent of the tumor and identify benign vs. malignant features. Options include ultrasound, CT, and MRI. Ultrasound is highly specific but is limited in identifying tumor extent to the deep lobe of the parotid; typically would show a hypoechoic mass. MRI is more sensitive in distinguishing malignant features.
- Diagnosis is confirmed by sampling tissue via FNA or core needle biopsy showing mixed epithelial and myoepithelial components consistent with a pleomorphic adenoma (see image).

Management:

The entire involved lobe of the parotid gland should be resected with facial nerve preservation. If the mass alone is resected without removing the associated lobe of the parotid, the adenoma has a 30% chance of recurring due to residual pseudopods.

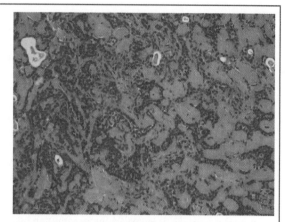

Pleomorphic adenoma. The background is a variably eosinophilic and myxoid acellular matrix. Interspersed within the background matrix are myoepithelial cells. The third component of pleomorphic adenomas is ductules. Hematoxylin and eosin, 40×. (Reproduced with permission from Kemp WL, Burns DK, Brown TG. Pathology: The Big Picture. Copyright 2008 McGraw-Hill Education.)

Mini-Case

Recurrent Respiratory Papillomatosis	**Hx:** Typically diagnosed between ages 2 and 3, the primary risk factor is a mother with a history of HPV. Child will present with hoarseness, occasional respiratory distress, intermittent respiratory obstruction, or aphonia.

Hx: Typically diagnosed between ages 2 and 3, the primary risk factor is a mother with a history of HPV. Child will present with hoarseness, occasional respiratory distress, intermittent respiratory obstruction, or aphonia.

PE: Multiple finger- or grape-like, verrucous, polypoid growths overlying true vocal folds, false vocal folds, subglottic region, and/or trachea.

Diagnostics: Laryngoscopy showing irregular, exophytic growths on the vocal cord (see image below).

Management: Microlaryngeal surgery to debulk the lesions; usually multiple treatments needed before puberty.

Discussion: Also known as laryngeal papillomatosis, this is the most common *benign* laryngeal tumor in children. It is believed to be caused by HPV (strains 6 and 11) acquired during passage of the birth canal of an infected mother or through vertical transmission prior to delivery. Benign squamous papillomas proliferate in the larynx affecting both the respiratory and digestive tracts.

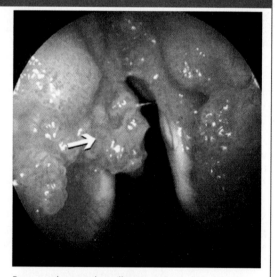

Recurrent laryngeal papillomatosis (*arrow*). (Reproduced with permission from Grippi MA, Elias JA, Fishman JA, Kotloff RM, Pack AI, Senior RM, Siegel MD. Fishman's Pulmonary Diseases and Disorders, 5e. Copyright 2015 McGraw-Hill Education.)

TRANSPLANT SURGERY

Transplantation can be both a life-altering and life-saving operation, and includes both solid organ transplantation (e.g., kidney, liver) and hematopoietic stem cell (i.e., bone marrow) transplantation. Patients can receive tissue from themselves (autologous), another individual (allogeneic), from a genetically identical recipient such as a twin (isograft), or from a different species, such as pig (xenograft).

To understand the risks and benefits of transplantation, knowledge of basic immunology is essential. Donor and recipient patients should be ABO blood type compatible and have matching major histocompatibility complex (MHC) or human leukocyte antigen (HLA) alleles (i.e., typed and cross-matched). In humans, MHC Class I includes HLA-A, HLA-B, and HLA-C, while MHC Class II includes HLA-DR, HLA-DP, and HLA-DQ. If patients do not have matching HLA alleles, the HLA peptides on the graft will be recognized as foreign by the recipient's adaptive immune system (largely T lymphocytes), which can result in acute rejection of the graft. Cross-matching involves screening recipient serum for preformed antibodies against donor lymphocytes that could result in hyperacute rejection.

Because of the requirement for lifelong immunosuppression to prevent rejection of the transplanted organ following surgery, care must be taken when evaluating patients pre-operatively to ensure the success of their graft. Patients on immunosuppressants are at increased risk for infection. Careful assessment should also be performed post-operatively for evidence of organ rejection.

CASE 43 | Renal Transplant

A 64-year-old man with diabetes, hypertension, and end-stage renal disease (ESRD) not yet on dialysis presents for pre-operative planning for a living relative renal transplant. The patient's son is the donor. He also has depression that is well controlled with sertraline. Both the patient and donor have no history of prior blood transfusions. The patient has no past or current substance use, has received all his childhood and adult vaccinations, and had an unremarkable colonoscopy 4 years ago. The patient has a good support system including his spouse and two adult children. The patient's BMI is 33 kg/m². He has an estimated glomerular filtration rate of 14 mL/min and serum creatinine of 5.4 mg/dL. A hepatitis panel is negative for active infection with evidence of hepatitis B immunity. Urinalysis is normal and urine culture is sterile, HIV serology is negative, and interferon-γ; release assay is negative. He has adequate antibody titers to measles, mumps, rubella, and varicella. Both the patient and the donor are seropositive for cytomegalovirus. They are ABO compatible with blood type O⁺ and have a negative donor-recipient complement-dependent cytotoxicity crossmatch. His prostate specific antigen is 3.1 ng/mL.

Considerations	• This patient is undergoing pre-operative evaluation for consideration of a renal transplant. Given his poor kidney function, this can be a life-saving operation. If the patient is ineligible for renal transplant, the alternative, less-preferred option for a patient with ESRD would be to initiate dialysis. • Access for **hemodialysis** is often done through surgical creation of an **arteriovenous (AV) fistula**, connecting an artery typically in the forearm or upper arm to a large vein, bypassing the high-resistance arterioles and allowing some volume to pass directly into the low-resistance venous system. Once created by a vascular surgeon, it typically takes a few months before the AV fistula has fully developed and is ready for use. An alternative to an AV fistula is an AV graft, which involves placement of synthetic tubing to connect the arterial and venous systems.
Initial Diagnostic Tests	• Check ABO and HLA compatibility between donor and recipient; complement-dependent cytotoxicity crossmatch • Obtain: CBC, CMP, PT/INR, aPTT, PTH, pregnancy test (if applicable), serology for measles, mumps, rubella, varicella, HIV, HBV, HCV, HSV, syphilis, and CMV; drug screen; TB testing; CXR; ECG • Also check age- and sex-appropriate cancer screening; psychological assessment
Next Steps in Management	• If the patient has no active, uncontrolled infection, malignancy, substance use, psychiatric condition, or medication nonadherence, they can proceed with the transplantation. • If an underlying condition is detected, care should be taken to optimize the patient medically prior to transplantation.
Discussion	Renal transplant is the most common solid-organ transplant and the preferred treatment for ESRD (CKD stage 5) as it offers better long-term outcomes and survival than dialysis. Living-related renal transplant portends the best outcomes, as it allows for better HLA matching. This is followed by living-unrelated renal transplant and then deceased donor transplantation. Diabetic nephropathy is the number one cause of ESRD and subsequent renal transplant in the United States.

CASE 43 | Renal Transplant *(continued)*

Discussion	**History:**
	• Assess history of medical conditions that caused or may lead to recurrence of renal failure, such as diabetes mellitus, hypertension, and lupus.
	• Determine if there is a history of blood transfusions or prior transplantation that may have caused immunologic sensitization in the recipient therefore increasing the risk of graft failure.
	• Ask about any symptoms or risk factors indicative of active infection or malignancy, immunization and cancer screening history, prior abdominal surgeries, and any medical comorbidities, especially cardiovascular and peripheral arterial disease, which may complicate the procedure.
	• Perform a psychosocial assessment to identify any barriers to long-term success of the transplantation. Any psychological conditions should be adequately managed prior to transplantation.
	• Patients who undergo renal transplantation require lifelong immunosuppression, and any barriers to accomplishing this, such as financial or cognitive barriers, must be addressed.
	• Absolute contraindications to renal transplant include unsuitable vascular anatomy, active infections, and recent malignancy.
	Physical Exam:
	• The physical exam is the same as that for all potential elective surgical candidates as outlined in the pre-operative risk assessment section of this chapter.
	• Additionally, the femoral pulses should be palpated to assess for peripheral vascular disease that may complicate the procedure. The renal graft is anastomosed to the external iliac artery, and vein and calcification or claudication of this artery puts the patients at higher risk for graft failure and peri-surgical embolization.
	• BMI is also assessed, as many centers will not perform renal transplantation in patients with a BMI >35 due to increased graft failure and peri-operative complications (i.e., wound infections).
	Diagnostics:
	• ABO and HLA compatibility between the donor and recipient—important to reduce graft failure rates. The fewer HLA mismatches, the better the graft survival.
	• Complement-dependent cytotoxicity (CDC) crossmatch— this test for preformed anti-HLA antibodies against donor organ. The presence of these antibodies is associated with hyperacute rejection.
	• Pregnancy test—routine in all patients with childbearing potential. If pregnant, postpone until the patient is no longer pregnant.
	• Infectious serologies—for vaccine-preventable infections (e.g., mumps, measles, rubella) given risk of severe infection following transplantation and immunosuppression. Also test for syphilis, HIV, hepatitis B and C, and treat if positive. Finally, test for CMV, a common virus dormant in people with healthy immune systems that may cause active disease in an immunocompromised patient. Donors are also screened for CMV to match with recipient. Recipients who have negative CMV serology are more likely to experience severe disease if they receive a transplant from a seropositive donor.
	• Assess for latent TB—tuberculin skin test or interferon-γ release assay, treat prior to immunosuppression if positive.
	• Ensure patient is up to date with age- and sex-appropriate cancer screenings.
	• CBC with differential, CMP, PT/INR, aPTT, parathyroid hormone level, CXR and ECG to assess for any comorbid conditions that may increase the surgical risk for the candidate.
	Management:
	• Address any concerns found in the pre-operative evaluation and initial diagnostics prior to transplantation.
	• The left kidney is preferred in living-donor transplants due to the longer left renal vein. A living donor must have two healthy functioning kidneys in order to be eligible to donate one of their kidneys.
	• Patients should be placed on immunosuppressive therapy, initially an induction regimen to prevent acute rejection, followed by maintenance regimens which are continued long-term. Induction regimens include high-dose glucocorticoids and biological antibodies. Maintenance regimens may include glucocorticoids, calcineurin inhibitors such as tacrolimus or cyclosporine, antimetabolite agents (e.g., mycophenolate, azathioprine), and mTOR inhibitors (e.g., sirolimus, everolimus). Careful attention should be paid for symptoms and signs of drug toxicity from these agents.
	• Patients should ideally follow with a transplant nephrologist and their transplant surgeon for a minimum of 3–6 months (ideally 6–12 months) following the procedure.
	• At each visit, the following laboratory analyses should be performed: serum creatinine and eGFR, glucose, and electrolytes; trough levels for immunosuppressant medications; CBC with differential; urinalysis; spot urine protein-to-creatinine ratio.
	• Additional testing that should be performed at regular intervals includes fasting plasma glucose, lipid panel, PTH and vitamin D levels, screening for BK polyomavirus, and PCR testing for HIV, HBV, HCV, and CMV.
	• If patients begin to display any evidence of allograft dysfunction, consider performing a biopsy of the graft kidney.

CASE 43 | Renal Transplant *(continued)*

Additional Considerations	**Complications:**
	• **Graft failure due to transplant rejection** has decreased over time as immunosuppressive regimens have been refined and pre-operative assessments identify risk for incompatibility. Chronic rejection is the most common and occurs months to years after transplant. In general, the longer the patient has the donor organ, the longer time the cellular and humoral immune systems have to mount a response and overcome immunosuppressive medications, which can decrease in efficacy over time due to increased tolerance. See discussion below for more detail on organ transplant rejection.
	• **Urologic:** After renal transplant, potential urologic complications include urinary obstruction and ureteral anastomotic leak. Urinary tract or bladder infection is also possible due to prolonged catheter use or long-term ureteral stent implantation. Urinary tract infection is more common in diabetic patients.
	• **Fluid/electrolyte imbalances:** After transplantation, patients may develop alterations in intravascular volume and/or electrolytes. Care should be taken to prevent dehydration, as inadequate perfusion to the transplanted kidney could lead to failure; conversely, patients are also susceptible to fluid overload. Electrolyte abnormalities include hyperkalemia, hyperphosphatemia, and metabolic acidosis. This is particularly important, as the transplanted kidney can take 5 (living donor) or even 15 days (cadaveric donor) to return to normal function after the procedure.
	• **Cardiovascular/hemodynamics:** Post-operatively, there is the possibility of arterial or venous thrombosis or dissection near the anastomotic sites. Intraabdominal hemorrhage or hematuria are also possible. Patients with history of renal disease due to hypertension and/or diabetes (such as the patient in this case) are at increased risk of peri- or post-operative myocardial infarction, clotting abnormalities, and renal artery stenosis.
	• **Infection:** Infection is a common complication and can be acquired from the donor, during the surgical procedure, during post-op recovery, or following recovery due to immunosuppression. Patients are particularly susceptible to opportunistic pathogens, such as CMV or BK polyomavirus.

Mini-Case

Infection after Lung Transplant	**Hx:** Patients who undergo lung transplant are at high risk of infectious complications. The most common infection is pneumonia. Symptoms include cough, fever, dyspnea and characteristic timeline is as follows:
	• <1 month: bacterial infections (e.g., transmitted with donor allograft, derived from recipient, infectious complications of surgery and hospitalization)
	• 1-6 months: opportunistic infections (e.g., fungal, CMV)
	• >6 months: extended range of bacteria (e.g., *Pneumococcus*, gram-negative bacilli, *Legionella*, etc.)
	PE: Abnormal lung exam with crackles, dullness to percussion, increased fremitus, and egophony may occur and are less likely with viral infections than bacterial infections.
	Diagnostics:
	• Chest imaging may reveal interstitial infiltrates, ground-glass opacities, nodules, or airspace consolidation.
	• Sputum and blood cultures to identify organism and antibiotic susceptibility should be performed.
	• However, bronchoscopy with bronchoalveolar lavage is most sensitive. Transbronchial biopsy is performed at the same time to rule out rejection due to overlapping presentation.
	Management: Initial empiric antibiotics given, subsequently narrowed based on culture and antibiotic susceptibilities. All lung transplant patients should be vaccinated against pneumococcus.
	Discussion: Candidates for lung transplant are individuals with advanced pulmonary disease refractory to medical management, disabling symptoms, and high risk of death over next 2 years without transplant. Pneumonia, particularly bacterial pneumonia, is the most common type of infection in lung transplant recipients.
	Bacterial Infections
	• Pneumonia: highest risk during early post-transplant phase (<1 month). Often caused by hospital-acquired bacteria (e.g., *Pseudomonas*, *Enterobacteriaceae*, MRSA).
	• Bloodstream infections: risks include central venous catheters, mechanical ventilation, and cystic fibrosis.
	• Patients undergoing lung transplant for cystic fibrosis are at increased risk for multi-drug resistant *Pseudomonas aeruginosa* and *Burkholderia cepacia*.
	Viral Infections
	• Community respiratory viruses (influenza, parainfluenza, RSV, hMPV).
	• CMV (very common), VZV, HSV, SARS-CoV-2.
	• Acute or chronic rejection can mimic viral infection and is diagnosed by lung biopsy.
	Fungal Infections
	• Most commonly: *Aspergillus*, *Candida*, and *Pneumocystis*.
	• Others include endemic mycoses (e.g., *Histoplasma*, *Coccidioides*, *Blastomyces*).

Organ Rejection

Rejection is a common complication in patients receiving transplanted organs. Some cases, such as acute rejection, are preventable by ensuring that the patient has proper support and access to their immunosuppressants. However, some patients develop chronic rejection despite adequate immunosuppression.

Organ Rejection: Presentation, Pathology, and Treatment

Rejection Type	Presentation	Pathology	Treatment
Hyperacute	Within first 24 hours following transplantation. May even be evident while the operation is still underway, with widespread thrombosis leading to ischemia throughout the graft.	Due to preformed recipient cytotoxic antibodies (Type II hypersensitivity reaction) against donor.	Remove affected organ immediately Prevented with proper pre-operative HLA and antibody screening and match
Acute	During first weeks to months post-operatively. May be asymptomatic and only recognized due to post-operative lab testing (e.g., rising serum creatinine after a renal transplant). Results in vasculitis of graft vessels with interstitial lymphocyte infiltrates.	Can be humoral (formation of antibodies post-operatively, Type II hypersensitivity) or T-cell-mediated (activation of $CD4^+$ and $CD8^+$ T cells against donor HLA complexes, Type IV hypersensitivity). It is due to an immune response over time.	Increase dose of (or restart if nonadherent) immunosuppressant regimen *Humoral:* IVIG, plasmapheresis, or anti-CD20 antibody ± corticosteroids *T-cell-mediated:* Corticosteroids Can be prevented with proper immunosuppression
Chronic	Months to years. Gradual decline in function of the graft with proliferation of vascular smooth muscle, arteriosclerosis, parenchymal atrophy, and interstitial fibrosis.	Recipient antigen-presenting cells present donor proteins to $CD4^+$ T cells. This leads to a mixed cellular and humoral response (Types II and IV hypersensitivity) as well as immune complex deposition (Type III hypersensitivity).	Eventual re-transplantation when the graft has failed Cannot be prevented with adequate immunosuppression
Graft-versus-host disease (GVHD)	Varied timeline. Common in bone marrow and liver transplants (donor organs with a lot of lymphocytes). Presents with maculopapular rash, jaundice, diarrhea, hepatosplenomegaly Graft-versus-host disease. A. Grade IV graft versus host disease involving skin with diffuse erythroderma and bullae formation. B. Resolution of graft versus host reaction after therapy with high-dose glucocorticoids and antithymocyte globulin. (Reproduced with permission from MA L, MS S, RE F, N W. Lichtman's Atlas of Hematology. Copyright 2016 McGraw-Hill Education.)	Donor T cells attack the recipient's own cells (Type IV hypersensitivity), resulting in severe organ dysfunction.	Optimize level of calcineurin inhibitors and systemic corticosteroids Prevent prior to transfusion by irradiating blood products

CASE 44 | Acute Transplant Rejection (Renal Transplant)

A 56-year-old woman with hypertension and anuric ESRD secondary to polycystic kidney disease presents for follow-up 5 months after receiving a deceased-donor renal transplant. Her surgery was uncomplicated, and she began producing urine on post-operative day 0. Her medications include tacrolimus and mycophenolate mofetil for immunosuppression. She has been taking her medications regularly up until last week. She had gone to visit her daughter in Ohio for 5 days and forgot to pack her medications. She feels fine and reports no symptoms. Her temperature is 37.2°C, pulse 72/min, blood pressure 142/93 mmHg. Her physical exam is unremarkable. Her serum creatinine is 2.4 mg/dL and she has an eGFR of 50 mL/min, changed from 1.1 mg/dL and 65 mL/min 2 weeks ago, respectively. Urinalysis (UA) reveals specific gravity 1.016, protein 1+, red blood cells 0/hpf, leukocytes 1–2/hpf, no casts, negative leukocyte esterase and nitrites.

Conditions with Similar Presentations	**Acute calcineurin inhibitor (e.g., tacrolimus) nephrotoxicity:** Can also present in asymptomatic patients as increasing serum creatinine. As this patient missed her medications for 5 days and given that the half-life of tacrolimus can reach up to 36–38 hours, this is unlikely. **Chronic rejection of renal graft:** Also presents with worsening renal function but is a more gradual process, occurring over months to years. **Other considerations:** Acute kidney injury due to other nephrotoxic drugs, UTI, hydronephrosis due to infection, kidney stone, or blood clot.
Initial Diagnostic Tests	• Confirm diagnosis: Check BMP and UA. If ↑serum creatinine, ↓eGFR, proteinuria, check serology for donor-specific antibodies, and consider renal biopsy for immunologic evidence of rejection and to differentiate between antibody-mediated vs. T-cell-mediated rejection. • Consider: Serum calcineurin inhibitor levels (may be low in acute rejection), urine culture, and renal ultrasound to rule out other causes of renal dysfunction.
Next Steps in Management	• **Antibody-mediated acute rejection:** Removal of existing antibodies with IVIG, plasmapheresis, anti-CD20 antibody, or lymphocyte-depleting antibody ± addition of corticosteroids. • **T-cell–mediated acute rejection:** Corticosteroids. If prednisone is not already part of the patient's maintenance therapy (as in this patient), add it to their regimen.
Discussion	The incidence of acute rejection in transplantation has decreased as immunosuppressive regimens have improved. However, acute rejection does still occur, especially in patients who may have trouble accessing or taking their medications. Acute rejection is the only type of rejection for which proper immunosuppression is both preventative and the treatment. When assessing for acute rejection, it is also important to consider calcineurin inhibitor nephrotoxicity. Calcineurin inhibitors have drastically decreased acute rejection in transplant recipients, but their use can lead to both acute and chronic nephrotoxicity. Acute graft rejection occurs due to an immunologic response by the recipient's immune system against the donor organ. This response can be either antibody- or T-cell–mediated in acute rejection, which can be determined based on biopsy findings. The etiology is important to distinguish because the recommended treatment differs. Rejection is more likely to occur in poorly HLA-matched patients, so optimal HLA matching is the first preventative step. **History:** Disruption in immunosuppressive regimen occurs weeks to months following transplant; most patients are otherwise asymptomatic (although if severe, may have decreased urine output). Most often, discovered on routine post-operative laboratory surveillance. **Physical Exam:** Most patients will not show evidence of rejection on physical exam. However, if they have severe proteinuria, they may exhibit peripheral edema. **Diagnostics:** • An increase in serum creatinine and decrease in eGFR raises suspicion for transplant rejection. • Perform serology for donor-specific antibodies. • Ultrasound is performed prior to renal biopsy to rule out other causes for the decreased renal function, such as vascular or anastomotic complications (e.g., renal vein thrombosis, urinary leak, compression due to hematoma). • Renal biopsy is required for confirmation of acute rejection. Biopsy will show microvascular inflammation, acute tubular injury, intimal arteritis, or acute thrombotic microangiopathy in the case of antibody-mediated acute rejection or tubulitis and interstitial inflammation in T-cell–mediated acute rejection (see image).

CASE 44 | Acute Transplant Rejection (Renal Transplant) (continued)

Discussion	• Serum calcineurin inhibitor levels should be drawn and may indicate whether a patient is more likely to have acute rejection (low serum levels) or calcineurin inhibitor nephrotoxicity (high serum levels). **Management:** Acute rejection should be treated with corticosteroids and in the case of this patient, resumption of immunosuppressive regimen. If the rejection is antibody-mediated, it is important to remove the antibodies from circulation to prevent further damage, which is accomplished by modalities such as IVIG and plasmapheresis. Prednisone may be added to the maintenance regimen to prevent recurrence. The importance of the immunosuppression regimen following transplant procedures highlights the need for adequate patient/caregiver education about these medications, an accessible interdisciplinary follow-up care team, and frequent check-ins and screening. 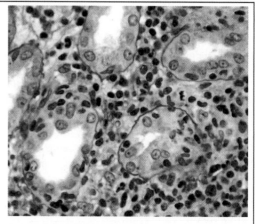 Acute cellular tubulointerstitial rejection. Light microscopy demonstrating tubulointerstitial inflammation with tubulitis with lymphocytes on the epithelial side of tubular basement membranes and focal disruption of tubular basement membranes (PAS stain). (Reproduced with permission from Reisner HM. Pathology: A Modern Case Study, 2e. Copyright 2020 McGraw-Hill Education.)
Additional Considerations	**Screening:** Surveillance of renal function at regular intervals with serum creatinine and eGFR is recommended post-transplantation to screen for early signs of rejection. A typical time course is twice a week for the first month, weekly for the next month, then every 2 weeks for a month, then every 3 months for the first year post-transplant. **Complications:** • Untreated acute rejection may lead to graft failure and need for re-transplantation and/or dialysis. • **Immunosuppressants:** Acute rejection is typically treated with high-dose pulses of immunosuppressants, which can have their own dose-dependent adverse reactions. The most notable in the short-term may be the effects of glucocorticoids on blood sugar and blood pressure, the neutrophil- and thrombocyte-depleting effects of anti-thymocyte biologics, and leukopenia from mycophenolate mofetil. Further, high-dose pulses of immunosuppressants could put patients at risk for hospital-acquired infections. • **Impaired Renal Function:** Decreased renal function during acute rejection events can lead to fluid and electrolyte imbalances, acidosis, and drug metabolite buildup. The loss of these regulatory roles that the kidneys normally perform can lead to cardiovascular arrhythmias, blood pressure extremes, respiratory distress, neuromuscular abnormalities, and neurologic signs, among other complications across organ systems.

Maintenance Immunosuppressants for Renal Transplantation

Class	Drugs	Mechanism of Action	Adverse Reactions
Induction Therapies (Used Prior to Transplant)			
Anti-T-cell antibodies	Polyclonal horse anti-thymocyte antibody, polyclonal rabbit anti-thymocyte antibody	Depletes T cells via antibody neutralization mechanisms, also depletes B and NK cells	Mild flu-like effects (e.g., fever, chills, malaise), transient neutropenia, and thrombocytopenia Rarely, may cause serum sickness
Anti-CD3 antibodies	Muromonab: mouse anti-CD3 monoclonal antibody	Inhibits naïve and cytotoxic T-cell function via blocking CD3-T-cell receptor (TCR) binding and thereby cytotoxicity	High risk of acute cytokine release syndrome; mitigate with glucocorticoids
Anti-IL-2 receptor antibodies	Basiliximab: monoclonal chimeric murine-human anti-IL-2 antibody Daclizumab: monoclonal humanized anti-IL-2 antibody	Blocks T-cell activation and B-cell differentiation via antagonism of TCR for IL-2 to prevent response to donor antigens	Diabetogenic (particularly in combination with maintenance drugs), risk of lymphoproliferative disorders, opportunistic infections

Maintenance Immunosuppressants for Renal Transplantation

Class	Drugs	Mechanism of Action	Adverse Reactions
Anti-CD52 antibodies	Alemtuzumab: humanized anti-CD52 monoclonal antibody	Depletes mature lymphocytes via binding to surface CD52	Risk for autoimmune disorders, (e.g., Hashimoto thyroiditis)
Glucocorticoids (high-dose)	Prednisone, methylprednisolone	Blocks T-cell function and proliferation and B-cell clonal expansion via inhibiting NF-KB and cytokine (IL-1, IL-6, prostaglandins, TNF) transcription	Cushing syndrome (weight gain, hypertension, lipodystrophy, hyperglycemia), osteoporosis, psychosis, adrenal insufficiency can occur if stopped abruptly
Maintenance Therapies (To Prevent Acute Rejection)			
Glucocorticoids (low-dose)	See earlier for drug examples, mechanism, and side effects. May be withdrawn at 1-week post-transplantation for patients at low rejection risk.		
Calcineurin inhibitors	Cyclosporine, tacrolimus	Block T-cell activation and proliferation via inhibition of IL-2 transcription; inhibit of IL-2 release by macrophages; inhibit B-cell proliferation	*Calcineurin:* Nephrotoxicity, neurotoxicity (tremors), hypertension, increased risk non-Hodgkin lymphoma *Tacrolimus:* Milder nephrotoxicity, headaches, tremors, hypertension, nausea, diarrhea, diabetogenic
Antimetabolite agents	Mycophenolate mofetil (MMF), azathioprine	*MMF:* Reduces lymphocyte proliferation and clonal expansion via inhibiting purine synthesis enzyme *Azathioprine:* Reduces lymphocyte proliferation and clonal expansion via blocking purine synthesis for DNA/RNA	*MMF:* Leukopenia, nausea, vomiting, diarrhea, constipation, abdominal pain *Azathioprine:* Frequent pancytopenia/myelosuppression, nausea, vomiting, diarrhea, liver dysfunction; can be used during pregnancy
mTOR inhibitors	Sirolimus, everolimus	Block lymphocyte proliferation, T-cell activation, and B-cell differentiation via FKBP12 binding, blunting IL-2 signaling	Hypogonadism, GI upset, oral ulcers, impaired wound healing, pancytopenia, insulin resistance, anti-tumor effect, hyperlipidemia
Costimulation blocker	Belatacept: fusion of antibody Fc domain and CTLA-4	Inhibits T-cell activation via binding of CD28 homolog CTLA-4 to B7	Increased risk of lymphoproliferative disease in EBV-negative patients, greater patient/graft survival but increased risk acute rejection
Rescue Therapies (To Treat Acute Rejection)			
High-dose glucocorticoids, anti-T-cell antibodies, mycophenolate mofetil, and alemtuzumab can be used. Other, more recently studied treatments are listed as follows.			
Anti-CD20 antibodies	Rituximab	Depletes B-cells by binding to CD20 on their surface, causing complement-dependent cytotoxicity	Bowel obstruction, myocardial infarction, arrhythmias, pancytopenia, hepatitis B reactivation and other infections
Proteasome inhibitor	Bortezomib	Blocks lymphocyte proliferation via inhibiting proteasome 26S chymotrypsin-like activity, causing apoptosis	GI upset, pancytopenia, herpes virus reactivation
Complement inhibitor	Eculizumab: humanized monoclonal anti-C5 antibody	Prevents formation of complement C5b-9 aka membrane attack complex (MAC) via blocking C5 cleavage	High risk of serious meningococcal, pneumonia, influenza, and other infections, risk of thrombotic complications after stopping

20
Emergency Medicine

Lead Author: Vinay Mikkilineni, MD
Contributor: Brittany Kotek, MD

RESUSCITATION AND SHOCK

The **ABC**s approach is part of the immediate management and stabilization of a critically ill patient and is *always* the first step of management:

- **Airway:** Ensure open airway, can use head tilt + chin lift, oropharyngeal airway, or intubation if necessary
- **Breathing:** Assess for respiratory distress, spontaneous respirations, O_2 saturation
- **Circulation:** Check pulse and blood pressure

Abnormal Breathing Patterns

Breathing Patterns	Findings	Causes
Hypopnea	Shallow breath and low RR Causes hypoxemia	Sedatives, alcohol, neuromuscular disease (daytime hypopnea)
Orthopnea	Dyspnea worsens with lying down	CHF, late stages of COPD
Platypnea	Dyspnea worsens with sitting or standing	Cardiac right-left shunts, hepatopulmonary syndrome
Cheynes-Stokes breathing	Alternating cycles of tachypnea and apnea	Increased circulatory time resulting in delay of chemoreceptors receiving timely information about $PaCO_2$—CHF, stroke, brainstem injury, dying patients
Kussmaul breathing	Deep respirations with rapid RR	Metabolic acidosis (e.g. DKA)
Biot (ataxic) breathing	Chaotic breathing with irregular depth and frequency	Damage to the respiratory center in the medulla from stroke or herniation

RR, respiratory rate; CHF, congestive heart failure; COPD, chronic obstructive pulmonary disease; DKA, diabetic ketoacidosis.

Shock

Shock is a life-threatening clinical syndrome characterized by inadequate tissue perfusion in the setting of hypotension, leading to end-organ dysfunction. Evidence of organ dysfunction can include:

- Altered mental status (AMS)
- Acute kidney injury (AKI)
- Thrombocytopenia
- Elevated bilirubin and transaminases
- Hypoxemia

Shock must be recognized quickly for rapid treatment (e.g., fluids, vasopressors, inotropes) as well as identifying and treating the underlying cause (e.g., infection, MI, hemorrhage). The table below provides an overview of the four main types of shock.

Types of Shock

Type of Shock	Cause	Cardiac Output (CO)	Afterload = SVR[*]	Preload = PCWP[**]
Hypovolemic	Hemorrhage, severe dehydration	↓	↑	↓
Obstructive	Tension pneumothorax, PE, Cardiac Tamponade	↓	↑	↓, but may vary depending on etiology
Distributive	Sepsis, anaphylaxis, neurogenic, adrenal crisis	↑	↓	↓
Cardiogenic	CHF, myocarditis, MI, arrhythmia	↓	↑	↑

[*]Systemic Vascular Resistance (SVR)

[**]Pulmonary Capillary Wedge Pressure (PCWP)

CASE 1 | Septic Shock

An 82-year-old man with hypertension and BPH is brought to the ED from a nursing home after the staff noted altered mental status (AMS). The patient had a low-grade fever yesterday but did not report any other symptoms. This morning he was confused and lethargic. He has an indwelling bladder catheter and his urine output was 200 mL over the last 12 hours. On exam, his blood pressure is 84/42 mmHg (mean arterial pressure [MAP] 56), temperature 39.2°C, heart rate 110/min, respirations 24/min, and SpO$_2$ 92% on room air. Physical exam is notable for warm skin and extremities. Serum creatinine is 2.8. After 2L of crystalloid, his BP is 88/48 (MAP 61) and norepinephrine is started.

Conditions with Similar Presentations	**Cardiogenic shock:** Will also present with hypotension but is due to decreased cardiac output; physical exam will have cool skin/extremities with signs of volume overload.
	Anaphylactic shock: Is also a type of distributive shock and would also present with hypotension; however, patients display respiratory distress, angioedema, wheezing, and/or urticarial rash.
	Neurogenic shock: Is also a type of distributive shock and the result of brain or spinal cord injury; patients exhibit loss of sympathetic tone and can exhibit hypotension, bradycardia, and temperature dysregulation.
	Adrenal crisis: Is also a type of distributive shock; consider this diagnosis in patients with hypotension without signs of infection, cardiovascular disease, or hypovolemia. Most common cause is sudden cessation of glucocorticoids.
Initial Diagnostic Tests	• Clinical diagnosis with sepsis (suspected infection) and, despite adequate fluid resuscitation, requires vasopressors to maintain MAP ≥65 mmHg • Check: Blood cultures, UA, CXR, lactic acid, CBC, electrolytes, creatinine, transaminases, bilirubin • Imaging to locate source of infection if unclear from history and physical
Next Steps in Management	• Address ABCs (Airway, Breathing, Circulation) • IV fluid resuscitation and vasopressors • Broad-spectrum antibiotics
Discussion	Shock is a life-threatening clinical syndrome characterized by inadequate tissue perfusion often in the setting of hypotension that leads to end-organ dysfunction. Septic shock is a type of distributive shock characterized by abnormal and excessive peripheral vasodilation. **Sepsis** is defined as suspected or proven infection and associated organ dysfunction. **Septic shock** is identified by sepsis that despite adequate fluid resuscitation requires vasopressors to maintain a MAP ≥65 mmHg and has a serum lactate level greater than 2 mmol/L. The diagnosis carries a high mortality rate, and early detection and intervention is critical to improve prognosis. **History:** • AMS; may have symptoms related to underlying infection (e.g., dysuria, back pain, and chills from pyelonephritis) • Risk factors include: Advanced age (>65 years), diabetes, obesity, immunosuppression, malignancy, and previous hospitalization **Physical Exam:** • Signs of systemic infection (fever, tachycardia, tachypnea) • Hypotension • Initially warm extremities, then cold and clammy • Signs of end-organ hypoperfusion may be evident, including AMS, hypoxemia **Diagnostics:** Clinical diagnosis with: 1. Sepsis: Suspected/proven infection with associated organ dysfunction (criteria such as systemic inflammatory response syndrome [SIRS] can help identify) 2. In spite of adequate fluid resuscitation, requires vasopressors to maintain MAP ≥ 65mmHg and have serum lactate >2 mmol/L Infectious Workup: • Peripheral blood cultures from at least two different sites, urinalysis/urine culture, and chest x-ray • Serum lactate elevated **Management:** • Address ABCs, admit to ICU • Aggressive fluid resuscitation with boluses of IV crystalloids (Lactated Ringers preferred) • Initiate empiric broad-spectrum antibiotics immediately on recognition of septic shock and ensure that blood cultures are obtained prior to antibiotic administration • Source control if possible (drainage of abscess, removal of infected lines or catheters) • Vasopressors (e.g., norepinephrine) to maintain MAP ≥65

CASE 1 | Septic Shock *(continued)*

Additional Considerations	**Complications:** Multiorgan failure, ARDS, DIC, death.
	SIRS (Systemic inflammatory response syndrome) **Criteria:** Not always caused by infection, so no longer formally used in definition of sepsis but still can be helpful clinically. SIRS is the presence of two or more of the following: • Temperature >38°C or <36°C • Heart rate >90/min • Respiratory rate >20/min or PaCO$_2$ <32 mmHg • WBC >12000/mm^3 or <4000/m^3

Distributive Shock Mini-Cases

Cases	Key Findings
Anaphylaxis	**Hx:** • Symptoms: Urticaria, dyspnea, palpitations, mucosal swelling, and gastrointestinal symptoms (nausea, vomiting, dysphagia, abdominal cramping, diarrhea) • Exposure to trigger: Medications, stinging insect venoms, foods, and contrast media, but the cause can be unidentified in up to one-fifth of cases **PE:** Hypotension, tachypnea, tachycardia, wheezing, urticaria, and angioedema **Diagnostics:** Clinical diagnosis • Elevated serum tryptase levels can support diagnosis **Management:** • Address ABCs • Immediate removal of trigger • Intramuscular epinephrine • After epinephrine administration, consider adjunctive therapies (e.g., antihistamines, corticosteroids, inhaled beta-2 agonists, and glucagon) • Observe for biphasic reaction (return of symptoms after initial improvement) which is seen in 20% of patients up to 72 hours (observe 1 hour if mild symptoms, 6 hours if severe symptoms) • Discharge patient with injectable epinephrine kit **Discussion:** • Anaphylaxis is a systemic allergic reaction that can be fatal • Risk factors for severe anaphylaxis include age older than 50, cardiovascular disease, asthma, drug-induced reactions, peanut or tree nut allergy, and mast cell disorders
Adrenal Crisis (Acute Adrenal Insufficiency)	**Hx:** May present with AMS, fever, fatigue, weakness, nausea, vomiting, abdominal pain, myalgias, or lethargy **PE:** Hypotension, possible signs of hypovolemia **Diagnostics:** • Low serum cortisol in state of stress, inadequate increase in serum cortisol after ACTH administration • Possible hyperkalemia and hyponatremia **Management:** • Address ABCs • Immediate IV glucocorticoid (hydrocortisone) • Aggressive IV fluid resuscitation **Discussion:** • Acute adrenal insufficiency is a life-threatening clinical syndrome • The most common cause is sudden cessation of glucocorticoid treatment • It can also present in patients with primary adrenocortical failure (Addison's disease) that is undiagnosed or undertreated during periods of stress such as acute infection or major illness • May develop due to bilateral adrenal infarction/hemorrhage (Waterhouse–Friderichsen syndrome) during sepsis • Less commonly due to secondary or tertiary adrenal disease due to impaired adrenal regulation by the pituitary gland or hypothalamus, respectively • Patients with borderline adrenal function may develop an adrenal crisis during an increased metabolic demand from a medical or surgical stress

Shock Mini-Cases

Cases	Key Findings

Cardiogenic Shock	**Hx:**
	• Symptoms of myocardial infarction (acute onset chest pain and dyspnea) or arrhythmia (palpitations)
	• Other signs of heart failure may be present, including orthopnea, lower extremity edema, decreasing urine output
	
	PE:
	• Hypotension, signs of poor tissue perfusion (e.g., oliguria, cyanosis, cool extremities, AMS, faint peripheral pulses, decreased capillary refill)
	• Signs of heart failure/volume overload: JVD, S3 and S4, pulmonary crackles, and tachycardia
	
	Diagnostics:
	• ECG and troponin (to evaluate for acute coronary syndrome), lactic acid, and BNP
	• Emergent echocardiography to evaluate ventricular function
	
	Management:
	• Address ABCs
	  • Administer oxygen to hypoxic patients
	  • May need IV inotropic support
	• Treat underlying cause (e.g., acute MI requires revascularization)
	
	Discussion:
	• Characterized by persistent hypotension and inadequate tissue perfusion due to reduced cardiac output due to myocardial disease and/or arrhythmia.
	• Acute myocardial infarction is the most common cause, although worsening heart failure, myocarditis, pulmonary embolism, and arrhythmia are other causes. These should receive prompt treatment and emergency revascularization if appropriate.

Advanced Cardiac Life Support (ACLS) Algorithm

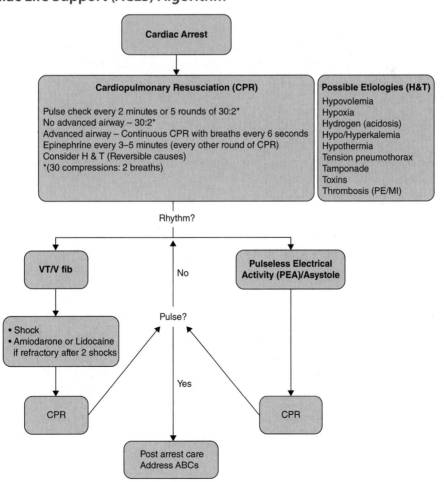

TOXICOLOGY

Toxicology examines how chemicals adversely affect humans. While this area of study is vastly encompassing of pharmacology, environmental medicine, and other areas, we will look at some high-yield ingestions and their treatments. Diagnosis is often reliant on "toxidromes," which are a constellation of symptoms and findings (physical exam and laboratory) that can point toward a cause. Below are some high-yield ingestions, presentations, and antidotes.

Overdoses/Adverse Reactions

Substance	Presentation	Treatment
Acetaminophen	Abdominal pain, nausea/vomiting, elevated transaminases	Acetylcysteine
Alcohol	AMS, slurred speech, aggression, unsteady gait	Supportive care
Anticholinergics	Dilated pupils, dry mouth, urinary retention, flushed skin, AMS	Physostigmine
Benzodiazepines	AMS, respiratory depression, nystagmus	Flumazenil
Beta-blockers	Bradycardia, hypotension	Glucagon
Calcium channel blockers	Bradycardia, hypotension	Calcium, high dose insulin
Cannabis	Pupil constriction, conjunctival injection, paranoia, anxiety, nausea, tachycardia, tachypnea, dry mouth, slurred speech	Benzodiazepines for agitation and antipsychotics for severe psychosis
Carbon monoxide	Headache, paresthesias, AMS	Oxygen
Cholinesterase inhibitors (organophosphates, found in insecticides)	Diaphoresis, salivation, lacrimation, miosis, bradycardia	Atropine + pralidoxime
Cyanide	AMS, vomiting, flushed (cherry-red skin), bitter almond breath odor, lactic acidosis	Hydroxycobalamin, sodium thiosulfate, sodium nitrite
Digoxin	Nausea and vomiting, hyperkalemia, arrhythmias	Digoxin FAB antibodies
Dopamine antagonists: antipsychotics (haloperidol), metoclopramide, promethazine	Neuroleptic malignant syndrome (NMS)—Hyperthermia, muscle rigidity, autonomic instability (tachycardia, labile BP), hyperreflexia, AMS, and mydriasis	IV fluids, benzodiazepines, dantrolene
Ethylene glycol, methanol	AMS, AKI (ethylene glycol), decreased visual acuity (methanol)	Fomepizole
Heavy metals (arsenic, lead, mercury)	Nausea, vomiting, diarrhea, AMS, paresthesias	Dimercaprol, dimercaptosuccinic acid
In susceptible patients after volatile anesthetics or neuromuscular blockers (halothane, succinylcholine)	Malignant hyperthermia—muscle rigidity, tachypnea, tachycardia, hyperthermia	Dantrolene
Iron	Abdominal pain, nausea/vomiting	Deferoxamine
Isoniazid	Neuropathy, seizures	Pyridoxine
Lidocaine	Metallic taste, tinnitus, arrhythmias	Intralipids
Methemoglobinemia (congenital or acquired (e.g., benzocaine, phenazopyridine, dapsone, and nitrates/nitrites)	Cyanosis, headache, dizziness, AMS, dyspnea	Methylene blue
Opioids	Miosis, respiratory depression, slurred speech, AMS	Naloxone
Phencyclidine/hallucinogens	Tachycardia, hypertension, nystagmus, ataxia, AMS, delusions, dilated pupils, combative	Benzodiazepines, antihypertensives, antihistamines, antipsychotics

Overdoses/Adverse Reactions

Substance	Presentation	Treatment
SSRIs and 5HT-agonists (antidepressants, ondansetron, metoclopramide)	Serotonin syndrome = altered mental status (AMS), hyperreflexia, clonus, autonomic hyperactivity (tachycardia, hypertension, hyperthermia, flushing, diarrhea)	Cyproheptadine
Stimulants: Amphetamine, methamphetamine, cocaine	Anxiety, tachycardia, pupillary dilation, hypertension, AMS, arrhythmias	Benzodiazepines, antipsychotics, antihypertensives
Warfarin	Bleeding	Phytonadione (Vitamin K), clotting factors

CASE 2 | Tricyclic Antidepressant (TCA) Overdose

A 36-year-old woman with generalized anxiety disorder presents with lethargy and vomiting. She was brought in by her boyfriend who says she has been getting progressively sleepy over the last 2 hours and started vomiting 30 minutes ago. She is minimally responsive to her name and unable to answer questions. He denies any illicit drug use or known medical problems, stating that she "just takes a daily pill for her mood" but doesn't know the name. He is worried that she has been more depressed lately and notes she has had one suicide attempt in the past. Vitals are T 99.9°F, HR 130, BP 80/60, RR 15, SpO_2 96%. She is warm, flushed, lethargic, and responds to her name. She opens her eyes to her name, pupils are dilated, and oropharynx is clear with dry mucous membranes. She is tachycardic with clear lung sounds; abdominal exam is notable for a large, soft, suprapubic mass, normal bowel sounds, no tenderness or guarding. She withdraws her extremities to pain.

Conditions with Similar Presentations	**AEIOU TIPS** is a common acronym used when considering a quick differential for AMS: **A**lcohol, **E**pilepsy/**E**ndocrine, **I**nfection, **O**verdose, **U**remia, **T**rauma/**T**umor, **I**nsulin, **P**sychiatric, **S**troke/**S**hock. **Overdose/Ingestion:** Includes drugs such as opiates, benzodiazepines, alcohol, antiepileptics, and antipsychotics. Drugs that can cause anticholinergic symptoms include antihistamines, TCAs, procainamide, quinidine, clozapine, and carbamazepine.
Initial Diagnostic Testing	• Clinical Diagnosis • Check Point-of-care (POC) glucose, CBC, CMP, ECG, UA, blood alcohol (BAC), salicylate and acetaminophen levels, urine tox, CT head, ABG to rule out other causes
Next Steps in Management	• ABCs • Administer IV fluids and sodium bicarbonate to prevent further cardiotoxicity and cardiac arrhythmias • Consider oral activated charcoal therapy if awake and cooperative
Discussion	TCA overdose presents with sedation, flushed skin, abnormal vitals, ECG changes, and anticholinergic signs (dilated pupils, dry mouth, urinary retention). TCAs inhibit fast sodium channel conductivity in cardiac myocytes, leading to decreased conduction velocity, increased refractory period, and ECG changes. Further, they exhibit antagonistic properties at histamine, acetylcholine, GABA-A, and alpha-1 adrenergic receptors. **History:** • Identify substance, how much, over what time period, and how long ago prior to presentation via patient or collateral (family, friends, EMS) **Physical Exam:** • Alerted mental status • Hypotension and tachycardia • Anticholinergic symptoms: Dry, flushed skin and mucous membranes, myopia, delirium, urinary retention **Diagnostics:** • POC glucose for hypoglycemia • ECG may show signs of TCA sodium channel inhibition, including QRS prolongation >100 msec, deep, slurred S waves in leads I and aVL, R wave in AVR >3 mm, and requires urgent intervention • Drug levels including blood alcohol (BAC), acetaminophen, salicylate, or anti-epileptics to evaluate for co-ingestion • TCA levels not useful in acute setting

CASE 2 | Tricyclic Antidepressant (TCA) Overdose *(continued)*

Discussion	**Management:** • Address ABCs • Sodium bicarbonate to prevent arrhythmias and stabilize cardiac membrane • Charcoal if within 1 hour of overdose and patient is awake and cooperative • Monitor closely for worsening signs of toxicity or respiratory/neurologic depression • Monitor for seizures due to GABA-A antagonism, treat with benzodiazepines
Additional Considerations	**Pediatric Considerations:** Pediatric toxic ingestions of TCAs should be managed and treated in the same manner as adult patients. Additional investigation into the child's access to such medications is warranted along with counseling for guardians on proper safe storage and handling.

Toxicology Mini-Cases

A 71-year-old man is brought to the ED for AMS. His daughter says he is generally healthy except for chronic knee pain which had recently worsened. She states that her father recently switched from acetaminophen to larger doses of aspirin. On exam, patient is confused, unable to follow commands, and is tachypneic and has hyperpnea. His vital signs are T 38.7°C, BP 100/50 mmHg, HR 108/min, RR 30/min, SpO$_2$ 97% on room air.

Salicylate (Aspirin) Toxicity	**Hx:** May have vomiting, abdominal pain, fever, confusion, tinnitus, seizures, or coma
	PE: AMS, hyperpnea (abnormally deep breathing), tachypnea, tachycardia, hyperthermia
	Diagnostics:
	• BMP and ABG with mixed acid-base disorder:
	  • Anion-gap metabolic acidosis (low bicarb, elevated anion gap)
	  • Respiratory alkalosis (low pCO$_2$) from hyperventilation
	• Elevated serum salicylate levels
	Management:
	• Address ABCs
	• IV fluids and alkalinization of serum and urine with IV sodium bicarbonate
	• Oral activated charcoal therapy if awake and cooperative
	• Dialysis for severe cases, such as those with AMS, seizures, pulmonary edema, or high ASA levels
	Discussion:
	• Toxic salicylate levels stimulate respiratory drive directly in the CNS, which causes hyperpnea (earliest finding).
	• Patients may present with hyperthermia as ASA uncouples oxidative phosphorylation in mitochondria and generates heat.
	• Alkalinizing the serum creates a concentration gradient for non-ionized salicylate to diffuse out of affected tissues (e.g., CNS) and into the extracellular space. Bicarbonate excreted in the urine creates an environment more basic than serum, leading to ionized salicylates trapped in the urine and increased overall excretion.

A 17-year-old girl presents with blurry vision, labored breathing, and hematuria after being dared to ingest various car fluids found in the garage at a party she had attended. On exam, she is alert and oriented to person, place, time, and situation. Her temperature is 37.1°C, BP is 94/50 mmHg, pulse is 60/min, and she has Kussmaul respirations at a rate of 28/min. She has dilated pupils, retinal edema, and flank tenderness.

Methanol/ Ethylene Glycol Toxicity	**Hx:** • Ingestion of toxic alcohols produces similar CNS effects as ethanol: AMS, slurred speech, ataxic gait • Visual complaints (methanol toxicity): Burning, decreased visual acuity (scotomata) • Flank pain, hematuria, oliguria (ethylene glycol toxicity) **PE:** • Similar to ethanol intoxication, AMS • Tachypnea and Kussmaul respirations may be present • Methanol toxicity may lead to an afferent pupillary defect, mydriasis, or retinal edema

Toxicology Mini-Cases (*continued*)

Methanol/ Ethylene Glycol Toxicity	**Diagnostics:** • Toxic alcohol levels to confirm diagnosis • BMP will show anion gap metabolic acidosis and elevated serum osmolar gap (measured osmolarity – calculated osmolarity) • Ethylene glycol ingestion may present with hematuria, acute renal failure, and oxalate crystals in the urine **Management:** • Address ABCs • IV sodium bicarbonate to maintain pH >7.3 • Inhibit metabolism of the toxic alcohols using a competitive inhibitor of alcohol dehydrogenase (ADH): Fomepizole (preferred) or ethanol • Severe cases require hemodialysis to rapidly clear toxic alcohols and their metabolites **Discussion:** • Toxic alcohols are found in antifreeze, air coolant, and other automotive/industrial cleaners, solvents, or fuels. • Investigate timing of ingestion to guide therapy and management while monitoring lab values. • Methanol is metabolized by alcohol dehydrogenase to formaldehyde and the formic acid. The latter inhibits cytochrome C oxidase, disrupting mitochondrial function and causing hypoxia to tissues, especially the retina. • Ethylene glycol is metabolized to glycolate, glyoxylate, and oxalate, which cause direct renal tubular injury and may precipitate in renal tubules causing obstructive uropathy.
	A 42-year-old jeweler is found unresponsive and apneic at home. EMS found a half-empty bottle of chemicals near the patient. The patient was intubated and transferred to the ED. Exam is notable for sluggishly reactive pupils bilaterally, and temperature is 36.5°C, blood pressure is 90/47 mmHg, and pulse is 60/min.
Cyanide Poisoning	**Hx:** Headache, cyanosis, dyspnea, AMS, vomiting, flushed skin **PE:** Findings dependent on timing, route, and dosing of exposure • Vitals signs may show tachycardia with hypertension and eventually bradycardia with hypotension • Similarly, tachypnea occurs early and bradypnea eventually occurs • Flushed skin is present in a minority of patients **Diagnostics:** • Clinical diagnosis • Severe anion gap metabolic acidosis due to elevated lactic acid (cyanide inhibits mitochondrial function; as a result, cells must then use anaerobic metabolism to generate ATP, which produces lactic acid) **Management:** • Address ABCs • Hydroxocobalamin directly binds cyanide • Sodium thiosulfate catalyzes the metabolism of cyanide to thiocyanate • Sodium nitrite creates methemoglobin, which has iron in the Fe^{3+} state, which binds cyanide **Discussion:** • Cyanide toxicity is rapidly fatal if not treated immediately and should be suspected in a patient with AMS, anion gap metabolic acidosis, and lactic acidosis of unclear etiology • Most common cause = smoke inhalation (due to its inclusion in many manufactured products and plastics) but can also occur due to ingestion (used to create jewelry) or absorption through mucous membranes

ENVIRONMENTAL INJURIES

Environmental injuries include extremes of temperature to encounters with animals and insects.

CASE 3 | Hypothermia

A 45-year-old man found unconscious on a cold snowy night on the side of the road is brought in by EMS. He is unable to provide a history. Temperature is 31°C, pulse is 50/min, blood pressure is 80/50, respirations are 14/min, and SpO$_2$ is 98% on bag mask ventilation (intubated by EMS). On exam, he is lethargic, slightly shivering; his digits, nose, and lips are dusky. He is making incomprehensible sounds, not moving his extremities to pain or command, his eyes do not open to command.

Conditions with Similar Presentations	**Drugs or toxins:** Substances that decrease sympathetic tone (and therefore decrease cutaneous vasoconstriction) can lead to inappropriate vasodilation, heat loss, and hypothermia. Beta-blockers and clonidine overdose can cause hypothermia by this mechanism. Ethanol suppresses sympathetic tone, and in excess may also be associated with loss of consciousness and inability to seek warmth in a cold environment. **Sepsis:** Many of the cytokines, as well as nitric oxide, released during sepsis cause cutaneous vasodilation and heat loss that can result in hypothermia. The presence of hypothermia in sepsis is a poor prognostic sign. **Sympathetic injury:** Patients with diseases of, or injury to, the sympathetic nervous system may have inappropriate cutaneous vasodilation with heat loss and hypothermia. This can be seen in patients with spinal cord injury or severe peripheral neuropathy. **Hypothyroidism:** Body temperatures causing hypothermia are usually only seen in severe hypothyroidism (myxedema coma). **Hypoadrenalism:** If due to total loss of function of the gland including the medulla, can lead to inadequate catecholamines to prevent heat loss through the skin. **Hypoglycemia:** If severe may cause hypothermia by causing temporary or permanent injury to the hypothalamus, thus inhibiting sympathetic outflow.
Initial Diagnostic Tests	• Clinical Diagnosis • In unresponsive patients, should check: glucose, CBC, BMP, TSH, UA, CXR, EKG, CT head, CK, BAC, toxicology screen
Next Steps in Management	• Remove all clothing, begin external rewarming with heated blankets, heating pads, and warm forced air • Warmed IV fluids • Intubate and ventilate with warm humidified air • Treat any determined non-environmental underlying causes
Discussion	Hypothermia is defined as a body temperature <35°C (95°F). Hypothermia typically occurs in exposure to cold climates but can occur in temperate environments, especially when exposed to significant evaporative cooling (i.e., rafting trips with continued cold water exposure) or thermal dysregulation (see conditions with similar presentations above). Patients who are undomiciled are at greater risk because of lack of shelter from such elements. **History:** Obtain history from patient, bystanders, family including information on medical conditions and toxic ingestions. **Physical Exam:** Always get a core temperature • Temperature <35°C • Initially tachycardiac and tachypneic, but progress to bradycardia, hypoventilation, and hypotension • AMS • Shivering on exam is less likely at core temperatures <30°C • Evaluate the skin for any sign of burns or breakdown **Diagnostics:** • Fingerstick glucose to evaluate for hypoglycemia • ECG to evaluate for arrhythmia; Osborn waves (a positive deflection at the beginning of the ST segment) may be seen • CBC and PT/INR, PTT may show leukocytosis or DIC • CMP for identifying electrolyte abnormalities, liver injury, or renal dysfunction • CXR may show pulmonary edema • TSH to assess for hypothyroidism

CASE 3 | Hypothermia *(continued)*

Discussion	**Management:** • Address ABCs • Ventricular fibrillation is common, but defibrillation can be ineffective at very low core temperatures, thus rewarming is prioritized as arrhythmias may resolve without other interventions after the patient is adequately rewarmed. • Treatment depends on stage of hypothermia: • **Mild hypothermia** 32–35°C (90–95°F): Treat with passive external rewarming by removing wet clothing, using blankets or other insulation, and maintaining a warm room temperature. • **Moderate hypothermia** 28–32°C (82–90°F): Treat with active external rewarming—heated blankets, heating pads, forced warm air. • **Severe hypothermia** <28°C (82°F): The above methods are used, in addition to active internal rewarming with heated lavage (thoracic or peritoneal) and IV warmed fluids. Severe hypothermia warrants ICU admission.
Additional Considerations	**Complications:** **Rhabdomyolysis and DIC** are common in hypothermic patients. **Failure to respond to rewarming:** Look for additional causes other than environmental exposure, such as infection, thyroid abnormalities, neurologic injury, endocrine dysfunction, or toxic ingestion. **Surgical Considerations:** Extracorporeal membrane oxygenation (ECMO) is considered for patients with severe hypothermia who fail to rewarm despite aggressive active internal and external methods.

CASE 4 | Hyperthermia

A 64-year-old woman with anxiety is found unconscious in her home after a welfare call is made to the local police station at her family's request. She lives in an older home with no updated heating or cooling units. It is 98°F outside and only a few windows are open. Other than a fully closed bottle of paroxetine 10 mg, no opened medications, bottles, or illicit drugs were found at the scene. Patient's temperature is 41°C, pulse is 130/min, respirations are 20/min, blood pressure is 90/65, and SpO_2 is 98% on room air. On exam, she is diaphoretic, flushed, and lethargic. Pupils are equal, round, and reactive to light; mucous membranes are dry, capillary refill is brisk, reflexes are normal, there is no muscular rigidity on exam.

Conditions with Similar Presentations	**Infections:** Present similarly with elevated temperature due to cytokine-mediated resetting of the hypothalamic temperature setpoint. This is unlike hyperthermia, where the hypothalamus is not the reason for the elevated temperature. If temperature is >40°C, treat hyperthermia while workup for infection is ongoing. **Serotonin syndrome:** Occurs in patients taking 5HT-agonists (antidepressants, ondansetron, metoclopramide) and presents with AMS, hyperreflexia, clonus, autonomic hyperactivity (tachycardia, hypertension, hyperthermia, flushing, diarrhea) **Thyroid storm:** Presents with hyperthermia, tachycardia, atrial fibrillation, and AMS (agitation, psychosis, coma). Patients may have a history of anti-thyroid medication (that was discontinued), thyroid surgery, or exposure to iodine therapy. **Neuroleptic malignant syndrome (NMS):** Presents with hyperthermia, muscle rigidity, autonomic instability (tachycardia and hypertension), hyperreflexia, AMS, and mydriasis following exposure to a dopamine antagonist (antipsychotics, metoclopramide, promethazine). **Malignant hyperthermia:** Is a genetic derangement in skeletal muscle receptors that malfunction in response to volatile anesthetics (halothane) or neuromuscular blockers (succinylcholine), typically occurring postoperatively with muscle rigidity, tachycardia, arrhythmias, and hyperthermia (a later finding)
Initial Diagnostic Tests	• Clinical diagnosis • Also check CBC, PT/INR, PTT, BMP, transaminases, TSH, CK, blood and urine cultures
Next Steps in Management	• Rapid cooling with ice packs, cool water sprays, and fans • IV fluids to address hypotension, kidney injury, and rhabdomyolysis

CASE 4 | Hyperthermia (continued)

Discussion	**Heat stroke** is a cause of hyperthermia and is defined as severe hyperthermia with neurologic dysfunction, after exposure to extreme heat. Elevated temperature is most commonly due to cytokine-induced resetting of the hypothalamus temperature setpoint, which is the definition of fever. Hyperthermia, however, is an increase in temperature not mediated by cytokine-induced changes. Severe hyperthermia (as in this case) is a core temperature >40°C. Medical comorbidities, medications, and older age predispose certain populations to hyperthermia as a result of impaired vasodilation, thermal dysregulation, and the impaired delivery of heat to the skin surface. Social isolation is another risk factor for those to suffer worse effects during heat waves.
	History:
	• May describe feeling lightheaded or dizzy prior to collapse
	• Obtain history including age, time of exposure, time since last known normal, medical history, and medication and allergy list
	Physical Exam:
	• Elevated core body temperature, tachycardia, tachypnea, flushed skin, diaphoresis, and hypotension
	• CNS findings include lethargy, dizziness, ataxia, seizures
	Diagnostics:
	• Obtain core body temperature (rectal or esophageal)
	• CBC and PT/INR; PTT may show evidence of infection or DIC
	• BMP to evaluate for AKI, hypo/hypernatremia, transaminases for hepatic injury, CK for rhabdomyolysis
	• Consider head CT to rule out CNS pathology (stroke, bleed)
	Management:
	• Address ABCs
	• Rapid cooling: Ice water immersion is best, but ice packs to neck, axillae, and groin, with water sprayed over the body, and fans is practical.
	• Treat hypovolemia with IV fluids and correct any electrolyte derangements
	• Address other complications, rhabdomyolysis, liver injury, kidney injury, DIC, as indicated
Additional Considerations	**Complications:**
	May develop **multisystem organ failure** leading to a variety of complications including:
	• **Rhabdomyolysis**
	• **Disseminated intravascular coagulation (DIC)**
	• **Seizures**
	• **Cerebral edema** is a common complication, and administration of IV fluids and correction of hypernatremia should be done carefully
	• **Acute kidney injury**
	Inpatient Considerations: All patients with heat stroke should be hospitalized for ongoing management and monitoring of vital signs.

Environmental/Envenomation Injuries

Species	Signs/Symptoms	Treatment
Bees and wasps	Painful, itchy, red; can lead to anaphylaxis if sensitized	• Antihistamines, steroids, or topical creams for itch and pain relief • IM epinephrine if anaphylaxis
Animal bites	Risk of infection: human > cat > dog	• Thoroughly irrigate and cleanse the wound • Consider x-ray to assess for retained foreign body (i.e., tooth) or joint/bone injury • Prophylactic amoxicillin-clavulanate for human bites, and other bites if patient is immunocompromised, bite is near joint or bone (such as on the hand), or there is evidence of crush injury or edema • Rabies prophylaxis with human rabies immunoglobulin (HRIG) should be given depending on the biting animal; lower risk in rodents and domesticated animals that can be observed

Environmental/Envenomation Injuries

Species	Signs/Symptoms	Treatment
Crotalids (vipers— rattlesnake, copperhead, cottonmouth)	Severe burning, soft tissue edema, necrosis, bullae; abnormal metallic taste sensation; tingling in the mouth, face, extremities; fasciculations; can result in DIC, thrombocytopenia, rhabdomyolysis, or renal injury	• Remove tight-fitting or restrictive clothing, jewelry, or accessories • Immobilize and elevate the affected area • DO NOT use a tourniquet, try to suck out the venom, use aspirin (may worsen bleeding), or try to catch and kill the snake • Monitor for compartment syndrome • Crotalidae polyvalent-immune Fab is FDA-approved antivenin for North American crotalid envenomation
Elapids (coral snake)	Nausea, vomiting, headache, abdominal pain, diarrhea, diaphoresis, pallor, paresthesias, descending paralysis	• Elapid venom is a potent neurotoxin; monitor and maintain airway closely • Treat with coral snake antivenom
Black Widow	Muscle stiffness, cramps, headache, chills, fever, dizziness, nausea, vomiting, severe abdominal pain	• Cold compresses and medications for pain relief • Antivenom is available but has a high allergic rate
Brown Recluse	Tissue ulceration and necrosis; minimal systemic signs; toxin may cause hemolysis which might result in anemia, hemoglobinuria, or kidney injury	• Cold compresses and medications for pain relief
Scorpion	Neuromuscular dysfunction and autonomic hyperactivity including, fasciculations, muscle spasms, respiratory depression, swallowing difficulty	• Cold compress for pain relief and benzodiazepines for muscle spasms • Scorpion-specific antivenom indicated for severe cases

Index